Gynecologic Pathology

Commissioning Editor: Bill Schmitt
Project Development Manager: Helen Sofio (HS Publishing Services)
Project Manager: Bryan Potter
Design Manager: George Ajayi
Marketing Manager(s) (UK/USA): Clara Toombs/Brenna Christiansen

Gynecologic Pathology

A Volume in the Series

Foundations in Diagnostic Pathology

Edited by

Marisa R Nucci, MD
Division of Women's and Perinatal Pathology
Department of Pathology
Brigham and Women's Hospital
Boston, MA

Esther Oliva, MD
Pathology Department
Massachusetts General Hospital
Boston, MA

Series Editor

John R Goldblum, MD, FCAP, FASCP, FACG
Chairman, Department of Anatomic Pathology
The Cleveland Clinic Foundation
Cleveland Clinic Lerner College of Medicine
Case Western Reserve University
Cleveland, Ohio

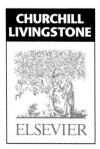

CHURCHILL
LIVINGSTONE

ELSEVIER

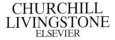

CHURCHILL
LIVINGSTONE
ELSEVIER

ELSEVIER CHURCHILL LIVINGSTONE
© 2009, Elsevier Inc. All rights reserved.

ISBN: 978-0-443-06920-8

NOTICE

Pathology is constantly changing. Standard safety precautions must be followed, but as new research and clinical experience broaden our knowledge, changes in treatment and drug therapy may become necessary or appropriate. Readers are advised to check the most current product information provided by the manufacturer of each drug to be administered to verify the recommended dose, the method and duration of administration, and contraindications. It is the responsibility of the practitioner, relying on experience and knowledge of the patient, to determine dosages and the best treatment for each individual patient. Neither the Publisher nor the author assume any liability for any injury and/or damage to persons or property arising from this publication.

The Publisher

First published 2009

British Library Cataloguing in Publication Data
A catalogue record for this book is available from the British Library

Library of Congress Cataloging in Publication Data
A catalog record for this book is available from the Library of Congress

Printed in China

Last digit is the print number: 9 8 7 6 5 4 3 2 1

Contents

The goal of this volume in the series Foundations in Diagnostic Pathology is to offer a textbook with a novel perspective on the many aspects of gynecologic pathology as reflected by the diversity of the contributors, who not only represent the "younger generation" in this field, but also have a breadth of experience from around the world. This book is not meant to be all inclusive, but rather focuses on the most common as well as some of the most challenging entities of gynecologic pathology. In contrast to other gynecologic pathology textbooks which cover diseases of the female genital tract in a traditional manner, the most notable and defining feature of this book is the accompanying Clinical and Pathologic Fact Sheets, which allow quick access to the main highlights of a particular disease. This textbook is aimed primarily at pathology residents and fellows in training as well as all who would like a comprehensive, "user-friendly" overview of this discipline.

The book is divided into seventeen chapters with coverage of both non-neoplastic and neoplastic conditions of the female genital tract. Even though each entity has a discussion of immunohistochemistry, this book devotes a separate chapter to this topic, focusing on the most useful markers in the differential diagnosis of challenging lesions. All of the chapters are richly illustrated and contain numerous informational boxes and tables, which will provide the reader with practical information on all the aspects of a given entity.

We are indebted to our many excellent contributors. In our opinion, the strength of a diverse and international collaboration far outweighed the difficulties in creating a uniform style throughout this book. Therefore, any errors or omissions are entirely our responsibility. We wish to extend our warm appreciation to John Goldblum for the trust and encouragement that has enabled us to undertake this work. It has been a long but fruitful journey, and in the end, it has not only resulted in a practical textbook of gynecologic pathology, but has also cemented a friendship.

Marisa R. Nucci
Esther Oliva
Boston, 2008

Isabel Alvarado-Cabrero MD
Chief of the Pathology Department
Mexican Oncology Hospital
National Medical Center
Mexico

Patricia M Baker MD
Associate Professor
Department of Pathology
Faculty of Medicine
University of Manitoba
Winnipeg, Manitoba, Canada

Kumarasen Cooper MBChB, DPhil, FRC Path
Professor of Pathology
Department of Pathology
University of Vermont College of Medicine
Fletcher Allen Health Care
Burlington, Vermont, USA

Michael T Deavers MD
Professor
UT MD Anderson Cancer Center
Departments of Pathology and Gynecologic Oncology
Houston, TX, USA

C Blake Gilks MD
Professor of Pathology
Department of Pathology and Laboratory Medicine
Vancouver General Hospital
Vancouver, BC, Canada

Maureen L Harmon MD
Associate Professor of Pathology
Department of Pathology
University of Vermont College of Medicine
Fletcher Allen Health Care
Burlington, Vermont, USA

David W Kindelberger MD
Associate Pathologist
Division of Women's and Perinatal Pathology
Department of Pathology
Boston, MA, USA

Sanjay Logani MD
Associate Professor
Pathology and Laboratory Medicine
Emory University School of Medicine
Atlanta, GA, USA

Teri A Longacre MD
Associate Professor
Department of Pathology
Stanford University School of Medicine
Stanford, California, USA

Anais Malpica MD
Professor
Departments of Pathology and Gynecologic Oncology
UT MD Anderson Cancer Center
Houston, TX, USA

W Glenn McCluggage FRCPath
Professor of Gynecological Pathology
Department of Pathology
Royal Group of Hospitals Trust
Belfast, Northern Ireland

Xavier Matias-Guiu MD, PhD
Chairman of Pathology and Molecular Genetics
Professor of Pathology
Hospital Universitari Arnau de Vilanova
University of Lleida
Lleida, Spain

Marisa R Nucci, MD
Associate Professor of Pathology
Harvard Medical School
Associate Pathologist
Division of Women's and Perinatal Pathology
Department of Pathology
Brigham and Women's Hospital
Boston, MA, USA

Esther Oliva, MD
Associate Professor
Department of Pathology, Harvard Medical School
Massachusetts General Hospital
Boston, MA, USA

Victor G Prieto MD PhD
Director of Dermatopathology
Professor of Pathology and Dermatology
Department of Pathology
University of Texas - MD Anderson Cancer Center
Houston, TX, USA

Brigitte M Ronnett MD
Professor
Departments of Pathology (Division of Gynecologic
    Pathology) and Gynecology & Obstetrics
The Johns Hopkins University School of Medicine
Baltimore, MD, USA

Timothy R. Quinn MD CM
Associate Dermatopathologist
Pathology Services Inc.
Cambridge, MA, USA

Christopher R Shea MD
Chair of Dermatology (Department of Medicine)
University of Chicago
Chicago, IL, USA

Ie-Ming Shih MD PhD

Associate Professor
Departments of Pathology, Gynecology and Obstetrics
The Johns Hopkins University School of Medicine
Baltimore, MD, USA

Robert A Soslow MD

Attending Pathologist
Memorial Sloan-Kettering Cancer Center
Professor of Pathology and Laboratory Medicine
Weill Medical College of Cornell University
New York, NY, USA

Russell Vang MD

Associate Professor
Departments of Pathology (Division of Gynecologic
    Pathology) and Gynecology & Obstetrics
The Johns Hopkins University School of Medicine
Baltimore, MD, USA

Acknowledgments

I am indebted to Dr. Belur S. Bhagavan who introduced me to the field of pathology; Dr. Stanley Hamilton for his guidance; Dr Ramzi Cotran for his vision; Dr. Christopher D.M. Fletcher for his mentorship; and most of all to Dr. Christopher P. Crum for everything.

Marisa R. Nucci, MD

To Dr Jaime Prat, the teacher and mentor who first taught me how to learn and enjoy pathology; who then gave me the opportunity to deepen my experience in the field of gynecologic pathology. To Dr Robert H Young for his teaching over the years, and to Dr Robert E Scully, who I consider the father and master of modern gynecologic pathology, and from whom I learned not only about pathology, but also about humanity, talking and looking at slides together.

Esther Oliva, MD

Dedications

To my loving husband, Branch, and to my two beautiful
boys, Julian and Cole, and my dear mother.
Marisa

Als meus pares, amb tota la meva estimació
To my parents, with gratitude
Esther

1

Inflammatory Diseases of the Vulva
Timothy R Quinn

The initial approach to any inflammatory disorder of the skin or mucosa requires knowledge of the precise anatomic location from which the biopsy was taken, an appreciation of the alterations in the regional mucocutaneous anatomy, effects of occlusion (e.g., clothing, skin folds, etc), and the dynamic changes effected by chronicity, and partial treatment. The mons pubis/labia majora closely resembles skin from other anatomic regions of the body and is composed of a slightly rugose, keratinizing, stratified epithelium, containing all of the cutaneous adnexal structures and a richly vascular dermis. The labia minora, in contrast, has a stratified, glycogen-rich squamous epithelium. Adnexal structures are absent. The subjacent dermis is highly vascular and contains erectile tissue.

The next step in evaluating an inflammatory process is the identification at low power of the *major tissue reaction pattern*, followed by the *pattern of inflammation*. Detailed description of this approach, championed initially in the teachings of Wallace Clark, has been further popularized and refined by Ackerman, Weedon, and LeBoit. The *tissue reaction pattern* is a distinctive group of morphologic findings which allows the observer to place a biopsy within a group of cutaneous diseases (Table 1.1). The *pattern of inflammation* refers to the distribution of the inflammatory infiltrate within the dermis and subcutis (Box 1.1). This approach will be applied to the most common inflammatory disorders of the vulva, and should allow the observer to categorize and generate a rational histopathologic and clinically relevant differential that allows the clinician to develop a meaningful treatment plan.

THE LICHENOID REACTION PATTERN (INTERFACE DERMATITIS)

This tissue reaction pattern is characterized by basal keratinocyte damage via T-cell-mediated cytotoxic damage or the induction of apoptosis. By convention, the damaged keratinocytes are termed *dyskeratotic cells* (Civatte bodies) if they are confined to the epidermis, and *colloid bodies* when they descend into the papillary dermis. In addition to basal keratinocyte damage, vacuolar change may also be present, and may be more prominent than cell death in certain dermatoses. *Vacuolar change* consists of intracellular keratinocyte vacuole

formation and edema with separation from the basement membrane zone. The *distribution of the inflammatory infiltrate* is the next feature to assess. The infiltrate may appose the undersurface of the basal layer or obscure the dermoepidermal junction (DEJ). The density and composition of the infiltrate also vary according to the specific disorder. The presence and quantity of melanin incontinence should also be noted. Lastly, classification of the lichenoid epidermal reaction pattern (Table 1.2) is of paramount importance in realizing a specific histopathologic diagnosis. The epidermis may be minimally affected in acute cytotoxic reactions, as in the early lesions of erythema multiforme (erythema multiforme-like epidermal reaction pattern). In more chronic lesions, such as found in lichen planus, where the epidermis has time to react to the inflammatory assault, the epidermis undergoes premature terminal differentiation (lichen planus-like epidermal reaction pattern). Over time, there may be supervening epidermal hyperplasia, which may be regular (psoriasiform epidermal reaction pattern) as in secondary syphilis, or irregular, as observed in discoid lupus erythematosus. The final or end-stage epidermal reaction pattern is found in those dermatoses featuring epidermal atrophy (lichen sclerosus). Integration of all these findings will allow the observer, in most cases, to generate a specific histopathologic diagnosis and differential diagnosis in one of the most important reaction patterns in genital skin. The following discussion will examine the most common dermatoses of the lichenoid reaction pattern.

LICHEN PLANUS

CLINICAL FEATURES

Lichen planus (LP) is an idiopathic dermatosis characterized clinically by purple polygonal papules which classically contain thin white lines – Wickham's striae. Mucosal involvement may appear as reticulate lacy lesions; however, erosive lesions are a more common presentation at anogenital sites, and may eventuate in scarring. Several clinical variants exist, including papular, erosive, hypertrophic, atrophic, and bullous.

TABLE 1.1
Major tissue reaction patterns

PATTERN	CHARACTERISTIC MORPHOLOGIC FEATURE
Lichenoid	Basal keratinocyte damage
Psoriasiform	Regular epidermal hyperplasia
Spongiotic (eczematous)	Intraepidermal edema
Vesiculobullous	Subepidermal or intraepidermal blister formation
Granulomatous	Granulomatous inflammation
Vasculopathic	Vascular injury

BOX 1.1
PATTERNS OF INFLAMMATION

Superficial perivascular inflammation
Superficial and deep perivascular inflammation
Folliculitis and perifolliculitis
Panniculitis

LICHEN PLANUS – FACT SHEET

Definition
▸ Idiopathic prototypical disorder of the lichenoid tissue reaction characterized clinically by purple pruritic papules and histologically by a band-like lymphohistiocytic infiltrate at the dermoepidermal junction, basal cell damage, and a characteristic epidermal reaction pattern

Incidence
▸ Uncommon; prevalence 0.3–0.8% worldwide

Morbidity
▸ Occasionally, scarring of mucous membranes and scalp, or, rarely, squamous dysplasia or carcinoma (in chronic lesions)

Gender, Race, and Age Distribution
▸ Female predominance
▸ No racial predisposition
▸ Rare in childhood; most cases in the 30–60-year range

Clinical Features
▸ Predilection for wrists, ankles, and genitalia, but may be widespread, including mucous membranes, nails, and hair
▸ Purple polygonal papules with white lines – "Wickham's striae"
▸ Lacy or reticulate and often eroded appearance of mucosal lesions

Prognosis and Treatment
▸ Generally self-limited disorder (12–18 months)
▸ Topical or intralesional steroids for regionally confined lesions
▸ Systemic steroids, retinoids, or cyclosporine for widespread involvement

TABLE 1.2
Lichenoid epidermal reaction patterns

PATTERN	DISORDER
I Premature terminal differentiation	Lichen planus Lichenoid keratosis Lichenoid drug eruption
II Acute cytotoxic type	Erythema multiforme Fixed drug eruption
III Psoriasiform epidermal hyperplasia	Secondary syphilis Early lichen sclerosus
IV Irregular epidermal hyperplasia	Hypertrophic lichen planus Some lichenoid drug eruptions
V Epidermal atrophy	Lichen sclerosus Plasmacytosis mucosae

MICROSCOPIC FEATURES

Evolved lesions of LP feature a band-like infiltrate composed of lymphocytes with an admixture of macrophages, which adhere to the undersurface of the epidermis (Figure 1.1). Basal cell damage results in dyskeratosis within the epidermis, and eosinophilic colloid bodies within the papillary dermis. Although the basal keratinocytes exhibit "squamatization," the infiltrate does not obscure the interface, nor extend into the suprabasilar epidermis. Plasma cells may be prominent in, or adjacent to, mucosal surfaces. Other hallmarks of LP include hyperkeratosis, "wedge-shaped" hypergranulosis (adjacent to acrosyringia or acrotrichia), and clefts which appear at the DEJ ("Max–Joseph" spaces) (Figure 1.2). Over time, there is subsequent dermal fibrosis and the epidermis becomes progressively flattened and thinned.

DIFFERENTIAL DIAGNOSIS

As all lichenoid dermatitides feature a band-like infiltrate, attention should be drawn to the epidermal reaction pattern and composition of the infiltrate. Although uncommon in flexural or mucosal sites, *lichenoid drug eruptions* may be histologically indistinguishable from LP. The presence of eosinophils within the infiltrate, involvement of the deep vascular plexus, and the presence of parakeratosis and focal dyskeratotic cells within the stratum corneum are all clues to a lichenoid drug eruption. *Lichen sclerosus* (LS), *fixed drug eruptions* (FDEs), *plasmacytosis mucosae* (PM), and *syphilis* may all exhibit a lichenoid tissue reaction and will be discussed individually below. *Neoplastic proliferations* may also exhibit a lichenoid host response, and may be mistaken clinically for inflammatory conditions. *Lichenoid*

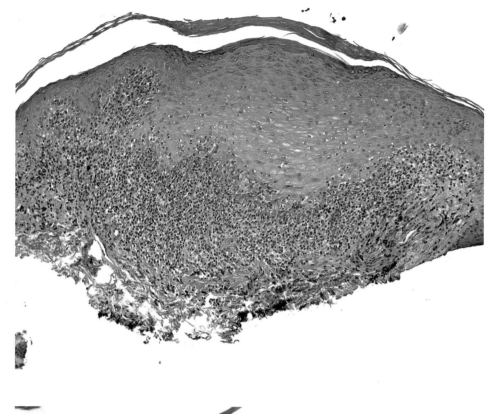

FIGURE 1.1

Lichen planus. A band-like infiltrate is present at the dermoepidermal junction with resultant dyskeratosis and squamatization of the basal keratinocytes. The overlying epidermis is acanthotic with hyperkeratosis and hypergranulosis.

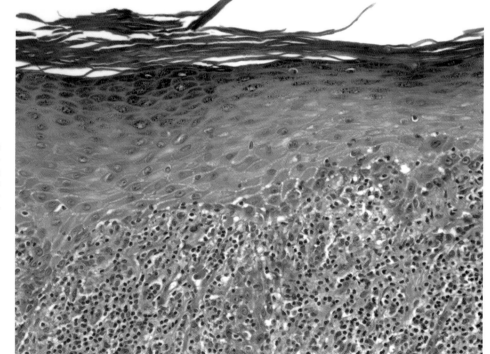

FIGURE 1.2

Lichen planus. Colloid bodies are present at the dermoepidermal junction. The infiltrate does not obscure the interface, nor extend into the suprabasilar epidermis. There is characteristic "wedge-shaped" hypergranulosis and hyperkeratosis.

keratosis or lichen planus-like keratosis is a solitary lesion that is essentially a T-cell-mediated regression of a variety of benign "keratoses" including warts, seborrheic keratoses, and lentigines. These may be present alongside the inflammatory infiltrate, and be a helpful histologic clue to the diagnosis. Unfortunately, inflammatory regression of pigmented lesions, including melanoma, and atypical keratinocytic proliferations, including squamous cell carcinoma in situ and basal cell carcinoma, may be mediated by a lichenoid infiltrate. Lichenoid infiltrates containing numerous melanophages should be treated with suspicion, and additional level sections and immunohistochemical stains for melanocytic markers may be useful in evaluating a clinically ambiguous lesion.

LICHEN PLANUS – PATHOLOGIC FEATURES

Microscopic Findings
▸ Prototypical lichenoid tissue reaction pattern
▸ Band-like lymphohistiocytic infiltrate at the dermoepidermal junction accompanied by basal keratinocyte damage and squamatization
▸ Infiltrate does not obscure the dermoepidermal junction or extend into the epidermis
▸ Other epidermal changes include hyperkeratosis, "wedge-shaped" hypergranulosis, and clefting at the dermoepidermal junction

Differential Diagnosis
▸ Lichenoid drug eruption
▸ Lichen sclerosus (early lesions)
▸ Fixed drug eruption
▸ Plasmacytosis mucosae
▸ Regression of benign or atypical keratinocytic or melanocytic proliferations

PROGNOSIS AND TREATMENT

Lichen planus is generally self-limited with spontaneous remission occurring in 12–18 months in over two-thirds of patients. Treatment is largely symptomatic and consists of agents that suppress the immune response. Topical or intralesional steroids are the mainstay for local to regionally confined lesions. In cases of widespread involvement, systemic corticosteroids, retinoids, and cyclosporine have been used.

ERYTHEMA MULTIFORME

Erythema multiforme (EM) consists of a clinical spectrum of disorders which affect the skin, and may at times involve the mucous membranes. The importance of recognizing the EM epidermal reaction pattern in genital skin is its association with herpes simplex virus (HSV) infection. Atypical presentations of EM in genital and paragenital sites may herald HSV reactivation.

CLINICAL FEATURES

Erythema multiforme typically presents as urticarial papules/papulovesicles often assuming a classical targetoid morphology, favoring acral rather than axial locations (EM minor). In some cases, there is additional involvement of one or more mucous membranes with epidermal detachment affecting < 10 % of the total body surface area (EM major). In the Stevens–Johnson syndrome and in toxic epidermal necrolysis, now separated by most experts from the EM spectrum, mucosal sites are involved, usually following ingestion of a drug.

ERYTHEMA MULTIFORME – FACT SHEET

Definition
▸ Prototype disorder of acute cytotoxic vacuolar interface dermatitis

Incidence
▸ Uncommon

Morbidity
▸ Typically self-limited, resolving in 2–4 weeks

Gender, Race, and Age Distribution
▸ Slight male preponderance
▸ No racial predilection
▸ Predominantly young adults

Clinical Features
▸ Urticarial papules/papulovesicles with a "targetoid" morphology, most commonly in acral locations (erythema multiforme minor)
▸ Erythema multiforme major if there is involvement of one or more mucous membranes
▸ Atypical presentations in genital sites may herald herpes simplex virus reactivation

Prognosis and Treatment
▸ Excellent prognosis, particularly if etiologic trigger is identified
▸ Prophylactic acyclovir may be required if linked to herpesvirus infection
▸ Supportive skin care for active cutaneous and mucocutaneous lesions

ERYTHEMA MULTIFORME – PATHOLOGIC FEATURES

Microscopic Findings
▸ Vacuoles both above and below the basement membrane
▸ Lymphocytes present at the dermoepidermal junction
▸ Necrotic keratinocytes in the epidermis, as clusters or whorls
▸ Secondary subepidermal vesicles

Differential Diagnosis
▸ Fixed drug eruption
▸ Evolving or recurrent herpesvirus infection

MICROSCOPIC FEATURES

Erythema multiforme is the prototype of acute cytotoxic vacuolar interface dermatitis. Early lesions feature perivascular lymphocytes which ascend, and decorate the DEJ, inciting vacuoles both above and below the basement membrane (Figure 1.3). As the lesions progress,

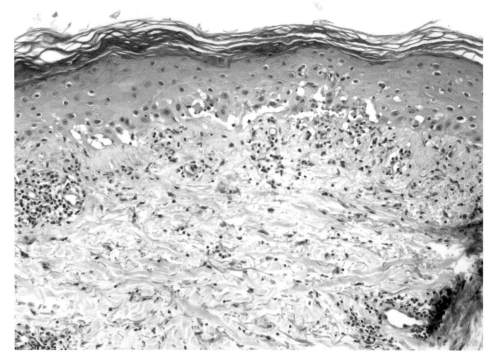

FIGURE 1.3

Erythema multiforme. A perivascular lymphohistiocytic infiltrate decorates the dermoepidermal junction inciting vacuoles both above and below the epidermal basement membrane.

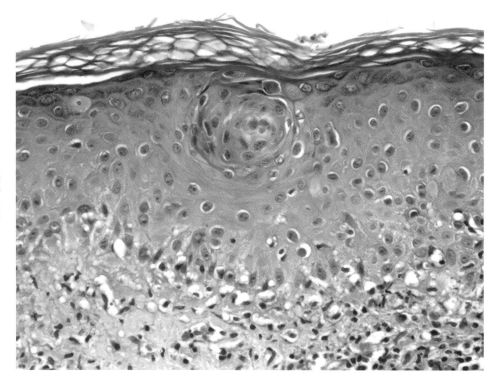

FIGURE 1.4

Erythema multiforme, late phase. Whorls of necrotic keratinocytes are present in the spinous layer. Note the preservation of the "basket-weave" pattern of the cornified layer.

keratinocyte necrosis ensues, eventuating in whorls of necrotic keratinocytes (Figure 1.4). When fully evolved, subepidermal vesiculation may occur following the confluence of clefting at the DEJ. The acute nature of this process typically allows preservation of the normal "basket-weave" cornified layer.

DIFFERENTIAL DIAGNOSIS

The epidermal changes are similar to that of a *FDE*; however, the presence of eosinophils, neutrophils, and deep extension of the infiltrate in FDE, and extension

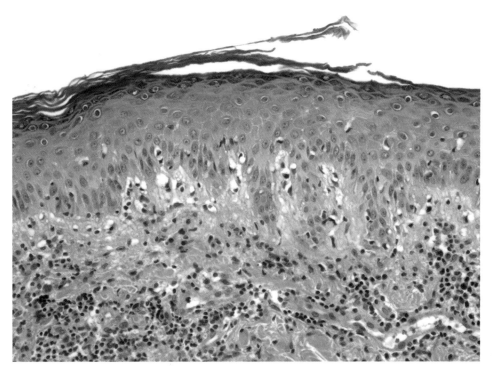

FIGURE 1.5

Acute herpes simplex virus infection. There is acute vacuolar interface dermatitis similar to that observed in an early lesion of erythema multiforme. No viral cytopathic changes are seen within the epidermis.

of lymphocytes into the upper layer of the epidermis, should allow separation in most cases.

Evolving lesions of HSV may have histologic features identical to EM (Figure 1.5). For this reason, level sections are important in evaluating EM if clinical suspicion for a herpes infection is high, as viral cytopathic changes may be focal, or confined to hair follicles (Figure 1.6).

PROGNOSIS AND TREATMENT

Most cases of EM are self-limited, and resolve spontaneously in 2–4 weeks. Treatment is directed at the identification and elimination of the etiologic trigger. In those cases of EM that have been linked to herpesvirus infection, prophylactic acyclovir may be required if recurrences are frequent or debilitating. Skin care of active lesions is supportive.

FIXED DRUG ERUPTION

CLINICAL FEATURES

Following exposure to an inciting agent, this eruption occurs repetitively in the same area after each exposure to the drug. Commonly implicated agents include phenolphthalein, tetracycline, and barbiturates. Genital

---

FIXED DRUG ERUPTION – FACT SHEET

Definition
▶ Characteristic eruption occurring in the same anatomic area each time an inciting agent is ingested

Incidence
▶ Uncommon

Morbidity
▶ Mild or absent local and constitutional symptoms
▶ Persistent hyperpigmentation in some cases

Gender, Race, and Age Distribution
▶ No specific predilection

Clinical Features
▶ Erythematous ovoid patches or edematous plaques which may blister in acute lesions
▶ Persistent areas of gray or brown hyperpigmentation in late-stage lesions

Prognosis and Treatment
▶ Withdrawal of offending agent and patient education regarding avoidance of the drug to prevent recurrence

---

sites are frequently involved. Acute lesions are erythematous ovoid patches and edematous violaceous to brown plaques which may blister. Late-stage lesions resolve as persistent areas of gray or brown hyperpigmentation.

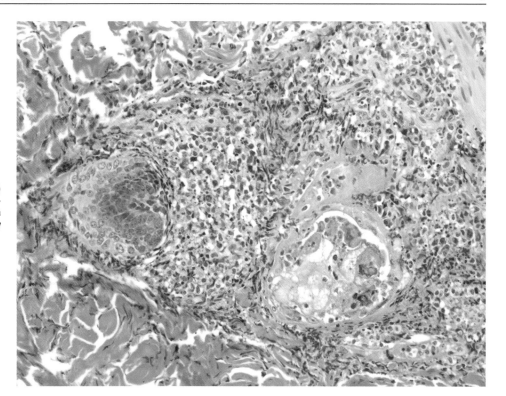

FIGURE 1.6
Acute herpes simplex virus (HSV) infection. Characteristic HSV cytopathic changes are confined within a follicular unit. This finding was only detected on level sections.

FIXED DRUG ERUPTION – PATHOLOGIC FEATURES

Microscopic Findings
▸ Vacuolar change at the dermoepidermal junction
▸ Formation of single and clustered necrotic keratinocytes at the dermoepidermal junction and within the spinous layer
▸ Secondary subepidermal blisters if there is extensive vacuolar change
▸ Conspicuous melanophages, particularly following repeat exposure to the inciting agent

Differential Diagnosis
▸ Erythema multiforme

MICROSCOPIC FEATURES

Unlike LP, there is usually vacuolar change at the DEJ with the formation of single and clustered necrotic keratinocytes both at the DEJ and within the spinous layer (Figures 1.7 and 1.8). Progression to subepidermal blister formation may result from extensive vacuolar change. The perivascular and interstitial dermal infiltrate is frequently mixed, containing eosinophils, and not infrequently, some neutrophils, and involves the deep dermis. Melanophages are frequently conspicuous, particularly if previous episodes have occurred.

DIFFERENTIAL DIAGNOSIS

The principal differential consideration is *EM*. Although in some cases it is histologically indistinguishable from FDE, the clinical distribution (i.e., single or few lesions), history (recurrent lesions at the same site) and presence of a mixed infiltrate (eosinophils, neutrophils) associated with melanophages would favor a FDE over EM.

PROGNOSIS AND TREATMENT

Withdrawal of the offending agent and symptomatic treatment are generally all that is necessary. Patient education regarding avoidance of the offending drug or agent will prevent further occurrence.

LICHEN SCLEROSUS

CLINICAL FEATURES

Lichen sclerosus (LS) is a fibrosing dermatitis with a predilection for the anogenital skin of women (women/

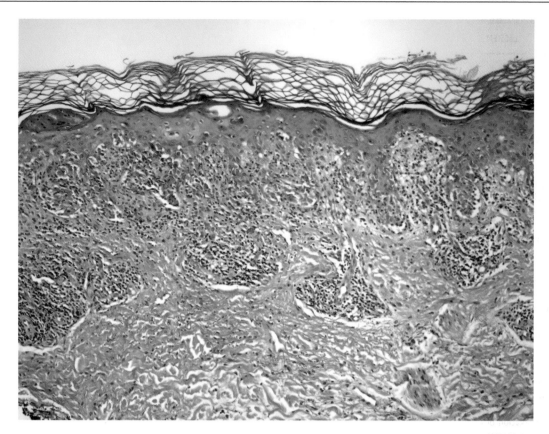

FIGURE 1.7

Fixed drug eruption. The lichenoid infiltrate is accompanied by basal vacuolization and abundant necrotic keratinocytes present both singly and in clusters at the dermoepidermal junction and in the spinous layer.

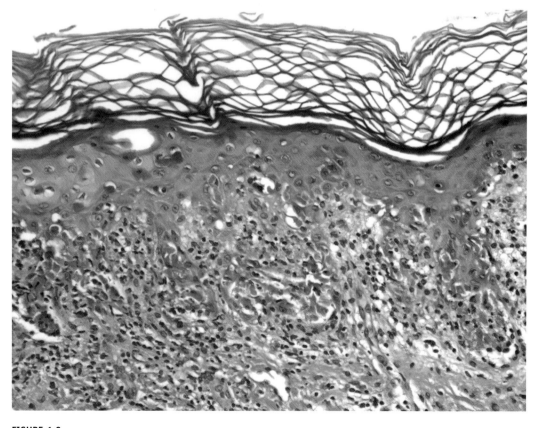

FIGURE 1.8

Fixed drug eruption. On higher power, dyskeratotic cells are present at all levels of the epidermis. The stratum corneum retains its open "basket-weave" appearance.

men 10 : 1). Classical lesions appear in a "figure-of-eight" distribution as "porcelain-white" plaques with a wrinkled surface and follicular plugs, often with intralesional ecchymoses. Long-standing lesions result in vanishing of the labia minora, and urethral stenosis.

MICROSCOPIC FEATURES

Early lesions feature psoriasiform epidermal hyperplasia accompanied by a band-like lymphocytic infiltrate, papillary dermal fibrosis, and hyperkeratosis (Figure 1.9). As the lesions develop, the hallmark findings of papillary dermal homogenization, pallor, and vascular

---

LICHEN SCLEROSUS – FACT SHEET

Definition
▶ Fibrosing dermatitis with a predilection for the anogenital skin in women

Incidence
▶ Uncommon

Morbidity
▶ Vanishing of the labia minora and urethral stenosis may occur in long-standing lesions
▶ Secondary epithelial dysplasia and squamous cell carcinoma (4%)

Gender, Race, and Age Distribution
▶ Female predominance (10 : 1)
▶ More common in Caucasians
▶ More common in fifth decade (perimenopausal)

Clinical Features
▶ "Figure-of-eight" distribution and "porcelain-white" plaques with a wrinkled surface and follicular plugging

Prognosis and Treatment
▶ Chronic waxing and waning clinical course
▶ Topical steroids and calcineurin inhibitors for local control, but uncommon complete resolution
▶ Regular observation of dysplastic areas with conservative treatment (cryotherapy)
▶ Surgery for severe introital stenosis or if carcinoma evolves within dysplastic areas

---

LICHEN SCLEROSUS – PATHOLOGIC FEATURES

Microscopic Findings
▶ Psoriasiform epidermal hyperplasia with band-like lymphohistiocytic infiltrate, papillary dermal fibrosis, and hyperkeratosis in early lesions
▶ Papillary dermal homogenization, pallor, and vascular drop-out with epidermal atrophy in mature lesions

Differential Diagnosis
▶ Lichen planus
▶ Morphea
▶ Chronic radiation dermatitis

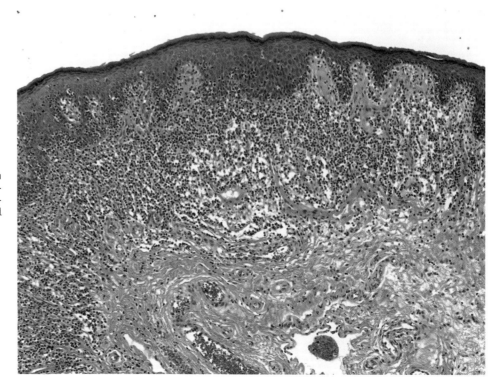

FIGURE 1.9
Early lichen sclerosus. Psoriasiform epidermal hyperplasia is accompanied by a dense band-like lymphocytic infiltrate, papillary dermal fibrosis, and hyperkeratosis.

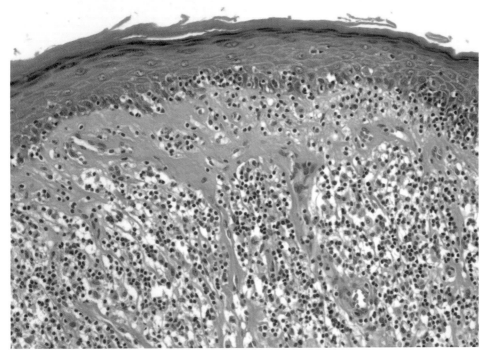

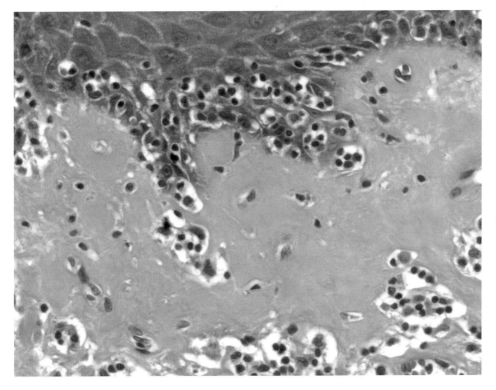

"drop-out" become apparent (Figure 1.10). As the homogenization of the papillary dermis progresses, the inflammatory infiltrate is pushed downward, and the overlying epidermis undergoes rete effacement and eventuates in pronounced epidermal atrophy (Figure 1.11). Shear injury to the epidermis may result in hemorrhagic subepidermal bullae.

DIFFERENTIAL DIAGNOSIS

While early lesions of LS may resemble *LP*, the presence of pointed rete, basal layer squamatization, wedge-shaped hypergranulosis, and preservation of the superficial elastic tissue favors a diagnosis of LP over LS. In some cases of *morphea*, there is homogenization of the papillary dermis similar to that observed in LS. The preservation of the superficial elastic tissue and presence of thickened collagen bundles in the subjacent reticular dermis will favor morphea over LS. *Late-stage radiation dermatitis* may exhibit an almost identical histomorphology to that seen in LS; however, observation of atypical endothelial cells and fibroblasts, perivascular fibrin deposition, and elastotic material admixed with zones containing sclerotic collagen in late-stage radiation dermatitis should allow separation of these two entities.

PROGNOSIS AND TREATMENT

Control of symptomatic pruritic lesions with conservative use of topical corticosteroids may be useful; however, lesions seldom resolve completely. Calcineurin inhibitors have been reported as a steroid-sparing maintenance therapy. Surgery may be required to prevent stricture, and it is necessary in the event of supervening squamous cell carcinoma, which occurs in approximately 4% of cases as a long-term complication.

PLASMACYTOSIS MUCOSAE (ZOON VULVITIS)

CLINICAL FEATURES

This is an uncommon condition which most frequently affects the glans of older men, but also has been reported in women under a variety of terms (Zoon vulvitis, vulvitis circumscripta plasmacellularis). Lesions appear as solitary, asymptomatic, sharply defined red/brown patches, which frequently exhibit a speckled and hemorrhagic surface. Ulceration commonly supervenes.

MICROSCOPIC FEATURES

A dense plasma cell-rich band-like infiltrate is present in the papillary and upper reticular dermis. The infiltrate may contain lymphocytes, histiocytes, and an occasional neutrophil and eosinophil (Figure 1.12). The overlying epidermis is usually spongiotic with an absent stratum granulosum and stratum corneum. The superficial keratinocytes often take on a "lozenge"-shaped configuration within the spongiotic foci. Extravasated red blood cells and hemosiderin deposits are frequently found in the superficial dermis (Figure 1.13).

PLASMACYTOSIS MUCOSAE (ZOON VULVITIS) – FACT SHEET

Definition
▶ A plasma cell-rich inflammatory lesion which affects the vulva in adult women and glans of older men

Incidence
▶ Rare

Morbidity
▶ Chronic erosive and ulcerative vulvitis

Gender, Race, and Age Distribution
▶ Much more common in men; rare in adult women
▶ No racial predilection

Clinical Features
▶ Solitary, initially asymptomatic, sharply defined red/brown patches with speckled and hemorrhagic surface
▶ Frequent ulceration

Prognosis and Treatment
▶ Chronic condition recalcitrant to therapy
▶ Variable results with topical steroids
▶ Excision for circumscribed lesions

DIFFERENTIAL DIAGNOSIS

Given an appropriate clinical history and morphologic description, the differential diagnosis is very narrow. Lesions of *secondary syphilis* are widespread, and are accompanied by psoriasiform epidermal hyperplasia and involve the deep vascular plexus. Occasionally, *lichenoid drug eruptions* may have a plasma cell-rich infiltrate, although the clinical appearance is much different. Resolving lesions of *herpesvirus infections* may feature a plasma cell-rich infiltrate. Interestingly, herpesvirus antigen has been detected in occasional cases of PM; therefore, if clinical suspicion for HSV infection exists, additional level sections may be useful in ruling out this latter possibility.

PLASMACYTOSIS MUCOSAE (ZOON VULVITIS) – PATHOLOGIC FEATURES

Microscopic Findings
▶ Dense plasma cell-rich band-like infiltrate in papillary and upper reticular dermis
▶ Spongiotic epidermis with absent stratum granulosum and stratum corneum
▶ "Lozenge"-shaped configuration of the superficial keratinocytes

Differential Diagnosis
▶ Syphilis
▶ Lichenoid drug eruption (uncommon)
▶ Resolving herpesvirus infection

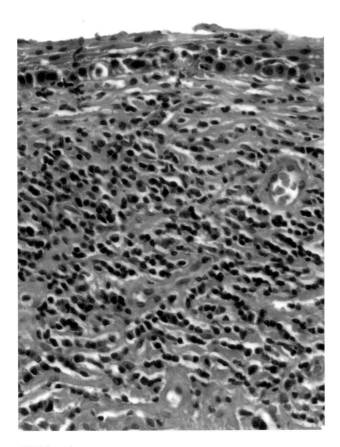

FIGURE 1.12

Plasmacytosis mucosae. A plasma cell-rich band-like infiltrate is present in the upper dermis. The overlying epidermis is spongiotic with loss of the stratum granulosum and corneum.

PROGNOSIS AND TREATMENT

Lesions are frequently recalcitrant to local therapies. Symptomatic treatment with a topical steroid is frequently employed. Circumscribed lesions have been treated by excision.

SECONDARY SYPHILIS

The lesions of primary syphilis and condyloma lata are discussed under infectious agents as they do not exhibit a lichenoid histomorphology.

CLINICAL FEATURES

Secondary syphilis develops weeks to months following infection by the spirochete *Treponema pallidum*, and is a reaction to the bacteria following systemic dissemination. Cutaneous lesions of secondary syphilis generally occur between 6 weeks and 6 months following the appearance of a primary chancre. The morphologic appearance is broad, and may be pustular, hyperkeratotic, or macular.

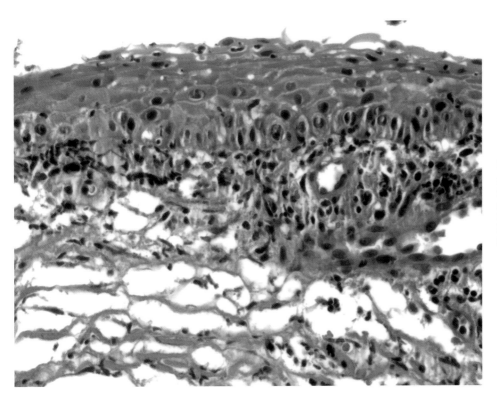

FIGURE 1.13

Plasmacytosis mucosae. The superficial keratinocytes focally exhibit a "lozenge"-shaped configuration. Note red blood cell extravasation and hemosiderin deposition in the superficial dermis.

SYPHILIS – FACT SHEET

Definition
▸ Sexually transmitted infection caused by the spirochete *Treponema pallidum*

Incidence
▸ 2.7 cases/100 000 overall rate of infection in United States

Morbidity
▸ Disfiguring nodules or progressively destructive ulcers may occur in late mucocutaneous lesions
▸ Neurosyphilis may lead to paralysis, numbness, blindness, and dementia

Gender, Race, and Age Distribution
▸ 84% of syphilitic infections occur in men
▸ 9.0 cases/100,000 in African Americans
▸ 14/100,000 in African American men
▸ 4.3/100,000 in African American women (2004)
▸ Ratio of African American to white: 9.0:1.6
▸ Increasing rates in homosexual men
▸ More common between 20 and 39 years

Clinical Features

Primary Syphilis
▸ Initial lesion (chancre): indurated, "punched-out," painless ulcer, 20–30 days postexposure

Condyloma Lata
▸ Elevated flat-topped red-brown to gray papules on mucosal surfaces of the labia

Secondary Syphilis
▸ Lesions with broad morphology, including pustules, macules, or hyperkeratotic lesions (weeks to months following infection)

Prognosis and Treatment
▸ Excellent prognosis if early treatment with penicillin
▸ If untreated, tertiary syphilis is associated with skin, bone, central nervous system, heart, and great vessel abnormalities

MICROSCOPIC FEATURES

Early lesions are often nonspecific, exhibiting plasma cell-rich perivascular dermatitis without significant epidermal alteration. As the lesions evolve, there is psoriasiform epidermal hyperplasia, with a band-like infiltrate composed of lymphocytes, plasma cells, and macrophages at the DEJ, often accompanied by a deep perivascular infiltrate (Figures 1.14 and 1.15). Keratinocyte necrosis is uncommon. In spirochete-rich lesions, neutrophilic spongiform pustules similar to those found in psoriasis may be present in the epidermis. Neutrophil-rich crusts may also surmount such lesions. Other features include endothelial swelling, and, in older lesions, a more granulomatous infiltrate.

SECONDARY SYPHILIS – PATHOLOGIC FEATURES

Microscopic Features
▸ Highly variable histology
▸ Psoriasiform epidermal hyperplasia more common
▸ Band-like infiltrate with plasma cells often involving deep vascular plexus
▸ Spirochete-rich lesions, often containing neutrophils
▸ Slender "left-handed" spiral spirochetes, 6-16 μm in length
▸ Variable endothelial swelling
▸ Epithelioid granulomas may be present in late stage lesions

Differential Diagnosis
▸ Any inflammatory response involving mucosal or paramucosal sites
▸ Plasmacytosis mucosae

HISTOCHEMICAL AND IMMUNOHISTOCHEMICAL FEATURES

Traditionally, silver stains (Warthin–Starry, Steiner) are used to demonstrate the organisms; however, their sensitivity and high background limit their application. Immunoperoxidase stains will increase sensitivity as they become more widely available.

DIFFERENTIAL DIAGNOSIS

The presence of psoriasiform epidermal hyperplasia accompanied by plasma cell-rich lichenoid infiltrates is strongly supportive of a diagnosis of syphilis. Some *long-standing lichenoid hypersensitivity eruptions* (drug, herpesvirus, *Borrelia* infection) may contain plasma cells; however, the clinical setting is quite different, and significant epidermal hyperplasia is generally absent. Likewise, *plasmacytosis mucosae* exhibits an atrophric epidermis with sponfiosis, and in long-standing lesions hemosiderin is present. *Mycosis fungoides* may show a similar low-power appearance to that seen in syphilis; however, the finding of atypical lymphocytes within the epidermis allows separation from lue. Lastly, correlation with the patient's serology is helpful if diagnostic uncertainty remains.

PROGNOSIS AND TREATMENT

Thankfully, syphilis remains exquisitely sensitive to penicillin therapy. When treated early, the prognosis is excellent. Following clinical cure, the patient is monitored for reversion to seronegativity. If left untreated, tertiary syphilis produces widespread manifestations in the skin, bone, central nervous system, heart, and great vessels.

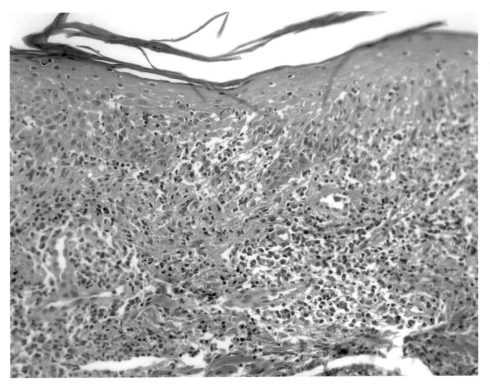

FIGURE 1.14

Secondary syphilis. Psoriasiform epidermal hyperplasia with a band-like infiltrate composed of lymphocytes, plasma cells, and histiocytes is observed.

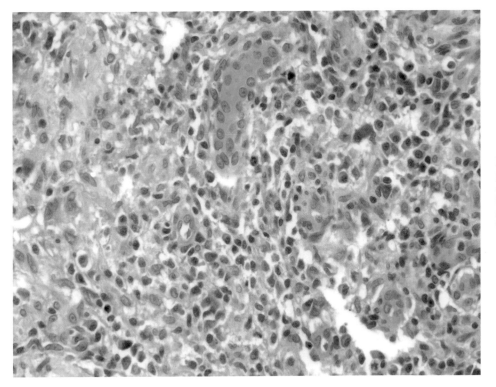

FIGURE 1.15

Secondary syphilis. A mixed plasma cell and histiocytic inflammatory infiltrate is present in the superficial dermis associated with mild endothelial swelling.

THE SPONGIOTIC (ECZEMATOUS) EPIDERMAL REACTION PATTERN

The characteristic feature of the spongiotic (eczematous) epidermal reaction pattern is the presence of intercellular edema (spongiosis), histologically manifest as an increase in the intercellular space between keratinocytes. In most cases, there is at least focal exocytosis of lymphocytes into the epidermis. Eosinophil and neutrophil exocytosis is much less common, and their presence invokes additional diagnostic considerations. If the severity of the response increases, there is widening of the intercellular space, eventuating in desmosomal rupture, followed by formation of vesicles within the epidermis. These vesicles may contain fluid, lymphocytes, and Langerhans cells, as well as acantholytic or ruptured keratinocytes.

All eczematous dermatitides demonstrate epidermal spongiosis during their evolution, clinically seen as crusted patches and plaques, papules and vesicles, and, at the far end of the spectrum, frank bullous lesions. Although absolute histologic distinction between the various categories of spongiotic dermatitis is not possible, there are some features that may be utilized to favor a more specific clinical-pathologic correlate. The most important differential considerations in genital skin will be discussed below.

ATOPIC DERMATITIS

CLINICAL FEATURES

Atopic dermatitis is a chronic, pruritic dermatitis which occurs in individuals with a personal or family history of an atopic diathesis (atopic dermatitis, asthma, allergic rhinitis). Generally, onset is in infancy or childhood. Findings include an erythematous papulovesicular rash involving the flexural and extensor surfaces of the arms and legs. Over time, scaly lichenified patches and plaques appear. The vulva is sometimes involved, particularly in children.

MICROSCOPIC FEATURES

Atopic dermatitis exhibits the full spectrum of epidermal changes observed in most spongiotic processes, and may be used as a model to study the evolution of a typical spongiotic tissue reaction. In acute lesions, there is both intercellular, and, to some extent, intracellular edema of the lower epidermis with exocytosis of lymphocytes. A perivascular lymphohistiocytic infiltrate is present, usually with occasional eosinophils. Subacute lesions exhibit increasing psoriasiform epidermal hyperplasia and parakeratosis (Figures 1.16 and 1.17), and as increased lichenification supervenes, the degree of spongiosis generally decreases. Chronic lesions display more marked psoriasiform epidermal hyperplasia with variable, but often very mild to absent spongiosis. Further lichenification produces prominent hyperkeratosis with "vertical streaking" of collagen in the papillary dermis. These later changes are recognized as lichen simplex chronicus (LSC). Unlike the regular pattern of epidermal hyperplasia found in psoriasis, the rete ridges in the later stages of a chronic eczematous dermatitis are generally irregular in both length and width.

DIFFERENTIAL DIAGNOSIS

The distinction between atopic dermatitis, *allergic contact dermatitis*, and *irritant contact dermatitis* is difficult without clinicopathologic correlation.

ATOPIC DERMATITIS – FACT SHEET

Definition
▶ Chronic pruritic dermatitis which occurs in individuals with a personal or family history of an atopic diathesis (atopic dermatitis, asthma, allergic rhinitis)

Incidence
▶ Common
▶ Symptoms in approximately 20% of infants and young children, 90% before age 5

Morbidity
▶ Chronic hand dermatitis may complicate occupational performance
▶ Predisposition to infection due to compromised cutaneous barrier

Gender and Race
▶ Increased risk in males
▶ Increased risk in those of black and Asian ethnicity

Clinical Features
▶ Erythematous papulovesicular rash in flexural and extensor surfaces of arms and legs
▶ Sometimes vulvar involvement, particularly in children
▶ Scaly lichenified patches and plaques

Prognosis and Treatment
▶ Generally spontaneous remission throughout childhood
▶ Few cases persist over age 30
▶ Treatment includes hydration of skin, minimizing trigger factors, relief of pruritus, and decreasing inflammation
▶ Topical steroids and nonsteroidal immune modulators

ATOPIC DERMATITIS – PATHOLOGIC FEATURES

Microscopic Findings

Acute Lesion
▶ Intercellular edema of lower epidermis
▶ Exocytosis of lymphocytes
▶ Perivascular lymphohistiocytic infiltrate with occasional eosinophils

Subacute Lesion
▶ Psoriasiform epidermal hyperplasia with parakeratosis
▶ Variable lymphocyte exocytosis

Chronic Lesion
▶ Marked psoriasiform epidermal hyperplasia
▶ Mild to absent spongiosis and lymphocyte exocytosis

Differential Diagnosis
▶ Contact dermatitis
▶ Spongiotic hypersensitivity reaction (drug, ingestant, scabetic infestation, others)

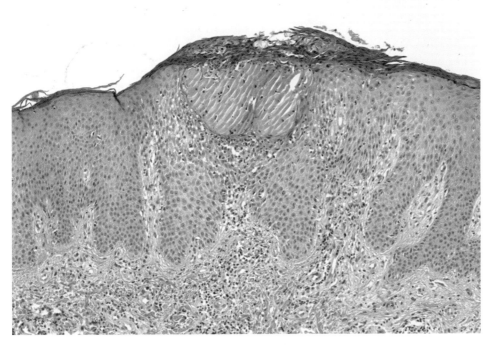

FIGURE 1.16

Subacute spongiotic dermatitis (atopic dermatitis). Psoriasiform epidermal hyperplasia and parakeratosis are accompanied by spongiotic microvesicles, lymphocyte exocytosis, and a perivascular lymphohistiocytic infiltrate.

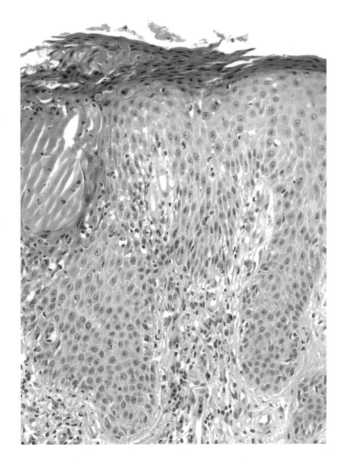

FIGURE 1.17

Subacute spongiotic dermatitis (atopic dermatitis). There is intracellular edema of the epidermis with formation of spongiotic microvesicles containing mononuclear cells. A perivascular lymphohistiocytic infiltrate is accompanied by occasional eosinophils.

PROGNOSIS AND TREATMENT

Atopic dermatitis tends to resolve spontaneously throughout childhood, with few cases persisting over age 30. Therapeutic management is directed towards hydration of the skin, minimizing triggering factors, relief of pruritus, and decreasing inflammation. Topical steroids have traditionally been the treatment choice. Recently, nonsteroidal agents such as tacrolimus have been utilized as a powerful immune modulator without the disadvantages of chronic steroid use.

ALLERGIC CONTACT DERMATITIS

Allergic contact dermatitis (ACD) is a hypersensitivity reaction initiated by contact with an allergen to which an individual has been previously sensitized. Lesions typically develop within 48 hours following exposure to the allergen. Numerous agents, including cosmetics, plants, preservatives, textile dyes, chemicals associated with rubber and plastic production, and metals, may elicit this reaction pattern.

CLINICAL FEATURES

In acute contact dermatitis, common findings include a pruritic papulovesicular eruption, discretely patterned crusted plaques, or, occasionally, bizarre-appearing pat-

---

ALLERGIC CONTACT DERMATITIS – FACT SHEET

Definition
▶ Type IV hypersensitivity reaction initiated by contact with an allergen to which an individual has been previously sensitized

Incidence
▶ Common (4–7% of all dermatologic consultations)

Morbidity
▶ Relapse and chronicity from re-exposure to offending antigen, particularly occupational exposure, may impact individual occupational choices

Gender and Race
▶ Approximately twice as common in females as in males
▶ More frequent in whites than in other racial groups

Clinical Features
▶ Pruritic papulovesicular eruption
▶ Circumscribed crusted plaques
▶ Occasionally bizarre-appearing patterns

Prognosis and Treatment
▶ Excellent prognosis if removal or protection from the offending agent
▶ Emollients and short-term topical steroid therapy to reduce inflammation and allow re-establishment of cutaneous barrier

terns, depending on the extent of contact with the agent.

MICROSCOPIC FEATURES

Following the appearance of lower epidermal spongiosis, spongiotic microvesicles form within various levels of the epidermis, imparting a "Swiss-cheese" appearance (Figure 1.18). There is exocytosis of lymphocytes, as well as eosinophils in some cases. In an acute allergic contact, the stratum corneum remains unchanged. If the allergen persists, there is subsequent epidermal hyperplasia with a diminution of spongiosis.

ALLERGIC CONTACT DERMATITIS – PATHOLOGIC FEATURES

Microscopic Findings
▶ Spongiotic microvesicles within various levels of epidermis ("Swiss-cheese" appearance)
▶ Exocytosis of lymphocytes and eosinophils (eosinophilic spongiosis)
▶ Unchanged stratum corneum in acute reaction
▶ Epidermal hyperplasia and diminution of spongiosis if persistent allergen

Differential Diagnosis
▶ Atopic dermatitis
▶ Eczematous hypersensitivity reaction (drug, ingestant, scabetic infestation, others)

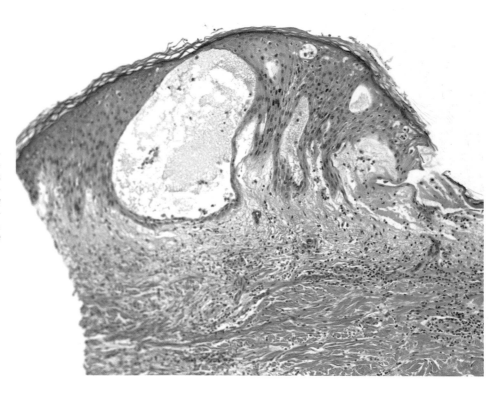

FIGURE 1.18
Spongiotic dermatitis (allergic contact dermatitis). Spongiotic microvesicles are formed within various levels of the epidermis, imparting a "Swiss-cheese" appearance, accompanied by exocytosis of lymphocytes. The stratum corneum remains unchanged, reflecting the acute nature of the insult.

DIFFERENTIAL DIAGNOSIS

See atopic dermatitis section.

PROGNOSIS AND TREATMENT

Removal of, or protection from the offending agent is paramount. Short-term topical corticosteroid therapy to reduce inflammation, and emollients to allow the re-establishment of the barrier function of the skin, are employed.

IRRITANT CONTACT DERMATITIS

Irritant contact dermatitis (ICD) is initiated by the direct effect of an irritant compound on an epithelial surface, and therefore occurs rapidly after exposure to the agent. Offending agents include soaps and detergents, feces and urine, solvents, wool, and other fibers.

CLINICAL FEATURES

A large range of clinical appearances may be seen, including erythema, eczematous changes, vesiculobullous lesions, and epidermal necrosis.

MICROSCOPIC FEATURES

In contrast to ACD, the agent responsible for ICD produces direct injury to the epidermis. The degree and severity of the epidermal injury vary based on the nature and concentration of the irritant. Frequently, there is ballooning degeneration of the surface keratinocytes with subsequent necrosis and surrounding epidermal spongiosis. Neutrophil exocytosis is frequently observed in the areas of epidermal necrosis. The subjacent dermis contains a superficial perivascular infiltrate of lymphocytes, macrophages and, frequently, neutrophils. Interstitial edema and vasodilatation are also present (Figure 1.19).

DIFFERENTIAL DIAGNOSIS

See atopic dermatitis section.

PROGNOSIS AND TREATMENT

Removal of, or protection from, the offending agent will prevent recurrence of symptoms. The treatment of ICD is directed towards the re-establishment of the skin's barrier function. Topical applications containing ceramides may be particularly helpful. Corticosteroids and immune modulators have an unproven role in the treatment of ICD.

IRRITANT CONTACT DERMATITIS – FACT SHEET

Definition
▶ Dermatitis initiated by direct effect of an irritant compound on an epithelial surface

Incidence
▶ Common

Morbidity
▶ Significant long-term sequelae possible if chronic occupational exposure

Gender, Race, and Age Distribution
▶ More common in women than in men, secondary to environmental rather than genetic factors
▶ No age or racial predilection

Clinical Features
▶ Wide range of clinical appearances, including erythema, eczematous changes, vesiculobullous lesions, and epidermal necrosis

Prognosis and Treatment
▶ Excellent prognosis if removal of, or protection from the offending agent
▶ Emollients re-establish cutaneous barrier function
▶ Topical steroids and immune modulators not helpful

IRRITANT CONTACT DERMATITIS – PATHOLOGIC FEATURES

Microscopic Findings
▶ Ballooning degeneration and necrosis of surface keratinocytes
▶ Neutrophil exocytosis in areas of epidermal necrosis
▶ Interstitial edema and vasodilatation may occur

Differential Diagnosis
▶ Allergic contact dermatitis
▶ Eczematous hypersensitivity reaction (Drug, ingestant, scabetic infestation, others)

SEBORRHEIC DERMATITIS

CLINICAL FEATURES

Seborrheic dermatitis is a common eczematous dermatitis occurring in areas of the skin that have the greatest number of sebaceous glands (scalp, face, chest, upper back, axillae, and anogenital skin). The affected skin is erythematous, with scaling papules and plaques having a "greasy yellow" appearance.

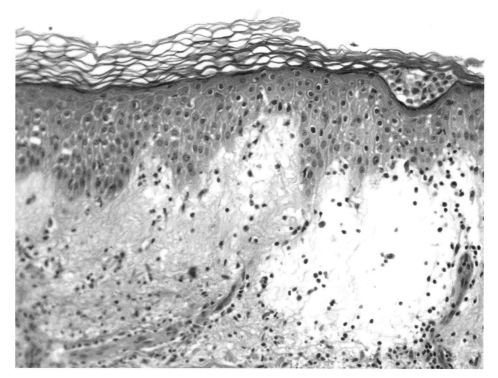

FIGURE 1.19
Spongiotic dermatitis (irritant contact dermatitis). This case exhibits only mild spongiosis with the formation of Langerhans cell microabscesses. Marked edema and vasodilatation are present in the papillary dermis.

SEBORRHEIC DERMATITIS – FACT SHEET

Definition
▸ Common eczematous dermatitis occurring on skin with greatest number of sebaceous glands

Incidence
▸ Common; approximate 5% prevalence

Morbidity
▸ Cosmetic

Gender, Race, and Age Distribution
▸ More common in men than women
▸ No racial predisposition
▸ Common in fourth to fifth decade
▸ Self-limited infantile form in first 3 months of life

Clinical Features
▸ Erythematous skin, with papules and plaques with a bran-like scale and a "greasy yellow" appearance
▸ Extensive therapy-resistant seborrheic dermatitis may indicate underlying human immunodeficiency virus infection

Prognosis and Treatment
▸ Mild clinical course with little discomfort other than cosmetic concerns
▸ Removal of scale with keratolytics followed by sparing use of corticosteroids and antifungal agents

---

SEBORRHEIC DERMATITIS – PATHOLOGIC FEATURES

Microscopic Findings

Acute Lesion
▸ Mild spongiosis with neutrophil parakeratosis
▸ Papillary dermal edema and lymphohistiocytic perivascular infiltrate

Advanced Lesion
▸ Substantial psoriasiform hyperplasia and "shoulder parakeratosis" (perifollicular accentuation of parakeratosis)

Differential Diagnosis
▸ Psoriasis
▸ Dermatophyte infection
▸ Impetiginized eczema

MICROSCOPIC FEATURES

In acute lesions, there is mild spongiosis with a parakeratotic scale crust frequently containing a few neutrophils (Figure 1.20). The papillary dermis may be slightly edematous, and a perivascular dermatitis composed of lymphocytes, histiocytes and, rarely, neutrophils is present in the superficial plexus. As lesions progress, there is more substantial psoriasiform hyperplasia, as well as parafollicular accentuation of the parakeratotic

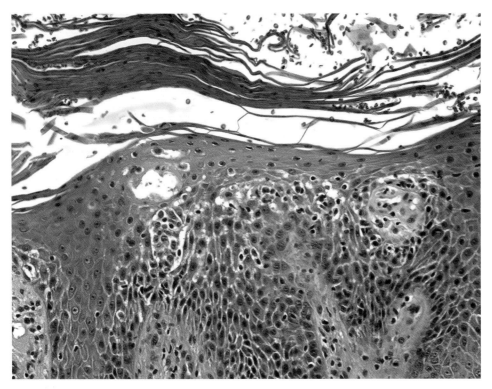

FIGURE 1.20

Seborrheic dermatitis. There is psoriasiform epidermal hyperplasia with spongiosis, a parakeratotic scale crust, mild papillary dermal edema, and a perivascular dermatitis composed of lymphocytes and histiocytes.

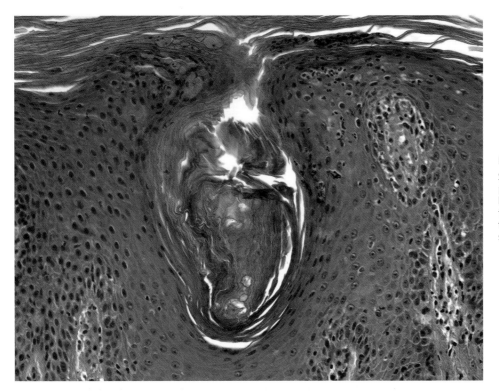

FIGURE 1.21

Seborrheic dermatitis. Characteristic parafollicular accentuation of parakeratosis ("shoulder parakeratosis") is accompanied by exocytosis of neutrophils into the scale crust and spongiotic foci.

scale ("shoulder parakeratosis"). Neutrophils are commonly observed within the scale crust and within spongiotic foci (Figure 1.21). In chronic lesions, there is increasing psoriasiform hyperplasia, and the parakeratosis and scale crust may extend into the interfollicular epidermis.

DIFFERENTIAL DIAGNOSIS

The presence of neutrophil parakeratosis and psoriasiform epidermal hyperplasia raises consideration of a diagnosis of *psoriasis*. While differentiation between these possibilities may at times be difficult, the irregular elongation of the epidermal rete, accentuation of parakeratosis and scale crusts about the follicular ostia, and predilection of the follicular and epidermal spongiosis to be more concentrated toward the upper layers of the epidermis all favor a diagnosis of seborrheic dermatitis over psoriasis. Neutrophil-rich parakeratosis is also a feature observed in many impetiginized eczematous dermatitis and in cutaneous fungal infections (see below). A tissue gram stain ("Brown and Hopps") and periodic acid-schiff, diastase resistant (PAS-D) stain are helpful adjuncts in excluding these respective possibilities.

PROGNOSIS AND TREATMENT

Seborrheic dermatitis generally exhibits a mild chronic clinical course with little discomfort. Treatment is directed towards removal of scale with keratolytics, followed by sparing use of topical corticosteroids. Topical antifungal agents constitute an important adjunct in therapy and reduce or eliminate the need for steroid therapy over time when used consistently.

PSORIASIFORM EPIDERMAL REACTION PATTERN

Psoriasis is the prototype of a group of dermatoses which characteristically exhibit regular epidermal hyperplasia.

PSORIASIS

CLINICAL FEATURES

Psoriasis is a chronic dermatitis characterized by a hyperproliferative epidermis. Lesions consist of circumscribed patches and plaques with a "silvery" scale. When removed, this scale produces focal bleeding (*Auspitz sign*). The anatomic distribution is wide; however, lesions concentrate in areas of persistent trauma or friction (elbows, knees, sacrum, scalp, and intertriginous areas). The occurrence of lesions in response to trauma has been termed the *Koebner phenomenon*. Other triggers include drugs and infections. *Inverse psoriasis* is the label given to psoriasis affecting the intertriginous areas. Secondary changes of friction and maceration may cause loss of the characteristic fine scale of psoriasis. Superinfection by yeast, fungi, and bacteria is possible. Linkage studies suggest a polygenic inheritance model for this disease, with the major gene, *PSORS1*, being mapped to 6p21.3.

PSORIASIS – FACT SHEET

Definition
▸ Chronic dermatitis characterized by a hyperproliferative epidermis and regular epidermal hyperplasia

Incidence
▸ 2–4% prevalence rate in Caucasian population

Morbidity
▸ Significant cosmetic impact on quality of life
▸ Hand and foot involvement may limit certain occupational pursuits
▸ Psoriatic arthritis complicates 5–30% of patients

Gender, Race, and Age Distribution
▸ No gender predisposition
▸ Low prevalence in patients of Asiatic, Native American, and African descent
▸ Earlier onset in females than males
▸ Onset before age 40 in about 75% of patients

Clinical Features
▸ Circumscribed patches and plaques with a "silvery" scale
▸ Wide anatomic distribution, but mostly in areas of persistent trauma or friction
▸ "Inverse psoriasis" if it affects intertriginous areas

Prognosis and Treatment
▸ Long-term management discouraging due to chronic course of disease
▸ Topical therapies for localized disease
▸ Systemic therapies for severe disease, including methotrexate, retinoids, cyclosporine, phototherapy, and photochemotherapy (psoralen with ultraviolet A)

MICROSCOPIC FEATURES

Psoriasis exhibits a range of histologic appearances which are dependent upon the duration of the lesion. Early lesions exhibit a spongiotic epidermal reaction pattern with papillary dermal vascular congestion, edema, and a sparse perivascular dermatitis. As lesions progress, characteristic mounds of neutrophil-rich parakeratosis form, with subsequent loss of the granular cell layer (hypogranulosis). There is increased mitotic activity in the basal unit associated with regular acanthosis (Figure 1.22). Mature lesions exhibit confluent neutrophil-rich parakeratosis. The intracorneal collections of neutrophils have been termed *Munroe microabsecesses,* whereas those in the spinous layer are called *spongiform pustules of Kogoj.* The epidermis may show marked regular psoriasiform epidermal hyperplasia with intervening thinned suprapapillary plates and subjacent dilated capillaries, frequently in immediate apposition to the overlying epidermis (Figure 1.23). A lymphocyte-rich perivascular infiltrate is present in the superficial vascular plexus. Neutrophils are uncommon, and eosinophils are usually absent.

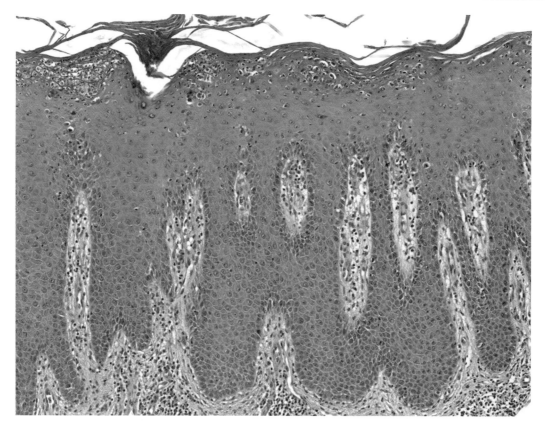

FIGURE 1.22

Psoriasis. This well-developed lesion exhibits regular psoriasiform epidermal hyperplasia surmounted by mounds of neutrophil-rich parakeratosis and loss of the granular cell layer.

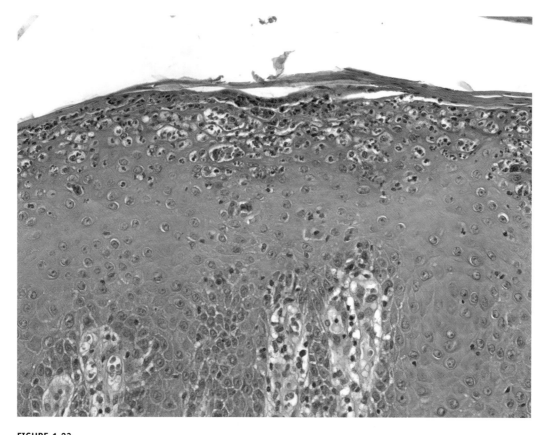

FIGURE 1.23

Psoriasis. The suprapapillary plates are thinned and contain dilated capillaries, often in immediate apposition to the overlying epidermis.

PSORIASIS – PATHOLOGIC FEATURES

Microscopic Findings

Early Lesion
▶ Epidermal spongiosis
▶ Papillary dermal vascular congestion and edema
▶ Sparse perivascular dermatitis

Advanced Lesion
▶ Regular acanthosis with increased basal mitotic activity
▶ Mounds of neutrophil-rich parakeratosis
▶ Hypogranulosis

Mature Lesion
▶ Marked regular psoriasiform epidermal hyperplasia with thinned suprapapillary plates
▶ Confluent neutrophil-rich parakeratosis, "Munroe microabscesses", and "spongiform pustules of Kogoj"
▶ Papillary dermal vascular ectasia
▶ Lymphocytic-rich perivascular dermatitis

Differential Diagnosis
▶ Lichen simplex chronicus
▶ Seborrheic dermatitis
▶ Dermatophytosis and candidiasis

LICHEN SIMPLEX CHRONICUS – FACT SHEET

Definition
▶ Idiopathic condition in which scaly plaques are formed in response to repetitive rubbing of affected sites

Incidence
▶ Common

Morbidity
▶ Cosmetic
▶ Superinfection if abraded and ulcerated lesions

Gender, Race, and Age Distribution
▶ More common in women than men
▶ No racial predilection
▶ Peak incidence between 30 and 50 years

Clinical Features
▶ Hyperpigmented scaly plaques at sites of repetitive rubbing
▶ Perianal and genital regions, posterior neck, forearms, and pretibial areas are anatomic sites of predilection

Prognosis and Treatment
▶ Cessation of the itch–scratch cycle
▶ Emollients, topical steroids, and barrier occlusion
▶ Behavior modification and psychopharmacologic agents may be beneficial in select patients

DIFFERENTIAL DIAGNOSIS

Late-stage lesions of *LSC* (see below) can usually be differentiated from psoriasis by the presence of thicker suprapapillary plates, hypergranulosis, and the presence of thickened vertically oriented collagen bundles within the papillary dermis. Differentiation from *seborrheic dermatitis* is sometimes very difficult. Attention to the anatomic location and the presence of spongiosis involving the rete ridges will often allow the observer to exclude psoriasis. *Chronic candidiasis and dermatophytoses* may feature neutrophil exocytosis and psoriasiform epidermal hyperplasia. Therefore, a PAS-D or methenamine silver stain is recommended to exclude the presence of fungal elements.

PROGNOSIS AND TREATMENT

The frustrating chronic course requires long-term management focused on balancing the extent of disease involvement with the potential side-effects of therapy. Topical therapies are utilized for localized plaques. They include emollients, corticosteroids, tars, and, more recently, vitamin D analogs and tacrolimus. Systemic therapies for severe disease include methotrexate, retinoids, and cyclosporine. Phototherapy and photochemotherapy (psoralen with ultraviolet A) are also frequently used in these cases.

LICHEN SIMPLEX CHRONICUS

CLINICAL FEATURES

Lichen simplex chronicus is an idiopathic condition in which scaly plaques are formed in response to repetitive rubbing of affected sites. Anatomic sites of predilection include the perianal and genital regions, as well as the posterior neck, forearms, and pretibial areas. The cause of the apparent underlying pruritus is unknown, although patients with underlying atopic dermatitis appear to be at increased risk.

MICROSCOPIC FEATURES

There is broad compact orthokeratosis with subjacent hypergranulosis. Focal parakeratosis is often present (Figure 1.24). There is irregular psoriasiform epidermal hyperplasia composed of thick rete ridges without suprapapillary plate thinning. The lesions may demonstrate focal abrasions or ulceration. A characteristic feature is the presence of thickened eosinophilic bundles of colla-

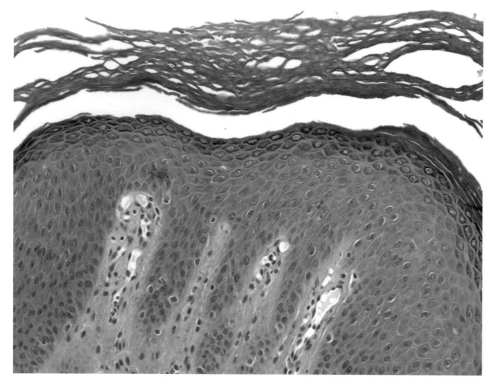

FIGURE 1.24
Lichen simplex chronicus. There is broad compact orthokeratosis and hypergranulosis. The psoriasiform epidermal hyperplasia does not exhibit suprapapillary plate thinning.

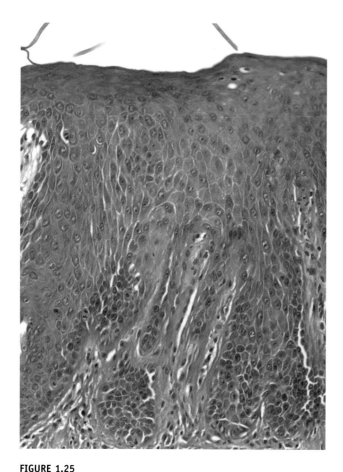

FIGURE 1.25
Lichen simplex chronicus. Thick eosinophilic bundles of collagen are arranged in vertical streaks within the papillary dermis.

LICHEN SIMPLEX CHRONICUS – PATHOLOGIC FEATURES

Microscopic Findings

▸ Compact orthokeratosis and focal parakeratosis
▸ Hypergranulosis with subjacent irregular psoriasiform epidermal hyperplasia
▸ Thick eosinophilic bundles of collagen in "vertical streaks" in papillary dermis

Differential Diagnosis

▸ Lichen simplex chronicus may be superimposed on virtually all dermatoses
▸ Frequently present in patients with an underlying atopic diathesis

gen arranged in vertical streaks within the papillary dermis (Figure 1.25), although this feature is less well developed in the mucocutaneous surfaces of the vulva and perineum.

DIFFERENTIAL DIAGNOSIS

Superimposed changes of LSC can be observed in virtually all dermatoses, therefore careful evaluation to exclude a primary dermatosis is essential before rendering a diagnosis of idiopathic LSC.

PROGNOSIS AND TREATMENT

Cessation of the traumatic perpetuation of this condition is one of the greatest barriers to resolution of these lesions. Emollients, topical steroids, and simple barrier occlusion may help halt the itch–scratch cycle. If no underlying etiologic factor is identified, behavioral modification is paramount in the prevention of relapse. Psychopharmacologic agents may also be beneficial in select patients.

INFECTIONS

SYPHILIS

CLINICAL FEATURES

After years of diminishing incidence following the introduction of antimicrobial therapy, syphilis is undergoing resurgence, particularly among drug users, and in individuals who participate in high-risk sexual behavior. A close relationship between human immunodeficiency virus (HIV) infection and syphilis exists. The presence of genital ulceration in syphilis likely provides a portal of entry for HIV infection.

The organism, *Treponema pallidum*, is a slender "left-handed" spiral spirochete, 6–16 μm in length. The initial lesion (chancre) typically appears on the labia 20–30 days following direct exposure. The lesion characteristically appears as an indurated, "punched-out," painless ulcer. This resolves without scarring in 1–4 weeks. The lesions of secondary syphilis are discussed under lichenoid dermatitis. Condyloma lata affect the mucosal surfaces of the host and appear as elevated flat-topped red-brown to gray papules.

MICROSCOPIC FEATURES

Primary lesions occur at the site of inoculation, and characteristically exhibit epidermal hyperplasia with a neutrophil- and plasma cell-rich lymphohistiocytic infiltrate. Ulceration ensues, frequently with adjacent pseudoepitheliomatous hyperplasia. Vascular endothelial swelling has frequently been described.

Condyloma lata appear histologically as papillary epithelial hyperplasia with an associated plasma cell-rich lymphohistiocytic infiltrate. The number of organisms is usually quite large.

DIFFERENTIAL DIAGNOSIS

See discussion of secondary syphilis.

PROGNOSIS AND TREATMENT

See discussion of secondary syphilis.

CANDIDIASIS

Candida albicans is the most common species of *Candida* found in the gastrointestinal tract, but is not commonly isolated from the skin surface. Many host factors may contribute to clinical infection. These include local factors such as skin moisture level, heat, and maceration; metabolic factors such as endocrinopathies, immunocompromised states, and pregnancy; and lastly, iatrogenic factors such as antibiotic or topical steroid therapy. The two clinical variants observed in the vulva will be discussed.

CLINICAL FEATURES

Acute superficial candidiasis is characterized by a pruritic vesiculopustular eruption ("satellite pustulation")

CANDIDIASIS – FACT SHEET

Definition
▸ Infection caused by the yeast *Candida albicans*

Incidence
▸ Common

Morbidity
▸ Superficial infections of mucosa are numerically most important; however, extension into soft tissue, septicemia, endocarditis, and meningitis may occur, particularly in immunocompromised patients

Gender, Race, and Age Distribution
▸ No gender or racial predilection
▸ Very young, elderly, and immunocompromised patients commonly affected

Clinical Features
▸ Acute superficial candidiasis: pruritic vesiculopustular eruption "satellite pustulosis" with crusted erosions involving intertriginous areas
▸ Chronic mucocutaneous candidiasis: mild erythema or lichenified plaques

Prognosis and Treatment
▸ Topical or oral agent antifungal therapy depending on extent of involvement
▸ Alteration of local and generalized susceptibility factors necessary to prevent relapse

---

CANDIDIASIS – PATHOLOGIC FEATURES

Microscopic Findings

Acute Superficial Candidiasis
- Spongiform or subcorneal pustulation
- Variable acanthosis and hyperkeratosis
- Variable neutrophil-rich perivascular and interstitial lymphohistiocytic infiltrate

Chronic Mucocutaneous Candidiasis
- Greater acanthosis and scale crust formation in comparison to acute superficial candidiasis

Ancillary Studies
- Periodic acid–schiff-D stain highlights the presence of yeast and pseudohyphal forms

Differential Diagnosis
- Psoriasis
- Impetiginized eczema

---

with crusted erosions and a "beefy-red" appearance involving the intertriginous areas, particularly in humid environments and the obese.

Chronic infection of the vulva by candida and is thought to be caused by a defect in cytokine production in response to certain candidal antigens. Immunodeficient states, endocrinopathies, and nutritional deficiency may also contribute to the pathogenesis of this disorder. These patients present with lichenified plaques, or may exhibit only erythema, mild edema, and minimal discharge.

MICROSCOPIC FEATURES

The presence of neutrophils in the epidermis is characteristic of acute superficial candidiasis and may manifest as spongiform and/or subcorneal pustulation within a variable acanthotic epidermis. Hyperorthokeratosis or parakeratosis may be present. A neutrophil-rich perivascular and interstitial lymphohistiocytic infiltrate is found in the superficial dermis accompanied by variable edema. A PAS-D stain will highlight the predominantly pseudohyphal forms which are often aligned perpendicular to the surface of the skin.

Chronic lesions are similar to those seen in acute superficial candidiasis, but tend to have greater acanthosis and scale crust formation. A PAS-D preparation highlights the presence of yeast and pseudohyphal forms.

DIFFERENTIAL DIAGNOSIS

Psoriasis frequently demonstrates neutrophil exocytosis and spongiform pustulation but lacks fungal elements. An *impetiginized eczematous dermatitis* will contain

intraepidermal and intracorneal neutrophils; however, fungal forms are absent on special stains.

PROGNOSIS AND TREATMENT

Topical antifungal therapy remains the mainstay of treatment. Oral agents are now widely available and effective in single-dose and short-course regimens.

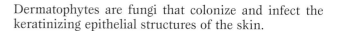

DERMATOPHYTOSES

Dermatophytes are fungi that colonize and infect the keratinizing epithelial structures of the skin.

CLINICAL FEATURES

Although quite variable, the classical appearance is that of an erythematous annular plaque with peripheral scale, and a central zone of clearing. Hair involvement is not uncommon. Atypical iatrogenic presentations, particularly following the use of topical steroids, have sometimes been given the appellation "tinea incognito." Underlying diseases may predispose individuals to infection, especially immunocompromised patients, or those having a history of diabetes mellitus or other endocrinopathies. Local factors such as sweating, abrasion, and maceration also contribute to the development of infection.

MICROSCOPIC FEATURES

Unfortunately, dermatophyte infection may produce almost every epidermal inflammatory reaction pattern. Classically, neutrophils and compact orthokeratosis and/or parakeratosis are present ("sandwich" sign of Ackerman) in the stratum corneum. The epidermis is frequently spongiotic, progressing to epidermal pustulation in some cases. The dermal infiltrate is usually sparse, but may be dense and contain both neutrophils and eosinophils. Liberal evaluation of vulvar biopsies with a PAS-D stain is recommended in the vast majority of cases of inflammatory vulvar disease, particularly when a lesion appears "nonspecific" upon initial evaluation (Figure 1.26).

PROGNOSIS AND TREATMENT

Topical antifungal agents are generally effective for uncomplicated superficial dermatophyte infections. Oral systemic therapy is now widely available and useful for cases in which there is extensive involvement, folliculitis, or in immunocompromised patients.

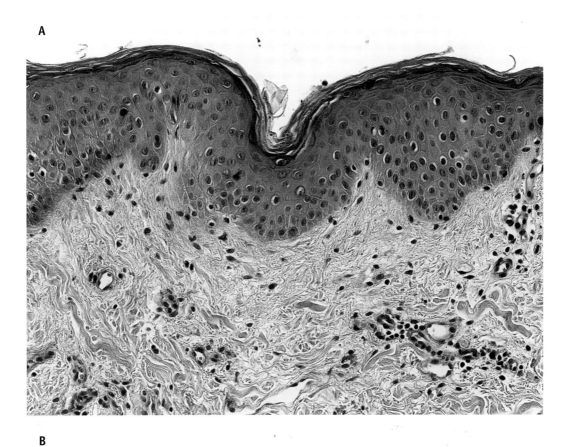

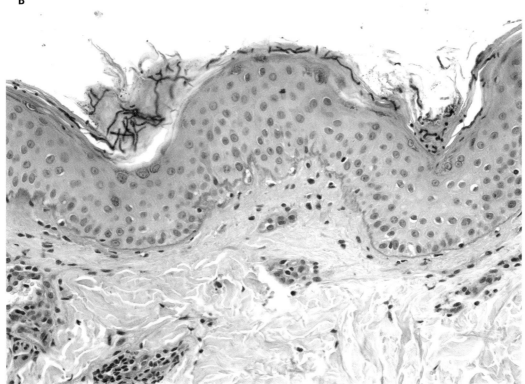

FIGURE 1.26

Dermatophytoses. A "nonspecific" perivascular dermatitis associated with focal parakeratosis is observed. No fungal pathogens are identified on the hematoxylin and eosin stain (A). Fungal hyphal forms in the stratum corneum are highlighted by a periodic acid–Schiff-D stain (B).

DERMATOPHYTOSES – FACT SHEET

Definition
▸ Fungi that colonize and infect the keratinizing epithelial structures of the skin

Incidence
▸ Common

Morbidity
▸ Cosmetic concerns
▸ Alopecia

Gender, Race, and Age Distribution
▸ No specific gender or racial predilection
▸ May occur at any age
▸ Greater risk of infection in prepubertal children and immunocompromised patients

Clinical Features
▸ Erythematous annular plaque with peripheral scale and central clearing

Prognosis and Treatment
▸ Generally self-limited infection
▸ Topical antifungal agents effective for uncomplicated superficial infections
▸ Oral systemic therapy useful if there is extensive involvement, folliculitis, or in immunocompromised patients

DERMATOPHYTOSES – PATHOLOGIC FEATURES

Microscopic Findings
▸ Typical lesion:
  ▸ Neutrophils and compact orthokeratosis and/or parakeratosis in stratum corneum ("sandwich" sign of Ackerman)
  ▸ Subjacent epidermal spongiosis
  ▸ Sparse perivascular lymphohistiocytic infiltrate which may contain neutrophils and eosinophils
▸ Dermatophyte infection may produce almost every epidermal inflammatory reaction pattern

Ancillary Studies
▸ Periodic acid–Schiff-D stain

Differential Diagnosis
▸ Impetiginized eczema
▸ Psoriasis

SUGGESTED READING

General References

Ackerman AB, Chongchitnant N, Sanchez J, et al. Histologic Diagnosis of Inflammatory Skin Diseases. An Algorithmic Method Based on Pattern Analysis, 2nd edn. Baltimore: Williams and Wilkins, 1997.
Bolognia JL, Jorizzo JL, Rapini RP (eds) Dermatology. St. Louis: Mosby, 2003.
Burns T, Breathnach S, Cox N, et al. (eds) Rook's Textbook of Dermatology, 7th edn. Oxford: Blackwell, 2004.

Maize JC, Burgdorf WH, Hurt Mark A, et al. Cutaneous Pathology. Philadelphia, PA: Churchill Livingstone, 1998.
McKee PH, Calonje E, Granter SR. Pathology of the Skin, 3rd edn. Philadelphia, PA: Mosby, 2005.
Weedon D, Strutton G. Skin Pathology, 2nd edn. London: Churchill Livingstone, 2002.

Lichenoid Dermatitis

LeBoit PE. Interface dermatitis. How specific are its histopathologic features? Arch Dermatol 1993;129:1324–1328.

Lichen Planus

Lewis FM, Shah M, Harrington CI. Vulval involvement in lichen planus: a study of 37 women. Br J Dermatol 1996;135:89–91.
Ragaz A, Ackermann AB. Evolution, maturation, and regression of lesions of lichen planus. New observations and correlations of clinical and histologic findings. Am J Dermatopathol 1981;3:5–25.
Lewis FM, Harrington CI. Squamous cell carcinoma arising in vulvar lichen planus. Br J Dermatol 1994;131:703–705.

Erythema Multiforme

Huff SC, Weston WL, Tonnesen MG. Erythema multiforme: a critical review of characteristics, diagnostic criteria, and causes. J Am Acad Dermatol 1983;8:763–775.

Fixed Drug Eruption

Korkij W, Soltani K. Fixed drug eruption. A brief review. Arch Dermatol 1984;120:520–524.
Shiohara T. What is new in fixed drug eruption? Dermatology 1995;1:185–187.

Lichen Sclerosus

Fung MA, LeBoit PE. Light microscopic criteria for the diagnosis of early vulvar lichen sclerosus. A comparison with lichen planus. Am J Surg Pathol 1998;22:473–478.
Meffert JJ, Davis BM, Grimwood RE. Lichen sclerosus. J Am Acad Dermatol 1995;32:393–416.

Plasmacytosis Mucosae (Zoon Vulvitis)

Davis J, Schapiro L, Baral J. Vulvitis circumscripta plasmacellularis. J Am Acad Dermatol 1983;8:413–416.
Kavanagh GM, Burton PA, Kennedy CTG. Vulvitis chronica plasmacellularis (Zoon's vulvitis). Br J Dermatol 1993;129:92–93.

Syphilis

Brown TJ, Yen-Moore A, Tyring SK. An overview of sexually transmitted diseases. Part I. J Am Acad Dermatol 1999;41:511–529.
Felman YM. Syphilis. From 1945 Naples to 1989 AIDS. Arch Dermatol 1989;125:1698–1700.

Atopic Dermatitis

Hurwitz RM, DeTrana C. The cutaneous pathology of atopic dermatitis. Am J Dermatopathol 1990;12:544–551.
Rothe MJ, Grant-Kels JM. Atopic dermatitis: an update. J Am Acad Dermatol 1996;35:1–13.

Contact Dermatitis

Taylor RM. Histopathology of contact dermatitis. Clin Dermatol 1986;4:18–22.

Irritant Contact Dermatitis

Rietschel RL. Irritant contact dermatitis. Dermatol Clin 1984;2:545–551.
Willis CM, Stephens CJM, Wilkinson JD. Epidermal damage induced by irritants in man: a light and electron microscopic study. J Invest Dermatol 1989;93:695–699.

Seborrheic Dermatitis

Barr RJ, Young EM Jr. Psoriasiform and related papulosquamous disorders. J Cutan Pathol 1985;12:412–425.
Webster G. Seborrheic dermatitis. Int J Dermatol 1991;30:843–844.

Psoriasis

Fry L. Psoriasis. Br J Dermatol 1988;119:445–461.
Ragaz A, Ackerman AB. Evolution, maturation, and regression of lesions of psoriasis. Am J Dermatopathol 1979;1:199–214.

Lichen Simplex Chronicus

Shaffer B, Beerman H. Lichen simplex chronicus and its variants. Arch Dermatol 1951;64:340–351.

Candidiasis

DeCastro P, Jorizzo JL. Cutaneous aspects of candidiasis. Semin Dermatol 1985;4:165–172.
Odds FC. Pathogenesis of Candida infections. J Am Acad Dermatol 1994;31: S2–S5.

Dermatophytoses

Elewski BE, Hazen PG. The superficial mycoses and the dermatophytes. J Am Acad Dermatol 1989;21:655–673.
Ollague J. Ackerman AB. Compact orthokeratosis as a clue to chronic dermatophytosis and candidiasis. Am J Dermatopathol 1982;4: 359–363.

2 Vulvar Neoplasia

2a Mesenchymal Lesions
Marisa R Nucci

Mesenchymal lesions that occur in the vulva can be separated into two general categories: (1) those that are relatively site-specific, i.e., they may occasionally occur at extragenital sites; and (2) those that occur more commonly at other sites but which may also involve this region. The former group includes deep "aggressive" angiomyxoma, angiomyofibroblastoma, cellular angiofibroma, and fibroepithelial stromal polyp; the latter group comprises the remainder of entities discussed in this chapter.

FIBROEPITHELIAL STROMAL POLYP

CLINICAL FEATURES

Fibroepithelial stromal polyps typically occur in women of reproductive age (most commonly during pregnancy), but may be seen in postmenopausal women on hormonal replacement therapy. They are often incidental findings discovered during routine gynecologic examination. Symptoms, when present, may include bleeding, discharge, or the sensation of a mass. Fibroepithelial polyp usually presents as a solitary lesion; however, multiple polyps may occur during pregnancy, following which they typically will regress.

PATHOLOGIC FEATURES

GROSS FINDINGS

Fibroepithelial stromal polyps are usually < 5 cm, typically polypoid or pedunculated, and may project from a thin connecting stalk. Occasionally, they may have multiple finger-like projections, which can mimic a condyloma.

FIBROEPITHELIAL STROMAL POLYP – FACT SHEET

Definition
▶ Benign polypoid growth that arises from the distinctive subepithelial stroma of the distal female genital tract

Incidence and Location
▶ Most common during pregnancy
▶ May occur in the vulva, vagina, and, rarely, cervix

Morbidity and Mortality
▶ If large, may be disfiguring and cause pain and bleeding

Gender, Race, and Age Distribution
▶ Typically in reproductive-aged women
▶ May occur in postmenopausal women on hormone replacement therapy
▶ There is an association with pregnancy

Clinical Features
▶ Typically polypoid or pedunculated
▶ Usually < 5 cm
▶ May have thin connecting stalk
▶ Multiple polyps may occur during pregnancy

Prognosis and Treatment
▶ Benign lesion
▶ May regress following pregnancy
▶ Complete local excision treatment of choice
▶ Potential for local recurrence if incompletely excised or if continued hormonal stimulation

---

MICROSCOPIC FINDINGS

Fibroepithelial stromal polyps are polypoid lesions with a variably cellular stroma, central fibrovascular core, and overlying squamous epithelium. The most characteristic feature is the presence of stellate and multinucleate stromal cells, which are most commonly seen near the epithelial–stromal interface or adjacent to the

FIBROEPITHELIAL STROMAL POLYP – PATHOLOGIC FEATURES

Gross Findings

▸ Usually < 5 cm
▸ Polypoid or pedunculated with thin connecting stalk

Microscopic Findings

▸ Polypoid with variably cellular stroma, central fibrovascular core, and overlying squamous epithelium
▸ Stellate and multinucleate stromal cells are characteristic; typically located at the epithelial–stromal interface and around blood vessels
▸ Some polyps may exhibit stromal hypercellularity, stromal cell nuclear pleomorphism, and increased mitotic activity (so-called pseudosarcoma botryoides)

Immunohistochemical Findings

▸ Desmin, vimentin, ER and PR typically positive
▸ Actin less frequently positive

Differential Diagnosis

▸ Sarcoma, not otherwise specified
▸ Embryonal rhabdomyosarcoma
▸ Aggressive angiomyxoma

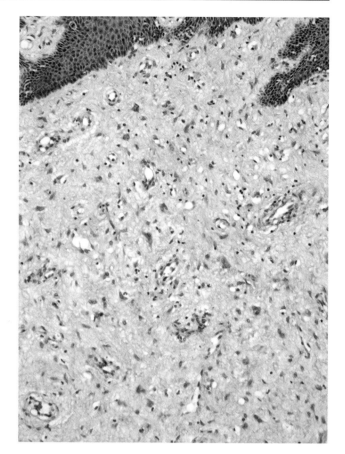

FIGURE 2a.1

Fibroepithelial stromal polyp. Characteristic stellate and multinucleated stromal cells are prominent near the stromal–epithelial interface.

prominent central vasculature (Figure 2a.1). The variably cellular stromal component, which may exhibit a significant degree of cellularity, nuclear pleomorphism, and mitotic activity (including > 10 mitoses/10 HPFs and atypical mitoses), thereby mimicking a malignant process (Figure 2a.2), has no clearly defined margin and extends up to the epithelial–stromal interface.

ANCILLARY STUDIES

IMMUNOHISTOCHEMISTRY

The stromal cells of these lesions are often positive for desmin, vimentin, estrogen and progesterone receptors (ER and PR), and less frequently for actin.

DIFFERENTIAL DIAGNOSIS

Fibroepithelial stromal polyps, particularly those with increased cellularity and atypical stromal cells, must be distinguished from a malignant process. *Sarcomas* typically have an identifiable lesional margin, show homogeneous cellularity throughout, and lack the stellate and multinucleate stromal cells near the epithelial–stromal interface. In contrast, even the most floridly pseudosarcomatous examples of fibroepithelial stromal polyps characteristically show stellate multinucleated cells and tend to exhibit a greater degree of cellularity in the center of the lesion. Fibroepithelial stromal polyps are readily distinguished from *botryoid embryonal rhab-*

domyosarcoma, as fibroepithelial stromal polyps are rare before puberty and lack the characteristic hypercellular subepithelial (cambium) layer as well as specific markers of skeletal muscle differentiation.

PROGNOSIS AND THERAPY

These lesions have the potential to recur locally, particularly if incompletely excised or if there is continued hormonal stimulation (e.g., pregnancy).

DEEP (AGGRESSIVE) ANGIOMYXOMA

CLINICAL FEATURES

Deep (aggressive) angiomyxoma typically occurs in the pelvis and perineum of women in the fourth decade, although it has also been described in the male inguinoscrotal region. When it involves the perineum, it is often

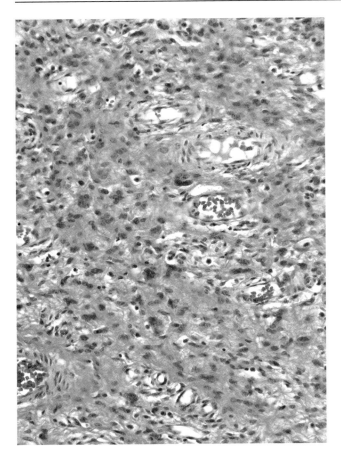

FIGURE 2a.2
Fibroepithelial stromal polyp. Increased stromal cellularity and atypia are present. Note the presence of the characteristic multinucleated cells.

DEEP AGGRESSIVE ANGIOMYXOMA – PATHOLOGIC FEATURES

Gross Findings
▸ Poor demarcation
▸ Soft, gelatinous cut surface

Microscopic Findings
▸ Poorly marginated
▸ Hypocellular with copious myxoid matrix
▸ Bland spindled cells with round/ovoid nuclei and palely eosinophilic cytoplasmic processes
▸ Medium to large-sized, often hyalinized, blood vessels
▸ Condensation of fibrillary collagen around vessels
▸ Occasional collections of smooth-muscle cells in bundles

Immunohistochemical Features
▸ Desmin, smooth-muscle actin, ER and PR positive
▸ S-100 and CD34 may be positive

Differential Diagnosis
▸ Fibroepithelial stromal polyp
▸ Angiomyofibroblastoma
▸ Superficial angiomyxoma

DEEP AGGRESSIVE ANGIOMYXOMA – FACT SHEET

Definition
▸ Infiltrative, nonmetastasizing, hypocellular myxoid tumor of the pelvic–perineal region with potential for local, sometimes destructive, recurrence

Incidence and Location
▸ Uncommon
▸ Pelvis and perineum

Morbidity and Mortality
▸ Potential for local destructive recurrence may result in repeat surgeries leading to distorted anatomy and secondary loss of function of infiltrated structures
▸ Nonmetastasizing

Gender and Age Distribution
▸ Reproductive-aged women with a median in the fourth decade

Clinical Features
▸ Clinical impression is often a Bartholin's gland cyst

Prognosis and Treatment
▸ Wide local excision with 1-cm margins recommended treatment
▸ 30–40% risk of local recurrence if incompletely excised

clinically mistaken for a labial cyst, most commonly a Bartholin's gland cyst. It is a locally infiltrative neoplasm but it does not have metastatic potential.

PATHOLOGIC FEATURES

GROSS FINDINGS

Tumors can be of varying size but are often relatively large (> 10 cm). They are typically poorly demarcated and characteristically have a soft, gelatinous appearance, but occasionally may show a white and rubbery cut surface in a recurrence, presumably due to involvement of surgical scar tissue.

MICROSCOPIC FINDINGS

Deep (aggressive) angiomyxoma is composed of bland spindled cells with round to ovoid nuclei and palely eosinophilic cytoplasmic processes set within a copious myxoid matrix that typically contains medium-sized, thick, and often hyalinized blood vessels (Figure 2a.3), although they may also display small and/or large vessels. The presence of bundles of smooth-muscle cells and condensation of delicate fibrillary collagen around blood vessels is characteristic. Because the tumor is deceptively bland and poorly marginated, it is often difficult to distinguish between neoplastic cells and non-neoplastic vulvovaginal mesenchyme.

ANCILLARY STUDIES

IMMUNOHISTOCHEMISTRY

Similar to nonneoplastic vulval mesenchyme, the neoplastic stromal cells of deep (aggressive) angiomyxoma are usually positive for desmin, smooth-muscle actin, vimentin, ER and PR and they may be S-100-positive. Much less frequently they may stain for CD34.

DIFFERENTIAL DIAGNOSIS

Deep (aggressive) angiomyxoma must be distinguished from other relatively site-specific mesenchymal lesions such as fibroepithelial stromal polyp and angiomyofibroblastoma, as well as other myxoid neoplasms that occur in the vulva, particularly superficial angiomyxoma. Deep location, poor circumscription, lack of superficial polypoid growth associated with a fibrovascular core, and bland cytomorphologic features distinguish deep (aggressive) angiomyxoma from *fibroepithelial stromal polyp*. Deep angiomyxoma can be dis-

tinguished from *angiomyofibroblastoma* because of its deep location, infiltrative margin, uniform paucicellularity, wide-range caliber vessels, and lack of clustering of the neoplastic cells around blood vessels. Finally, *superficial angiomyxoma* has a distinctive lobulated growth, in contrast to the diffuse growth of deep angiomyxoma. Furthermore, it lacks the medium to large-sized vessels seen in deep angiomyxoma and it is frequently associated with acute inflammatory cells.

PROGNOSIS AND THERAPY

Local recurrence occurs in up to 30–40% of deep (aggressive) angiomyxomas, sometimes many years (often decades) after the initial excision. Recurrence usually only occurs if the tumor is initially incompletely excised. Wide local excision with 1-cm margins is therefore considered optimal.

ANGIOMYOFIBROBLASTOMA

CLINICAL FEATURES

This is a benign neoplasm that occurs in the vulvovaginal region of reproductive-aged women but it may also occur in the inguinoscrotal region in males. Similar to deep angiomyxoma, it is often thought to represent a cyst on clinical examination.

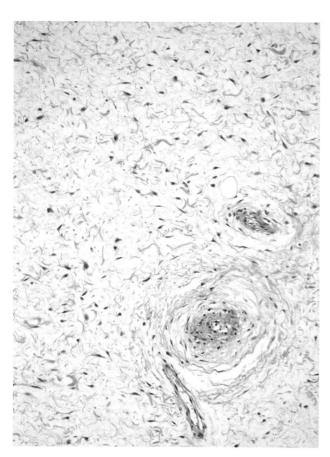

FIGURE 2a.3
Deep (aggressive) angiomyxoma. The tumor is paucicellular and it is composed of bland spindle-shaped cells set within a striking myxoid matrix. Note the condensation of collagen around the vessels and the presence of bundles of smooth muscle (upper right).

ANGIOMYOFIBROBLASTOMA –
FACT SHEET

Definition
▶ Benign nonrecurring tumor composed of myofibroblasts and thin-walled capillaries, which principally occurs in vulvovaginal soft tissues

Incidence and Location
▶ Uncommon
▶ Vulvovaginal region

Morbidity and Mortality
▶ Benign, nonrecurring neoplasm

Gender and Age Distribution
▶ Reproductive-aged women

Clinical Features
▶ Often thought to represent a vulvar cyst

Prognosis and Treatment
▶ Excellent prognosis
▶ Local excision with clear margins

ANGIOMYOFIBROBLASTOMA – PATHOLOGIC FINDINGS

Gross Findings

▸ Usually < 5 cm
▸ Well circumscribed
▸ Tan-white, rubbery cut surface

Microscopic Findings

▸ Well circumscribed, nonencapsulated
▸ Alternating zones of cellularity
▸ Plump (plasmacytoid) to spindle-shaped cells
▸ Numerous delicate thin-walled capillaries
▸ Clustering of stromal cells around vasculature
▸ Variably edematous to collagenous matrix

Immunohistochemical Features

▸ Desmin typically positive
▸ ER and PR, S-100 and CD34 variably positive
▸ Smooth-muscle actin usually negative

Differential Diagnosis

▸ Deep "aggressive" angiomyxoma
▸ Cellular angiofibroma

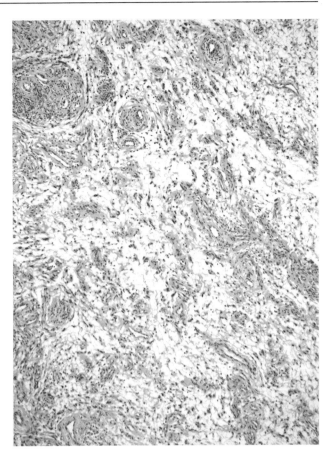

FIGURE 2a.4

Angiomyofibroblastoma. Alternating hypocellular and hypercellular areas are seen. Tumor cells tend to cluster around numerous capillary-sized vessels.

PATHOLOGIC FEATURES

GROSS FINDINGS

The tumors are typically small (usually < 5 cm) and well circumscribed and they display a tan/white and rubbery cut surface.

MICROSCOPIC FINDINGS

Angiomyofibroblastoma, although not encapsulated, is well demarcated from the surrounding nonneoplastic vulval soft tissues. It is composed of plump, ovoid (plasmacytoid) to spindle-shaped cells that may be multinucleated and tend to cluster around the numerous small- to medium-caliber blood vessels. The cells are set within a variably edematous to collagenous matrix with alternating zones of cellularity (Figure 2a.4). Mitotic activity is uncommon and occasionally intratumoral adipose tissue may be present.

ANCILLARY STUDIES

IMMUNOHISTOCHEMISTRY

The tumor cells are typically positive for desmin. Smooth-muscle actin positivity is variable but usually negative. They may also exhibit immunoreactivity for CD34, S-100, and ER and PR.

DIFFERENTIAL DIAGNOSIS

The main differential diagnostic consideration is the distinction of angiomyofibroblastoma from *deep (aggressive) angiomyxoma*, particularly since these two tumors have differing clinical behavior. Unlike deep angiomyxoma, angiomyofibroblastoma is well circumscribed and has alternating zones of cellularity as well as more prominent vascularity composed of small to medium-sized vessels, in contrast to the infiltrative growth, homogeneous hypocellularity and medium to large-sized vessels typically seen in deep angiomyxoma. Angiofibroma is more uniformly *cellular*, contains fewer vessels which are larger and more commonly hyalinized, and it is typically positive for CD34.

PROGNOSIS AND THERAPY

Angiomyofibroblastoma is a benign tumor without recurrent potential; therefore, local excision with clear margins is adequate treatment. Rarely, this tumor may undergo sarcomatous transformation.

CELLULAR ANGIOFIBROMA

CLINICAL FEATURES

Cellular angiofibroma is a benign tumor that occurs in the vulva or perineum of middle-aged women (mean 54 years), although it also occurs in the inguinoscrotal region in men as well as at extragenital sites. In the vulva, they most commonly present as a small, well-circumscribed, painless, subcutaneous mass.

PATHOLOGIC FEATURES

GROSS FINDINGS

Tumors are typically small (average 2.7 cm) with a well-demarcated border. On cut section, they have a firm, rubbery gray-white surface.

MICROSCOPIC FINDINGS

Most cellular angiofibromas also have a well-demarcated border on low-power examination; however a few may exhibit focal limited infiltration of surrounding soft tissues. It is a cellular neoplasm composed of short, intersecting fascicles of bland spindle-shaped cells with scant pale-staining cytoplasm and ovoid nuclei (Figure 2a.5). These tumors may show brisk mitotic activity. The vascular component is prominent, with numerous small to medium-sized, thick-walled (and often hyalinized) blood vessels. Interspersed wispy collagen bundles are also characteristic and mast cells are a common associated finding. In addition, most tumors also have a small component of adipose tissue, often located at the periphery. Entrapped small nerves may also be seen at the periphery of the tumor.

ANCILLARY STUDIES

IMMUNOHISTOCHEMISTRY

The tumor cells can be positive for CD34 (in 60% of cases), smooth-muscle actin (20%), and desmin (8%). ER and PR may also be positive ($\sim$50% of cases) whereas S-100 is negative.

DIFFERENTIAL DIAGNOSIS

Because of the presence of short intersecting fascicles, cellular angiofibroma may be confused with a benign smooth-muscle tumor. It is distinguished from a *leiomyoma* by its shorter fascicles, more prominent vascular component, less abundant eosinophilic cytoplasm, and lack of blunt-ended nuclei. Less frequently, *cellular angiofibroma* may be confused with *angiomyofibroblastoma*, and *deep angiomyxoma* (discussed earlier), and *solitary fibrous tumor*. In contrast to cellular angiofi-

---

CELLULAR ANGIOFIBROMA – FACT SHEET

Definition
▸ Benign tumor of vulval mesenchyme composed of bland spindled cells admixed with a prominent vascular component

Incidence and Location
▸ Relatively uncommon
▸ Vulvovaginal region
▸ Can occur at extragenital sites

Morbidity and Mortality
▸ Benign, nonrecurring tumor

Gender and Age Distribution
▸ Middle-aged women (mean 54 years)

Clinical Features
▸ Small, well-circumscribed subcutaneous mass
▸ Patients may present with pain

Prognosis and Treatment
▸ Local excision with clear margins
▸ Excellent prognosis

CELLULAR ANGIOFIBROMA – PATHOLOGIC FEATURES

Gross Findings
▸ Typically small (< 3 cm) and well circumscribed
▸ Firm, rubbery consistency
▸ Gray-white cut surface

Microscopic Findings
▸ Usually well-demarcated border
▸ Short intersecting fascicles of bland spindle-shaped cells
▸ Cells with ovoid nuclei and scant, pale eosinophilic cytoplasm with indistinct borders
▸ No cytologic atypia but mitotic activity may be brisk
▸ Prominent vascular component with small to medium-sized vessels, often thick-walled and hyalinized
▸ Interspersed wispy collagen bundles
▸ Entrapped fat and nerves at the periphery
▸ Abundant mast cells

Immunohistochemical Features
▸ CD34 positive in 60%, smooth muscle actin in 20%, and desmin in 8% of cases
▸ ER and PR positive in ~50% of cases
▸ S-100 negative

Differential Diagnosis
▸ Leiomyoma
▸ Deep (aggressive) angiomyxoma
▸ Angiomyofibroblastoma
▸ Solitary fibrous tumor

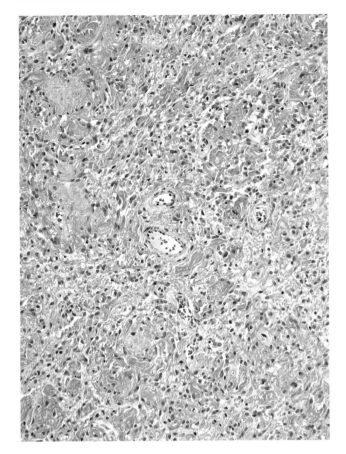

FIGURE 2a.5
Cellular angiofibroma. Short intersecting fascicles of bland spindle-shaped cells and numerous small to medium-sized vessels are present in a collagenous background.

broma, solitary fibrous tumor is characterized by a "patternless" architecture, heterogeneous cellularity, hemangiopericytoma-like vasculature, and frequent presence of keloid-type collagen.

PROGNOSIS AND THERAPY

Cellular angiofibroma is a benign tumor. Incomplete excision may lead to regrowth of tumor; therefore, local (conservative) excision with negative margins appears to be adequate treatment.

SUPERFICIAL ANGIOMYXOMA

CLINICAL FEATURES

Although superficial angiomyxoma more typically involves the head, neck, and trunk region, it does occasionally occur in the vulva. Patients are usually in their fourth decade and typically present with a single, slowly growing, painless, polypoid mass. Multiple lesions may be associated with Carney's complex.

SUPERFICIAL ANGIOMYXOMA – FACT SHEET

Definition
▸ Superficially located, multilobulated, myxoid neoplasm

Incidence and Location
▸ Rare
▸ Typically in head and neck region but may involve vulva

Morbidity and Mortality
▸ 30–40% risk of local nondestructive recurrence

Gender and Age Distribution
▸ Usually reproductive-aged women in fourth decade

Clinical Features
▸ Slowly growing and painless
▸ Typically polypoid
▸ Multiple lesions may be associated with Carney's complex

Prognosis and Treatment
▸ Complete excision with negative margins
▸ 30–40% risk of local nondestructive recurrence

SUPERFICIAL ANGIOMYXOMA – PATHOLOGIC FEATURES

Gross Findings
▸ Polypoid lesion
▸ Usually < 5 cm
▸ Gelatinous cut surface

Microscopic Findings
▸ Well demarcated
▸ Multilobulated growth pattern
▸ Myxoid stroma
▸ Slender spindle and stellate-shaped stromal cells
▸ Thin-walled vessels
▸ Scattered inflammatory cells, particularly polymorphonuclear leukocytes
▸ Associated epithelial component in 10–20% of cases

Immunohistochemical Features
▸ Vimentin positive
▸ Smooth-muscle actin, desmin, and S-100 negative

Differential Diagnosis
▸ Deep "aggressive" angiomyxoma

PATHOLOGIC FEATURES

GROSS FINDINGS

These tumors are typically polypoid, usually < 5 cm in diameter, and may have a gelatinous appearance on cut section.

MICROSCOPIC FINDINGS

Superficial angiomyxoma is a relatively well-demarcated, multilobulated myxoid neoplasm centered in the dermis and superficial subcutaneous tissues. The tumor lobules are composed of slender spindle and stellate-shaped cells and thin-walled curvilinear vessels set within a myxoid matrix (Figure 2a.6). The cells show bland cytologic features and mitotic activity is very low. Scattered inflammatory cells are present, particularly acute inflammatory cells. In 10–20% of cases, an epithelial component is present which may be the result of entrapped adnexal structures or stimulation of the overlying epithelium by the tumor.

ANCILLARY STUDIES

IMMUNOHISTOCHEMISTRY

Superficial angiomyxomas are typically positive for vimentin but, unlike the other mesenchymal tumors presented herein, these tumors are typically negative for smooth-muscle actin, desmin, and S-100.

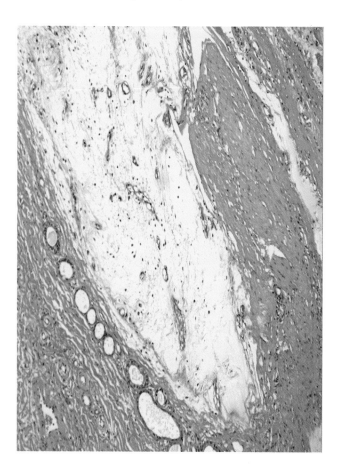

FIGURE 2a.6
Superficial angiomyxoma. The tumor has a lobulated growth and it is composed of bland spindle cells within a myxoid matrix and show a lobulated growth. Note the presence of adnexal structures adjacent to the tumor, signifying a dermal location.

DIFFERENTIAL DIAGNOSIS

As superficial angiomyxoma is myxoid, it should be distinguished from *deep (aggressive) angiomyxoma*. Superficial angiomyxoma does not involve deep soft tissues, it has a characteristic lobulated growth pattern and delicate blood vessels, which is in contrast to the infiltrating margin and medium to large-sized vessels of deep angiomyxoma. In addition, superficial angiomyxoma is typically desmin-negative.

PROGNOSIS AND THERAPY

Complete excision with negative margins is considered appropriate as these tumors have the potential for local, nondestructive recurrence in approximately one-third of cases.

LEIOMYOMA

CLINICAL FEATURES

Vulvar leiomyomas occur over a wide age range but are most common in the fourth and fifth decades. They usually present as a painless, subcutaneous mass and at the time of surgical excision appear well demarcated from the surrounding soft tissues. Similar to the other entities described herein, they are often thought to represent a vulvar cyst.

LEIOMYOMA – FACT SHEET

Definition
▸ Benign smooth-muscle tumor

Incidence and Location
▸ Infrequent
▸ Vulvovaginal region

Morbidity and Mortality
▸ If large can be disfiguring

Gender and Age Distribution
▸ Wide age range but most common in fourth and fifth decades

Clinical Features
▸ Typically painless mass
▸ Often thought to represent a cyst

Prognosis and Treatment
▸ Excellent prognosis
▸ Local excision with clear margins

LEIOMYOMA – PATHOLOGIC FEATURES

Gross Findings
▸ Well circumscribed
▸ White/tan whorled appearance
▸ Firm, rubbery consistency
▸ Bulging cut section

Microscopic Findings
▸ Intersecting fascicles of spindle-shaped cells with moderate amount of eosinophilic cytoplasm and blunt-ended nuclei
▸ Variable amounts of myxohyaline matrix imparting a "lacy" growth pattern
▸ Epithelioid morphology may be prominent
▸ No cytologic atypia and minimal to absent mitotic activity
▸ No tumor cell necrosis

Immunohistochemical Features
▸ Desmin, smooth-muscle actin, h-caldesmon typically positive

Differential Diagnosis
▸ Leiomyosarcoma; in order to classify a smooth-muscle tumor as malignant it should have three of the five following criteria:
  1. > 5 cm
  2. Infiltrative margin
  3. Moderate to severe cytologic atypia
  4. > 5 mitoses/10 HPFs
  5. Tumor cell necrosis
▸ Cellular angiofibroma

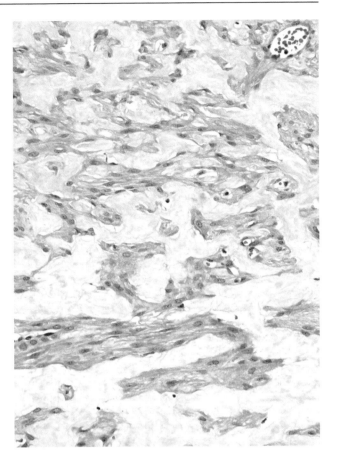

FIGURE 2a.7
Leiomyoma. Benign-appearing smooth cells show a lacy growth pattern secondary to the abundant myxohyaline matrix associated with the tumor.

PATHOLOGIC FEATURES

GROSS FINDINGS

The tumors are typically small (usually < 3 cm) and well circumscribed. On sectioning they show a homogeneous firm, white, whorled, and bulging cut surface with no areas of hemorrhage or necrosis, an appearance that closely overlaps with that seen in uterine leiomyomas. Some vulvar leiomyomas, however, have a more homogeneous cut surface with less obvious whorling, related to the amount of extracellular matrix deposition.

MICROSCOPIC FINDINGS

Vulvar leiomyomas are typically well circumscribed and they are composed of intersecting fascicles of spindle-shaped cells with moderate amounts of eosinophilic cytoplasm forming bipolar processes and blunt-shaped (or "cigar"-shaped) nuclei admixed with variable amounts of collagen. However, somewhat unique to smooth-muscle tumors of the distal female genital tract (vulvovaginal) is the finding of an extensive epithelioid component or the presence of varying amounts of myxohyaline matrix, which when extensive may impart a lacy or plexiform growth pattern of the tumor cells (Figure 2a.7). No significant nuclear atypia (defined as nuclear atypia notable upon 10×-power examination,

usually moderate to severe) or tumor cell necrosis is present and mitotic activity is low to absent.

ANCILLARY STUDIES

IMMUNOHISTOCHEMISTRY

Tumor cells are typically positive for smooth-muscle markers such as smooth-muscle actin, desmin, and h-caldesmon. They are also frequently positive for ER and PR.

DIFFERENTIAL DIAGNOSIS

The principal differential diagnostic consideration is with *leiomyosarcoma* and a *smooth-muscle tumor with recurrent potential*. Because smooth-muscle tumors of the vulva are uncommon, there are few long-term studies that assess histologic criteria associated with recurrence and/or malignant behavior. In order to diagnose a smooth-muscle tumor as malignant, three of the following five criteria must be present: (1) > 5 cm in size; (2) infiltrative margin; (3) significant (moderate to severe) cytologic atypia; (4) mitotic activity exceeding

5/10 HPFs; and (5) tumor cell necrosis. For practical purposes, smooth-muscle tumors with any of the following are considered as having recurrent potential: (1) mitotic activity; (2) significant cytologic atypia; (3) infiltrative margin; or (4) necrosis. *Cellular angiofibroma* is another important entity in the differential diagnosis as this tumor has a fascicular growth of spindle-shaped cells. It is important to separate these two tumors as cellular angiofibroma may show brisk mitotic activity and, if confused with a smooth-muscle tumor, it may be misdiagnosed as a leiomyosarcoma. In contrast to smooth-muscle tumors, blood vessels are more prominent; the tumor cells have scant cytoplasm and lack the blunt-shaped nuclei seen in leiomyomas, and desmin is negative in most cases.

PROGNOSIS AND THERAPY

Vulvar leiomyomas are benign tumors and local excision with clear margins is the treatment of choice.

SUGGESTED READING

Fibroepithelial Stromal Polyp

Burt RL, Prichard RW, Kim BS. Fibroepithelial polyp of the vagina. A report of five cases. Obstet Gynecol 1976;47:52S–54S.

Chirayil SJ, Tobon H. Polyps of the vagina: a clinicopathologic study of 18 cases. Cancer 1981;47:2904–2907.

Elliott GB, Reynolds HA, Fidler HK. Pseudo-sarcoma botryoides of cervix and vagina in pregnancy. J Obstet Gynaecol Br Commonw 1967;74:728–733.

Hartmann CA, Sperling M, Stein H. So-called fibroepithelial polyps of the vagina exhibiting an unusual but uniform antigen profile characterized by expression of desmin and steroid hormone receptors but no muscle-specific actin or macrophage markers. Am J Clin Pathol 1990;93:604–608.

Maenpaa J, Soderstrom KO, Salmi T, et al. Large atypical polyps of the vagina during pregnancy with concomitant human papilloma virus infection. Eur J Obstet Gynecol Reprod Biol 1988;27:65–69.

Miettinen M, Wahlstrom T, Vesterinen E, et al. Vaginal polyps with pseudosarcomatous features. A clinicopathologic study of seven cases. Cancer 1983;51:1148–1151.

Mucitelli DR, Charles EZ, Kraus FT. Vulvovaginal polyps. Histologic appearance, ultrastructure, immunocytochemical characteristics, and clinicopathologic correlations. Int J Gynecol Pathol 1990;9:20–40.

Norris HJ, Taylor HB. Polyps of the vagina. A benign lesion resembling sarcoma botryoides. Cancer 1966;19:227–232.

Nucci MR, Fletcher CD. Fibroepithelial stromal polyps of vulvovaginal tissue: from the banal to the bizarre. Pathol Case Rev 1998;3:151–157.

Nucci MR, Young RH, Fletcher CD. Cellular pseudosarcomatous fibroepithelial stromal polyps of the lower female genital tract: an underrecognized lesion often misdiagnosed as sarcoma. Am J Surg Pathol 2000;24:231–240.

O'Quinn AG, Edwards CL, Gallager HS. Pseudosarcoma botryoides of the vagina in pregnancy. Gynecol Oncol 1982;13:237–241.

Ostöir AG, Fortune DW, Riley CB. Fibroepithelial polyps with atypical stromal cells (pseudosarcoma botryoides) of vulva and vagina. A report of 13 cases. Int J Gynecol Pathol 1988;7:351–360.

Deep "Aggressive" Angiomyxoma

Begin LR, Clement PB, Kirk ME, et al. Aggressive angiomyxoma of pelvic soft parts: a clinicopathologic study of nine cases. Hum Pathol 1985;16:621–628.

Fetsch JF, Laskin WB, Lefkowitz M, et al. Aggressive angiomyxoma: a clinicopathologic study of 29 female patients. Cancer 1996;78:79–90.

Granter SR, Nucci MR, Fletcher CD. Aggressive angiomyxoma: reappraisal of its relationship to angiomyofibroblastoma in a series of 16 cases. Histopathology 1997;30:3–10.

Iezzoni JC, Fechner RE, Wong LS, et al. Aggressive angiomyxoma in males. A report of four cases. Am J Clin Pathol 1995;104:391–396.

Nucci MR, Weremowicz S, Neskey DM, et al. Chromosomal translocation t(8;12) induces aberrant HMGIC expression in aggressive angiomyxoma of the vulva. Genes Chromosomes Cancer 2001;32:172–176.

Steeper TA, Rosai J. Aggressive angiomyxoma of the female pelvis and perineum. Report of nine cases of a distinctive type of gynecologic soft-tissue neoplasm. Am J Surg Pathol 1983;7:463–475.

Tsang WY, Chan JK, Lee KC, et al. Aggressive angiomyxoma. A report of four cases occurring in men. Am J Surg Pathol 1992;16:1059–1065.

Angiomyofibroblastoma

Fletcher CD, Tsang WY, Fisher C, et al. Angiomyofibroblastoma of the vulva. A benign neoplasm distinct from aggressive angiomyxoma. Am J Surg Pathol 1992;16:373–382.

Hisaoka M, Kouho H, Aoki T, et al. Angiomyofibroblastoma of the vulva: a clinicopathologic study of seven cases. Pathol Int 1995;45:487–492.

Laskin WB, Fetsch JF, Tavassoli FA. Angiomyofibroblastoma of the female genital tract: analysis of 17 cases including a lipomatous variant. Hum Pathol 1997;28:1046–1055.

Nielsen GP, Rosenberg AE, Young RH, et al. Angiomyofibroblastoma of the vulva and vagina. Mod Pathol 1996;9:284–291.

Nielsen GP, Young RH, Dickersin GR, et al. Angiomyofibroblastoma of the vulva with sarcomatous transformation ("angiomyofibrosarcoma"). Am J Surg Pathol 1997;21:1104–1108.

Ockner DM, Sayadi H, Swanson PE, et al. Genital angiomyofibroblastoma. Comparison with aggressive angiomyxoma and other myxoid neoplasms of skin and soft tissue. Am J Clin Pathol 1997;107:36–44.

Cellular Angiofibroma

Iwasa Y, Fletcher CD. Cellular angiofibroma: clinicopathologic and immunohistochemical analysis of 51 cases. Am J Surg Pathol 2004;28:1426–1435.

Laskin WB, Fetsch JF, Mostofi FK. Angiomyofibroblastomalike tumor of the male genital tract: analysis of 11 cases with comparison to female angiomyofibroblastoma and spindle cell lipoma. Am J Surg Pathol 1998;22:6–16.

McCluggage WG, Perenyei M, Irwin ST. Recurrent cellular angiofibroma of the vulva. J Clin Pathol 2002;55:477–479.

Nucci MR, Granter SR, Fletcher CD. Cellular angiofibroma: a benign neoplasm distinct from angiomyofibroblastoma and spindle cell lipoma. Am J Surg Pathol 1997;21:636–644.

Superficial Angiomyxoma

Allen PW, Dymock RB, MacCormac LB. Superficial angiomyxomas with and without epithelial components. Report of 30 tumors in 28 patients. Am J Surg Pathol 1988;12:519–530.

Calonje E, Guerin D, McCormick D, et al. Superficial angiomyxoma: clinicopathologic analysis of a series of distinctive but poorly recognized cutaneous tumors with tendency for recurrence. Am J Surg Pathol 1999;23:910–917.

Fetsch JF, Laskin WB, Tavassoli FA. Superficial angiomyxoma (cutaneous myxoma): a clinicopathologic study of 17 cases arising in the genital region. Int J Gynecol Pathol 1997;16:325–334.

Leiomyoma

Newman PL, Fletcher CD. Smooth muscle tumours of the external genitalia: clinicopathological analysis of a series. Histopathology 1991;18:523–529.

Nielsen GP, Rosenberg AE, Koerner FC, et al. Smooth-muscle tumors of the vulva. A clinicopathological study of 25 cases and review of the literature. Am J Surg Pathol 1996;20:779–793.

Nucci MR, Fletcher CD. Vulvovaginal soft tissue tumours: update and review. Histopathology 2000;36:97–108.

Tavassoli FA, Norris HJ. Smooth muscle tumors of the vulva. Obstet Gynecol 1979;53:213–217.

Squamous Neoplasia
Sanjay Logani

CONDYLOMA ACUMINATUM

This is a sexually transmitted benign proliferative lesion of the squamous epithelium of the genital area caused by the human papillomavirus (HPV), most often HPV 6 and 11. It is present in approximately 1% of sexually active adults in the United States and is clinically recognized as "genital wart."

CONDYLOMA ACUMINATUM – FACT SHEET

Definition
▶ Sexually transmitted benign proliferative lesion of squamous epithelium of genital area caused by human papillomavirus (HPV) infection, most often HPV types 6 and 11

Incidence and Location
▶ Present in approximately 1% of sexually active adults in the United States (US)
▶ Most common in vulva, vagina, cervix, anal canal, and perianal skin

Morbidity and Mortality
▶ Benign disease with potential for recurrence
▶ Rarely progression to vulvar intraepithelial neoplasia and invasive squamous cell carcinoma

Race and Age Distribution
▶ No racial predilection
▶ Most common in patients of child-bearing age

Clinical Features
▶ Most commonly asymptomatic
▶ Less commonly pruritus, irritation, or bleeding
▶ Usually multiple, either small or exophytic
▶ Predilection for introitus, perineal, and perianal skin
▶ Association with cervical HPV infection in 30–50% of patients

Prognosis and Treatment
▶ Benign lesion with protracted course
▶ Small lesions treated with podophyllin therapy
▶ Large lesions treated with surgical removal, laser, or cryotherapy
▶ May recur after excision

CLINICAL FEATURES

Patients are typically asymptomatic but may have pruritus, irritation, or bleeding. Lesions have a predilection for moist surfaces, including introitus, perineal and perianal skin, and, less commonly, vagina and cervix. They have a very distinct clinical appearance, showing multiple papillary projections and a granular surface. An association with cervical HPV infection is noted in 30–50% of the patients. Risk factors are similar to those for cervical HPV infection (e.g., sexual activity with multiple partners).

PATHOLOGIC FEATURES

GROSS FINDINGS

The lesions are typically exophytic and may range from small papillomatous excrescences to extensive and coalescent cauliflower-like masses involving the vulva and perianal skin (Figure 2b.1).

MICROSCOPIC FINDINGS

On low power examination, there is a striking papillary architecture. Papillae of different sizes and shapes are lined by acanthotic squamous epithelium, and they have a fibrovascular stroma, often containing scattered chronic inflammatory cells. Hyperkeratosis, parakeratosis, hypergranulosis, and basal cell hyperplasia are commonly seen. Koilocytic atypia is present in the most superficial layers of the squamous epithelium, facilitating the diagnosis (Figure 2b.2). Koilocytosis is typically identified by the finding of rigid perinuclear halos, binucleated nuclei, and nuclei with irregular contours and coarse chromatin. It is important to be aware that koilocytic change may be focal. Mitotic figures are typically confined to the lower third of the epithelium and may be numerous in lesions that have been pretreated with podophyllin. Atypical mitotic figures are not usually identified. Other features seen with podophyllin treatment include superficial apoptotic keratinocytes with a range of nuclear degenerative changes.

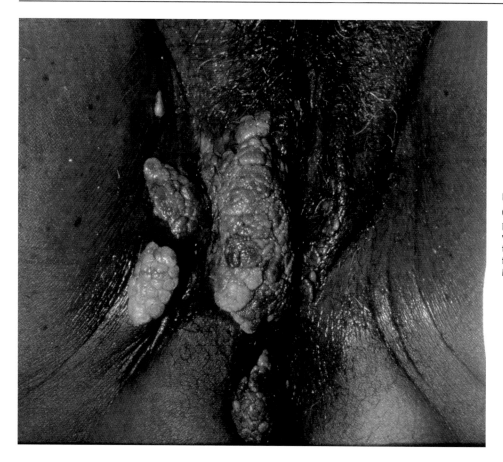

FIGURE 2b.1
Condyloma acuminatum. Exophytic polypoid lesion involves the vulvo-vaginal mucosa and extends to the perianal skin and gluteal folds. (Courtesy of Dr. Bhagirath Majmudar.)

**CONDYLOMA ACUMINATUM –
PATHOLOGIC FEATURES**

Gross Findings

▸ Typically exophytic
▸ Small papillomatous excrescences or extensive and coalescent cauliflower-like-masses

Microscopic Findings

▸ Striking papillary architecture with +/− hyalinized fibrovascular cores
▸ Acanthotic squamous epithelium with hyper- and parakeratosis and hypergranulosis
▸ Koilocytic atypia in the most superficial layers
▸ Basal cell hyperplasia
▸ Scattered mitoses confined to the lower third of the epithelium; no abnormal mitoses
▸ Numerous mitoses, superficial apoptotic keratinocytes with a range of nuclear degenerative changes if pretreated with podophyllin

Immunohistochemical Features

▸ MIB-1 positivity in the upper third of the epithelium
▸ Human papillomavirus antigen detection

Differential Diagnosis

▸ Fibroepithelial polyp
▸ Seborrheic keratosis
▸ Warty vulvar intraepithelial neoplasia

ANCILLARY STUDIES

Some authors have used the proliferation index as measured by the presence of MIB-1-positive nuclei in the upper third of the epithelium as an adjunct test to confirm the diagnosis of condyloma, especially in lesions that lack prominent koilocytic atypia. The presence of MIB-1 staining has been further correlated with the detection of HPV DNA by polymerase chain reaction (PCR) analysis. In situ hybridization for HPV can also be performed on paraffin-fixed tissue to confirm the diagnosis of a condyloma; however, this test lacks sensitivity.

DIFFERENTIAL DIAGNOSIS

One of the diagnostic challenges is the differentiation of condyloma acuminatum from *fibroepithelial polyp*. This problem arises because some condylomata acuminata may not demonstrate appreciable koilocytotic atypia, thus mimicking a fibroepithelial polyp. However, the latter typically shows atypical multinucleated cells in the stroma and the overlying squamous epithelium does not show HPV changes. Based on PCR detection of HPV DNA, lesions without koilocytic atypia showing other

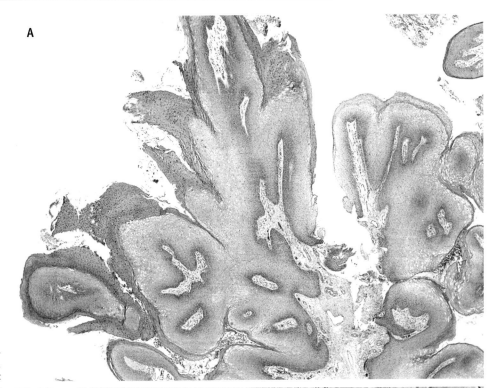

FIGURE 2b.2

Condyloma acuminatum. A prominent papillary architecture is seen. The papillae are lined by hyperplastic squamous epithelium showing hyper- and parakeratosis (A). Notice prominent koilocytotic atypia with perinuclear halos and binucleated cells (B).

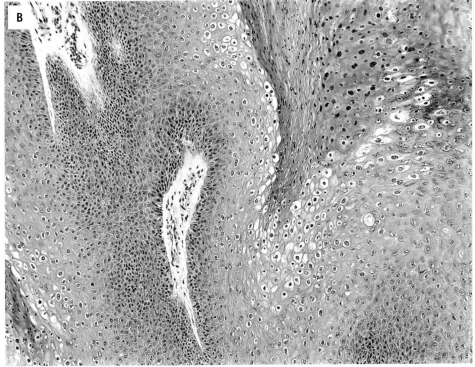

features of condyloma (papillary frond-like projections) have been referred to as "regressed condylomas" (Figure 2b.3). Although both fibroepithelial polyp and regressed condyloma acuminatum are benign, it is important to distinguish between the two because of the social and emotional implications associated with the diagnosis of condyloma. Some condylomata histologically show features overlapping with *seborrheic keratosis*. In the vulva, these are discrete lesions composed of a predomi-

nant population of basaloid cells with minimal cytologic atypia and horn pseudocyst formation. However, they show hyperkeratosis, papillomatosis, and acanthosis, as seen in typical condylomata acuminata, and they may be associated with HPV. Condyloma acuminatum also needs to be distinguished from a *high-grade vulvar intraepithelial lesion of the warty type*, as the latter also shows papillary growth and koilocytic changes, but the presence of significant nuclear atypia and mitotic

A

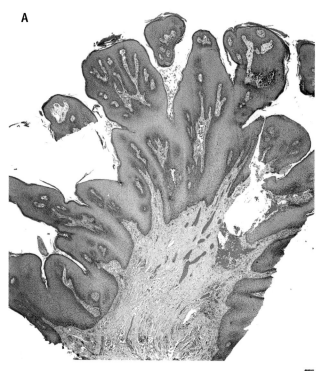

B

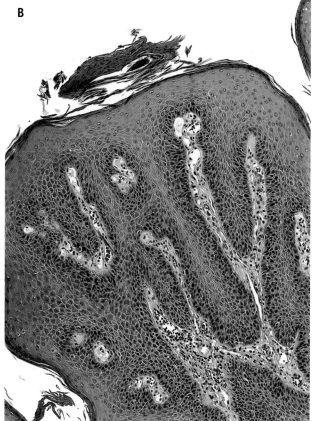

FIGURE 2b.3

Condyloma acuminatum with regressed changes. A typical polypoid architecture is associated with focal hyperparakeratosis (A) but lacks koilocytic changes (B).

activity throughout the full-thickness epithelium distinguishes it from a condyloma (Figure 2b.4).

PROGNOSIS AND THERAPY

Condyloma acuminatum is a benign lesion with a protracted course punctuated by periods of remission and recurrence. Most untreated lesions eventually resolve spontaneously, but it is likely that latent or subclinical infection persists indefinitely. The natural history of anogenital HPV infection is influenced by the cell-mediated immune system. Progression to vulvar intraepithelial neoplasia (VIN) and invasive squamous cell carcinoma is rare but has been documented. Small lesions may be treated with topical application of podophyllin. Surgical removal, cryotherapy, and laser ablation are all accepted methods of treatment for large lesions.

VULVAR INTRAEPITHELIAL NEOPLASIA

The term "vulvar intraepithelial neoplasia" or VIN was endorsed by the International Society for the Study of Vulvar Disease (ISSVD) in 1986 to describe intraepithelial neoplastic proliferations of the vulvar epithelium with the goal of replacing the atypia–carcinoma in situ terminology. Previously, some other terms in the literature that had been used to describe these lesions included Bowen's disease, erythroplasia of Queyrat, bowenoid papulosis, and bowenoid dysplasia. Similar to their counterpart in the cervix, most of the vulvar lesions are etiologically related to HPV infection (more commonly HPV 16), except the simplex or differentiated type of VIN. This permits the classification of VIN into classic types (with further grading into VIN1, VIN2, and VIN3) and the simplex type which is considered a high-grade lesion (VIN3).

CLINICAL FEATURES

The average age at the time of diagnosis of the classic type of VIN has been decreasing in the past two decades, and it is currently diagnosed at the age of approximately 40 years. Considering that classical VIN lesions are caused by HPV infection, the risk factors are similar to those for cervical intraepithelial neoplasia (CIN). Indeed, a significant percentage of patients with VIN have associated CIN or vaginal intraepithelial neoplasia. Other risk factors include smoking, and patients who are human immunodeficiency virus-positive. In contrast, the differentiated type of VIN is characteristically seen in postmenopausal women (sixth to seventh decades). However, this type of VIN accounts for fewer than 10% of cases and, typically, it is not associated with cervical or vaginal squamous neoplasia. In general, VIN is asymptomatic in more than 50% of patients, and in the remainder, pruritus is the most common complaint.

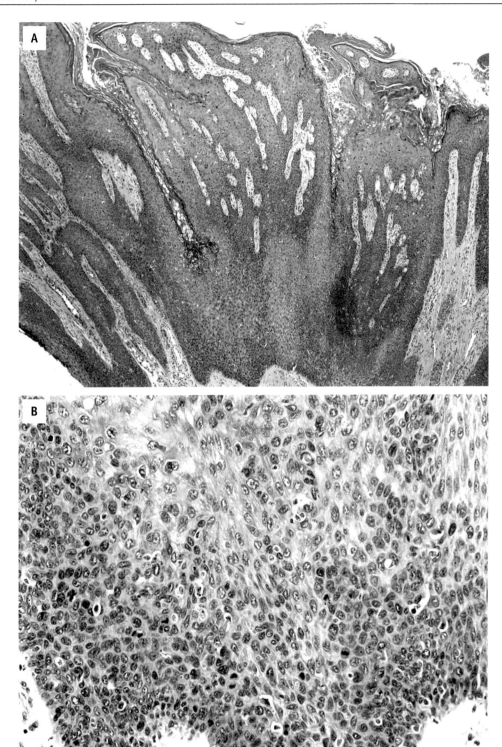

FIGURE 2b.4

High-grade vulvar intraepithelial neoplasia, warty type. A prominent papillary architecture is associated with hyper- and parakeratosis and focal koilocytic change mimicking a condyloma acuminatum (A). However, appreciable nuclear atypia with brisk mitotic activity is seen throughout the epithelium at high-power magnification (B).

VULVAR INTRAEPITHELIAL NEOPLASIA (VIN) – FACT SHEET

Definition

▶ Intraepithelial neoplastic proliferation of the vulvar epithelium with disordered maturation and nuclear abnormalities

Incidence and Location

▶ 2.1 per 100,000 women/year
▶ Increased incidence (× 3) in last two decades in white women < 35 years
▶ Vulvar, perineal, and perianal skin and mucosa

Morbidity and Mortality

▶ Recurrences common
▶ May be difficult to control in immunocompromised patients

Race and Age Distribution

▶ No racial predilection
▶ Classic VIN: reproductive age women
▶ Differentiated (simplex) VIN: postmenopausal women

Clinical Features

▶ More commonly pruritus
▶ Risk factors: smoking, immunosuppression

Prognosis and Treatment

▶ Low-grade lesions have minimal or no potential to progress to high-grade VIN
▶ Surgical excision with clear margins for high-grade VIN
▶ Cautery, laser, or cryotherapy, especially if there is multifocal disease
▶ High-recurrence rate after surgical treatment, especially in smokers and immunocompromised patients
▶ Multiple recurrences may progress to invasive carcinoma (interval for progression approximately 4 years; higher frequency for differentiated VIN)

PATHOLOGIC FINDINGS

GROSS FINDINGS

Typical low-grade VIN appears as pale areas, whereas typical high-grade VIN lesions appear as conspicuous white or erythematous papules or macules that frequently coalesce or show a verrucous growth (Figure 2b.5). Approximately 10–15 % of the lesions are hyperpigmented. Well-differentiated/simplex VIN can be seen as focal discoloration, ill-defined white plaque(s), or discrete elevated nodules, but they are typically less bulky than typical VIN lesions. Both typical and well-differentiated VIN are frequently multifocal. Bleeding and infection may occur due to scratching, with secondary scar formation. Clinically, a high degree of suspicion is necessary to avoid misdiagnosis since the lesions may be subtle.

VULVAR INTRAEPITHELIAL NEOPLASIA (VIN) – PATHOLOGIC FEATURES

Gross Findings

▶ Low-grade classic VIN: single or multiple pale areas
▶ High-grade classic VIN: coalescent white or erythematous papules or macules or verrucous growth with hyperpigmentation in 10–15%
▶ Well-differentiated/simplex VIN: focal discoloration, ill-defined white plaque(s) or discrete elevated nodules

Microscopic Findings

1. Classica (bowenoid) VIN

▶ Epithelial thickening with hyperkeratosis and parakeratosis
▶ Loss of cell maturation, cellular crowding, and dyskeratosis
▶ Nuclear pleomorphism, hyperchromatism, and increased mitoses, including abnormal forms
▶ Involvement of pilosebaceous units, follicles, and Bartholin's glands

1A. Warty ("condylomatous")

▶ Papillary or "spiky" appearance and prominent koilocytic changes

1B. Basaloid

▶ Flat surface and homogeneous growth of "parabasal" cells with uncommon koilocytosis

2. Differentiated (simplex) VIN

▶ Epidermal hyperplasia with frequent elongation of rete ridges and parakeratosis
▶ Abnormal keratinocytes in all layers
▶ Cells with abundant bright eosinophilic cytoplasm and prominent intercellular bridges
▶ Enlarged nuclei with vesicular chromatin and very prominent nucleoli
▶ Whorls including keratin pearls in deeper layers of the epithelium and rete ridges
▶ Smaller cells with high nuclear/cytoplasmic ratio and cytologic atypia in basal layer
▶ No koilocytosis
▶ Lichen sclerosus or squamous hyperplasia commonly nearby

Immunohistochemical Features

▶ Increased MIB-1 staining
▶ p16 extensively positive in classic VIN
▶ p53 overexpression in differentiated/simplex VIN

Differential Diagnosis

Classic VIN

▶ Yeast infections
▶ Chronic dermatoses
▶ Multinucleated atypia of the vulva
▶ Bowenoid papulosis (now included as classic VIN)
▶ Paget disease

Differentiated VIN

▶ Squamous hyperplasia
▶ Lichen sclerosus

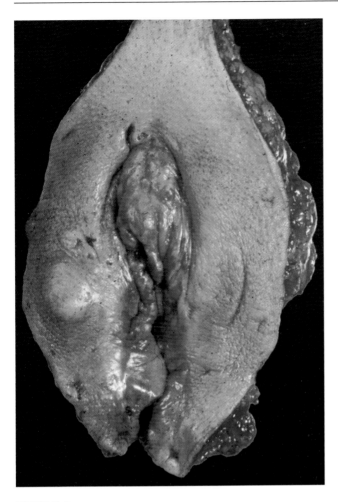

FIGURE 2b.5
Vulvar intraepithelial neoplasia. The lesion appears as a variegated nodular growth, raising concern for an associated invasive process. (Courtesy of Dr. Bhagirath Majmudar.)

MICROSCOPIC FINDINGS

Classic (bowenoid)-type VIN is characterized by epithelial thickening and surface hyperkeratosis frequently accompanied by parakeratosis. Dysplastic squamous cells with scant cytoplasm and hyperchromatic nuclei are accompanied by dyskeratotic cells with eosinophilic cytoplasm and pyknotic nuclei. Loss of cell maturation, cellular crowding, nuclear pleomorphism and hyperchromatism, and increased mitotic activity, including abnormal mitotic figures, are the histologic parameters utilized to classify these lesions. Based on the level of involvement of the thickness of the epithelium by the dysplastic cells, the lesion is graded as follows: (1) low-grade (VIN1) if the abnormal cells involve the lower third of the epithelium; (2) moderate (VIN2) when the abnormal cells are present in the lower two-thirds of the epithelium; and (3) high-grade (VIN3) if there is full-thickness involvement of the epithelium by the atypical cells (Figures 2b.6 and 7). VIN3 is synonymous with carcinoma in situ. This grading scheme is similar to the one employed for classifying cervical dysplasia (CIN). However, as there is poor

inter- and intraobserver reproducibility in distinguishing VIN2 from VIN3, and biologically it is likely that VIN2 and VIN3 confer the same risk and rate of progression to invasive carcinoma if untreated, the ISSVD Vulvar Oncology Subcommittee has recently recommended that the term "VIN" be used exclusively to define high-grade lesions and that VIN2 and VIN3 be combined into a single diagnostic category of high-grade VIN. At the other end of the spectrum, due to the uncertainty regarding the risk of progression of low-grade lesions, it has been recommended that the term "VIN" be dropped to describe low-grade lesions. It is recommended that histologic changes previously diagnosed as VIN1 be described as flat condyloma acuminatum or HPV effect (Figure 2b.8). It is interesting to note that, if carefully selected cases of VIN1 are evaluated for HPV DNA by PCR, the admixture of low- and high-risk HPV encountered in these so-called "flat condylomata acuminata" is distinctly different from the exclusive finding of HPV 6 and 11 found in exophytic condyloma acuminatum. This suggests that flat lesions are etiologically closer to classic-type VIN than to condyloma acuminatum. The ISSVD states that VIN classification should be performed on the basis of morphologic criteria only and not based on HPV type or clinical appearance. If this proposal is widely accepted, the category of low-grade VIN would likely be excluded from the spectrum of VIN.

Some authors subclassify classic VIN into warty ("condylomatous") and basaloid types based on the architecture and appearance of the proliferating squamous cells. The warty type shows a striking papillary or "spiky" appearance at low power, with hyper- and parakeratosis and prominent koilocytic changes (Figure 2b.4), whereas the basaloid type has a flat surface, and is composed of a homogeneous population of small "parabasal" cells, and, even though koilocytosis can be seen on the most superficial areas, it is uncommon (Figure 2b.7). However, not infrequently, the two types are present within the same lesion. Classic/bowenoid VIN frequently shows involvement of the pilosebaceous units and follicular epithelium; it may also involve Bartholin's glands, but rarely affects sweat glands.

Differentiated (simplex) VIN is an important precursor lesion of well-differentiated squamous cell carcinoma of the vulva. It is classified as high-grade VIN due to the associated risk for progression to invasive carcinoma. On low-power examination, the abnormality is subtle because of the differentiated nature of the abnormal cell population. It shows epidermal hyperplasia with associated parakeratosis, and its appearance is reminiscent of hyperplastic squamous epithelium. It may also show elongated rete ridges. Cytologically, the key histologic feature is the finding of squamous cells with abundant bright eosinophilic cytoplasm and prominent intercellular bridges (Figure 2b.9). These keratinocytes also show marked cytologic abnormalities. The nuclei are enlarged, with vesicular chromatin and very prominent nucleoli. These abnormal keratinocytes are present in the basal as well as mid layers of the epithelium. However, the most basal layer contains smaller

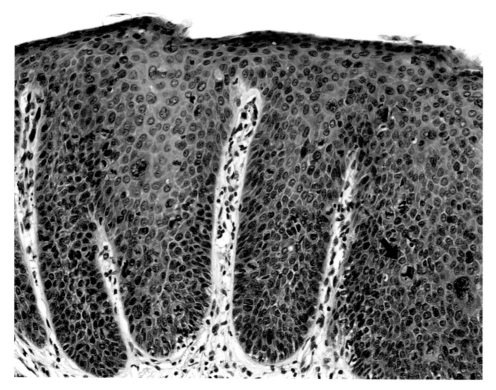

FIGURE 2b.6

Classic-type high-grade vulvar intraepithelial neoplasia (VIN3). Note full-thickness involvement by highly atypical cells with brisk mitotic activity, including an abnormal mitotic figure (arrow).

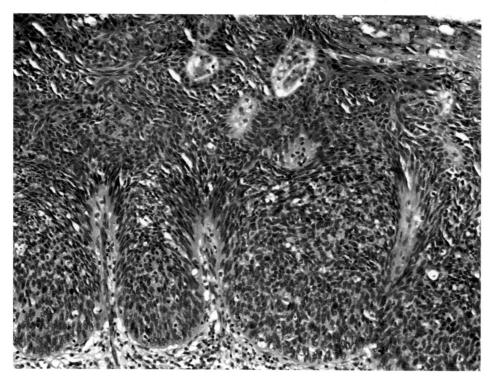

FIGURE 2b.7

Basaloid high-grade vulvar intraepithelial neoplasia. There is a uniform growth of "basaloid" cells with scant cytoplasm, nuclear hyperchromasia and brisk mitotic activity.

cells with a higher nuclear-to-cytoplasmic ratio and greater degree of cytologic atypia. Mitotic activity is also more common at the base of the epithelium. In the deeper layers of the epithelium and in the rete ridges, the abnormal keratinocytes tend to form whorls, including the formation of keratin pearls. Importantly, no HPV changes are identified. This lesion is frequently seen in the vicinity of lichen sclerosus or squamous hyperplasia.

ANCILLARY STUDIES

p16, a surrogate marker of HPV, can be used to detect HPV infection. Diffuse and intense nuclear and cytoplasmic staining typically correlates with high-risk HPV infection. However, focal and weak positivity should be interpreted with caution, as it is nonspecific. Detection of increased proliferative activity in the upper

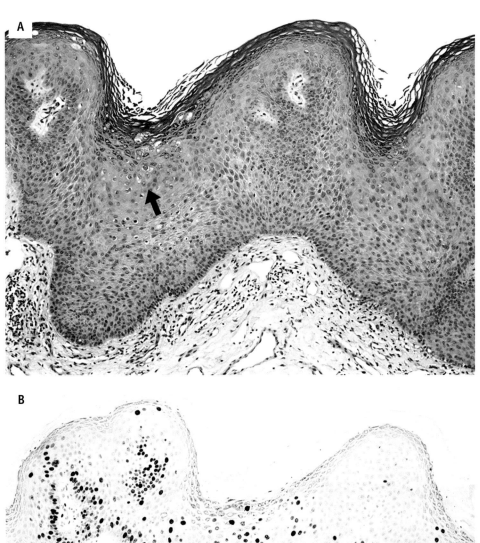

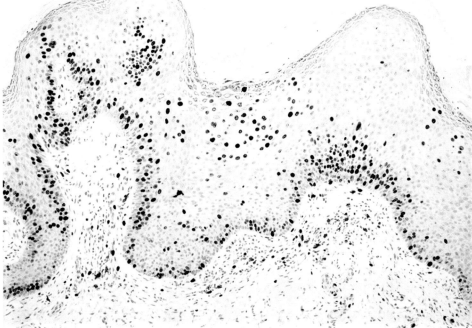

FIGURE 2b.8

Low-grade vulvar intraepithelial neoplasia (VIN1). Only subtle nuclear changes with focal slight disorganization and koilocytosis (arrow) are seen (A). A MIB-1 stain is positive in the upper third of the epithelium, confirming the diagnosis of VIN1 (B).

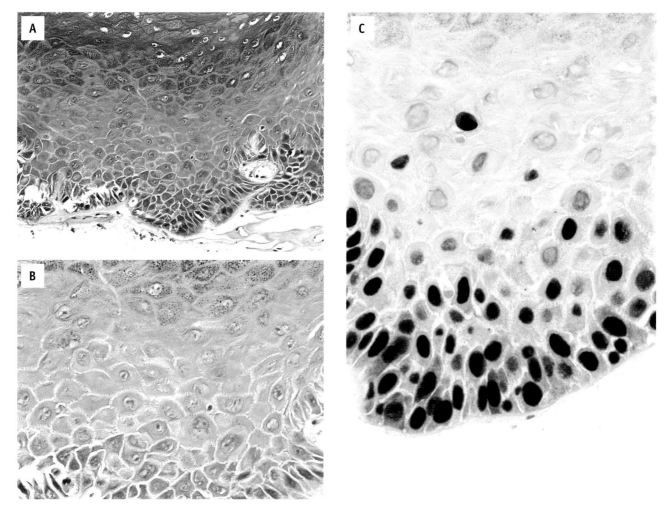

FIGURE 2b.9

Differentiated/simplex vulvar intraepithelial neoplasia. Abnormal keratinocytes with abundant eosinophilic cytoplasm and enlarged nuclei with prominent nucleoli are seen (A). Notice the prominent and well-developed intercellular bridges (B). p53 overexpression is seen in the basal and suprabasilar layers (C).

layers of the epithelium using MIB-1 staining has been shown to have a good correlation with the presence of HPV DNA by molecular analysis (Figure 2b.6). Interpretation of MIB-1 staining needs well-oriented specimens, since a tangentially sectioned biopsy may appear to show MIB-1-positive basal cells in the upper third of the epithelium. HPV in situ hybridization can also be used and is more specific than MIB-1 staining, however, this test suffers from low sensitivity. HPV DNA can be demonstrated in the majority of classic VIN lesions. PCR analysis of VIN1 lesions has shown a mixture of low- and high-risk HPV serotypes whereas VIN2 and VIN3 are generally associated with high-risk HPV, most commonly HPV 16 and 18.

p53 staining can be used as a marker to identify differentiated VIN; normal squamous mucosa and lichen sclerosus show low p53 labeling index with positive staining confined to the basal epithelium. In contrast, differentiated VIN demonstrates a high p53 index in the

basilar epithelium along with suprabasilar extension of p53-positive nuclei (Figure 2b.9C). Whether this corresponds to mutations in the *p53* gene and indicates a pathogenetic pathway for vulvar carcinoma remains to be shown. Molecular studies have failed to demonstrate any HPV DNA in well-differentiated VIN.

DIFFERENTIAL DIAGNOSIS

The main differential diagnosis for low-grade VIN is reactive nonspecific atypia associated with inflammation. *Yeast infection* and *chronic dermatoses* can show reactive nuclear changes that may raise the possibility of a low-grade lesion. On the other hand, morphologic changes of HPV infection in the skin as opposed to cervical mucosa can be subtle, and distinguishing nonneo-

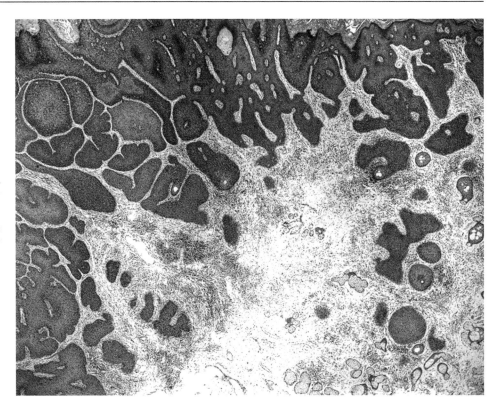

FIGURE 2b.10

High-grade vulvar intraepithelial neoplasia with hair follicle involvement. A tangential section of VIN3 raises suspicion for broad invasion. Notice the spatial orientation of the squamous nests and partial involvement of benign hair follicles.

plastic dermatosis from VIN1 remains a challenge. Ancillary studies including proliferative index (MIB-1) can be used to distinguish true low-grade VIN from chronic dermatoses. The lesion described as *"multinucleated atypia of the vulva"* is characterized by the presence of scattered multinucleated squamous cells without nuclear enlargement or atypia confined to the lower to middle layers of an otherwise normal-appearing squamous epithelium; it is not associated with HPV infection. Extension of the dysplastic cells in high-grade VIN to the underlying hair follicles is not uncommon, and in a tangentially sectioned biopsy it may be misinterpreted as the broad pattern of invasion often seen in *squamous cell carcinoma of the vulva* (Figure 2b.10). However, it is important to notice the spatial orientation of the squamous nests in the stroma and the partial involvement of benign hair follicles and sebaceous glands. *Bowenoid papulosis* histologically very closely resembles classic VIN, although it frequently shows less cytologic atypia and pleomorphism. Clinical correlation is important, as this lesion is typically seen as multiple hyperpigmented lesions in pregnant or postpartum women. Even though it seems to be associated with a lower risk of progression to invasive squamous cell carcinoma when compared to VIN, the ISSVD does not recommend the use of the term "bowenoid papulosis," classifying the lesion within the category of classic VIN. Finally, high-grade VIN can also mimic *Paget disease* due to a prominent nested pattern (pagetoid Bowen disease), a feature seen in approximately 5% of cutaneous squamous cell carcinomas in situ. Cytokeratin 7 is not a helpful marker in this differential diagnosis.

However, the nested pagetoid Bowen disease cells are negative for mucin stains, gross cystic disease fluid protein 15 (GCDFP-15), carcinoembryonic antigen (CEA), and CAM5.2.

The main differential diagnosis of differentiated VIN is *squamous hyperplasia*. Hyperplastic squamous epithelium lacks the nuclear atypia seen in differentiated VIN. Moreover, the epithelium shows orderly maturation, a feature lacking in differentiated VIN. *Lichen sclerosus* may be confused with differentiated VIN, as it may look somewhat similar on low-power examination. However, it lacks the prominent nuclear atypia seen in differentiated VIN; it may have basal layer damage and shows associated dermal changes characteristic of lichen sclerosus. Other dermatoses like psoriasis or *Candida* vulvitis may show some overlapping features with differentiated VIN, but careful attention to the nuclear features should permit their distinction.

PROGNOSIS AND THERAPY

The biologic potential of low-grade lesions (VIN1) is virtually unknown, since prospective long-term follow-up studies to ascertain the natural history of these lesions have not been performed. However, it is likely that it is a lesion with minimal or no potential to progress to high-grade VIN, as invasive carcinoma has not been observed in association with low-grade lesions.

High-grade classic VIN has a high rate of recurrence after surgical treatment, especially if clear margins could not be obtained at the time of initial surgery. It also has a significant potential to progress to invasive carcinoma if untreated. In a recent long-term prospective follow-up study, the mean interval for progression to invasive carcinoma for untreated VIN3 was 4 years. A small percentage of high-grade VIN has been reported to undergo spontaneous regression. These lesions tend to be preferentially pigmented. Surgical excision with negative margins is the preferred treatment for high-grade VIN. Other treatment modalities include cryoablation and laser ablation. The latter are particularly useful in cases of multifocal extensive disease where surgery would be mutilating or primary closure difficult after a wide local excision. Differentiated VIN seems to show a higher frequency to progression to invasive squamous cell carcinoma when compared to classic VIN. In one study, one-third of patients with simplex VIN developed invasive keratinizing squamous cell carcinoma. Clinically evident lesions should be excised, otherwise careful clinical follow-up is warranted.

SUPERFICIALLY INVASIVE SQUAMOUS CELL CARCINOMA

This type of squamous cell carcinoma represents 7–17% of all squamous cell carcinomas. Early stromal invasion is noted in about 6–7% of lesions excised with a preoperative clinical or biopsy diagnosis of high-grade VIN. For this reason, the importance of careful sampling and examination of multiple levels from the excised tissue cannot be overemphasized. Evaluation of invasion requires well-oriented histologic sections because tangential sectioning creates unique artifacts that can lead to overdiagnosis of invasion. Measurement of the depth of invasion is also critical, as it has important prognostic implications.

CLINICAL FEATURES

The clinical profile of patients with superficially invasive squamous cell carcinoma is similar to that of patients with VIN. The disease may be asymptomatic, but frequently patients complain of pruritus. The lesions appear red and may be associated with ulceration and bleeding. Over the last few decades, patients have presented at an earlier age, mirroring the epidemiology of classic VIN. Patients with early invasive carcinoma in a background of differentiated VIN tend to be in their sixth or seventh decades. Finally, as approximately 20% of squamous cell carcinomas are multifocal, it is important to evaluate the vulvar and perianal regions carefully to identify other lesions.

SUPERFICIALLY INVASIVE SQUAMOUS CELL CARCINOMA – FACT SHEET

Definition

▶ Single squamous lesion with a diameter of < 2 cm and a depth of invasion ≤ 1 mm (T1a)

Incidence and Location

▶ 7–17% of all squamous cell carcinomas
▶ Early stromal invasion in about 6–7% of lesions excised with a preoperative diagnosis of VIN
▶ Vulvar, perineal, and perianal skin and mucosa

Morbidity and Mortality

▶ No increased morbidity compared to VIN
▶ Very rare reports of inguinal nodal metastases

Race and Age Distribution

▶ No racial predilection
▶ Fourth decade if background of classic VIN
▶ Sixth to seventh decades if background of differentiated VIN

Clinical Features

▶ Asymptomatic or pruritus

Prognosis and Treatment

▶ Excellent prognosis with a 5-year survival with negative lymph nodes close to 95%
▶ Wide local excision with free margins
▶ Minimal risk of nodal metastases; groin dissection not recommended
▶ Sentinel lymph node excision may be performed if lymphovascular invasion present

---

PATHOLOGIC FEATURES

GROSS FINDINGS

There are no gross features that can reliably predict the presence of microscopic invasion, and therefore this assessment is entirely based on the microscopic evaluation of the specimen.

MICROSCOPIC FINDINGS

The American Joint Commission on Cancer (AJCC) defines a T1 tumor as a single lesion < 2 cm in greatest dimension, with further subdivision into T1a and T1b based on the depth of invasion being 1 mm, or > 1 mm, respectively. There is, however, no universally agreed-upon definition of what constitutes superficially invasive squamous cell carcinoma. This is in part due to problems related to correctly determining the important dimensions of the lesions clinically and how these dimensions should be measured in order to define stage 1a lesions. The ISSVD has proposed tumor size < 2 cm and depth of invasion ≤1 mm to define superficially invasive squamous cell carcinoma. Accordingly, the depth of invasion should be measured from the epithe-

SUPERFICIALLY INVASIVE SQUAMOUS CELL CARCINOMA – PATHOLOGIC FEATURES

Gross Findings

▸ Frequently indistinguishable from VIN
▸ White or erythematous papule or raised ulcerated area
▸ Tumor size < 2 cm

Microscopic Findings

▸ Predominant in situ disease
▸ Small squamous nests with paradoxical keratinization budding off from base
▸ Depth of invasion ≤ 1 mm (measured from epithelial–stromal junction of most superficial adjacent dermal papilla to deepest point of invasion)
▸ Depth of invasion and tumor thickness (from tumor surface or base of granular layer to deepest point of invasion) most important parameters

Immunohistochemical Features

▸ Dual staining with cytokeratin and collagen IV/laminin potentially useful

Differential Diagnosis

▸ Tangentially sectioned VIN
▸ Extension of vulvar intraepithelial neoplasia into hair follicles

lial–stromal junction of the most superficial adjacent dermal papillae to the deepest point of invasion (Figure 2b.11). This measurement is not significantly influenced by the presence of hyperkeratosis, tumor ulceration, or adjacent epidermal hyperplasia. The importance of defining 1 mm as the cutoff for depth of invasion is based on the risk of nodal metastases. Depth of invasion needs to be differentiated from "tumor thickness," which is defined as the measurement from the surface of the tumor or the base of the granular layer to the deepest point of invasion (Figure 2b.11). In the pathology report, both measurements should be mentioned along with the presence or absence of lympovascular space invasion. The identification of lymphovascular space invasion, however, does not preclude classifying the lesion as stage 1a, as defined above. Superficial invasion can be identified as small foci of squamous epithelium showing paradoxical keratinization budding from the base of a papilla involved by high-grade VIN (Figure 2b.12). In well-oriented specimens, it is not difficult to recognize such foci and ascertain that the depth of invasion is ≤1 mm. In some instances, superficial invasion is more difficult to differentiate from the in situ component and determining the landmarks for accurate assessment of superficial invasion may also be problematic. To optimize accurate identification of superficial invasion and correct interpretation of the depth of invasion,

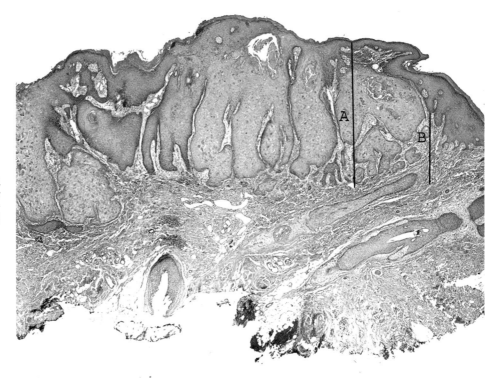

FIGURE 2b.11

Superficially invasive squamous cell carcinoma. This well-oriented biopsy is helpful in illustrating the landmarks to assess tumor thickness (A) and depth of invasion (B).

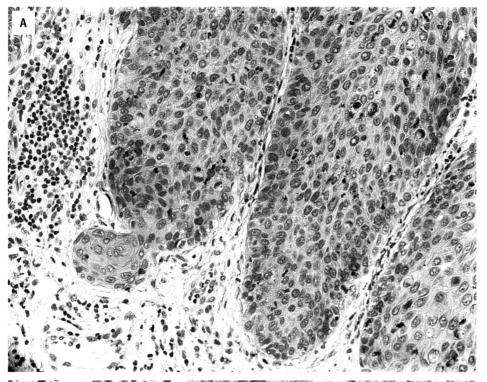

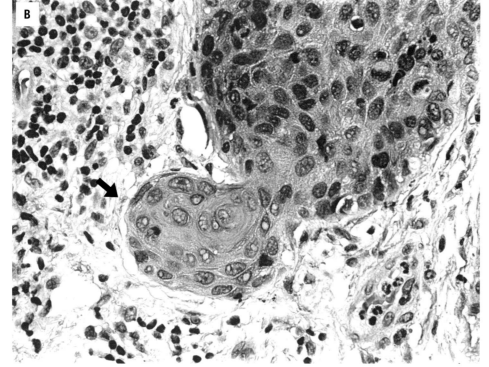

FIGURE 2b.12

High-grade vulvar intraepithelial neoplasia with early stromal invasion (superficially invasive squamous carcinoma). A small atypical squamous nest breaches the basement membrane (A). Paradoxical keratinization is an important feature in the recognition of superficial invasion (arrow) (B).

all wide local excision specimens should be thinly sliced and properly oriented. As squamous cell carcinomas are frequently associated with VIN lesions, it is important to keep in mind that the VIN component should not be included in the measurement of the tumor diameter.

ANCILLARY STUDIES

Generally, staining for the presence or absence of basement membrane components has not been proven to be useful in equivocal cases where superficial invasion is suspected because of the documented focal absence of basement membrane in carcinoma in situ and the demonstrated ability of invasive carcinoma to generate secondary basement membrane surrounding invasive nests. Dual staining with cytokeratin and collagen IV/laminin has been advocated in a recent study to be potentially helpful in some cases. For practical purposes, if serial sectioning and levels on the block are unable to provide definitive evidence of invasion, the recommendation is to follow a conservative approach.

DIFFERENTIAL DIAGNOSIS

On a biopsy specimen, *tangential sectioning of VIN* and *involvement of the hair follicles by VIN* may be overdiagnosed as superficially invasive squamous cell carcinoma. It is important to recognize the evenly spaced distribution of the nests in the stroma as well as the focal identification of sebaceous glands in deeper sections to avoid the diagnosis of invasion. Ulceration and previous biopsy site changes can also compound the problem of assessing superficial invasion. If serial sectioning and levels cannot resolve the differential diagnosis, invasion should not be diagnosed. The concern for invasion can be communicated to the clinician in the report and further evaluated on the resection specimen. On a resection specimen, a similar cautionary approach is advocated. Given that the risk for lymph node involvement in patients with superficial invasion is extremely low, it is prudent to exercise caution when diagnosing superficially invasive carcinoma.

PROGNOSIS AND THERAPY

There are data to support that the size of the lesion and the depth of invasion correlate with the risk of nodal metastases in vulvar cancer. The risk of nodal metastases in lesions 2 cm in maximum size is approximately 19%, increasing to 54% for lesions 3–4 cm. The risk of nodal metastases is about 11% if the cutoff for depth of invasion is 5 mm, and drops to 4.8% when the depth of invasion is 3 mm. A review of the literature reveals that only two stage 1a tumors as defined above harbored lymph node metastases. Thus, at the present time, for patients with tumors invading ≤ 1 mm, a groin lymph node dissection is not recommended. These patients can be adequately treated with wide local excision of the lesion. In selected patients where lymph node metastasis is suspected because of the presence of lymphovascular invasion near the invasive front of the tumor, a sentinel node excision may be performed. The 5-year survival rate with negative lymph nodes is close to 95%.

INVASIVE SQUAMOUS CELL CARCINOMA

An estimated 4000 new cases and 870 deaths from vulvar cancer were recorded in the United States in 2005. The majority of vulvar cancers are squamous in origin and they represent 5–8% of all gynecologic cancers. The current understanding of the clinicopathologic features of two distinct types of high-grade VIN as precursor lesions has contributed to our understanding of the clinical features, pathogenesis, and epidemiology of their invasive counterparts.

INVASIVE SQUAMOUS CELL CARCINOMA – FACT SHEET

Definition
▶ Invasive carcinoma of the vulva with squamous differentiation and dimensions greater than superficially invasive tumors

Incidence and Location
▶ Approximately 4000 new cases in US in 2005
▶ Approximately 5–8% of all gynecologic cancers
▶ Labia minora or majora more commonly involved

Morbidity and Mortality
▶ 870 deaths from vulvar cancer in US in 2005
▶ Local recurrence
▶ Metastasis to inguinal lymph nodes; rarely distant metastasis

Race and Age Distribution
▶ No racial predilection
▶ Higher incidence in patients of low socioeconomic status
▶ Bimodal age distribution:
  ▶ Fifth decade for tumors associated with classic VIN
  ▶ Sixth to seventh decades for tumors associated with differentiated VIN

Clinical Features
▶ Pruritus or mass in approximately 50% of cases
▶ Bleeding, dyspareunia, dysuria, and unpleasant odor

Prognosis and Treatment
▶ Prognosis stage dependent
▶ Overall 5-year survival > 95% for stage I tumors and 29% for stage IV tumors
▶ Stage, tumor size, depth of invasion, lymphovascular invasion, and lymph node involvement important prognostic factors
▶ Wide local excision with 1 cm gross margin with inguinal lymph node dissection mainstay of treatment
▶ Increased risk of recurrence if positive margins (< 8 mm), lymphovascular invasion, size > 5 cm and depth of invasion ≥ 11 mm and high-grade VIN at margin

INVASIVE SQUAMOUS CELL CARCINOMA – PATHOLOGIC FEATURES

Gross Findings

▶ Typically solitary (multifocal in < 10%)
▶ Exophytic cauliflower-like growth or endophytic ulcerated lesion

Microscopic Findings

Subtypes

1. Keratinizing squamous cell carcinoma, not otherwise specified
▶ Conspicuous evidence of keratinization with pearl formation
▶ Neoplastic cells with abundant eosinophilic cytoplasm
▶ Considerable nuclear atypia and mitotic activity, including abnormal forms
▶ Invasion as irregular nests and single cells in a desmoplastic stroma
▶ Adjacent lichen sclerosus or differentiated high-grade VIN

2. Nonkeratinizing squamous cell carcinoma
▶ Minimal evidence of keratinization with no pearl formation

3. Basaloid carcinoma
▶ Broad bands, large or small irregular nests and cords
▶ Immature uniform basaloid cells with scant cytoplasm
▶ Evenly distributed granular chromatin with no evident nucleoli
▶ Occasional focal abrupt keratinization within the tumor nests
▶ Hyalinized or markedly desmoplastic stroma

4. Warty (condylomatous) carcinoma
▶ Multiple papillary projections with fibrovascular cores
▶ Papillae lined by keratinized squamous epithelium with koilocytic changes
▶ Considerable cytologic atypia including brisk mitotic activity
▶ Irregular jagged nests of keratinized squamous cells infiltrating stroma
▶ Keratin pearl formation in invasive nests helpful clue in excluding pseudoinvasion

5. Verrucous carcinoma
▶ Deceptive pushing broad pattern of invasion
▶ Bulbous nests of neoplastic cells pushing into underlying stroma
▶ Hyperplastic squamous proliferation with prominent hyper- and parakeratosis
▶ Cells with abundant eosinophilic cytoplasm, but typically lacking nuclear atypia and koilocytosis

Immunohistochemical Features

▶ p16 strongly positive in basaloid and warty squamous cell carcinomas
▶ p53 typically positive in keratinizing squamous cell carcinomas
▶ Cytokeratin, S-100, and HMB-45 and neuroendocrine markers useful in differential diagnosis

Differential Diagnosis

▶ Condyloma acuminatum (vs warty carcinoma)
▶ Squamous cell carcinoma with verrucous growth pattern (vs verrucous carcinoma)
▶ Warty carcinoma (vs verrucous carcinoma)
▶ Amelanotic malignant melanoma (vs squamous carcinoma with giant cells)
▶ Small cell carcinoma (vs basaloid squamous cell carcinoma)
▶ Merkel cell carcinoma (vs basaloid squamous cell carcinoma)
▶ Basal cell carcinoma (vs basaloid squamous cell carcinoma)

CLINICAL FEATURES

Basaloid and warty squamous cell carcinomas tend to occur in younger patients, are associated with classic high-grade VIN, and HPV DNA can be demonstrated in most of these lesions. In contrast, well-differentiated squamous cell carcinoma is most often seen in patients in their sixth to seventh decades; it is associated with differentiated (simplex) VIN and does not seem to be associated with HPV infection. Women with invasive vulvar squamous cell carcinoma may present with a variety of complaints. Pruritus and the presence of a lump or mass occur in up to 50% of patients. Other symptoms include bleeding, dyspareunia, dysuria, and unpleasant odor.

PATHOLOGIC FEATURES

GROSS FINDINGS

Invasive squamous cell carcinoma may appear grossly as an exophytic cauliflower-like growth or an endophytic ulcerated lesion (Figure 2b.13). The labia majora and minora are preferentially involved, and the majority of tumors are solitary. Multifocal disease may be seen in < 10% of the patients.

MICROSCOPIC FINDINGS

The current World Health Organization (WHO) classification of vulvar carcinoma lists several morphologic variants of invasive squamous carcinoma. Salient histologic features of these subtypes of invasive squamous cell carcinoma are discussed below.

Keratinizing squamous cell carcinoma, not otherwise specified. This is the most common histologic subtype of squamous cell carcinoma. The neoplastic cells are mature with abundant eosinophilic cytoplasm and show conspicuous evidence of keratinization with keratin pearl formation. The nuclei are enlarged with prominent nucleoli, and features readily identified in most cases include considerable nuclear atypia, mitotic activity, including abnormal forms, and perineural invasion. The tumor invades as irregular nests and single cells, eliciting a desmoplastic response (Figure 2b.14). The adjacent skin may show evidence of either lichen sclerosus or differentiated VIN.

Nonkeratinizing squamous cell carcinoma. The cells in this subtype of invasive squamous carcinoma show minimal evidence of keratinization with scattered keratinized cells providing evidence of its histogenesis. Keratin pearl formation is not seen.

Basaloid carcinoma. This tumor subtype arises in association with high-grade classic VIN and comprises broad bands, large or small irregular nests, and cords of immature "basaloid" cells with scant cytoplasm (Figure 2b.15). The cells are relatively uniform in size and the nuclei show evenly distributed granular chromatin with no evident nucleoli. Focal keratinization

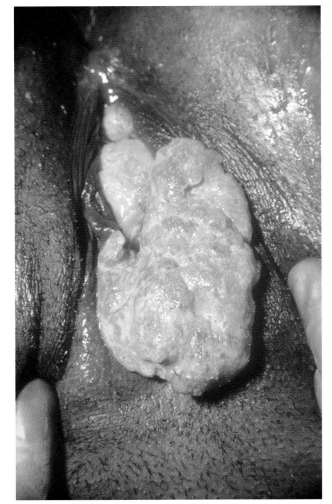

FIGURE 2b.13

Invasive squamous cell carcinoma. A large polypoid and ulcerated tumor involves both the labium minor and major on the left side and crosses over the right labium minor. (Courtesy of Dr. Bhagirath Majmudar.)

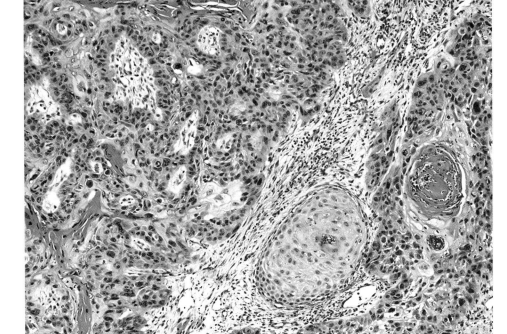

FIGURE 2b.14

Invasive keratinizing squamous cell carcinoma. Irregular tongues of well to moderately differentiated and keratinizing neoplastic squamous cells infiltrate the stroma in a haphazard pattern.

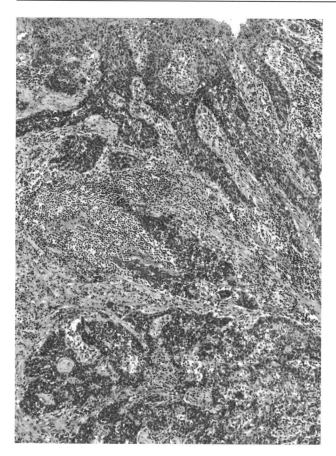

FIGURE 2b.15

Basaloid carcinoma. Wide anastomosing bands of small "basaloid" blue cells are deeply infiltrating the stroma.

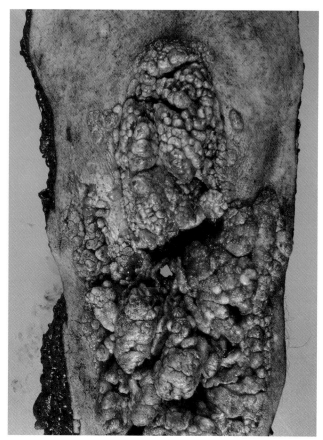

FIGURE 2b.16

Warty high-grade vulvar intraepithelial neoplasia with associated invasive squamous cell carcinoma. This rather extreme example resulted in a total vulvectomy and vaginectomy for the patient. The majority of the lesion showed warty high-grade VIN with foci of invasion noted near the vaginal margin.

within the tumor nests may be seen occasionally, but formation of keratin pearls is unusual, and when it occurs, the transition is typically abrupt. Hyalinized or markedly desmoplastic stroma surrounding the infiltrating nests of tumor cells is characteristic. HPV 16 DNA can be demonstrated in the majority of these tumors.

Warty (condylomatous) carcinoma. This histologic subtype is architecturally characterized by the presence of multiple papillary projections with fibrovascular cores (Figure 2b.16). The papillae are lined by keratinized squamous epithelium showing koilocytic changes on the surface reminiscent of a condyloma acuminatum, hence the morphologic descriptor. However, there is considerable cytologic atypia, including brisk mitotic activity as well as invasion into the underlying stroma, usually in the form of irregular jagged nests of atypical keratinized squamous epithelium. Keratin pearl formation in the invasive nests is often seen and it is a helpful clue in excluding pseudoinvasion, an artifact created by the tangential sectioning of hair follicle structures that have been colonized by the neoplastic squamous epithelium. This lesion is frequently associated with HPV 16.

Verrucous carcinoma. This highly differentiated variant of squamous cell carcinoma is characterized by bulbous nests of neoplastic cells that appear to push their way into the underlying stroma (Figure 2b.17). This broad pattern of invasion is deceptive in that it may not be recognized as an invasive process, especially

in a poorly oriented specimen. The neoplastic squamous epithelium is hyperplastic and associated with prominent hyper- and parakeratosis. The tumor cells have abundant cytoplasm; however, nuclear atypia is not significant and koilocytosis is usually absent.

Squamous carcinoma with tumor giant cells. This is a rare and aggressive variant of invasive squamous cell carcinoma characterized by the presence of numerous multinucleated tumor giant cells. Large atypical nuclei with prominent nucleoli and brisk mitotic activity are usually seen.

Keratoacanthoma-like carcinoma. This variant has been included in the latest WHO classification of vulvar squamous cell carcinoma. It has an appearance reminiscent of keratoacanthoma as occurs elsewhere on hair-bearing skin. These tumors are characterized by the presence of a central crater filled with proliferating squamous epithelium and anucleated masses of keratin. Invading nests and cords of squamous epithelium are noted in the dermis. These tumors may regress spontaneously by a poorly understood immune mechanism.

There is no universally accepted grading system for vulvar squamous cell carcinoma. The AJCC recommends a four-grade system: well-differentiated (G1), moderately differentiated (G2), poorly differentiated

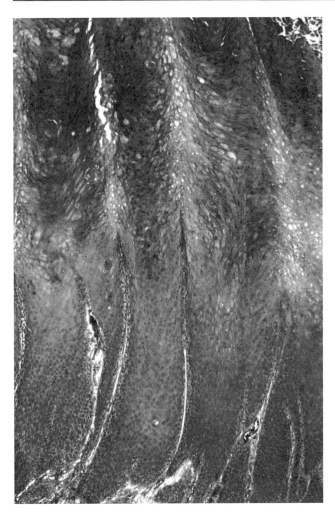

FIGURE 2b.17
Verrucous carcinoma. Notice marked squamous hyperplasia associated with hyper- and parakeratosis and a striking pushing border of the neoplastic proliferation.

(G3), and undifferentiated (G4). However, it does not provide definitions of the grading scheme. The grading system recommended by the Gynecologic Oncology Group (GOG) is based on the percentage of undifferentiated cells (small cells with scant cytoplasm infiltrating the stroma). Due to the lack of a uniform grading system, it is difficult to evaluate the importance of grade as an independent prognostic factor in vulvar squamous cell carcinoma.

ANCILLARY STUDIES

The role of immunohistochemistry in the diagnosis of squamous cell carcinoma of the vulva is limited. However, it has recently been shown that p16 immunostaining is a good adjunct in separating HPV-related from HPV-unrelated vulvar carcinomas. p16 is strongly positive in basaloid and warty squamous cell carcinomas but is usually negative in verrucous and keratinizing squamous cell carcinomas. In contrast, p53 is typically positive in keratinizing squamous cell carcinomas but not in basaloid and warty squamous cell carcinomas.

DIFFERENTIAL DIAGNOSIS

Some specific diagnostic considerations may arise when one of the following variants of vulvar carcinoma are encountered. Warty carcinoma can be confused with *condyloma acuminatum* at low-power magnification due to overlapping architecture and koilocytic changes, especially if the lesion shows minimal infiltration. However, at high power, there is noticeable cytologic atypia and mitotic activity throughout the tumor. Verrucous carcinoma may be confused with a *squamous cell carcinoma with verrucous growth pattern*. The distinction is important because verrucous carcinoma, once adequately excised, has an excellent prognosis and a clinical course that includes local recurrence but not lymph node or distant metastasis. The presence of cytologic atypia and/or irregular infiltration favors a diagnosis of well-differentiated squamous cell carcinoma with prominent verrucous growth. Less frequently, verrucous carcinoma may be confused with *warty carcinoma*. However, the latter typically shows koilocytic atypia and an irregular infiltrative growth. The rare squamous carcinoma with giant cells may mimic an *amelanotic malignant melanoma*. The finding of focal squamous differentiation, adjacent VIN, or a melanocytic precursor lesion may help in this differential diagnosis. In difficult cases, HMB-45, Melan-A, S-100, and keratin can be performed. Finally, basaloid squamous cell carcinoma can be confused with small cell carcinoma, Merkel cell carcinoma, and basal cell carcinoma. *Small cell carcinoma* frequently shows nuclear molding, brisk mitotic activity, and absence of squamous differentiation; this tumor is typically positive for TTF-I. *Merkel cell carcinoma* is composed of small blue cells with high mitotic index and frequent apoptosis arranged in diffuse or trabecular patterns. Squamous differentiation is extremely rare. The tumor cells are characteristically positive for neuron-specific enolase (NSE), chromogranin, and keratin 20 in a dot-like pattern. *Basal cell carcinoma* may show central keratinization, but, in contrast to basaloid squamous cell carcinoma, the tumor cells show bland cytologic features and peripheral palisading. p16 is not helpful in differentiating basaloid squamous from basal cell carcinoma.

PROGNOSIS AND THERAPY

The prognosis of invasive vulvar squamous cell carcinoma is stage-dependent (Table 2b.1). The overall 5-year survival is greater than 95 % for stage I tumors, dropping to about 29 % for stage IV disease. Stage, tumor size, depth of invasion, lymphovascular invasion, and involvement of lymph nodes have been reported to be highly correlated with survival. Patients with positive lymph nodes relapse earlier than those without lymph node involvement; it has been shown that lymph node metastases closely correlate with clinical node status, depth of invasion, size of the primary tumor, and lymphovascular invasion. Local recurrence is related to positive margins (< 8 mm), presence of lymphovascular invasion, size ≥ 5 cm, and depth of invasion ≥ 11 mm.

TABLE 2b.1

Carcinomas of the vulva: TNM and FIGO staging system

TNM	FIGO	
Tis	0	Carcinoma in situ (preinvasive carcinoma)
T1	I	Tumor confined to vulva or vulva and perineum, ≤ 2 cm in greatest dimension
T1a	IA	Tumor confined to vulva or vulva and perineum, ≤ 2 cm in greatest dimension, with stromal invasion <1 mm
T1b	IB	Tumor confined to vulva or vulva and perineum, ≤ 2 cm in greatest dimension, with stromal invasion ≥ 1 mm
T2	II	Tumor confined to vulva or vulva and perineum, > 2 cm in greatest dimension
T3	III	Tumor invades any of the following: lower urethra, vagina, or anus
T4	IVA	Tumor invades any of the following: bladder mucosa, rectal mucosa, upper urethra; or is fixed to pubic bone

Patients with high-grade VIN at the margin also have a higher risk of recurrence. The standard of treatment for patients with vulvar squamous cell carcinoma consists of wide local excision with a 1-cm gross margin. If tumors invade to a depth > 1 mm, groin (ipsi- or bilateral) dissection is advocated, with sentinel node examination. Radical vulvectomy is rarely used.

SUGGESTED READING

Condyloma Acuminatum

Bai H, Cviko A, Granter S, et al. Immunophenotypic and viral (human papilloma virus) correlates of vulvar seborrheic keratosis. Hum Pathol 2003;34:559–564.

Gall SA. Female genital warts: global trends and treatments. Infect Dis Obstet Gynecol 2001;9:149–154.

Hammarlund K, Nystrom M. The lived experience of genital warts: the Swedish example. Health Care Women Int 2004;25:489–502.

Li J, Ackerman AB. "Seborrheic keratoses" that contain human papillomavirus are condyloma acuminata. Am J Dermatopathol 1994;16:398–405.

Medeiros F, Nascimento AF, Crum CP. Early vulvar squamous neoplasia. Advances in classification, diagnosis and differential diagnosis. Adv Anat Pathol 2005;12:20–26.

Nucci MR, Genest DR, Tate JE, et al. Pseudobowenoid vulvar change: untreated condyloma acuminatum. Mod Pathol 1995;9:375–379.

O'Mahony C. Genital warts: current and future management options. Am J Clin Dermatol 2005;6:239–243.

Pirog EC, Chen YT, Isacson C. MIB-1 immunostaining is a beneficial adjunct test for accurate diagnosis of vulvar condyloma acuminatum. Am J Surg Pathol 2000;24:1393–1399.

Vulvar Intraepithelial Neoplasia

Chang DY, Wu MY, Huang SC. Bowen's disease and bowenoid papulosis of the vulva. Int J Gynaecol Obstet 1995;48:227–229.

Fox H, Wells M. Recent advances in the pathology of the vulva. Histopathology 2003;42:209–216.

Haefner HK, Tate JE, McLachlin CM, et al. Vulvar intraepithelial neoplasia: age, morphological phenotype, papillomavirus DNA, and coexisting invasive carcinoma. Hum Pathol 1995;26:147–154.

Hart WR. Vulvar intraepithelial neoplasia: historical aspects and current status. Int J Gynecol Pathol 2001;20:16–30.

Jones RW, Rowan DM, Steward AW. Vulvar intraepithelial neoplasia. Aspects of the natural history and outcome in 405 women. Obstet Gynecol 2005;106:1319–1326.

Logani S, Lu D, Quint WGV, et al. Low grade vulvar and vaginal intraepithelial neoplasia: correlation of histologic features with human papilloma virus detection and MIB-1 immunostaining. Mod Pathol 2003;16:735–741.

McLachlin CM, Mutter GL, Crum CP. Multinucleated atypia of the vulva. Report of a distinct entity not associated with human papillomavirus. Am J Surg Pathol 1994;18:1233–1239.

Raju RR, Goldblum JR, Hart WR. Pagetoid squamous cell carcinoma in situ (pagetoid Bowen's disease) of the external genitalia. Int J Gynecol Pathol 2003;22:127–135.

Rausch D, Angermeiyer M, Capaldi L, et al. Multinucleated atypia of the vulva. Cutis 2005;75:118–120.

Santos M, Montagut C, Mellado B, et al. Immunohistochemical staining for p16 and p53 in premalignant and malignant epithelial lesions of the vulva. Int J Gynecol Pathol 2004;23:206–214.

Sideri M, Jones RW, Wilkinson EJ, et al. Squamous vulvar intraepithelial neoplasia, 2004 modified terminology, ISSVD Vulvar Oncology Subcommittee. J Reprod Med 2005;50:807–810.

Sykes P, Smith N, McCormick P, et al. High-grade vulvar intraepithelial neoplasia (VIN 3): a retrospective analysis of patient characteristics, management, outcome and relationship to squamous cell carcinoma of the vulva 1989–1999. Aust NZ J Obstet Gynaecol 2002;42:69–74.

Yang B, Hart WR. Vulvar intraepithelial neoplasia of the simplex (differentiated) type: a clinicopathologic study including analysis of HPV and p53 expression. Am J Surg Pathol 2000;24:429–441.

Superficially Invasive Squamous Cell Carcinoma

Burke TW, Levenback C, Coleman RL, et al. Surgical therapy of T1 and T2 vulvar carcinoma: further experience with radical wide excision and selective inguinal lymphadenectomy. Gynecol Oncol 1995;57:215–220.

Kelley JL 3rd, Burke TW, Tornos C, et al. Minimally invasive vulvar carcinoma: an indication for conservative surgical therapy. Gynecol Oncol 1992;44:240–244.

Magrina JF, Gonzalez-Bosquet J, Weaver AL, et al. Squamous cell carcinoma of the vulva stage 1A: long term results. Gynecol Oncol 2000;76:24–27.

Scheistroen M, Nesland JM, Trope C. Have patients with early squamous carcinoma of the vulva been overtreated in the past? The Norwegian experience 1977–1991. Eur J Gynaecol Oncol 2002;23:93–103.

Wilkinson EJ. Superficially invasive carcinoma of the vulva. Clin Obstet Gynecol 1991;34:651–661.

Invasive Squamous Cell Carcinoma

Chiesa-Vottero A, Dvoretsky PM, Hart WR. Histopathologic study of thin vulvar squamous cell carcinomas and associated cutaneous lesions. A correlative study of 48 tumors in 44 patients with analysis of adjacent vulvar intraepithelial neoplasia types and lichen sclerosus. Am J Surg Pathol 2006;30:310–318.

Crum CP, McLachlin CM, Tate GE, et al. Pathobiology of vulvar squamous neoplasia. Curr Opin Obstet Gynecol 1997;9:63–69.

Kurman RJ, Toki T, Schffman MH. Basaloid and warty carcinomas of the vulva. Distinctive types of squamous cell carcinoma frequently associated with human papillomaviruses. Am J Surg Pathol 1993;17:133–145.

Lerma E, Matias-Guiu X, Lee SJ, et al. Squamous cell carcinoma of the vulva: study of ploidy, HPV, p53, and pRb. Int J Gynecol Pathol 1999;18:191–197.

Maggino T, Landoni F, Sartori E, et al. Patterns of recurrence in patients with squamous cell carcinoma of the vulva. A multicenter CTF study. Cancer 2000;89:116–122.

Oonk MH, Hollema H, de Hullu JA, et al. Prediction of lymph node metastases in vulvar cancer: a review. Int J Gynecol Cancer 2006;16:963–971.

Santos LD, Krivanek MJ, Chan F, et al. Pseudoangiosarcomatous squamous cell carcinoma of the vulva. Pathology 2006;38:581–584.

Santos M, Landolfi F, Olivella A, et al. p16 overexpression identifies HPV-positive vulvar squamous cell carcinomas. Am J Surg Pathol 2006;30:1347–1356.

Stehman FB, Look KH. Carcinoma of the vulva. Obstet Gynecol 2006;107:719–733.

Trimble CL, Hildesheim A, Brinton LA, et al. Heterogeneous etiology of squamous carcinoma of the vulva. Obstet Gynecol 1996;87:59–64.

Wilkinson EJ, Teixeira MR. The World Health Organization Classification of Tumours. Pathology and Genetics of Tumours of the Breast and Female Genital Organs. Lyon: IARC Press, 2003:316–318.

Extramammary Paget Disease and Melanocytic Lesions

Victor G Prieto · Christopher R Shea · Esther Oliva

EXTRAMAMMARY PAGET DISEASE

Extramammary Paget disease (EMPD) can be defined as an intraepithelial adenocarcinoma that primarily involves the epidermis outside the breast.

CLINICAL FEATURES

This tumor accounts for only 1% of vulvar cancers. EMPD typically appears as an eczematous-type plaque, sometimes with erosion (Figure 2c.1), more commonly in the anogenital region, and less commonly it involves the axillae, ears (ceruminal glands), and eyelids (Moll glands). Itching is the most frequent presenting symptom. Due to its erythematous appearance EMPD is frequently confused clinically with *Candida* infection.

EXTRAMAMMARY PAGET DISEASE – FACT SHEET

Definition
▶ Intraepidermal adenocarcinoma

Incidence and Location
▶ Rare (< 1% of the population)
▶ Anogenital region (also axilla, ear, eyelid)

Morbidity and Mortality
▶ Pruritus, ulceration, and superinfection
▶ High recurrence rate if incompletely excised
▶ If associated with internal malignancy, mortality rate related to primary tumor

Clinical Features
▶ Eczematous, itchy plaque
▶ 25% associated with internal malignancy (colorectal, cervical, bladder/urethra)

Prognosis and Treatment
▶ Poor prognosis if more than minimal invasion (> 1 mm) or association with internal malignancy
▶ Radical resection treatment of choice
▶ Radiotherapy or chemotherapy in nonsurgical cases (poor response)

Unlike Paget disease of the breast, in which an associated mammary ductal carcinoma is almost invariably present, an underlying carcinoma (colorectal, cervical, bladder/urethra, or prostatic) is identified in only approximately 25% of EMPD. The remainder of cases probably represent in situ malignant transformation of the cutaneous sweat ducts.

PATHOLOGIC FEATURES

GROSS FINDINGS

EMPD appears as an ill-defined, diffuse red plaque that may occasionally become ulcerated.

EXTRAMAMMARY PAGET DISEASE (EMPD) – PATHOLOGIC FEATURES

Gross Findings
▶ Ill-defined, diffuse red plaque with rare ulceration

Microscopic Findings
▶ Nests, isolated large cells, or even rare glands mainly located in basal and parabasal layers "compressing" basal keratinocytes
▶ Atypical cells may be present in upper layers
▶ Cells with abundant pale cytoplasm with frequent intracytoplasmic vacuoles and large nuclei
▶ Variable mitotic activity
▶ Rare intracytoplasmic melanin pigment

Immunohistochemical Features
▶ CAM5.2, CEA, epithelial membrane antige (EMA) positive and ER/PR receptor negative
▶ Primary EMPD: CK7+/CK20–/gross cystic disease fluid protein 15 (GCDFP-15)+/MUC1 and MUC5+
▶ Secondary EMPD (anorectal): CK7–/CK20+/GCDFP15–/MUC2+
▶ Secondary EMPD (urothelial): CK7+/CK20+/GCDFP15–/uroplakin III+

Differential Diagnosis
▶ In situ or invasive squamous cell carcinoma with pagetoid growth
▶ Melanoma
▶ Sebaceous carcinoma
▶ Pagetoid dyskeratosis

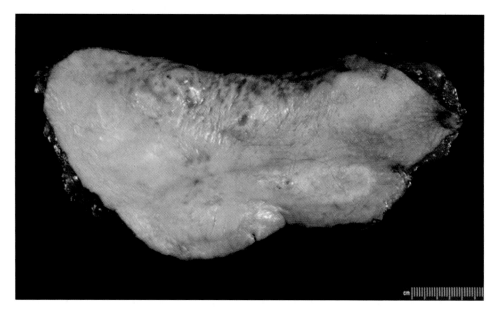

FIGURE 2c.1

Extramammary Paget disease. An eczematous plaque in the groin area is surrounded by normal skin. (Courtesy of Drs Anais Malpica and Michael Deavers, UT-MDACC.)

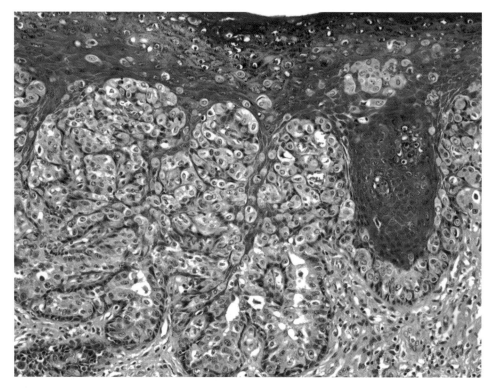

FIGURE 2c.2

Extramammary Paget disease. Neoplastic cells with abundant cytoplasm are arranged in confluent nests and as single cells throughout the epidermis.

MICROSCOPIC FINDINGS

Extramammary Paget disease shows nests and isolated large cells typically involving the epidermis and epithelium of related adnexal structures, predominantly with a basal and parabasal location (Figure 2c.2). There is preservation of the normal basal-layer keratinocytes which frequently become displaced downward or later-ally by the tumor cells (Figure 2c.3). Rarely, the tumor cells form glands within the epidermis. Paget cells have abundant pale cytoplasm with occasional intracytoplasmic vacuoles and large vesicular nuclei with prominent nucleoli. They only infrequently may contain melanin pigment (Figure 2c.4), due to melanin transfer from melanocytes to the Paget cells.

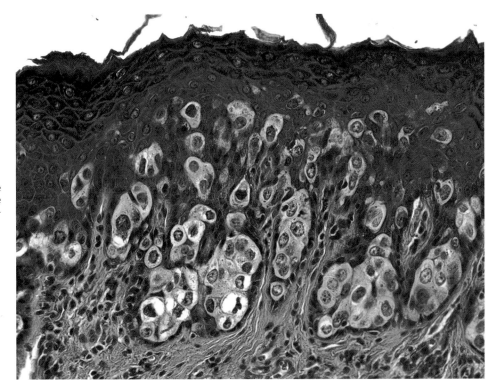

FIGURE 2c.3

Extramammary Paget disease. The clusters of Paget cells compress the basal keratinocytes against the basement membrane.

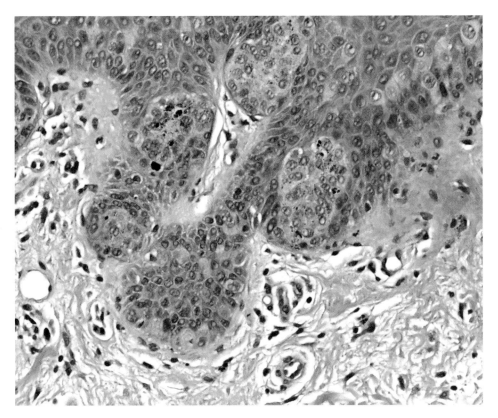

FIGURE 2c.4

Extramammary Paget disease. Paget cells show some intracytoplasmic melanin transferred by epidermal melanocytes.

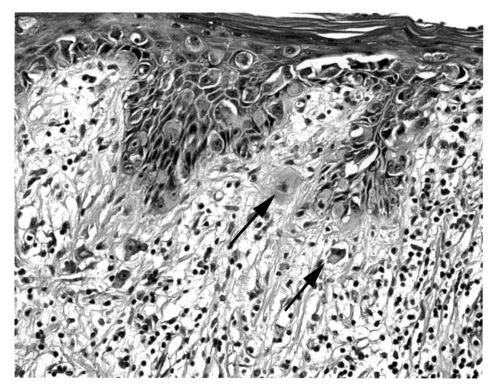

FIGURE 2c.5

Extramammary Paget disease. Single neoplastic cells (arrows) are infiltrating the superficial dermis (< 0.1 cm).

EMPD is associated with proliferative epidermal lesions in one-third of cases, including squamous hyperplasia not otherwise specified, fibroepithelioma-like hyperplasia, and papillomatous hyperplasia. Invasion is seen in < a third of cases, more commonly as single cells (Figure 2c.5) or small nests in the most upper dermal layer; overt invasion is uncommon.

ANCILLARY STUDIES

IMMUNOHISTOCHEMISTRY

Intracytoplasmic mucin (neutral and acidic) is found in the majority of tumor cells, and can be highlighted by special stains (Alcian blue, mucicarmine). Furthermore, there seems to be differential expression of mucin core proteins (MUC) between primary intraepidermal and invasive EMPD, as the former coexpresses MUC1 and MUC5 while invasive EMPD usually lacks MUC5 expression, both being MUC2-negative. EMPD secondary to rectal carcinoma is typically MUC2 positive with variable expression of MUC1 and MUC5. In difficult cases, immunoperoxidase studies are useful, as most EMPD cells express low-molecular-weight cytokeratin, CEA (Figure 2c.6a), epithelial membrane antigen (EMA) and gross cystic disease fluid protein 15 (GCDFP-15). CK7 (Figure 2c.6b), CK20, and GCDFP15 are helpful in the distinction between primary and secondary EMPD. The immunoprofile of primary EMPD shows CK7+/CK20−/GCDFP15+. EMPD secondary to urothelial carcinomas is CK7+/CK20+/GCDFP15− and uroplakin III+ whereas EMPD secondary to rectal carcinoma is typically CK7−/CK20+/GCDFP15−. S100 expression is usually negative in contrast to 25 % positivity in Paget disease of the breast. Androgen receptor (but not ER and PR) are detected in approximately 50 % of cases. Finally, immunohistochemistry may help determine the status of surgical margins and possible dermal invasion since it allows detection of isolated Paget cells and it may also be helpful in investigating and determining the possible cell of origin for cases of primary EMPD. Possible origins of EMPD include Bartholin glands and Toker cells. Bartholin glands are small apocrine-like structures located in the introitus. Toker cells are mononuclear cells that can be seen in multiple anatomic areas, including the vulva. These cells are large and arranged as single units at all levels of the epidermis. The fact that the immunophenotype of Toker cells, Bartholin glands cells, and EMPD is very similar (CK7, low-molecular-weight cytokeratin, MUC1, and MUC5AC-positive) would support the possible origin of EMPD from these two sites. Very recently, it has been hypothesized that EMPD may represent a proliferation of adnexal stem cells residing in the infundibulosebaceous unit of hair follicles and adnexal structures as the EMPD cells stain for markers typically seen in follicular stem cells located in the hair follicle bulge region, including CK15 and CK19.

DIFFERENTIAL DIAGNOSIS

In situ and invasive squamous cell carcinoma may show intraepidermal tumor cells distributed in a pagetoid pattern (so-called pagetoid Bowen disease). However, the atypical cells are usually present at all levels of the epidermis and, unlike EMPD, they also occupy the basal layer and contain keratohyaline granules within tumor

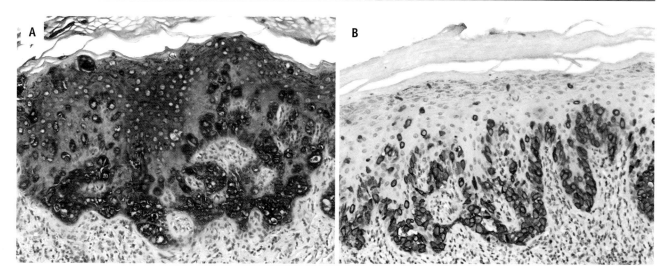

FIGURE 2c.6
Primary extramammary Paget disease. The neoplastic cells are positive for CEA (A) and CK7 (B).

cells. Of note, CK7 is not helpful in this differential diagnosis as it is positive in both entities. However, neoplastic squamous cells are GCDFP-15- and CEA-negative. *Melanoma* should also be considered in the differential diagnosis as both entities may have a pagetoid growth and melanin may be secondarily present in the cytoplasm of Paget cells. Thus, the presence of a melanocytic proliferation along the basal layer of the adjacent epidermis should therefore be sought in every case of putative EMPD. Immunohistochemistry can be useful; however, as EMPD cells may occasionally be S-100-positive, a panel of antibodies is recommended in problematic cases (e.g., cytokeratins, CEA, HMB-45, tyrosinase, MART-1). *Sebaceous carcinoma* typically shows involvement of the overlying epidermis in a pattern similar to EMPD. However, the cells exhibit multiple cytoplasmic vacuoles with the typical indentation of nuclei and, unlike Paget disease, the neoplastic cells lack CEA and GCDFP-15 expression. In addition, involvement of the perineum by sebaceous carcinoma is exceptional. Finally, *pagetoid dyskeratosis* is characterized by the presence of small papules in intertriginous areas. It is considered a reactive process in which a small part of the normal population of keratinocytes is induced to proliferate or develop dyskeratosis. These cells spread in the epidermis in a pagetoid manner and express low-molecular-weight cytokeratin (e.g., detected with CAM5.2). In contrast to EMPD, pagetoid dyskeratosis cells are small in size, display small pyknotic nuclei and are negative for CEA.

PROGNOSIS AND THERAPY

"Primary" EMPD is associated with an overall good prognosis; however, there is a relatively high recurrence rate even after wide local excision which can be explained by the presence of frequent microscopic

extension beyond the clinically involved area and the presence of multifocal disease; thus, status of resection margins is not predictive of local recurrence. Cases with more than minimally invasive disease (> 1 mm) are associated with a worse prognosis, and may result in nodal or distant metastases and secondary death. Chemotherapy and radiotherapy have been used in non-surgical cases, with diverse results. The prognosis of EMPD associated with an underlying carcinoma is poor, and related to the prognosis of that particular carcinoma.

MELANOCYTIC LESIONS

MUCOSAL LENTIGO (GENITAL "MELANOTIC" MACULE, VULVAR LENTIGO, GENITAL MELANOSIS)

Mucosal lentigo is a benign lesion defined as a pigmented patch on a mucous membrane. In the vulva, it typically presents as a large and asymmetric area of brown to blue-black hyperpigmentation with irregular borders which not infrequently can cause clinical concern for melanoma. On rare occasions, it may be associated with Carney's complex. Histologically, the epithelium displays hyperpigmentation of the basal keratinocytes predominantly involving the tips of the elongated rete (Figure 2c.7). Other associated findings include mild acanthosis, slightly increased number of melanocytes, and increased melanin pigment present within melanophages in the papillary dermis. However, in contrast to malignant melanoma, melanocytes are cytologically benign and they are arranged as evenly distributed single cells in the epidermis without pagetoid upward migration.

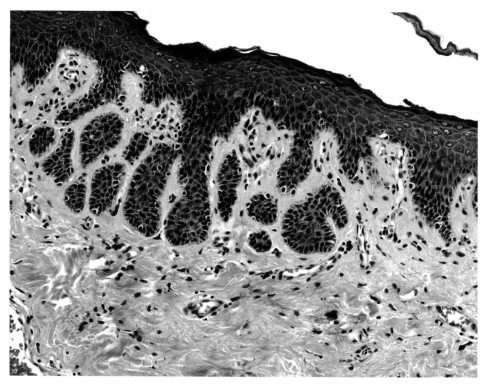

FIGURE 2c.7
Lentigo. Mild acanthosis with hyperpigmentation of keratinocytes is seen with no increase in number of melanocytes.

ATYPICAL MELANOCTIC NEVI OF THE GENITAL TYPE

Vulvar melanocytic nevi are uncommon and occur in approximately 2–3% of women. In the genital region, nevi often show clinical and histologic features somewhat different from those seen in other anatomic locations. As a group, some authors refer to melanocytic nevi occurring in the genital area, flexural sites (inguinal folds, scrotum, perineal area, and axilla) and acral regions as nevi of "special sites." It is important to recognize these types of nevi in order to avoid a misdiagnosis of dysplastic nevus or melanoma.

ATYPICAL MELANOCYTIC NEVI OF THE GENITAL TYPE – FACT SHEET

Definition
▶ Benign melanocytic neoplasm of the external female genitalia

Incidence and Location
▶ Relatively uncommon (3% of women)

Morbidity
▶ Rare malignant transformation

Clinical Features
▶ Usually asymptomatic
▶ Symmetrical, uniformly pigmented

Prognosis and Treatment
▶ Complete surgical excision

CLINICAL FEATURES

The lesions occur in young women (mean 25 years) and are typically asymptomatic. They are frequently discovered during routine gynecologic examination, at the time of delivery, or during pregnancy.

ATYPICAL MELANOCYTIC NEVI OF THE GENITAL TYPE – PATHOLOGIC FEATURES

Gross findings
▶ Small (usually < 1 cm)
▶ Well circumscribed
▶ Uniform coloration

Microscopic Findings
▶ Enlarged junctional nests, with variation in size and shape
▶ Junctional nests located at tips as well as at sides of rete tips
▶ Junctional nests with prominent retraction artifact
▶ Maturation of melanocytes in dermal nests
▶ Melanocytes with enlarged nuclei, prominent nucleoli, and abundant cytoplasm with fine melanin pigment (more common in junctional component)
▶ No mitotic activity or necrosis
▶ Fine delicate dermal fibrosis

Differential Diagnosis
▶ Lentigo
▶ Dysplastic nevus
▶ Melanoma
▶ Epithelioid histiocytoma

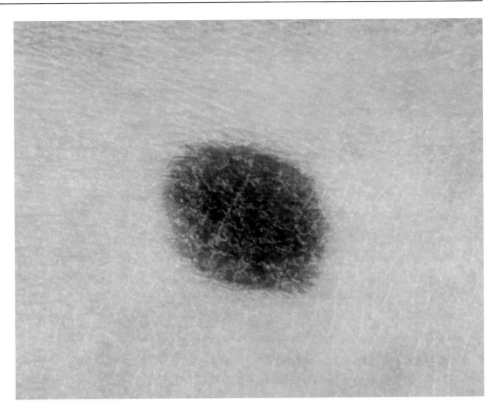

FIGURE 2c.8
Atypical melanocytic nevus of the genital type. A small, symmetrical macule shows brown pigmentation with only slight variation in color.

PATHOLOGIC FEATURES

GROSS FINDINGS

Most of the lesions are located in the labium majus or minus, and less commonly in the clitoral area. Most genital-type nevi are typically macular or papular symmetrical small lesions (usually < 1 cm) with well-defined margins (Figure 2c.8). They typically exhibit evenly distributed tan to brown pigment.

MICROSCOPIC FINDINGS

On low-power examination, genital nevi are relatively well circumscribed. Whereas most nevi show the morphologic appearance of common nevi outside the genital area (Figure 2c.9), a minority may have unusual morphologic features. Atypical features include striking enlargement of junctional melanocytic nests, and variation in size, shape, and location of the nests. The nests in the junctional component are located at the tips as well as at the sides of the rete tips (the latter feature not seen in typical nevi), and are associated with prominent retraction artifact (Figure 2c.10). The size of the junctional nests may vary from two or three cells to large clusters, with some nests being confluent ("bridging"). Reflecting the striking nested nature of the junctional component, pigment is arranged in columns in the stratum corneum; however, it is not associated with prominent pagetoid spread of single cells or nests of melanocytes. The dermal component usually has clusters of melanocytes in the papillary dermis showing maturation, whereby the cells become smaller and lose

melanin pigment the deeper they are in the dermis, as seen in common compound nevi (Figure 2c.11). The melanocytes are larger than those seen in common nevi; they display enlarged nuclei, prominent nucleoli, and abundant cytoplasm with fine melanin pigment – features more commonly seen in the junctional component. Mitotic figures and single cell necrosis are not present. The dermis may show a slight increase in collagen when compared with the adjacent dermis; however, this delicate fibrosis is different from the coarser lamellar/concentric or regression fibrosis seen in either dysplastic nevi or melanomas. Similar to dysplastic nevi, genital nevi may contain a lymphocytic infiltrate in the dermis. Therefore, as nevi arising in the genital region share histologic features with dysplastic nevi (bridging, fibrosis, and lymphocytic infiltrate), most authors agree that the threshold to diagnose a nevus as "dysplastic" in the genital region should be higher than in other regions of the skin (see below).

DIFFERENTIAL DIAGNOSIS

The main differential diagnosis includes dysplastic nevi and malignant melanoma. *Dysplastic nevi* have a prominent lentiginous growth pattern with regular rete ridge elongation, features that are lacking in genital nevi. *Malignant melanoma* has a peak incidence around the sixth decade, in contrast to genital-type nevi that typically occur in young women. Unlike most mucosal malignant melanomas, genital nevi are small and well circumscribed with uniform pigmentation and no necrosis or ulceration. Additionally there is a small

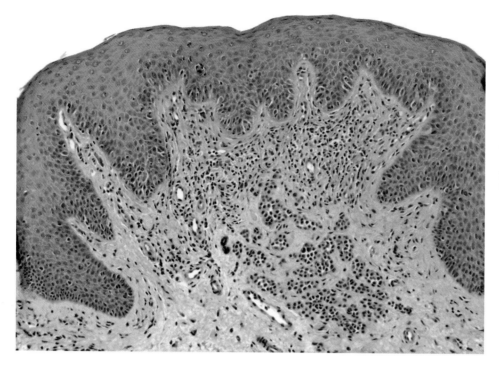

FIGURE 2c.9

Typical nevus in the genital area. Proliferation of small melanocytes is present, mainly in the papillary dermis.

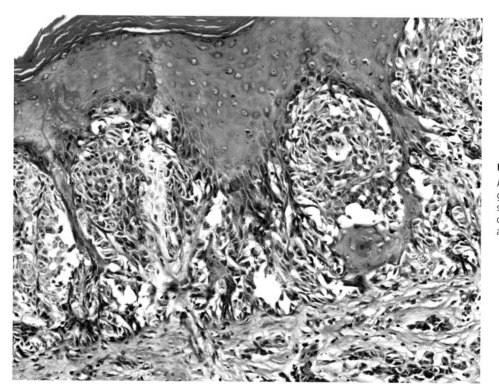

FIGURE 2c.10

Atypical melanocytic nevus of the genital type. Variable-sized and shaped nests of melanocytes at the dermoepidermal junction are associated with retraction artifact.

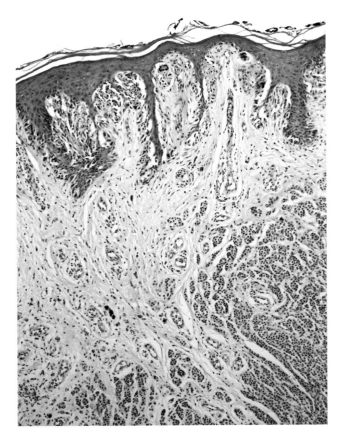

FIGURE 2c.11
Atypical melanocytic nevus of the genital type. Small nests of melanocytes in the dermis undergo maturation. There is delicate fibrosis in the upper dermis.

"shoulder" component, little or no pagetoid spread of melanocytes, larger melanin granules than the "dusty" melanin of the malignant melanoma, no single cell necrosis, and no mitotic activity in the dermal component. The finding of pagetoid spread, diffuse cytologic atypia associated with mitotic activity, and absence of cell maturation should strongly raise the suspicion for malignant melanoma. Finally, nevi arising in the context of genital dermatoses, particularly lichen sclerosus, may be histologically worrisome and cause concern for melanoma. Such lesions may have marked architectural atypia (single cells, irregular nests) secondary to the epithelial and dermal changes associated with the chronic nature of lichen sclerosus. Although melanomas associated with lichen sclerosus have been reported, it seems that most melanocytic lesions arising in this context are, in fact, common genital nevi. As a general rule, exercise caution before rendering a diagnosis of melanoma in vulvar skin of a young woman.

PROGNOSIS AND THERAPY

Complete excision is the treatment of choice as genital nevi may recur after incomplete excision. It is widely recommended that any incompletely excised pigmented lesion with atypical features should be completely excised to exclude the diagnosis of malignant melanoma and avoid recurrence. Finally, it has been shown that patients with genital nevi do not have an increased risk of dysplastic nevi at other sites.

DYSPLASTIC NEVI

These are defined as melanocytic neoplasms with atypical (dysplastic) features occurring in the female external genitalia.

CLINICAL FEATURES

Dysplastic nevi occur on the vulva of women of all ages. It is important to keep in mind that patients with dysplastic nevi have an increased risk of developing malignant melanoma, this risk being higher if there is a clinical history of melanoma in any first-degree relatives. In a large series, there was approximately one dysplastic nevus for every three common genital nevi. These lesions have irregular borders and asymmetrical pigmentation, and are usually larger than nondysplastic nevi (> 6 mm in diameter).

VULVAR DYSPLASTIC NEVI – FACT SHEET

Definition
▶ Neoplasm of melanocytes in the external female genitalia with atypical architectural and cytologic (dysplastic) features

Incidence
▶ Relatively rare (< 1% of women)

Morbidity
▶ Possibly increased risk of malignant transformation
▶ Higher risk of malignant melanoma if first-degree family history of melanoma

Clinical Features
▶ Usually asymptomatic
▶ Irregular borders
▶ Asymmetrical pigmentation, usually > 6 mm

Prognosis and Treatment
▶ Complete surgical excision to avoid recurrence

PATHOLOGIC FEATURES

GROSS FINDINGS

They appear as irregular, poorly circumscribed macules or papules with areas of hyper- and hypopigmentation.

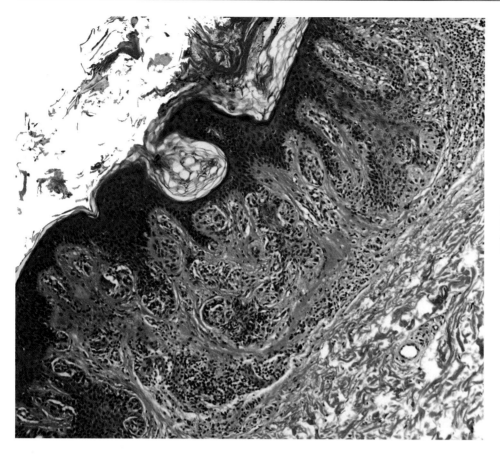

FIGURE 2c.12
Dysplastic nevus. Prominent fusion of rete ridges ("bridging") as well as lamellar fibrosis.

VULVAR DYSPLASTIC NEVI – PATHOLOGIC FEATURES

Gross Findings

▸ Irregular coloration and border

Microscopic Findings

▸ Asymmetric proliferation with prominent lentiginous growth
▸ Junctional component with irregular nests and single cells
▸ Intraepidermal "shoulder"
▸ Bridging of rete ridges
▸ Rare pagetoid migration limited to the center of lesion
▸ Dermal lamellar fibrosis
▸ Lymphocytic infiltrate
▸ Prominent vasculature in papillary dermis
▸ "Dusty" melanin in cytoplasm
▸ Cytologic atypia from mild to severe

Differential Diagnosis

▸ Melanoma
▸ Genital nevus
▸ Lentigo

MICROSCOPIC FINDINGS

On low-power examination, there is an asymmetric proliferation of melanocytes with a prominent lentiginous growth. The junctional (intraepidermal) component typically extends beyond three rete ridges from any dermal component ("shoulder"). The melanocytes appear either singly or form irregularly shaped and sized nests with prominent secondary fusion of the rete ridges ("bridging") (Figure 2c.12). Pagetoid migration may be seen, although it is limited to the central portion of the lesion. The dermal component usually shows small or large clusters of melanocytes in the papillary region associated with lamellar/concentric (eosinophilic) fibrosis, a lymphocytic infiltrate, and prominent vascularity of the papillary dermis (Figure 2c.12). Many melanocytes, particularly in the junctional component, display abundant cytoplasm with fine "dusty" melanin pigment and associated cytologic atypia which ranges from mild to severe based on: (1) nuclear size; (2) degree of hyperchromasia and pleomorphism; and (3) nucleolar prominence. Severely atypical melanocytes show nuclei at least twice the size of nuclei of spinous keratinocytes as well as irregular contours and prominent nucleoli.

DIFFERENTIAL DIAGNOSIS

Mucosal melanoma is the most important entity in the differential diagnosis, as it also shows irregular margins, areas of hyper- and hypopigmentation, as well as pagetoid spread of the melanocytes and cytologic atypia. However, in dysplastic nevi, the pagetoid spread of melanocytes is limited to the center of the lesion; and necrosis, ulceration, or dermal mitoses are exceptional. As a rule, due to morphologic overlap between dysplastic nevi and malignant melanoma, melanocytic lesions with cytologic atypia and prominent single cell growth should be completely excised.

Although there seem to be some overlapping features between *genital nevi* and dysplastic nevi, the diagnosis of dysplastic nevus in the genital region should be rendered when there is significant single cell growth in the epidermis (> 50 % of the lesion), extension beyond the dermal component, associated lamellar/concentric fibrosis, and dense lymphocytic infiltrate in the papillary dermis. Finally, the last entity that may be included in this differential diagnosis is *lentigo* as it appears clinically as a hyperpigmented lesion. However, by definition, lentigo only shows hyperpigmentation of the epidermis with minimal increase in numbers of single, nonatypical melanocytes, lacking well-formed melanocytic nests.

PROGNOSIS AND THERAPY

Dysplastic nevi may recur after incomplete excision. As at least 25 % of melanomas have an associated dysplastic nevus when examined histologically. Complete excision is recommended.

MALIGNANT MELANOMA

Malignant melanoma of the vulva is defined as a malignant melanocytic neoplasm arising in a sun-protected region and therefore not related to ultraviolet light. It is the second most common malignant neoplasm of the vulva following squamous cell carcinoma. The vulvar region is the most common site for malignant melanoma in the female genital tract. Approximately 3 % of all melanomas in women arise in the genital region with an overall world incidence of 0.26–0.52 cases per million, with 71 : 1 ratio skin to vulvar melanoma and an average calculated age-standardized incidence of approximately 0.10 per 100,000 females per year in the United States.

CLINICAL FEATURES

Patients typically present at an older age when compared to malignant melanoma arising in sun-exposed areas (sixth to seventh decades). Most vulvar malignant melanomas arise in the clitoris (31 %) and labia majora (27 %), followed by labia minora. The most common clinical presentation is that of a pigmented, flat, or polypoid (approximately 40 % for the latter) asymmetrical lesion (Figure 2c.13), followed by bleeding and itching, and 20 % of patients will have more than one lesion at presentation (satellite lesions). In contrast to cutaneous melanomas, which usually display pigmentation, up to 35 % of vulvar melanomas are amelanotic.

VULVAR MELANOMA – FACT SHEET

Definition

▸ Malignant melanocytic neoplasm arising on the external female genitalia, either hair-bearing skin or mucosa

Incidence and Location

▸ 0.10 per 100,000 females per year in US
▸ Second most common malignant vulvar neoplasm
▸ 3% of melanomas in women
▸ Most common location in the female genital tract
▸ More common in mucosal–epidermal junction (clitoris and labia majora)

Morbidity and Mortality

▸ Median survival of 41 months

Clinical Features

▸ Sixth or seventh decade
▸ Pigmented flat or polypoid asymmetrical lesion most common presentation, followed by bleeding and itching
▸ 35% amelanotic
▸ 20% satellite lesions

Prognosis and Treatment

▸ Worse prognosis than cutaneous melanoma
▸ Overall 27–60% survival rate
▸ 90% 5-year survival rate if < 1 mm in thickness
▸ Treatment of choice complete surgical excision with 2-cm free margins
▸ Tumor thickness and ulceration main prognostic factors
▸ Overall 60% recurrence rate
▸ Sentinel lymph node status may be indicated if tumor thickness of ≥ 1 mm

---

PATHOLOGIC FEATURES

GROSS FINDINGS

The lesions are typically asymmetrical, flat, or polypoid, with ill-defined borders that display irregular pigmentation and frequently exceed 6 mm in largest diameter.

MICROSCOPIC FINDINGS

Most vulvar melanomas are histologically similar to acral lentiginous melanomas (hence the term "mucosal-lentiginous" melanomas), while superficial spreading and nodular subtypes are less common and desmoplastic melanoma is exceedingly rare at this site. The intraepidermal component of the "mucosal-lentiginous" melanomas is characterized by a diffuse proliferation of large, epithelioid atypical melanocytes arranged in irregular nests and single cells along the basal layer of the epidermis (Figure 2c.14). Pagetoid upward migration is common (Figure 2c.15) and can be extensive. If the vulvar melanoma is of the nodular type it lacks a radial growth phase. The overlying epidermis may have normal

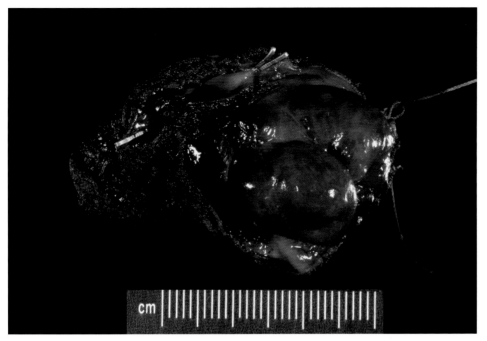

FIGURE 2c.13
Vulvar melanoma. A large polypoid tumor is focally pigmented. (Courtesy of Dr. Jinsong Liu, UT-MDACC.)

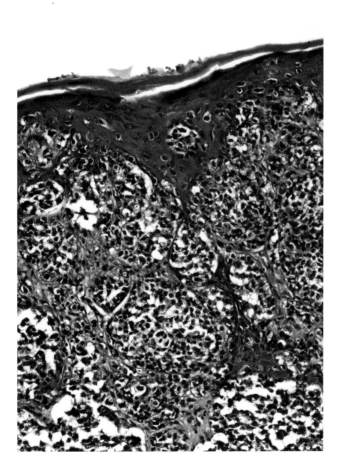

FIGURE 2c.14
Vulvar melanoma. A striking proliferation of large, epithelioid atypical melanocytes arranged in irregular nests is present along the basal layer of the epidermis.

VULVAR MELANOMA – PATHOLOGIC FEATURES

Gross Findings
▸ Flat or polypoid and asymmetrical
▸ Ill-defined borders
▸ Irregular pigmentation
▸ Usually > 6 mm in diameter

Microscopic Findings
▸ Acral-lentiginous pattern most common
▸ Prominent pagetoid migration
▸ Nests or single epithelioid cells in the intraepidermal component
▸ Fascicular growth of the invasive dermal component
▸ Absence of "cell" maturation
▸ Frequent marked cytologic atypia
▸ Common extension to adnexa and nerves
▸ Regression and vascular invasion

Immunohistochemical Features
▸ S-100, HMB-45, MART1 (Melan A) typically positive

Differential Diagnosis
▸ Dysplastic genital nevi
▸ Squamous cell carcinoma, including squamous cell carcinoma in situ
▸ Extramammary Paget disease

---

thickness or be acanthotic and ulceration is a common finding. The dermal component is similar to that seen in acral lentiginous melanoma and it is characterized by a proliferation of spindle-shaped cells forming fascicles as well as nests of cells and single cells. Epithelioid cells can also be seen. The tumor cells have a tendency to track along nerves and adnexal structures. In the intraepidermal component the tumor cells have abundant eosinophilic cytoplasm, enlarged round nuclei, and

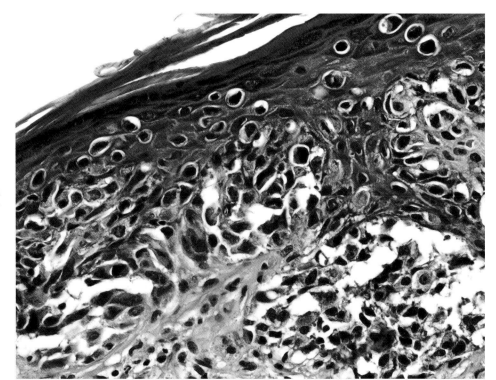

FIGURE 2c.15

Vulvar melanoma. The highly atypical tumor cells show a prominent pagetoid growth.

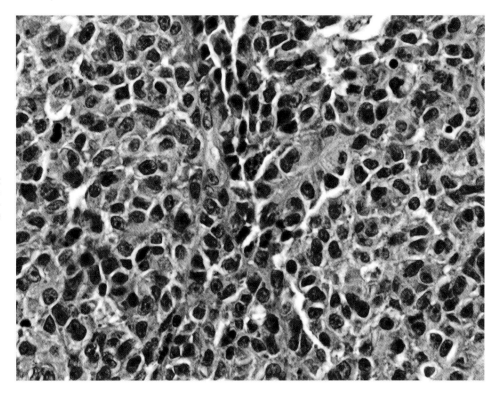

FIGURE 2c.16

Vulvar melanoma. The neoplastic cells have enlarged nuclei with prominent nuclei and abundant eosinophilic cytoplasm. Notice the presence of pigment in scattered cells.

prominent nucleoli, while in the invasive component the cells have less abundant cytoplasm and fusiform nuclei with no maturation. Both components frequently display marked cytologic atypia associated with variable mitotic activity (Figure 2c.16). The dermis usually shows a myxoid or desmoplastic response to the invasive tumor. Regression and vascular invasion are more common than in cutaneous melanoma.

When evaluating vulvar melanomas, it is recommended to report the same histologic features as done for cutaneous melanomas, including histologic subtype, Clark anatomic level (if occurring in skin), tumor thickness (Breslow), ulceration, radial and vertical growth phases, precursor lesion if present, margins, mitotic rate, tumor infiltrating lymphocytes, vascular or perineural invasion, regression, and microsatellite lesions.

DIFFERENTIAL DIAGNOSIS

Malignant melanoma should be distinguished from *dysplastic melanocytic nevus* (already discussed), squamous cell carcinoma, including carcinoma in situ, and EMPD. *Poorly differentiated squamous cell carcinoma* may show overlapping histologic features with an invasive malignant melanoma, especially in biopsy specimens, as both share epithelioid and spindle-shaped morphologies. Furthermore, 5% of *squamous cell carcinomas in situ* have a nested growth with pagetoid spread simulating melanoma in situ or the intraepidermal growth of invasive melanoma. Extensive sampling when possible will help in identifying typical areas of squamous cell carcinoma or malignant melanoma. Moreover, squamous cell carcinomas are positive for keratin but negative for HBM-45 and Melan-A. *EMPD* may also show overlapping histologic features with in situ malignant melanoma, including striking pagetoid growth, prominent "junctional" distribution of malignant cells with nests of cells and single cells, and the finding of intracytoplasmic melanin. In contrast to malignant melanoma, most cells of EMPD have abundant mucin, some of the cells may have intracytoplasmic vacuoles, and the nests of cells may show poorly formed central lumens. Histochemical and immunohistochemical stains are also helpful in this differential diagnosis, as Paget cells are positive for mucicarmin, Alcian Blue, low-molecular-weight cytokeratin, CEA, EMA, and GCDFP-15, whereas they are negative for Melan-A and HMB-45.

PROGNOSIS AND THERAPY

The overall survival rates for patients with vulvar melanoma range from 27% to 60%, with a median survival rate of 41 months, and survival is typically worse than other melanomas. However, the 5-year survival for patients with melanomas invading < 1 mm and with negative lymph nodes is 90%. The main histologic prognostic factors in vulvar melanomas are tumor thickness (Breslow's) measured from the top of the granular layer or from the base of the ulcerated tumor to the deepest point of invasion accompanied by Clark levels in hair-bearing skin and ulceration. The importance of ulceration is reflected in the current American Joint Commission on Cancer staging system, indicating that the presence of ulceration upstages the disease. As the extent of the surgical excision (vulvectomy versus wide local resection) does not seem to impact survival, the treatment of choice is complete surgical excision with 2-cm free margins. Overall, there is a high recurrence rate despite complete surgical resection (approximately 60%). Inguinal node metastases are commonly detected ipsilaterally (15%) but may also be bilateral (7%) and there is controversy regarding the advantage of elective lymph node dissection in these patients. However, as nodal metastases are associated with high mortality, sentinel lymph node status in patients with vulvar melanomas may be useful to stratify patients at risk, may become an important prognostic factor, and is usually indicated for melanomas with a thickness of ≥ 1 mm. The analysis requires specialized methodology, includ-

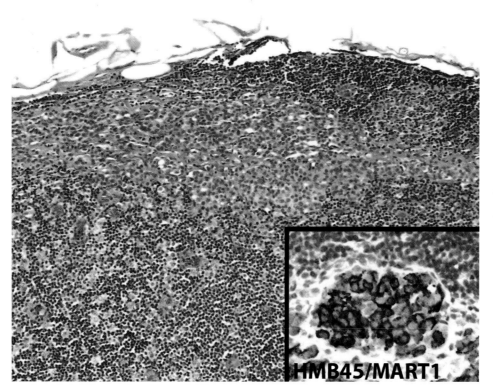

FIGURE 2c.17

Metastatic vulvar melanoma to sentinel lymph node. A small subcapsular deposit of metastatic melanoma is highlighted by HMB-45 and anti-MART1 staining cocktail.

ing serial sectioning of the node, routine histologic evaluation, and, in apparently negative cases, subsequent immunohistochemical analysis (e.g., with an antimelanocytic cocktail: HMB-45 and anti-MART1) (Figure 2c.17). Although the prognostic significance of isolated melanoma cells in the sentinel lymph nodes is unclear at present, their presence should be reported and may be used for staging.

SUGGESTED READING

Paget Disease

Bacchi CE, Goldfogel GA, Greer BE, et al. Paget's disease and melanoma of the vulva. Use of a panel of monoclonal antibodies to identify cell type and to microscopically define adequacy of surgical margins. Gynecol Oncol 1992;46:216–221.

Brainard JA, Hart WR. Proliferative epidermal lesions associated with anogenital Paget's disease. Am J Surg Pathol 2000;24:543–552.

Brown HM, Wilkinson EJ. Uroplakin-III to distinguish primary vulvar Paget disease from Paget disease secondary to urothelial carcinoma. Hum Pathol 2002;33:545–548.

Crawford D, Nimmo M, Clement PB, et al. Prognostic factors in Paget's disease of the vulva: a study of 21 cases. Int J Gynecol Pathol 1999;18:351–359.

Diaz de Leon E, Carcangiu ML, Prieto VG, et al. Extramammary Paget disease is characterized by the consistent lack of estrogen and progesterone receptors but frequently expresses androgen receptor. Am J Clin Pathol 2000;113:572–575.

Kuan SF, Montag AG, Hart J, et al. Differential expression of mucin genes in mammary and extramammary Paget's disease. Am J Surg Pathol 2001;25:1469–1477.

Pandolfino TL, Cotell S, Katta R. Pigmented vulvar macules as a presenting feature of the Carney complex. Int J Dermatol 2001;40:728–730.

Raju RR, Goldblum JR, Hart WR. Pagetoid squamous cell carcinoma in situ (pagetoid Bowen's disease) of the external genitalia. Int J Gynecol Pathol 2003;22:127–135.

Regauer S. Extramammary Paget's disease – a proliferation of adnexal origin? Histopathology 2006;48:723–729.

Willman JH, Golitz LE, Fitzpatrick JE. Vulvar clear cells of Toker: precursors of extramammary Paget's disease. Am J Dermatopathol 2005;27:185–188.

Yoshii N, Kitajima S, Yonezawa S, et al. Expression of mucin core proteins in extramammary Paget's disease. Pathol Int 2002;52:390–399.

Genital Nevi

Blickstein IE, Feldberg E, Dgani R, et al. Dysplastic vulvar nevi. Obstet Gynecol 1991;78:968–970.

Carlson JA, Mu XC, Slominski A, et al. Melanocytic proliferations associated with lichen sclerosus. Arch Dermatol 2002;138:77–87.

Clark WH Jr, Hood AF, Tucker MA, et al. Atypical melanocytic nevi of the genital type with a discussion of reciprocal parenchymal–stromal interactions in the biology of neoplasia. Hum Pathol 1998;29:S1–24.

Gleason BC, Hirsch MS, Nucci MR, et al. Atypical genital nevi. A clinicopathologic analysis of 56 cases. Am J Surg Pathol 2008;32:51–57.

Vulvar Melanoma

Cohen Y, Rosenbaum E, Begum S, et al. Exon 15 BRAF mutations are uncommon in melanomas arising in nonsun-exposed sites. Clin Cancer Res 2004;10:3444–3447.

Hassanein AM, Mrstik ME, Hardt NS, et al. Malignant melanoma associated with lichen sclerosus in the vulva of a 10-year-old. Pediatr Dermatol 2004;21:473–476.

Jiveskog S, Ragnarsson-Olding B, Platz A, et al. N-ras mutations are common in melanomas from sun-exposed skin of humans but rare in mucosal membranes or unexposed skin. J Invest Dermatol 1998;111:757–761.

Prieto VG, Clark SH. Processing of sentinel lymph nodes for detection of metastatic melanoma. Ann Diagn Pathol 2002;6:257–264.

Ragnarsson-Olding BK. Primary malignant melanoma of the vulva – an aggressive tumor for modeling the genesis of non-UV light-associated melanomas. Acta Oncol 2004;43:421–435.

Ragnarsson-Olding BK, Nilsson BR, Kanter-Lewensohn LR, et al. Malignant melanoma of the vulva in a nationwide, 25-year study of 219 Swedish females: predictors of survival. Cancer 1999;86:1285–1293.

Raspagliesi F, Ditto A, Paladini D, et al. Prognostic indicators in melanoma of the vulva. Ann Surg Oncol 2000;7:738–742.

Verschaegen CF, Benjapibal M. Supakarapongkul W, et al. Vulvar melanoma at the M. D Anderson Cancer Center: 25 years later. Int J Gynecol Cancer 2001;11:359–364.

Wechter ME, Gruber SB, Haefner HK, et al. Vulvar melanoma: A report of 20 cases and review of the literature. J Am Acad Dermatol 2004;50:554–562.

3

Benign Diseases of the Vagina
Anais Malpica

CONGENITAL ANOMALIES

VAGINAL AGENESIS AND ATRESIA

Complete agenesis of the vagina is rare, affecting 1 in 4000–5000 female births. In its isolated form, it is the result of incomplete caudal development and fusion of the lower portion of the müllerian ducts (müllerian dysgenesis). In these cases, the external genitalia appear normal, the uterus is present but affected by complications secondary to retrograde menstruation, and at the level of the introitus, a small blind pouch may be present. In contrast, vaginal agenesis associated with the absence of the uterus and with other skeletal and somatic anomalies (Mayer–Rokitansky–Küster–Hauser syndrome) is the result of müllerian agenesis. These patients have a normal 46XX karyotype, normal external genitalia, functional ovaries, and absence or severe hypoplasia of the upper two-thirds of the vagina, as well as frequent uterine agenesis. Due to a different embryonic origin, the lower third of the vagina is always present. Two subtypes of the Mayer–Rokitansky–Küster–Hauser syndrome have been described: (1) the typical form, in which only the caudal part of the müllerian duct is affected (upper vagina and uterus, which appear as symmetric muscular buds with normal fallopian tubes); and (2) the atypical form, in which there is asymmetric hypoplasia of one or both müllerian buds (with or without development abnormalities of the fallopian tubes), common association with somatic (mainly kidney defects), skeletal (mostly cervicothoracic), and to a minor extent hearing abnormalities. Vaginal atresia may also be seen as part of the Winter syndrome, characterized by renal agenesis and deafness, and the Vater syndrome, associated with renal and skeletal malformations, single umbilical artery, anal atresia, tracheoesophageal fistula, and cardiac defects. Treatment consists of creation of a neovagina through progressive use of vaginal dilators or surgery.

IMPERFORATE HYMEN

Although it represents the most common obstructive anomaly of the female genital tract, this congenital disorder is rare, with an estimated frequency of 0.1% in female newborns.

CLINICAL FEATURES

Patients diagnosed before 4 years of age are usually asymptomatic and the diagnosis is made incidentally, whereas those diagnosed after age 10 are usually symptomatic and present with abdominal or back pain, constipation, peritonitis, primary amenorrhea, or urinary symptoms (i.e., dysuria or urinary retention).

PATHOLOGIC FEATURES

GROSS FINDINGS

The hymenal membrane appears as homogeneous white elastic tissue with variable vascularity.

MICROSCOPIC FINDINGS

The hymen consists of connective tissue covered by stratified squamous epithelium.

PROGNOSIS AND THERAPY

Imperforate hymen has been traditionally treated with a stellate or cruciate incision through the hymenal membrane. More recently, the intravaginal use of a Foley catheter for 2 weeks after puncture of the hymen with a sterile injector needle has been advocated to preserve the normal architecture of the hymen.

INFECTIOUS VAGINITIS

BACTERIAL VAGINOSIS

This is the most common cause of acute vaginitis, representing 15–50% of all symptomatic cases. It is the result of a shift in the vaginal flora from lactobacilli-dominant to mixed flora, including genital *Mycoplasma*, *Gardnerella vaginalis*, and anaerobes (i.e., peptostreptococci, *Prevotella*, and *Mobiluncus* species).

CLINICAL FEATURES

Bacterial vaginosis is a clinical diagnosis that requires at least three of the following features: (1) vaginal pH > 4.5; (2) thin, watery, fishy-smelling discharge; (3) wet mount showing > 20% clue cells, and (4) positive "amine" odor test (performed by adding 10% potassium hydroxide to a drop of vaginal discharge on a slide and smelling the distinctive odor that results from released volatilized amines). Risk factors for bacterial vaginosis include: black ethnicity, cigarette smoking, use of intrauterine device, oral sex, new or multiple sexual partners, having a female sexual partner, frequent douching, sexual activity during menses, and lack of hydrogen peroxide-producing lactobacilli.

PATHOLOGIC FEATURES

MICROSCOPIC FINDINGS

No specific histopathologic changes have been described. Wet mount shows > 20% clue cells (i.e., squamous cells with numerous adherent coccobacilli) and an altered background vaginal flora with numerous cocci, bacteria of different shapes, and few, if any, lactobacilli. Clue cells can also be detected on Papanicolaou (Pap) smears (Figure 3.1).

PROGNOSIS AND THERAPY

Bacterial vaginosis is treated with a 7-day course of oral metronidazole, a 5-day course of vaginal metronidazole gel, or a 7-day course of vaginal clindamycin cream. This infection is associated with an increased risk of upper genital tract infections (i.e., endometritis after cesarean section, vaginal delivery, or abortion), wound infection, infection after hysterectomy, pelvic inflammatory disease, preterm delivery, chorioamnionitis, spontaneous abortion, and decreased success with in vitro fertilization.

CANDIDA INFECTION

Only 15–30% of acute vaginitis are caused by *Candida*, mainly *C. albicans*, a commensal organism in many asymptomatic women.

CLINICAL FEATURES

Vaginal candidiasis is characterized by white, thick vaginal discharge accompanied by pruritus and a burning sensation. Dysuria may be present. Risk factors include pregnancy, being in the luteal phase of the menstrual cycle, nulliparity, use of spermicides, young age (15–19 years), and recent therapy with broad-spectrum antibiotics.

BACTERIAL VAGINOSIS – FACT SHEET

Definition
▶ A clinical diagnosis requiring at least three of the following features:
  ▶ Vaginal pH > 4.5
  ▶ Thin, watery, fishy-smelling discharge
  ▶ Wet mount showing > 20% clue cells
  ▶ Positive "amine" odor test

Clinical Features
▶ Most common cause of vaginitis
▶ Thin, watery, fishy-smelling discharge

Prognosis and Treatment
▶ 7 days of oral metronidazole, 5 days of vaginal metronidazole gel, or 7 days of vaginal clindamycin cream

Morbidity
▶ Increased risk of upper genital tract infections

BACTERIAL VAGINOSIS – PATHOLOGIC FEATURES

Microscopic Findings
▶ No specific histopathologic changes
▶ Clue cells (i.e., squamous cells with numerous adherent coccobacilli) on wet mount or Papanicolaou (Pap) smear
▶ Altered vaginal flora with numerous cocci, bacteria of different shapes and a few, if any, lactobacilli on wet mount

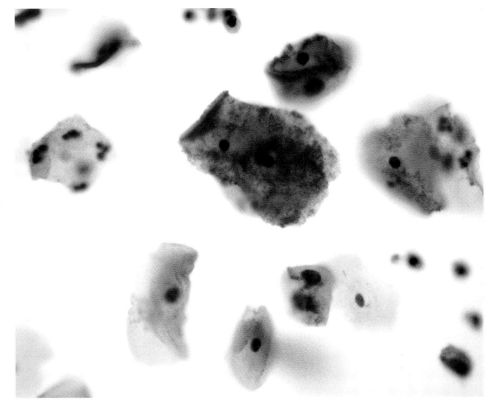

FIGURE 3.1
Bacterial vaginosis. Clue cells are present in a vaginal Pap smear.

CANDIDA VAGINITIS – FACT SHEET

Clinical Features

▶ Represents up to 30% of acute vaginitis
▶ White, thick vaginal discharge
▶ Pruritus and burning sensation

Prognosis and Treatment

▶ If uncomplicated, single dose of oral fluconazole or topical antifungal agents
▶ If complicated (immunosuppressed patients), tailored treatment

---

CANDIDA VAGINITIS – PATHOLOGIC FEATURES

Gross Findings

▶ Mucosal erythema

Microscopic Findings

▶ Marked inflammation and reactive changes of squamous epithelium
▶ Hyphae or spores identified in the epithelial surface or within detached squamous cells in potassium hydroxide wet mount or Pap smear

---

PATHOLOGIC FEATURES

GROSS FINDINGS

The vaginal mucosa frequently appears erythematous.

MICROSCOPIC FINDINGS AND ANCILLARY STUDIES

Hyphae or spores are visible on a potassium hydroxide wet mount or Pap smear (Figure 3.2). Tissue sections show marked acute inflammation, reactive changes in the squamous epithelium, and fungal forms within the superficial layers of the squamous epithelium or within the detached squamous cells. A vaginal culture is also useful if a wet mount is negative.

PROGNOSIS AND THERAPY

Uncomplicated vaginal candidiasis (defined as three or fewer episodes per year) with mild to moderate symptoms, most likely caused by *C. albicans*, and occurring in an immunocompetent host, is treated with a single dose of oral fluconazole or a variety of topical antifungal agents, typically for 1 to 3 days. In complicated cases (i.e., pregnant patients, immunocompromised or debilitated patients or those who have uncontrolled diabetes, severe symptoms, infections by other species other than *C. albicans*, or four or more episodes in 1 year), treatment is tailored accordingly.

TRICHOMONAS VAGINALIS

This intracellular parasite is responsible for the most common sexually transmitted disease in the United States. It is the cause of acute vaginitis in 5–50% of patients, depending on the population studied.

CLINICAL FEATURES

Symptoms associated with *Trichomonas vaginalis* infection include yellow vaginal discharge, malodor, pruritus, and dysuria. On colposcopic examination, the vaginal mucosa shows erythema with variable punctate hemorrhages.

PATHOLOGIC FEATURES

MICROSCOPIC FINDINGS

The diagnosis is made by identifying pear-shaped cyanophilic organisms, 10–20 μm in diameter, showing polar flagellae in a saline preparation. *Trichomonas* can also be detected on a Pap smear, where they are also pear-shaped and show a "lancet"-shaped nucleus and red cytoplasmic granules (Figure 3.3). The vaginal squamous epithelium is usually spongiotic with numerous neutrophils that can form intraepithelial abscesses.

TRICHOMONAS VAGINALIS – FACT SHEET

Clinical Features
▸ 5–50% of acute vaginitis
▸ Most common sexually transmitted disease in US
▸ Yellow vaginal discharge, malodor, pruritus, and dysuria

Treatment
▸ Oral nitroimidazole or tinidazole
▸ Treatment of patient's partner

TRICHOMONAS VAGINALIS – PATHOLOGIC FEATURES

Gross Findings
▸ Mucosal erythema and variable punctate hemorrhage

Microscopic Findings
▸ Spongiotic squamous epithelium with numerous neutrophils that may form intraepithelial abscesses

Ancillary Techniques
▸ *Trichomonas* can be identified in a saline preparation or in a Pap smear (pear-shaped cells with "lancet"-shaped nucleus and red intracytoplasmic granules)

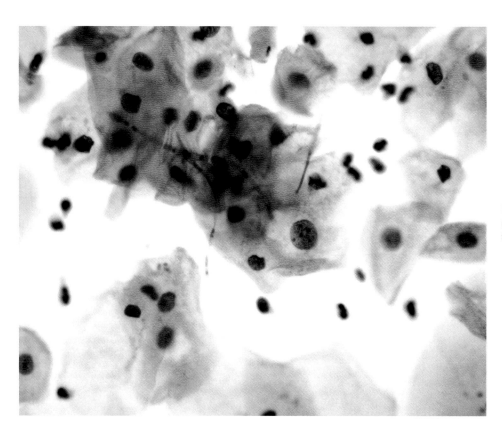

FIGURE 3.2
Candida infection. Hyphal forms are seen on a Pap smear.

ANCILLARY STUDIES

A test for *T. vaginalis* antigen can be rapidly performed (10 minutes). It has a sensitivity and specificity of 83% and 98.8% respectively.

THERAPY

Oral nitroimidazole or tinidazole is the treatment of choice. Treatment of the patient's partner increases cure rates.

GROUP B STREPTOCOCCUS

Approximately 25% of women are carriers of this organism. In asymptomatic patients, vaginal group B streptococcus does not require treatment. Patients with symptoms and a positive culture should be treated with antibiotics. When it is detected during pregnancy, the patient should be treated, as group B streptococcus is a common cause of sepsis and meningitis in newborns.

ACTINOMYCOSIS

This is a Gram-positive, non-acid-fast anaerobic bacterium, found in up to 27% of asymptomatic women without an intrauterine device. However, symptomatic cases tend to be seen in patients with vaginal foreign bodies such as an intrauterine device or permanent

---

ACTINOMYCOSIS – FACT SHEET

Clinical Features

▸ Postcoital bleeding, malodorous vaginal discharge, and pruritus
▸ Abdominal/pelvic pain due to abscess formation
▸ If symptomatic, vaginal foreign bodies (permanent suture material or intrauterine devices) usually present

Prognosis and Treatment

▸ Removal of foreign body and penicillin

ACTINOMYCOSIS – PATHOLOGIC FEATURES

Microscopic Findings

▸ *Actinomyces* detected as tangled filaments, "sulfur granules," within a background of neutrophils

---

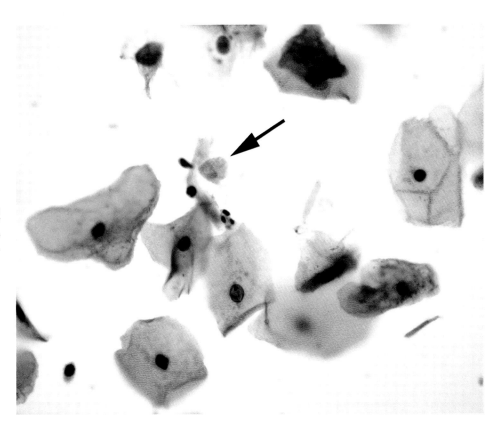

FIGURE 3.3
Trichomonas vaginalis infection. An organism showing a "lancet-shaped" nucleus and fine cytoplasmic granules is seen (arrow) on a Pap smear.

suture material. Symptoms related to *Actinomyces* infection include postcoital bleeding, malodorous vaginal discharge, pruritus, or abdominopelvic pain due to abscess formation. Microscopically, these bacteria are seen as tangled filaments or "sulfur granules" within a background of neutrophils. Treatment involves removal of the foreign body and use of penicillin.

TOXIC SHOCK SYNDROME (TSS)

This systemic disease is characterized by acute onset of fever, myalgia, headache, confusion, hypotension, rash followed by desquamation of hands and feet, and multiple organ failure. When initially described, TSS was primarily associated with menstruation and tampon usage. Currently, the incidence of menstrual TSS has decreased significantly due to multiple factors, including increased public awareness, changes in tampon usage and composition, and withdrawal of superabsorbent tampons from the market. Menstrual TSS is caused by *Staphylococcus aureus*, whereas both *S. aureus* and *Streptococcus pyogenes* may be implicated in the nonmenstrual TSS (i.e., TSS seen in postpartum, following surgical procedure, or skin, bone, or respiratory infections). Four factors appear to be required for the development of menstrual TSS: (1) vaginal colonization with a toxigenic strain of *Staphylococcus aureus*; (2) production of toxic shock syndrome toxin-1 (TSST-1); (3) penetration of sufficient concentrations of TSST-1 across the epithelium; and (4) absence or insufficient titers of neutralizing antibodies.

Microscopically, fresh ulcerations with Gram-positive cocci are present on the surface, and are associated

with phlebitis. In other organs, phlebitis is also identified in addition to edema, necrotizing capillaritis, and inflammation. Treatment includes use of beta-lactamase-resistant antistaphylococcal antibiotics and supportive measures for shock-related manifestations.

PARASITIC VAGINITIS

These infections are very rare in the United States. Vaginal amebiasis is caused by *Entamoeba histolytica* and seen in countries where this infection is endemic. Patients usually present with bloody vaginal discharge and ulcerated and friable lesions. Microscopically, the ulcerated areas show a fibrinopurulent exudate containing trophozoites measuring 15–60 µm in diameter that stain with PAS stain. Trophozoites can also be identified on wet smears from vaginal discharge. Metronidazole is the treatment of choice.

Schistosoma mansoni and *haematobium* can be found in the vagina. The most common symptoms are vaginal discharge, pruritus, and dyspareunia. Gross lesions include polyps, ulcers, or a granular appearance of the mucosa. Microscopically, viable or nonviable eggs are usually seen in the submucosa and are associated with a prominent inflammatory response, including eosinophils, that ultimately results in marked fibrosis (Figure 3.4). Multiple doses of praziquantel are required to treat this infection. Eggs and worms of *Enterobius vermicularis* have also been found in the vagina, where they elicit a granulomatous reaction associated with central necrosis (Figure 3.5). Finally, eggs of *Trichuris trichiura* can be seen in the vagina as contamination in cases of intestinal infestation.

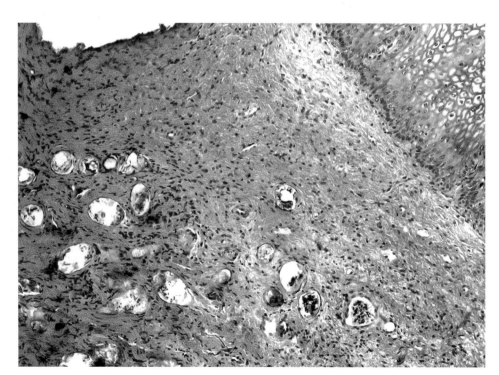

FIGURE 3.4

Schistosomiasis. Viable and nonviable eggs are surrounded by fibrosis in the vaginal submucosa.

VIRAL INFECTIONS

The vagina can be involved as part of a genital herpes simplex infection. Usually, the causative agent is herpes simplex virus type 2 (HSV-2) and, less frequently, HSV-1. "Classic" outbreaks of this infection begin with a prodrome lasting 2–24 hours that includes regional pain or a burning sensation. In addition, patients may have fever, headache, malaise, lymphadenopathy, and anorexia. Subsequently, papules, vesicles, and erosions/ulcers appear over hours to days. The vesicles are usually asymptomatic, whereas the ulcers are very painful. In addition to the vagina, the ulcers can involve the vulva, cervix, bladder, urethra, and anus. Some patients can have intermittent bleeding and vaginal discharge. Microscopically, the vesicles involve the entire squamous epithelium. The infected cells contain one or more nuclei

with "ground-glass" chromatin, and may or may not have intranuclear inclusions (Figure 3.6). Primary lesions last 2–6 weeks, tend to be very painful, and contain large quantities of infectious HSV particles. Recurrent HSV episodes are usually milder than the initial episode, typically with fewer lesions, and viral shedding occurs at a lower concentration and with shorter duration. The diagnosis is based on the identification of the epithelial/nuclear changes described above either on a cytology preparation of the scraping of the base and edges of a fresh ulcer (Tzanck preparation) or in tissue sections. In the latter, the characteristic viral cytopathic changes are more commonly identified at the edge of the lesion. In situ hybridization for HSV can be used to confirm the diagnosis (Figure 3.7). Other diagnostic tools include viral culture and polymerase chain reaction. Acyclovir and related compounds such as valacyclovir and famciclovir are used in the treatment of this infection.

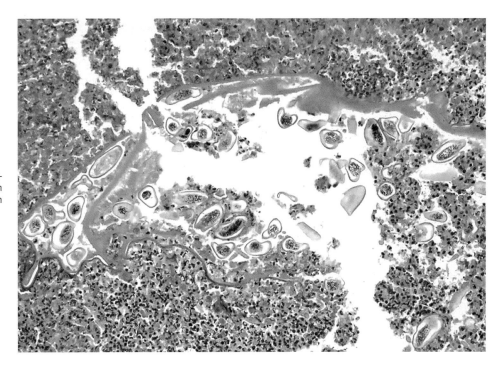

FIGURE 3.5

Enterobiasis. Multiple eggs of *Enterobius vermicularis* are associated with necrosis and acute inflammation (Courtesy of Dr. RC Neafie).

VIRAL INFECTIONS – FACT SHEET

Clinical Features

▶ Herpes simplex virus type 2, and, less frequently, type 1
  ▶ Pain or burning sensation, vaginal discharge, or intermittent vaginal bleeding
  ▶ Fever, malaise, lymphadenopathy, and anorexia may be seen
▶ Cytomegalovirus-associated ulcers may be painful in HIV-positive patients

Prognosis and Treatment

▶ Acyclovir and related compounds for herpes
▶ Topical or systemic steroids for aphthous ulcers in AIDS patients

---

VIRAL INFECTIONS – PATHOLOGIC FEATURES

Gross Findings

▶ Papules, vesicles, and erosions/ulcers in herpesvirus infection
▶ Ulcers in cytomegalovirus (CMV) infection in HIV-positive patients

Microscopic Findings

▶ Vesicles involving the entire epithelium
▶ Infected cells display:
  ▶ One enlarged nucleus (CMV)
  ▶ Bi- or multinucleation (Herpes)
  ▶ Ground-glass chromatin (Herpes)
  ▶ Intranuclear inclusions (Both)
  ▶ Intracytoplasmic inclusions (CMV)

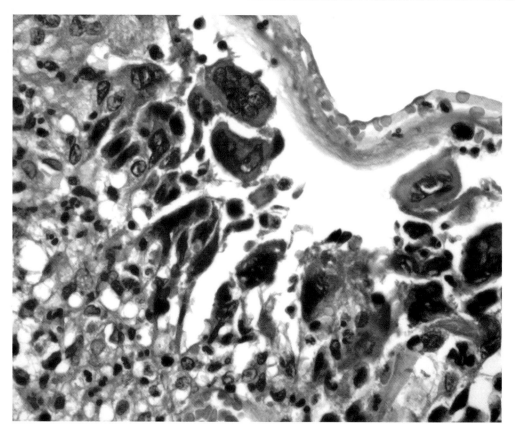

FIGURE 3.6
Herpesvirus. Infected squamous cells show multinucleation, nuclei with ground-glass chromatin, and intranuclear inclusions.

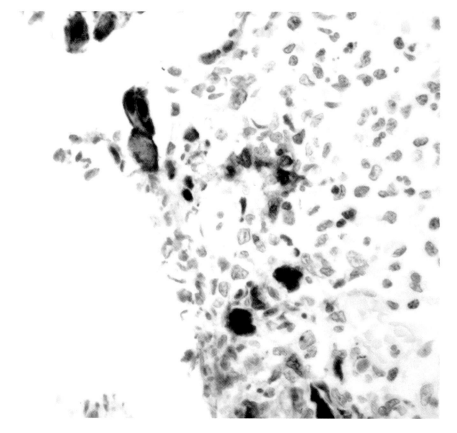

FIGURE 3.7
Herpesvirus. In situ hybridization highlights the infected cells.

Cytomegalovirus infection produces vaginal ulcers in addition to ulcers involving the cervix and vulva in human immunodeficiency virus (HIV)-positive patients. Women markedly immunosuppressed secondary to HIV infection can develop aphthous genital ulcers. Such ulcers, either single or multiple, may be confined to the lower genital tract or coexist with oroesophageal ulcers. They are painful, range in size from 1 to 6 cm, are often deep, and occasionally progress to form fistulas. The infected cells (epithelial and endothelial) are enlarged and contain intranuclear and intracytoplasmic inclusions. Peripheral clearing of the chromatin imparts an "owls eye" appearance to the nucleus. They respond to treatment with topical or systemic steroids.

EMPHYSEMATOUS VAGINITIS

This rare, benign, self-limited disease of unknown cause is usually seen in the vagina, although occasionally can affect the cervix.

CLINICAL FEATURES

Patients range in age from 17 to 77 years. Symptoms, when present, include vaginal discharge or bleeding, pressure, and a "popping" sound with intercourse or physical examination due to rupture of the gas-filled cysts. Associations with pregnancy, infection with either *Trichomonas vaginalis* or *Gardnerella vaginalis*, or cardiopulmonary disease have been described.

RADIOLOGIC FEATURES

Anteroposterior abdominal and lateral X-rays show air bubbles of variable size within the soft tissues above the symphysis pubis and oriented in a tubular fashion between the expected position of the urinary bladder and rectum, respectively. CT scan also shows cystic collections of gas measuring up to several millimeters within the vaginal wall. Transvaginal US examination shows dot-like or linear echogenicities in the vaginal wall.

PATHOLOGIC FEATURES

GROSS FINDINGS

The lesions are usually seen in the upper two-thirds of the vagina, although they can involve the entire vagina and cervix. They tend to be evenly distributed but can form clusters. Individual lesions are tense, smooth, and discrete, although as they aggregate, the vaginal mucosa shows a pebbled or granular appearance, and on occasion may resemble a nabothian cyst. Lesions range in size from a few millimeters to 2 cm.

MICROSCOPIC FINDINGS

The hallmark of emphysematous vaginitis is the finding of variably sized cystic spaces within the lamina propria. The cyst walls are composed of fibroconnective tissue that may or may not contain multinucleated giant cells (Figure 3.8). The cysts are usually empty but may occasionally contain eosinophilic material. The overlying squamous epithelium is intact and may show acanthosis. In some cases, there may be associated chronic inflammation.

PROGNOSIS AND THERAPY

This benign lesion regresses after treatment of the underlying infection (trichomoniasis or *G. vaginalis*), or after pregnancy.

INFLAMMATORY DISEASES OF THE VAGINA

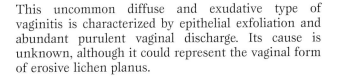

DESQUAMATIVE INFLAMMATORY VAGINITIS

This uncommon diffuse and exudative type of vaginitis is characterized by epithelial exfoliation and abundant purulent vaginal discharge. Its cause is unknown, although it could represent the vaginal form of erosive lichen planus.

CLINICAL FEATURES

This disease affects women from adolescence to postmenopause, but tends to be more frequent in peri- or

---

DESQUAMATIVE INFLAMMATORY VAGINITIS – FACT SHEET

Definition
▸ Inflammatory process of unknown etiology, possibly vaginal form of erosive lichen planus

Clinical Features
▸ More common in premenopausal or postmenopausal women, during postpartum, or women on antiestrogen therapy
▸ Purulent vaginal discharge or malodor
▸ Vulvovaginal burning sensation, pruritus, dyspareunia
▸ Elevated vaginal pH (> 4.5)

Prognosis and Treatment
▸ Vaginal clindamycin
▸ Up to 29% relapse rate
▸ In relapses, additional antibiotic treatment (topical clindamycin, oral ampicillin, or cephalexin) or estrogen therapy (in postmenopausal women) required

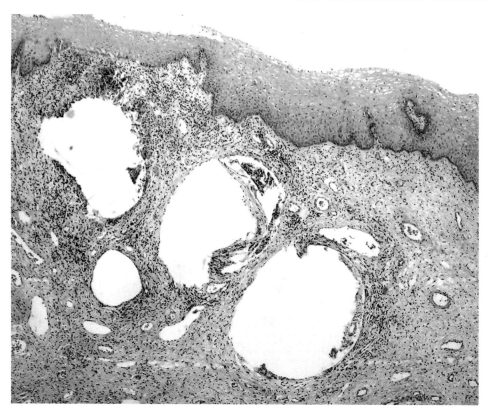

FIGURE 3.8

Emphysematous vaginitis. Several irregular cystic spaces lack an epithelial lining and are surrounded by marked chronic inflammation (Courtesy of Dr. Michael Stamatako).

postmenopausal women, during the postpartum, or women receiving antiestrogen therapy. Symptoms include purulent vaginal discharge, a vulvovaginal burning sensation, dyspareunia, malodor, and vulvar pruritus. These symptoms have a variable duration, ranging from a few months to years. The vaginal pH is also typically elevated (> 4.5).

PATHOLOGIC FEATURES

GROSS FINDINGS

There is mucosal erythema and ecchymotic spots; the latter can also be seen in the vulva and cervix.

DESQUAMATIVE INFLAMMATORY VAGINITIS – PATHOLOGIC FEATURES

Gross Findings
▶ Erythema and ecchymotic spots

Microscopic Findings
▶ Dense acute and chronic inflammation involving squamous epithelium and submucosa with a nonspecific pattern

Ancillary Techniques
▶ Increased number of acute inflammatory cells, numerous parabasal cells and naked nuclei on wet mount (ratio of PMN to epithelial cells > 1:1 in at least 4 HPFs)

Differential Diagnosis
▶ Infectious vaginitis

MICROSCOPIC FINDINGS

The squamous epithelium and submucosa are associated with a dense acute and chronic inflammatory infiltrate with a non-specific pattern. There may be thinning or ulceration of the overlying epithelium.

ANCILLARY STUDIES

Wet mount shows an increase in polymorphonuclear (PMN) leukocytes, defined as the ratio of PMN to epithelial cells > 1:1 in at least 4 HPFs, numerous parabasal cells, and naked nuclei. There is also an absence of lactobacilli which is confirmed on a Gram stain, which may also show Gram-positive cocci in up to 92 % of patients.

DIFFERENTIAL DIAGNOSIS

Infectious vaginitis may show some overlapping features with desquamative inflammatory vaginitis; however, identification of the histopathological features described above and the presence of specific microorganisms will establish the correct diagnosis.

PROGNOSIS AND THERAPY

The use of vaginal clindamycin is successful, although up to 29 % of patients may relapse. In these cases, additional treatment with vaginal clindamycin or oral ampicillin or cephalexin is required. Postmenopausal patients who relapse after clindamycin treatment may obtain long-term remission following estrogen therapy.

LIGNEOUS VAGINITIS

This is a rare form of chronic pseudomembranous inflammation, originally described in the conjunctiva, that can affect the vagina and cervix in addition to the oral cavity, respiratory tract, and middle ear. Involvement of the gynecological tract can be isolated or coexist with involvement of other anatomical sites. The pathogenesis of this disease is poorly understood, but may be secondary to absent or very low plasminogen levels resulting in overaccumulation of fibrin and delayed healing.

CLINICAL FEATURES

Patients range in age from 2 to 65 years, and symptoms include dysmenorrhea, chronic vaginal discharge, and postcoital bleeding, besides gingival disease or conjunctivitis. Infertility may also occur if the upper genital tract is involved. On colposcopic exam, plaques or ulcers may be seen.

PATHOLOGIC FEATURES

MICROSCOPIC FINDINGS

Fibrin deposition, seen as amorphous eosinophilic amyloid-like material, is admixed acute and chronic inflammation and it is associated with alternating

---

LIGNEOUS VAGINITIS – PATHOLOGIC FEATURES

Gross Findings
▶ Plaques or ulcers

Microscopic Findings
▶ Alternating areas of denuded and hyperplastic squamous epithelium
▶ Underlying fibrin deposition (amorphous eosinophilic amyloid-like material) ± acute and chronic inflammation

Ancillary Techniques
▶ PAS positive
▶ Congo red/negative

Differential Diagnosis
▶ Lichen sclerosus
▶ Amyloidosis

---

denuded and hyperplastic patches of squamous epithelium (Figure 3.9). The fibrin deposits stain with PAS but do not stain with Congo red.

DIFFERENTIAL DIAGNOSIS

Ligneous vaginitis is distinguished from *lichen sclerosus* by the presence of deposits of fibrin rather than hyalinization of the stroma. The lack of Congo-red deposits excludes *amyloidosis*.

PROGNOSIS AND THERAPY

Surgery, anti-inflammatory agents, and antibiotics, have been used with limited or no success to treat this disease. Plasminogen activity is decreased in these patients; therefore, hematologic surveillance is required.

MALAKOPLAKIA

The vagina is the most frequently involved site within the gynecological tract for this rare chronic inflammatory disease. It appears to be caused by an acquired defect in macrophage function that results in an impaired histiocytic response to common pathogens. *Escherichia coli* has been the most commonly isolated organism; however, a wide variety of bacteria and mycobacteria also have been identified.

LIGNEOUS VAGINITIS – FACT SHEET

Clinical Features
▶ 2–65 years
▶ Dysmenorrhea, infertility, chronic vaginal discharge, postcoital bleeding
▶ Frequently associated gingival disease or conjunctivitis

Prognosis and Treatment
▶ Surgery, anti-inflammatory agents, and antibiotics used with limited
▶ Hematologic surveillance required as plasminogen activity is decreased

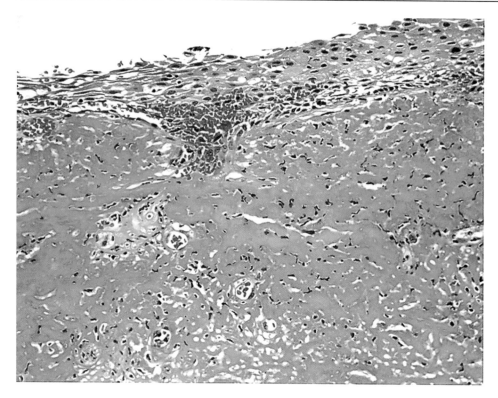

FIGURE 3.9
Ligneous vaginitis. Compact deposits of fibrin are seen as amorphous eosinophilic amyloid-like material admixed with inflammation (Courtesy of Dr. Elvio G Silva).

CLINICAL FEATURES

Patients range in age from 29 to 84 years, but they are more commonly postmenopausal. Symptoms include bleeding or malodorous vaginal discharge, or it may present as a vaginal mass. On physical examination and imaging studies, this lesion may therefore mimic a malignancy.

MALAKOPLAKIA – FACT SHEET

Definition
▶ Acquired defect in macrophage function resulting in impaired histiocytic response to common pathogens, most frequently *Escherichia coli*

Frequency
▶ Most common affected organ in the female gynecologic tract

Clinical Features
▶ More common in postmenopausal patients, but wide age range (29–84 years)
▶ Vaginal bleeding or malodorous vaginal discharge
▶ Vaginal mass

Prognosis and Treatment
▶ Benign
▶ Surgery and/or antibiotics
▶ Recurrences may occur if treated with surgery alone

PATHOLOGIC FEATURES

GROSS FINDINGS

Malakoplakia can result in the formation of small nodules or fungating necrotic masses that may reach up to 7 cm in greatest dimension.

MICROSCOPIC FINDINGS

This lesion is characterized by the presence of numerous histiocytes intermixed with variable amounts of lymphocytes, neutrophils, and plasma cells. Michaelis–Gutmann bodies are the hallmark of malakoplakia; they are seen as spherules with concentric lamination ranging from 5 to 10 µm, located within the cytoplasm of the histiocytes or extracellularly (Figure 3.10).

ANCILLARY STUDIES

The calcified nature of the Michaelis–Gutmann bodies is highlighted with a von Kossa stain. By electron microscopy, Michaelis–Gutmann bodies have an electron-lucent core surrounded by a thin layer of electron-dense hydroxyapatite spicules oriented radially.

DIFFERENTIAL DIAGNOSIS

Recognition of Michaelis–Gutmann bodies will allow the correct diagnosis of this condition which can otherwise be misinterpreted as *severe chronic inflammation*.

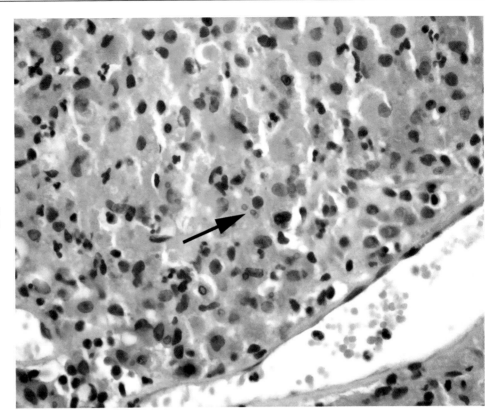

FIGURE 3.10

Malakoplakia. Michaelis–Gutmann bodies (arrow) are seen within the cytoplasm of histiocytes.

MALAKOPLAKIA – PATHOLOGIC FEATURES

Gross Findings

▸ Small nodules to large fungating necrotic masses

Microscopic Findings

▸ Dense histiocytic infiltrate admixed with variable numbers of lymphocytes, neutrophils, and plasma cells
▸ Concentrically laminated spherules present extracellularly or in the cytoplasm of the histiocytes (Michaelis–Gutmann bodies)

Ancillary Techniques

▸ von Kossa stain for Michaelis–Gutmann bodies
▸ Electron-lucent core surrounded by a thin layer of electron-dense hydroxyapatite spicules oriented radially characteristic of Michaelis–Gutmann bodies

Differential Diagnosis

▸ Severe chronic inflammation

PROGNOSIS AND THERAPY

This benign lesion is treated with surgery and/or antibiotics, but may recur if treated exclusively with surgery.

CROHN DISEASE

This chronic intestinal inflammatory disorder can result in the formation of fistulas from the bowel to the vagina (mainly from the rectosigmoid) and vaginal granulomas. Vaginal involvement may represent the first manifestation of the disease. Rectovaginal and anovaginal fistulas occur in up to 25% of patients. Symptoms include fecal or clear vaginal discharge, passage of gas vaginally, or repeated episodes of vaginal infection. Patients are treated with antibiotics or monoclonal antibodies, tumor necrosis factor-alpha, or surgery in nonresponsive cases. Patients with long-standing Crohn disease and rectal or anal/vaginal fistulas may develop a mucinous adenocarcinoma.

OTHER INFLAMMATORY CONDITIONS OF THE VAGINA

Mucosal genital lichen planus can affect the vagina, although it typically involves the labia minora. Patients are usually perimenopausal, may present with vaginal bleeding, and may or may not have oral lesions. Grossly, erythema surrounded by a lacy border may be seen. The latter is the best area to biopsy in order to confirm the diagnosis. Erosions may develop but are secondary, thus the commonly used term "erosive lichen planus" is inaccurate. Microscopically, there is a band-like inflammatory infiltrate with alteration of the basal epithelial layer and Civatte bodies. Treatment of this disease is mandatory because its natural course will lead to fusion of the labia minora and vagina. However, there is no standard effective treatment.

PSEUDONEOPLASTIC LESIONS OF THE VAGINA

VAGINAL PROLAPSE

Prolapse occurs as a consequence of loss of support of the ligaments that suspend the vagina, usually secondary to multiple vaginal deliveries. Symptoms include lower abdominal discomfort, backache, "heaviness" in the perineum, vaginal discharge, and frequent micturition. Microscopic examination of the vaginal mucosa demonstrates acanthosis and hyperkeratosis with or without parakeratosis (Figure 3.11). Erosion and reparative changes may also be seen.

POSTOPERATIVE SPINDLE CELL NODULE

This is an uncommon benign proliferative mesenchymal lesion typically involving the lower genitourinary tract, occurring at the site of previous surgery, 2.5–12

weeks later. Although the vagina is the most commonly involved site in the female genital tract, it can also occur in the vulva, cervix, or even endometrium.

CLINICAL FEATURES

Patients range in age from 29 to 75 years. These lesions are frequently asymptomatic, and they are usually detected during a follow-up (post-surgical) physical examination.

POSTOPERATIVE SPINDLE CELL NODULE – FACT SHEET

Definition
▸ Benign proliferative mesenchymal lesion detected in a previous surgery site involving the lower genitourinary tract, occurring 2.5–12 weeks after a surgical procedure

Frequency
▸ Vagina most common location in the female genital tract

Clinical Features
▸ 29–75 years
▸ Commonly asymptomatic
▸ Incidental finding during gynecologic examination

Prognosis and Treatment
▸ Local excision
▸ Recurrences treated successfully with re-excision

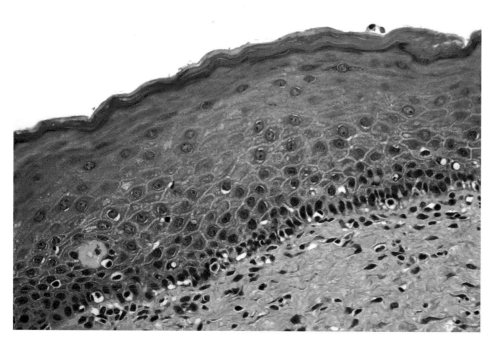

FIGURE 3.11
Vaginal prolapse. Prominent compact and homogeneous hyperkeratosis is seen.

PATHOLOGIC FEATURES

GROSS FINDINGS

Postoperative spindle cell nodule frequently appears as a polypoid, soft mass measuring up to 4 cm.

MICROSCOPIC FINDINGS

Spindle cells are arranged in a fascicular pattern, often with a delicate network of small blood vessels (Figure 3.12). The cells can have plump nuclei with vesicular chromatin and one or two enlarged nucleoli; however, pleomorphism is not seen. The mitotic index is brisk and can be as high as 25 mitoses/10 HPFs, but no atypical forms are found. Surface ulceration, acute and chronic inflammatory cells, small foci of hemorrhage, and edema are commonly detected. The lesion may infiltrate the adjacent tissue to a limited degree, simulating a malignant process.

ANCILLARY STUDIES

The cells may be positive for desmin and keratin and ultrastructurally show features of fibroblasts and myofibroblasts.

POSTOPERATIVE SPINDLE CELL NODULE – PATHOLOGIC FEATURES

Gross Findings
▸ Soft, polypoid mass up to 4 cm

Microscopic Findings
▸ Spindle cells arranged in a fascicular pattern, often with a delicate network of small blood vessels
▸ Cells with plump nuclei, vesicular chromatin, one or two enlarged nucleoli, and minimal cytologic atypia
▸ High mitotic index (up to 25/10 HPFs) without atypical mitoses
▸ Limited infiltration into adjacent tissue

Ancillary Studies
▸ Desmin and keratin positive
▸ Fibroblasts and myofibroblasts by electron microscopy

Differential Diagnosis
▸ Leiomyosarcoma

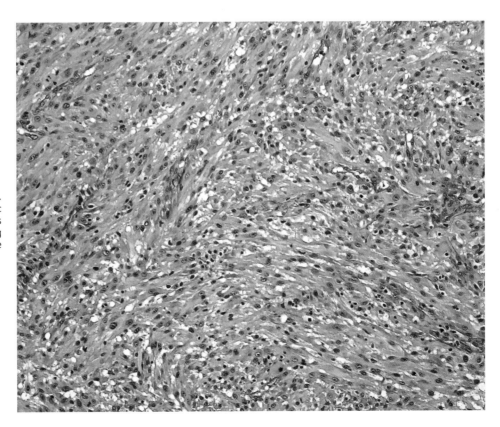

FIGURE 3.12
Postoperative spindle cell nodule. Fusiform cells with bland cytologic features form intersecting fascicles and are associated with a sprinkling of lymphocytes and a delicate network of small blood vessels.

DIFFERENTIAL DIAGNOSIS

Leiomyosarcoma is the main entity in the differential diagnosis. Attention to the clinical setting (i.e., a previous history of surgery at the involved site and absence of symptoms) as well as the presence of inflammatory cells, delicate blood vessels, and absence of nuclear pleomorphism will allow the distinction of postoperative spindle cell nodule from leiomyosarcoma. Immunohistochemical stains may not be useful, as postoperative spindle cell nodule may be positive for smooth muscle markers.

PROGNOSIS AND THERAPY

These lesions have an excellent prognosis. Treatment consists of local excision; however, recurrences can occur, which are successfully treated with re-excision.

VAGINAL VAULT GRANULATION TISSUE

This is a common finding after hysterectomy. Grossly, it appears as one or more small, red, granular, polypoid lesions in the upper vagina near or within the sutured cuff. Microscopically, it shows the typical features of granulation tissue with prominent small blood vessels, edema, and marked acute and chronic inflammation (Figure 3.13). It can contain scattered bizarre stromal cells. It heals over time, although a biopsy may be required to exclude recurrence or metastasis if a previous hysterectomy was performed for a malignant condition. Alternatively, cauterization may be performed.

FALLOPIAN TUBE PROLAPSE

Prolapse of the fallopian tube most commonly occurs following a vaginal hysterectomy, but it can also occur after abdominal hysterectomy or colpotomy. Predisposing factors include significant bleeding after surgery, incomplete peritoneal closure, drains left in the Douglas pouch as well as postoperative infections.

CLINICAL FEATURES

The most common symptoms include vaginal bleeding, lower abdominal pain, watery or foul-smelling vaginal discharge, and dyspareunia. Some patients are asymp-

---

FALLOPIAN TUBE PROLAPSE – FACT SHEET

Frequency
- Most commonly seen following vaginal hysterectomy, but also after abdominal hysterectomy or colpotomy (from 2 weeks to 28 years)

Clinical Features
- Most frequently vaginal bleeding and lower abdominal pain
- Watery or foul-smelling vaginal discharge, and dyspareunia
- Less frequently asymptomatic

Treatment
- Excision

---

tomatic. Symptoms may occur from 2 weeks up to 28 years after surgery; however, they often appear within 6 months postoperatively. On vaginal examination, an erythematous mass is seen in the vaginal vault. The diagnosis of fallopian tube prolapse can be suspected if a probe can be passed through a discernible lumen, or if traction of the mass induces pain.

PATHOLOGIC FEATURES

GROSS FINDINGS

The lesions tend to be relatively small, red or gray to tan granular and polypoid, measuring up to 2 cm.

FALLOPIAN TUBE PROLAPSE – PATHOLOGIC FEATURES

Gross Findings
- Small red, gray or tan, granular to polypoid, measuring up to 2 cm
- Occasionally prolapsed fallopian tube fimbria is identified

Microscopic Findings
- Clubbed folds (plicae) at the surface of the lesion or rounded or slit-like structures containing luminal spaces that are buried in fibroconnective tissue or granulation tissue
- Fallopian tube epithelium with variable degrees of hyperplasia (cribriforming and papillary formation)
- Loss of cilia, and loss of the secretory and intercalated cells
- Variable degree of cytologic atypia with cell enlargement and nuclear hyperchromasia
- Numerous thick-walled blood vessels and variable amounts of smooth muscle fibers deeper in the lesion
- Frequently admixed with numerous plasma cells

Differential Diagnosis
- Granulation tissue
- Adenocarcinoma

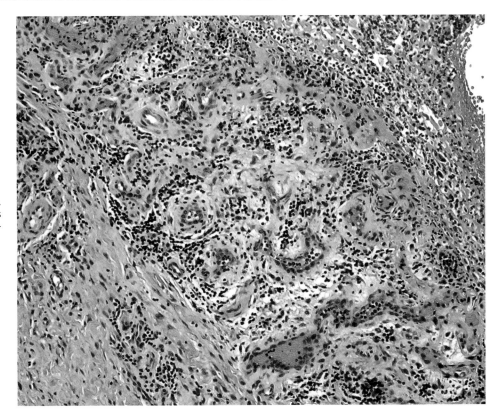

FIGURE 3.13
Vaginal vault granulation tissue. Prominent chronic inflammation is associated with small vessels, reactive fibroblasts and mild edema.

Sometimes, the prolapsed fallopian tube fimbria may be identified.

MICROSCOPIC FINDINGS

The hallmark of fallopian tube prolapse is the finding of tubal-type epithelium either forming clubbed folds (plicae) at the surface of the lesion or rounded or slit-like structures with luminal spaces buried in fibroconnective or granulation tissue (Figure 3.14). The fallopian tube epithelium may show variable degrees of proliferation with cribriforming and papillary formation, and some degree of cytologic atypia (i.e., enlargement of the cells, nuclear hyperchromasia). It may also exhibit lack of cilia, and loss of the secretory and intercalated cells. Numerous plasma cells can be seen. Deeper in the lesion, there are numerous thick-walled blood vessels and variable amounts of smooth-muscle fibers.

DIFFERENTIAL DIAGNOSIS

Although the gross appearance of fallopian tube prolapse overlaps with that seen in *granulation tissue*, on microscopic examination, this distinction is easy. Rarely, on low-power scrutiny, an *adenocarcinoma with papillary features* may be confused with fallopian tube prolapse, as complex architecture as well as occasional

cytologic atypia may be seen in the latter. It is important to recognize that the complex infolding of papillae corresponds to the plicae covered by tubal-type epithelium.

PROGNOSIS AND THERAPY

Treatment consists of excision with complete resolution of the symptoms. It does not recur.

ENDOMETRIOSIS

The vagina is a relatively uncommon location for endometriosis. It can occur superficially or deep in the vaginal wall. Symptoms include vaginal bleeding or the presence of a mass. Grossly, it can appear as a blue-colored area or a polypoid lesion. On microscopic examination, endometrial-type glands which may be mitotically active, are admixed with endometrial stroma, recent hemorrhage and/or hemosiderin (Figure 3.15). The endometrial-type glands may display metaplastic as well as hyperplastic changes, as can be seen in the endometrium. Rarely, clear cell carcinoma, low-grade müllerian adenosarcoma,

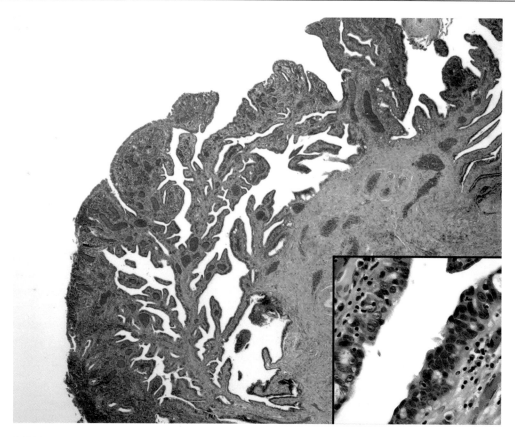

FIGURE 3.14

Fallopian tube prolapse. Bulbous clubbed-like folds (plicae) are present on the surface. They are lined by tubal epithelium, some containing cilia (inset) (Courtesy of Dr. Bojana Djordjevic).

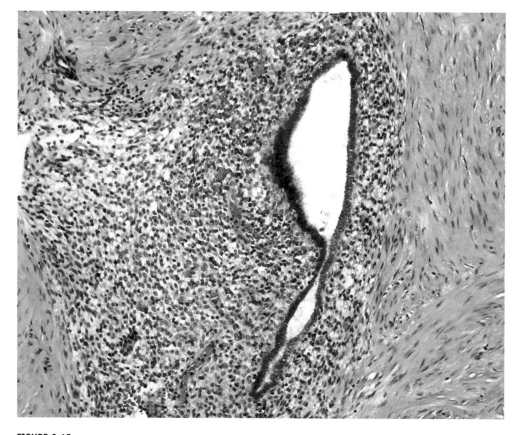

FIGURE 3.15

Endometriosis. An endometrial-type gland is surrounded by endometrial stroma accompanied by recent hemorrhage.

ENDOMETRIOSIS – FACT SHEET

Definition
▶ Presence of endometrial-type glands and stroma ± hemorrhage

Location and Frequency
▶ Relatively uncommon location
▶ Superficial or deep

Clinical Features
▶ Vaginal bleeding
▶ Occasionally forms a mass

Prognosis and Treatment
▶ Laser vaporization for small lesions
▶ Excision for large lesions
▶ 3–11% rate of malignant transformation (clear cell carcinoma, low-grade müllerian adenosarcoma, low-grade endometrioid stromal sarcoma)

ENDOMETRIOSIS – PATHOLOGIC FEATURES

Gross Findings
▶ Blue discoloration or polypoid lesion

Microscopic Findings
▶ Endometrial-type glands which may be mitotically active, admixed with endometrial stroma +/− recent hemorrhage and/or hemosiderin
▶ Metaplastic and/or hyperplastic changes (variable degree of architectural and cytologic atypia)

Differential Diagnosis
▶ Adenocarcinoma

---

and low-grade endometrioid stromal sarcoma may arise in vaginal endometriosis (3 to 11% rate of malignant transformation). As florid endometriosis may have a striking pseudoinfiltrative growth into the vaginal wall, it may be misinterpreted as invasive carcinoma. Recognizing the presence of endometrial stroma around the glands will facilitate the diagnosis of endometriosis. Excision is the treatment of choice for large areas of endometriosis, while smaller lesions can be treated with laser vaporization.

VAGINAL ADENOSIS

Adenosis is defined by the finding of benign glandular endocervical or tuboendometrioid epithelium either replacing the surface squamous epithelium or forming glands in the lamina propria of the vagina. It almost always occurs in the upper third of the vagina in reproductive-age and postmenopausal patients. Although this lesion is associated with a history of prenatal diethylstilbestrol (DES) exposure, vaginal adenosis can also occur following 5-fluorouracil therapy and carbon dioxide laser treatment, as well as transverse septum resection. Symptoms include mucoid vaginal discharge and postcoital and vaginal bleeding.

ADENOSIS – FACT SHEET

Definition
▶ Benign endocervical or tuboendometrioid epithelium replacing the squamous epithelium or forming glands in the lamina propria of the vagina

Frequency and Location
▶ 20–40% in women exposed to DES in utero
▶ Most frequently upper third of the vagina

Morbidity and Mortality
▶ Risk of developing secondary clear cell carcinoma

Clinical Features
▶ Mucoid vaginal discharge
▶ Postcoital and vaginal bleeding

Prognosis
▶ Follow-up or excision

The glandular epithelium is present either replacing the surface squamous epithelium or in the nearby stroma. It can be of endocervical (Figure 3.16) or tuboendometrioid type, the latter being less common. The glands can be associated with squamous metaplasia, which can obscure the glandular elements. In these cases, adenosis can be recognized by the immaturity and scant amount of glycogen present in the squamous epithelium, the finding of residual gland openings, and scattered mucin-filled cells within the surface epithelium or center of the glands. Adenosis can undergo metaplastic as well as hyperplastic (premalignant) changes, and it is associated with a higher risk of malignant transformation, most commonly clear cell carcinoma.

ADENOSIS – PATHOLOGIC FEATURES

Microscopic Findings
▶ Endocervical or tuboendometrioid-type epithelium replacing surface squamous epithelium or forming glands in stroma
▶ Squamous metaplasia may fill and obscure glandular elements
▶ Metaplastic and hyperplastic changes (with variable degrees of architectural and cytologic atypia)

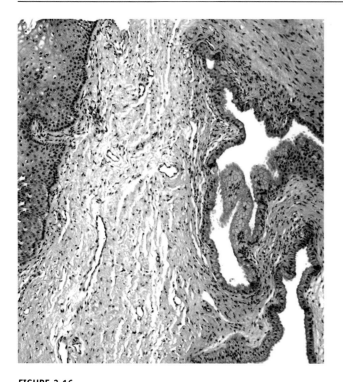

FIGURE 3.16

Vaginal adenosis. Glands lined by endocervical-type epithelium are present in the superficial vaginal wall.

CYSTS OF THE VAGINA

The prevalence of vaginal cysts is estimated to be 1 in 200 women; however, this number is probably inaccurate, since most cysts are not reported. They are more common in women in their third and fourth decades and are usually detected incidentally. When symptomatic, patients may present with mild vaginal discomfort, vaginal pressure or fullness, vaginal mass or swelling, dyspareunia, vaginal bleeding, or urinary symptoms. Ultrasound, voiding cystourethrogram, CT-scan, and especially MRI are useful to characterize these lesions. Vaginal cysts are treated with excision. The most common types of vaginal cysts discussed herein include: (1) müllerian cyst; (2) epidermal inclusion cyst; and (3) Gartner's cyst.

MÜLLERIAN CYST

This is the most common type of vaginal cyst. They can be located anywhere in the vagina but have a predilection for the anterolateral wall. The cysts are usually small, ranging from 0.1 to 2 cm, although they may measure > 4 cm. They are lined predominantly by endocervical-like columnar mucinous epithelium (Figure 3.17). However, cuboidal mucinous, endometrioid, or tubal-type epithelium can also be seen.

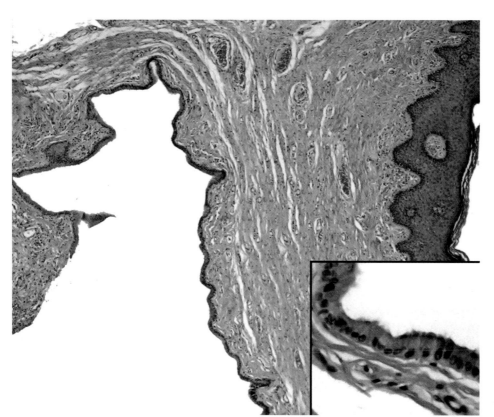

FIGURE 3.17

Müllerian cyst. A cyst is lined by columnar mucin-producing epithelium (inset) (Courtesy of Dr. Michael Stamatakos).

ous surgical site. They range in size from a few millimeters to several centimeters and tend to be asymptomatic. The cysts are lined by benign squamous epithelium (Figure 3.18) and may have luminal keratinous contents that on gross examination may impart a "cheese-like" appearance.

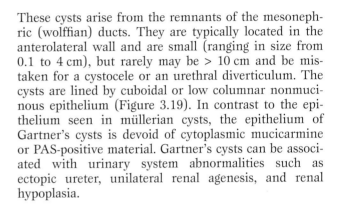

GARTNER'S CYST

These cysts arise from the remnants of the mesonephric (wolffian) ducts. They are typically located in the anterolateral wall and are small (ranging in size from 0.1 to 4 cm), but rarely may be > 10 cm and be mistaken for a cystocele or an urethral diverticulum. The cysts are lined by cuboidal or low columnar nonmucinous epithelium (Figure 3.19). In contrast to the epithelium seen in müllerian cysts, the epithelium of Gartner's cysts is devoid of cytoplasmic mucicarmine or PAS-positive material. Gartner's cysts can be associated with urinary system abnormalities such as ectopic ureter, unilateral renal agenesis, and renal hypoplasia.

ATROPHY

Vaginal atrophy occurs in the postmenopausal years, during lactation, or following hypothalamic amenorrhea, as a consequence of estrogen deprivation.

CLINICAL FEATURES

Although vaginal atrophy is seen in most postmenopausal women, not all of them will be symptomatic. Symptoms may also occur in perimenopausal patients without signs of atrophic vaginitis. Symptoms include vaginal dryness and irritation, pruritus, and dyspareunia.

EPIDERMAL INCLUSION CYST

These cysts form secondarily to displacement of epithelial fragments following episiotomy or other surgical procedures, and their location correlates with a previ-

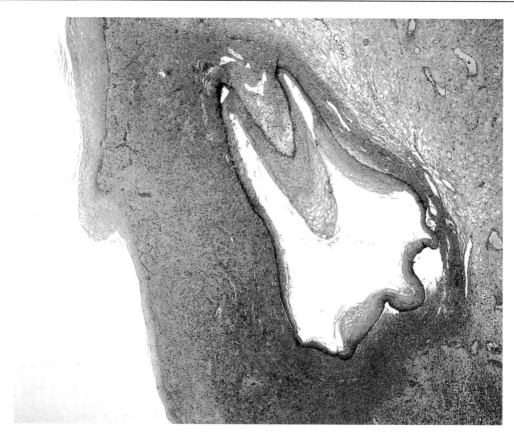

FIGURE 3.18
Epithelial inclusion cyst. The cyst is lined by mature multilayered squamous epithelium.

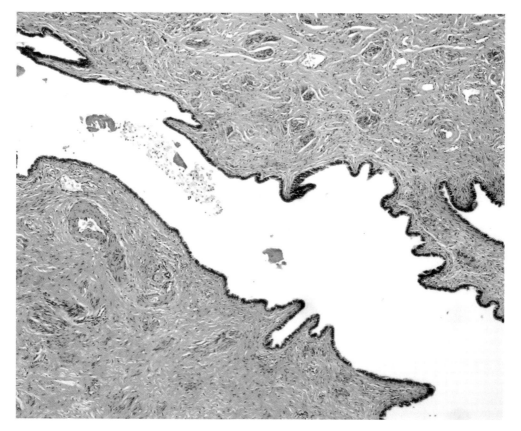

FIGURE 3.19
Gartner's cyst. The cyst has an irregular outline and is lined by a single layer of cuboidal cells.

PATHOLOGIC FEATURES

GROSS FINDINGS

There is frequent loss of rugal folds and a pale, dry appearance of the mucosa that may be associated with petechiae.

VAGINAL ATROPHY – PATHOLOGIC FEATURES

Gross Findings
▶ Loss of rugal folds
▶ Pale and dry mucosa
▶ Petechiae may be present

Microscopic Findings
▶ Reduced or normal-thickness squamous epithelium
▶ Loss or variable reduction of superficial and intermediate squamous cells
▶ Lack of glycogenated squamous epithelium
▶ Transitional cell metaplasia (variant of atrophy)
  ▶ Epithelial thickness > 10 cells
  ▶ Main axis of the cells often parallel to basement membrane
  ▶ Oval or spindle nuclei with frequent nuclear grooves
▶ Increased nuclear/cytoplasmic ratio
▶ Absent or minimal cytologic atypia and/or mitoses

Differential Diagnosis
▶ High-grade vaginal intraepithelial neoplasia

MICROSCOPIC FINDINGS

These is loss or variable reduction of superficial and intermediate squamous cells, usually resulting in an epithelium with 7–10 cell layers (Figure 3.20A); however, in some cases the squamous epithelium displays a normal thickness. The squamous epithelium lacks cytoplasm glycogen, resulting in an increased nuclear to cytoplasmic ratio. However, no cytologic atypia or mitotic activity are seen. In transitional cell metaplasia, considered to be a variant of atrophy, the epithelium is > 10 cells thick, it shows oval or elongated nuclei with frequent grooves, with the main axis of the cells being often parallel to the basement membrane. The very superficial cells may resemble umbrella cells (Figure 3.21). Mitotic figures are absent or rare.

ANCILLARY STUDIES

The vaginal pH is > 5.0 and there is a change of the maturation index with a predominance of parabasal cells.

DIFFERENTIAL DIAGNOSIS

Atrophy and transitional cell metaplasia may be confused with *high-grade vaginal intraepithelial neoplasia*, as all show lack of cell maturation in the mid and upper layers of the epithelium, with the cells showing marked increased nuclear to cytoplasmic ratio. Absence of nuclear pleomorphism, mitoses in upper layers, and Ki-67 immunopositivity limited to scattered basal/parabasal cells favor the diagnosis of atrophy or transitional cell metaplasia (Figure 3.20B).

PROGNOSIS AND THERAPY

Treatment includes use of vaginal moisturizers, and/or topical or systemic hormone replacement.

ECTOPIC DECIDUAL REACTION (DECIDUOSIS)

Ectopic decidual reaction is not an infrequent finding in the vagina. Rarely, it may mimic carcinoma, since it can cause vaginal bleeding or form a mass. This lesion can be detected any time during pregnancy, undergoes spontaneous regression after parturition, and requires no specific treatment. Microscopically, it is characterized by the presence of polygonal or spindle-shaped cells with eosinophilic cytoplasm and nuclei that can display

---

ECTOPIC DECIDUAL REACTION (DECIDUOSIS) – FACT SHEET

Clinical Features
▶ Detected from the sixth week of gestation to term
▶ Very rarely vaginal bleeding or mass

Prognosis and Treatment
▶ Spontaneous regression after parturition

ECTOPIC DECIDUAL REACTION (DECIDUOSIS) – PATHOLOGIC FEATURES

Microscopic Findings
▶ Polygonal or spindle cells with abundant eosinophilic cytoplasm and round nuclei with or without conspicuous nucleoli
▶ No mitotic activity

Differential Diagnosis
▶ Carcinoma

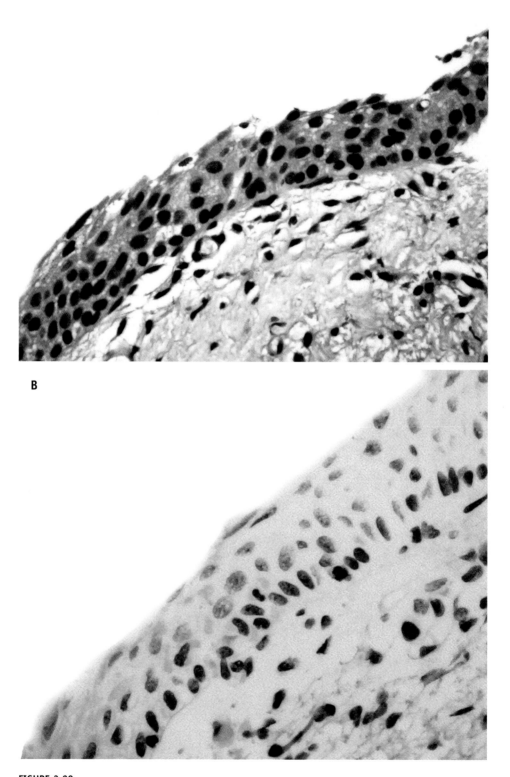

FIGURE 3.20

Vaginal atrophy. The squamous epithelium appears flattened with decreased to absent intracytoplasmic glycogen (A). Ki-67 immunostain demonstrates rare positivity in the basal layer (B).

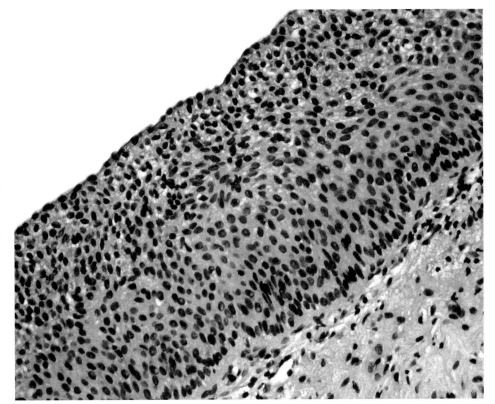

FIGURE 3.21

Transitional cell metaplasia. The thickened epithelium is composed of cells with oval to elongated nuclei. The main axis of the superficial cells tends to be oriented in parallel to the basement membrane.

conspicuous nucleoli. Ectopic decidual reaction should not be mistaken for carcinoma and in difficult cases a negative immunostain for keratin will facilitate the diagnosis.

vessels, and hyperplastic endothelial cells, as well as stromal hyalinization with scattered enlarged fibroblasts showing enlarged and hyperchromatic nuclei. The differential diagnosis includes *high-grade vaginal intraepithelial neoplasia* characterized by an increased nuclear to cytoplasmic ratio, nuclei with coarse chromatin, and conspicuous mitotic activity.

RADIOTHERAPY-ASSOCIATED CHANGES

Radiation therapy may cause atrophy, necrosis, erosion, ulceration, and stenosis of the vagina. Grossly, the mucosal changes evolve from erythema and congestion with possible ulceration to mucosal thinning, friability, and the presence of telangiectasias. Microscopically, the squamous epithelium becomes atrophic and the cells display cytoplasmic vacuolization, nuclear enlargement, but with a low nuclear to cytoplasmic ratio, multinucleation, and rare to absent mitotic activity (Figure 3.22). There are vascular changes such as thrombosis and vascular obliteration, hyalinization of vessels walls, ectatic

---

RADIOTHERAPY-ASSOCIATED CHANGES – PATHOLOGIC FEATURES

Gross Findings

▶ Erythema, congestion, ulceration, mucosal thinning, friability, and telangiectasias

Microscopic Findings

▶ Atrophic or reactive squamous epithelium
▶ Squamous cells with enlarged nuclei, low nuclear/cytoplasmic ratio, cytoplasmic vacuolization as well as multinucleated cells.
▶ Rare mitosis
▶ Stromal hyalinization with variable inflammatory infiltrate
▶ Stromal fibroblasts with plump hyperchromatic nuclei
▶ Vascular changes, including thrombosis, vascular obliteration, hyalinization of vessels walls, ectatic vessels, and hyperplastic endothelial cells

Differential Diagnosis

▶ High-grade vaginal intraepithelial neoplasia

RADIOTHERAPY-ASSOCIATED CHANGES – FACT SHEET

Clinical Features

▶ Atrophy, erosion, ulceration, necrosis, or stenosis of the vagina

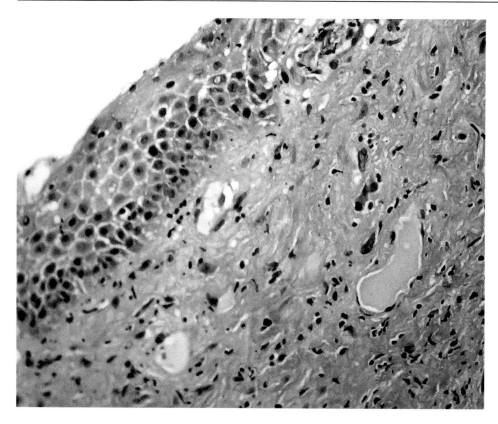

FIGURE 3.22

Radiation changes. Reactive fibroblasts with enlarged and hyperchromatic nuclei are admixed with chronic inflammation and ectatic vessels.

SUGGESTED READING

Congenital Anomalies

Ali A, Cetin C, Nedim C, et al. Treatment of imperforate hymen by application of Foley catheter. Eur J Obstet Gynecol Reprod Biol 2003;106:72–75.

Berkowitz CD, Elvik SL, Logan M. A simulated "acquired" imperforate hymen following the genital trauma of sexual abuse. Clin Pediatr (Phila) 1987;26:307–309.

Botash AS, Jean-Louis F. Imperforate hymen: congenital or acquired from sexual abuse? Pediatrics 2001;108:E53.

Guerrier D, Mouchel T, Pasquier L, et al. The Mayer–Rokitansky–Kuster–Hauser syndrome (congenital absence of uterus and vagina) – phenotypic manifestations and genetic approaches. J Negat Results Biomed 2006;5:1.

Posner JC, Spandorfer PR. Early detection of imperforate hymen prevents morbidity from delays in diagnosis. Pediatrics 2005;115:1008–1012.

Bacterial and Parasitic Vaginitis

Cory J, Schrag S, Dinsmoor MJ, et al. Group B strep; successful model of "from science to action." Available online from http://www.cdc.gov/ncidod/EID/vol10no11/04-gov/ncidod/EID/vol100623_03.htm.

Cox RA, Slack MP. Clinical and microbiological features of *Haemophilus influenzae* vulvovaginitis in young girls. J Clin Pathol 2002;55:961–964.

de Mundi Zamorano A, del Alamo CM, de Blas LL, et al. Egg of *Trichuris trichiura* in a vaginal smear. Acta Cytol 1978;22:119–120.

Eckert LO. Acute vulvovaginitis. N Engl J Med 2006;355:1244–1252.

Nopdonrattakoon L. Amoebiasis of the female genital tract: a case report. J Obstet Gynaecol Res 1996;22:235–238.

Poggensee G, Feldmeier H. Female genital schistosomiasis: facts and hypotheses. Acta Trop 2001;79:193–210.

Shukla S, Saini P, Smriti, et al. Functional characterization of *Candida albicans* ABC transporter Cdr1p. Eukaryot Cell 2003;2:1361–1375.

Sinniah B, Leopairut J, Neafie RC, et al. Enterobiasis: a histopathological study of 259 patients. Ann Trop Med Parasitol 1991;85:625–635.

Wai CY, Nihira MA, Drewes PG, et al. *Actinomyces* associated with persistent vaginal granulation tissue. Infect Dis Obstet Gynecol 2005;13:53–55.

Toxic Shock Syndrome

Davis D, Gash-Kim TL, Heffernan EJ. Toxic shock syndrome: case report of a postpartum female and a literature review. J Emerg Med 1998;16:607–614.

Parsonnet J, Hansmann MA, Delaney ML, et al. Prevalence of toxic shock syndrome toxin 1-producing *Staphylococcus aureus* and the presence of antibodies to this superantigen in menstruating women. J Clin Microbiol 2005;43:4628–4634.

Reiss MA. Toxic shock syndrome. Prim Care Update Obstet Gynecol 2000;7:85–90.

Viral Infections

Anderson J, Clark RA, Watts DH, et al. Idiopathic genital ulcers in women infected with human immunodeficiency virus. J Acquir Immune Defic Syndr Hum Retrovirol 1996;13:343–347.

Beauman JG. Genital herpes: a review. Am Fam Physician 2005;72:1527–1534.

Friedmann W, Schäfer A, Kretschmer R, et al. Disseminated cytomegalovirus infection of the female genital tract. Gynecol Obstet Invest 1991;31:56–57.

Emphysematous Vaginitis

Kramer K, Tobon H. Vaginitis emphysematosa. Arch Pathol Lab Med 1987;111:746–749.

Sherer DM, Hellmann M, Gorelick C, et al. Transvaginal sonographic findings associated with emphysematous vaginitis at 32 weeks' gestation. J Ultrasound Med 2006;25:515–517.

Desquamative Inflammatory Vaginitis

Oates JK, Rowen D. Desquamative inflammatory vaginitis. A review. Genitourin Med 1990;66:275–279.
Sobel JD. Desquamative inflammatory vaginitis: a new subgroup of purulent vaginitis responsive to topical 2% clindamycin therapy. Am J Obstet Gynecol 1994;171:1215–1220.

Ligneous Vaginitis

Deen S, Duncan TJ, Hammond RH. Ligneous cervicitis; is it the emperor's new clothes? Case report and different analysis of aetiology. Histopathology 2006;49:198–199.
Pantanowitz L, Bauer K, Tefs K, et al. Ligneous (pseudomembranous) inflammation involving the female genital tract associated with type-1 plasminogen deficiency. Int J Gynecol Pathol 2004;23:292–295.

Malakoplakia

Chen KT, Hendricks EJ. Malakoplakia of the female genital tract. Obstet Gynecol 1985;65(Suppl):84S–87S.
Fishman A, Ortega E, Girtanner RE, et al. Malacoplakia of the vagina presenting as a pelvic mass. Gynecol Oncol 1993;49:380–382.
Kogulan PK, Smith M, Seidman J, et al. Malakoplakia involving the abdominal wall, urinary bladder, vagina, and vulva: case report and discussion of malakoplakia-associated bacteria. Int J Gynecol Pathol 2001;20:403–406.

Crohn Disease

Feller ER, Ribaudo S, Jackson ND. Gynecologic aspects of Crohn's disease. Am Fam Physician 2001;64:1725–1728.
Moore-Maxwell CA, Robboy SJ. Mucinous adenocarcinoma arising in rectovaginal fistulas associated with Crohn's disease. Gynecol Oncol 2004;93:266–268.

Other Inflammatory Conditions of the Vagina

Kirtschig G, Wakelin SH, Wojnarowska F. Mucosal vulval lichen planus: outcome, clinical and laboratory features. J Eur Acad Dermatol Venereol 2005;19:301–307.
Lotery HE, Galask RP. Erosive lichen planus of the vulva and vagina. Obstet Gynecol 2003;101:1121–1125.

Postoperative Spindle Cell Nodule

Guillou L, Gloor E, De Grandi P, et al. Post-operative pseudosarcoma of the vagina. A case report. Pathol Res Pract 1989;185:245–248.
Proppe KH, Scully RE, Rosai J. Postoperative spindle cell nodules of genitourinary tract resembling sarcomas. A report of eight cases. Am J Surg Pathol 1984;8:101–108.
Young RH, Clement PB. Pseudoneoplastic lesions of the lower female genital tract. Pathol Annu 1989;24:189–226.

Endometriosis

Parker RL, Dadmanesh F, Young RH, et al. Polypoid endometriosis: a clinicopathologic analysis of 24 cases and a review of the literature. Am J Surg Pathol 2004;28:285–297.
Shah C, Pizer E, Veljovich DS, et al. Clear cell adenocarcinoma of the vagina in a patient with vaginal endometriosis. Gynecol Oncol 2006;103:1130–1132.

Adenosis

Goodman A, Zukerberg LR, Nikrui N, et al. Vaginal adenosis and clear cell carcinoma after 5-fluorouracil treatment for condylomas. Cancer 1991;68:1628–32.
Robboy SJ, Noller KL, O'Brien P, et al. Increased incidence of cervical and vaginal dysplasia in 3980 diethylstilbestrol-exposed young women. Experience of the National Collaborative Diethylstilbestrol Adenosis project JAMA 1984;252:2979–2983.

Cysts of the Vagina

Eilber KS, Raz S. Benign cystic lesions of the vagina: a literature review. J Urol 2003;170:717–722.
Pradhan S, Tobon H. Vaginal cysts: a clinicopathological study of 41 cases. Int J Gynecol Pathol 1986;5:35–46.

Vaginal Atrophy

Nilsson K, Risberg B, Heimer G. The vaginal epithelium in the postmenopause-cytology, histology and pH as methods of assessment. Maturitas 1995;21:51–56.
SOGC clinical practice guidelines. The detection and management of vaginal atrophy. Number 145, May 2004. Int J Gynaecol Obstet 2005;88:222–228.
Weir MM, Bell DA, Young RH. Transitional cell metaplasia of the uterine cervix and vagina: an underrecognized lesion that may be confused with high-grade dysplasia. A report of 59 cases. Am J Surg Pathol 1997;21:510–517.

Ectopic Decidual Reaction (Deciduosis)

Mathie JG. Vaginal deciduosis simulating carcinoma. J Obstet Gynaecol Br Emp 1957;64:720–721.

Radiotherapy-associated Changes

Mazeron JJ, Gerbaulet A. Late effects of ionizing radiations on the vulva, vagina and uterus. Cancer Radiother 1997;1:781–789.
Shield PW. Chronic radiation effects: a correlative study of smears and biopsies from the cervix and vagina. Diagn Cytopathol 1995;13:107–119.

4

Vaginal Neoplasia

Anais Malpica

Primary neoplasms of the vagina, whether benign or malignant, are rare. Primary carcinomas are the most common malignant tumors and account for approximately 2% of all gynecological malignancies. Among vaginal carcinomas, in situ and invasive squamous carcinomas are the most frequent. As a general rule, when evaluating a primary malignant tumor in the vagina, it is essential to exclude the possibility of a metastasis, especially if it is an epithelial neoplasm. This chapter will focus on the most common tumors occurring at this site.

BENIGN NEOPLASMS

MÜLLERIAN PAPILLOMA

This uncommon lesion was initially designated "mesonephric papilloma," as it was thought to be of mesonephric origin. However, it is now considered to be of müllerian origin based on its morphologic appearance and immunophenotype.

CLINICAL FEATURES

Müllerian papilloma typically occurs in girls under 10 years of age, although it has occasionally been described in adults. Patients usually present with vaginal bleeding or an exophytic mass.

PATHOLOGIC FEATURES

GROSS FINDINGS

This lesion can be found in the anterior, posterior, or lateral walls of the vagina. It appears as a polypoid to papillary, well circumscribed lesion up to 5 cm.

MICROSCOPIC FINDINGS

It is characterized by papillary fronds lined by columnar or cuboidal epithelium (Figure 4.1). The papillary cores are composed of fibroconnective tissue, which can show edematous or myxoid change. The lining epithelial cells are cuboidal to columnar and have eosinophilic cytoplasm, uniform, bland nuclei, and absent or rare mitotic figures. The cells can form solid nests with scattered glandular lumina containing eosinophilic PAS positive and diastase-resistant globules.

ANCILLARY STUDIES

The epithelial cells are positive for EMA, CEA, CAM 5.2, and EP4, and focally positive for CA125. By electron microscopy, the cells contain luminal microvilli, perinuclear arrays of microfilaments, abundant lysosomes, complex cytoplasmic interdigitations, and pseudoinclusions of "cytoplasmic" collagen, features that have been associated with müllerian-type epithelium.

DIFFERENTIAL DIAGNOSIS

Fibroepithelial polyp, condyloma acuminatum, embryonal rhabdomyosarcoma, and clear cell adenocarcinoma may enter into the differential diagnosis because they all share a papillary to polypoid growth pattern. *Fibroepithelial polyp* and *condyloma acuminatum* are lined by squamous as opposed to cuboidal to columnar epithelium, with the latter also exhibiting koilocytotic atypia. *Embryonal rhabdomyosarcoma* characteristically exhibits condensation of relatively undifferentiated neoplastic cells underneath the mucosal surface (so-called cambium layer) in addition to spindled or strap-shaped cells with brightly eosinophilic cytoplasm within a loose myxoid stroma; these neoplastic cells are also positive for skeletal muscle markers, including MyoD1 and myogenin, antibodies directed against skeletal muscle-

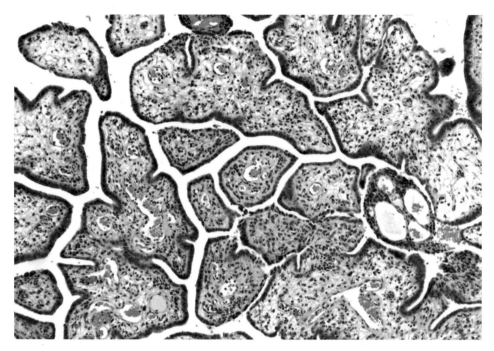

FIGURE 4.1
Müllerian papilloma. Papillary fronds are lined by bland cuboidal epithelium.

specific nuclear transcription factors. *Clear cell carcinoma* is distinguished by its nuclear atypia and mitotic activity as well as the presence of other characteristic growth patterns (e.g., tubulocystic, papillary and solid).

PROGNOSIS AND TREATMENT

Müllerian papilloma is treated with local excision. These lesions can recur, and rarely, may progress to a border-line-type neoplasm (i.e., cytologic atypia and conspicuous mitotic activity) and ultimately, a clear cell carcinoma may develop.

SPINDLE CELL EPITHELIOMA (MIXED TUMOR)

This uncommon tumor, characterized by a predominance of stromal-type cells with a minor component of glandular and/or squamous elements, lacks true myoepithelial differentiation as seen in neoplasms designated as mixed tumor at other anatomical sites. Therefore, the alternative designation of "spindle cell epithelioma" has been accepted.

CLINICAL FEATURES

Patients range in age from 20 to 80 (mean 40) years at presentation. Most cases are detected incidentally during

---

SPINDLE CELL EPITHELIOMA (MIXED TUMOR) – FACT SHEET

Definition
▸ Benign tumor with a predominance of stromal-type cells and a minor component of glandular/squamous elements

Incidence and Location
▸ Uncommon
▸ Usually lower posterior vaginal wall

Age Distribution
▸ 20–80 years

Clinical Features
▸ Most frequently an incidental finding
▸ Rarely, vaginal bleeding

Prognosis and Treatment
▸ Surgical excision
▸ Long-term follow-up required, as late recurrences can occur

routine pelvic examination as a submucosal mass typically located in the distal vagina.

PATHOLOGIC FEATURES

GROSS FINDINGS

Most tumors are located in the posterior wall close to the hymenal ring. They range in size from 1 to 9 cm,

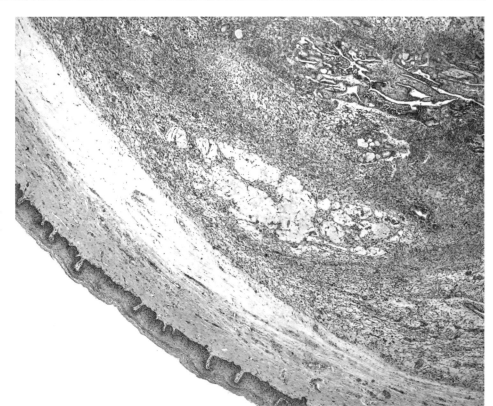

FIGURE 4.2
Spindle cell epithelioma (mixed tumor). A well-circumscribed tumor shows stromal-like and epithelial components (upper right).

SPINDLE CELL EPITHELIOMA (MIXED TUMOR) – PATHOLOGIC FEATURES

Gross Findings
▸ Well circumscribed
▸ Gray or white, gelatinous, soft, or rubbery
▸ 1 to 9 cm

Microscopic Findings
▸ Well-circumscribed, nonencapsulated, with an expansile margin
▸ Stromal component with diffuse, fascicular, nested, reticular, or cording patterns
▸ Myxomatous background may be present
▸ Bland, oval, round, or spindle shape stromal-like cells with rare or absent mitoses
▸ Minor epithelial component, either glandular or squamous (including morules) or both

Immunohistochemical Features
▸ Keratin AE1/E3 and CD10 positive in stromal-like cells
▸ Keratins 7 and 20, EMA, and muscle markers variably positive in stromal-like cells
▸ S-100 negative in stromal-like cells
▸ ER and PR can be positive in both the stromal-like and epithelial components

Ultrastructural Features
▸ Stromal-like cells lack myofibrils, pinocytotic vesicles, and basal lamina

Differential Diagnosis
▸ Smooth muscle tumor

---

and on sectioning they are well circumscribed, gray or white, and have a gelatinous, soft, or rubbery consistency.

MICROSCOPIC FINDINGS

The tumors are typically well circumscribed but not encapsulated (Figure 4.2). They are located within a few millimeters of the overlying squamous epithelium, but are not connected to it. The neoplastic stromal-like cells have scant cytoplasm and bland nuclei that range from oval or round to spindled. They can be arranged in sheets, fascicles, nests, or cords, or have a reticulate growth pattern (Figures 4.3 and 4.4); the background can appear myxomatous. Hyaline globules may be seen and are secondary to condensation of the stromal matrix. Mitotic figures are usually rare or absent. A minor epithelial component either glandular or squamous, is generally present (Figure 4.5). The glands are lined by cuboidal or columnar epithelium; they can have areas of squamous metaplasia or contain PAS-positive, diastase-sensitive luminal material. In some cases, there are no glandular elements but only numerous squamous morules.

ANCILLARY FEATURES

The spindle cells are usually positive for keratin AE1/E3 and CD10, and can be positive for keratin 7, keratin 20, and EMA, with a variable number of cells expressing

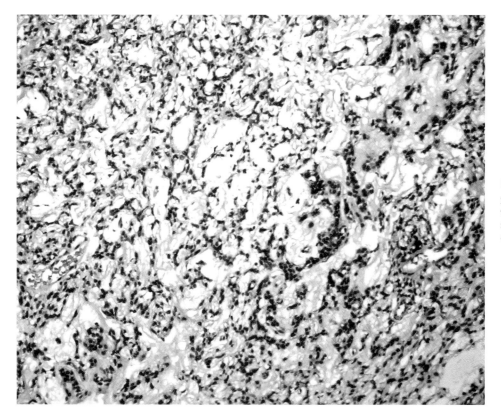

FIGURE 4.3

Spindle cell epithelioma (mixed tumor). A reticular pattern of the stromal-like cells is associated with a myxoid background.

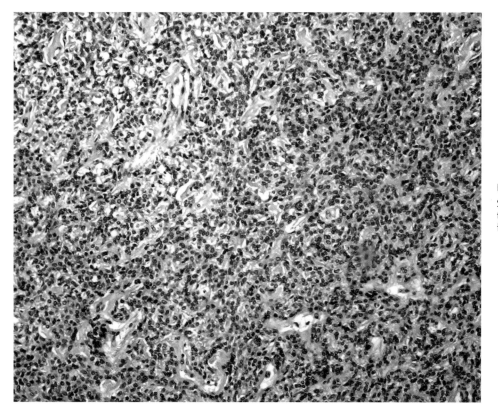

FIGURE 4.4

Spindle cell epithelioma (mixed tumor). The stromal-like cells form irregular anastomosing cords.

these markers. These cells can also express muscle actin, smooth-muscle actin, h-caldesmon, and desmin, but they are negative for S-100. Based on these findings, it has been suggested that this tumor may arise from a primitive pluripotential cell. Estrogen and progesterone receptors have been found to be positive in both components of the tumor. By electron microscopy, the stromal-like cells lack myofibrils with dense bodies, pinocytotic vesicles, and basal lamina, features typically seen in myoepithelial cells.

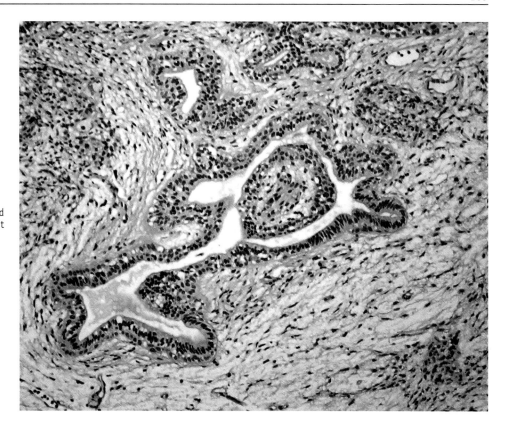

FIGURE 4.5
Spindle cell epithelioma (mixed tumor). The epithelial component shows irregularly shaped glands.

DIFFERENTIAL DIAGNOSIS

Mixed tumors may only have a focal epithelial component, thus mimicking a *smooth muscle tumor*. Extensive sampling is necessary to identify the epithelial and spindled components. A reticular growth pattern and a nonhomogeneous staining for smooth muscle markers favor a diagnosis of mixed tumor.

PROGNOSIS AND TREATMENT

This is a benign neoplasm that can recur locally even years after the initial diagnosis. Treatment consists of excision with re-excision if it recurs. Although rare cases of malignant mixed tumor have been reported, most of these tumors are best classified as malignant mesonephric tumors.

LEIOMYOMA

Leiomyoma is the most common benign mesenchymal tumor of the vagina.

CLINICAL FEATURES

Patients have a median age of 40 years at presentation and most are asymptomatic. When present, symptoms include vaginal bleeding or discharge, lower abdominal or vaginal pain, dyspareunia, frequency, dysuria, urinary retention, or a vaginal mass.

LEIOMYOMA – FACT SHEET

Definition
▶ Benign smooth muscle tumor

Incidence and Location
▶ Most common benign mesenchymal tumor of the vagina
▶ Typically submucosal

Age Distribution
▶ Mean age 40 years

Clinical Features
▶ Most often asymptomatic
▶ Vaginal bleeding or discharge
▶ Lower abdominal or vaginal pain
▶ Urinary symptoms

Prognosis and Treatment
▶ Benign
▶ Surgical excision
▶ Long time follow-up as recurrences may occur

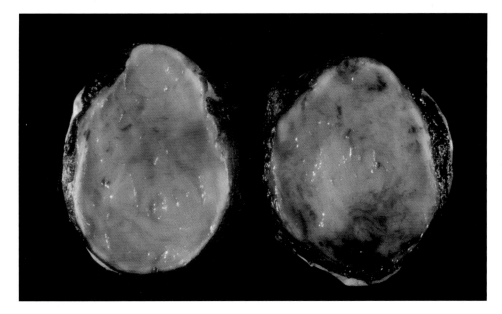

FIGURE 4.6

Leiomyoma. A well-circumscribed tumor displays a homogeneous rubbery and tan cut surface.

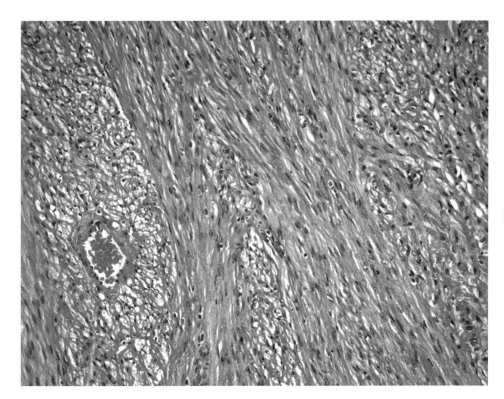

FIGURE 4.7

Leiomyoma. Elongated and bland-appearing smooth-muscle cells form intersecting fascicles.

PATHOLOGIC FEATURES

GROSS FINDINGS

Most leiomyomas are submucosal, but if large, they can become pedunculated. They usually range in size from 0.5 to 20 (median 3) cm. Leiomyomas may enlarge during pregnancy and partially involute postpartum. They are well-circumscribed with a firm cut surface (Figure 4.6); however, they may be soft or have cystic changes. Areas of hemorrhage or calcification can be seen.

MICROSCOPIC FINDINGS

Most tumors are composed of bland spindle-shaped cells arranged in intersecting fascicles (Figure 4.7) Histologic variants similar to those occurring in the uterus may be seen.

LEIOMYOMA – PATHOLOGIC FEATURES

Gross Findings
▸ Usually single, well circumscribed
▸ 0.5–20 (mean 3) cm
▸ Firm consistency
▸ Soft, cystic, calcified, or hemorrhagic areas may be seen

Microscopic Findings
▸ Intersecting fascicles of bland spindle-shaped cells
▸ Cells with eosinophilic cytoplasm and elongated nuclei with blunt ends
▸ Mitotic activity < 5/10 HPFs
▸ Mitoses and myxoid change more frequent in pregnant women
▸ Leiomyoma variants may be seen

Immunohistochemical Features
▸ Desmin, smooth muscle actin, and h-caldesmon positive

Differential Diagnosis
▸ Leiomyosarcoma
▸ Spindle cell epithelioma (mixed tumor)

ANCILLARY STUDIES

IMMUNOHISTOCHEMISTRY

The tumor cells stain with smooth-muscle markers including desmin, h-caldesmon, and smooth-muscle actin.

DIFFERENTIAL DIAGNOSIS

Leiomyosarcoma is the main entity to consider in the differential diagnosis. A tumor is considered benign if it: (1) shows no evidence of infiltration; (2) lacks significant cytologic atypia; (3) has a low mitotic index (< 5 mitoses/10 HPFs); and (4) lacks necrosis (see section on leiomyosarcoma for criteria of malignancy). As discussed earlier, *spindle cell epithelioma (mixed tumor)* may enter in the differential diagnosis if the epithelial component has not been sampled.

PROGNOSIS AND TREATMENT

This tumor is benign but has the potential to recur if incompletely excised. Thus, complete excision is the treatment of choice.

RHABDOMYOMA

In the female genital tract, the vagina is the most common site for this uncommon benign mesenchymal tumor showing skeletal muscle differentiation.

CLINICAL FEATURES

Patients range in age from 25 to 54 years and symptoms are typically related to the presence of a mass, including vaginal bleeding and pain.

RHABDOMYOMA – FACT SHEET

Definition
▸ Benign tumor of striated muscle

Incidence and Location
▸ Rare
▸ Most common location in the female gynecologic tract

Age Distribution
▸ Reproductive age and perimenopausal women

Clinical Features
▸ Vaginal bleeding
▸ Dyspareunia

Prognosis and Treatment
▸ Benign
▸ Local excision
▸ Rare recurrences

PATHOLOGIC FEATURES

GROSS FINDINGS

The neoplasms are frequently polypoid, measuring up to 3 cm with a white to gray elastic cut surface.

RHABDOMYOMA – PATHOLOGIC FEATURES

Gross Findings
▸ Polypoid (1–3 cm)
▸ White to gray elastic cut surface

Microscopic Findings
▸ Spindle cells with abundant eosinophilic cytoplasm containing cross-striations and no cytologic atypia or mitoses
▸ Background of loose connective tissue

Immunohistochemical Features
▸ Desmin, myoglobin, actin, and myosin positive

Differential Diagnosis
▸ Rhabdomyosarcoma botryoides

MICROSCOPIC FINDINGS

The tumor is composed of spindle-shaped muscle cells with abundant eosinophilic cytoplasm containing cross-striations within loose connective tissue (Figure 4.8). The cells have regular vesicular nuclei with conspicuous nucleoli but with no cytologic atypia or mitotic activity (Figure 4.9).

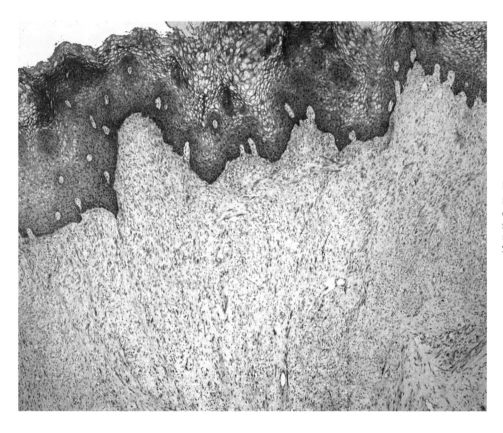

FIGURE 4.8

Rhabdomyoma. Elongated and eosinophilic rhabdomyoblasts are seen in a background of loose connective tissue (Courtesy of Dr. Elvio Silva).

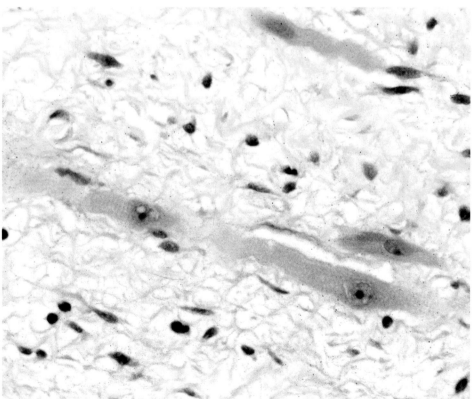

FIGURE 4.9

Rhabdomyoma. Rhabdomyoblasts show prominent cross-striations. (Courtesy of Dr. Elvio Silva).

ANCILLARY STUDIES

IMMUNOHISTOCHEMISTRY

The cells stain with actin, desmin, myoglobin, and myosin.

DIFFERENTIAL DIAGNOSIS

This neoplasm can be histologically differentiated from *rhabdomyosarcoma botryoides* by the lack of a cambium layer, cytologic atypia and mitoses. In addition, rhabdomyosarcoma occurs at a younger age, grows rapidly, and is associated with an infiltrative growth.

PROGNOSIS AND TREATMENT

Rhabdomyoma is treated with local excision. It may very rarely recur years aften excision.

PREMALIGNANT AND MALIGNANT EPITHELIAL NEOPLASMS

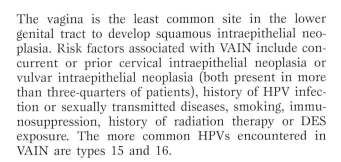

VAGINAL INTRAEPITHELIAL NEOPLASIA (VAIN)

The vagina is the least common site in the lower genital tract to develop squamous intraepithelial neoplasia. Risk factors associated with VAIN include concurrent or prior cervical intraepithelial neoplasia or vulvar intraepithelial neoplasia (both present in more than three-quarters of patients), history of HPV infection or sexually transmitted diseases, smoking, immunosuppression, history of radiation therapy or DES exposure. The more common HPVs encountered in VAIN are types 15 and 16.

CLINICAL FEATURES

Patients range in age from 16 to 84 years, with a mean age varying from 35 to 55 years, according to different series. Most patients are asymptomatic. The abnormality is frequently detected after colposcopic examination and biopsy for an abnormal Pap smear. Less commonly, a vaginal lesion is found during routine gynecologic examination, or patients present with symptoms such as recurrent vaginal discharge or vaginal bleeding.

VAGINAL INTRAEPITHELIAL NEOPLASIA (VAIN) – FACT SHEET

Definition
▶ Lesion characterized by variable degrees of atypia and maturation of the keratinocytes which is confined to the epithelium

Incidence and Location
▶ 0.2–0.3 per 100,000 women in US
▶ Upper third of the vagina most common location

Morbidity and Mortality
▶ 10–42% overall recurrence rate
▶ 2–12% rate of development of invasive squamous carcinoma

Age Distribution
▶ 16–84 (mean 35–55) years

Clinical Features
▶ Commonly asymptomatic
▶ Detection typically following Pap smear
▶ Rarely, vaginal bleeding or discharge

Prognosis and Treatment
▶ If untreated, ≤ 9% of patients followed ≥ 3 years develop invasive squamous carcinoma
▶ Low risk of progression in VAIN I; close observation suffices
▶ Treatment with either carbon dioxide laser or topical 5-fluorouracil if persistent VAIN I
▶ Surgical excision if VAIN II or III
▶ Treatment with carbon dioxide laser or topical 5-fluorouracil if invasion can be excluded in high-grade VAIN

PATHOLOGIC FEATURES

GROSS FINDINGS

Vaginal intraepithelial neoplasia is more common in the upper third of the vagina and is multifocal in approximately 50 % of cases. Usually, there is no grossly identifiable lesion; however, sometimes there are mucosal irregularities or color changes. The most common colposcopic abnormality is acetowhite epithelium followed by punctation and, rarely, mosaicism.

MICROSCOPIC FINDINGS

The lesion can be flat or exophytic, and depending on the degree and extent of the squamous atypia, is classified as VAIN I, VAIN II, and VAIN III. VAIN I (low-grade squamous intraepithelial lesion or mild dysplasia) encompasses lesions demonstrating koilocytosis (cells with thickened cell membranes, rigid and clear perinuclear halo, irregular nuclear contours, hyperchromatic nuclei, and binucleation) in the upper third of the epithelium and mild squamous atypia (i.e., mild nuclear variation and disorganization) confined to the lower third of the epithelium (Figure 4.10). VAIN II (high-grade squamous intraepithelial lesion or moderate dysplasia) encompasses lesions demonstrating moderate

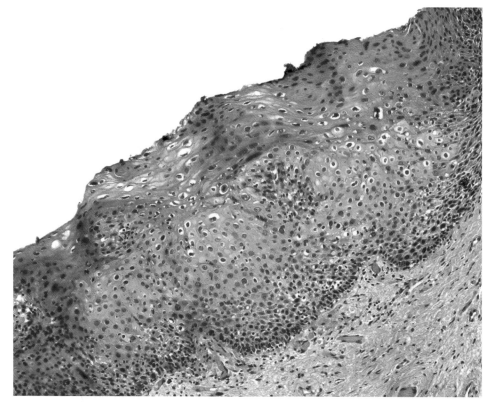

FIGURE 4.10
Vaginal intraepithelial neoplasia I. Prominent superficial koilocytosis with minimal squamous atypia of the basal layers is seen.

VAGINAL INTRAEPITHELIAL NEOPLASIA (VAIN) – PATHOLOGIC FEATURES

Gross Findings
▶ Often multifocal
▶ Commonly no gross lesion
▶ Less frequently, mucosal irregularities or color changes
▶ Acetowhite epithelium, punctation, and mosaicism by colposcopy

Microscopic Findings
▶ Exophytic or flat
▶ VAIN I: susperficial koilocytosis and mild squamous atypia confined to the lower third of the epithelium
▶ VAIN II: moderate squamous atypia confined to the lower two-thirds of the epithelium or marked atypia confined to the lower third of the epithelium. Koilocytes may be seen
▶ VAIN III: moderate to marked squamous atypia involving the full thickness of the epithelium. Koilocytes may be seen

Immunohistochemical Features
▶ VAIN I: Ki-67 positivity in the superficial two-thirds of the epithelium
▶ VAIN II and III: Ki-67 positivity throughout the entire epithelial thickness

Differential Diagnosis
▶ Nonspecific squamous hyperplasia
▶ Immature squamous metaplasia
▶ Reactive inflammatory atypia
▶ Atrophy
▶ Transitional cell metaplasia
▶ Pseudokoilocytosis
▶ Micropapillomatosis
▶ Radiation atypia

---

nuclear atypia (i.e., cell crowding, high nuclear-to-cytoplasmic ratio, significant variability in nuclear size, coarse chromatin, and frequent mitotic activity, including atypical mitoses) as well as cellular disorganization involving the lower two-thirds of the epithelium (Figure 4.11). Lesions with severe atypia or atypical mitotic figures confined to the lower third of the epithelium are also included in this category. VAIN III (high-grade squamous intraepithelial lesion or severe dysplasia/squamous carcinoma in situ) encompasses lesions demonstrating moderate to severe atypia reaching the upper third of the squamous epithelium with or without maturation of the surface epithelium (Figure 4.12). Koilocytosis can also be seen in VAIN II or III.

ANCILLARY STUDIES

IMMUNOHISTOCHEMISTRY

Ki67 or MIB-1 is a useful adjunct in the diagnosis of VAIN. In normal vaginal mucosa, Ki67 is only expressed in the parabasal nuclei of the squamous epithelium, whereas in VAIN I, Ki67 is positive in the upper two-thirds of the epithelium, and in VAIN II and III shows nuclear positivity throughout the entire thickness of the epithelium.

DIFFERENTIAL DIAGNOSIS

Nonspecific squamous hyperplasia displays acanthosis, hyperkeratosis and/or parakeratosis without evidence

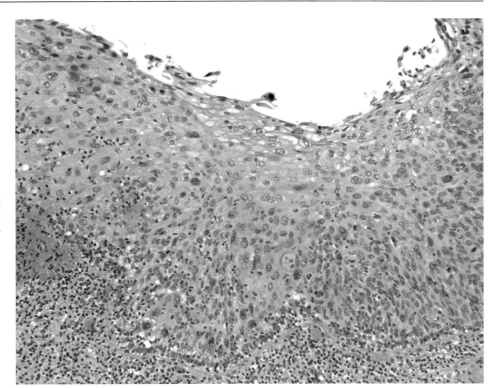

FIGURE 4.11

Vaginal intraepithelial neoplasia II. Cellular crowding, nuclear enlargement and hyperchromasia of the lower two thirds of the epithelium are associated with superficial maturation.

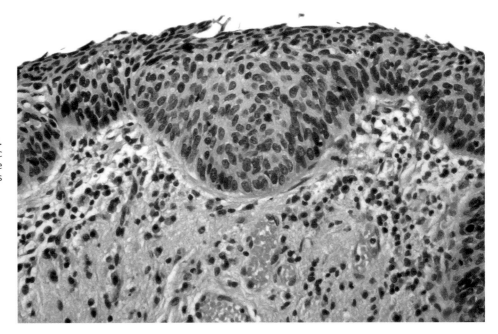

FIGURE 4.12

Vaginal intraepithelial neoplasia III. Severe cytologic atypia, mitotic activity, and loss of maturation are seen throughout the full thickness of the squamous epithelium.

of koilocytosis or cytologic atypia. *Immature squamous metaplasia* involving adenosis may show nuclear enlargement, but the chromatin is evenly distributed and there is no significant variation in nuclear shape or conspicuous mitotic activity. In *reactive inflammatory atypia*, the epithelial cells show increased nuclear/cytoplasmic ratio, nuclear hyperchromasia, and scattered

mitoses; however, the nuclei have evenly distributed chromatin and may have prominent nucleoli. No unequivocal koilocytosis is seen, and there is variable exocytosis as well as spongiosis associated with the squamous epithelium. *Atrophy* is characterized by loss of maturation, cells showing increased nuclear-to-cytoplasmic ratio, as well as dark evenly distributed chromatin. In contrast to VAIN, it lacks significant nuclear pleomorphism or mitotic activity. *Transitional cell metaplasia* may be confused with VAIN because it is associated with hypercellularity, lack of cellular maturation, and perinuclear halos. However, nuclei in the upper third of the epithelium are perpendicularly oriented to the basal epithelium nuclei (so-called streaming pattern), and they display frequent nuclear grooves, low nuclear-to-cytoplasmic ratio, and no mitotic activity. *Pseudokoilocytosis* is frequently seen with atrophic changes and is characterized by the presence of cytoplasmic clearing without significant nuclear enlargement or variation in shape. *Vaginal micropapillomatosis (mucosal excrescences)* has a papillomatous appearance, but shows no evidence of koilocytosis. Finally, in *radiation atypia*, the nuclei are enlarged, vary in size and shape, and display dark chromatin, but the nuclear-to-cytoplasmic ratio is low, mitoses are absent or rare, and the stroma and vessels appear hyalinized.

PROGNOSIS AND TREATMENT

The overall recurrence rate of VAIN ranges from 10 to 42%. The associated rate of development of invasive squamous cell carcinoma in patients treated for this condition ranges from 2 to 12%, whereas up to 9% of patients with untreated VAIN and followed for at least 3 years develop invasive squamous cell carcinoma. Since patients with VAIN I have a low risk of progression to high-grade lesions, they should be followed. Patients with persistent disease are treated with either carbon dioxide (CO_2) laser or topical 5-fluorouracil. High-grade VAIN (II and III) is usually treated with surgical excision, especially for lesions located in the upper vagina, since the incidence of occult carcinoma arising in high-grade VAIN at this site can be as high as 12%. If invasion is excluded, patients can be treated with CO_2 laser ablation or topical 5-fluorouracil.

SQUAMOUS CELL CARCINOMA

This tumor represents only 1% of all malignant tumors of the female genital tract, but accounts for 80% of those arising in the vagina. According to the International Federation of Gynecologists and Obstetrics (FIGO), a tumor should be classified as a vaginal primary if this organ is the primary site of growth. Thus, a tumor that involves the vagina and cervix should be considered as a cervical primary; a tumor that involves the vagina and the vulva should be considered primary in the vulva, and a tumor that affects the vagina and the urethra should be considered a primary urethral carcinoma. Furthermore, a squamous cell carcinoma occurring in the vagina within 5 years of treatment for cervical/vulvar cancer is considered to be a recurrence of the cervical/vulvar tumor rather than a new primary.

Risk factors include trauma to the vagina associated with parity, prolapse, or chronic use of pessary, HPV infection, low socioeconomic status, smoking, previous pelvic radiation therapy or hysterectomy, history of cervical neoplasia or vaginal intraepithelial lesion, and immunosuppression, as seen in patients with HIV infection.

CLINICAL FEATURES

Vaginal squamous carcinoma can occur in patients ranging in age from 16 to 95 years. However, it is most commonly seen in patients in the sixth and seventh

---

SQUAMOUS CELL CARCINOMA – FACT SHEET

Definition
- A carcinoma demonstrating squamous differentiation (i.e., keratin formation and/or intercellular bridges)
- Diagnosis after exclusion of cervical, vulvar, and urethral origin

Incidence and Location
- 80% of malignant vaginal tumors
- Relatively infrequent (0.42–0.93 per 100,000 women)
- 1000 new cases per year in the US
- Predominantly involves the upper third of the vagina

Race and Age Distribution
- Higher incidence among Caucasians
- Most common in postmenopausal women (range 16–95 years)

Morbidity and Mortality
- Tumor behavior depends on stage
- 73% relative 5-year survival rate for stage I disease
- 58% relative 5-year survival rate for stage II disease, and 36% for stages III–IV
- Risk factors: trauma, HPV, low social economical status, smoking, pelvic radiation, previous hysterectomy, history of cervical neoplasia or VAIN, and immunosuppression

Clinical Features
- Vaginal bleeding, discharge, dyspareunia, or pain
- Urinary symptoms
- Rarely asymptomatic; may be detected by routine Pap smear or physical examination

Radiologic Features
- T1- or T2-predominant images of medium or high signal intensity on MRI
- Higher detection of vaginal tumor and abnormal lymph nodes by fluorodeoxyglucose positron emission tomography than CT-scan

Prognosis and Treatment
- Radiotherapy, including brachytherapy and external-beam radiation treatment of choice
- Surgery in selected cases

decades. The most common symptom at presentation is vaginal bleeding, followed by vaginal discharge or pain, urinary symptoms, and dyspareunia. Some patients are asymptomatic and the tumor is detected by routine Pap smear or physical examination. The tumor can occasionally occur during pregnancy and in patients with neovagina.

SQUAMOUS CELL CARCINOMA – PATHOLOGIC FEATURES

Gross Findings

▸ Exophytic, ulcerating, or infiltrative
▸ Variable size (millimeters to > 10 cm)

Microscopic Findings

▸ Well, moderately, or poorly differentiated
▸ Keratinizing or nonkeratinizing
▸ Spindle, verrucous, and warty subtypes

Differential Diagnosis

▸ Tangentially sectioned squamous cell carcinoma in situ
▸ Radiation-induced atypia
▸ Epithelioid trophoblastic tumor and placental site trophoblastic tumor
▸ Melanoma
▸ Sarcomas composed of epithelioid cells

RADIOLOGIC FEATURES

These tumors can be detected on MRI as T1- or T2-predominant images of medium or high signal intensity (i.e., loss of the normal low signal intensity of the vaginal wall). Positron emission tomography and F-19 fluorodeoxyglucose detect a vaginal tumor and abnormal lymph nodes more often than CT-scan.

PATHOLOGIC FEATURES

GROSS FINDINGS

Invasive squamous cell carcinomas can be exophytic, ulcerating, or infiltrative, and they are most frequently seen in the upper third of the vagina involving the posterior wall. Tumor size varies from a few millimeters to > 10 cm.

MICROSCOPIC FINDINGS

The neoplasms are composed of malignant squamous cells, and depending on the degree of differentiation, they are classified as well (Figure 4.13), moderately, or poorly differentiated (Figure 4.14); they can also be keratinizing or nonkeratinizing. Verrucous, warty, and spindle squamous cell carcinomas may occur in the

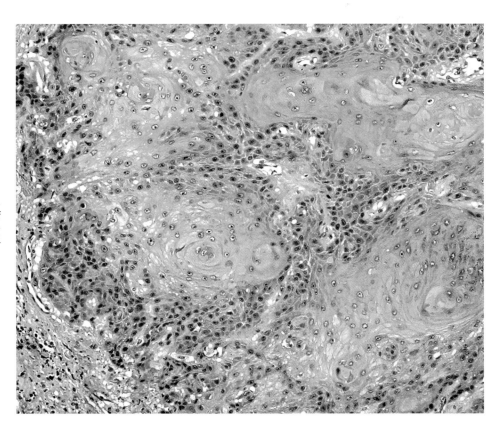

FIGURE 4.13
Invasive well-differentiated squamous cell carcinoma. Nests of tumor cells with abundant eosinophilic cytoplasm show central keratinization.

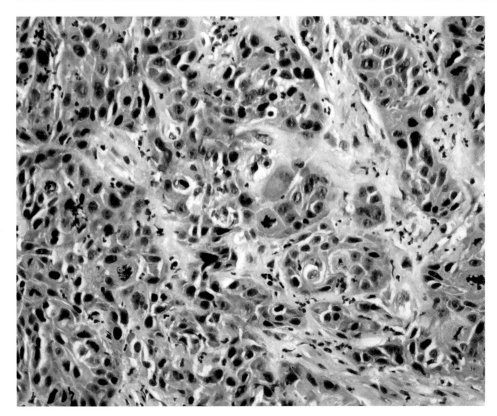

FIGURE 4.14

Invasive poorly differentiated squamous cell carcinoma. The tumor cells have scant eosinophilic cytoplasm, high-grade cytologic features, and lack keratinization.

vagina, but much less frequently than in the vulva. Tumors with papillary architecture represent a diagnostic challenge in small biopsies, since invasion cannot be assessed and complete removal is required for a definitive diagnosis of invasive squamous carcinoma.

DIFFERENTIAL DIAGNOSIS

Tangential sectioning of a *squamous cell carcinoma in situ* may represent an important diagnostic challenge, as the undulating architecture at the base of the neoplastic proliferation may be interpreted as invasive nests secondary to poor orientation (pseudoinvasion). To establish a definitive diagnosis of invasive squamous cell carcinoma, one of the following features must be identified: (1) excessive reduplication of the neoplastic squamous epithelium; (2) desmoplastic stromal response; or (3) irregularly shaped/ragged nests of neoplastic squamous epithelium in the stroma. The pseudoinvasive nests in carcinoma in situ are regular in shape and size and do not elicit a stromal response. *Radiation-induced atypia* of the squamous epithelium may also cause concern for either in situ or invasive carcinoma. Attention to the cytologic features typically seen in radiation atypia, including squamous cells with enlarged nuclei and abundant cytoplasm, as well as atypical spindle stromal cells with smudgy chromatin that lack mitotic activity which may be associated with dense fibrosis/hyalinization, will facilitate the correct diagnosis. *Trophoblastic tumors (epithelioid trophoblastic tumor and*

placental-site trophoblastic tumor) may simulate a squamous cell carcinoma because they are composed of cells with abundant eosinophilic cytoplasm and are associated with eosinophilic material that may simulate keratin. However, in contrast to squamous cell carcinoma, trophoblastic tumors are negative for p16 (or only focally positive), but are positive for inhibin and CK18. They also show variable expression of human placental lactogen, human chorionic gonadotropin and Mel-Cam. Much less frequently, *melanoma and sarcomas* composed of epithelioid cells may enter into the differential diagnosis. The finding of more conventional areas of squamous cell neoplasia as well as immunoperoxidase studies will help to establish the correct diagnosis.

PROGNOSIS AND TREATMENT

The behavior of squamous cell carcinoma is related to FIGO stage (Table 4.1) and the overall survival rate is relatively poor (approximately 46%). The relative 5-year survival rate for stage I disease is 73%, whereas for stages II and III–IV tumors it drops to 58% and 36% respectively. Tumors with superficial invasion (< 2.5 mm) and no vascular/lymphatic invasion appear to have a low risk of nodal metastases. Recently, only three factors have been proved to independently predict poor survival: (1) older age at diagnosis; (2) large size (≥ 4 cm); and (3) advanced stage. Tumors located at the vaginal apex appear to have a better prognosis. Radia-

TABLE 4.1

Carcinoma of the vagina: International Federation of Gynecologists and Obstetrics staging nomenclature

Stage	Description
0	Carcinoma in situ
I	Carcinoma is limited to the vaginal wall
II	Carcinoma has involved the subvaginal tissue but has not extended to the pelvic wall
III	Carcinoma has extended to the pelvic wall
IV	Carcinoma has extended beyond the true pelvis or has involved the mucosa of the bladder or rectum; bullous edema as such does not permit a case to be allotted to stage IV
IVa	Tumor invades bladder and/or rectal mucosa and/or direct extension beyond the true pelvis
IVb	Spread to distant organs

tion therapy, including brachytherapy and external-beam radiation, is the primary treatment of choice. Surgical treatment may be indicated in selected cases, such as in early-stage tumors or those with central recurrence following radiotherapy.

ADENOCARCINOMA

Primary adenocarcinomas of the vagina are uncommon, representing at the most 14 % of all carcinomas at this site. Of note, < 20 % of adenocarcinomas involving the vagina are primaries in this organ. Therefore, the diagnosis of adenocarcinoma in the vagina should raise the possibility of metastasis or local spread from a neoplasm arising in an adjacent organ. Associations with adenosis, endometriosis, endocervicosis, and mesonephric remnants, or with 5-fluorouracil treatment for condyloma may occur.

CLINICAL FEATURES

In patients with a history of intrauterine DES exposure, adenocarcinomas of the vagina are of the clear cell type with a peak incidence around 20 years. The risk of developing adenocarcinoma is higher when the drug was initiated before the 18th week of gestation. If there is no history of DES exposure, vaginal adenocarcinoma is usually seen in women between 46 and 67 years; however, it rarely can occur in patients as young as 5 years. Symptoms at presentation are not specific and include vaginal bleeding or discharge, and dyspareunia.

ADENOCARCINOMA – FACT SHEET

Definition
▶ A carcinoma demonstrating glandular differentiation

Incidence and Location
▶ Extremely uncommon
▶ 14% of all vaginal carcinomas
▶ < 20% of adenocarcinomas are primary at this site
▶ Commonly anterior wall of upper third of vagina in clear cell adenocarcinoma
▶ May be centered in vaginal wall with secondary mucosal extension in endometrioid, mucinous and mesonephric carcinomas

Morbidity and Mortality
▶ Poor relapse-free survival (48% versus 72% for squamous cell carcinoma)

Age Distribution
▶ Clear cell carcinoma:
  ▶ If intrauterine DES, patients in their 20s
  ▶ If no intrauterine DES, 46–67 years

Clinical Features
▶ Vaginal bleeding, discharge, or dyspareunia

Prognosis and Treatment
▶ Tumor stage most important prognostic factor
▶ Overall 5-year survival rate of 60–80% for clear cell carcinoma, increasing to 100% for patients with stage I tumors
▶ Better prognosis if association with DES
▶ Pelvic or para-aortic lymph node involvement in 15%
▶ Metastases to lungs in 20%
▶ Radiotherapy treatment of choice
▶ Very limited experience with endometrioid, mucinous and mesonephric adenocarcinomas

PATHOLOGIC FEATURES

GROSS FINDINGS

Clear cell carcinomas arise more commonly in the anterior wall of the upper third of the vagina and they may range from large, polypoid to papillary or ulcerated masses (Figure 4.15). Endometrioid, mucinous, and mesonephric carcinomas may be centered in the vaginal wall and secondarily extend to the mucosa.

MICROSCOPIC FINDINGS

The most common histologic subtypes of adenocarcinoma include clear cell, endometrioid, mucinous, and mesonephric carcinoma.

Clear cell adenocarcinoma has a histologic appearance that overlaps with that seen in its more common uterine and ovarian counterparts. It typically shows several architectural patterns, including tubulocystic (Figure 4.16), papillary, and solid, either as a single pattern or

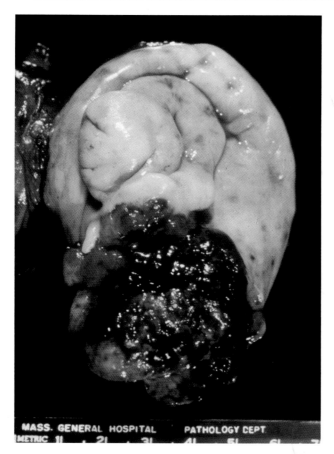

FIGURE 4.15
Clear cell carcinoma. A large exophytic mass associated with extensive ulceration and hemorrhage is arising from the vaginal wall.

more commonly admixed. The neoplastic cells have clear or eosinophilic cytoplasm and hobnail cells may be seen in the tubulocystic and papillary patterns. These tumors frequently show moderate to severe cytologic atypia and brisk mitotic activity (Figure 4.17). The tumor may be seen next to areas of adenosis.

Endometrioid adenocarcinoma closely resembles the morphology of endometrioid carcinomas seen in the endometrium. It is composed of endometrioid-type glands with variable degrees of complexity lined by columnar to cuboidal cells lacking intracellular mucin. It may be seen in association with adenosis or endometriosis (Figure 4.18).

Mucinous adenocarcinoma is very rare in the vagina and can be either of endocervical or enteric type, the latter being characterized by the presence of goblet cells. It may be seen in association with adenosis, endocervicosis, or intestinal-type adenoma or may arise in a neovagina.

Mesonephric adenocarcinoma is commonly composed of tightly packed glands or tubules lined by flat to cuboidal to columnar cells (ductal pattern) with variable degrees of cytologic atypia that frequently contain dense eosinophilic luminal material (Figure 4.19). Mesonephric remnants can be detected at the periphery and are centered in the vaginal wall.

ADENOCARCINOMA – PATHOLOGIC FEATURES

Gross Findings

▶ Polypoid to papillary +/− ulceration
▶ Variable size

Microscopic Findings

Clear Cell Adenocarcinoma

▶ Tubulocystic, papillary, or solid patterns
▶ Clear and/or eosinophilic cells and variable number of hobnail cells
▶ Moderate to severe cytologic atypia and brisk mitotic activity
▶ Association with adenosis

Endometrioid Adenocarcinoma

▶ Glands with variable complexity lined by columnar to cuboidal epithelium similar to that seen in endometrial endometrioid carcinoma
▶ Association with adenosis or endometriosis

Mucinous Adenocarcinoma

▶ Glands with variable complexity lined by endocervical or enteric type (including goblet) cells
▶ Association with adenosis, endocervicosis, or intestinal-type adenoma

Mesonephric Adenocarcinoma

▶ Tightly packed tubules or glands usually filled with eosinophilic material and showing variable degrees of cytologic atypia
▶ Frequent association with mesonephric remnants

Immunohistochemical Features

▶ Leu-M1 (CD15) and CK7 positive in clear cell adenocarcinoma
▶ ER and PR negative in clear cell adenocarcinoma
▶ Vimentin and keratin 7 positive in endometrioid adenocarcinoma
▶ Variable CD10 and calretinin expression in endometrioid adenocarcinoma
▶ Variable expression of CEA and keratins 7 and 20 in mucinous adenocarcinoma
▶ Vimentin, CD10, and calretinin positive in mesonephric adenocarcinoma
▶ ER and PR negative in mesonephric adenocarcinoma

Differential Diagnosis

▶ Metastases
▶ Clear cell adenocarcinoma (vs mesonephric adenocarcinoma)
▶ Endometrioid adenocarcinoma (vs mesonephric adenocarcinoma)
▶ Direct extension from colonic carcinoma (vs intestinal-type mucinous adenocarcinoma)

ANCILLARY STUDIES

IMMUNOHISTOCHEMISTRY

Clear cell adenocarcinoma stains for a variety of keratins, including CK7; it is also positive for Leu-M1 (CD-15), but is negative for ER and PR. Endometrioid adenocarcinoma is typically positive for cytokeratin 7, vimentin, ER, and PR. Mucinous adenocarcinoma shows variable expression of CEA and keratins 7 and 20. Mesonephric adenocarcinoma is typically positive for CD10, calretinin, and vimentin, but negative for ER and PR.

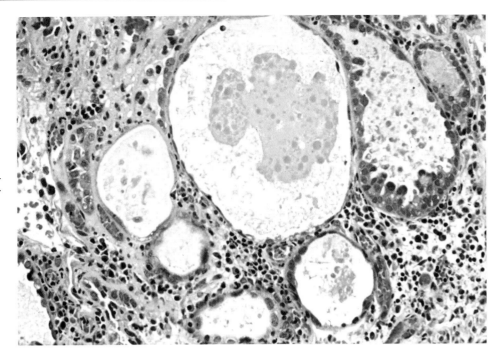

FIGURE 4.16

Clear cell adenocarcinoma. A tubulocystic pattern is seen. Note the presence of hobnail cells.

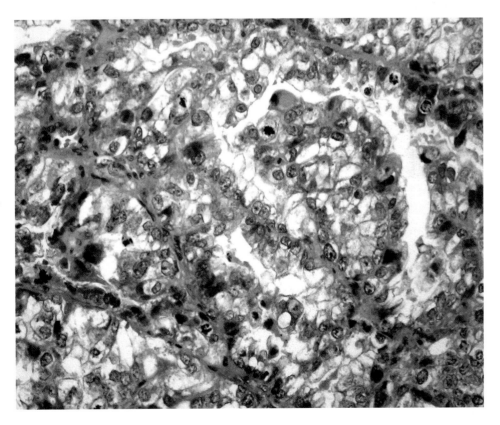

FIGURE 4.17

Clear cell adenocarcinoma. Tumor cells with abundant clear cytoplasm display marked cytologic atypia and brisk mitotic activity.

DIFFERENTIAL DIAGNOSIS

Exclusion of *metastases* is the main consideration in the differential diagnosis. However, in most cases, it is not possible on histological grounds alone to determine with certainty if the tumor arises in the vagina or represents a metastasis. Therefore, clinical correlation is required to make this distinction. Among primary adenocarcino-

mas of the vagina, *clear cell adenocarcinoma* may be confused with mesonephric adenocarcinoma. However, the former usually occurs in younger women with a history of intrauterine exposure to DES. It shows different architectural patterns with clear cells and hobnail cells, as well as a different immunohistochemical profile. *Endometrioid adenocarcinoma* may also be difficult to distinguish from mesonephric adenocarcinoma, as both

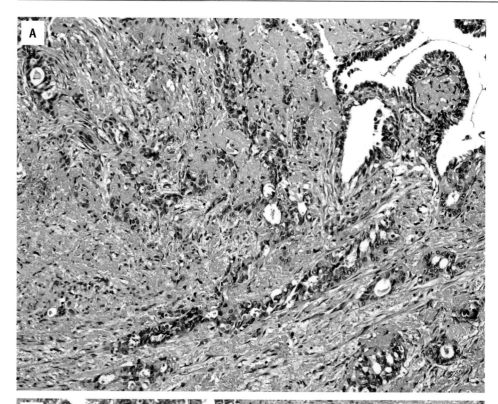

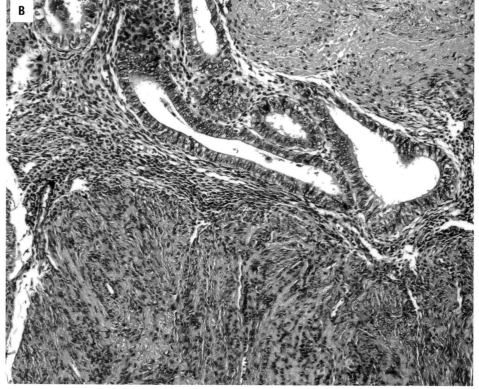

FIGURE 4.18

Endometrioid adenocarcinoma. Irregularly shaped glands have an infiltrative growth pattern (A). The adenocarcinoma is adjacent to an area of endometriosis (B) (Courtesy of Dr. Michael T. Deavers).

show prominent glandular architecture, and endometrioid adenocarcinoma may also display the eosinophilic secretions seen in mesonephric adenocarcinomas and may be positive for calretinin or CD10. The finding of endometriosis or mesonephric remnants as well as the use of a panel of antibodies including ER may be helpful in their distinction. The rare mucinous enteric-type adenocarcinoma should be distinguished from direct extension of a *colonic adenocarcinoma*. As immunohistochemistry is not helpful, clinical correlation and/or the finding of an intestinal-type adenoma are needed to definitively categorize the site of origin.

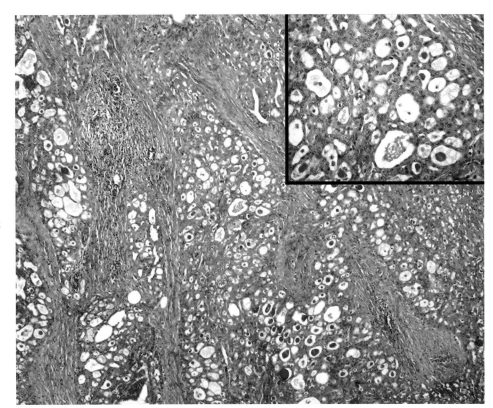

FIGURE 4.19
Mesonephric adenocarcinoma. The tumor shows back to back and cribriform glands containing abundant eosinophilic material (inset).

PROGNOSIS AND TREATMENT

Patients with clear cell adenocarcinoma have an overall 60–80% 5-year survival rate, increasing to 100% for patients with stage I tumors. Prognosis is primarily determined by tumor stage, but patients with carcinomas associated with DES exposure have a better prognosis. Tumors tend to exhibit local extension or spread to pelvic or para-aortic lymph nodes (15%) and/or lungs (20%). Radiotherapy is the treatment of choice. Surgery is indicated in selected cases. Experience with the other subtypes of adenocarcinoma is very limited.

MALIGNANT MESENCHYMAL NEOPLASMS

EMBRYONAL RHABDOMYOSARCOMA

This is the most common vaginal neoplasm in children. When the tumor has a polypoid configuration, it is referred to as "sarcoma botryoides."

CLINICAL FEATURES

Most patients are children, usually under 5 years of age; however, it can rarely occur in postmenopausal women.

EMBRYONAL RHABDOMYOSARCOMA – FACT SHEET

Definition
▶ Malignant tumor of striated muscle
▶ "Sarcoma botryoides" if polypoid

Incidence and Location
▶ Most common vaginal tumor in children
▶ Usually anterior vaginal wall

Morbidity and Mortality
▶ Recurrences usually within 5 years after diagnosis

Age Distribution
▶ Most patients children < 5 years
▶ Rarely in postmenopausal patients

Clinical Features
▶ Vaginal bleeding
▶ Mass that may protrude from introitus

Prognosis and Treatment
▶ Overall survival ≥ 90%
▶ Surgery in combination with chemotherapy treatment of choice

Patients present with vaginal bleeding and/or a vaginal mass that may protrude from the introitus.

PATHOLOGIC FEATURES

GROSS FINDINGS

This tumor frequently arises in the anterior vaginal wall. It is usually soft and polypoid, with multiple nodules having a grape-like configuration.

MICROSCOPIC FINDINGS

Embryonal rhabdomyosarcoma is characterized at low-power magnification by a cambium layer that is defined as a subepithelial layer of condensed rhabdomyoblasts separated from an intact epithelium by a zone of loose connective tissue (Figure 4.20). This feature must be present in at least one microscopic field to make the diagnosis of rhabdomyosarcoma of the botryoid subtype. The tumor has alternating hypo- and hypercellular areas, the former being typically edematous and/or myxoid. The neoplastic cells range from small and primitive in appearance with scanty cytoplasm, to cells with definitive rhabdomyoblastic differentiation and cross-striations. Mitotic activity is brisk and easy to identify in areas containing less-differentiated cells. Small islands of cartilage may be present, similar to its cervical counterpart.

EMBRYONAL RHABDOMYOSARCOMA – PATHOLOGIC FEATURES

Gross Findings
▸ Soft, polypoid with a grape-like configuration

Microscopic Findings
▸ Subepithelial layer of condensed small blue cells (rhabdomyoblasts) separated from an intact epithelium by a zone of loose stroma (cambium layer)
▸ Alternating hypo- and hypercellular areas, the former typically edematous/myxoid
▸ Cells ranging from small and primitive to those with definitive evidence of rhabdomyoblastic differentiation (cross-striations)
▸ Brisk mitotic activity, especially in less differentiated cells
▸ Small islands of cartilage may be seen

Immunohistochemical and Ultrastructural Features
▸ Desmin, myogenin, and myo-D1 positive
▸ Cytoplasmic thin and thick fibrils as well as Z-bands

Differential Diagnosis
▸ Fibroepithelial polyp
▸ Rhabdomyoma

ANCILLARY STUDIES

Desmin, myogenin, and myo-D1 are helpful in determining the rhabdomyoblastic nature of the tumor cells

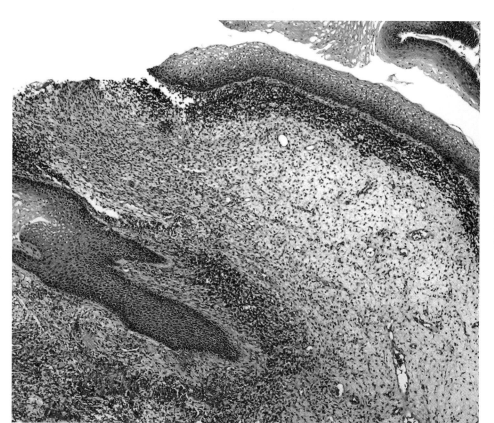

FIGURE 4.20
Embryonal rhabdomyosarcoma. A dense subepithelial "cambium layer" is present.

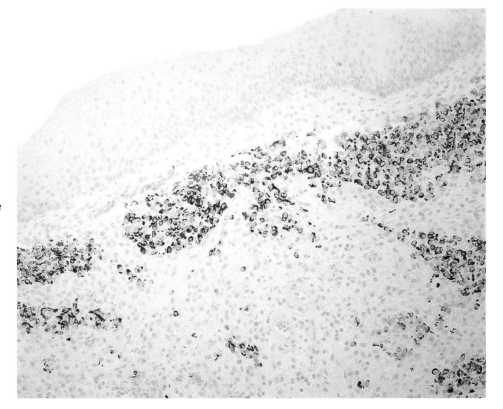

FIGURE 4.21
Embryonal rhabdomyosarcoma. The tumor cells are desmin-positive.

(Figure 4.21). By electron microscopy, this tumor is characterized by the presence of cytoplasmic thin and thick fibrils as well as Z-bands.

DIFFERENTIAL DIAGNOSIS

Fibroepithelial polyp with atypical cells and *rhabdomyoma* are the main entities in the differential diagnosis. However, both lack the "cambium layer" as well as the primitive small cells. Fibroepithelial polyp also lacks cells with cross-striations and is frequently seen in pregnant women, while rhabdomyoma is composed of mature rhabdomyoblasts.

PROGNOSIS AND TREATMENT

The overall survival of patients with vaginal rhabdomyosarcoma is currently 90% or higher. It has improved notably with the use of surgery in combination with chemotherapy. Recurrences usually occur within the first 5 years after diagnosis.

LEIOMYOSARCOMA

CLINICAL FEATURES

This is an uncommon tumor, accounting for < 1% of all vaginal neoplasms; however, it represents the most common vaginal sarcoma of adults. Patients' ages range from 25 to 86 (average 47) years. They more commonly present with vaginal bleeding and pain, but may be asymptomatic.

PATHOLOGIC FEATURES

GROSS FINDINGS

Leiomyosarcomas tend to occur more frequently in the posterior wall, can be exophytic or intramural, and range in size from 2 to > 10 cm.

MICROSCOPIC FINDINGS

The histologic appearances are similar to those encountered in uterine leiomyosarcoma. The criteria used to diagnose a malignant smooth muscle tumor

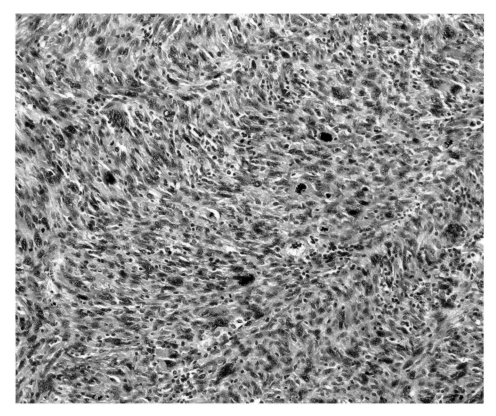

FIGURE 4.22
Leiomyosarcoma. The tumor cells form intersecting fascicles and show marked cytologic atypia.

include the presence of moderate or marked cytologic atypia and the finding of at least 5 mitoses/10 HPFs (Figure 4.22); coagulative tumor cell necrosis and infiltrative margins are also associated with malignant behavior.

ANCILLARY STUDIES

IMMUNOHISTOCHEMISTRY

The tumor cells variably express h-caldesmon, desmin, and/or smooth muscle actin, depending on the degree of differentiation.

DIFFERENTIAL DIAGNOSIS

The principal differential diagnostic considerations include *spindle squamous cell carcinoma and melanoma*. The finding of an in situ component, areas indicative of squamous (keratinization) or melanocytic (melanin pigment) differentiation are useful histologic features. In addition, melanoma is positive for melanoma marker (S-100, HMB-45, Melan-A, Mart-1) and squamous cell carcinoma typically shows diffuse keratin and EMA expression. Although smooth muscle tumors may be positive for keratin and EMA, they stain for smooth muscle markers, which are negative in squamous cell carcinoma.

PROGNOSIS AND TREATMENT

The overall 5-year survival rate for patients with leiomyosarcoma is 43%. Pulmonary metastases as well as local recurrences are common. Surgery is the treatment of choice, and adjuvant radiotherapy with or without chemotherapy has not improved patient survival.

OTHER PRIMARY MALIGNANT VAGINAL TUMORS

MELANOMA

This neoplasm accounts for < 3% of all malignant tumors of the vagina, < 10% of melanomas of the female genital tract, and < 0.3% of melanomas overall.

CLINICAL FEATURES

Patients range in age from 36 to 91 years, but are more commonly postmenopausal. Most patients are Caucasian and present with vaginal bleeding, discharge, or a

---

MELANOMA – FACT SHEET

Definition

‣ Malignant tumor composed of melanocytes

Incidence and Location

‣ < 3.0% of malignant tumors of the vagina
‣ < 10% of melanomas of the female genital tract
‣ < 0.3% of melanomas overall
‣ More frequent in anterior and lateral walls and lower third of vagina

---

Race and Age Distribution

‣ Commonly Caucasian
‣ Predominance in postmenopausal women (range 36–91 years)

Clinical Features

‣ Vaginal bleeding or discharge
‣ Pigmented lesion

Prognosis and Treatment

‣ Overall 5-year survival 13–21% with a median survival of 20 months
‣ Stage most important factor
‣ No standard treatment
‣ Improved clinical outcome if surgical removal of gross disease
‣ Sentinel lymph node biopsy adopted as a less morbid alternative to determine lymph node status
‣ Radiotherapy in patients with unresectable disease

MELANOMA – PATHOLOGIC FEATURES

Gross Findings

‣ Usually polypoid, may be flat or ulcerated
‣ Commonly pigmented (> 90%)
‣ Variable size, from 0.5 cm to involve entire vagina
‣ Satellite nodules and concurrent vaginal melanosis may be seen

---

Microscopic Findings

‣ Solid, nested, and trabecular patterns
‣ Epithelioid or spindle cells (less frequent)
‣ Rarely pleomorphic cells, signet-ring cells, and small cells mimicking lymphocytes and cells with cytoplasmic clearing
‣ Melanin pigment present at least focally
‣ Brisk mitotic activity (> 5 mitoses per mm^2)
‣ Radial growth phase (i.e., neoplastic melanocytes in or near the basal layer) usually seen

---

Immunohistochemical Features

‣ S-100 most sensitive marker
‣ Tyrosinase and Melan-A useful if S-100 negative
‣ Up to 23% of cases HMB-45 negative
‣ Spindle cell melanomas usually positive for S-100 but negative for other melanocytic markers

---

Differential Diagnosis

‣ Carcinoma, poorly differentiated or small cell
‣ Sarcoma
‣ Metastatic melanoma

---

vaginal mass. Occasionally, the tumor can be detected on a Pap smear.

PATHOLOGIC FEATURES

GROSS FINDINGS

Melanoma more frequently involves the anterior and lateral walls, and often is located in the lower third of the vagina. It ranges from 0.5 cm to very large lesions that may involve the length of the vagina. It is usually polypoid, although it can be flat or ulcerated. Non-pigmented tumors are uncommon (< 10%). Satellite nodules can be seen, as well as concurrent vaginal melanosis.

MICROSCOPIC FINDINGS

The tumor is composed of epithelioid cells (Figure 4.23), epithelioid and spindle cells or, less frequently, of spindle cells exclusively. The tumor cells can be arranged in a variety of patterns, including solid, nested, and trabecular, but frequently they are admixed. Pleomorphic cells, signet-ring cells, cells with cytoplasmic clearing, and small cells mimicking lymphocytes can be seen. At least some of the cells will contain melanin pigment.

Mitotic activity tends to be high (> 5 mitoses per mm^2) and a radial growth phase (i.e., neoplastic melanocytes in or near the basal layer) is usually identified. According to the Chung's level (i.e., tumor thickness measured from the outermost point of the mucosa to the point of deepest invasion), most tumors are level IV.

ANCILLARY STUDIES

IMMUNOHISTOCHEMISTRY

S-100 is the most sensitive marker for the diagnosis of vaginal melanoma (Figure 4.24). Tyrosinase and Melan-A (Mart-1) are useful when S-100 is negative or only focally positive. Up to 23% of these tumors can be negative for HMB-45. Melanomas composed of spindle cells are likely to be positive for S-100 but negative for other melanocytic markers.

DIFFERENTIAL DIAGNOSIS

The main differential diagnosis includes *carcinoma* (either poorly differentiated or small cell), *high grade-*

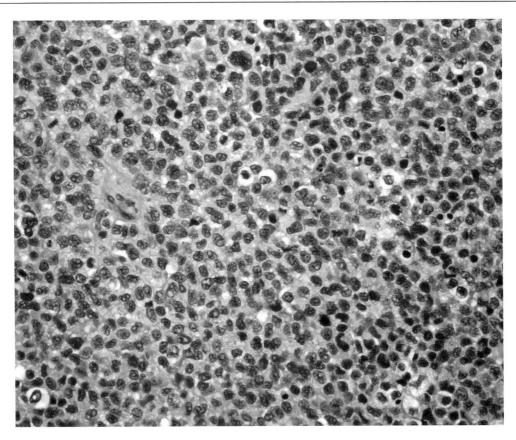

FIGURE 4.23
Malignant melanoma. The tumor cells grow in sheets and have an epithelioid appearance.

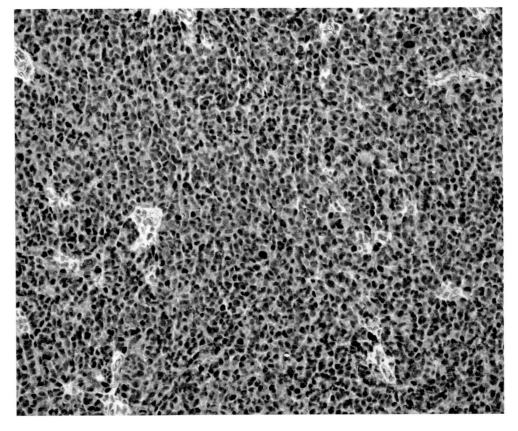

FIGURE 4.24
Malignant melanoma. The tumor cells show diffuse S-100-positivity.

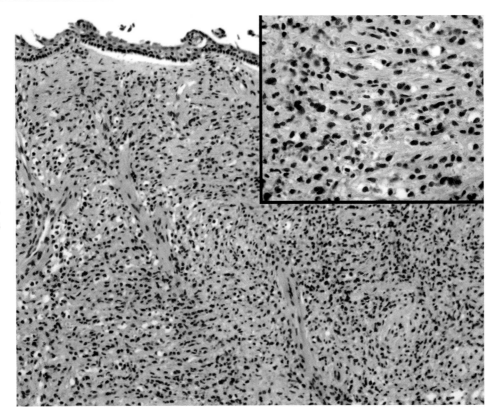

FIGURE 4.25
Secondary involvement by leukemia. Diffuse and monotonous infiltrate of medium-sized myeloid cells (inset).

sarcoma, and, very rarely, *metastatic melanoma*. Immunohistochemistry as well as extensive sampling, when possible, will facilitate a correct diagnosis, except in metastatic melanoma, in which clinical history is key to the diagnosis.

PROGNOSIS AND TREATMENT

Patients with vaginal melanoma have a poor prognosis, with an overall 5-year survival rate ranging from 13 to 21% and a median survival of 20 months, partly because most cases remain undetected until late in the natural evolution of the disease. Stage is the most important prognostic factor. The most appropriate treatment for vaginal melanoma is still a matter of debate. Improved clinical outcome has been associated with surgical removal of gross disease. Lymphadenectomy is not considered an obligatory component of the surgical management of these patients. Sentinel lymph node biopsy has been adopted as a less morbid alternative to determine the status of the lymph nodes. In patients with unresectable disease, primary radiation therapy is indicated. Chemotherapy appears not to be useful.

LYMPHOMA AND LEUKEMIA, INCLUDING GRANULOCYTIC SARCOMA

Primary lymphomas of the vagina are rare, although secondary involvement in advanced disease is found in about 40% of cases. Involvement of the vagina in patients with advanced leukemia is not uncommon (Figure 4.25), although clinically significant involvement is rare. Vaginal tumors characterized by an infiltrate of neoplastic myeloid cells (known as granulocytic sarcoma, chloroma, or myeloid sarcoma) are unusual and can be seen in patients with known acute myeloid leukemia, chronic myeloproliferative disorder, or in those with no other clinical evidence of hematologic disease at the time of presentation.

CLINICAL FEATURES

Patients with vaginal lymphoma range in age from 19 to 66 (mean 42) years. Most patients present with a vaginal mass, bleeding or pelvic pain, although some patients are asymptomatic and the tumor may be detected during routine physical examination. Patients with granulocytic sarcoma of the vagina tend to be post-menopausal and present either with vaginal bleeding or a mass, or with abnormal cells on a Pap smear. Bone marrow biopsy, peripheral blood count and smear can be normal or show evidence of leukemia.

PATHOLOGIC FEATURES

GROSS FINDINGS

Vaginal lymphoma typically forms an ill-defined, white to gray mass or firm thickening of the vaginal walls. It commonly presents as bulky pelvic disease with frequent involvement of adjacent tissues/organs (i.e., cervix, rectovaginal septum, pelvic sidewall, or rectum). Regional lymph node involvement can also be seen. Granulocytic sarcoma involving the vagina can form small fleshy nodules to large ill-defined tumors and can have a green discoloration on cut section.

MICROSCOPIC FINDINGS

Most vaginal lymphomas are of the diffuse large B-cell type, they are frequently associated with prominent sclerosis and are composed of sheets of large or inter-mediate-size neoplastic cells extensively infiltrating the stroma (Figure 4.26). The cells are typically round but

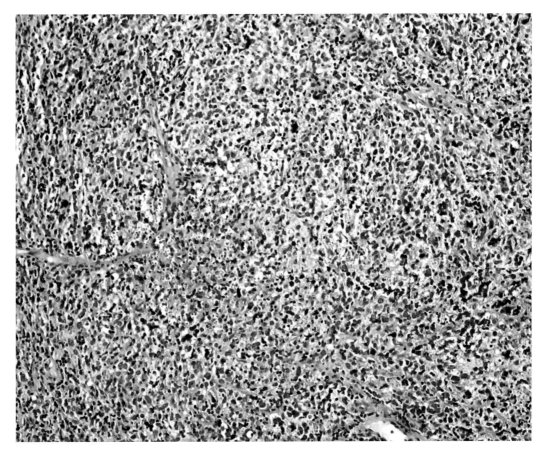

FIGURE 4.26
Large cell B-cell lymphoma. Sheets of large or intermediate-sized neoplastic cells extensively infiltrate the stroma.

may be spindled, and occasionally the presence of retraction artifact can give a clear cell-like appearance. The cells have round or multilobed nuclei with vesicular chromatin and small nucleoli. Mitotic activity is conspicuous. The neoplastic cells lack tropism for the overlying epithelium and lymphoepithelial lesions are not seen. Granulocytic sarcoma is composed of a diffuse, monotonous infiltrate of noncohesive, medium to large immature myeloid cells with scant cytoplasm, oval or round nuclei, evenly distributed chromatin, and inconspicuous nucleoli. A variable number of more mature myeloid cells can be seen, including eosinophilic myelocytes, lymphocytes, and tingible body macrophages, as well as rare megakaryocytes. Other features include sclerosis, involvement of vascular walls, cells with cytoplasmic vacuoles mimicking signet-ring cells, and the presence of pseudoalveolar and trabecular patterns.

ANCILLARY STUDIES

IMMUNOHISTOCHEMISTRY

In diffuse large B-cell lymphoma, the neoplastic cells are CD20 (L26) positive (Figure 4.27) and CD3 nega-

tive. Granulocytic sarcoma stains with CD45, myeloperoxidase, CD4, CD68, and CD117. The tumor cells in granulocytic sarcoma also stain with naphtholarylsulfatase D-chloroacetate esterase in most cases; however, this staining correlates with the extent of tumor differentiation.

DIFFERENTIAL DIAGNOSIS

Lymphoma in the vagina should be distinguished from *secondary involvement* at this site, which is diagnosed if the tumor is detected concurrently in lymph nodes and/or extragenital organs. In addition, *lymphoma-like lesions* may simulate lymphoma, especially in biopsy specimens. A lymphoma-like lesion is characterized by: (1) a heterogeneous population of plasma cells, histiocytes, polymorphonuclear cells, and lymphocytes without atypia, (2) a superficial location, and (3) a band-like distribution of the inflammatory infiltrate. Moreover, it is not associated with sclerosis, it does not form a mass, and it is polyclonal by immunohistochemistry. Much less commonly, *poorly differentiated carcinoma*, including small cell carcinoma, *poorly differentiated sarcoma*, including primitive neuroectodermal

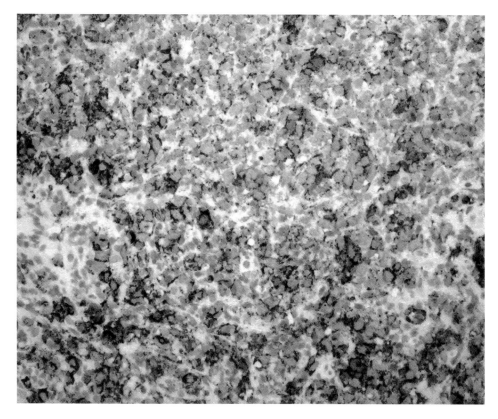

FIGURE 4.27
Large cell B-cell lymphoma. The neoplastic cells are CD20 (L-26) positive.

tumor, and *melanoma* may enter in the differential diagnosis, especially when there is prominent "crush artifact" or cell compartmentalization. Attention to the histological features of the tumor and the use of immunohistochemical studies will allow the correct diagnosis.

PROGNOSIS AND TREATMENT

Patients with primary lymphoma of the vagina have an overall favorable prognosis with a 5-year survival rate of 88%. In patients with low-stage disease, complete remission has been obtained with radiation alone, chemotherapy, or a combination thereof. In contrast, only one-third of patients with high-stage disease have long-term disease-free survival. The prognosis of patients with granulocytic sarcoma who develop leukemia is poor.

ENDODERMAL SINUS TUMOR (YOLK SAC TUMOR)

This tumor is rare in the vagina and is seen exclusively in children under 3 years of age. Only 8% of endodermal sinus tumors originate in the vagina.

CLINICAL FEATURES

Patients typically present with vaginal bleeding. A polypoid mass protruding through the introitus may be seen under vaginal examination. Serum alpha-fetoprotein (AFP) is typically elevated.

YOLK SAC TUMOR – FACT SHEET
Definition
▶ Subtype of malignant germ cell tumor
Incidence
▶ Only 8% primary in the vagina
Age Distribution
▶ Exclusive of children < 3 years
Clinical Features
▶ Vaginal bleeding
▶ Polypoid mass protruding through the introitus
▶ Elevated serum AFP
Prognosis and Treatment
▶ 95% disease-free survival at 2 years with combination chemotherapy
▶ Chemotherapy (cisplatin, etoposide, and bleomycin) with or without partial vaginectomy treatment of choice
▶ AFP to monitor recurrences

PATHOLOGIC FEATURES

GROSS FINDINGS

The tumor usually appears as a friable mass of variable size.

MICROSCOPIC FINDINGS

Endodermal sinus tumor is characterized by a combination of histological patterns that overlap with those seen at other anatomical sites, including reticular, microcystic, papillary, and solid (Figures 4.28–4.30). The cells are either flat, cuboidal or polygonal, they have clear cytoplasm and primitive, hyperchromatic nuclei with prominent nucleoli. Schiller–Duval bodies (Figure 4.30) and hyaline globules may be seen (see Chapter 13).

ANCILLARY STUDIES

IMMUNOHISTOCHEMISTRY

The tumor cells stain with AFP and keratin cocktail, although they do not usually stain with keratin 7.

YOLK SAC TUMOR – PATHOLOGIC FEATURES

Gross Findings
▸ Friable mass of variable size

Microscopic Findings
▸ Reticular, microcystic, papillary, and solid pattens as seen in yolk sac tumors at other sites
▸ Flat, cuboidal, or polygonal cells with clear cytoplasm
▸ Primitive, hyperchromatic nuclei with prominent nucleolus and brisk mitotic activity
▸ Schiller–Duval bodies can be present typically within reticular areas
▸ Hyaline globules common

Immunohistochemical Features
▸ AFP and keratin cocktail positive
▸ CK7 negative

Differential Diagnosis
▸ Embryonal rhabdomyosarcoma (grossly)
▸ Clear cell carcinoma

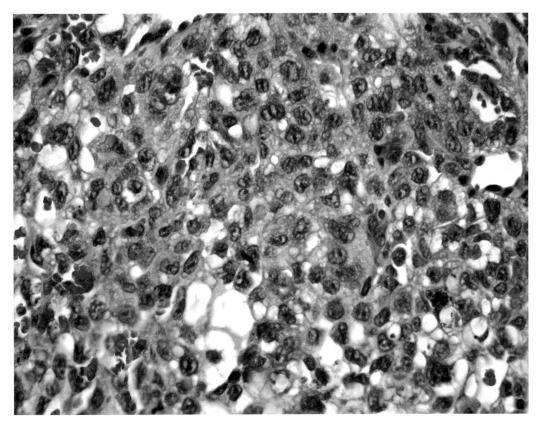

FIGURE 4.28
Endodermal sinus tumor. Primitive tumor cells with abundant clear cytoplasm grow in a solid pattern.

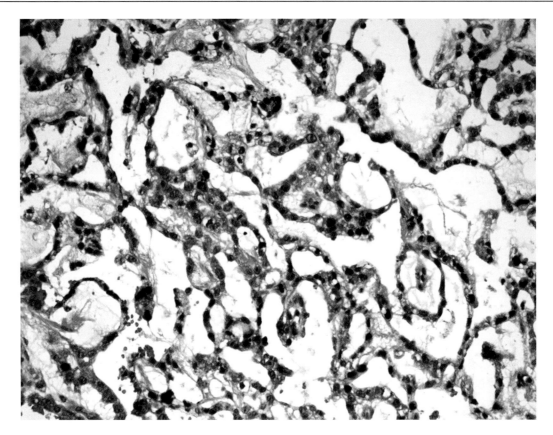

FIGURE 4.29
Endodermal sinus tumor. A reticular pattern merges with small cysts.

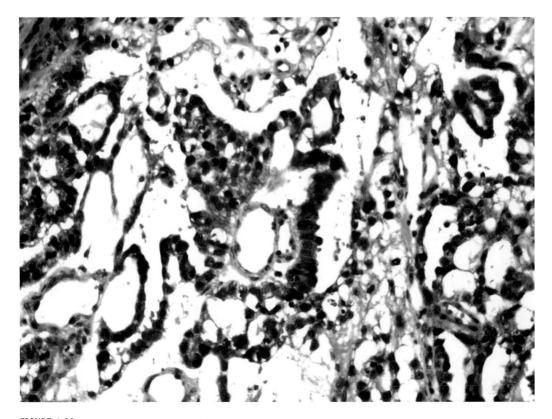

FIGURE 4.30
Endodermal sinus tumor. A Schiller–Duval body is composed of a central blood vessel surrounded by loose stroma with an outer mantle of cuboidal to columnar neoplastic cells present in a space lined by flattened tumor cells.

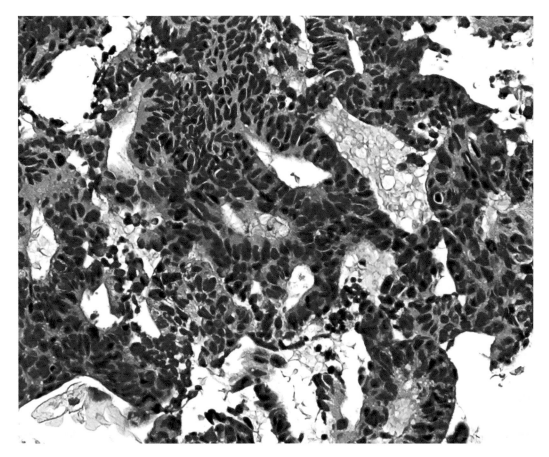

FIGURE 4.31
Metastatic colonic adenocarcinoma. The neoplastic cells form cribriform glands and show cytologic atypia.

DIFFERENTIAL DIAGNOSIS

The main entities in the differential diagnosis include *embryonal rhabdomyosarcoma (sarcoma botryoides)* on gross examination, and *clear cell carcinoma* on microscopic examination because of the finding of clear cells. However, the latter occurs in older women (≥ 20 years), shows characteristic architectural patterns, and may be associated with adenosis.

PROGNOSIS AND TREATMENT

The survival of patients with vaginal endodermal sinus tumor has improved notably during the past two decades. In the past, untreated patients died within 2–4 months, as these tumors are associated with early hematogenous and lymphatic spread. Chemotherapy, more commonly including a combination of cisplatin, etoposide, and bleomycin, with or without partial vaginectomy, is the treatment of choice resulting in a 95% disease free survival rate at 2 years. Pelvic exenteration, chemotherapy, and autologous bone marrow transplant have been used in the treatment of recurrent disease. Alpha fetoprotein can be used to monitor recurrent disease.

METASTASES

Adenocarcinomas involving the vagina are usually metastatic. The most common primary sites include endometrium, cervix, colon (Figures 4.31 and 4.32), and ovary. Less common origins include pancreas, stomach, breast, urinary bladder, and kidney (Figure 4.33). Other tumors that have been described to metastasize to the vagina are melanoma, trophoblastic tumors, alveolar soft-part sarcoma, and uterine leiomyosarcoma. In some cases, the vaginal metastasis represents the first manifestation of the disease.

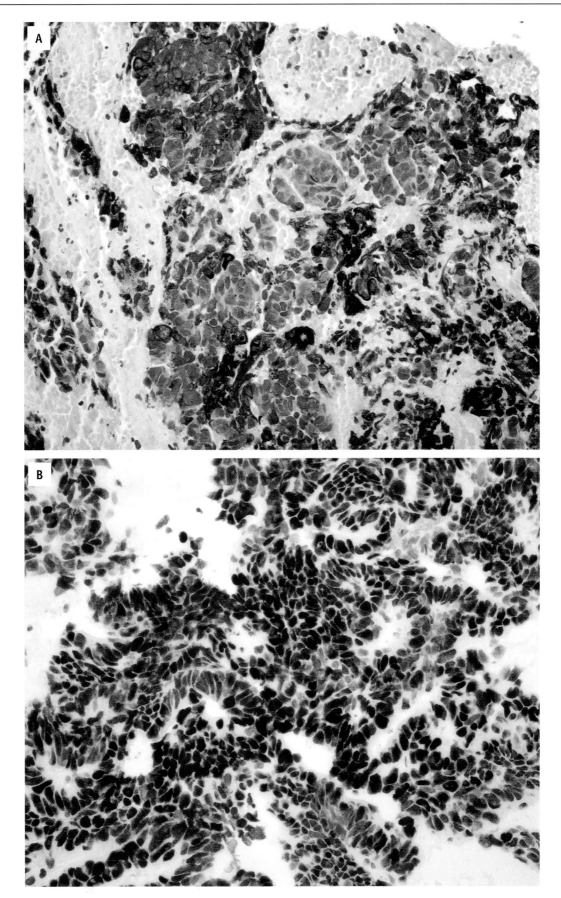

FIGURE 4.32

Metastatic colonic adenocarcinoma. The tumor cells show strong cytokeratin 20 (A) and CDX2 (B) positivity.

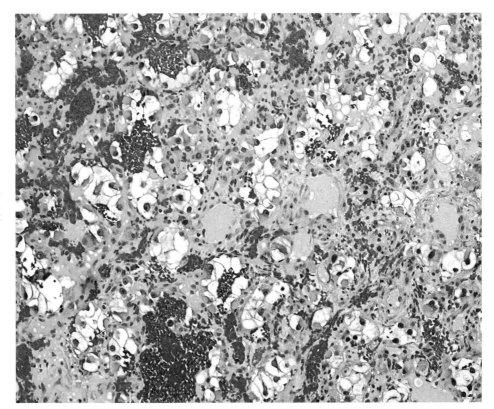

FIGURE 4.33

Metastatic renal cell carcinoma. The neoplastic clear cells display a nested growth associated with prominent hemorrhage.

SUGGESTED READING

Müllerian Papilloma

Abu J, Nunns D, Ireland D, et al. Malignant progression through borderline changes in recurrent Müllerian papilloma of the vagina. Histopathology 2003;42:510–511.

Cohen M, Pedemonte L, Drut R. Pigmented müllerian papilloma of the vagina. Histopathology 2001;39:540–547.

Lüttges JE, Lübke M. Recurrent benign Müllerian papilloma of the vagina. Immunohistochemical findings and histogenesis. Arch Gynecol Obstet 1994;255:157–160.

McCluggage WG, Nirmala V, Radhakumari K. Intramural müllerian papilloma of the vagina. Int J Gynecol Pathol 1999;18:94–95.

Spindle Cell Epithelioma (Mixed Tumor)

Branton PA, Tavassoli FA. Spindle cell epithelioma, the so-called mixed tumor of the vagina. A clinicopathologic, immunohistochemical, and ultrastructural analysis of 28 cases. Am J Surg Pathol 1993;17:509–515.

Oliva E, Gonzalez L, Dionigi A, et al. Mixed tumors of the vagina: an immunohistochemical study of 13 cases with emphasis on the cell of origin and potential aid in differential diagnosis. Mod Pathol 2004;17:1243–1250.

Sirota RL, Dickersin GR, Scully RE. Mixed tumors of the vagina. A clinicopathological analysis of eight cases. Am J Surg Pathol 1981;5:413–422.

Van den Broek N, Emmerson C, Dunlop W. Benign mixed tumor of the vagina: an unusual cause for postmenopausal bleeding. Eur J Obstet Gynecol Reprod Biol 1996;69:143–144.

Leiomyoma

Biankin SA, O'Toole VE, Fung C, et al. Bizarre leiomyoma of the vagina: report of a case. Int J Gynecol Pathol 2000;19:186–187.

Gowri R, Soundararaghavan S, Oumachigui A, et al. Leiomyoma of the vagina: an unusual presentation. J Obstet Gynaecol Res 2003;29:395–398.

Sesti F, La Marca L, Pietropolli A, et al. Multiple leiomyomas of the vagina in a premenopausal woman. Arch Gynecol Obstet 2004;270:131–132.

Tavassoli FA, Norris HJ. Smooth muscle tumors of the vagina. Obstet Gynecol 1979;53:689–693.

Rhabdomyoma

Chabrel CM, Beilby JO. Vaginal rhabdomyoma. Histopathology 1980;4:645–651.

Hanski W, Hagel-Lewicka E, Daniszewski K. Rhabdomyomas of female genital tract. Report on two cases. Zentralbl Pathol 1991;137:439–442.

Iversen UM. Two cases of benign vaginal rhabdomyoma. APMIS 1996;104:575–578.

Vaginal Intraepithelial Neoplasia (VAIN)

Diakomanolis E, Stefanidis K, Rodolakis A, et al. Vaginal intraepithelial neoplasia: report of 102 cases. Eur J Gynaecol Oncol 2002;23:457–459.

Dodge JA, Eltabbakh GH, Mount SL, et al. Clinical features and risk of recurrence among patients with vaginal intraepithelial neoplasia. Gynecol Oncol 2001;83:363–369.

Indermaur MD, Martino MA, Fiorica JV, et al. Upper vaginectomy for the treatment of vaginal intraepithelial neoplasia. Am J Obstet Gynecol 2005;193:577–581.

Logani S, Lu D, Quint WGV, et al. Low-grade vulvar and vaginal intraepithelial neoplasia: correlation of histologic features with human papillomavirus DNA detection and MIB-1 immunostaining. Mod Pathol 2003;16:735–741.

Rome RM, England PG. Management of vaginal intraepithelial neoplasia: a series of 132 cases with long-term follow-up. Int J Gynecol Cancer 2000;10:382–390.

Srodon MH, Stoler M, Baber GB, et al. The distribution of low and high-risk HPV types in vulvar and vaginal intraepithelial neoplasia (VIN and VaIN). Am J Surg Pathol 2006;30:1513–1518.

Squamous Cell Carcinoma

Chang YC, Hricak H, Thurnher S, et al. Vagina: evaluation with MR imaging. Part II. Neoplasms. Radiology 1988;169:175–179.

Creasman WT, Phillips JL, Menck HR. The National Cancer Database report on cancer of the vagina. Cancer 1998;83:1033–1040.

Fujita K, Aoki Y, Tanaka K. Stage I squamous cell carcinoma of the vagina complicating pregnancy: successful conservative treatment. Gynecol Oncol 2005;98:513–515.

Hellman K, Silfversward C, Nilsson B, et al. Primary carcinoma of the vagina: factors influencing the age at diagnosis. The Radiumhemmet series 1956–96. Int J Gynecol Cancer 2004;14:491–501.

Hellman K, Lundell M, Silfversward C, et al. Clinical and histopathologic factors related to prognosis in primary squamous cell carcinoma of the vagina . Int J Gynecol Cancer 2006;16:1201–1211.

Lamoreaux WT, Grigsby PW, Dehdashti F, et al. FDG-PET evaluation of vaginal carcinoma. Int J Radiat Oncol Biol Phys 2005;62:733–737.

Pecorelli S, Benedet JL, Creasman WT, et al. FIGO staging of gynecologic cancer. 1994–1997 FIGO Committee on Gynecologic Oncology. International Federation of Gynecology and Obstetrics. Int J Gynaecol Obstet 1999;65:243–249.

Peters WA, Kumar NB, Morely GW. Microinvasive carcinoma of the vagina: a distinct clinical entity? Am J Obstet Gynecol 1985;153:505–507.

Pingley S, Shrivastava SK, Sarin R, et al. Primary carcinoma of the vagina: Tata Memorial Hospital experience. Int J Radiat Oncol Biol Phys 2000;1:101–108.

Rubin SC, Young J, Mikuta JJ. Squamous carcinoma of the vagina: treatment, complications, and long-term follow-up. Gynecol Oncol 1985;20:346–353.

Rutledge F. Cancer of the vagina. Am J Obstet Gynecol 1967;97:635–655.

Tjalma WA, Monaghan JM, de Barros A, et al. The role of surgery in invasive squamous carcinoma of the vagina. Gynecol Oncol 2001;81:360–365.

Adenocarcinoma

Bagué, S, Rodriguez IM, Prat J. Malignant mesonephric tumors of the female genital tract. A clinicopathologic study of 9 cases. Am J Surg Pathol 2004;28:601–607.

Donnelly LF, Gylys-Morin VM, Warner BW, et al. Case report: clear cell carcinoma of the vagina in a 5-year old girl: imaging findings. Clin Radiol 1998;53:69–72.

Ebrahim S, Daponte A, Smith TH, et al. Primary mucinous adenocarcinoma of the vagina. Gynecol Oncol 2001;80:89–92.

Fox H, Wells M, Harris M, et al. Enteric tumours of the lower female genital tract a report of three cases. Histopathology 1988;12:167–176.

Goodman A, Zukerberg LR, Nikrui N, et al. Vaginal adenosis and clear cell carcinoma after 5-fluorouracil treatment for condylomas. Cancer 1991;68:1628–1632.

Kondi-Pafitis A, Kairi E, Kontogianni KI, et al. Immunopathological study of mesonephric lesions of cervix uteri and vagina. Eur J Gynaecol Oncol 2003;24:154–156.

Lee SE, Park NH, Park IA, et al. Tubulo-villous adenoma of the vagina. Gynecol Oncol 2005;96:556–558.

McCluggage WG, Price JH, Dobbs SP. Primary adenocarcinoma of the vagina arising in endocervicosis. Int J Gynecol Pathol 2001;20:399–402.

McNall RY, Nowicki PD , Miller B, et al. Adenocarcinoma of the cervix and vagina in pediatric patients. Pediatr Blood Cancer 2004;43:289–294.

Mortensen BB, Nielsen K. Tubulo-villous adenoma of the female genital tract: a case report and review of literature. Acta Obstet Gynecol Scand 1991;70:161–163.

Mudhar HS, Smith JHF, Tidy J. Primary vaginal adenocarcinoma arising from an adenoma: case report and review of the literature. Int J Gynecol Pathol 2001;20:204–209.

Shah C, Pizer E, Veljovich DS, et al. Clear cell adenocarcinoma of the vagina in a patient with vaginal endometriosis. Gynecol Oncol 2006;103:1130–1132.

Staats PN, Clement PB, Young RH. Primary endometrioid adenocarcinoma of the vagina: a clinicopathologic analysis of 18 cases. Am J Surg Pathol 2007;31:1490–1501.

Tjalma WA, Colpaert CG. Primary vaginal adenocarcinoma of intestinal type arising from a tubulovillous adenoma. Int J Gynecol Cancer 2006;16:1461–1465.

Waggoner SE, Mittendorf R. Influence of in utero diethylstilbestrol exposure on the prognosis and biologic behavior of vaginal clear-cell adenocarcinoma. Gynecol Oncol 1994;55:238–244.

Werner D, Wilkinson EJ, Ripley D, et al. Primary adenocarcinoma of the vagina with mucinous-enteric differentiation: a report of two cases with associated vaginal adenosis without history of diethylstilbestrol exposure. J Low Genit Tract Dis 2004;8:38–42.

Embryonal Rhabdomyosarcoma

Gonzalez Montalvo P, Jaffe N, Farzin E. Relapse eighteen and one-half years after apparent cure of sarcoma botryoides of the vagina. Med Pediatr Oncol 2003;41:178–179.

Hays DM, Shimada H, Raney B, et al. Sarcomas of the vagina and uterus: the Intergroup Rhabdomyosarcoma Study. J Pediatr Surg 1985;20:718–724.

Leuschner I, Harms D, Mattke A, et al. Rhabdomyosarcoma of the urinary bladder and vagina. A clinicopathologic study with emphasis on recurrent disease: a report from the Kiel Pediatric Tumor Registry and the German CWS study. Am J Surg Pathol 2001;25:856–864.

Qualman SJ, Coffin CM, Newton WA, et al. Intergroup Rhabdomyosarcoma Study: update for pathologists. Pediatr Dev Pathol 1998;1:550–561.

Shy SW, Lee WH, Chen D, et al. Rhabdomyosarcoma of the vagina in a postmenopausal woman: report of a case and review of the literature. Gynecol Oncol 1995;58:395–399.

Weiss SW, Goldblum JR. Embryonal rhabdomyosarcoma, botryoid type. In: Strauss M (ed.) Rhabdomyosarcomas. Enzinger and Weiss' Soft Tissue Tumors, 4th edn. St. Louis, MO: Mosby, 2001:800–803.

Leiomyosarcoma

Ahram J, Lemus R, Schiavello HJ. Leiomyosarcoma of the vagina: case report and literature review. Int J. Gynecol Cancer 2006;16:884–891.

Ciaravino G, Kapp DS, Vela AM, et al. Primary leiomyosarcoma of the vagina. A case report and literature review. Int J Gynecol Cancer 2000;10:340–347.

Tavassoli FA, Norris, HJ. Smooth muscle tumors of the vagina. Obstet Gynecol 1979;53:689–693.

Melanoma

Chung AF, Casey MJ, Flannery JT, et al. Malignant melanoma of the vagina – report of 19 cases. Obstet Gynecol 1980;55:720–727.

Cobellis L, Calabrese E, Stefano B, et al. Malignant melanoma of the vagina. A report of 15 cases. Eur J Gynaecol Oncol 2000;21:295–297.

Gupta D, Malpica A, Deavers MT, et al. Vaginal melanoma. A clinicopathologic and immunohistochemical study of 26 cases. Am J Surg Pathol 2002;26:1450–1457.

Gupta D, Neto AG, Deavers MT, et al. Metastatic melanoma to the vagina: clinicopathologic and immunohistochemical study of three cases and literature review. Int J Gynecol Pathol 2003;22:136–140.

Miner TJ, Delgado Zeisler J, Busam K, et al. Primary vaginal melanoma: a critical analysis of therapy. Ann Surg Oncol 2004;11:34–39.

Lymphoma and Leukemia (Including Granulocytic Sarcoma)

Freeman C, Berg JW, Cutler SJ. Occurrence and progression of extranodal lymphomas. Cancer 1972;29:252–260.

Lagoo AS, Robboy SJ. Lymphoma of the female genital tract: current status. Int J Gynecol Pathol 2006;25:1–21.

Oliva E, Ferry JA, Young RH, et al. Granulocytic sarcoma of the female genital tract: a clinicopathologic study of 11 cases. Am J Surg Pathol 1997;21:1156–1165.

Vang R, Medeiros LJ, Silva EG, et al. Non-Hodgkin's lymphoma involving the vagina. A clinicopathologic analysis of 14 patients. Am J Surg Pathol 2000;24:719–725.

Endodermal Sinus Tumor

Davidoff AM, Hebra A, Bunin N, et al. Endodermal sinus tumor in children. J Pediatr Surg 1996;31:1075–1079.

Handel LN, Scott SM, Giller RH, et al. New perspectives on therapy for vaginal endodermal sinus tumors. J Urol 2002;168:687–690.

Lopes LF, Chazan R, Sredni ST, et al. Endodermal sinus tumor of the vagina in children. Med Pediatr Oncol 1999;32:377–381.

Mauz-Körholz C, Harms D, Calaminus G, et al. Primary chemotherapy and conservative surgery for vaginal yolk sac tumor. Lancet 2000;355:625.

Shinkoda Y, Tanaka S, Ijichi O, et al. Successful treatment of an endodermal sinus tumor of the vagina by chemotherapy alone: a rare case of an infant diagnosed by pathological examination of discharged tumor fragment. Pediatr Hematol Oncol 2006;23:563–569.

Metastases

Allard JE, McBroom JW, Zahn CM, et al. Vaginal metastasis and thrombocytopenia from renal cell carcinoma. Gynecol Oncol 2004;92:970–973.

Cantisani V, Koenraad J, Kalantari BN, et al. Vaginal metastasis from uterine leiomyosarcoma. Magnetic resonance imaging features with pathological correlation. J Comput Assist Tomogr 2003;27:805–809.

Guidozzi F, Sonnendecker EWW, Wright C. Ovarian cancer with metastatic deposits in the cervix, vagina, or vulva preceding primary cytoreductive surgery. Gynecol Oncol 1993;49:225–228.

Mazur MT, Hsueh S, Gersell DJ. Metastases to the female genital tract. Analysis of 325 cases. Cancer 1984;53:1978–1984.

Ohira S, Yamazaki T, Hatano H, et al. Epithelioid trophoblastic tumor metastatic to the vagina: an immunohistochemical and ultrastructural study. Int J Gynecol Pathol 2000;19:381–386.

Yingna S, Yang X, Xiyu Y, et al. Clinical characteristics and treatment of gestational trophoblastic tumor with vaginal metastasis. Gynecol Oncol 2002;84:416–419.

5

Cervical Neoplasia

Maureen L Harmon · Kumarasen Cooper

SQUAMOUS COLUMNAR JUNCTION AND TRANSFORMATION ZONE

The squamous columnar junction (SCJ) is defined as the border between the stratified squamous epithelium of the exocervix and the glandular epithelium of the endocervix. The SCJ is constantly subjected to hormonal influences, and as a consequence, its anatomic location varies with age. At birth, most female neonates have endocervical epithelium present in the portio because of intrauterine exposure to maternal hormones but it rapidly moves back into the endocervical canal until menarche. During puberty, pregnancy, or progesterone therapy, the presence of endocervical glandular epithelium in the exocervix results in what is clinically known as physiologic cervical *eversion* or *ectropion* (Figure 5.1). Throughout the reproductive years, the endocervical epithelium is continuously replaced by metaplastic squamous epithelium due to exposure of the ectropion to the acidity of the vagina and other environmental factors. The degree of ectropion decreases with increasing age and time from onset of sexual activity. During menopause, the transformation zone recedes into the endocervical canal, and in postmenopausal women may be located completely within the endocervical canal. Hence, the transformation zone is the remodeled area of ectropion which undergoes active squamous metaplasia and represents the region between the original and the functional SCJ. It is important to note that the transformation zone is a very dynamic area, which is changing under hormonal and environmental influences. Remodeling of the ectropion does not occur in a uniform fashion, and, in fact, squamous metaplasia can, and often does, occur anywhere within the exposed endocervical columnar epithelium in a patchy fashion. This area is the one most susceptible to HPV infection for several reasons, including higher susceptibility of the advancing edge of the immature squamous epithelium to infection.

The terms "transformation zone" and "SCJ" are *not* synonymous, even though experienced pathologists frequently and erroneously interchange them.

HUMAN PAPILLOMAVIRUS AND THE PATHOGENESIS OF PRECURSOR LESIONS AND CERVICAL CARCINOMA

It is now well established that HPV infection plays an essential role in the development of precancers and cancers of the cervix, as > 99% of all cervical cancers are HPV-related which is independent of racial origin. HPV, a double-stranded DNA virus and a member of the Papovaviridae family, is sexually transmitted disease that predominantly infects squamous epithelia of skin and mucosae. Risk factors associated with HPV infection include early age at first intercourse, early age at first pregnancy, number of sexual partners, cigarette smoking, oral contraceptive use, low socioeconomic class, interval since previous Pap test, increasing parity, nutritional status, immunosuppression (particularly HIV infection), and other sexually transmitted infections. Use of barrier methods of contraception, including condoms and diaphragms, is associated with a decreased risk of HPV infection. The different subtypes of HPV are divided into "low-risk" and "high-risk" depending on the associated risk of carcinoma. Low-risk subtypes include 6, 11, 42, 43, 44, and 53, whereas high-risk subtypes are 16, 18, 31, 33, 35, 39, 45, 51, 52, 56, 58, 59, and 68.

The human papilloma virus enters the basal cells or immature squamous metaplastic cells through defects in the mucosa at the transformation zone. It usually infects the squamous epithelium; however, the virus can also infect subcolumnar reserve cells. The virus can cause either a nonproductive (latent) or a productive infection. In the latter, large amounts of free DNA virus (episomal) are produced in the intermediate and superficial cell layers, which are nonproliferating terminally differentiated squamous cells. As the virally infected cells mature and migrate towards the surface, the characteristic cytopathic effect – the so-called koilocytic atypia – becomes apparent.

Integration of HPV DNA into the host cell genome, with covalent binding of viral genome into host DNA, is thought to be a critical event in the progression to

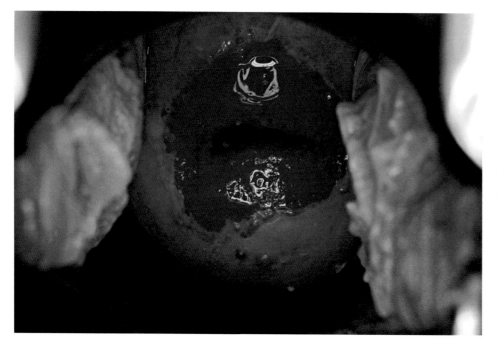

FIGURE 5.1

Ectropion. By colposcopy, the endo-cervical mucosa has a rough, red appearance, in sharp contrast to the smooth pink surface of the native squamous epithelium.

high-grade squamous intraepithelial lesions (HSIL). High-risk HPVs produce E6 and E7, two proteins with growth-stimulating and transforming properties. Viral integration into host cell genome results in disruption of the viral DNA with overexpression of E6/E7 genes. Excessive levels of E6/E7 viral oncoproteins result in abrogation of p53/Rb tumor suppressor proteins, with resultant uncontrolled cell cycling and proliferative activity of the squamous epithelium.

It has been stated that low-risk HPV is almost always associated with low-grade squamous intraepithelial lesions (LSIL), frequently regresses, and its association with cervical carcinoma is exceedingly rare, whereas high-risk HPV subtypes can result in either LSIL or HSIL. Moreover, if untreated, HSIL may subsequently progress to invasive carcinoma. However, a recent multi-center study ("Atypical squamous cells/Low grade squamous intraepithelial lesion Triage Study (ALTS)") has shown that 83 % of women with a LSIL on Pap test had a high-risk HPV subtype, challenging to some extent the previous findings. Nevertheless, there is agreement in that at least high-grade subtypes are usually associated with high-grade lesions. Persistent or recurrent HPV infections can occur with both low- and high-risk subtypes, but lesions associated with low-risk subtypes are not known to progress to cancer.

In recent years, widespread cytology screening programs have allowed detection and treatment of high-grade lesions before they progress to cancer. Half of all cervical cancers in the US arise in women who have never been screened and 10 % occur in women who have not been screened in the previous 5 years. Finally, although currently only one HPV assay approved by the Food and Drug Administration is commercially available, which uses the 13 most common high-risk HPV subtypes in a single probe mixture, it can be used as an extra tool in the screening of patients.

TERMINOLOGY

In 1975, for the first time, the World Health Organization (WHO) proposed unified terminology to describe and report cervical carcinoma precursor lesions in cervical biopsy specimens. Squamous dysplasia was defined as a "lesion in which part of the thickness of the epithelium is replaced by cells showing varying degrees of atypia," and it was divided into mild, moderate, and severe. However, there were no widely accepted criteria for separating grades of dysplasia and the separation of each lesion into one of the categories was subjective. Dysplasia was considered a distinct entity from carcinoma in situ, which was described by the WHO as a "lesion in which all or most of the epithelium shows the cellular features of carcinoma." The separation of dysplasia from carcinoma in situ implied two distinct disease processes rather than a spectrum of severity of what is now known to be a single disease process.

In the 1980s, the International Society of Gynecological Pathologists (ISGYP) introduced nomenclature that replaced the term "dysplasia" with "cervical intraepithelial neoplasia" (CIN) and eliminated the category of carcinoma in situ. The CIN terminology was similarly divided into three categories, CIN I, CIN II, and CIN III, with carcinoma in situ being incorporated into the CIN III category. One advantage of this terminology is that it eliminates the concept of two distinct disease processes inherent in the WHO classification. The CIN classification system is still used today, but not without criticism. Many have pointed out that the CIN terminology may not accurately reflect the immense knowledge gained about cervical cancer and its precursor lesions since the 1980s. Central to the controversy is the designation of CIN I as a neoplastic lesion, since it is now known that the vast majority of these lesions are transient and spontaneously regress, even if untreated. Hence, labeling these lesions "neoplastic" may be an overstatement.

The most recently proposed nomenclature for reporting cervical lesions on biopsy specimens is based on the Bethesda System, which has been used for many years in the reporting of cervical cytology. The Bethesda System is a two-tiered system, which divides dysplasia into LSIL and HSIL. This terminology incorporates CIN II and CIN III into the single category of HSIL. The Bethesda System also places condyloma acuminatum into the LSIL category, whereas both the WHO and CIN terminologies kept condyloma acuminatum as a separate category. The Bethesda classification more closely reflects the biology of cervical cancer precursor lesions and also unifies the nomenclature used for reporting both cervical cytology and biopsy specimens, resulting in less confusion amongst clinicians, pathologists, and patients.

The Bethesda System is widely used in the US, but the CIN and SIL terminologies are not infrequently combined when reporting cervical biopsies. For example, low-grade lesions are reported as LSIL (CIN I) and high-grade lesions as either HSIL (CIN II) or HSIL (CIN III).

COLPOSCOPY

This method allows examination of the cervix with a colposcope, a binocular instrument with a magnification up to 40×. The entire transformation zone can easily be examined in women of reproductive age, both before and after 5 % acetic acid is applied to the surface of the cervix. In postmenopausal women, the transformation zone may be located completely within the endocervical canal, which results in an unsatisfactory or indeterminate colposcopic examination (Figure 5.2). Abnormal colposcopic findings include acetowhite epithelium (squamous epithelium that becomes white after acetic acid application), leukoplakia, punctation, mosaicism, and abnormal vessels.

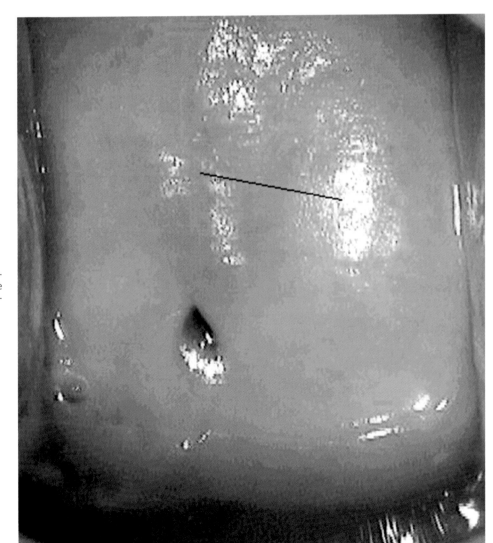

FIGURE 5.2

Indeterminate colposcopy. The transformation zone has receded into the endocervical canal in a postmenopausal woman.

LOW-GRADE SQUAMOUS INTRAEPITHELIAL LESION

This category includes flat condyloma, condyloma acuminatum (also known as exophytic condyloma), and CIN I. All of these low-grade lesions are the result of productive viral infections in which large numbers of viral particles are generated. They are usually self-limited and all display koilocytic atypia. Among them, condyloma acuminatum is strongly associated with low-risk HPV subtypes 6 and 11.

CLINICAL FEATURES

Low-grade squamous intraepithelial lesions typically occur in reproductive age women, with a peak incidence

in the third decade, as most young women are exposed to HPV sometime after becoming sexually active. The incidence decreases with age, as < 0.1% of postmenopausal women have LSIL on a Pap test. While the true prevalence of squamous intraepithelial lesions is not known, a large study conducted by the College of American Pathologists in 1997, including 300 US laboratories, showed that only 1.97% and 0.5% of 16 132 Pap tests were diagnosed as LSIL and HSIL, respectively. Most women will develop transient infections which regress spontaneously. However, women infected with HIV have a seven times greater risk of developing squamous intraepithelial lesions involving the lower genital tract compared to non-HIV-infected women. Condyloma acuminata tend to recur and grow in size and number in otherwise healthy non-HIV-infected pregnant women, but typically regress during postpartum.

COLPOSCOPIC FEATURES

These lesions may be seen as white plaques (leukoplakia) or acetowhite lesions after the administration of 5% acetic acid (Figure 5.3). Nonetheless, these colposcopic changes are not specific for LSIL, as squamous metaplasia, inflammatory/reactive changes, and HSILs may have a similar appearance. Condyloma acuminatum may be seen under colposcopic exam as a raised polypoid or papillary lesion with prominent vasculature.

PATHOLOGIC FEATURES

GROSS FINDINGS

The majority of LSILs are not apparent on gross examination; however, some may be identified as white irregular plaques (leukoplakia). Low-grade SILs can occur anywhere in the transformation zone, tend to be smaller than HSIL, and only infrequently involve the endocervical canal. Condyloma acuminatum is typically multifocal and can involve the transformation zone as well as the exocervix. The lesion is white and exophytic, but may be papillary.

MICROSCOPIC FINDINGS

On low-power examination, condyloma acuminatum shows distinctive architectural changes, including epithelial hyperplasia (acanthosis) and papillomatosis (Figure 5.4A and B). Often atypical parakeratosis and hyperkeratosis are present. Incipient condyloma acuminatum may only have an undulating appearance of the epithelium. Other forms of LSIL lack the papillomatosis of condyloma, but may show acanthosis with variable degree of cellular disorganization at or near the surface (Figure 5.4C). Cytologic alterations associated with

---

LOW-GRADE SQUAMOUS INTRAEPITHELIAL LESION (LSIL) – FACT SHEET

Definition
- Cervical cancer precursor lesion associated with both low- and high-risk HPV subtypes
- The category of LSIL includes flat and exophytic condyloma and CIN I

Prevalence and Location
- Reproductive age women
- Unknown true prevalence; however, up to 3.0% of Pap smear reported as SIL
- Mostly at the transformation zone
- Exocervix can also be involved if condyloma acuminatum

Race and Age Distribution
- No race predilection, but greater frequency in Caucasians than blacks, reflecting less screening in black women
- Peak incidence in mid-20s, decreasing thereafter (approximately 5% of women < 30 have LSIL on Pap smear, versus < 0.1% of women ≥ 65 years)

Clinical Features
- Asymptomatic

Colposcopic Features
- Leukoplakia or acetowhite epithelium
- Cerebriform or papillary raised lesion with prominent vasculature (condyloma acuminatum)

Prognosis and Treatment
- Only 15% of LSIL progress to HSIL
- Following a diagnosis of LSIL on Pap smear, colposcopic exam is performed with biopsy of any lesion to confirm the diagnosis
  - If confirmatory biopsy, follow-up with Pap smears every 4–6 months
  - If discordant biopsy, additional sampling may be necessary

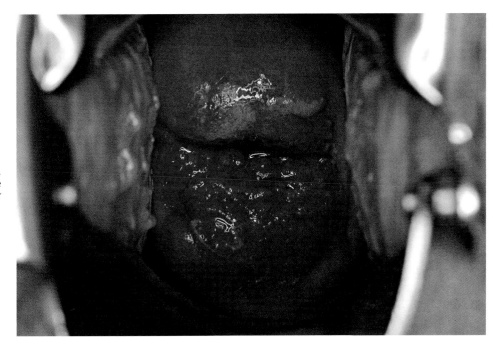

FIGURE 5.3

Low-grade intraepithelial lesion. Colposcopic exam shows acetowhite epithelium involving the anterior lip.

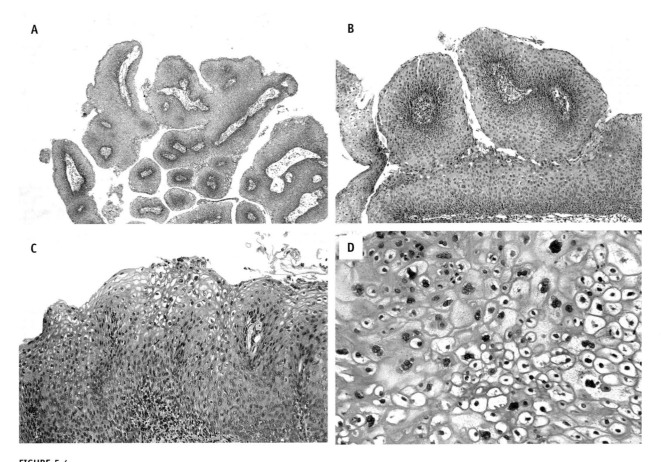

FIGURE 5.4

Condyloma acuminatum. The lesion has a striking exophytic papillary growth (A). The lining squamous epithelium shows koilocytic atypia (B). Low-grade squamous intraepithelial lesion. The squamous epithelium shows cellular disorganization and koilocytic atypia is most prominent at the surface (C and D).

LOW-GRADE SQUAMOUS INTRAEPITHELIAL LESION (LSIL) – PATHOLOGIC FEATURES

Gross Findings

▶ May be uncommonly seen as white irregular plaques (leukoplakia)
▶ Tan-white raised papillary or cerebriform lesion (condyloma acuminatum)

Microscopic Findings

▶ Koilocytic atypia (nuclear enlargement, nuclear membrane irregularities, coarse chromatin, hyperchromasia, multinucleation, and peripheral cytoplasm condensation) in superficial layers
▶ Epithelial hyperplasia may be present

Categories of LSIL

In Condyloma acuminatum:

▶ Epithelial hyperplasia with acanthosis and papillomatosis
▶ Parakeratosis and hyperkeratosis
▶ Koilocytic atypia

In Papillary immature metaplasia:

▶ Epidermal hyperplasia with slender filiform papillae
▶ Immature metaplastic squamous cells with regular nuclear spacing +/– nucleoli
▶ Minimal to absent koilocytic atypia

Cytology Correlation

▶ Nuclear but not cytoplasmic changes in mature superficial squamous cells required for diagnosis of LSIL
▶ Nuclear enlargement > three times that of a normal intermediate-sized squamous cell, with nuclear hyperchromasia, coarse or smudgy chromatin, frequent binucleation and multinucleation, and inconspicuous nucleoli

Differential Diagnosis

▶ Mature glycogenated squamous epithelium
▶ Postmenopausal squamous atypia
▶ Metaplastic squamous epithelium with reactive changes
▶ High-grade squamous intraepithelial lesion

show nucleoli. Focal koilocytic atypia may be seen in the upper layers of the squamous epithelium. The lack of overt koilocytotic atypia likely reflects the dependence of viral cytopathic effect on maturation, which is limited in these lesions. Similar to exophytic condyloma, papillary immature metaplasia is associated with HPV types 6 and 11, which supports their inclusion in the LSIL category.

ANCILLARY STUDIES

CYTOLOGY

Findings diagnostic of LSIL include nuclear enlargement more than three times the size of a normal intermediate size squamous cell nucleus associated with nuclear hyperchromasia. The chromatin pattern is either coarse or smudgy and opaque. Binucleation and multinucleation are frequent and nucleoli are inconspicuous. Cytoplasmic changes include clearing of the central cytoplasm (perinuclear cavitation) with condensation at the periphery of the cell (Figure 5.5), but in some cases, the cytoplasm may be densely eosinophilic. However, cytoplasmic changes are not necessary to establish the diagnosis of LSIL.

Pap smears displaying squamous cells with borderline changes that do not fully meet the criteria for LSIL are placed in the category of "atypical squamous cells of undetermined significance" (ASCUS). According to current treatment recommendations, patients with Pap tests interpreted as ASCUS should undergo HPV testing for high-risk subtypes; if present, the patient may be referred for colposcopy.

DIFFERENTIAL DIAGNOSIS

Several studies, most recently including the multicenter ALTS, have shown high interobserver variability in the diagnosis of LSIL. Although the architectural changes in LSIL can be subtle, the cytologic abnormalities, particularly the nuclear changes, must be present to establish a diagnosis of LSIL. *Mature glycogenated squamous epithelium* has a basket-weave architecture with regular cytoplasmic halos and small and pyknotic nuclei without viral nuclear changes. Prominent cytoplasmic perinuclear clearing alone without the characteristic virally induced nuclear changes is nonspecific and can be seen in atrophy, infections (such as trichomoniasis, candidiasis, and bacterial vaginosis), and reactive squamous epithelium.

Postmenopausal squamous atypia may be confused with koilocytic atypia because of the finding of cytoplasmic halos, some degree of nuclear enlargement, hyperchromasia, and occasional binucleated cells. However, in contrast to LSIL, there is epithelial maturation, the

HPV infection affect both the cytoplasm and nucleus. Cytoplasmic changes include irregular perinuclear clearing with condensation of the cytoplasm at the periphery of the cell. Nuclear changes include enlargement, membrane irregularities ("raisinoid" appearance), coarse chromatin, hyperchromasia, and multinucleation. These cytologic features are pathognomonic of HPV infection and are collectively termed "koilocytic atypia" or "koilocytic change" (Figure 5.4D). A prominent nucleolus is not a feature of either LSIL or HSIL. There may be few or no mitotic figures, and if present, they are normal in appearance and are located in the basal/parabasal layers.

An uncommon entity included in the LSIL category is *papillary immature metaplasia*, characterized by slender filiform papillae lined by acanthotic metaplastic squamous cells with only minimal to absent cytologic atypia. The nuclei are often evenly spaced and may

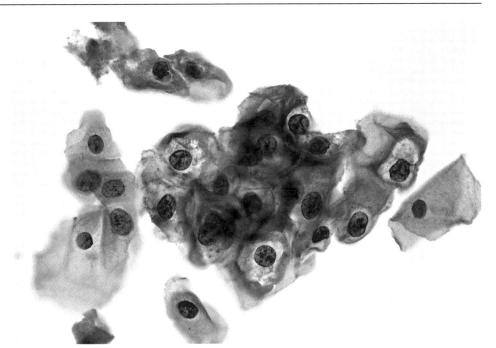

FIGURE 5.5
Low-grade squamous intraepithelial lesion. A Pap smear shows koilocytic atypia with clearing of central cytoplasm, condensation of peripheral cytoplasm, nuclear enlargement, and hyperchromasia.

nuclei are evenly spaced, the cytoplasmic halos have uniform contours, and mitotic activity is absent.

Squamous metaplasia associated with reactive changes may exhibit lack of maturation, binucleated cells, hyperchromatic nuclei, and scattered mitotic activity mainly in the basal layers. However, the cells appear monotonous, the nuclei are not crowded, have smooth contours, and frequently show nucleoli that may be prominent. Moreover, cytoplasmic halos are round and regular in shape.

High-grade squamous intraepithelial neoplasia may be difficult to distinguish from LSIL, especially in flat epithelium. LSIL typically shows cell maturation in the upper two-thirds of the epithelium and koilocytic change within the superficial cell layers. Only minimal nuclear atypia is present in the lower one-third of the epithelium. If there is parabasal cell anisokaryosis, abnormal mitoses, or more extensive abnormal maturation, the lesion should be diagnosed as HSIL.

PROGNOSIS AND THERAPY

The majority of lesions will regress within 1 year, and only approximately 15% will progress to HSIL. Clinical management partially depends upon factors such as age, compliance, and immune status of the patient, and requires close communication between clinician and pathologist. Following an abnormal Pap test, the patient will be referred for colposcopy, at which time the cervix is thoroughly evaluated and any suspicious areas are biopsied. If the biopsy shows a benign process that cor-

relates with the colposcopic findings (squamous metaplasia, inflammation with reactive squamous changes, etc.), the patient will undergo a second Pap test in 4–6 months. If the biopsy shows LSIL and the entire transformation zone is visualized at colposcopy with findings consistent with LSIL, no further therapy is necessary, and the patient is followed with a repeat Pap test in 4–6 months. If, however, the colposcopic examination is indeterminate or reveals a lesion more worrisome than the biopsy findings, and/or the Pap test is concerning for a high-grade lesion, treatment of the entire transformation zone may be necessary.

HIGH-GRADE SQUAMOUS INTRAEPITHELIAL LESION

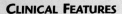

CLINICAL FEATURES

High-grade squamous intraepithelial lesions are relatively frequent with an estimated incidence of up to 31 per 100,000 women, without racial differences.

These lesions are seen in a slightly older age group than LSIL, with the highest prevalence in women between 35–39 years. However, over the past 20 years, the frequency of HSIL has increased in younger women, in part secondary to changing sexual habits in recent years. The lesions are frequently clinically asymptomatic.

COLPOSCOPIC FEATURES

In addition to acetowhite epithelium and leukoplakia, additional colposcopic abnormalities include alterations in small superficial stromal vessels that result in changes termed "mosaicism" and "punctations" (Figure 5.6). Although these vascular changes are occasionally seen in LSIL, they are more prominent in HSIL. The mosaic pattern is a result of anastomosing vessels branching portions of epithelium and displaying a basket-like pattern. Punctations are created by vessels which form a hairpin turn as they approach the surface and then return to the underlying stroma. The further apart the vessels, the coarser the punctations, and consequently the more worrisome the colposcopic appearance.

PATHOLOGIC FINDINGS

GROSS FINDINGS

Other than the colposcopic findings described above, the changes associated with HSIL usually cannot be visualized on gross examination. Occasionally, HSIL may be seen as an area of leukoplakia.

MICROSCOPIC FINDINGS

On low-power examination, HSIL demonstrates loss of maturation with increased nuclear density and nuclear atypia involving both the upper and lower epithelial layers. The dysplastic cells frequently show a syncytial growth with no distinct intercellular borders, secondary to crowding in the parabasal layers. The atypical cells appear immature, with high nuclear-to-cytoplasmic ratio, irregular nuclear membranes, coarse and irregularly distributed chromatin, and inconspicuous nucleoli. Mitoses are present in the upper half of the epithelium, and abnormal mitotic figures may be present. Although most HSILs show variation in nuclear size, in some cases the nuclei are quite uniform in size. However, they still exhibit crowding, high nuclear-to-cytoplasmic ratio, hyperchromasia, and increased mitotic activity.

Cervical intraepithelial neoplasia II and III are distinguished from one another by the degree of discernible cell maturation. In CIN II, immature cells occupy the lower two-thirds of the epithelium but some degree of maturation or koilocytic atypia is present towards the surface (Figure 5.7A). However, koilocytes usually have smaller halos. In addition, mitotic figures are usually confined to the lower two-thirds of the epithelium. In CIN III, there is absence of maturation, as immature cells occupy the full-thickness epithelium, often associated with a layer of atypical parakeratotic cells on the surface. Mitoses can be seen at all levels of the epithelium (Figures 5.7B and C).

High-grade squamous intraepithelial lesion coexists with LSIL in approximately 15% of cases, and not infrequently involves the endocervical glands, which may result in complete luminal obliteration (Figures 5.8 and 5.9).

ANCILLARY STUDIES

IMMUNOHISTOCHEMISTRY

p16 protein, a surrogate marker for HPV infection, is overexpressed in cervical cancers and precursor lesions associated with high-risk HPV subtypes. p16 typically shows diffuse and strong nuclear and cytoplasmic immunostaining in HSIL involving two-thirds or full-thickness squamous epithelium in the majority of

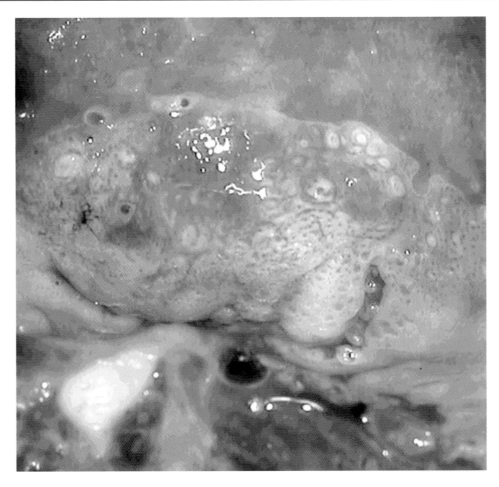

FIGURE 5.6

High-grade squamous intraepithelial lesion. Acetowhite epithelium with mosaicism (note the blocks of varying size) and punctations (coarse stippling of the epithelium) is seen with green filter colposcopy.

A

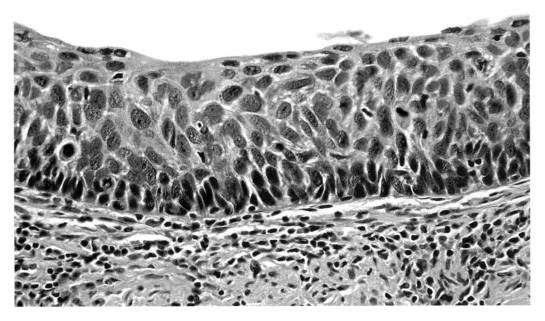

FIGURE 5.7

High-grade squamous intraepithelial lesion. (A) CIN II shows immature-appearing cells in the lower two-thirds of the epithelium associated with some maturation in the upper one-third (A).

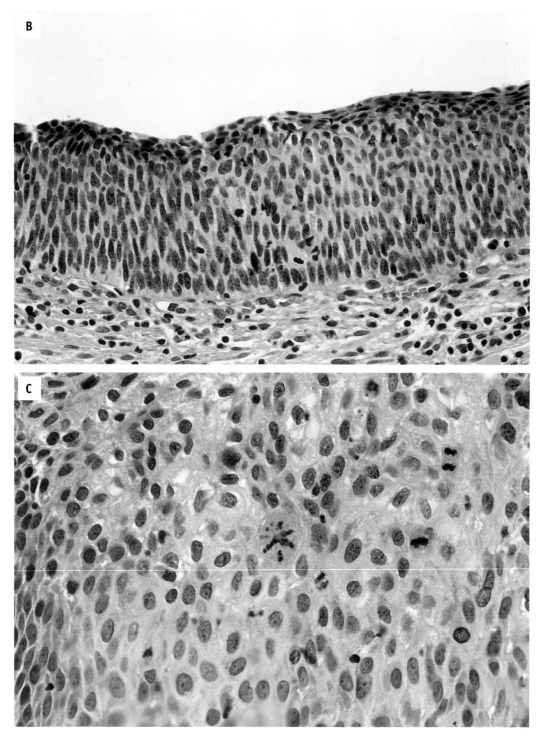

FIGURE 5.7—cont'd
CIN III shows dysplastic cells lacking maturation throughout all layers associated with atypical parakeratosis (B) and prominent syncytial growth in basal layers accompanied by increased nuclear-to-cytoplasmic ratio and brisk mitotic activity, including an abnormal form (C).

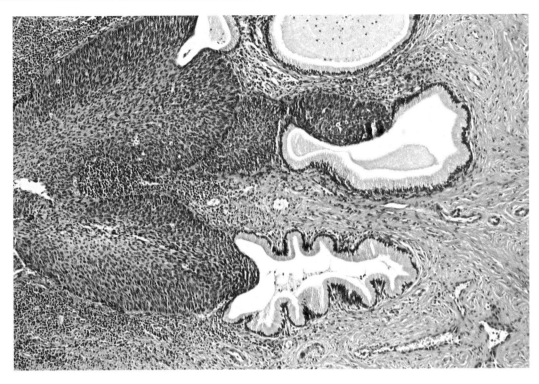

FIGURE 5.8
High-grade squamous intraepithelial lesion. Partial involvement of endocervical glands.

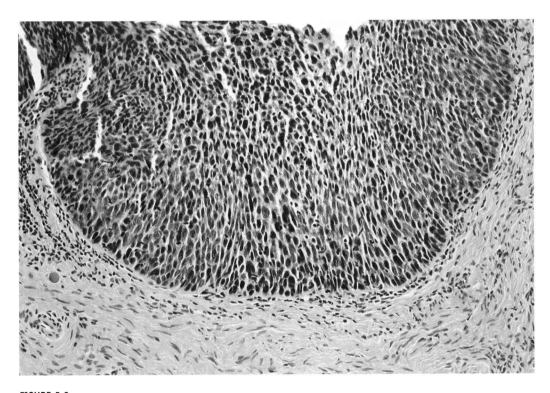

FIGURE 5.9
High-grade squamous intraepithelial lesion, with prominent endocervical gland involvement. There is a smooth rounded contour of the gland with an intact basement membrane, and no associated desmoplasia.

HIGH-GRADE SQUAMOUS INTRAEPITHELIAL LESION (HSIL) – PATHOLOGIC FEATURES

Gross Findings
▸ Typically not visible
▸ Occasionally leukoplakia

Microscopic Findings
▸ Loss of maturation and cytologic atypia in the lower two-thirds (CIN II) to the full thickness (CIN III) epithelium
▸ Syncytial growth with lack of distinct intercellular borders in basal and parabasal layers
▸ Immature cells with high nuclear-to-cytoplasmic ratio, irregular nuclear membrane contour, coarse chromatin, and inconspicuous nucleoli
▸ Superficial layers may show lower nuclear-to-cytoplasmic ratio and koilocytic change; however, halos are small
▸ Frequent mitoses, including atypical forms:
  ▸ CIN II: mitoses in lower two-thirds of epithelium
  ▸ CIN III: mitoses in all levels of epithelium

Immunohistochemical Features
▸ Strong and diffuse positive nuclear and cytoplasmic p16 in at least two-thirds of the epithelial thickness
▸ Positive nuclear Ki67 staining in the upper two-thirds of the dysplastic squamous epithelium

Cytology Correlation
▸ Single cells or crowded, syncytial groups
▸ Cell size similar to squamous metaplastic or parabasal cells and smaller and less mature than LSIL cells
▸ Increased nuclear-to-cytoplasmic ratio
▸ Irregular nuclear membranes ("boulder"-like)
▸ Hyperchromatic nuclei with coarse chromatin
▸ Lacy and delicate, to dense and metaplastic, to orangophilic and keratinized cytoplasm

Differential Diagnosis
▸ Atypia of repair
▸ Radiation changes
▸ Atrophy
▸ Immature squamous metaplasia
▸ Transitional metaplasia
▸ Low-grade squamous intraepithelial lesion
▸ Invasive squamous cell carcinoma (vs HSIL with florid glandular involvement)

---

lesions (Figure 5.10). Ki-67 (MIB-1) immunoreactivity is present in the nuclei of the upper two-thirds of the epithelium in HSIL (Figure 5.11).

CYTOLOGY

On Pap smears, HSIL cells are smaller and less mature than those of LSIL, having the size of metaplastic squamous or parabasal cells. They can occur singly or in crowded, syncytial groups. The nuclear-to-cytoplasmic ratio is markedly increased. Nuclear membrane irregularities are present and may be prominent, so that the nuclei may take on a three-dimensional "boulder"-like configuration. Nuclei are hyperchromatic with a coarse

chromatin pattern. Nucleoli are inconspicuous, and if prominent, should raise the possibility of microinvasion. Finally, the scant cytoplasm may be delicate and lacy, dense and metaplastic, or orangophilic and keratinized (Figure 5.12).

DIFFERENTIAL DIAGNOSIS

High-grade squamous intraepithelial lesion should be distinguished from atypia of repair, radiation changes, atrophy, immature squamous metaplasia, transitional metaplasia, LSIL, and invasive squamous cell carcinoma.

In *atypia of repair*, the squamous epithelium may be disorganized, atypical basal-like cells may be present up to the mid-zone, and there may be nuclear atypia with nuclear enlargement causing confusion with HSIL. In contrast to HSIL, in repair there should be some maturation of the squamous epithelium towards the surface, the cells have well-defined cell borders without crowding, and there is no variation in cell size or shape. There is no coarse chromatin but prominent nucleoli, and if cytoplasmic halos are present, they are small and uniform secondary to accelerated cell maturation. Frequently, there is acute inflammation, spongiosis, and mitoses are limited to the parabasal layers of the epithelium. Ki-67 can be helpful in distinguishing SIL from reactive epithelium as staining should be confined to the lower third of the epithelium in atypia of repair. However, reactive changes can occasionally coexist with SIL. In these cases, a clue to the diagnosis may be the finding of nuclei with HPV effect in the superficial layers.

Radiation changes are distinguished from HSIL by an increase not only of the nuclear size but also of the amount of cytoplasm. Therefore, there is a proportionate or decreased nuclear-to-cytoplasmic ratio. Nuclear spacing is uniform with minimal nuclear crowding and the chromatin is smudgy, rather than coarse. Mitoses are rare and cytoplasmic vacuolization may be present.

Atrophic squamous epithelium may be seen in postmenopausal women or those on Depo-Provera. Distinguishing atrophy from HSIL can be very difficult as: (1) the epithelium lacks maturation; (2) the cells have increased nuclear-to-cytoplasmic ratio; and (3) the nuclei are small with coarse and hyperchromatic chromatin. However, in atrophy, the nuclei are uniform in size and spacing, and there is minimal nuclear pleomorphism and absent to rare mitoses (Figure 5.13). Ki-67 can be helpful in this distinction, as atrophy should show minimal to absent staining, while HSIL shows strong positive staining involving at least the upper two-thirds of the epithelium.

Immature squamous metaplasia can be difficult to distinguish from HSIL, as immature squamous cells with increased nuclear-to-cytoplasmic ratio may occupy almost the full thickness epithelium, and maturation may only be seen towards the surface. However, there is no cell crowding and, unlike HSIL, cell membranes

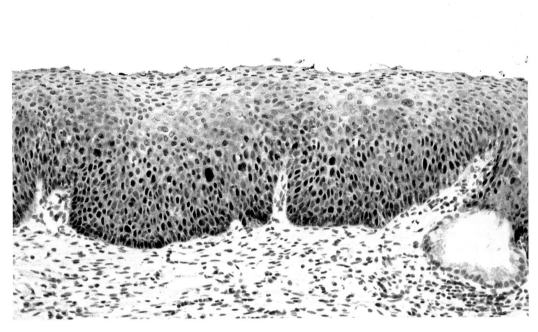

FIGURE 5.10
High-grade squamous intraepithelial lesion. Strong and diffuse nuclear and cytoplasmic p16 staining of the lower two-thirds of the epithelium is seen.

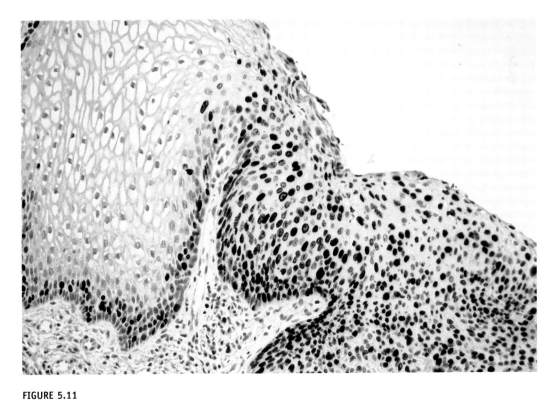

FIGURE 5.11
High-grade squamous intraepithelial lesion. MIB-1 immunoreactivity is present in nuclei at all levels of the epithelium, whereas in normal epithelium it is limited to the basal layer.

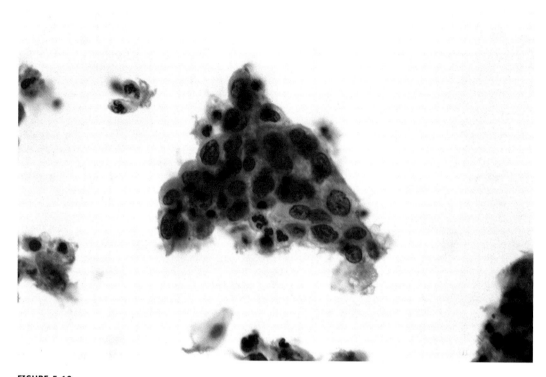

FIGURE 5.12

High-grade squamous intraepithelial lesion. Increased nuclear-to-cytoplasmic ratio, hyperchromatic nuclei, and coarse chromatin are seen on a Pap smear. Some nuclei have a "boulder-like" configuration.

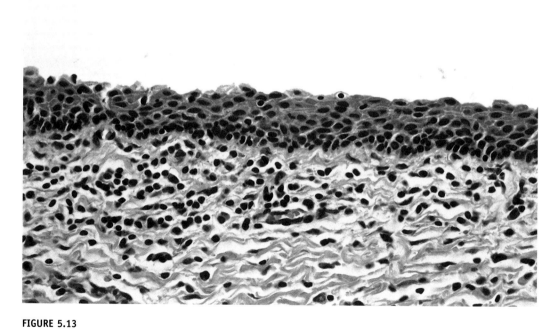

FIGURE 5.13

Atrophy. Cells with increased nuclear-to-cytoplasmic ratio and hyperchromatic nuclei mimic HSIL. However, nuclei are uniform in size and evenly spaced, and mitoses are absent.

are usually well defined. The nuclei are uniform in size and shape, they have fine chromatin, and small nucleoli may be seen. Even though mitoses may be present, abnormal mitoses are lacking. Columnar cells may be present on the surface overlying the metaplastic epithelium but are only rarely present overlying dysplastic epithelium, and thus is a helpful feature. Differentiating atypical immature squamous metaplasia from HSIL is even more difficult and sometimes not possible. The degree of nuclear atypia is usually less prominent than HSIL and although mitotic figures may be present, they are not abnormal, as they can be in HSIL. p16 immunohistochemistry may be useful in some of these cases.

Transitional metaplasia occurs predominantly in postmenopausal women and it can involve the transformation zone the exocervix as well as the vagina. It can be confused with HSIL as: (1) this lesion has > 10 cell layers; (2) there is absence of maturation; and (3) the nuclei are oval to spindle and have irregular contours. However, in contrast to HSIL, the cells in the superficial layers are oriented horizontally with a streaming pattern, the nuclei are elongated with prominent grooves, there is fine granular chromatin, and mitoses are rare. Nevertheless, it is important to keep in mind that transitional cell metaplasia may show superimposed dysplastic changes.

Finally, *florid HSIL with extensive glandular involvement* should be distinguished from invasive squamous cell carcinoma. The distinction is not difficult when the endocervical gland is only partially replaced and native endocervical glandular epithelium is appreciated adjacent to HSIL (Figure 5.8). When HSIL completely replaces and expands endocervical glands, the distinction may be more difficult. However, glands involved by HSIL maintain a smooth, rounded contour (Figure 5.9), rather than the irregular, angular configuration of invasive carcinoma. The basement membrane is intact and the surrounding stroma, although sometimes associated with inflammation, does not show desmoplasia (Figure 5.9). Occasionally, dysplastic epithelium may be artifactually displaced into the stroma during a surgical procedure, thus mimicking invasive carcinoma (Figure 5.14). However, the fragmented and distorted appearance of the epithelium is apparent, and the lack of "paradoxical maturation" where the carcinoma cells acquire more abundant, eosinophilic cytoplasm, prominent nucleoli, and well-defined cell borders helps in this distinction (Figure 5.15).

PROGNOSIS AND THERAPY

If untreated, HSIL, particularly CIN III, has a much greater risk of progressing to invasive carcinoma compared to LSIL, ranging from 22 to 72%. Studies with the longest follow-up had the highest rates of progression to carcinoma.

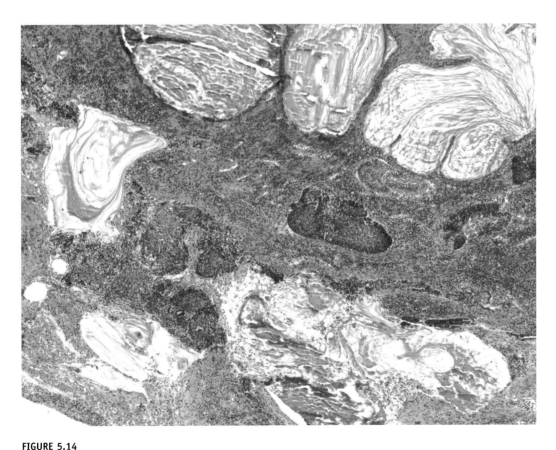

FIGURE 5.14
Pseudoinvasion. Distorted fragments of highly dysplastic squamous epithelium are present within the cervical stroma, but are not associated with desmoplasia.

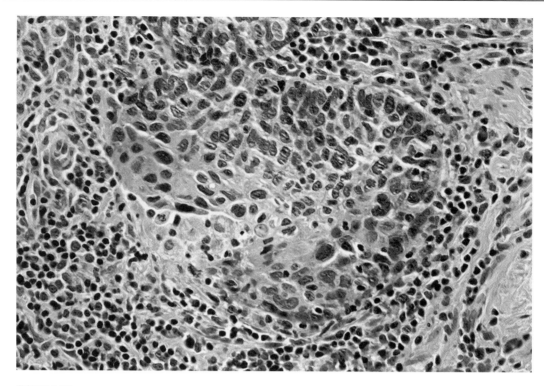

FIGURE 5.15
Early invasive squamous cell carcinoma. Paradoxical maturation associated with marked inflammation and desmoplasia are seen.

According to the current American Society for Clinical Colposcopists and Pathologists treatment guidelines, the preferred treatment for biopsy-confirmed HSIL is excision of the entire transformation zone, either by laser conization, cold-knife conization, loop electrosurgical excisional procedure, or loop electrosurgical conization. The mode of treatment utilized varies depending upon age of the patient, fertility issues, size of the transformation zone, compliance of the patient (risk of loss to follow-up), and grade of the lesion (CIN II versus CIN III).

In most cases, the excised tissue is received intact and is easy to orient. However, it may be received in more than one fragment for the following reasons: (1) the transformation zone is wide and requires two or more passes of the loop for complete excision; or (2) a loop electrosurgical conization is performed, which consists of an exocervical portion and a separate endocervical "top hat." In these cases, orientation is impossible in the pathology laboratory if the gynecologist has not oriented the specimens previously. If both the endocervical margin and the endocervical curettage (which is performed following excision) are positive for HSIL, the patient may undergo a repeat excisional procedure. Despite a negative endocervical curettage, the presence within the excision of: (1) extensive HSIL involving all four quadrants; (2) positive endocervical margins; and (3) endocervical gland extension are indicative of greater recurrence risk. In such cases, the patient will be followed more closely.

Since many of these specimens are removed using electrocautery, thermal artifact is often present at the margins. Within the thermal zone, there is loss of cellular detail, making assessment of SIL difficult within that zone. However, the zone of thermal artifact should be thin in an electrocautery excision that is performed correctly. If the SIL extends into the zone of cautery upon which ink is visible, the margin is considered positive. Less frequently, SIL may involve the deep stromal margin within an endocervical gland and, since these patients are also at risk for residual/recurrent disease and subsequent development of invasive carcinoma, they must also be closely followed or have a repeat excision.

SQUAMOUS CELL CARCINOMA

This is the second most common cancer in women worldwide following breast cancer. In developing countries, squamous cell carcinoma of the cervix is the most common cancer in women. In the US, cervical carcinoma follows endometrial and ovarian carcinomas in prevalence in the female genital tract. Squamous cell carcinoma is the most common type of carcinoma of the cervix. Although previously accounting for > 90 % of all cervical cancers, the overall frequency has decreased due to the implementation and success of national cervical smear screening programs. This has also resulted in the detection of otherwise asymptomatic small, early invasive lesions, which offers the possibility of conservative management due to the negligible (but not absent) risk of metastases.

CLINICAL FEATURES

Invasive squamous cell carcinoma accounts for approximately 4% of all newly diagnosed cancers and it is responsible for 18% of all deaths from genital tract cancers in women in the US. However, the incidence has declined with the implementation of widespread cervical screening programs. In fact, in countries with modern health care systems, the majority of patients with early invasive carcinoma present with an abnormal Pap smear. In contrast, grossly evident carcinoma presents with postcoital or intermenstrual bleeding. With growth into parametria and involvement of ureters, obstructive uropathy and renal failure herald the natural course of untreated cervical cancer. Pain is usually indicative of pelvic wall or lumbosacral nerve root invasion. In advanced stages, hematuria, rectal bleeding, or constipation indicates bladder or rectal involvement.

COLPOSCOPIC FEATURES

Early invasive carcinoma may have a colposcopic appearance similar to that seen in HSIL (punctations and mosaicism); however, the presence of atypical vessels is highly suggestive of early invasion. The atypical vessels run parallel to the surface and often have irregular shapes such as spirals and commas.

Small invasive carcinoma of the cervix appears as a raised, red, granular lesion on colposcopic exam. More advanced tumors tend to be exophytic, involve the ectocervix, and thus, are clinically apparent with speculum examination (Figure 5.16). Tumors confined to the endocervical canal are more commonly endophytic, resulting in a barrel-shaped expansion of the cervix.

PATHOLOGIC FEATURES

GROSS FINDINGS

Squamous cell carcinoma may either present as an exophytic friable polypoid or papillary tumor (more

---

SQUAMOUS CELL CARCINOMA – FACT SHEET

Definition
▶ Malignant epithelial neoplasm of the cervix showing squamous differentiation

Incidence and Location
▶ Approximately 4% of all newly diagnosed cancers in women in the US
▶ Decline by almost 75% in the last 50 years in the US due to cervical screening programs
▶ Vast majority in transformation zone

Morbidity and Mortality
▶ Approximately 4800 deaths each year in the US (2.6 deaths/100,000 women)
▶ 18% of all deaths from genital tract cancer in women in the US

Race and Age Distribution
▶ 7.3/100,000 for Caucasian women and 11.7/100,000 for African American women in the US
▶ Currently 25% of stage IB tumors occur in women < 40 years and 5% in women ≤ 30 years

Clinical Features
▶ Abnormal Pap smear in early invasive carcinoma (stage IA) in developed countries
▶ Postcoital or intermenstrual bleeding in stage IB or higher
▶ Obstructive uropathy, pain, hematuria, or rectal bleeding in advanced stages

Prognosis and Treatment
▶ Stage single most important determinant of outcome
▶ Size, depth of invasion, lymphovascular involvement, direct spread to parametrium, and presence and number of lymph node metastases are all adverse prognostic factors
▶ Frequency of distant metastases increases with stage
▶ Cone biopsy for selected stage IA tumors
▶ Radiotherapy or surgery for early invasive tumors (IB to IIA)
▶ Combined radiation and chemotherapy for advanced tumors

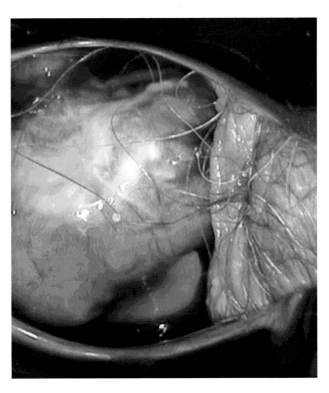

FIGURE 5.16
Squamous cell carcinoma. A large exocervical mass obliterates the exocervix on colposcopy.

SQUAMOUS CELL CARCINOMA – PATHOLOGIC FEATURES

Gross Findings

▸ Raised, red granular lesion if early but grossly visible
▸ Polypoid/papillary (ectocervical) or barrel-shaped (endocervical) in large tumors

Microscopic Findings

▸ Early invasive carcinoma:
 – maximum depth of 5 mm and maximum width of 7 mm (FIGO)
 – maximum depth of 3 mm and maximum width of 7 mm without lymphovascular invasion (SGO)
▸ Heterogeneity in growth pattern, cell type, and degree of differentiation
▸ Nests, cords, islands, individual cells with oval to polygonal shape, eosinophilic cytoplasm, intercellular bridges, and variable degree of nuclear pleomorphism
▸ Keratin pearls or individual keratinized cells may be seen
▸ Variants:
 1. Basaloid
 2. Verrucous
 3. Warty or condylomatous
 4. Papillary
 5. Squamotransitional
 6. Lymphoepithelioma-like

Immunohistochemical Features

▸ p16 diffuse nuclear and cytoplasmic positivity
▸ p63 nuclear positivity

Ultrastructural Features

▸ Tonofilaments, desmosome complexes, and intercellular microvilli in well-differentiated tumors

Cytology Correlation

▸ Bizarre "tadpole" cells with eosinophilic cytoplasm
▸ Large irregular hyperchromatic nuclei
▸ Necrotic debris with inflammatory changes: "tumor diathesis"

Differential Diagnosis

▸ Squamous metaplasia with extensive glandular involvement
▸ Postbiopsy entrapped squamous epithelium
▸ Marked decidualized reaction
▸ Placental-site nodule
▸ Clear cell adenocarcinoma
▸ Small cell neuroendocrine carcinoma

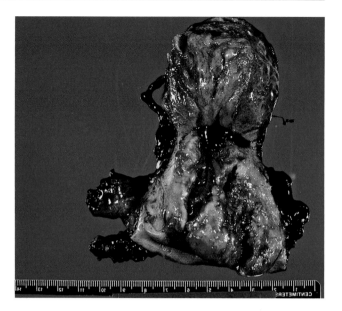

FIGURE 5.17
Squamous cell carcinoma. A large fungating mass is centered in the transformation zone and grows into the endocervical canal.

frequently in the exocervix) (Figure 5.17), as a nodular, ulcerated, endophytic mass (more frequently involving the endocervix) with extensive infiltration of the cervical wall resulting in a barrel-shaped configuration, or as an ulcerative lesion.

MICROSCOPIC FINDINGS

Early invasive carcinoma is defined by the International Federation of Gynecology and Obstetrics (FIGO) as microscopically identified carcinoma with invasion to a maximum depth of 5 mm and a width of 7 mm (stage IA) (Table 5.1). Although lymphovascular invasion does not alter stage, its presence should be recorded. If the tumor is grossly visible, the lesion is upstaged regardless of size (stage IB) (Table 5.1). However, the Society of Gynecologic Oncologists (SGO) defines early invasive carcinoma as a lesion with ≤ 3 mm stromal invasion that is ≤ 7 mm wide without evidence of lymphovascular invasion. Stromal invasion should be measured from the base of HSIL involving either the surface or gland crypts, and it is seen as small tongues of malignant cells detached from the underlying HSIL. The invasive cells appear more differentiated than those of the adjacent HSIL, with abundant eosinophilic cytoplasm and even keratinization. A useful diagnostic clue to early invasion is the presence of accompanying desmoplastic stroma, edema, and marked chronic inflammation (Figure 5.18).

Overt invasive squamous cell carcinomas usually display considerable morphologic heterogeneity in growth pattern, cell type, and degree of cellular differentiation. The majority form anastomosing cords or nests or irregular, rounded, or angulated and spiked islands (Figures 5.19A and B). The cells are oval to polygonal, often with eosinophilic cytoplasm, cell borders are usually sharp but may be indistinct, and intercellular bridges may be apparent. The nuclei are relatively uniform but may display considerable pleomorphism, with coarse and granular chromatin (Figure 5.19C). Mitoses are common, with frequent atypical forms. The desmoplastic stroma present in some tumors may be heavily infiltrated by inflammatory cells, with eosinophils or lymphocytes often predominating.

TABLE 5.1

TNM and International Federation of Gynecology and Obstetrics (FIGO) classification of carcinoma of the cervix (abbreviated)

TNM categories	FIGO stages	
Primary tumor (T)		
TX		Primary tumor cannot be assessed
T0		No evidence of primary tumor
Tis	0	Carcinoma in situ
T1	I	Carcinoma confined to uterus (extension to corpus should be disregarded)
T1a*	IA	Invasive carcinoma diagnosed only by microscopy. Stromal invasion with a maximum depth of 5.0 mm measured from the base of the epithelium and a horizontal spread ≤ 7.0 mm. Vascular space involvement, venous or lymphatic, does not affect classification
T1b	IB	Clinical visible lesion confined to the cervix or microscopic lesion greater than T1a/IA
T2	II	Carcinoma invades beyond uterus but not to pelvic wall or to lower third of vagina
T2a	IIA	Tumor without parametrial invasion
T2b	IIB	Tumor with parametrial invasion
T3	III	Tumor extends to pelvic wall and/or involves lower third of vagina, and/or causes hydronephrosis or nonfunctioning kidney
T3a	IIIA	Tumor involves lower third of vagina
T3b	IIIB	Tumor extends to pelvic wall and/or causes hydronephrosis or nonfunctioning kidney
T4	IVA	Tumor invades mucosa of bladder or rectum, and/or extends beyond true pelvis
Regional lymph nodes (N)		
NX		Regional lymph nodes cannot be assessed
N0		No regional lymph node metastasis
N1		Regional lymph node metastasis
Distant metastasis (M)		
MX		Distant metastasis cannot be assessed
M0		No distant metastasis
M1	IVB	Distant metastasis

*All macroscopically visible lesions – even with superficial invasion – are T1b/IB.

Grading squamous cell carcinomas of the cervix has poor clinical correlation. Nevertheless, the following system may be used:

1. Well-differentiated (grade 1: mature squamous cells with abundant keratin pearl formation and intercellular bridges).
2. Moderately differentiated (grade 2: less cytoplasm, less distinct cell borders, nuclear pleomorphism, and mitoses). Approximately 60% of squamous cell carcinomas belong to this group.
3. Poorly differentiated (grade 3: primitive-appearing small cells with scant cytoplasm and hyperchromatic nuclei with increased mitoses).

Squamous cell carcinomas have also been subtyped according to both cell type and degree of differentiation (Box 5.1). This system subdivides these tumors into three categories:

1. Large cell nonkeratinizing carcinoma (most common). It lacks keratin pearls but can have keratinization of individual cells.
2. Keratinizing carcinoma. By definition, it requires the presence of keratin pearl formation. A keratin pearl is composed of a nest of squamous epithelium in which the cells are arranged in concentric circles surrounding central acellular keratin.
3. Small cell nonkeratinizing carcinoma. It is composed of small cells with scant cytoplasm and small nuclei reminiscent of HSIL cells. There may be isolated cells with abundant eosinophilic cytoplasm or nests of cells with keratinization. It should not be confused

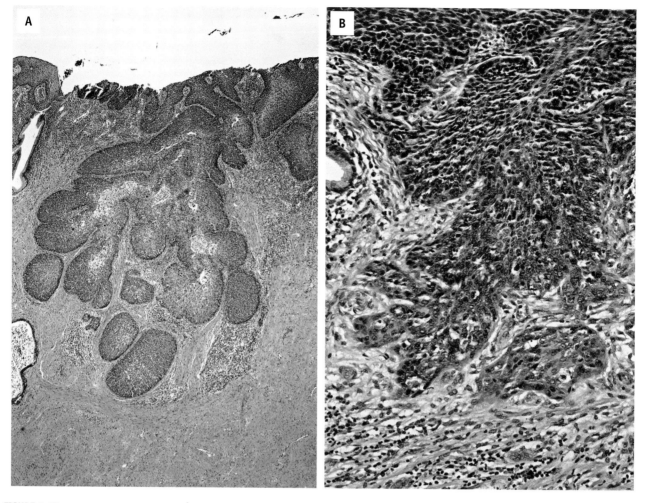

FIGURE 5.18

Early invasive squamous cell carcinoma. At the base of a crypt, focal prominent stromal reaction is seen in a background of extensive HSIL involving endocervical glands (A). At high power, small irregular nests of malignant squamous epithelium invade the surrounding stroma (B).

with basaloid carcinoma or small cell neuroendocrine carcinoma (discussed below).

However, although these classifications exist, no grading system has been widely accepted, and the WHO recommends the use a two-tiered system separating squamous cell carcinomas into keratinizing and nonkeratinizing.

Several variants of cervical carcinoma have been described (Box 5.1), including:

Basaloid squamous cell carcinoma is composed of nests of small oval-shaped basaloid cells with scant cytoplasm. The cells resemble those of squamous cell carcinoma in situ; they have hyperchromatic nuclei and are associated with brisk mitotic activity. Foci of squamous differentiation may be present, but keratin pearls are not seen.

Verrucous carcinoma is a highly differentiated squamous cell carcinoma that has a propensity to recur but not to metastasize. It typically has a papillary growth with an undulating, hyperkeratotic surface and prominent acanthosis. It invades the underlying stroma with

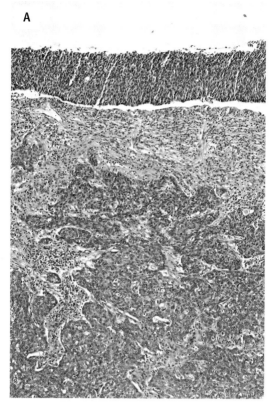

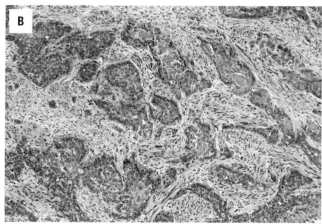

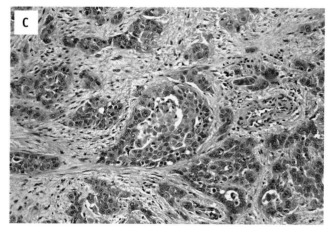

FIGURE 5.19
Moderately differentiated squamous cell carcinoma. The tumor is deeply invasive and is associated with HSIL (A); it is composed of irregular, angulated, or spiked islands of tumor cells associated with a prominent desmoplastic reaction (B); and the tumor cells have abundant eosinophilic cytoplasm with individual keratinization and prominent nuclear pleomorphism (C).

a wide-front, bulbous pushing border. The cells have abundant eosinophilic cytoplasm, minimal cytologic atypia and no koilocytosis. It is distinguished from common squamous cell carcinoma by the absence of both nuclear atypia and destructive stromal invasion.

Warty carcinoma is defined as an invasive squamous cell carcinoma with morphological features of HPV infection (Figure 5.20). It has also been called condylomatous squamous cell carcinoma.

Papillary squamous cell carcinoma is characterized by thick or thin papillae with fibrovascular cores covered by squamous epithelium that, seen in isolation, has the appearance of HSIL (Figure 5.21). Underlying features of typical squamous cell carcinoma are present, although a superficial biopsy may be misleading. Papillary squamous carcinoma is distinguished from warty carcinoma by inconspicuous keratinization and the absence of HPV effect, and from transitional cell carcinoma by its squamous cell differentiation.

Squamotransitional carcinoma is rare in the cervix and is indistinguishable from papillary transitional carcinomas of the urinary bladder. The fibrovascular

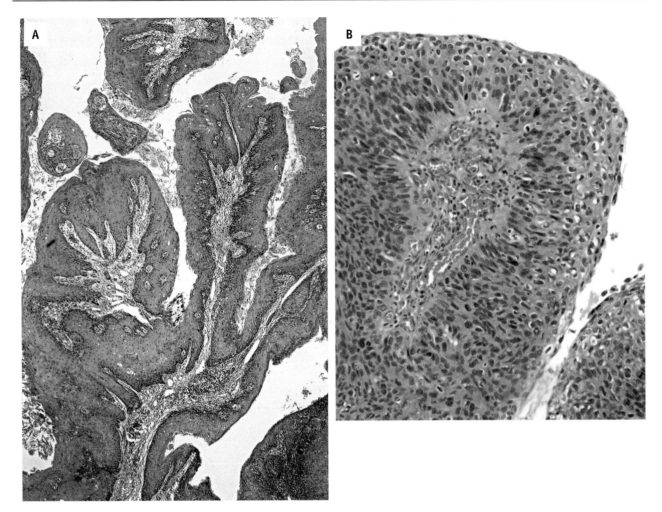

FIGURE 5.20

Warty carcinoma (condylomatous squamous cell carcinoma). The tumor has a prominent papillary architecture (A). HPV effect is present in some of the neoplastic cells (B).

cores are lined by multilayered epithelium resembling HSIL; however, it may have a purely transitional appearance.

Lymphoepithelioma-like carcinoma bears a striking resemblance to its nasopharyngeal counterpart. This tumor is characterized by ill-defined islands of undifferentiated cells associated with a marked lymphocytic background within the stroma. The tumor cells have a syncytial growth, with poorly defined cell borders and moderate pale eosinophilic cytoplasm. The nuclei are large and uniform with vesicular chromatin and prominent nucleoli.

ANCILLARY STUDIES

IMMUNOHISTOCHEMISTRY

Although immunohistochemistry plays a minor role in the diagnosis of conventional squamous cell carcinomas, it helps identify unusual variants and distinguish

them from other types of cervical tumors. p16 (a cyclin-dependent kinase inhibitor) is diffusely positive (nuclear and cytoplasmic staining) in squamous cell carcinomas which correlates with the presence of high-risk HPV. p63 (a homologue of p53) is an excellent marker of squamous cell carcinomas and its expression highly correlates with HPV 16. It is useful in the distinction of squamous cell carcinoma from adenocarcinoma, adenosquamous carcinoma, and neuroendocrine tumors.

Neuroendocrine markers (synaptophysin and chromogranin, among others) are essential to exclude small cell carcinoma, as it is important to distinguish the latter from small cell nonkeratinizing squamous cell carcinoma and basaloid squamous carcinoma, both of which may also be composed of small dark blue cells.

ULTRASTRUCTURAL EXAMINATION

Nowadays, electron microscopy is rarely used in the diagnosis of squamous cell carcinoma. Typical features

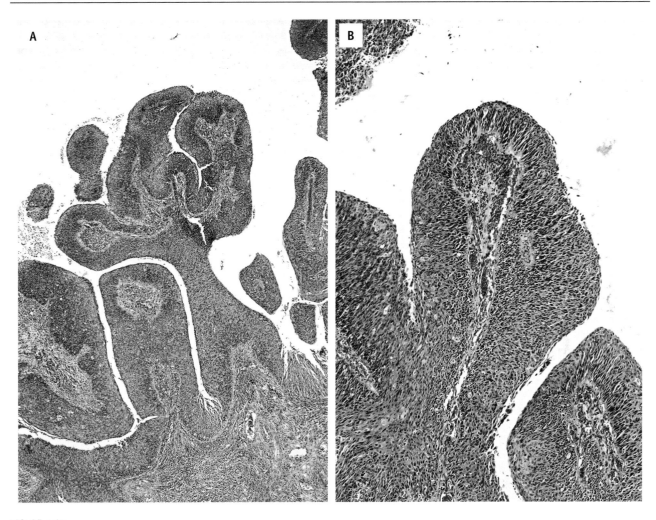

FIGURE 5.21

Papillary squamous cell carcinoma. Papillae with fibrovascular cores are lined by malignant epithelium that resembles HSIL (A). Lack of maturation of the neoplastic cells with increased nuclear-to-cytoplasmic ratio and absence of HPV effect distinguishes papillary squamous cell carcinoma from warty carcinoma (B).

in well-differentiated tumors include intracytoplasmic tonofilaments, desmosome–tonofilament complexes, and intercellular microvilli. However, these features are less frequent in tumors with decreasing differentiation. Importantly, dense core granules are absent, excluding small cell carcinoma.

CYTOLOGY

Cytologic preparations of keratinizing squamous cell carcinoma usually show bizarre-shaped and "tadpole" cells with eosinophilic cytoplasm and large irregular hyperchromatic nuclei (Figure 5.22A). In nonkeratinizing carcinoma, the cells show anisokaryosis that are either seen singly or arranged in syncytia. The nuclei are large, with coarsely granular chromatin and irregular nucleoli (Figure 5.22B). A dirty background (tumor diathesis) including necrotic debris and inflammation is present more commonly in nonkeratinizing squamous

cell carcinoma but can also be seen in keratinizing carcinoma; hence the background is as important as the cytologic features.

Cytologic findings of early invasive carcinoma are somewhat controversial as cells may lack sufficiently robust features to allow this diagnosis. Cytologic features such as cytoplasmic differentiation with cell elongation and presence of nucleolus can also be seen in squamous cell carcinoma in situ, particularly when the latter involves endocervical gland necks.

DIFFERENTIAL DIAGNOSIS

A benign lesion that enters the differential diagnosis of invasive squamous cell carcinoma is *florid squamous metaplasia with gland involvement* as it may impart

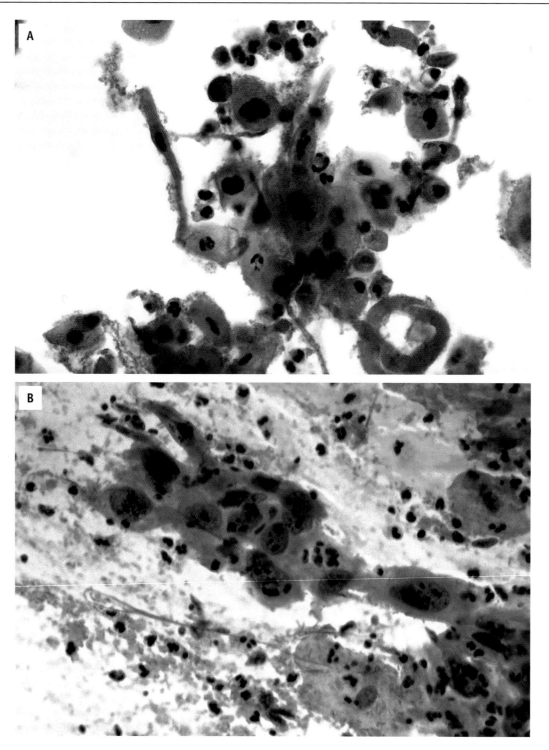

FIGURE 5.22

Squamous cell carcinoma. Neoplastic cells show cytoplasmic keratinization, cellular pleomorphism, and background tumor diathesis in a Pap smear (A). A group of malignant nonkeratinizing squamous cells shows prominent nucleoli and background tumor diathesis (B).

a false impression of invasion. However, the latter shows smooth outlines, evenly spaced nuclei, and absence of nuclear atypia and mitotic activity. *Benign squamous epithelium* may become entrapped deep in the cervical wall following a biopsy, giving the false impression of invasion, even more so because of an associated abnormal stromal reaction. However, the epithelial nests within the stroma have benign nuclear features and the overlying squamous epithelium is also unremarkable. The clinical history of a previous biopsy is helpful.

Marked decidualized reaction of the cervical stroma may also be mistaken for squamous cell carcinoma. Decidual cells lack mitotic activity and have no cytologic atypia. Cytokeratin is also helpful as it is strongly positive in squamous cell carcinoma, but negative in decidualized cells.

Placental-site nodule may be difficult to distinguish from squamous cell carcinoma on small biopsy specimens, as its small round projections from the main nodule consisting of eosinophilic cells admixed with eosinophilic, fibrinoid material similar to keratin may simulate invasion. However, there is extensive hyalinization, the intermediate trophoblast cells are arranged in a haphazard pattern, they have degenerated nuclei and abundant eosinophilic cytoplasm that may show vacuolization. Keratin and EMA are not helpful in this differential diagnosis. However, only intermediate trophoblast cells are positive for placental alkaline phosphatase, inhibin, human placental lactogen (HPL), and Mel-CAM.

Squamous cell carcinoma may occasionally have clear cytoplasm due to abundant glycogen, leading to confusion with *clear cell adenocarcinoma*. However, the latter typically has characteristic papillary or tubulocystic patterns, with hobnail cells in addition to clear cells. The poorly differentiated or small cell nonkeratinizing carcinoma has to be distinguished from *small cell neuroendocrine carcinoma*. Whilst the latter has distinctive morphological features (small nests, ribbons and trabeculae, cells with scant cytoplasm, hyperchromatic round to spindled nuclei and smudged chromatin and crush artifact), the diagnosis of small cell neuroendocrine carcinoma is confirmed by positivity for neuroendocrine markers (chromogranin and synaptophysin) and low-molecular-weight keratins (paranuclear dotlike pattern).

PROGNOSIS AND THERAPY

The single most important factor for determining outcome of cervical carcinoma is stage (Table 5.1). Hence, the 5-year survival rate for stage 1A tumors ranges from 97 to 100%; approximately 84% for stage 1B tumors, and from 65 to 73% for stage II tumors; it drops to 36% for stage III tumors; and < 15% for stage IV tumors. In addition, size and depth of the tumor also influence prognosis. In a recent Gynecologic Oncology Group study, the 3-year disease-free interval was 95%

for occult tumors and 88% for those < 3 cm, while it dropped to 68% for tumors > 3 cm. In the same study, when evaluating depth of invasion, the 3-year disease-free interval was 94% for tumors infiltrating < 5 mm, 84.5% for those invading 6–10 mm, and 73.6% when deeper invasion was present.

Some studies have shown that direct tumor spread to the parametrium is an adverse factor regardless of lymph node status, and that the frequency of distant metastases (most frequently lung, abdomen, liver, and gastrointestinal tract) increases with stage, ranging from 3% in stage I tumors to 75% in stage IV tumors. The finding of lymphovascular involvement is considered to be an adverse prognostic sign, as it is a significant predictor of lymph node metastases. The presence and number of lymph node metastases and the number of nodal groups involved are also parameters of prognostic significance. The primary lymphatic drainage of the cervix is to the paracervical and parametrial lymph nodes, then to the obturator, external iliac, and internal iliac nodes. Progressive involvement of common iliac, para-aortic and even supraclavicular nodes may be seen. Survival rates decrease with increasing number of involved lymph nodes. One study reported a 90% survival rate with negative lymph nodes, 70% with one to three lymph nodes involved by carcinoma, dropping to 38% with ≥ four positive lymph nodes.

Early invasive carcinoma (stage IA) may be treated with conservative surgery, especially if the patient wants to preserve fertility. Radiotherapy and surgery have similar results for stages IB and IIA early invasive cancer. More advanced tumors (IIB–IV) are treated with a combination of external and intracavitary radiation. Recent trials with chemotherapy (concurrent with radiotherapy) have shown significant overall and disease-free survival advantage. Hence, this combination is emerging as the new standard of care for advanced cervical cancer.

ADENOCARCINOMA IN SITU AND ENDOCERVICAL GLANDULAR DYSPLASIA

In contrast to the marked reduction in the incidence of invasive squamous cell carcinoma resulting from effective cervicovaginal screening, the incidence of cervical adenocarcinoma has increased over the last 30 years. In addition, both adenocarcinoma in situ (AIS) and invasive adenocarcinoma are being diagnosed more frequently in women under the age of 35 years. This increase may be partly a result of improved endocervical sampling devices as well as of increased recognition and refinement of criteria to diagnose glandular lesions both cytologically and histologically. The higher frequency of adenocarcinoma in younger women is similar to the trend seen in SIL and likely a result of changing sexual practices over recent years. Nevertheless, AIS is much less common than SIL, with AIS representing only 1% of all in situ carcinomas. AIS is a precursor lesion to invasive adenocarcinoma which is supported by several lines of evidence:

1. There is a temporal relationship between AIS and invasive adenocarcinoma; AIS is diagnosed in women 10–20 years younger than those with invasive adenocarcinoma (mean age of 29–35 years). This age difference is similar to the temporal relationship between SIL and invasive squamous carcinoma. Interestingly, however, unlike SIL, which is much more common than invasive squamous carcinoma, AIS is found less frequently than invasive adenocarcinoma. The reason for the difference is not entirely clear but may be related to the relative difficulty in detecting glandular lesions on Pap smears compared to SIL and the fact that AIS does not produce a visible lesion on colposcopic examination.
2. Adenocarcinoma in situ is frequently found adjacent to invasive adenocarcinoma.
3. Similar HPV subtypes are identified in both AIS and invasive adenocarcinoma, most frequently HPV 18 (70%), followed by 16 (30%). Similar to SIL, AIS is probably a result of HPV infection (the relationship of AIS to HPV has not been as extensively studied as SIL), with HPV DNA present in up to 89% of AIS.

Finally, SIL or invasive squamous carcinoma has been found in 25–85% of specimens containing AIS (Figure 5.23). It is currently unknown what percentage of AIS progresses to invasive adenocarcinoma and with what frequency it regresses.

CLINICAL FEATURES

Adenocarcinoma in situ is incidentally detected either on a Pap smear or a colposcopically obtained biopsy, endocervical curettage, or excisional procedure performed during clinical evaluation of SIL. If symptoms are present, the most common is abnormal bleeding.

COLPOSCOPIC FINDINGS

Adenocarcinoma in situ is difficult to detect by colposcopy because unlike SIL, it does not produce a characteristic lesion. As AIS is only slightly thicker than normal glandular surface epithelium, it would be difficult to see even with the magnification of a colposcope, despite the fact that the lesion involves the transformation zone in up to 65% of cases.

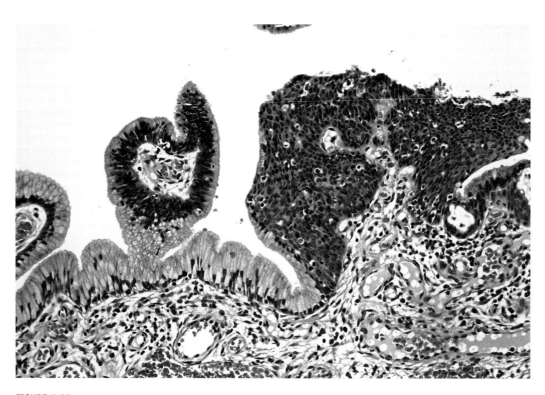

FIGURE 5.23
Adenocarcinoma in situ. A segment of normal glandular epithelium separates AIS (left) and HSIL (right) involving the surface epithelium.

PATHOLOGIC FINDINGS

GROSS FINDINGS

Adenocarcinoma in situ does not produce a grossly visible lesion, often occurs in the transformation zone, is usually unifocal, but through horizontal and lateral spread can involve multiple quadrants.

MICROSCOPIC FINDINGS

Both the surface epithelium and endocervical glands may be involved by AIS with preservation of the normal glandular architecture (Figure 5.24A), although occasionally intraglandular papillae or cribriforming are present. There is often an abrupt transition from neoplastic to normal epithelium (Figure 5.24B). AIS may involve a gland focally, multifocally, or in its entirety. The cells display crowding and pseudostratification, they have columnar morphology, and markedly increased

nuclear-to-cytoplasmic ratio with elongate, irregular nuclei and coarse chromatin (Figure 5.24C). Nucleoli are usually inconspicuous but may be multiple. Mitotic figures, particularly in an apical location, are frequent. Also present and characteristic are numerous apoptotic bodies (Figure 5.24D). The cytoplasm may be scant and eosinophilic with little or no mucin production, or, less frequently, may display abundant mucin.

Different subtypes of AIS may occur, including endocervical, intestinal (colonic), endometrioid, mixed adenosquamous, clear cell, and the most recently described type, tubal. Although there is no known difference in behavior amongst the different subtypes, knowledge and recognition of the varying morphologies allows the pathologist to establish the correct diagnosis.

Endocervical-type AIS is most common and occurs either alone or admixed with intestinal or endometrioid

---

ADENOCARCINOMA IN SITU (AIS) – FACT SHEET

Definition
▸ Precursor lesion to invasive adenocarcinoma mainly associated with high-risk HPV, particularly type 18

Prevalence and Location
▸ Unknown exact prevalence
▸ HSIL:AIS ratio varies from 1:26 to 1:237
▸ Transformation zone, frequently unifocal
▸ Association with HSIL in 24–75% of cases

Morbidity and Mortality
▸ Therapy related morbidity
▸ If untreated, may progress to invasive adenocarcinoma

Race and Age Distribution
▸ No known race predilection
▸ Reproductive-age women (mean age 29 years)

Clinical Features
▸ Typically asymptomatic
▸ Rarely abnormal vaginal bleeding

Prognosis and Treatment
▸ Initial step: colposcopy, biopsy of any visible lesion, and endocervical curettage
▸ Biopsy-proven AIS followed by cold-knife conization to evaluate extent of AIS and exclude invasive adenocarcinoma
▸ If fertility is an issue and cone shows negative margins and no invasion, patient followed closely with repeat endocervical curettage at defined intervals with consideration for hysterectomy following child-bearing
▸ If fertility is not an issue, hysterectomy preferred treatment

---

ADENOCARCINOMA IN SITU (AIS) – PATHOLOGIC FEATURES

Gross Findings
▸ No grossly visible lesion

Microscopic Findings
▸ Preservation of normal architecture; occasionally intraglandular papillae or cribriforming
▸ Crowding, pseudostratification, and columnar morphology of glandular cells
▸ Marked increased nuclear-to-cytoplasmic ratio with elongate, irregular nuclei, and coarse chromatin
▸ Frequent mitoses and apoptotic bodies
▸ Sparse, eosinophilic to abundant mucinous cytoplasm

Cytology Correlation
▸ Atypical glandular cells in strips and sheets with prominent nuclear crowding
▸ Feathering at group edges and rosette formation may be prominent
▸ Increased nuclear-to-cytoplasmic ratio, nuclear enlargement, elongation, and hyperchromasia with coarse nuclear chromatin
▸ Mitoses and apoptotic bodies

Immunohistochemical Features
▸ Cytoplasmic CEA (up to 67% AIS)
▸ High Ki-67 index
▸ Frequent p53 positivity
▸ Strong p16 positivity
▸ Decreased positivity for ER and PR

Differential Diagnosis
▸ Reactive/reparative atypia
▸ Arias–Stella reaction
▸ Radiation atypia
▸ Endometriosis
▸ Lower uterine segment epithelium
▸ Tubal metaplasia
▸ Cautery artifact
▸ Secondary involvement by HSIL

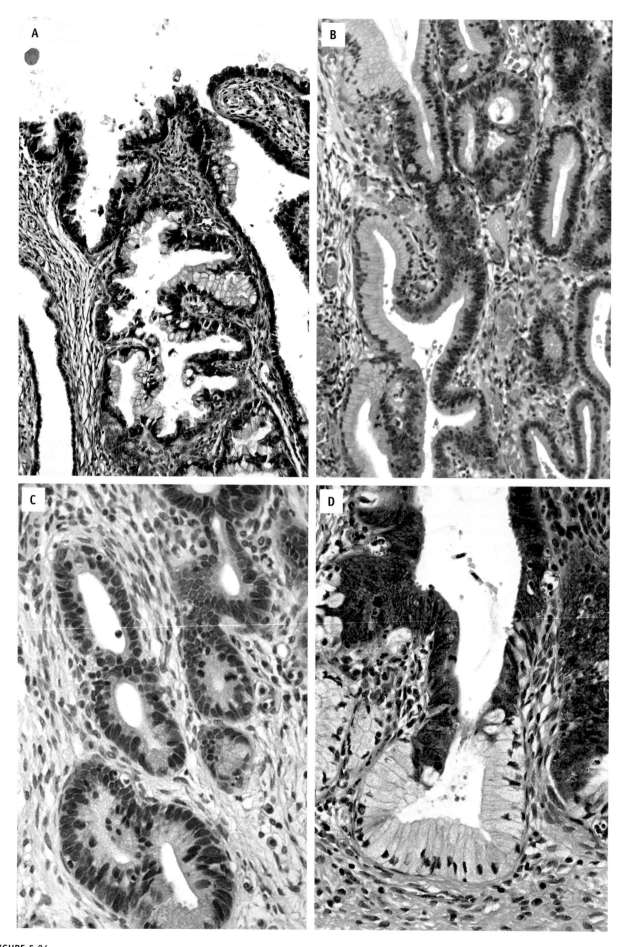

FIGURE 5.24

Adenocarcinoma in situ (AIS). Both surface epithelium and endocervical glands are involved by AIS. At this power, nuclear hyperchromasia and crowding can be appreciated (A). There is an abrupt transition between AIS and normal endocervical epithelium (B). The neoplastic cells have columnar morphology with crowding, pseudostratification, nuclear enlargement, and hyperchromasia (C). Note numerous mitotic figures and apoptotic bodies (D).

types. It most closely resembles normal endocervical glands. The intestinal type has prominent goblet cells and frequently shows less nuclear pseudostratification and mitotic activity than endocervical AIS. In the endometrioid type, the cells have densely eosinophilic, sparse cytoplasm with minimal to absent mucin. As its name implies, it resembles to some extent proliferative endometrial glands. Adenosquamous carcinoma in situ has two different appearances. It may have distinct populations of glandular and squamous cells. Alternatively, it may be composed of a population of neoplastic cells with features intermediate between glandular and squamous cells, with eosinophilic cytoplasm and polyhedral to columnar morphology intimately admixed with mucinous cells that show a stratified growth (stratified mucin-producing intraepithelial lesion). It is important to distinguish adenosquamous carcinoma in situ from AIS, which coexists but is separate from an adjacent SIL. The tubal type of AIS is diagnostically challenging because of its similarity to tubal metaplasia, including the presence of cilia and intercalated cells. Nevertheless, the cytologic features of AIS are present, including pseudostratification, nuclear enlargement and elongation, coarse chromatin, mitotic figures, and apoptotic bodies.

Lesser degrees of glandular atypia than seen in AIS have been identified. Various terminologies have been proposed for these lesions, including glandular atypia, glandular dysplasia, atypical hyperplasia, and low-grade and high-grade cervical glandular intraepithelial neoplasia. The latter terminology reflects an attempt to classify cervical glandular lesions in an analogous fashion to SIL. However, there are no well-defined criteria for recognizing and diagnosing glandular dysplasia, and not infrequently, lesions diagnosed as low-grade cervical glandular dysplasia show overlapping features with reactive processes. However, some lesions show variable degrees of pseudostratification, nuclear enlargement, nuclear coarsening, and apoptotic bodies but only occasional mitotic figures, changes that do not fulfil the diagnosis of AIS.

The relationship between glandular dysplasia and AIS is not well established. HPV DNA has been detected in glandular dysplasia at a significantly lower rate than in squamous dysplasia. It is assumed that, similarly to squamous lesions, glandular neoplasia progresses through a series of steps with distinct and reproducible morphology as it accumulates the genetic changes of carcinoma, but this has not yet been demonstrated.

ANCILLARY STUDIES

IMMUNOHISTOCHEMISTRY

Carcinoembryonic antigen is expressed in the cytoplasm of up to 67% of AIS. The cells show high Ki-67 index and express p53. p16 is diffusely positive (nuclear and cytoplasmic staining) in AIS, reflecting its association with high-risk HPV.

CYTOLOGY

Cervical cytology is primarily used as a screening test for SIL and early invasive squamous carcinoma. Its ability to detect glandular lesions is limited by both sampling and interpretation. The 2001 Bethesda System terminology for cervicovaginal cytology changed the reporting of glandular lesions to reflect better current knowledge of glandular neoplasia. The category "Atypical endocervical cells" is associated with an increased risk of AIS. Atypical glandular cells display nuclear atypia that exceeds obvious reactive/reparative changes, but lack definitive features of AIS or invasive adenocarcinoma. The category "atypical glandular cells, favor neoplastic" indicates increased suspicion for a significant lesion. The atypical cells are present in strips and sheets with prominent nuclear crowding. Feathering, where the atypical nuclei are arrayed perpendicular to the group's edge, may be focally present. Arrangement of the atypical cells in small glandular structures termer rosettes may also be focally seen. In this category, the atypical cells do not fully meet the criteria for AIS or invasive adenocarcinoma.

"Endocervical adenocarcinoma in situ" is a diagnostic category within the Bethesda System characterized by the presence of abnormal glandular cells in sheets, strips, and clusters with prominent nuclear crowding. Feathering and rosettes may also be prominent. Anisonucleosis, nuclear enlargement, elongation, and hyperchromasia are apparent, and mitoses and apoptotic bodies are frequent. Nucleoli remain inconspicuous and the background is clean (Figure 5.25). Coexistent HSIL may also be present.

DIFFERENTIAL DIAGNOSIS

Adenocarcinoma in situ should be distinguished from reactive/reparative atypia, Arias–Stella reaction, radia-

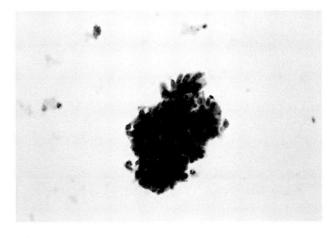

FIGURE 5.25

Adenocarcinoma in situ. A crowded group of neoplastic endocervical cells with increased nuclear-to-cytoplasmic ratio, nuclear hyperchromasia, feathering (superior edge of the group), and mitotic figures are seen in a monolayer Pap smear.

tion atypia, endometriosis, lower uterine segment (LUS) epithelium, tubal metaplasia, and cautery artifact.

In *reactive/reparative atypia*, nuclear enlargement, hyperchromasia, and pleomorphism may be present, but the chromatin pattern is smudgy rather than coarse, mitotic figures are rare or absent, apoptotic bodies are not seen, and there is no cellular stratification. Inflammatory cells are present in the stroma adjacent to, and frequently within, the atypical epithelium. In very difficult cases, high Ki-67 index in combination with positive CEA favors AIS over reactive epithelium.

The *Arias–Stella reaction* may involve endocervical glands of pregnant women. It is identical in appearance to the Arias–Stella reaction within the gravid endometrium. The glands, which may be only partially affected, are lined by pseudostratified glandular epithelium, that can form intraluminal papillary structures. There is marked cell enlargement with hyperchromatic and irregular nuclei. A characteristic and useful differentiating feature is the presence of hobnail cells. In addition, unlike AIS, the cytoplasm is abundant and vacuolated to clear, and the cells lack nuclear crowding or uniformly atypical nuclei, there are rare to absent mitotic figures, and no apoptotic bodies are found (Figure 5.26A).

Radiation atypia can show enlarged nuclei and marked nuclear atypia, but the nuclear-to-cytoplasmic ratio is preserved or reduced and the cytoplasm is often vacuolated. Pseudostratification, apoptotic bodies, and mitotic figures are absent.

Endometriosis can occur in the cervix and frequently shows the characteristic histologic triad, including endometrial glands surrounded by endometrial-type stroma and recent hemorrhage or hemosiderin-laden macrophages. It is important to recognize the associated endometrial stroma, as the endometrial glands typically have pseudostratified, hyperchromatic, and elongated nuclei that show mitotic activity thus, resembling AIS (Figure 5.26B).

Lower uterine segment (LUS) epithelium can occasionally be difficult to distinguish from AIS in cold-knife cone specimens as it can be pseudostratified with increased nuclear-to-cytoplasmic ratio. However, the nuclei are usually bland and uniform and mitotic figures are rare. In particularly difficult cases, LUS epithelium should be compared to the patient's known AIS.

Tubal metaplasia can occur in both the endocervix and LUS. The presence of cilia and intercalated cells, as well as the bland appearance of the nuclei, readily distinguishes tubal metaplasia from AIS (Figure 5.26C). Rarely, tubal metaplasia may be associated with tubal-type AIS in which nuclei show marked nuclear enlargement, pseudostratification, cytologic atypia, and mitotic activity.

Cauterized epithelium may show artifactual crowding, nuclear elongation, and hyperchromatism, but the degree of elongation is exaggerated and involves both cell nucleus and cytoplasm. No mitotic activity or apoptotic bodies are identified.

Colonization of endocervical glands by HSIL can mimic AIS, however, the cells tend to have more abundant cytoplasm, the nuclei are less pseudostratified and hyperchromatic, and there is no sharp transition to normal endocervical cells.

PROGNOSIS AND THERAPY

Similar to SIL, a diagnosis of at least atypical endocervical cells on a Pap smear should prompt immediate colposcopy. Any visible lesion is biopsied and an endocervical curettage is performed. Following a histologic diagnosis of AIS, the patient undergoes cold-knife conization to evaluate the extent of AIS and exclude invasive adenocarcinoma.

Until recently, the information obtained from a cone biopsy was utilized to plan further surgery. If no invasion was identified on cone biopsy, the patient underwent simple hysterectomy; however, if invasive adenocarcinoma was present, the patient underwent radical hysterectomy. This management strategy is based on several studies which have shown residual disease in up to 30% of women in subsequent hysterectomy specimens despite negative margins on the cone biopsy. However, since many women are delaying child-bearing into the fourth decade, AIS is frequently diagnosed in patients in whom preservation of fertility is important. Even though in these cases cone biopsy may currently be selected as sole therapy, the definitive therapy for AIS remains hysterectomy at present. If conization alone is selected, then the transformation zone, at least 2.5 cm of the adjacent endocervical canal, and the deepest aspect of the endocervical glands must be removed. Close clinical follow-up should be performed with repeat endocervical curettage at defined intervals and consideration for hysterectomy following child-bearing. A LEEP or laser conization is not considered an alternative therapy to cold-knife conization, as there is higher frequency of positive margins (up to 75%) compared to cold-knife conization, where positive margins may be present in up to 24% of cases (Figure 5.27). Women with positive endocervical margins are at increased risk for having an undiagnosed invasive adenocarcinoma or for developing recurrent AIS.

EARLY INVASIVE ADENOCARCINOMA

This type of adenocarcinoma is by far less common than its squamous counterpart, and accounts for 12% of early invasive carcinomas.

CLINICAL FEATURES

Early invasive adenocarcinoma occurs in patients with an average age of 39 years, approximately 7 years younger than the peak frequency of frankly invasive adenocarcinoma. Patients commonly present with an abnormal Pap smear that shows atypical glandular cells,

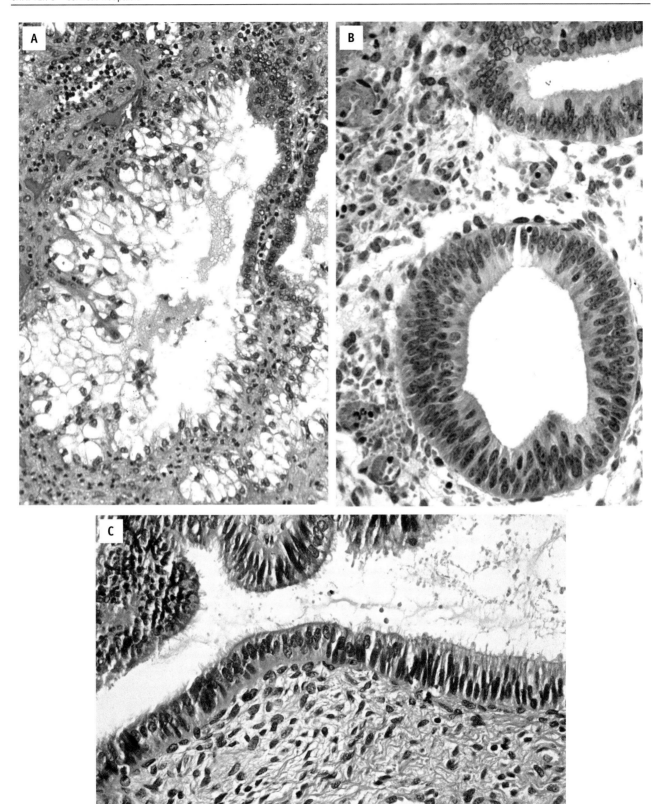

FIGURE 5.26

Arias–Stella reaction. There is focal nuclear enlargement and hyperchromasia of the lining epithelium. In contrast to AIS, the cells have abundant clear cytoplasm, smudgy chromatin, and no mitotic figures (A). Cervical endometriosis. There is nuclear crowding and hyperchromasia of the epithelial cells. Notice the accompanying edematous and focally hemorrhagic endometrial stroma and small vessels surrounding the endometrial-type gland (B). Tubal metaplasia. Nuclear pseudostratification and hyperchromasia are present. Of note, there is preservation of the nuclear-to-cytoplasmic ratio, absence of mitoses and apoptotic bodies, and presence of intercalated cells and cilia (C).

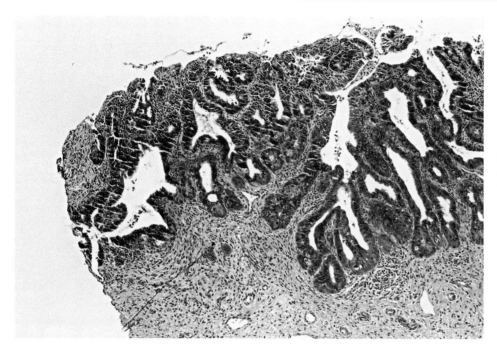

FIGURE 5.27
Adenocarcinoma in situ. Involvement of the inked endocervical margin in a cone excision.

but may also present with postcoital bleeding. It may represent an incidental finding in conization or hysterectomy specimens. These lesions cannot be seen on regular colposcopic exam. Similar to AIS and invasive adenocarcinoma, early invasive adenocarcinoma is associated with high-risk HPV (types 18 and 16).

PATHOLOGIC FEATURES

MICROSCOPIC FINDINGS

The pathologic definition of early invasive adenocarcinoma is the presence of stromal invasion, described as an effacement of the normal glandular architecture with tumor extending beyond the deepest normal crypt. Most studies define early invasive adenocarcinoma by depth of invasion (< 5 mm from base of surface epithelium) or by volume (< 500 mm^3). Measuring depth of invasion is often arbitrary and difficult, as the cells may invade the stroma either from the surface or from underlying glands, and consequently, the point of reference for measurement may not be clear. Furthermore, although it has been stated that in general normal endocervical glands do not extend deeper than 1 cm from the cervical surface, different benign glandular proliferations may be present further down in the cervical wall.

There are two unequivocal features that identify the presence of stromal invasion: (1) individual cells or incomplete glands lined by cytologically malignant-appearing cells; or (2) malignant-appearing glands surrounded by a desmoplastic and/or inflammatory response (Figure 5.28A). Unfortunately, in most early invasive adenocarcinoma, these features are lacking. In these cases, architecture is of paramount importance, and three additional features, although not entirely spe-

cific, may help to identify invasion. These include: (1) complex, branching, irregular, or small glands with a confluent growth; (2) cribriform growth pattern of malignant epithelium devoid of stroma within a single gland profile (Figure 5.28B); or (3) finding irregular bud-like projections, small glands, or uncommonly, solid nests that have a squamoid appearance with abundant eosinophilic cytoplasm and enlarged, rounded nuclei with cleared chromatin and prominent nucleoli. The presence of these squamoid cells within AIS glands should suggest the possibility of early stromal invasion, and deeper sections should be obtained.

CYTOLOGY

The Pap smear shows findings similar to those described in AIS.

DIFFERENTIAL DIAGNOSIS

Early invasive adenocarcinoma should be distinguished from *AIS*. AIS lacks florid architectural complexity and stromal reaction. Architecture is extremely important in distinguishing both entities, and, when possible, endocervical glands involved by adenocarcinoma should be compared with adjacent normal-appearing endocervical glands. Still, there will be a small percentage of cases where this distinction cannot be made with certainty.

PROGNOSIS AND THERAPY

Patients with early invasive adenocarcinoma have an excellent prognosis, especially when treated by hyster-

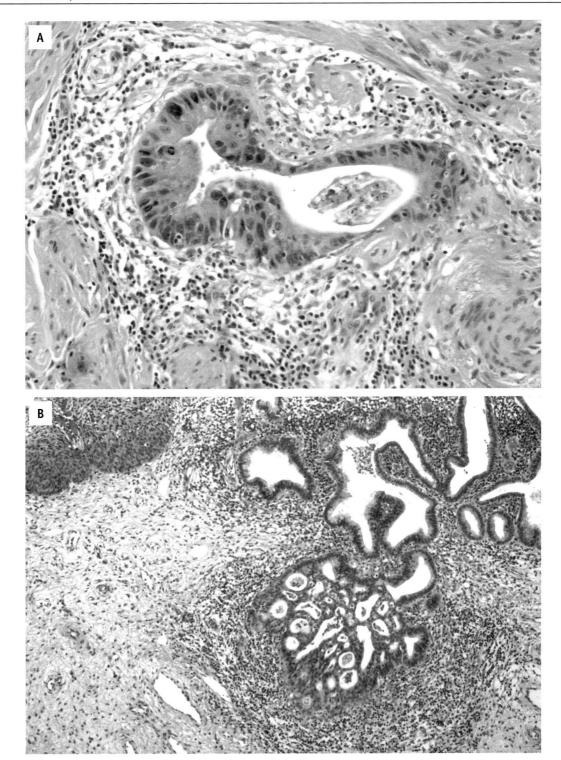

FIGURE 5.28

Early invasive adenocarcinoma. A focally incomplete gland is associated with marked stromal reaction (A). Cribriform growth of malignant epithelium devoid of stroma within a single gland profile is associated with a prominent inflammatory response (B).

ectomy or cone biopsy with negative margins. Tumors with 5 mm of invasion rarely recur or metastasize to lymph nodes.

CERVICAL ADENOCARCINOMA

This group of tumors is diverse, encompassing a variety of histologic types. Mucinous adenocarcinoma is the most common (60%), followed by endometrioid adenocarcinoma (30%). The remaining histologic subtypes include minimal-deviation adenocarcinoma, well-differentiated villoglandular, clear cell, serous, and mesonephric adenoarcinoma.

MUCINOUS ADENOCARCINOMA

CLINICAL FEATURES

The ratio of adenocarcinoma to squamous cell carcinoma has increased from 5% to 20% in the last half-century. This relative increase is a result of widespread screening, which detects squamous precursor lesions with a subsequent decrease in invasive squamous carcinomas; however, glandular precursor lesions are more difficult to detect on Pap smear and colposcopy. Therefore, many lesions are undetected until they progress to invasive adenocarcinoma.

Risk factors for the development of adenocarcinoma are similar to those for squamous carcinoma, including the association with squamous intraepithelial lesion, a > 5-year interval between Pap tests, multiple sex partners, and early age at first intercourse. In contrast to squamous carcinomas which are frequently associated with HPV type 16, the majority of adenocarcinomas have been linked to HPV type 18. There may also be an association between the use of hormone replacement therapy in postmenopausal women and the development of invasive cervical adenocarcinoma.

The mean age of patients diagnosed with adenocarcinoma is approximately 55 years. Abnormal vaginal bleeding is the most common sign, and, less frequently, vaginal discharge or pelvic pain. The majority of patients will have a mass detected on physical examination of the cervix, but in up to 15%, no lesion will be detected.

MUCINOUS ADENOCARCINOMA – FACT SHEET

Definition
▸ Malignant glandular neoplasm derived from reserve cells of endocervical columnar epithelium, frequently associated with HPV, particularly type 18

Incidence and Location
▸ 1.4–2.1 per 100,000 Caucasian women and 2.3–3.5 per 100,000 African American women in the US
▸ Approximately 25% of all cervical carcinomas
▸ Most common adenocarcinoma of the cervix
▸ Transformation zone

Morbidity and Mortality
▸ Treatment related morbidity
▸ Approximately 1200 women die each year in the US

Race and Age Distribution
▸ Higher rate in black Americans, probably due to less frequent screening
▸ Adult women between 45 and 54 years

Clinical Features
▸ Vaginal bleeding or discharge, and rarely, pelvic pain

Prognosis and Treatment
▸ Similar to slightly worse prognosis than squamous cell carcinoma
▸ Prognosis depends on stage, grade, tumor size, and lymph node involvement
▸ 93–100% 5-year survival for patients with stage IA tumors and 6% for patients with stage IV tumors

---

MUCINOUS ADENOCARCINOMA – PATHOLOGIC FEATURES

Gross Findings
▸ Exophytic, polypoid, or fungating mass in half of the cases
▸ Diffuse or nodular enlargement less frequent
▸ Occasionally, not grossly apparent

Microscopic Findings
▸ Complex architecture with cribriform and papillary growth
▸ Columnar cells with pseudostratified, basally located atypical nuclei and variable amount of mucinous cytoplasm
▸ Frequent mitoses and apoptotic bodies
▸ Desmoplastic stroma with occasional pools of mucin

Cytology Correlation
▸ Abnormal glandular cells in sheets, strips, and clusters, with prominent feathering and rosette formation
▸ Prominent nucleoli may be seen
▸ Background tumor diathesis and inflammatory debris

Immunohistochemical Features
▸ CEA and p16-positive
▸ Vimentin and ER typically negative

Differential Diagnosis
▸ Microglandular hyperplasia
▸ Adenocarcinoma in situ
▸ Endometrial endometrioid adenocarcinoma
▸ Endometrial mucinous adenocarcinoma
▸ Metastatic adenocarcinoma

PATHOLOGIC FEATURES

GROSS FINDINGS

The majority of invasive adenocarcinomas of the cervix originate in the transformation zone. In half of the cases, an exophytic, papillary, polypoid, or fungating mass is readily identifiable (Figure 5.29A). Less frequently, a diffuse (barrel-shaped) or nodular enlargement of the cervix with or without ulceration may be found. In 15% of cases, the lesion is located high up in the endocervical canal, is grossly inapparent, but may still invade deeply into the cervical wall.

MICROSCOPIC FINDINGS

Mucinous adenocarcinoma is the most common histologic subtype among invasive cervical adenocarcinomas. It is further divided into three morphologic variants that can exist in pure form or as an admixture:
Endocervical-type adenocarcinoma is the most common, where the malignant cells resemble endocervical columnar epithelium with at least some cells containing moderate amounts of mucin. Most of these tumors are moderately differentiated (Figure 5.29B and C). The glands may be closely packed or widely separated and may show cribriform, microglandular, papillary, or solid arrangements. Desmoplastic stroma is frequently present and pools of mucin are occasionally seen within the stroma. The tumor cells have basally located nuclei and at least some of them have abundant mucinous cytoplasm (Figure 5.29C). The nuclei are atypical with pseudostratification, loss of polarity, hyperchromasia, and coarse chromatin. Mitotic figures and apoptotic bodies are frequent.
Intestinal-type adenocarcinoma is the second most frequent mucinous adenocarcinoma, with morphologic features that overlap with colorectal adenocarcinoma. Goblet cells are frequent, whereas argentaffin cells and Paneth cells are uncommon.
Signet-ring cell type mucinous adenocarcinoma is very rare in pure form and is usually seen as a minor component of an endocervical or intestinal type adenocarcinoma.

ANCILLARY STUDIES

IMMUNOHISTOCHEMISTRY

The expected immunohistochemical profile for primary endocervical adenocarcinomas includes cytoplasmic positivity for CEA (Figure 5.30A) and strong nuclear and cytoplasmic staining for p16 (Figure 5.30B), while in most cases ER and vimentin are negative (Figure 5.30C).

CYTOLOGY

The cytologic features are similar to those of AIS, including the presence of abnormal glandular cells in sheets, strips, and clusters with prominent feathering and rosette formation. However, invasive cervical adenocarcinoma also shows tumor diathesis with inflammatory debris and nuclei with prominent nucleoli (Figure 5.31).

DIFFERENTIAL DIAGNOSIS

Among benign glandular proliferations of the cervix, *microglandular hyperplasia* may occasionally present as a polypoid lesion and show unusual histologic patterns including solid growth, irregular anastomosing glands, edematous to myxoid stroma or even mucin droplets, which may cause concern for invasive endocervical adenocarcinoma. Furthermore, some mucinous endocervical carcinomas may have a microglandular growth pattern. Helpful features in the diagnosis of microglandular hyperplasia include the finding of more typical areas, absence of significant cytologic atypia, and only rare mitotic figures.

Invasive endocervical adenocarcinoma may also be confused with *AIS*. In contrast to invasive adenocarcinoma, AIS does not extend beyond the depth of normal endocervical crypts, and it is not associated with desmoplasia. Although focal intraglandular papillary or cribriform growth may be present in AIS, normal endocervical glandular architecture is preserved, in contrast to invasive adenocarcinoma, where complex, back-to-back neoplastic glands are present.

The distinction between primary endocervical and *endometrial endometrioid adenocarcinomas* may be quite difficult, especially in biopsy specimens, as they may show overlapping histologic features. However, the distinction is important from both therapeutic and prognostic points of view. Helpful histologic findings in a curettage to establish an endometrial origin of the tumor include precancerous change of the endometrium (atypical complex hyperplasia/endometrial intraepithelial neoplasia), foamy histiocytes, and scant intervening stroma. Similarly, if the curettage shows coexistent AIS or HSIL, or abundant stroma between the neoplastic glands, then the most likely origin of the tumor is the cervix. An immunohistochemical panel to include CEA, vimentin, p16, and ER may also be helpful in distinguishing primary endocervical from endometrial tumors. Endometrial tumors are typically vimentin and ER positive, but CEA negative. p16 may be focally positive, but it does not show the strong diffuse nuclear and cytoplasmic positivity seen in endocervical adenocarcinomas.

Mucinous adenocarcinoma of the endometrium may be extremely difficult to distinguish from mucinous carcinomas of the cervix. The differential diagnosis should be based on clinical impression as well as histologic and immuno-histochemical findings. The presence of focal endometrioid areas or squamous differentiation and the absence of abundant intervening stroma associated with desmoplastic reaction is helpful. Moreover, mucinous carcinomas of the endometrium often express vimentin, ER and PR, but only infrequently CEA.

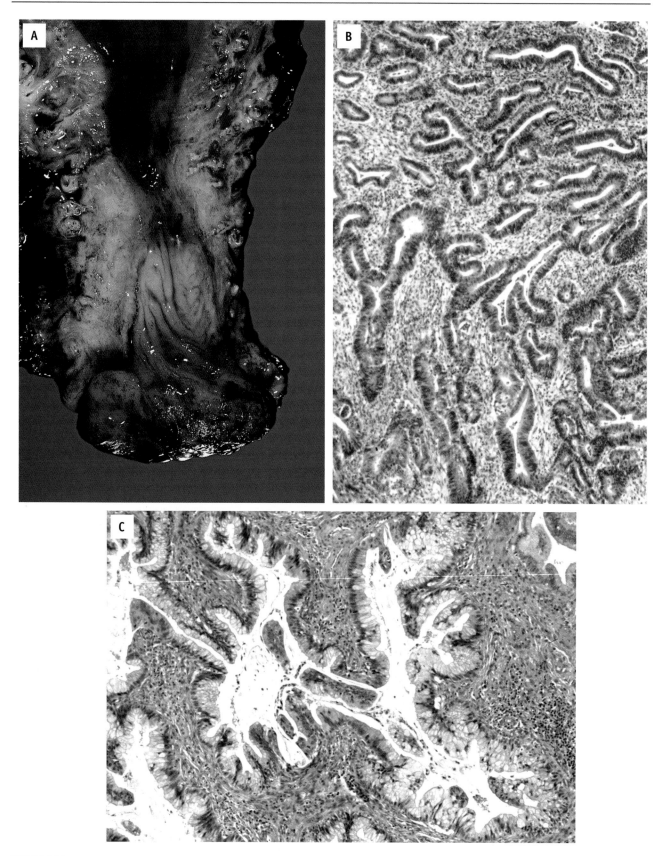

FIGURE 5.29

Mucinous adenocarcinoma, endocervical type. A large fungating, exophytic mass involves the transformation zone (A). The glands have irregular shapes and sizes and are associated with a desmoplastic stroma (B). The neoplastic glands are lined by cells with abundant mucinous cytoplasm resembling normal endocervical epithelium (C).

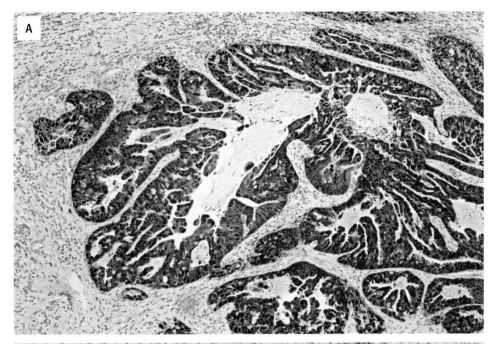

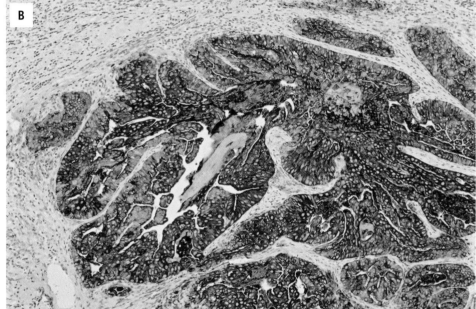

FIGURE 5.30

Mucinous adenocarcinoma, endocervical type. The tumor is CEA positive (A), it shows nuclear and cytoplasmic p16 (B), but it is negative for vimentin staining (C).

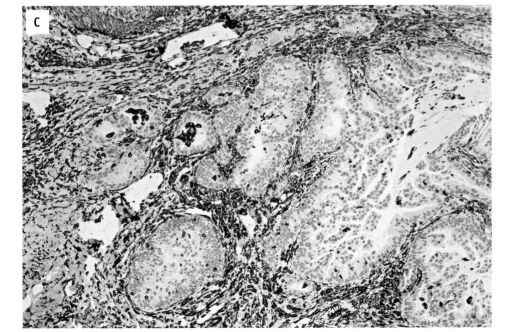

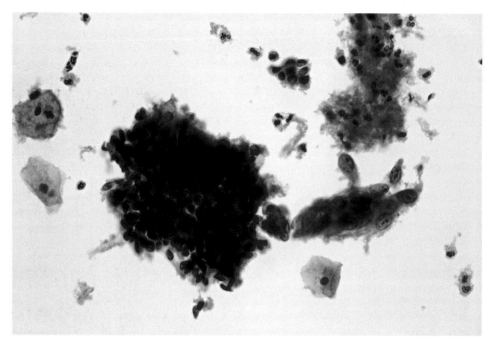

FIGURE 5.31

Mucinous adenocarcinoma, endocervical type. A monolayer Pap smear shows a crowded group of neoplastic glandular cells consistent with AIS (left), and a small group of malignant glandular cells (right) with prominent and multiple nucleoli associated with tumor diathesis.

Metastatic adenocarcinoma, especially from the gastrointestinal tract, should enter in the differential diagnosis whenever intestinal and/or signet-ring cells are present. Clinical findings as well as identification of areas of conventional endocervical adenocarcinoma are most useful as immunohistochemistry shows overlapping profiles.

PROGNOSIS AND THERAPY

For stage IA adenocarcinomas the survival rate is 93–100% at 5 years, while it decreases to 83% for stage IB, 50–59% for stage II, 13–31% for stage III, and 6% for stage IV tumors (Table 5.1). Adenocarcinoma of the cervix has a pattern of spread similar to squamous cell carcinoma. Thus, prognosis is affected by stage, grade, tumor size (> 3 cm is a poor prognostic sign), and presence of lymph node involvement, and overall, stage for stage, they have a similar or slightly worse prognosis. Histologic subtype does not generally affect prognosis.

Mucinous adenocarcinoma is treated similarly to squamous cell carcinoma, either with radiation alone, radiation and chemotherapy, or radiation followed by simple or radical hysterectomy, depending on tumor stage.

MINIMAL DEVIATION MUCINOUS ADENOCARCINOMA

Minimal deviation mucinous adenocarcinoma (MDA) is also known as adenoma malignum because of the

contrast between the highly differentiated appearance of the tumor and its very aggressive behavior. It accounts for only 1–3% of all cervical adenocarcinomas.

CLINICAL FEATURES

It is considered a variant of mucinous adenocarcinoma, but in contrast, patients are younger ($\simeq$ 40 years old), and often present with vaginal bleeding or abundant watery or mucoid discharge. MDA is associated with mucinous or sex cord tumors such as sex cord tumors with annular tubules (most common) or Sertoli cell tumors of the ovary. It may be part of the Peutz–Jeghers syndrome, as mutations of its gene, *SKT11*, are frequently detected in MDA.

PATHOLOGIC FEATURES

GROSS FINDINGS

In most cases, there is induration of the cervical wall, and the cervical mucosa varies from hemorrhagic and friable to mucoid. On sectioning, the cervix often appears abnormal; however, occasionally it may be grossly unremarkable.

MICROSCOPIC FINDINGS

Most, and rarely all, of the tumor is composed of tall mucinous epithelium which closely resembles normal endocervical columnar epithelium but lacks the characteristic cytologic features of malignancy. Architectural abnormalities are present, including complex variably sized glands, which are frequently irregular in shape

Definition
▶ Extremely well-differentiated variant of cervical mucinous adenocarcinoma

Incidence and Location
▶ Approximately 1–3% of cervical adenocarcinomas
▶ Endocervical canal

Morbidity and Mortality
▶ Difficulty in establishing the diagnosis may increase morbidity
▶ 30% overall survival at 2 years

Race and Age Distribution
▶ No apparent race predilection
▶ Younger age (mean 40 years) than typical mucinous adenocarcinomas

Clinical Features
▶ Vaginal bleeding or watery vaginal discharge
▶ Association with Peutz–Jeghers syndrome and ovarian mucinous and sex cord tumors

Prognosis and Treatment
▶ Worse prognosis than other well-differentiated adenocarcinomas
▶ 50% survival rate for stage I tumors
▶ Total abdominal hysterectomy with bilateral oophorectomy and lymph node dissection

MINIMAL-DEVIATION MUCINOUS ADENOCARCINOMA – PATHOLOGIC FEATURES

Gross Findings
▶ Friable, hemorrhagic, mucoid or indurated cervix
▶ Occasionally, no gross abnormality

Microscopic Findings
▶ Irregularly shaped glands with branching, papillary infoldings, and angular outpouchings deeply infiltrating the cervical wall
▶ Tall mucinous cells resembling normal endocervical epithelium
▶ Minimal cytologic atypia with mild nuclear enlargement and only occasional mitoses in most glands; however, cytologically malignant glands always present at least focally
▶ Focal stromal desmoplasia or edema
▶ Lymphovascular and perineural invasion

Immunohistochemical Features
▶ Variable CEA positivity
▶ ER and PR negative
▶ HPV and p16 negative

Cytology Correlation
▶ Pap smear not helpful

Differential Diagnosis
▶ Normal endocervical glands
▶ Tunnel clusters
▶ Lobular endocervical gland hyperplasia
▶ Deep nabothian cysts
▶ Adenomyoma, endocervical type

with papillary infoldings or angular outpouchings (Figure 5.32A). The malignant glands extend deeply into the cervical wall beyond the depth of normal endocervical crypts, which almost never extend beyond 8 mm in reproductive-age women (Figure 5.32A). Most of the neoplastic glands are lined by columnar mucin-producing cells with basally located nuclei, which may be normal in appearance or have slightly enlarged nuclei with only occasional mitoses (Figures 5.32B and C). At least focally, the well-differentiated glands elicit a desmoplastic response and atypical glands are also present (Figure 5.32D) usually adjacent to large vessels, deep in the stroma, or surrounding nerves. The diagnosis is difficult in a superficial cervical biopsy, and a cone biopsy or hysterectomy may be necessary to fully appreciate the diagnostic features. In essence, the diagnosis depends upon the recognition of the architectural abnormalities, including glandular irregularities and presence of glands deep in the cervical stroma.

ANCILLARY STUDIES

IMMUNOHISTOCHEMISTRY

CEA variably stains the cytoplasm of the malignant epithelium and is usually at least focally positive. ER and PR may also be helpful, since normal endocervical epithelium usually stains positively while MDA is typi-

cally negative. As these tumors are typically not associated with HPV, p16 is negative.

CYTOLOGY

The Pap smear shows a spectrum of atypical changes of the endocervical cells ranging from minimal atypia to frank carcinoma; however, in most instances it is impossible to establish this diagnosis solely based on the cytologic appearance.

DIFFERENTIAL DIAGNOSIS

Minimal deviation adenocarcinoma may be confused with normal endocervical glands and benign lesions of the cervix, including tunnel clusters, lobular endocervical glandular hyperplasia, deep glands, and adenomyoma (endocervical type).

Normal endocervical glands/crypts usually do not extend beyond 8 mm in the cervical wall in women of reproductive age, and they have a regular configuration.

Tunnel clusters may occasionally cause mucoid discharge, and on microscopic examination frequently show closely packed glands. In contrast to MDA, they show a striking lobular configuration and the glands are

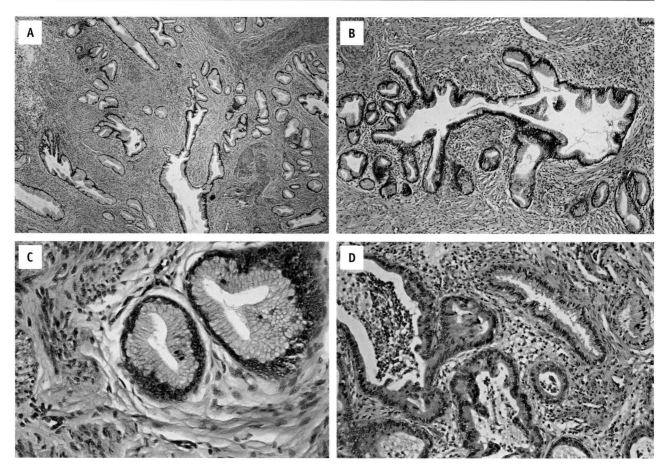

FIGURE 5.32

Minimal deviation endocervical adenocarcinoma. Complex, irregular glands infiltrate the cervical stroma in a disorderly fashion (A). An irregular branching gland is lined by cells with abundant intracellular mucin (B). The cells lining the neoplastic glands are columnar with small hyperchromatic nuclei and rare mitoses (C). However, notice the presence of overt malignant glands next to the better-differentiated areas (D).

uniform without complex architecture, appreciable cytologic atypia, or mitotic activity (Figure 5.33A).

Lobular endocervical glandular hyperplasia may be associated with mucoid discharge. However, on microscopic examination, it has a lobular pattern with a dilated gland in the center of a proliferation of smaller glands lined by cells with abundant eosinophilic cytoplasm, and it is usually confined to the inner one-half of the cervical wall (Figure 5.33B).

Deep glands or deep nabothian cysts can be distinguished from MDA, as they are usually much fewer in number and lack abnormal architecture, associated stromal reaction, or appreciable cytologic atypia.

Endocervical-type adenomyoma is a rare benign biphasic tumor that appears well circumscribed on gross examination. It is composed of endocervical glands and cysts and mature smooth muscle (Figure 5.33C and D). Similarly to MDA, the glands have irregular outlines with papillary infoldings; however, they may show a lobular arrangement. Endometrioid and tubal-type epithelium may be focally seen. Cytologic atypia and stromal desmoplasia around the glands are absent.

PROGNOSIS AND THERAPY

Because the tumor typically invades deeply into stroma and metastasizes early to lymph nodes, there is a 30% estimated overall survival at 2 years which increases up to 50% for stage I tumors. Treatment is similar to that of other endocervical adenocarcinomas.

WELL-DIFFERENTIATED VILLOGLANDULAR ADENOCARCINOMA

Villoglandular adenocarcinoma is a rare, well-differentiated variant of adenocarcinoma that occurs in young women and has an excellent prognosis in most cases. This tumor is associated with high-risk HPV and oral contraceptive use. Grossly, the tumor forms a papillary friable mass. On microscopic examination, elongate, thin papillary structures lined by cuboidal to columnar

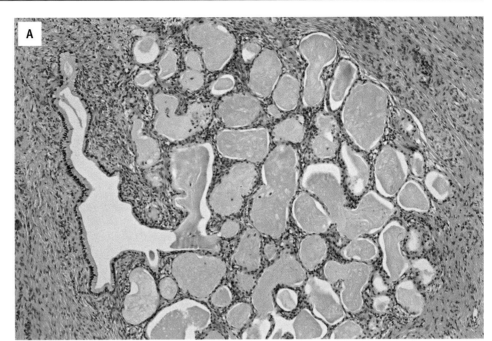

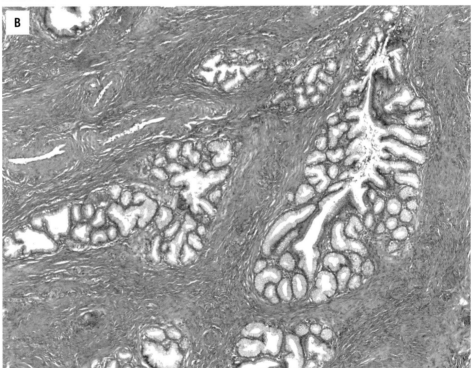

FIGURE 5.33

Pseudoneoplastic endocervical lesions. Type B tunnel clusters exhibit crowded glands that have a lobular arrangement and bland lining epithelium (A). Lobular endocervical gland hyperplasia is well demarcated and it is composed of a larger central duct surrounded by smaller acini. (B).

pseudostratified epithelium with mild cytologic atypia are seen. The lining epithelium usually resembles endocervical epithelium with some, but not all, cells containing intracellular mucin, but it can also have areas with an endometrioid or intestinal appearance. The fibrovascular cores are often sprinkled with acute and chronic inflammatory cells. The base of the tumor is usually well circumscribed, but it can show branching glands deeply infiltrating the cervical wall.

The tumors are frequently associated with HSIL or AIS. Some may be treated conservatively with cone biopsy if the interface between tumor and cervical

stroma can be seen and a conventional component of adenocarcinoma or an invasive component of the villoglandular carcinoma is not identified.

ENDOMETRIOID ADENOCARCINOMA

This tumor is histologically similar to its counterparts in the endometrium and ovary and accounts for approximately 10–30 % of all endocervical adenocarcinomas. The

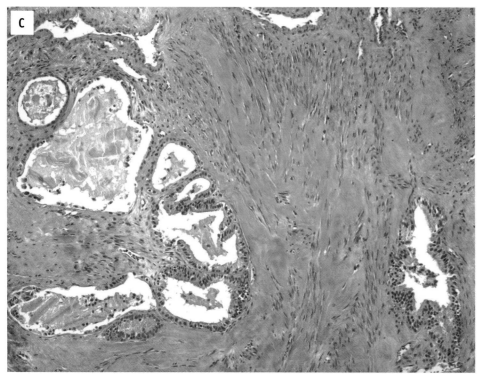

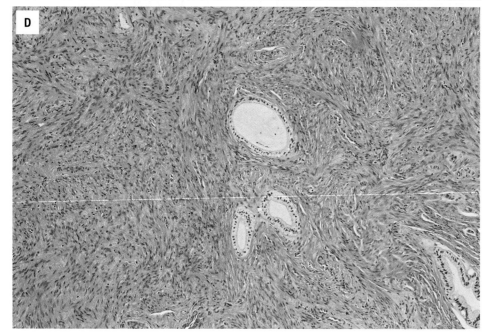

FIGURE 5.33—cont'd

Endocervical adenomyoma. Benign endocervical glands have irregular shapes and the smooth muscle is hyalinized simulating desmoplastic stroma (C); however, in some areas fascicles of banal smooth muscle cells are readily identified (D).

clinical presentation and gross appearance are similar to other cervical carcinomas. On microscopic examination, they usually show complex glandular architecture with cribriform and papillary patterns (Figure 5.34A). Squamous metaplasia may be present but it is less common than in endometrial endometrioid adenocarcinomas. The cytoplasm is less abundant than in endocervical-type adenocarcinoma and there is little or no mucin (Figure 5.34B). Included in this category is the endometrioid minimal deviation adenocarcinoma, an extremely well-differentiated variant characterized by deceptively bland glands deeply invading the cervical wall, associated at least focally with moderate cytologic atypia, mitotic activity, and some degree of stromal reaction.

Endometrioid adenocarcinoma of the cervix should be distinguished from *cervical extension of an endometrioid endometrial adenocarcinoma*. Helpful features in determining the origin of the tumor include the finding of a predominant mass in the uterine corpus or lower uterine segment, associated complex endometrial hyperplasia (endometrial intraepithelial neoplasia), and a negative staining for CEA and p16, but positive staining for ER, PR, and vimentin. p16, however, may be focally positive in endometrial adenocarcinomas.

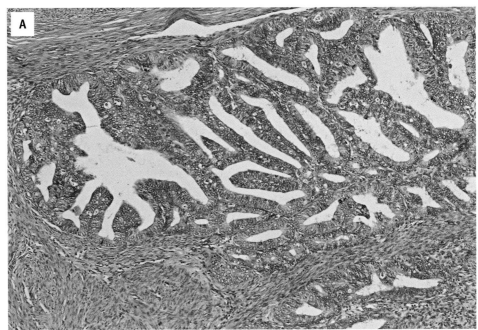

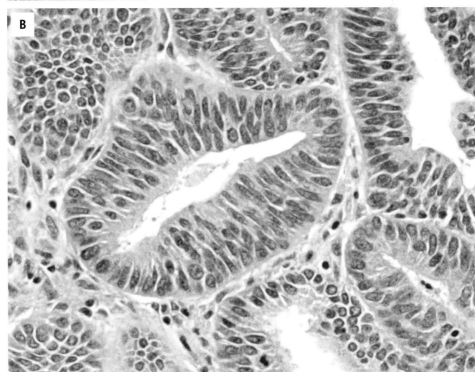

FIGURE 5.34

Endometrioid adenocarcinoma. The tumor shows complex glandular architecture with back-to-back glands (A). At high power, there is no mucin production, and pseudostratified oval and vesicular nuclei are seen (B).

CLEAR CELL ADENOCARCINOMA

This is a rare tumor, comprising up to 4% of all cervical adenocarcinomas, and is one of the few types that can occur in young women and older children. Similar to vaginal clear cell adenocarcinomas, there is an association with in utero DES exposure. However, in the cervix, they can also arise without exposure to DES. The tumors resemble clear cell adenocarcinomas that arise elsewhere in the female genital tract and similarly often demonstrate a variety of histologic patterns with solid, tubulocystic, and papillary areas. The tumor cells are usually pleomorphic with abundant clear cytoplasm and hyperchromatic, atypical nuclei. Hobnail cells, in which the atypical nucleus protrudes into a gland lumen, are characteristic of this tumor (Figure 5.35) but not always present. Extracellular but not intracellular mucin may be found. The most common differential diagnosis includes unusual forms of microglandular hyperplasia and Arias–Stella reaction. The latter tends to involve only a few glands and part of the glands, the nuclei have smudgy chromatin, and there is no mitotic activity.

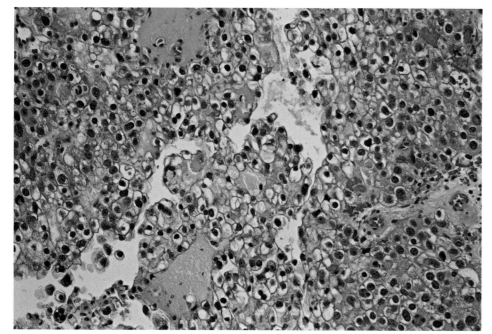

FIGURE 5.35

Clear cell adenocarcinoma. The tumor is composed of cells with abundant clear cytoplasm and hyperchromatic atypical nuclei.

SEROUS ADENOCARCINOMA

Primary serous adenocarcinoma of the cervix is extremely rare, accounting for 1% of cervical adenocarcinomas. It is histologically identical to papillary serous adenocarcinoma occurring in the ovary, endometrium, and percitoneum. Before establishing the diagnosis of primary serous carcinoma of the cervix, another origin within the female genital tract should be excluded. These tumors are associated with a very poor prognosis.

MESONEPHRIC ADENOCARCINOMA

Mesonephric adenocarcinoma is a rare tumor that originates from mesonephric remnants. It is usually found in the setting of mesonephric hyperplasia and is typically centered within the wall of the cervix; consequently these tumors are frequently bulky at the time of diagnosis, as they are deeply invasive. The microscopic appearance is highly variable; however the most common pattern shows a compact growth of small tubules, some of them containing eosinophilic PAS positive diastase-resistant secretions (Figure 5.36). These tumors can also show a complex glandular architecture with intraglandular papillae, so-called retiform pattern, and/or ductal (resembling endometrioid carcinoma) or solid patterns. Rarely, they may show a spindle cell component that resembles an endometrial stromal sarcoma or a nonspecific spindle cell sarcoma (mesonephric carcinosarcoma). These tumors are frequently positive for vimentin as well as for low-molecular-weight keratins, EMA, calretinin, and CD10. They can be positive for inhibin and androgen receptor whereas

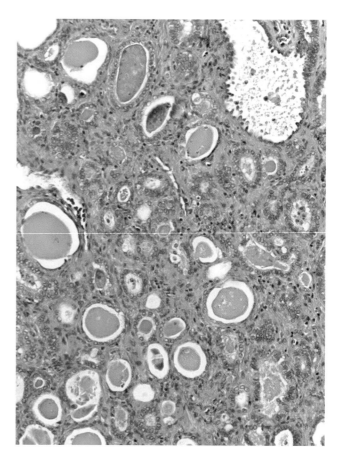

FIGURE 5.36

Mesonephric adenocarcinoma. Closely packed small to medium-sized tubules contain abundant intraluminal eosinophilic secretion. There is mild to moderate cytologic atypia.

they are negative for CEA, ER, and PR. These tumors generally have a better prognosis than their müllerian counterparts, as they present at earlier stages. Surgery alone appears to be the treatment of choice.

UNCOMMON CARCINOMAS AND NEUROENDOCRINE TUMORS

In the WHO histologic classification, this group of tumors includes adenosquamous carcinoma, adenoid cystic carcinoma, adenoid basal carcinoma, and neuroendocrine tumors, including small cell carcinoma.

ADENOSQUAMOUS CARCINOMA

This tumor is composed of malignant squamous and glandular elements, both of which can be distinctly identified on routinely stained sections. They likely arise from the reserve cell population of the endocervical epithelium, which probably undergoes biphasic differentiation. Poorly differentiated adenosquamous carcinoma is known as glassy cell carcinoma.

CLINICAL FEATURES

These tumors comprise 5–25 % of all cervical carcinomas. The average age of the patients is 57 years, similar to the most common forms of adenocarcinoma and squamous cell carcinoma, although they may occur in younger women, particularly when pregnant. Like pure squamous cell carcinoma and adenocarcinoma, adenosquamous carcinoma is also linked to HPV infection (types 16 and 18), and is therefore a sexually transmitted disease with similar risk factors.

PATHOLOGIC FEATURES

GROSS FINDINGS

Its gross appearance is similar to squamous cell carcinoma and the most common forms of adenocarcinoma, forming either an exophytic or ulcerating mass, or a nodular enlargement of the cervix (Figure 5.37A).

MICROSCOPIC FINDINGS

Both malignant squamous and glandular elements must be identified on routine stains in order to establish the diagnosis of adenosquamous carcinoma. The two components are usually intimately admixed (Figures 5.37B and C). The squamous component is moderately differentiated and squamous pearls may be seen, while the glandular component is typically of endocervical type. However, the cells in poorly differentiated tumors (glassy cell carcinoma) have a more hybrid appearance, with distinct cell borders, a "ground-glass" cytoplasm, and large nuclei with prominent nucleoli. There is typically a prominent inflammatory infiltrate composed mainly of eosinophils (Figure 5.37D).

ANCILLARY STUDIES

SPECIAL STAINS

In poorly differentiated tumors, a mucin stain may highlight the glandular component. However, the pres-

---

ADENOSQUAMOUS CARCINOMA – FACT SHEET

Definition
▶ Malignant tumor composed of squamous and glandular elements, both of which are identified on routine histologic examination

Incidence and Location
▶ 0.5–2.4 per 100,000
▶ 5–25% of all cervical carcinomas
▶ Transformation zone

Morbidity and Mortality
▶ Overall survival rate from 22 to 62% for all stages

Race and Age Distribution
▶ Slightly higher rates in black Americans, probably due to less screening
▶ Average age 57 years
▶ Can occur in younger women, particularly when pregnant

Clinical Features
▶ Vaginal bleeding
▶ HPV related, particularly types 16 and 18

Prognosis and Treatment
▶ Outcome similar to squamous cell carcinoma; however, metastases to regional lymph nodes may occur more frequently
▶ Total abdominal hysterectomy with bilateral salpingo-oophorectomy and lymph node dissection +/– adjuvant therapy

---

ADENOSQUAMOUS CARCINOMA – PATHOLOGIC FEATURES

Gross Findings
▶ Exophytic/ulcerating mass or nodular enlargement

Microscopic Findings
▶ Coexistence of malignant squamous and glandular elements
▶ Well-differentiated tumors: keratin pearls, intercellular bridges, and glands showing complex patterns
▶ Poorly differentiated tumors (glassy cell carcinoma): sheets and islands of malignant cells with ground-glass cytoplasm, large nuclei, prominent nucleoli, no keratinization, and associated stromal eosinophils

Cytology Correlation
▶ Groups of malignant squamous cells and glandular cells
▶ Tumor diathesis and inflammatory debris

Differential Diagnosis
▶ Endometrioid adenocarcinoma of the cervix with squamous differentiation
▶ Large cell nonkeratinizing squamous cell carcinoma

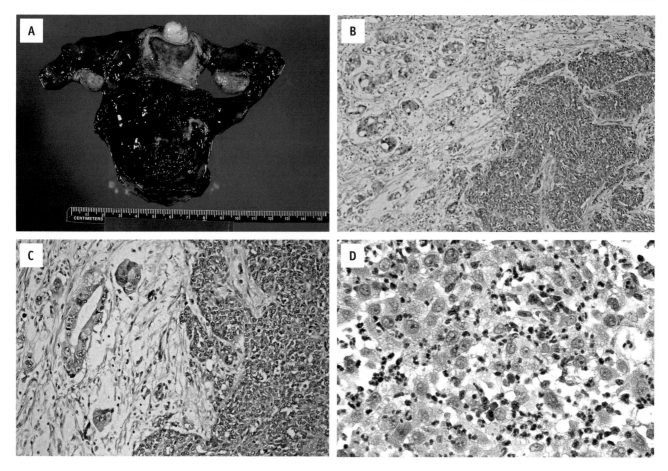

FIGURE 5.37

Adenosquamous carcinoma. A large, fungating, hemorrhagic mass occupies the cervix and extends into the lower uterine segment (A). Distinct squamous (right) and glandular (left) components are seen (B). Both elements have overt malignant cytologic features and focally merge (C). Glassy cell carcinoma. Cells with large vesicular nuclei and prominent nucleoli are admixed with an acute inflammatory infiltrate containing many eosinophils (D).

ence of adenocarcinoma must be strongly suspected on H&E examination in order to make the diagnosis of adenosquamous carcinoma.

CYTOLOGY

The Pap smear may show groups of malignant squamous and glandular cells. Tumor diathesis and inflammatory debris are usually present in the background.

DIFFERENTIAL DIAGNOSIS

Moderately to well-differentiated tumors should be distinguished from *endometrioid adenocarcinomas* of the cervix with squamous differentiation in which the squamous component is malignant. However, in adenosquamous carcinomas, the epithelial component is most often of endocervical type. In poorly differentiated carcinomas, where the glandular component may be less apparent, the main differential diagnosis is with *large cell nonkeratinizing squamous cell carcinoma.* In most cases, the latter shows small foci of discernible squamous differentiation while lacking the "ground-glass" appearance of the cytoplasm and the prominent nucleoli.

PROGNOSIS AND THERAPY

The most important prognostic factors include tumor volume, stage, and lymph node status. Although metastases to regional lymph nodes may occur more frequently in adenosquamous carcinoma, the overall survival rate for all stages ranges from 22 to 62 %, and there are no differences in prognosis with squamous cell carcinoma of similar size and stage. Thus, therapy is similar to squamous cell carcinoma and consists of total abdominal hysterectomy with bilateral salpingo-oophorectomy and lymph node dissection with or without adjuvant therapy.

ADENOID CYSTIC CARCINOMA

This tumor occurs more frequently in elderly non-Caucasian women (average 60 years). Patients typically present with postmenopausal bleeding, and on pelvic examination there is an obvious mass involving the cervix. On microscopic examination, the tumors are

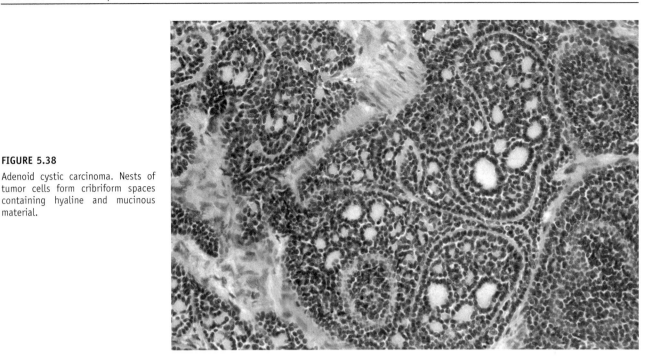

FIGURE 5.38

Adenoid cystic carcinoma. Nests of tumor cells form cribriform spaces containing hyaline and mucinous material.

reminiscent of their salivary gland counterpart. They are composed of sheets, islands, and nests of tumor cells, often arranged in a cribriform pattern. Cords and trabeculae can also be seen and, rarely, the tumors may be purely solid. The cells have scant cytoplasm, oval nuclei with mild to moderate cytologic atypia, inconspicuous nucleoli, and frequent mitotic figures. There may be focal palisading of the tumor cells at the periphery of the islands, and the cribriform spaces may contain mucin or hyaline material (Figure 5.38). They are associated with a desmoplastic stromal response. The main difference between these tumors and salivary tumors is the absence of myoepithelial cells in the cervical tumors. Adenoid cystic carcinoma may coexist with a component of adenoid basal carcinoma in approximately 20% of cases. They are positive for epithelial markers, including low-molecular-weight keratin, EMA, and CEA, and are associated with high-risk HPV. These are aggressive tumors, especially the solid variant that frequently presents at an advanced stage, often associated with local recurrences and distant metastases.

ADENOID BASAL CARCINOMA

This tumor occurs in postmenopausal, more commonly black, women (average age 64 years), who generally present with an abnormal Pap smear. The tumor may be an incidental finding in a uterus removed for a different reason.

On microscopic examination, the tumors are composed of small nests of cells with a lobular configuration resembling basal cell carcinoma of the skin, as the cells palisade at the periphery of the nests. Sometimes, the

nests may have a central lumen. The cells are small and uniform with scant cytoplasm, oval nuclei, inconspicuous nucleoli, and very low mitotic activity (Figure 5.39). It is always associated with a surface component of HSIL or early invasive squamous cell carcinoma, and the most superficial nests of adenoid basal carcinoma may show central squamous differentiation that appears cytologically bland. No stromal reaction is seen. Several studies have found high-risk HPV, especially type 16, as well as p53 abnormalities. Almost all patients present with stage I tumors and the prognosis is excellent.

NEUROENDOCRINE TUMORS

This group of tumors comprises carcinoid, atypical carcinoid, large cell neuroendocrine carcinoma, and small cell carcinoma. Typically, neuroendocrine differentiation is demonstrated with pan-neuroendocrine markers such as chromogranin and synaptophysin. Carcinoid tumors have the same morphological appearance as seen in other sites. However, distinction from atypical carcinoid is based on the presence of cytologic atypia with increased mitotic activity (5–10/HPF) associated with foci of necrosis present in the latter. Large cell neuroendocrine carcinoma is characterized by cells that have abundant cytoplasm, large nuclei, and prominent nucleoli and also show frequent mitotic activity. These tumors are aggressive and have a similar outcome to small cell carcinoma. In this section, only small cell carcinoma will be discussed, as it is the most common neuroendocrine tumor of the cervix.

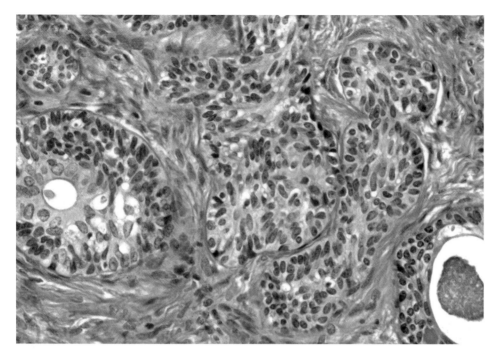

FIGURE 5.39
Adenoid basal carcinoma. Small nests, some of them with a central lumen, are composed of cytologically bland cells that palisade at the periphery of the nests.

SMALL CELL NEUROENDOCRINE CARCINOMA

These neuroendocrine tumors are histologically identical to small cell carcinoma of the lung. However, they differ from the latter in that up to 80% are related to high-risk HPV (more frequently HPV 18). They account for up to 5% of all cervical carcinomas.

CLINICAL FEATURES

Patients have an average age of 36–42 years and are typically younger than those with squamous cell carcinoma. They may present with vaginal bleeding or a paraneoplastic syndrome such as Cushing syndrome.

PATHOLOGIC FEATURES

GROSS FINDINGS

The tumors range from small and inconspicuous to large, ulcerated masses (Figure 5.40A). Since they often invade deeply into the cervical wall, advanced tumors may cause marked distortion, resulting in a "barrel-shaped" cervix.

MICROSCOPIC FINDINGS

Small cell neuroendocrine carcinoma is composed of small blue cells with solid, insular, trabecular, or nested patterns (Figure 5.40B). The cells have markedly increased nuclear-to-cytoplasmic ratio, inconspicuous nucleoli, and finely stippled chromatin. Nuclear molding is a prominent feature. Mitotic figures are numerous and apoptotic bodies are present (Figure 5.40C). Spindled cells and focal rosette-like or acinar formation may be seen. Crush artifact and necrosis may be prominent.

SMALL CELL NEUROENDOCRINE CARCINOMA – FACT SHEET

Definition
▶ Poorly differentiated neuroendocrine tumor histologically similar to its pulmonary counterpart, associated with high-risk HPV

Incidence and Location
▶ 0.5 per 100,000 in the US
▶ Mostly at the transformation zone

Morbidity and Mortality
▶ Highly aggressive disease; greater than 75% of patients are dead from disease within 1 year

Race and Age Distribution
▶ No race predilection
▶ Between 36 and 42 years

Clinical Features
▶ Vaginal bleeding or, less frequently, paraneoplastic syndrome
▶ Association with high-risk HPV, most frequently type 18

Prognosis and Treatment
▶ Poor outcome even in patients diagnosed at early stages, with low survival and highest rate of recurrence among cervical carcinomas
▶ Adjuvant chemotherapy widely employed with initial high response rate, but of short duration and minimal impact on final outcome

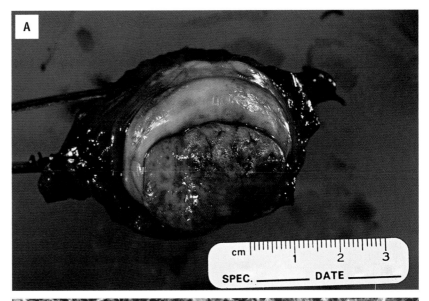

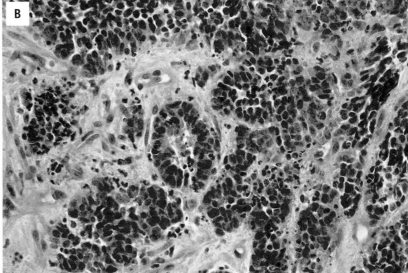

FIGURE 5.40

Small cell carcinoma. A large polypoid tumor is replacing the posterior cervical lip (A). It is composed of irregular nests of small cells (B). The cells have markedly increased nuclear-to-cytoplasmic ratio, nuclear hyperchromasia, finely stippled chromatin, and numerous apoptotic bodies (C).

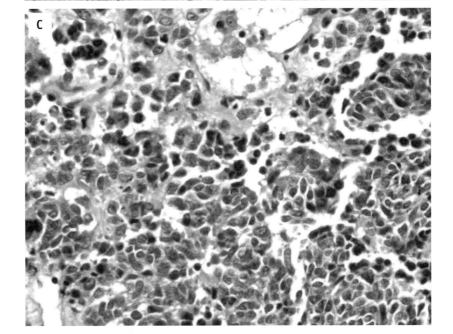

ANCILLARY STUDIES

IMMUNOHISTOCHEMISTRY

The tumors are positive for low-molecular-weight keratin, EMA, CEA, and neuroendocrine markers (including chromogranin, neuron-specific enolase, synaptophysin, and Leu 7).

ULTRASTRUCTURAL EXAMINATION

Although not routinely employed, in difficult cases electron microscopy will usually demonstrate round or oval dense-core granules 120–150 nm in diameter.

CYTOLOGY

Small cell carcinoma may be present on a Pap smear as small single cells and groups with inconspicuous cytoplasm, hyperchromatic nuclei, and nucleoli. Molding is usually prominent (Figure 5.41).

DIFFERENTIAL DIAGNOSIS

Before establishing the diagnosis of primary small cell carcinoma, a *small cell carcinoma metastatic to the cervix* must be excluded. The patient with small cell *carcinoma* metastatic to the cervix will often have widely metastatic disease. Small cell carcinoma should also be distinguished from poorly differentiated nonkeratinizing squamous cell carcinoma of the small cell type, basaloid squamous cell carcinoma, and lymphoma. Although *poorly differentiated squamous cell carcinoma and basaloid squamous cell carcinoma* may have small cells with increased nuclear-to-cytoplasmic ratio and nuclear hyperchromasia, nuclear molding and crush artifact are absent. In difficult cases, electron microscopy and immunohistochemistry may be helpful. *Lymphoma* may involve the cervix growing as diffuse sheets of small blue

---

SMALL CELL NEUROENDOCRINE CARCINOMA – PATHOLOGIC FEATURES

Gross Findings

▸ Small, inconspicuous to large, ulcerating masses
▸ If deeply invasive, may result in a barrel-shaped cervix

Microscopic Findings

▸ Sheets, islands, cords, and trabeculae of small ovoid, round to spindled cells
▸ Cells with markedly increased nuclear-to-cytoplasmic ratio, hyperchromatic nuclei with finely stippled chromatin, and inconspicuous nucleoli
▸ Rosette-like or acinar formation may be seen
▸ Mitotic figures and apoptotic bodies easily found
▸ Prominent nuclear molding and crush artifact
▸ Necrosis usually present

Immunohistochemical Features

▸ Epithelial markers, including low-molecular-weight keratin, EMA, CEA positive
▸ Chromogranin, NSE, synaptophysin, Leu-7 positive

Ultrastructural Features

▸ Round or oval dense core granules, 120–150 nm in diameter

Cytology Correlation

▸ Single small cells and small groups of cells with markedly increased nuclear-to-cytoplasmic ratio, nuclear hyperchromasia, nucleoli, and prominent molding
▸ Tumor diathesis with inflammatory debris

Differential Diagnosis

▸ Small cell carcinoma metastatic to cervix
▸ Poorly differentiated nonkeratinizing squamous cell carcinoma of small cell type
▸ Basaloid squamous cell carcinoma
▸ Lymphoma

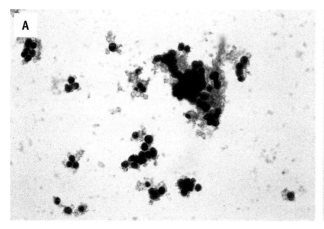 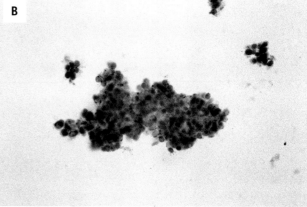

FIGURE 5.41

Small cell carcinoma. Small crowded groups and single malignant cells with markedly increased nuclear-to-cytoplasmic ratio, nuclear hyperchromasia, and molding associated with tumor diathesis are seen on a monolayer Pap smear (A). The malignant cells are positive for synaptophysin (B).

cells with brisk mitotic rate and prominent crush artifact. The tumors are frequently of B-cell lineage and they are associated with prominent sclerosis. Immunohistochemistry using neuroendocrine markers, leukocyte common antigen (LCA), as well as B-cell and T-cell markers, is helpful in this differential diagnosis.

PROGNOSIS AND THERAPY

Small cell carcinomas are highly aggressive tumors with a uniformly grim prognosis. In most large studies, over 75 % of patients are dead from this disease within 1 year of diagnosis. The poor prognosis is not stage-dependent since patients diagnosed with early-stage disease also do poorly compared to equivalent-stage squamous cell carcinomas. Patients are frequently treated with surgery and adjuvant chemotherapy, which results in an initial high response; however, it does not affect the final outcome.

MALIGNANT MESENCHYMAL TUMORS OF THE CERVIX

Whilst smooth-muscle tumors are the most common in this group of rare tumors, other mesenchymal tumors with skeletal muscle (sarcoma botryoides), endometrial stroma (endometrioid stromal sarcoma), vascular (angiosarcoma), and nerve sheath (malignant peripheral nerve sheath tumor) differentiation have been described in the

---

MALIGNANT MESENCHYMAL TUMORS – FACT SHEET

Definition
▸ Group of tumors that exhibit smooth muscle, skeletal muscle, endometrial stromal, vascular, peripheral nerve and other types of mesenchymal differentiation

Incidence
▸ Approximately 0.5% of cervical tumors
▸ Leiomyosarcoma most common primary sarcoma

Age Distribution
▸ Mostly in adults
▸ Sarcoma botryoides occurs in children and young women (mean age 18 years)

Clinical Features
▸ Vaginal bleeding
▸ Polypoid tumors may protrude through the cervical os
▸ Compression of adjacent organs if bulky tumors

Prognosis and Treatment
▸ Poor outcome
▸ Sarcoma botryoides carries a better prognosis
▸ Surgery mainstay of treatment, with adjuvant radiotherapy and/or chemotherapy

---

uterine cervix. The prognosis of cervical sarcomas as a group is poor, with the exception of sarcoma botryoides (embryonal rhabdomyosarcoma). Other sarcomas, such as alveolar soft-part sarcoma, alveolar rhabdomyosarcoma, liposarcoma, osteosarcoma, and so-called malignant fibrous histiocytoma, may occur, but they are exceedingly rare.

CLINICAL FEATURES

Patients with sarcomas of the cervix frequently present with vaginal bleeding and/or vaginal discharge. Bulky tumors may result in compression of adjacent organs. Not uncommonly, polypoid tumors protrude through the cervical os into the vagina. Less commonly, tissue may be passed via the vagina. These tumors typically affect adult patients, with the exception of sarcoma botryoides, which occurs in children and young women (mean age 18 years).

PATHOLOGICAL FINDINGS

GROSS FEATURES

These tumors expand and replace the cervix or, alternatively, form a polypoid mass with frequent areas of necrosis and hemorrhage.

MICROSCOPIC FINDINGS

Leiomyosarcoma resembles its uterine corpus counterpart, with hypercellular interlacing fascicles

---

MALIGNANT MESENCHYMAL TUMORS – PATHOLOGIC FEATURES

Gross Findings
▸ Typically expand and replace the cervix
▸ Sometimes polypoid
▸ Soft and fleshy with areas of necrosis and hemorrhage

Microscopic Findings
▸ Leiomyosarcoma: interlacing fascicles of spindle cells with nuclear atypia, high mitotic count, and tumor cell necrosis
▸ Sarcoma botryoides (embryonal rhabdomyosarcoma): small, round, or spindle cells showing skeletal muscle differentiation with subepithelial cambium layer and, in 50% of cases, cartilaginous differentiation

Immunohistochemical Features
▸ h-caldesmon and desmin in leiomyosarcoma
▸ Myogenin and myoD1 in rhabdomyosarcoma

Differential Diagnosis
▸ Leiomyoma (vs leiomyosarcoma)
▸ Low-grade mullerian adenosarcoma and rhabdomyoma (vs embryonal rhabdomyosarcoma)

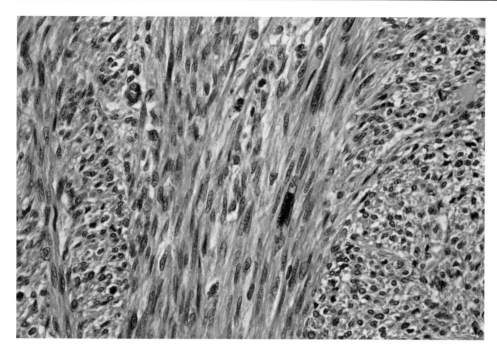

FIGURE 5.42

Leiomyosarcoma. Hypercellular interlacing fascicles of spindled cells show
moderate atypia and mitotic
activity.

of spindle cells with diffuse moderate to marked atypia, high mitotic count, and tumor necrosis (Figure 5.42). Myxoid and epithelioid variants can also occur.

Sarcoma botryoides (embryonal rhabdomyosarcoma), although occurring more commonly in the vagina, can also be seen in the cervix. It frequently has a polypoid configuration on gross and microscopic examination. It is composed of small, round, or spindle cells with variable evidence towards skeletal muscle differentiation. The neoplastic cells show the typical subepithelial condensation or "cambium layer" under the surface epithelium as well as around the nonneoplastic glands (Figure 5.43A and B). Nodules of cartilage may be seen in up to 50 % of tumors (Figure 5.43C).

Endometrioid stromal sarcoma typically arises from cervical endometriosis and is indistinguishable from uterine corpus tumors. Importantly, primary cervical stromal sarcoma should be distinguished from cervical extension of an endometrial stromal sarcoma arising in the corpus and stromal endometriosis. The latter is typically a microscopic incidental finding.

ANCILLARY STUDIES

IMMUNOHISTOCHEMISTRY

As with sarcomas elsewhere, immunohistochemistry plays a major role in arriving at the diagnosis of cervical sarcomas; h-Caldesmon and desmin in leiomyosarcoma, myogenin and myoD1 in rhabdomyosarcoma, and CD10 in endometrioid stromal sarcoma being most helpful. It is important to use a panel of antibodies, as

some overlap in expression may be seen among different sarcomas.

DIFFERENTIAL DIAGNOSIS

Criteria to distinguish *leiomyoma* from leiomyosarcoma in the cervix are the same as for the corpus and include diffuse marked nuclear atypia, mitotic activity (> 10/10 HPFs), and tumor necrosis.

Embryonal rhabdomyosarcoma should be separated from *low-grade müllerian adenosarcoma*, as 10 % of the latter originate in the cervix, may also be polypoid and show cartilaginous differentiation. However, this tumor has a biphasic growth of benign glands and malignant stroma, with the latter showing condensation and intraluminal protrusions around the glands, often resembling endometrial-type stroma without a cambium layer (Figure 5.44). *Cervical rhabdomyoma* has also been rarely reported as a polypoid lesion on the cervix. However, it lacks a cambium layer and it is composed of well-differentiated rhabdomyoblasts with small, uniform nuclei in an edematous stroma.

PROGNOSIS AND THERAPY

Prognosis of cervical sarcomas in general is poor, with the exception of sarcoma botryoides. Hence, correct subclassification of these tumors is critical. Treatment consists of surgery and radiotherapy (with or without concurrent chemotherapy), depending on grade and stage.

Embryonal Rhabdomyosarcoma

Low Grade Müllerian
Adenosarcoma
biphasic →
benign glds
& malig stroma
showing condensation
& intra luminal protrusion
around glds
resembling Endometrial
type stroma

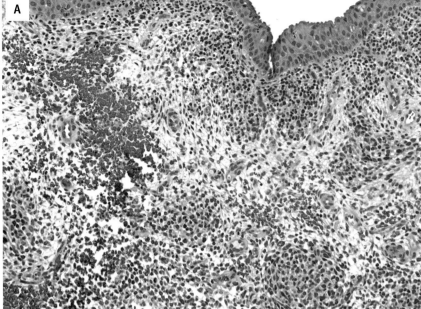

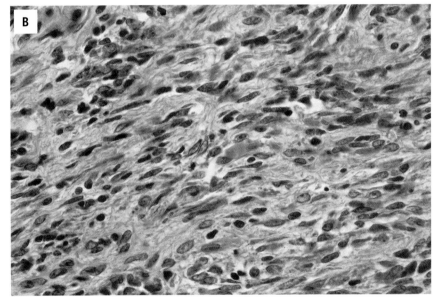

FIGURE 5.43

Sarcoma botryoides (embryonal rhabdomyosarcoma). There is subepithelial condensation of
primitive small cells resulting in the characteristic "cambium layer" (A). Focal skeletal muscle
differentiation is seen in the background of small
undifferentiated cells (B). A nodule of fetal-type
cartilage is also present (C).

IHC

Leiomyosarcoma
  — a Caldesmon
  — desmin

Rhabdomyosarcoma
  — myogenin
  — Myo D1

Endometrial Stromal
       Sarcoma
  — CD10

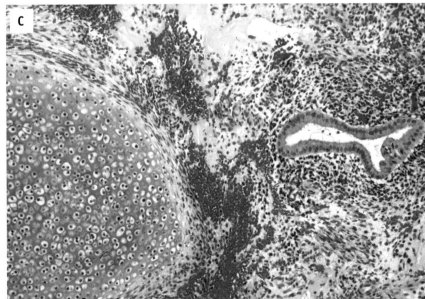

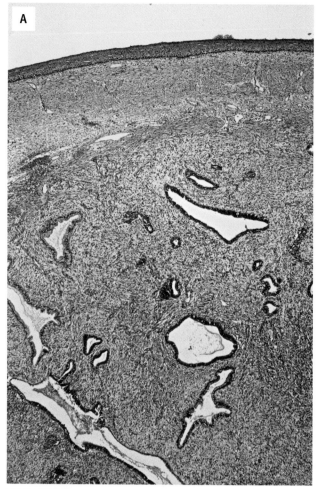

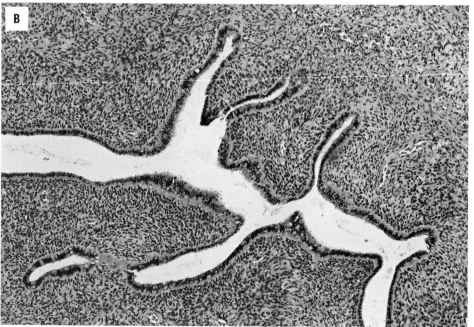

FIGURE 5.44

Low-grade müllerian adenosarcoma. The tumor has a biphasic growth of malignant mesenchymal and benign glandular components (A). Polypoid intraluminal protrusions and periglandular condensation of the malignant mesenchymal component is seen (B).

SUGGESTED READING

Squamous Neoplasia

Cooper K, Evans MF, Mount S. Biology and evolution of cervical squamous intraepithelial lesions: A hypothesis with diagnostic prognostic implications. Adv Anat Pathol 2003;10:200–203.

Geng L, Connolly DC, Isacson C, et al. Atypical immature metaplasia (AIM) of the cervix; is it related to high-grade squamous intraepithelial neoplasia (HSIL)? Hum Pathol 1999;30:345–351.

Kalof AN, Evans M, Simmons-Arnold L, et al. p16^{INK4A} expression and HPV in situ hybridization signal patterns: potential markers of high-grade cervical intraepithelial neoplasia. Am J Surg Pathol 2005;29:674–679.

Koenig C, Turnicky RP, Kankam CF, et al. Papillary squamotransitional cell carcinoma of the cervix: a report of 32 cases. Am J Surg Pathol 1997;21:915–921.

Kong CD, Balzer BL, Troxel ML, et al. p16^{INK4A} immunohistochemistry is superior to HPV in-situ hybridization for the detection of high-risk HPV in atypical squamous metaplasia. Am J Surg Pathol 2007;31:33–43.

Kurman RJ, Norris HJ, Wilkinson E. In: Atlas of Tumor Pathology: Tumors of the Cervix, Vagina and Vulva. AFIP Press, Bethesda, 1992, #4, p55–76.

Mount S, Evans MF, Wong C, et al. Human Papillomavirus induced lesions of the cervix: A review and update on the grading of cervical dysplasia. Pathology Case Reviews 2003;8:145–151.

Ng WK, Cheung LK, Li AS. Warty (condylomatous) carcinoma of the cervix. A review of 3 cases with emphasis on thin-layer cytology and molecular analysis for HPV. Acta Cytol 2003;47:159–166.

Nucci MR, Crum CP. Redefining early cervical neoplasia; recent progress. Adv Anat Pathol 2007;14:1–10.

Nuovo J, Melnikow J. Willan AR, et al. Treatment outcomes for squamous intraepithelial lesions. Int J Gynaecol Obstet 2000;68:25–33.

Ostör AG. Natural history of cervical intraepithelial neoplasia: A critical review. Int J Gynecol Pathol 1993;12:186–192.

Robboy SJ, Anderson MC, Russell P, et al. Malignant tumor of the cervix. In: Pathology of the Female Reproductive Tract. Ed. SJ Robboy, MC Anderson and P Russell, London, 2002;195–218.

Solomon D, Nayar R. The Bethesda System for Reporting Cervical Cytology. Definitions, criteria and explanatory notes. 2nd ed. Springer-Verlag, 2004.

Solomon D, Schiffman M, Tavone R. Comparison of three management strategies for patients with atypical squamous cells of undetermined significance: baseline results from a randomized trial. J Natl Cancer Inst 2001;93:293–299.

Sung HY, Kearney KA, Miller M, et al. Papanicolaou smear history and diagnosis of invasive cervical carcinoma among members of a large prepaid health plan. Cancer 2000;88:2283–2289.

Wells M, Ostör AG, Crum CP. In: Pathology & Genetics: Tumours of the Breast and Female Genital Organs. Ed. FA Tavassoli, P Devilee. WHO/IARCPress, Lyon 2003;260–272.

Wong WS, Ng CS, Lee CK. Verrucous carcinoma of the cervix. Arch Gynecol Obstet 1990;247:47–51.

Glandular Neoplasia

Biscotti CV, Hart WR. Apoptotic bodies: a consistent morphologic feature of endocervical adenocarcinoma in situ. Am J Surg Pathol 1998; 22:434–439.

Ceballos KM, Shaw D, Daya D. Microinvasive cervical adenocarcinoma (FIGO stage 1A tumors): results of surgical staging and outcome analysis. Am J Surg Pathol 2006;30:370–374.

Gilks CB, Young RH, Aguirre P, DeLellis RA, Scully RE. Adenoma malignum (minimal deviation adenocarcinoma) of the uterine cervix: a clinico-pathological and immunohistochemical analysis of 26 cases. Am J Surg Pathol 1989;13:717–729.

Gilks CB, Young RH, Clement PB, Hart WR, Scully RE. Adenomyomas of the uterine cervix of endocervical type: a report of ten cases of a benign cervical tumor that may be confused with adenoma malignum [corrected]. Mod Pathol 1996;9:220–224.

Grayson W, Taylor LF, Cooper K. Carcinosarcoma of the uterine cervix: a report of eight cases with immunohistochemical analysis and evaluation of human papillomavirus status. Am J Surg Pathol 2001;25:338–347.

Hart WR. Symposium Part II: Special types of adenocarcinoma of the uterine cervix. Int J Gynecol Pathol 2002;21:327–346.

Herbst AL, Cole P, Colton T, et al. Age-incidence and risk of diethylstilbestrol-related clear cell adenocarcinoma of the vagina and cervix. Am J Obstet Gynecol 1977;128:43–50.

Hirai Y, Takeshima N, Haga A, et al. A clinicocytopathologic study of adenoma malignum of the uterine cervix. Gynecol Oncol 1998; 70:219–223.

Ishikawa H, Nakanishi T, Indus T, et al. Prognostic factors of adenocarcinoma of the uterine cervix. Gynecol Oncol 1999;73:42–46.

Jones MW, Silverberg SG, Kurman RJ. Well-differentiated villoglandular adenocarcinoma of the uterine cervix: a clinicopathological study of 24 cases. Int J Gynecol Pathol 1993;12:1–7.

Krane JF, Granter SR, Trask CE, et al. Papanicolau smear sensitivity for the detection of adenocarcinoma of the cervix: a study of 49 cases. Cancer 2001;93:8–15.

Kuragaki C, Enomoto T, Ueno Y, et al. Mutations in the STK11 gene characterize minimal deviation adenocarcinoma of the uterine cervix. Lab Invest 2003;83:35–45.

Kurman RJ, Norris HJ, Wilkinson E. In: Atlas of Tumor Pathology: Tumors of the Cervix, Vagina and Vulva. AFIP Press, Bethesda, 1992; 253–381.

Lee KR, Flynn CE. Early invasive adenocarcinoma of the cervix: A histopathologic analysis of 40 cases with observations concerning histogenesis. Cancer 2000;89:1048–1054.

LiVolsi VA, Merino MJ, Schwartz PE. Coexistent endocervical adenocarcinoma and mucinous adenocarcinoma of ovary: a clinicopathologic study of four cases. Int J Gynecol Pathol 1983;1:391–402.

Michael H, Grawe L, Kraus FT. Minimal deviation endocervical adenocarcinoma: Clinical and histologic features, immunohistochemical staining for carcinoembryonic antigen, and differentiation from confusing benign lesions. Int J Gynecol Pathol 1984;3:261–276.

Miller BE, Flax SD, Arherat K, et al. The presentation of adenocarcinoma of the uterine cervix. Cancer 1993;72:1281–1285.

Nucci MR. Symposium part III: tumor-like glandular lesions of the uterine cervix. Int J Gynecol Pathol 2002;21:347–359.

Ostör AG. Early invasive adenocarcinoma of the uterine cervix. Int J Gynecol Pathol 2000;19:29–38.

Ostör AG, Duncan A, Quinn M, et al. Adenocarcinoma in situ of the uterine cervix: an experience with 100 cases. Gynecol Oncol 2000; 79:207–210.

Park JJ, Sun D, Quade BJ, et al. Stratified mucin-producing intraepithelial lesions of the cervix: adenosquamous or columnar cell neoplasia? Am J Surg Pathol 2000;24:1414–1419.

Poynor EA, Marshall D, Sonoda Y, et al. Clinicopathologic features of early adenocarcinoma of the cervix initially managed with cervical conization. Gynecol Oncol 2006;103:960–965.

Robboy SJ, Anderson MC, Russell P, et al. Malignant tumors of the cervix. In: Pathology of the Female Reproductive Tract. Ed. SJ Robboy, MC Anderson and P Russell, London, 2002;165–239.

Schorge JO, Lee KR, Flynn CE, et al. Stage IA1 cervical adenocarcinoma: definition and treatment. Obstet Gynecol 1999;93:219–222.

Silverberg SG, Hurt WG. Minimal deviation adenocarcinoma ("adenoma malignum") of the cervix. Am J Obstet Gynecol 1975;121:971–975.

Smith HO, Tiffany MF, Qualls CR, et al. The rising incidence of adenocarcinoma relative to squamous cell carcinoma of the uterine cervix in the United States: a 24-year population-based study. Gynecol Oncol 2000;78:97–105.

Wells M, Ostör AG, Crum CP. In: Pathology & Genetics: Tumours of the Breast and Female Genital Organs. Ed. FA Tavassoli, P Devilee. WHO/IARCPress, Lyon 2003;259–277.

Young RH, Scully RE. Villoglandular papillary adenocarcinoma of the uterine cervix. A clinicopathologic analysis of 13 cases. Cancer 1989;63:1773–1779.

Young RH, Clement PB. Endocervical adenocarcinoma and its variants: their morphology and differential diagnosis. Histopathol 2002; 41:185–207.

Zaino RJ. Symposium Part I: Adenocarcinoma in situ, glandular dysplasia and early invasive adenocarcinoma of the uterine cervix. Int J Gynecol Pathol 2002;21:314–326.

Uncommon Carcinomas and Neuroendocrine Tumors

Abeler VM, Holm R, Nesland JM, et al. Small cell carcinoma of the cervix: a clinicopathologic study of 26 patients. Cancer 1994;73:672–677.

Albores-Saavedra J, Gersell D, Gilks CB, et al. Terminology of endocrine tumors of the uterine cervix: results of a workshop sponsored by the College of American Pathologists and the National Cancer Institute. Arch Pathol Lab Med 1997;121:34–39.

Costa MJ, Kenny MB, Hewan-Lowe K, et al. Glassy cell features in adeno-squamous carcinoma of the uterine cervix: histologic, ultrastructural, immunohistochemical, and clinical findings. Am J Clin Pathol 1991;96:520–528.

Grayson W, Cooper K. A reappraisal of "basaloid carcinoma" of the cervix, and the differential diagnosis of basaloid cervical neoplasm. Adv Anat Pathol 2002;9:290–300.

Grayson W, Taylor LF, Cooper K. Adenoid cystic and adenoid basal carcinoma of the uterine cervix: comparative morphologic, mucin and immunohistochemical profile of two rare neoplasms of putative "reserve cell" origin. Am J Surg Pathol 1999;23: 448–458.

Gilks CB, Young RH, Gersell DJ, Clement PB. Large cell neuroendocrine carcinoma of the uterine cervix: a clinicopathologic study of 12 cases. Am J Surg Pathol 1997;21:905–914.

Mackay B, Osborne BM, Wharton JT. Small cell tumor of the cervix with neuroepithelial features: ultrastructural observations in 2 cases. Cancer 1979;43:1138.

Stoler MH, Mills SE, Gersell DJ, et al. Small-cell neuroendocrine carcinoma of the cervix. A human papillomavirus type 18-associated cancer. Am J Surg Pathol 1991;15:28–32.

Ulbright TM, Gersell DJ. Glassy cell carcinoma of the uterine cervix. A light and electron microscopic study of five cases. Cancer 1983;51:2255–2263.

Malignant Mesenchymal Tumors

Bell SW, Kempson RL, Hendrickson MR. Problematic uterine smooth muscle neoplasias: a clinicopathologic study of 213 cases. Am J Surg Pathol 1994;18:535–558.

Carcangiu ML. In: Pathology & Genetics: Tumours of the Breast and Female Genital Organs. Ed. FA Tavassoli, P Devilee. WHO/IARC Press, Lyon 2003;260–272.

Clement PB, Young RH, Scully RE. Stromal endometriosis of the cervix: a variant of endometriosis that may simulate a sarcoma. Am J Surg Pathol 1990;14:449–455.

Daya DA, Scully RE. Sarcoma botryoides of the uterine cervix in young women: a clinicopathological study of 13 cases. Gynecol Oncol 1988;29:290–304.

Ferguson SE, Gerald W, Barakat RR, et al. Clinicopathologic features of rhabdomyosarcoma of gynecologic origin in adults. Am J Surg Pathol 2007;31:382–389.

Jones MW, Lefkowitz M. Adenosarcoma of the uterine cervix: a clinico-pathological study of 12 cases. Int J Gynecol Pathol 1995; 14:223–229.

Kerner H, Lichtig C. Müllerian adenosarcoma presenting as cervical polyps: a report of seven cases and review of the literature. Obstet Gynecol 1993;81:655–659.

6 Benign Endometrium

David W Kindelberger · Marisa R Nucci

CYCLING ENDOMETRIUM

The key clinical issues that are being addressed when a pathologist is asked to evaluate an endometrial biopsy in a reproductive age woman are whether the patient has ovulated and if so, whether the luteal phase is progressing normally. The histologic criteria most commonly used by the pathologist to answer these questions were put forth by Noyes, Hertig, and Rock in 1950 whereby a "date" is assigned to endometrial biopsies, based on morphologic grounds. Several modifications have been made to their initial system, but the basic principles remain largely unchanged. The pathologist should approach the task of dating endometrial biopsies with the above questions in mind and attempt to assign a date as precisely as possible. To create a reproducible conceptual framework, cycling endometrium may be divided into six categories, based on morphologic features: (1) early proliferative endometrium with residual stromal breakdown (from the previous menstrual cycle); (2) 16-day endometrium; (3) early (vacuolar) secretory endometrium; (4) mid (exhausted) secretory endometrium; (5) late (predecidual) secretory endometrium; and (6) menstrual endometrium. A prototypical setting of a 28-day cycle is assumed, with day 1 representing the first day of menses. In reality, many women have cycles that differ from the standard 28-day cycle. These differences are most often accounted for within the preovulatory interval of the cycle (proliferative phase), while the postovulatory period (secretory phase to menses) remains remarkably constant at 14 days. When selecting fragments within an endometrial biopsy to use for assigning a date, basalis and lower uterine segment endometrium must be excluded, as these portions of the endometrium do not respond to hormonal stimuli with the same morphologic reproducibility as does the functionalis, which corresponds to the upper portions of the endometrium containing surface epithelium and subjacent glands and stroma.

CYCLING ENDOMETRIUM – PATHOLOGIC FEATURES

Proliferative Endometrium
▶ Round or tubular glands with pseudostratified nuclei
▶ Abundant mitoses in glands and stroma

Day-16 Endometrium
▶ Tubular glands with pseudostratified nuclei
▶ Frequent mitoses in glands and stroma
▶ Scattered basal cytoplasmic vacuoles
▶ Changes can be caused by estrogen alone and are *not* diagnostic of ovulation

Early Secretory Endometrium
▶ Day-17: Rows of subnuclear vacuoles (piano key) and scattered mitoses
▶ Day-18: Sub- and supranuclear vacuoles and apical discharge
▶ Day-19: Basal nuclei, scattered subnuclear vacuoles, and increased intraluminal secretions. *No* mitotic activity

Mid Secretory Endometrium
▶ Day-20: Rare subnuclear vacuoles and increased gland complexity; intraluminal secretions peak
▶ Day 21: Beginning of stromal edema
▶ Day 22: Maximal stromal edema with "naked" nuclei

Late Secretory Endometrium
▶ Day-23: Predecidual change limited to "cuffing" around spiral arterioles
▶ Day-24: Predecidual change extending from gland to gland, but *not* going to surface
▶ Day-25: *Thin* layer or patch of predecidual change just beneath the surface
▶ Day-26: *Thick* layer of predecidual change forming a band beneath the surface
▶ Day-27: Predecidual change extending deep into functionalis

Menstrual Endometrium
▶ Collapsing hemorrhagic stroma with aggregates of necrotic predecidua
▶ Exhausted secretory glands

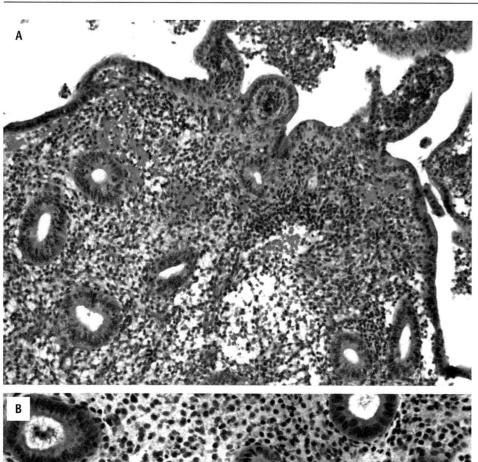

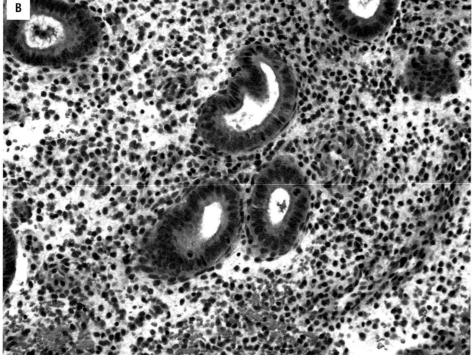

FIGURE 6.1

Proliferative endometrium. Residual stromal breakdown (upper right) may be seen in the early phase (A). Round to tubular glands show nuclear pseudostratification and mitotic activity (B).

EARLY PROLIFERATIVE ENDOMETRIUM WITH RESIDUAL STROMAL BREAKDOWN

This phase of the endometrial cycle has three characteristic morphologic features, which are invariably present. The endometrial glands are round to tubular with cells containing pseudostratified nuclei, rare subnuclear vacuoles, and frequent glandular and stromal mitoses. There is residual breakdown of the stroma, consisting of dense, discrete aggregates of predecidualized stromal cells admixed with blood and inflammatory cells (Figure 6.1A). Detachment of surface epithelium is also seen. At this stage of the cycle, it is not possible to histologically confirm that ovulation has occurred because none of the morphologic hallmarks of ovulation (predecidualized stroma and exhausted secretory glands) are still present.

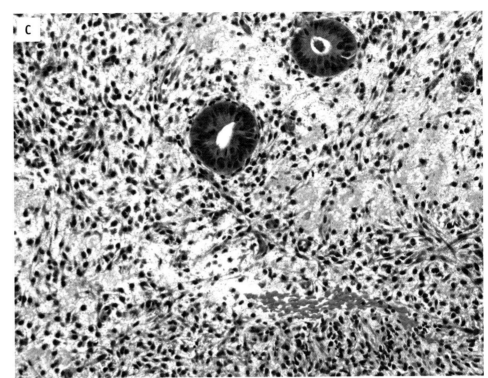

FIGURE 6.1—cont'd

Edematous stroma mimics predecidual change (C). Endometrial glands show "telescoping" artifact (gland inside gland) (D).

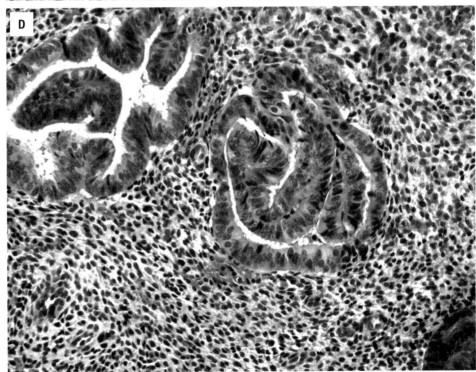

PROLIFERATIVE ENDOMETRIUM

In response to estrogen, endometrial glands are stimulated to proliferate and show the characteristic morphologic pattern of proliferative endometrium (Figure 6.1B) i.e. tubular glands with cells having pseudostratified, deeply basophilic nuclei with coarse chromatin, and numerous mitotic figures. The glands tend to be regularly spaced and relatively uniform in size and configuration. The stroma has a variable appearance during this phase and may be mildly edematous or spindled, mimicking predecidua (or progestin effect) (Figure 6.1C). The presence of abundant glandular and stromal mitoses and the lack of prominent spiral arterioles are both useful clues that argue against progestin effect. An additional pitfall which must be considered is the pres-

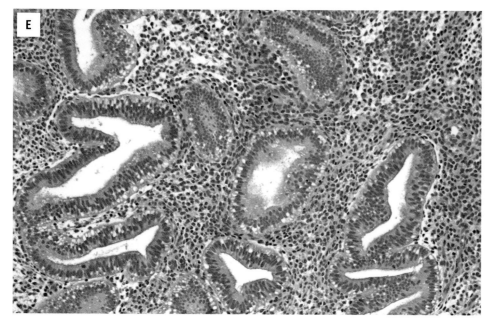

FIGURE 6.1—cont'd
Day 16 endometrium shows tubular glands with discontinuous and not well developed subnuclear vacuoles (E).

ence of "telescoping" of one gland tract into another (Figure 6.1D), which should not be interpreted as hyperplasia or neoplasia. For practical purposes, subdividing the proliferative phase has not been shown to have diagnostic or management utility as it is poorly reproducible.

DAY SIXTEEN ENDOMETRIUM

Day 16 endometrium is characterized by glands with cells displaying discontinuous and partially developed subnuclear vacuoles as well as mitotic figures (Figure 6.1E). The overall gland architecture is that of simple tubular glands of proliferative endometrium and, although mitoses are present, they are not as numerous as during the proliferative phase. Identification of at least one cluster of glands with cells showing confluent, uniform subnuclear vacuoles and no mitotic figures warrants a diagnosis of day 17 secretory endometrium. In day 16 endometrium, ovulation cannot be confirmed as the presence of occasional subnuclear vacuoles may be produced by estrogen alone.

EARLY (VACUOLE-PHASE) SECRETORY ENDOMETRIUM

Entry into the vacuole phase of the cycle suggests that ovulation has taken place. The "50% rule" is a good rule of thumb for confirming that ovulation has occurred. At least 50% of the cells in a given gland should contain vacuoles which are continuous and well developed. In general, when assigning a date to secretory-phase endometrium, during the first half of the phase, the date is determined by monitoring gland changes and during the second half, the date is determined by monitoring stromal changes.

At low power, secretory endometrium displays glands that are larger than those seen in proliferative endometrium. The cells also appear less basophilic during the secretory phase due to the loss of pseudostratified nuclei and the presence of prominent cytoplasmic vacuoles. Glands with cells showing uniform and continuous subnuclear vacuoles and rare mitotic figures warrant the diagnosis of day 17 secretory endometrium (Figure 6.2A). In day 18 secretory endometrium, the glandular cells have both sub- and supranuclear vacuoles and the nuclei occupy the center of the cell (Figure 6.2B). By day 19, the nuclei have nearly all returned to the base of the cell. The glands begin to show secretory exhaustion with low columnar to cuboidal cells, loss of vacuoles, prominent luminal secretions, and lack mitotic activity (Figure 6.2C).

MID (SECRETORY EXHAUSTION PHASE) SECRETORY ENDOMETRIUM

The loss of secretory vacuoles signals the end of the early secretory phase and the beginning of the mid-phase. From this point forward, the focus in assigning dates to endometrial samples is on stromal changes. Day 20 secretory endometrium exhibits maximal intraluminal secretions with only rare residual subnuclear vacu-

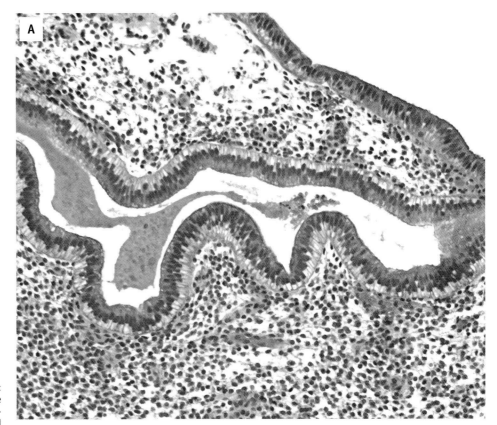

FIGURE 6.2

Early secretory endometrium. Day 17: Prominent subnuclear vacuoles are seen (A). Day 18: Sub- and supranuclear vacuoles with centrally located nuclei are present (B).

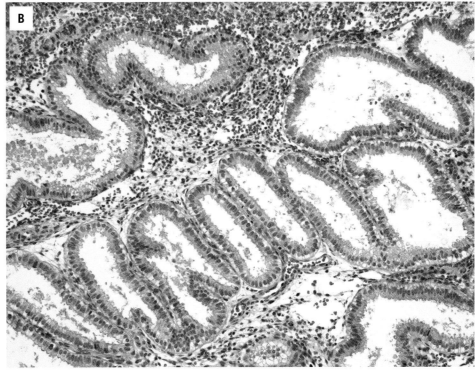

oles (Figure 6.3A). The stroma beneath the endometrial surface becomes more compact and can mimic predecidualized stroma. However, the stromal cells still have dark nuclei and a high nuclear-to-cytoplasmic ratio, unlike predecidualized cells. Day 21 secretory endome-trium shows increased stromal edema (Figure 6.3B), which peaks at day 22 (Figure 6.3C). The stromal cells may appear widely spaced and their high nuclear-to-cytoplasmic ratio make them appear as "naked nuclei." There are no conspicuous predecidual changes.

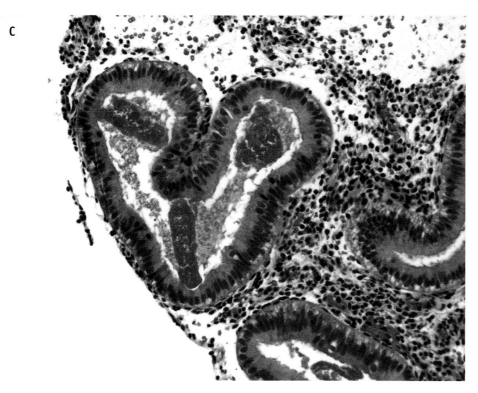

FIGURE 6.2—cont'd

(C) Day 19: Endometrial glands show prominent luminal secretion.

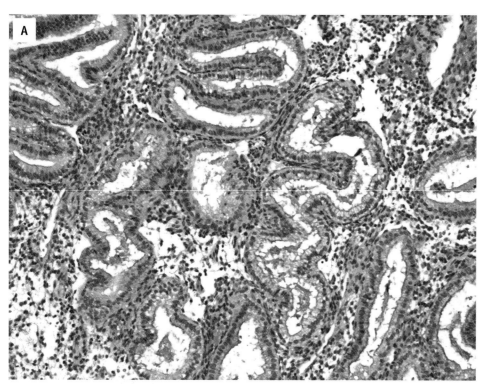

FIGURE 6.3

Mid-secretory endometrium. Day 20: Rare subnuclear vacuoles and increased gland complexity are associated with maximal intraluminal secretions (A).

LATE (PREDECIDUAL PHASE) SECRETORY ENDOMETRIUM

Identification of predecidual changes and then noting their location are key to assigning dates during the late secretory phase. There are three well-defined morpho-

logic alterations of predecidual change. Initially, stromal cells surrounding spiral arterioles become prominent. As the predecidual change develops, the stromal cells acquire distinct cell borders and slightly basophilic cytoplasm. Finally, the nuclei are less basophilic and the chromatin texture becomes finer. For day 23 secretory endometrium, the predecidua surrounds individual spiral arterioles (Figure 6.4A), and by day 24, it bridges

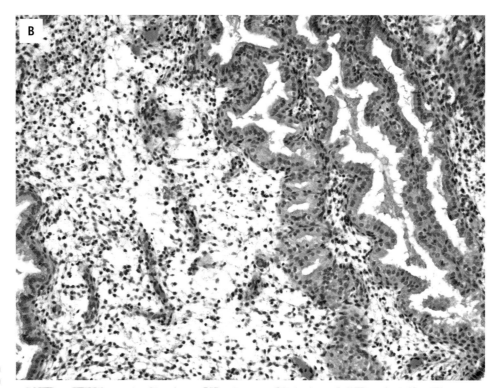

FIGURE 6.3—cont'd

Day 21: Endometrial glands with luminal secretion are associated with early stromal edema (B). Day 22: The endometrial stroma shows prominent edema (C).

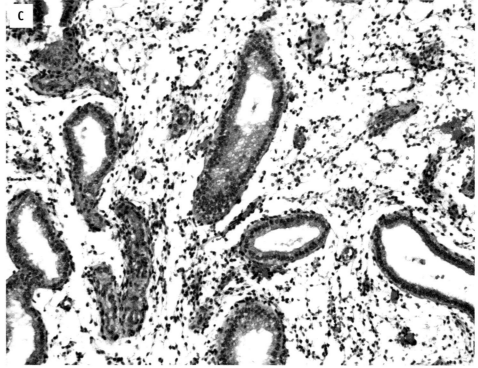

multiple vessels (Figure 6.4B). Day 25 secretory endometrium is characterized by thin aggregates of predecidua below the endometrial surface (Figure 6.4C) whereas a thick band of predecidua beneath the surface is present by day 26 (Figure 6.4D). Day 27 endometrium shows abundant predecidua expanding downward from the endometrial surface, with increased numbers of stromal granulocytes (Figure 6.4E).

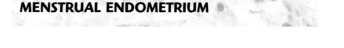

MENSTRUAL ENDOMETRIUM

The earliest feature of menstrual phase is defined by the presence of discrete aggregates of condensed predecidual cells (stromal breakdown), admixed with inflamma-

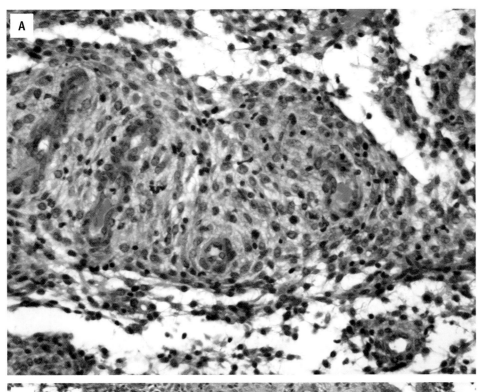

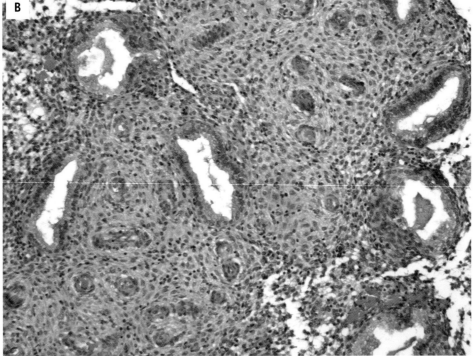

tory cells and blood. As the menstrual phase progresses, there is diffuse stromal breakdown with coordinated collapse of the functionalis. Interspersed with fragments of condensed stroma are glands that have a range of morphologic appearances. They vary in size and shape and are lined by cells displaying variable amounts of apical cytoplasm, ranging from abundant apical to minimal, the latter resulting in a delicate appearance of the glands (secretory exhaustion) (Figure 6.5). The presence of both components (stromal breakdown and

secretory exhausted glands) is evidence that ovulation has occurred.

DYSFUNCTIONAL UTERINE BLEEDING

A number of conditions may lead to dysfunctional uterine bleeding, which can be thought of as bleeding resulting from alterations in the normal cycling pattern of the endometrium. Dysfunctional uterine bleeding typically

C

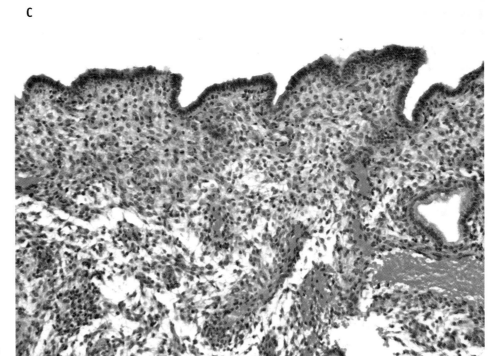

FIGURE 6.4—cont'd

Day 25: Predecidua is present as a thin layer beneath the surface (C). Day 26: A thick layer of predecidua forms a band beneath the surface (D).

D

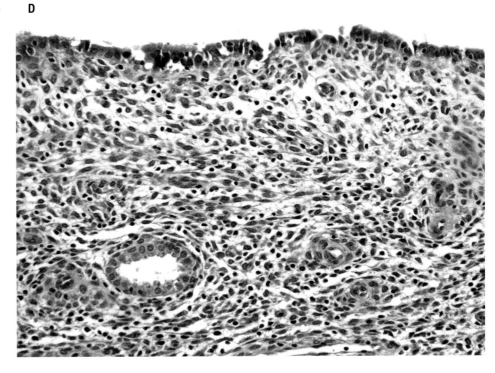

occurs in women from the third to the sixth decade and the most common causes include leiomyomata (particularly if submucosal), chronic endometritis, endometrial polyps, and anovulation. In addition to physical examination, clinical workup should include a variety of methods to identify structural abnormalities such as uterine imaging (either with ultrasonography or direct visualization through hysteroscopy) and/or endometrial sampling. As expected, direct visualization is most sensitive in identifying submucosal leiomyomata and endometrial polyps but it has essentially no role in detecting endometritis or anovulation.

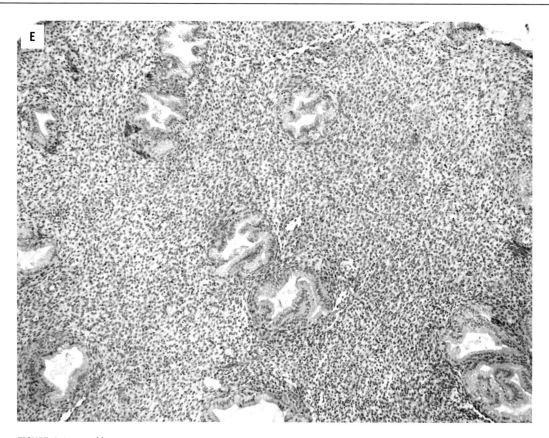

FIGURE 6.4—cont'd

(E) Day 27: Predecidual change extends deep into the functionalis.

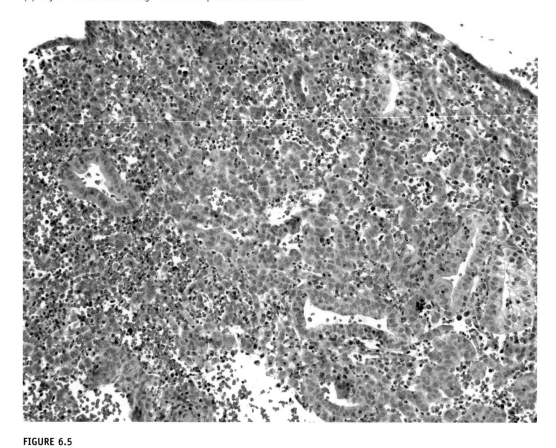

FIGURE 6.5

Ovulatory menstrual endometrium. Diffuse stromal breakdown with cord-like condensation of predecidua is associated with exhausted secretory glands.

SUBMUCOSAL LEIOMYOMATA

CLINICAL FEATURES

Uterine leiomyomata are extremely common, present in up to 80% of hysterectomy specimens, irrespective of the indication for surgery. However, they cause symptoms in only about one-quarter of reproductive-aged women, with symptomatic leiomyomata generally presenting after age 35. Symptoms, when present, typically include pelvic pain or pressure, abnormal uterine bleeding, and/or reproductive dysfunction. Type and severity of these symptoms are associated with tumor location and size; submucosal leiomyomata, which attenuate the overlying endometrium are commonly associated with abnormal bleeding.

LEIOMYOMATA – FACT SHEET

Definition
▸ Benign mesenchymal tumor of the uterus composed of fascicles of bland smooth-muscle cells

Incidence and Location
▸ Most common uterine neoplasm
▸ May be submucosal, intramural, or subserosal

Morbidity and Mortality
▸ Only 25% of tumors in reproductive-age women are symptomatic
▸ Most common indication for hysterectomy

Race and Age Distribution
▸ Reproductive-age women
▸ Symptomatic tumors generally present after age 35 years
▸ More common in black women

Clinical Features
▸ Pelvic pain, abdominal pressure, abnormal uterine bleeding, and reproductive dysfunction
▸ Severity of symptoms related to tumor size and location
▸ Bleeding common in submucosal tumors

Radiologic Features
▸ Well-circumscribed, homogeneous mass by ultrasound

Prognosis and Treatment
▸ Surgery mainstay of treatment
▸ Medical management possible in some cases
▸ Patients undergoing myomectomy require subsequent surgery in up to 26% of cases

---

RADIOLOGIC FEATURES

Ultrasonography, either transvaginal or transabdominal, is the preferred modality in the evaluation of uterine leiomyomata, which typically appear as well-circumscribed homogeneous masses. Associated calcifications may sometimes be evident on conventional radiographs obtained for other indications.

PATHOLOGIC FEATURES

GROSS FINDINGS

Leiomyomata are typically well circumscribed with a white, bulging cut surface and firm, rubbery texture, but these features are rarely identified in biopsy/curettage specimens. In hysterectomy specimens, submucosal leiomyomata may have a hemorrhagic or ulcerated surface secondary to compression.

MICROSCOPIC FINDINGS

Endometrial biopsies/curettages containing fragments of leiomyoma(s) seldom present diagnostic challenges. Histologically, they are composed of fascicles of bland tapered smooth-muscle cells with abundant eosinophilic cytoplasm and spindled nuclei having pale chromatin (Figure 6.6A). Occasionally, endometrial biopsies fail to sample the submucosal leiomyoma; however, an underlying leiomyoma may be associated with local effects, such as regions of functionalis having few or no glands (Figure 6.6B). The presence of two or more strips of aglandular functionalis at least 2 mm in length raises

---

SUBMUCOSAL LEIOMYOMATA – PATHOLOGIC FEATURES

Gross Findings
▸ Fragments of white, firm tissue

Microscopic Findings
▸ Fascicles of bland tapered smooth-muscle cells with abundant eosinophilic cytoplasm and spindled nuclei having pale chromatin
▸ Regions of functionalis having few or no glands (at least 2 mm in length) are suggestive of a submucosal leiomyoma in endometrial samplings

Immunohistochemical Findings
▸ h-caldesmon, smooth-muscle actin, and desmin positive
▸ ER and PR positive
▸ Variable positivity for CD10

Differential Diagnosis
▸ Myometrium
▸ Leiomyosarcoma
▸ Endometrial stromal sarcoma

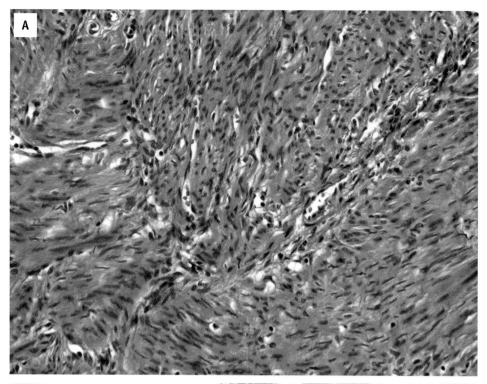

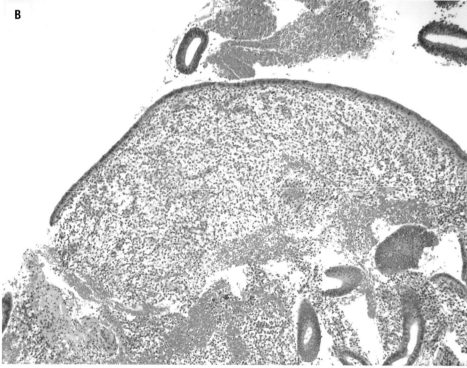

FIGURE 6.6

Submucosal leiomyoma. Intersecting bundles of benign-appearing smooth muscle cells (A). An area of functionalis lacks endometrial glands, suggesting an underlying submucosal leiomyoma (B).

the possibility of a submucosal leiomyoma. It is important to bear in mind that other conditions can lead to aglandular functionalis, including atrophic endometrium, polyps, hormone therapy, and endometrial stromal neoplasms; therefore, these possibilities should also be considered when fragments of aglandular stroma are present in an endometrial sampling.

ANCILLARY STUDIES

IMMUNOHISTOCHEMISTRY

Uterine smooth muscle tumors characteristically show strong, diffuse positivity for smooth muscle markers, including h-caldesmon, smooth-muscle actin, and desmin. These tumors may also express CD10, although in most cases not to the extent seen in endometrial stromal tumors. In addition, since they are hormonally dependent neoplasms, they are often positive for ER and PR.

DIFFERENTIAL DIAGNOSIS

Fragments of leiomyoma must be distinguished from sampling of normal myometrium, as well as, more importantly, from malignant conditions such as leiomyosarcoma and endometrial stromal sarcoma. The neoplastic cells of leiomyomata tend to be more tightly packed than *normal myometrium* and show intersecting fascicles without the organized and sometimes parallel bundle formation, seen in normal myometrium. *Leiomyosarcomas* typically have an infiltrative border (which may not be apparent in biopsy/curettage material), geographic tumor necrosis, increased mitotic activity, and cytologic atypia, whereas *endometrial stromal sarcomas* are typically more cellular, have cells with scant cytoplasm, display a whorled rather than fascicular architecture, and a characteristic vascular pattern of small to medium-sized spiral vessels.

PROGNOSIS AND THERAPY

Surgery is the mainstay of treatment (either myomectomy or hysterectomy), although medical therapy with a variety of hormone modulatory substances may be useful in certain clinical instances. Recently, uterine artery embolization has emerged as an alternative treatment. Patients undergoing myomectomy require a second operation for recurrent tumors in 10–26% of cases.

CHRONIC ENDOMETRITIS

CLINICAL FEATURES

Chronic endometritis is typically a disorder affecting reproductive-age women, although it may also occur in postmenopausal patients. It may accompany pelvic inflammatory disease of the upper genital tract; it may be associated with instrumentation or the presence of an intrauterine contraceptive device; or follow a recent pregnancy. Intermenstrual bleeding is the most common manifestation of endometritis; additionally, the disorder

---

CHRONIC ENDOMETRITIS – FACT SHEET

Definition
▸ Chronic inflammation including plasma cells (diagnostic), lymphocytes, eosinophils, and occasionally lymphoid aggeigates

Incidence
▸ May be present in up to 10% of endometrial samples obtained from women with irregular bleeding

Morbidity and Mortality
▸ Association with pelvic inflammatory disease
▸ Common cause of intermenstrual bleeding
▸ May be associated with infertility

Age Distribution
▸ Reproductive-age women

Clinical Features
▸ May accompany pelvic inflammatory disease of the upper genital tract, be associated with instrumentation or the presence of an intrauterine contraceptive device, or follow a recent pregnancy
▸ Intermenstrual bleeding most common symptom

Prognosis and Treatment
▸ Antibiotic therapy treatment of choice
▸ Improvement of symptoms within 48–72 hours following initiation of therapy in 90% of women

---

may be associated with infertility. The prevalence of chronic endometritis varies widely in different patient populations, ranging from < 1% to nearly 10% of all endometrial samples done for irregular bleeding. Causative agents include *Chlamydia trachomatis*, *Neisseria gonorrhoeae*, *Streptococcus agalactiae*, *Mycoplasma hominis*, and various viruses.

RADIOLOGIC FEATURES

Most cases are not associated with a radiologic correlate, although uterine luminal adhesions or a thickened endometrial stripe may be present on ultrasound examination.

PATHOLOGIC FEATURES

GROSS FINDINGS

Chronic endometritis typically is not detected on gross examination; however, in cases of uterine obstruction, most commonly seen in postmenopausal patients, pyometra may be present with a purulent, foul-smelling exudate occupying the endometrial cavity.

MICROSCOPIC FINDINGS

Chronic endometritis is defined by the presence of plasma cells within the functionalis of the endometrium. Plasma cells are most often found in the stroma just below the endometrial surface and in areas of stromal breakdown (Figure 6.7A). In some instances the presence of plasma cells is not synonymous with chronic endometritis, as they are occasionally encountered in endometrial polyps and in late menstrual endometrium. In these instances, their presence should be noted, but the diagnosis of chronic endometritis should not be made. Lymphocytes, eosinophils, and occasionally lymphoid aggregates (Figure 6.7B) may be found, but in the absence of plasma cells, are not sufficient to justify the diagnosis of chronic endometritis.

ANCILLARY STUDIES

HISTOCHEMISTRY AND IMMUNOHISTOCHEMISTRY

Plasma cells are readily identified by hematoxylin and eosin staining due to their characteristic cytomorphology. However, in difficult cases, methyl green pyronin or CD138 (syndecan) can be used.

DIFFERENTIAL DIAGNOSIS

As occasional plasma cells can be seen in late *menstrual endometrium* and in the stroma of *endometrial polyps*, their presence does not always signify an infectious etiology and the diagnosis of chronic endometritis should not be rendered in these cases. Uncommonly, primary *lymphoproliferative disorders* may occur in the uterus. They can also mimic chronic endometritis, but can usually be distinguished by diffuse involvement of the endometrium.

PROGNOSIS AND THERAPY

Antibiotic therapy is the treatment of choice; 90% of women experience improvement within 48–72 hours of institution of therapy.

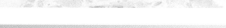

ENDOMETRIAL POLYP

CLINICAL FEATURES

Endometrial polyps are relatively common, being present in up to 25% of women; however, not all polyps are symptomatic. They more commonly occur in women ≥ 40 years of age. Less than 5% are associated with neoplasia and almost invariably occur in postmenopausal women. Of those that are symptomatic, the most common manifestation is abnormal bleeding (particularly postmenopausal or intermenstrual).

CHRONIC ENDOMETRITIS – PATHOLOGIC FEATURES

Gross Findings
▶ Not typically detectable

Microscopic Findings
▶ Plasma cells are most often found in the stroma just below the endometrial surface and in areas of stromal breakdown
▶ Lymphocytes, eosinophils, and lymphoid aggregates may be present

Immunohistochemical Features
▶ Plasma cells are methyl green pyronin or CD138 (syndecan) positive

Differential Diagnosis
▶ Endometrial polyp
▶ Late menstrual endometrium
▶ Lymphoproliferative disorder

ENDOMETRIAL POLYP – FACT SHEET

Definition
▶ Polypoid proliferation of endometrial stroma and glands with irregular architecture frequently associated with thick-walled blood vessels

Incidence and Location
▶ Most common in the fundus
▶ Relatively common; present in up to 25% of women

Age Distribution
▶ If symptomatic, most commonly affects women ≥ 40 years

Clinical Features
▶ If symptomatic, abnormal bleeding most common manifestation (particularly postmenopausal or intermenstrual)
▶ Less than 5% associated with neoplasia (almost invariably in postmenopausal women)

Radiologic Features
▶ Polypoid or sessile mass by ultrasound

Prognosis and Therapy
▶ Excellent prognosis if not associated with neoplasia
▶ Fractional dilatation and curettage, done in association with hysteroscopy or other imaging techniques, treatment of choice

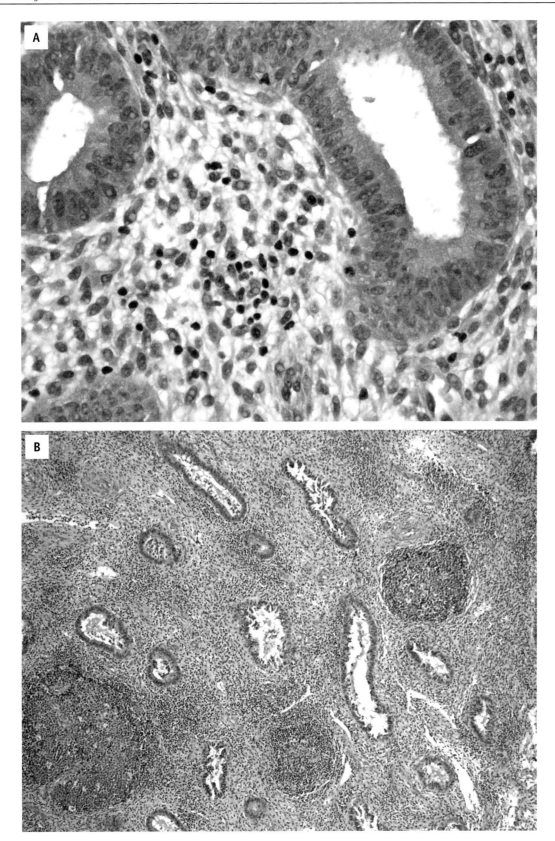

FIGURE 6.7

Chronic endometritis. Scattered plasma cells are present in the endometrial stroma (A). Lymphoid follicles may be seen (B).

RADIOLOGIC FEATURES

Transvaginal ultrasound, which is the preferred method for evaluation, typically reveals a polypoid or sessile mass occupying the endometrial cavity.

PATHOLOGIC FEATURES

GROSS FINDINGS

These lesions are frequently polypoid and may have either a thin connecting stalk or be broad based. They typically have a firm or fleshy appearance and, on cut section, cysts may be apparent.

MICROSCOPIC FINDINGS

As a result of endometrial sampling by biopsy or curettage, polyps are often removed piecemeal, leading to loss of several useful architectural features such as central vessels, surface lining epithelium, and a connecting stalk. In general, two of the three following features should be present before a diagnosis of endometrial polyp is rendered: thick-walled vessels, altered stroma (often with increased fibrosis and collagen deposition), and irregular gland architecture (Figure 6.8A). Infrequently, scattered cells with bizarre nuclei may be seen in the stroma.

ENDOMETRIAL POLYP – PATHOLOGIC FEATURES

Gross Findings
▸ Pedunculated, polypoid, or sessile
▸ Firm or fleshy
▸ Solid and/or cystic cut surface

Microscopic Findings
▸ Altered gland architecture with cysts and irregular gland outlines
▸ Altered stroma (often with increased fibrosis and collagen deposition)
▸ Thick-walled vessels

Differential Diagnosis
▸ Low-grade müllerian adenosarcoma
▸ Atypical polypoid adenomyoma
▸ Lower uterine segment/basalis

DIFFERENTIAL DIAGNOSIS

The differential diagnoses includes low-grade müllerian *adenosarcoma* (Figure 6.8B), which, in contrast to endometrial polyp, will exhibit periglandular condensation

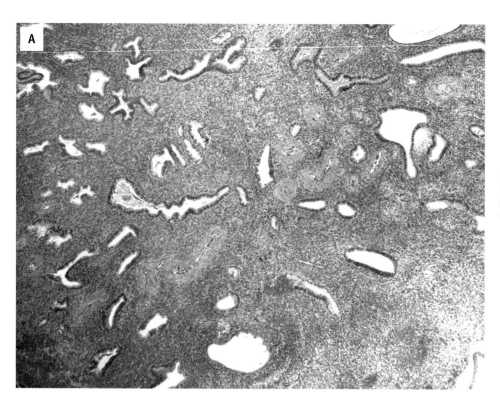

FIGURE 6.8
Endometrial polyp. Thick-walled vessels, dense stroma and irregularly-shaped glands are seen (A).

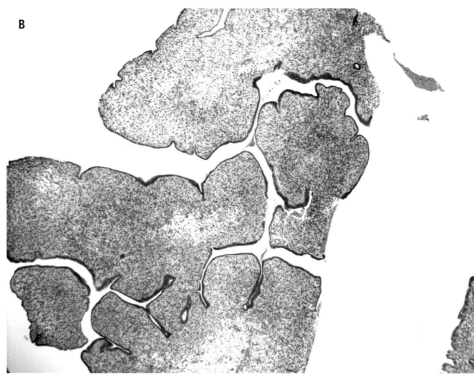

FIGURE 6.8—cont'd

Low-grade müllerian adenosarcoma. Fronds with a phyllodes architecture show hypercellular stroma that condenses under bland epithelium (B). Atypical polypoid adenomyoma. Fibromuscular stroma surrounds complex endometrial glands with squamous morular metaplasia (C).

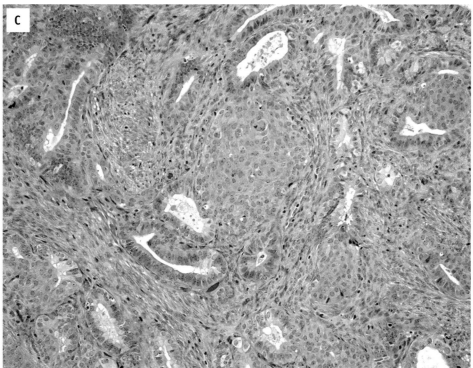

of endometrial stroma with increased stromal mitoses and stromal atypia; *atypical polypoid adenomyoma* (Figure 6.8C) characterized by fibromyomatous stroma admixed with a variably complex, often lobulated glandular component, typically with squamous morular metaplasia; and *lower uterine segment/basalis,* which often displays altered, compact stroma, but lacks the thick-walled vessels and irregularly shaped glands characteristic of endometrial polyp.

PROGNOSIS AND THERAPY

Fractional dilatation and curettage, done in association with hysteroscopy or other imaging techniques, is the treatment of choice. Polyps may be missed without the assistance of imaging. It is difficult to assess the rate of recurrence due to the variability in, and frequent lack of, symptoms.

ANOVULATION

CLINICAL FEATURES

Anovulatory cycles are one of the most common causes of abnormal uterine bleeding. When associated with menopause, anovulation is typically due to the declining functional capacity of the ovary. In younger patients, disorders in the hypothalamic–pituitary system may contribute to anovulatory bleeding. Whatever the ultimate cause, dysregulation of the balance between estrogens and progestins results in alterations in endometrial vascular homeostasis and leads to irregular bleeding.

RADIOLOGIC FEATURES

Transvaginal ultrasound may be useful in identifying endometrial and myometrial structural abnormalities. It allows for measurement of the thickness of the endometrium, which normally should not exceed 10 mm; however, this threshold may be exceeded in patients with anovulatory bleeding.

PATHOLOGIC FEATURES

GROSS FINDINGS

In hysterectomy specimens, the endometrial lining may be irregularly thickened. In biopsy/curettage specimens, an abundance of tissue may be the only finding.

MICROSCOPIC FINDINGS

Multiple histologic patterns may be seen depending on the presence or absence of elevated estrogen levels. Persistent estrogenic stimulation leads to formation of cystically dilated endometrial glands with an irregular distribution (Figure 6.9A). Stromal breakdown may be patchy due to ischemia from focal fibrin thrombi in spiral arterioles. In the absence of persistent estrogen elevation, two patterns may be seen depending on the duration of estrogen exposure. With longer exposure, the cystically dilated glands are not prominent, but other features of anovulation, including tubal metaplasia (Figure 6.9B), patchy breakdown and surface repair are present. With abrupt loss of estrogen (defect in follicular growth; "failed follicle"), uniform tubular glands with diffuse stromal breakdown are seen (Figure 6.9C). Another pattern that may be associated with disturbances in ovulation is a mixture of proliferative and secretory-pattern endometrium, which is composed of both tubular glands (proliferative pattern) and secretory changes (involving either or both glands and stroma) (Figure 6.10).

DIFFERENTIAL DIAGNOSIS

The identification of anovulation as the cause of abnormal bleeding is essentially a diagnosis of exclusion and based on clinicopathologic correlation. Once structural causes, cancer, and endometritis have been excluded, laboratory data such as serum hormone levels, determination of basal body temperature, and liver function tests may provide useful information as to the cause of the bleeding.

ANOVULATION – FACT SHEET

Definition
▸ Failure, cessation, or suppression of ovulation

Incidence
▸ Most common cause of dysfunctional uterine bleeding

Age Distribution
▸ Most common during perimenopausal period

Clinical Features
▸ Abnormal uterine bleeding

Radiologic Features
▸ Thickened endometrial stripe by transvaginal ultrasound

Prognosis and Therapy
▸ Cyclic hormonal therapy
▸ Endometrial ablation or hysterectomy

ANOVULATION – PATHOLOGIC FEATURES

Gross Findings
▸ Irregularly thickened endometrial lining
▸ Abundance of tissue may be the only finding in biopsy/curettage

Microscopic Findings
▸ Different patterns depending on estrogen levels:
  ▸ Irregularly distributed cystically dilated endometrial glands with tubal metaplasia, patchy stromal breakdown, focal fibrin thrombi in spiral arterioles, and surface repair
  ▸ Uniform tubular glands with diffuse stromal breakdown and absence of predecidual changes
  ▸ Mixed proliferative and secretory-pattern endometrium

Differential Diagnosis
▸ Endometrial polyp
▸ Ovulatory menstrual endometrium

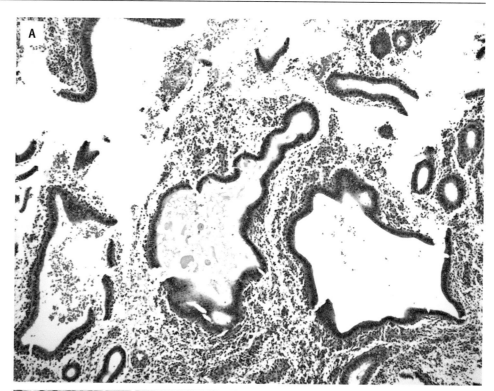

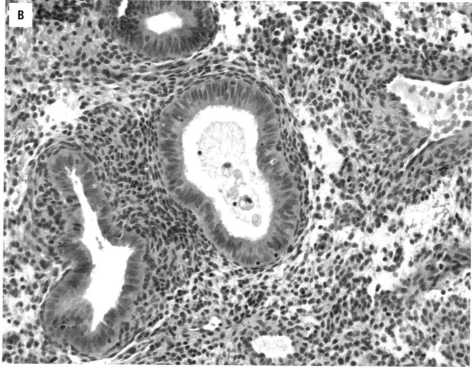

FIGURE 6.9

Anovulatory endometrium. Cystically dilated glands with irregular outlines (A). Some cells are ciliated (tubal metaplasia) (B).

The histologic differential diagnosis of anovulatory changes include endometical polyp and ovulatory menstrual endometrium. Similar to anovulatory endometrium, *endometrial polyps* may have cystically dilated glands; however, they are characterized by a frequent polypoid appearance, compact or collagenized stroma, and prominent vessels. The presence of diffuse stromal breakdown associated with a defect of follicular growth can be distinguished from diffuse stromal breakdown of *ovulatory endometrium* by the lack of both stromal predecidual and glandular secretory changes.

PROGNOSIS AND THERAPY

The most commonly used treatment for anovulatory bleeding is administration of cyclic estrogens with pro-

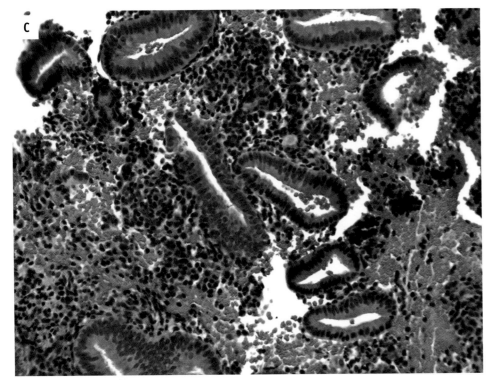

FIGURE 6.9—cont'd
Diffuse stromal breakdown in the presence of uniform tubular glands (C).

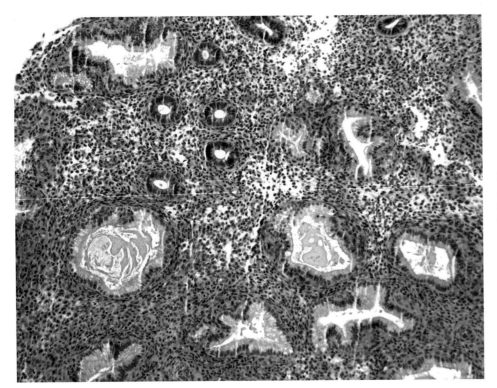

FIGURE 6.10
Mixed-pattern endometrium. Proliferative and secretory glands are seen.

gestins added in the last 10–15 days of a 25-day cycle. This regimen can be repeated for 3–6 months, followed by endometrial sampling. In older patients and those not desiring pregnancy, endometrial ablation may be an option; however, approximately 10% of patients continue to have bleeding following the procedure. Finally, vaginal hysterectomy may be appropriate for

patients who are refractory to other modes of treatment.

ENDOMETRIAL METAPLASIAS

The National Cancer Institute defines "metaplasia" as "a change of cells to a form that does not normally occur in the tissue in which it is found." Thus, strictly speaking, many examples of endometrial metaplasia are not true metaplasias, but rather alternative differentiation of the cells normally seen in the gynecologic tract. However, since the term has persisted in the literature, it will be used in this chapter.

Endometrial metaplasias may be associated with a wide spectrum of endometrial pathology, ranging from benign conditions to endometrial carcinoma. Not infrequently, the distinction between metaplasia and neoplasia can be challenging to the pathologist and the terms "atypical metaplasia" and "complex metaplasia" have been used to indicate uncertainty in the biologic potential of a given lesion.

SQUAMOUS METAPLASIA

CLINICAL FEATURES

Squamous metaplasia is most commonly encountered in menopausal women or in women who are undergoing evaluation in the context of infertility. The presenting clinical features reflect the associated underlying process associated with it.

PATHOLOGIC FEATURES

MICROSCOPIC FINDINGS

Squamous metaplasia is one of the most common metaplastic changes to involve the endometrium. It may be seen in association with a variety of histologic changes, ranging from benign reactive processes (e.g., chronic endometritis, intrauterine devices, and trauma) to adenocarcinoma. The most common pattern of squamous differentiation is nonkeratinizing, forming small clusters (termed morules), which have uniform cells with eosinophilic cytoplasm and round, centrally located nuclei (Figure 6.11). Morules typically are located within the gland lumens and may show central necrosis. Squamous morules may be an isolated finding in an otherwise normal appearing endometrium; however, they are more frequently associated with some degree of glandular crowding and complexity ranging from indeterminate to carcinoma.

DIFFERENTIAL DIAGNOSIS

Whenever squamous morules are identified, a coexisting neoplastic process (*atypical endometical hyperplasia/carcinoma*) should be excluded. It is important also to consider the possibility of an *atypical polypoid adenomyoma*, which can be recognized by the presence of polypoid fragments of tissue containing architecturally irregular glands with a lobulated distribution, set in a fibromuscular stroma.

PROGNOSIS AND THERAPY

The majority of patients with a diagnosis of isolated squamous morules have essentially no increased risk of finding adenocarcinoma on follow-up sampling (< 5%). The subset of squamous morular metaplasia associated with gland crowding does have a higher risk of being associated with carcinoma (14%) on follow-up sampling. Occasional cases of squamous morular metaplasia recur after a number of normal biopsies. In light of these observations, periodic endometrial sampling is warranted for patients with a diagnosis of squamous morular metaplasia.

SQUAMOUS METAPLASIA – FACT SHEET

Definition
▶ Squamous differentiation within the endometrium

Age Distribution
▶ Most common in menopausal women or in women undergoing evaluation for infertility

Clinical Features
▶ Typically asymptomatic
▶ If associated with preneoplastic or neoplastic conditions, irregular bleeding may occur

Prognosis and Treatment
▶ Marginal increased risk (< 5%) of adenocarcinoma on follow-up if isolated squamous morules
▶ Higher risk of carcinoma if associated with indeterminate lesions
▶ Periodic endometrial sampling warranted for isolated squamous morules or indeterminate lesions
▶ Hormonal or surgical treatment for precancerous or cancer lesions

---

SQUAMOUS METAPLASIA – PATHOLOGIC FEATURES

Microscopic Findings
▶ Nonkeratinizing squamous differentiation most common (squamous morules)
▶ Small clusters of cells with uniform round, centrally located nuclei and eosinophilic cytoplasm typically located within the gland lumens

Differential Diagnosis
▶ Endometrioid endometrial adenocarcinoma with extensive squamous differentiation
▶ Atypical polypoid adenomyoma

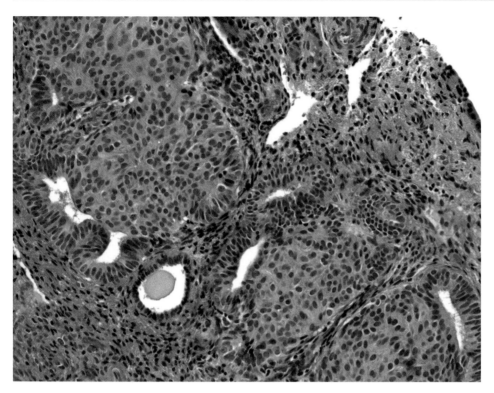

FIGURE 6.11
Squamous morular metaplasia. Aggregates of nonkeratinizing squamous cells show bland cytologic features.

MUCINOUS METAPLASIA

CLINICAL FEATURES

Mucinous metaplasia is most often encountered in menopausal women in the setting of hormone replacement therapy. It is one of the least commonly observed types of endometrial metaplasia.

PATHOLOGIC FEATURES

MICROSCOPIC FINDINGS

The morphologic appearance encountered in mucinous metaplasia ranges from simple cuboidal or columnar endocervical mucinous epithelium to complex proliferations consistent with adenocarcinoma (Figures 6.12A and B). These lesions are best classified by assessing the degree of architectural complexity, including the presence of papillary structures and cribriforming (the latter two features strongly suggestive of malignancy) as they typically show low-grade cytologic features.

DIFFERENTIAL DIAGNOSIS

One of the major diagnostic challenges associated with mucinous metaplasia of the endometrium is its distinction from *mucinous differentiation in an endometrial*

MUCINOUS METAPLASIA – FACT SHEET

Definition
▸ Presence of cuboidal or columnar mucinous epithelium within the endometrium

Age Distribution
▸ Most often in menopausal women in the setting of hormone replacement therapy

Clinical Features
▸ Typically asymptomatic

Prognosis and Treatment
▸ Low risk for associated carcinoma if no significant architectural complexity
▸ High risk of carcinoma if complex architecture (microacinar or papillary growth)
▸ Follow-up biopsy within 6 months recommended if any degree of architectural complexity

---

MUCINOUS METAPLASIA – PATHOLOGIC FEATURES

Microscopic Findings
▸ Range of morphologies from simple cuboidal or columnar endocervical-type mucinous epithelium to more complex proliferations (papillary and microacinar)

Differential Diagnosis
▸ Mucinous or mixed mucinous and endometrioid carcinoma
▸ Microglandular change in cervix

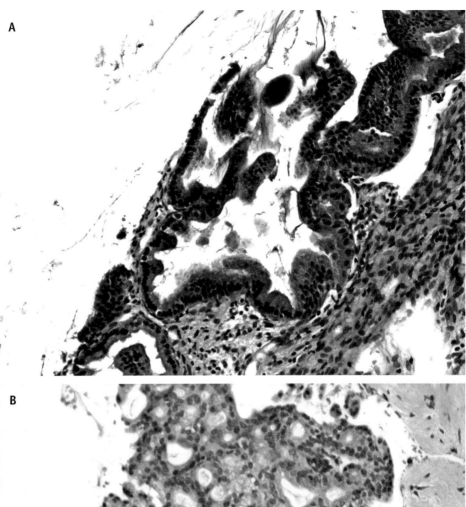

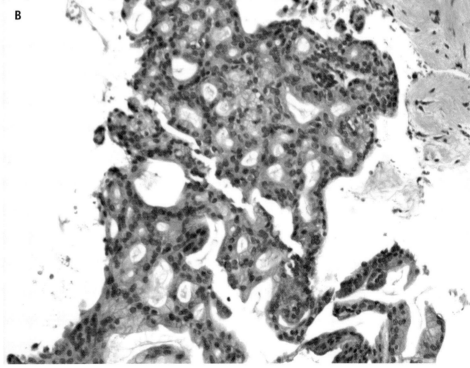

FIGURE 6.12

Mucinous metaplasia and mimics. Cells with abundant pale cytoplasm show minimal architectural complexity (A). A mucinous proliferation with severe architectural atypia is indicative of adenocarcinoma (B).

carcinoma (microglandular-like) (Figure 6.12B). Presence of the following features in biopsy specimens has been shown to favor the diagnosis of endometrial adenocarcinoma: stromal foam cells, other fragments of tissue with atypical hyperplasia/EIN and complex architecture. Complex (microglandular-like) mucinous proliferations may also be confused with *cervical microglandular hyperplasia*. However, in the latter, the glands have a very homogeneous architecture with subnuclear

vacuoles, minimal cytologic atypia and mitotic activity (Figure 6.12C).

PROGNOSIS AND THERAPY

Although the natural history of mucinous metaplasia is not well defined, in general, cases without significant

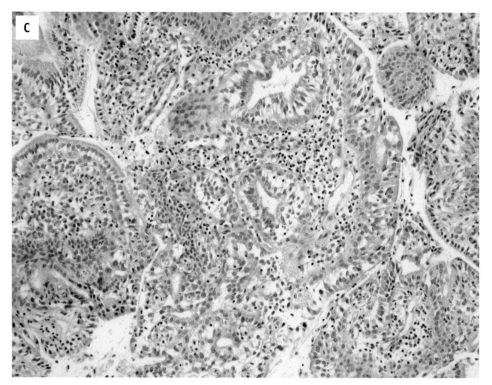

FIGURE 6.12—cont'd

Cervical microglandular change: Endo-cervical glands with abundant mucin and immature squamous metaplasia are closely apposed and may be confused with carcinoma with mucinous features. Notice the presence of striking subnuclear vacuoles (C).

architectural complexity are considered to have a low risk for associated carcinoma. However, a very high percentage of cases having complex architecture, such as microacinar or papillary growths, will show carcinoma on subsequent biopsy. Mucinous proliferations displaying any degree of architectural complexity should be followed with a biopsy within 6 months.

EOSINOPHILIC METAPLASIA

CLINICAL FEATURES

Similar to mucinous metaplasia, eosinophilic metaplasia is most often seen in menopausal women undergoing hormone replacement therapy.

PATHOLOGIC FEATURES

MICROSCOPIC FINDINGS

The cells are cuboidal to columnar and characterized by moderate amounts of pale pink cytoplasm, resembling that seen in ciliated cells of the fallopian tube. In fact, eosinophilic metaplasia often closely resembles tubal (or ciliated cell) metaplasia, except for the lack of cilia (Figure 6.13A). There is considerable variability in the appearance of the cytoplasm, ranging from distinctly granular (resembling Hürthle cells of the thyroid) to very dense and pink (squamous-like), which should not

---

EOSINOPHILIC METAPLASIA – FACT SHEET

Definition

▶ Presence of epithelium with abundant pink cytoplasm within the endometrium

Age Distribution

▶ Most often in menopausal women in the setting of hormone replacement therapy

Clinical Features

▶ Typically asymptomatic

Prognosis and Treatment

▶ Low risk for associated carcinoma if no significant architectural complexity

---

EOSINOPHILIC METAPLASIA – PATHOLOGIC FEATURES

Microscopic Findings

▶ Range of appearances from simple cuboidal or columnar cells with eosinophilic cytoplasm to more complex papillary and/or microacinar proliferations

Differertial Diagnosis

▶ Complex endometrial hyperplasia/carcinoma with eosinophilic metaplasia

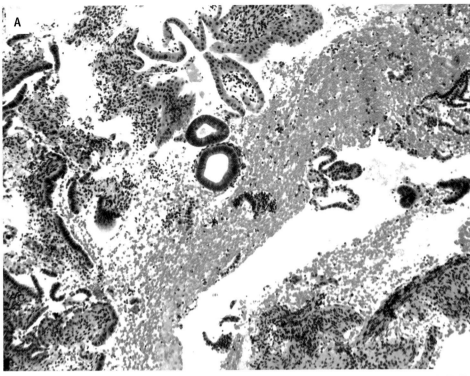

FIGURE 6.13

Eosinophilic metaplasia. Cells with abundant dense pink cytoplasm are seen (A). The eosinophilic cells have slightly enlarged round nuclei, some with visible nucleoli (B).

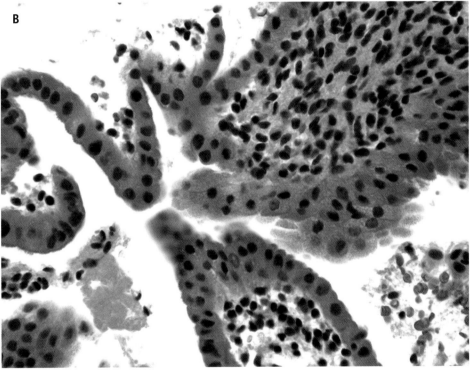

be confused with squamous metaplasia (Figure 6.13B). The nuclei are typically round and they may show degenerative changes including nuclear enlargement and smudgy chromatin. In parallel to mucinous and tubal metaplasias, eosinophilic change is associated with a variety of benign, premalignant and malignant conditions, and the degree and extent of architectural complexity stratifies patients at risk for carcinoma.

PROGNOSIS AND THERAPY

As with mucinous metaplasia, concern for associated carcinoma is greater as the level of architectural complexity increases. For lesions exhibiting any complex micropapillary or microglandular growth, follow-up within 6 months is recommended.

TUBAL (CILIATED CELL) METAPLASIA

CLINICAL FEATURES

Ciliated cells are normally present at various locations throughout the gynecologic tract, including the surface endometrium (particularly during the proliferative phase of the cycle). Endometrial glands lined by ciliated cells, however, are not a feature of normally cycling endometrium and extensive tubal metaplasia is often associated with anovulatory endometrium and hormone replacement therapy. Thus, there appears to be a link between tubal metaplasia and hyperestrogenic states.

TUBAL (CILIATED CELL) METAPLASIA – FACT SHEET

Definition
▸ Epithelium with eosinophilic cytoplasm and conspicuous cilia

Age Distribution
▸ Most often in menopausal women in the setting of hormone replacement therapy

Clinical Features
▸ Typically asymptomatic
▸ Associated with hyperestrogenic states

Prognosis and Treatment
▸ Low risk for associated carcinoma if no significant architectural complexity

---

PATHOLOGIC FEATURES

MICROSCOPIC FINDINGS

The cells of tubal metaplasia display conspicuous cilia and eosinophilic cytoplasm. Typically, there are accompanying clear round cells similar to those seen in fallopian tube epithelium (Figure 6.14). Tubal metaplasia, as with other metaplasias previously described, can be associated with a wide range of histologic entities, including carcinoma.

TUBAL (CILIATED) METAPLASIA – PATHOLOGIC FEATURES

Microscopic Findings
▸ Cells with eosinophilic cytoplasm and conspicuous cilia
▸ Can be seen in association with a range of endometrial abnormalities, including anovulation, endometrial polyp, premalignant and malignant processes

---

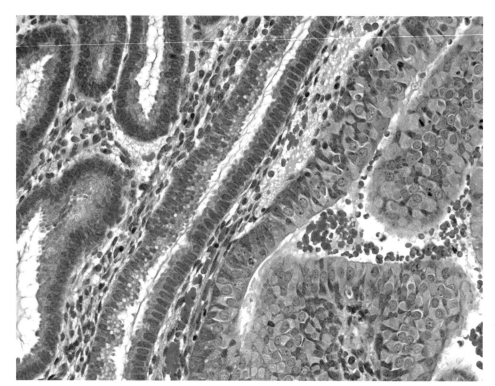

FIGURE 6.14

Tubal metaplasia. Ciliated cells with abundant eosinophilic cytoplasm and slightly enlarged nuclei with nucleoli (right).

PROGNOSIS AND THERAPY

As with other endometrial metaplasias, concern for associated risk of carcinoma increases with greater architectural complexity. For lesions exhibiting complex papillary or microglandular growth, follow-up within 6 months is recommended.

PAPILLARY SYNCYTIAL METAPLASIA

CLINICAL FEATURES

Papillary syncytial metaplasia is most often seen in menopausal women on hormone replacement therapy.

PATHOLOGIC FEATURES

MICROSCOPIC FINDINGS

Metaplasias that involve the endometrial surface epithelium are often associated with surface repair. The cells have indistinct cellular borders (syncytium), eosinophilic cytoplasm and loss of nuclear polarity imparting a disorganized pseudopapillary appearance. These changes are typically seen overlying stromal breakdown. However, no convincing papillary architecture or striking cytologic atypia is seen. Occasional apoptotic and acute inflammatory cells may also be present (Figure 6.15A). A morphologically different, although etiologically related, type of degenerative repair is seen in polyps that have undergone ischemic changes and

---

PAPILLARY SYNCYTIAL METAPLASIA – FACT SHEET

Definition
▸ Stratified syncytial epithelial process associated with endometrial stromal breakdown, thought to represent a reparative phenomenon

Incidence
▸ Associated with abnormal causes of stromal breakdown and hormone replacement therapy

Age Distribution
▸ Typically in perimenopausal and menopausal women

Clinical Features
▸ May be seen in association with abnormal uterine bleeding

Prognosis and Treatment
▸ Benign

---

necrosis (Figure 6.15B). The epithelium, instead of forming syncytia, forms small papillary clusters with cells having a hobnail appearance.

PAPILLARY SYNCYTIAL METAPLASIA – PATHOLOGIC FEATURES

Microscopic Findings
▸ Typically seen in surface epithelium and less commonly in superficial endometial glands
▸ Stratified cells with indistinct cell borders, eosinophilic cytoplasm, and loss of nuclear polarity, forming a syncytium
▸ Pseudopapillae without fibrovascular cores may be seen
▸ Bland nuclear features
▸ Associated stromal breakdown

Differential Diagnosis
▸ Endometrial carcinoma with papillary features

DIFFERENTIAL DIAGNOSIS

If little or no stromal breakdown is present, papillary syncytial metaplasia must be distinguished from *carcinoma* due to the presence of exfoliated cells in papillary clusters. In general, carcinoma must be seriously considered if any of the following are present: well-defined papillae having stromal cores, microglandular organization, or epithelium exhibiting significant cytologic atypia (Figure 6.15C).

PROGNOSIS AND THERAPY

Typically, surface reparative changes are benign self-limited processes; however, occasionally, atypical hyperplasia or adenocarcinoma may be also associated with stromal breakdown. In samples displaying a greater than anticipated degree of cytologic atypia or other worrisome architectural features, careful follow-up (including repeat sampling) is advised.

POSTMENOPAUSAL ENDOMETRIUM

CLINICAL FEATURES

In postmenopausal patients with abnormal bleeding, endometrial sampling is most often undertaken to rule out a malignant process as precancerous lesions and carcinoma may develop in the setting of unopposed estrogen associated with anovulation/menopause. Following menopause, however, ovarian estradiol levels usually fall to subfunctional levels and other sources of estrogenic stimulation of the endometrium (obesity, hormonal replacement therapy, or functioning ovarian tumors) may be at play.

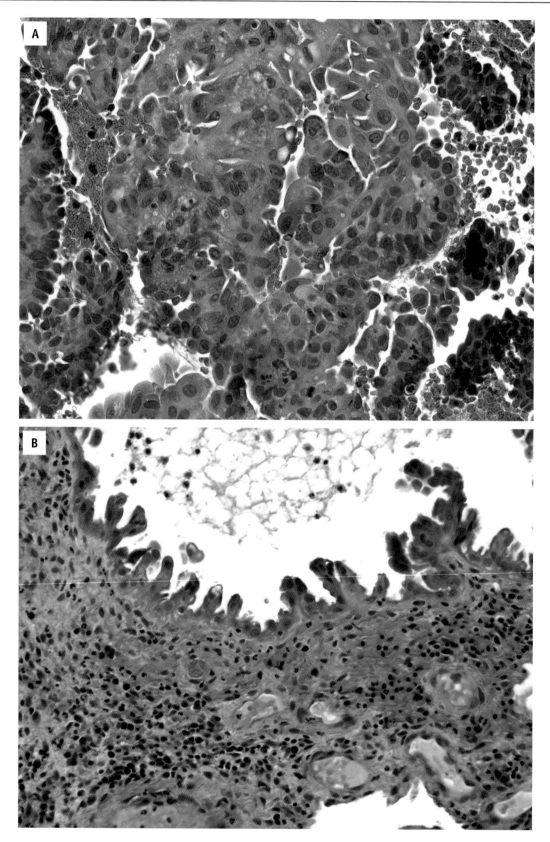

FIGURE 6.15

Papillary syncytial metaplasia. Papillary clusters of epithelial cells with eosinophilic cytoplasm and bland nuclei are focally associated with stromal breakdown (right) (A). Reparative changes associated with ischemia are seen in an endometrial polyp (B).

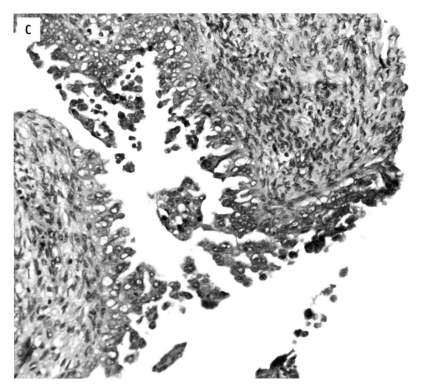

FIGURE 6.15—cont'd
Endometrial carcinoma with micro-papillary growth. Irregular buds of highly atypical cells are seen on the endometrial surface (C).

POSTMENOPAUSAL ENDOMETRIUM – FACT SHEET

Definition
▶ Alteration of the endometrial lining secondary to menopause

Age Distribution
▶ Following menopause (usually sixth decade and above)

Clinical Features
▶ Typically asymptomatic
▶ Postmenopausal bleeding

Prognosis and Treatment
▶ Consideration of hormone replacement therapy

PATHOLOGIC FEATURES

MICROSCOPIC FINDINGS

Frequently, endometrial samples taken from women older than 50 years fail to display typical proliferative or secretory patterns. These endometria are most commonly labeled as either "inactive" or "atrophic", although these terms are not synonymous. Inactive endometrium is defined as having sparse tubular glands which resemble those of proliferative endometrium, but show much less nuclear pseudostratification, lack mitotic activity, and are associated with inactive stroma

---

POSTMENOPAUSAL ENDOMETRIUM – PATHOLOGIC FEATURES

Microscopic Findings
▶ Typically atrophic-appearing, thin strips of surface epithelium with minimal or absent stroma

(Figure 6.16A). This is a descriptive term which may be applied to numerous clinical settings, including that seen at the conclusion of menstrual shedding, following hormone therapy (contraceptive or replacement), or at the transition to menopause.

Atrophic endometrium may present with one of several morphologic patterns, although all share the cardinal feature of markedly thinned epithelium. In curetting specimens, this is typically seen as thin strips of surface epithelium with minimal or absent underlying stroma (Figure 6.16B). In larger resections, including polypectomy specimens, atrophic endometrium often displays cystically dilated glands surrounded by dense or collagenous stroma (Figure 6.16C).

PROGNOSIS AND THERAPY

Until recently, hormone replacement therapy was widely prescribed for relief of menopausal symptoms;

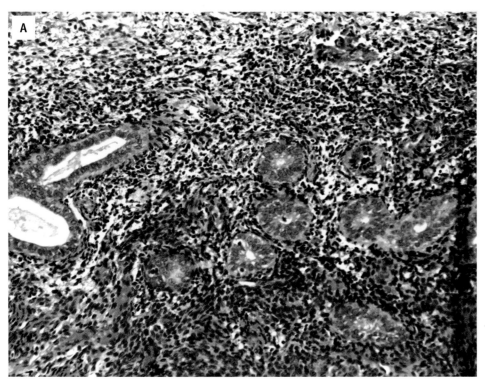

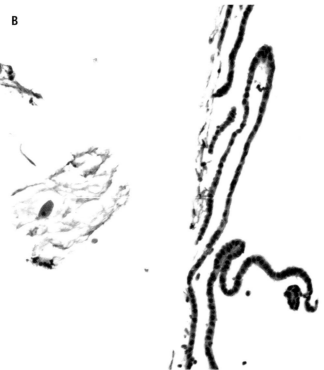

FIGURE 6.16

Postmenopausal endometrium. Inactive endometrial glands show slight pseudostratification but no mitotic activity (A). Atrophic endometrium shows superficial strips of cuboidal cells in the absence of supporting stroma (curetting) (B).

however, evidence now suggests that, although it does provide symptomatic relief, there is an increased risk of breast cancer in patients on long-term hormone replacement therapy. Current guidelines suggest tailoring hormone replacement therapy to patients' risk factors and re-evaluating the need for continued therapy at regular intervals.

PREGNANCY-RELATED CHANGES

A spectrum of morphologic changes occur in the endometrium during pregnancy, and their recognition is essential to correctly interpret endometrial biopsy specimens. Conceptually, the changes can be divided into those affecting the endometrial stroma (decidualiza-

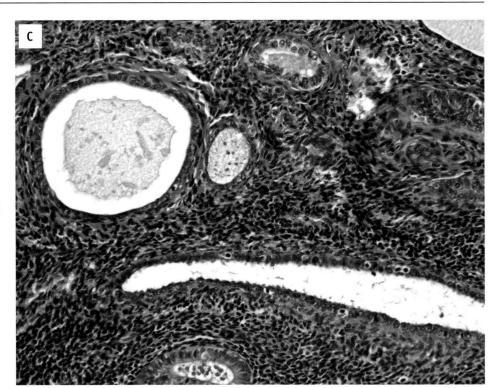

FIGURE 6.16—cont'd
Atrophic endometrium with dense stroma and cystically dilated glands (hysterectomy) (C).

PREGNANCY-RELATED CHANGES – FACT SHEET

Definition
▶ Pregnancy-induced morphologic changes of endometrial stroma (decidualization) and glands (Arias–Stella effect) secondary to placental implantation

Incidence and Location
▶ Associated with pregnancy
▶ Stromal decidualization and Arias–Stella effect may occur anywhere in the female genital tract

Microscopic Findings
▶ Decidual cells with abundant eosinophilic cytoplasm, central nuclei, and distinct cell borders
▶ Hypersecretory endometrium with complex luminal epithelial infoldings and increased intraluminal secretions
▶ Epithelial cells with abundant clear vacuolated cytoplasm and variably atypical, hyperchromatic nuclei with a hobnail appearance (Arias–Stella reaction)
▶ Immature chorionic villi with loose edematous stroma and conspicuous double layer of trophoblast
▶ Placental implantation site with intermediate trophoblast associated with a layer of fibrin (Nitabuch's fibrin) and decidua

Differential Diagnosis
▶ Decidua vera (vs stromal pseudodecidualization)
▶ Arias–Stella effect (vs clear cell carcinoma)
▶ Implantation site (vs degenerated decidualized cells)
▶ Implantation site (vs hyaline change in the endometrium secondary to scarring)
▶ Recent implantation site (vs old implantation site)

---

tion), those affecting the endometrial glands (hypersecretory endometrium and Arias–Stella effect), and changes associated with early placentation (immature chorionic villi and implantation site).

PATHOLOGIC FEATURES

MICROSCOPIC FINDINGS

Decidualization of the endometrial stroma is the response of the uterine lining to products of the corpus luteum (progestins). After fertilization, predecidualized cells are transformed into decidualized cells (or *decidua vera*). Decidual cells are large with ample cytoplasm, distinct cell borders and small, rounded nuclei (Figure 6.17A). Stromal decidualization is not diagnostic of intrauterine pregnancy, as similar-appearing changes may occur in response to exogenous progestin therapy and ectopic pregnancy (*pseudodecidualization*). Of note, these gestational stromal alterations are not confined to the endometrium and in fact are commonly seen in the cervix, upper genital tract, and peritoneum.

Hypersecretory endometrium (or *gestational hyperplasia*) is a late event in the luteal phase of the menstrual cycle. It displays complex glands with frequent intraluminal epithelial infoldings and increased secretions (Figure 6.17B). Morphologic changes to these hypersecretory glands in the presence of pregnancy-associated hormones produce the Arias–Stella effect.

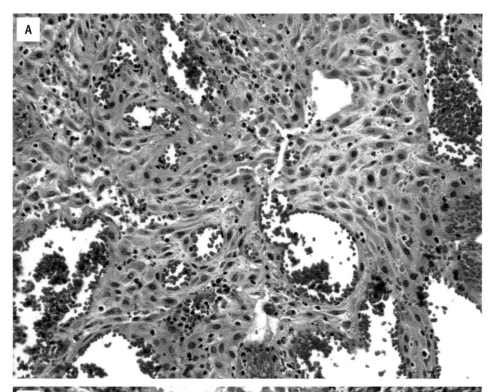

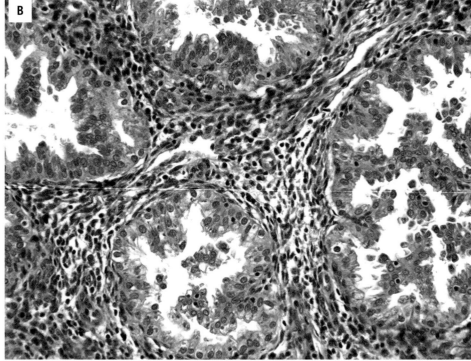

FIGURE 6.17

Pregnancy-related endometrial changes. Stromal decidualization: Stromal cells show abundant pink cytoplasm (A). Hypersecretory endometrium: Endometrial glands with multiple infoldings and pseudopapillary formation are lined by cells with vacuolated cytoplasm (B).

The resultant glands have cells with abundant clear vacuolated cytoplasm and often markedly enlarged, variably atypical, hyperchromatic nuclei. Pseudoinclusions and rare mitoses may be seen (Figure 6.17C). Not infrequently, the cells project into the gland lumens imparting a hobnail appearance. The Arias–Stella effect in secretory endometrium is not diagnostic of intrauterine pregnancy (as extrauterine gestations can lead to indistinguishable morphologic changes within the endometrium).

Finding immature chorionic villi in an endometrial sample is diagnostic of an early (first-trimester) intrauterine pregnancy. In the early stages of pregnancy, villi have loose, edematous stroma with few visible capillaries; they are surrounded by a double layer of trophoblasts, with the inner layer of cytotrophoblasts

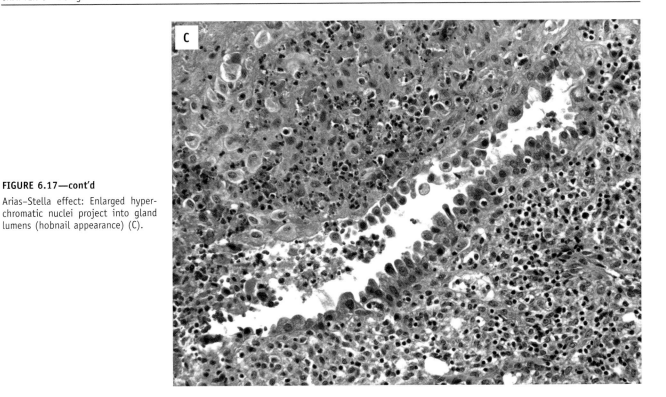

FIGURE 6.17—cont'd

Arias–Stella effect: Enlarged hyper-chromatic nuclei project into gland lumens (hobnail appearance) (C).

A

FIGURE 6.18

Intrauterine pregnancy. Immature chorionic villi with loose edematous stroma have nucleated red blood cells in villous capillaries (A).

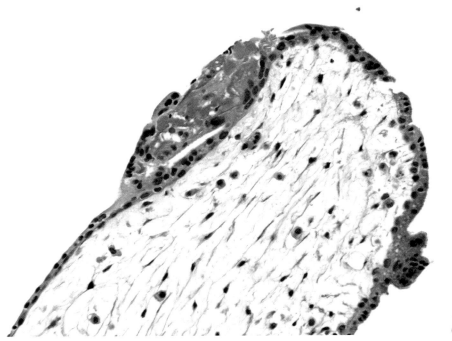

surrounded by an outer layer of syncytiotrophoblasts. Fetal nucleated red blood cells can frequently be found within the capillaries (Figure 6.18A). In the absence of chorionic villi or trophoblast, the finding of a recent implantation site in an endometrial sample is also sufficient for the diagnosis of intrauterine pregnancy. A recent implantation site is characterized by the presence of intermediate trophoblast cells which are intermingled with decidualized stroma, fibrinoid material in vessels, and Nitabuch's fibrin (Figure 6.18B). The intermediate trophoblast cells have variable shape with moderate amounts of amphophilic cytoplasm. Their nuclei are large, lobated, and hyperchromatic with irregular contours and often a "smudgy" appearance. Importantly, even though the intermediate trophoblast cells infiltrate the myometrium but they do not form a discrete mass.

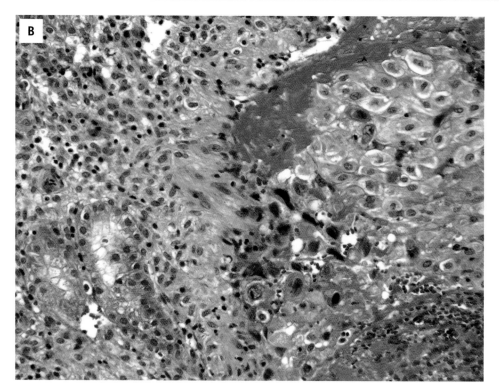

FIGURE 6.18—cont'd

Recent implantation site: Nitabuch's fibrin is juxtaposed to intermediate trophoblast (B).

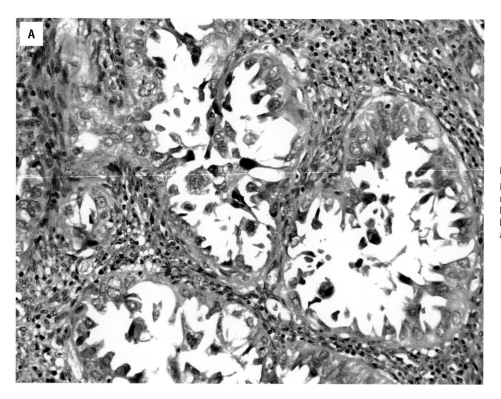

FIGURE 6.19

Differential diagnosis of pregnancy-related changes. Clear cell carcinoma: Neoplastic glands with focally papillary formation are lined by highly atypical cells (A)

ANCILLARY STUDIES

Intermediate trophoblast cells are positive for cytokeratins, inhibin, and HPL, which may be useful in distinguishing implantation site from decidual cells.

DIFFERENTIAL DIAGNOSIS

Extensive Arias–Stella reaction may be misinterpreted as endometrial *clear cell adenocarcinoma* (Figure 6.19A). In the latter, the neoplastic cells typically have high

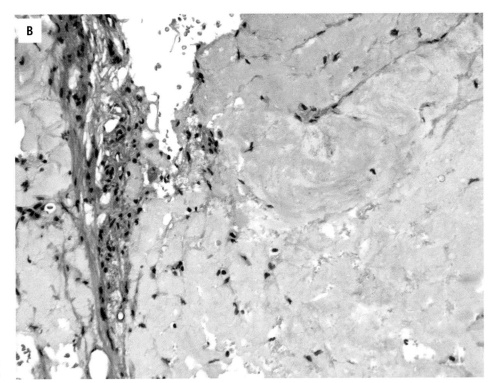

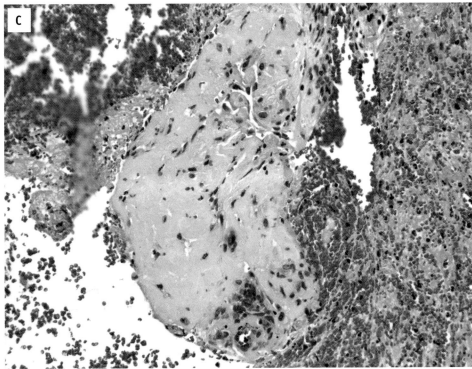

FIGURE 6.19—cont'd

Endometrial scarring: Dense collagen entraps scattered stromal cells. No trophoblastic proliferation is seen (B). Old implantation site: A nodular scar is no longer associated with trophoblast (C).

nuclear-to-cytoplasmic ratio, prominent nucleoli, and brisk mitotic activity. In contrast, Arias–Stella effect often leads to large cells with a normal nuclear-to-cytoplasmic ratio, absent mitotic activity, and a mixed population of normal-appearing and affected cells within the same gland.

Because of the implications for clinical management of identifying recent implantation site in biopsy specimens, before making this diagnosis, three common

mimics should be excluded. *Degenerated decidual cells* may have pyknotic nuclei that resemble those of intermediate trophoblast ("pseudoimplantation site"); however, they are not associated with Nitabuch's fibrin, which distinguishes them from true implantation site. Rarely, *hyaline change* in the endometrium secondary to injury may mimic the fibrinoid material of the implantation site; however, the absence of associated intermediate trophoblast cells is a useful negative finding in ruling out implantation site (Figure 6.19B). Finally, an *old implantation site* may mimic a recent implantation site. The most distinguishing feature of an old implantation site is the presence of nodular aggregates of hyaline material lacking intermediate trophoblast cells (Figure 6.19C).

SUGGESTED READING

Cycling Endometrium

Buckley CH, Fox H. Biopsy Pathology of the Endometrium, 2nd edn. London: Arnold, 2002.

Crum CP, Hornstein MD, Nucci MR, et al. Hertig and beyond. A systematic approach to the endometrial biopsy. Adv Anat Pathol 1993; 10:301–318.

Crum CP, Hornstein MD, Stewart EA. Evaluation of cyclic endometrium and benign endometrial disorders. In: Crum CP, Lee KR (eds) Diagnostic Gynecologic and Obstetric Pathology. Philadelphia: Saunders, 2006: 441–491.

Dallenbach-Hellweg G. Histopathology of the Endometrium, 4th edn. New York: Springer-Verlag, 1987.

Hendrickson MR, Longacre TA, Kempson RL. The uterine corpus. In: Sternberg SS (ed.) Diagnostic Surgical Pathology. Philadelphia: Lippincott, 1999:2203–2224.

Mazur MT, Kurman RJ. Diagnosis of Endometrial Biopsies and Curettings: A Practical Approach, 2nd edn. New York: Springer-Verlag, 2005.

Noyes FW, Hertig AT, Rock J. Dating the endometrial biopsy. Fertil Steril 1950;1:3–25.

Dysfunctional Uterine Bleeding

Mazur MT. Atypical polypoid adenomyomas of the endometrium. Am J Surg Pathol 1981;5:473–482.

Risse EK, Beerthuizen RJ, Voojis GP. Cytologic and histologic findings in women using an IUD. Obstet Gynecol 1981;58:569–573.

Tai LH, Tavassoli FA. Endometrial polyps with atypical (bizarre) stromal cells. Am J Surg Pathol 2002;26:505–509.

Vakiani M, Vavilis D, Agorastos T, et al. Histopathological findings of the endometrium in patients with dysfunctional uterine bleeding. Clin Exp Obstet Gynecol 1996;23:236–239.

Endometrial Metaplasias

Crum CP, Nucci MR, Mutter GL Altered endometrial differentiation (metaplasia). In: Crum CP, Lee KR (eds) Diagnostic Gynecologic and Obstetric Pathology. Philadelphia: Saunders, 2006:520–544.

Hendrickson MR, Kempson RL. Endometrial epithelial metaplasias: proliferations frequently misdiagnosed as adenocarcinoma. Report of 89 cases and proposed classification. Am J Surg Pathol 1980;4:525–542.

Hendrickson MR, Kempson RL. Ciliated carcinoma – a variant of endometrial adenocarcinoma: a report of ten cases. Int J Gynecol Pathol 1983;2:1–12.

Nucci MR, Prasad CJ, Crum CP, et al. Mucinous endometrial epithelial proliferations: a morphologic spectrum of changes with diverse clinical significance. Mod Pathol 1999;12:1137–1142.

Qiu W, Mittal K. Comparison of morphologic and immunohistochemical features of cervical microglandular hyperplasia with low grade mucinous adenocarcinoma of the endometrium. Int J Gynecol Pathol 2003; 22:261–265.

Quddus MR, Subg CJ, Zheng W, et al. (1999) p53 immunoreactivity in endometrial metaplasias with dysfunctional uterine bleeding. Histopathology 1999;35:44–49.

Vang R, Tavassoli FA. Proliferative mucinous lesions of the endometrium: analysis of existing criteria for diagnosing carcinoma in biopsies and curettings. Int J Surg Pathol 2003;11:261–270.

Postmenopausal Endometrium and Pregnancy-related Changes

Arias–Stella J. The Arias–Stella reaction: facts and fantasies four decades after. Adv Anat Pathol 2002;9:12–23.

Crum CP, Hornstein MD, Stewart EA. Evaluation of cyclic endometrium and benign endometrial disorders. In: Crum CP, Lee KR (eds) Diagnostic Gynecologic and Obstetric Pathology. Philadelphia: Saunders, 2006:479–481.

Hourihan HM, Sheppard BL, Bonnar J. The morphologic characteristics of menstrual hemostasis in patients with unexplained menorrhagia. Int J Gynecol Pathol 1989;8:221–229.

7

Endometrial Neoplasia

Xavier Matias-Guiu

The term "endometrial neoplasia" encompasses a spectrum of morphologic alterations that range from endometrial hyperplasia to the different varieties of endometrial carcinoma (EC). Hyperplasia and carcinoma represent only two different points along the spectrum of endometrial proliferations.

PRECURSOR LESIONS

ENDOMETRIAL HYPERPLASIA

Endometrial hyperplasia is defined by the 2003 World Health Organization (WHO) classification as a spectrum of morphologic alterations ranging from benign changes to premalignant disease, caused by an abnormal hormonal environment. Histologically, these lesions display a range of increasing architectural complexity and nuclear atypia. A group of investigators has proposed an alternative scheme to define precancerous lesions of the endometrium. They use the term "endometrial intraepithelial neoplasia (EIN)" to define premalignant endometrial lesions that show specific morphologic features, exhibit monoclonality, and share molecular alterations with EC. Since both approaches are used in daily practice, this chapter will present the criteria and advantages of each.

CLINICAL FEATURES

Endometrial hyperplasia occurs frequently; it is estimated that 150,000–200,000 new cases are diagnosed every year in western countries. It usually occurs in women around menopause; however, it may occur in young women and adolescents. The most significant etiologic factor is an unopposed estrogen source (endogenous or exogenous), which may occur under the following conditions: (1) successive prolonged periods of anovulation; (2) unopposed estrogen administration in the absence of progesterone; (3) peripheral conversion of androgens to estrone in adipose tissue in obese women

or in patients with polycystic ovarian syndrome; or (4) estrogen-secreting ovarian neoplasms.

Patients with endometrial hyperplasia most frequently present with abnormal vaginal bleeding, although a significant percentage are asymptomatic.

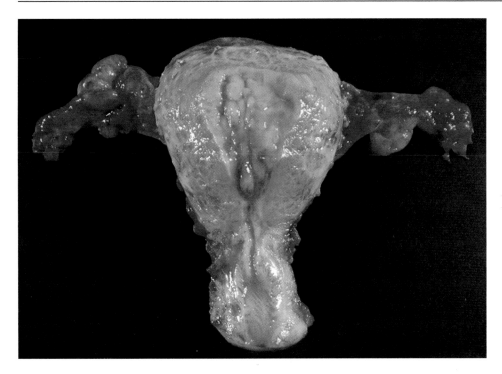

FIGURE 7.1
Endometrial hyperplasia. Irregular white to yellow tissue is protruding into the endometrial cavity.

ENDOMETRIAL HYPERPLASIA – PATHOLOGIC FEATURES

Gross Findings
▶ Irregular thickening of the endometrium

Microscopic Findings

World Health Organization Classification
▶ *Simple hyperplasia without atypia*: increased endometrial volume with balanced proliferation of both glands and stroma with absence of cytologic atypia
▶ *Complex hyperplasia without atypia*: increased volume of glands compared to stroma; glandular crowding with outpouching, papillary infoldings, and back-to-back arrangement
▶ *Simple and complex hyperplasia with atypia*: architectural features of simple and complex hyperplasia associated with nuclear atypia (loss of axial polarity, large, round nuclei with nucleoli and vesicular chromatin)

Endometrial Intraepithelial Neoplasia (EIN) System
▶ *EIN*: size > 1 mm; volume percentage stroma > 55%, cytologic features different from background glands
▶ *Benign hyperplasia sequence*: Generalized, non uniform proliferation of architecturally variably shaped glands +/− cysts, tubal metaplasia, and fibrin thrombi

---

Differential Diagnosis
▶ Variations/artifact of normal cycling endometrium
▶ Anovulatory cycles/disordered proliferative endometrium
▶ Postmenopausal cystic atrophy
▶ Endometrial polyps
▶ Metaplasias
▶ Chronic endometritis
▶ Well-differentiated endometrioid adenocarcinoma
▶ Endometrial intraepithelial carcinoma

PATHOLOGIC FEATURES

GROSS FINDINGS

Hyperplastic endometrium is often characterized by abundant white to tan tissue (Figure 7.1) that may have a diffuse or polypoid distribution, and may protrude into the endometrial cavity.

MICROSCOPIC FINDINGS

WHO Classification (2003)

The classification proposed by the International Society of Gynecological Pathologists (ISGP) and formulated by the WHO in 1994 and 2003 divides endometrial hyperplasia into four subtypes, according to the degree of architectural complexity and the presence or absence of nuclear atypia (Box 7.1). Although application of this system may seem simple, it is sometimes difficult to implement in routine practice. Some studies have demonstrated a considerable lack of reproducibility in the diagnosis and classification of endometrial hyperplasia, particularly in the recognition of cytologic atypia.

BOX 7.1

WORLD HEALTH ORGANIZATION CLASSIFICATION OF ENDOMETRIAL HYPERPLASIA (2003)

Simple hyperplasia without atypia
Complex hyperplasia without atypia
Simple hyperplasia with atypia
Complex hyperplasia with atypia

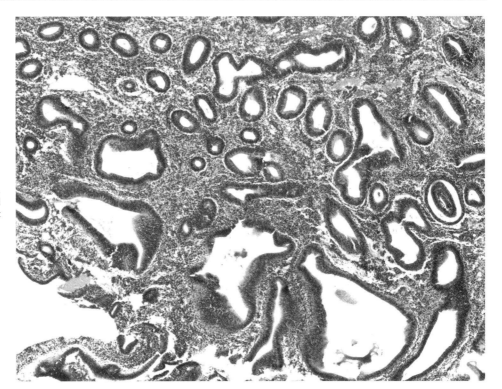

FIGURE 7.2

Simple hyperplasia without atypia. The endometrial glands are crowded and show irregular shapes and cystic change.

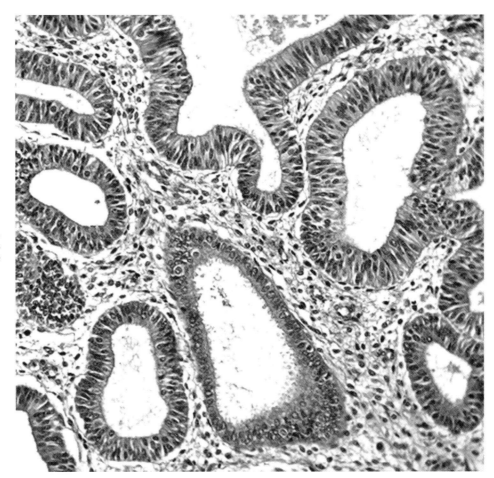

FIGURE 7.3

Simple hyperplasia without atypia. The glands show cytologic features similar to those seen in proliferative endometrium.

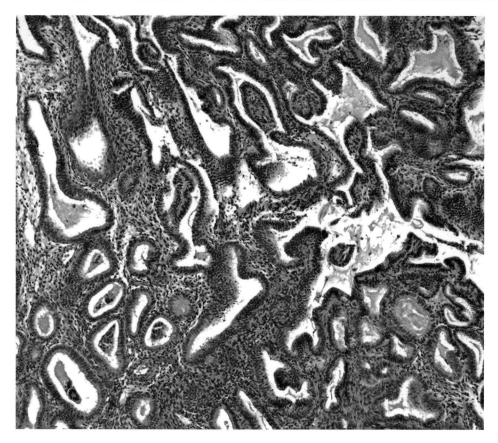

FIGURE 7.4
Complex hyperplasia without atypia. The lesion shows increased architectural complexity without significant cytologic atypia.

Simple Hyperplasia without Atypia (SH) is characterized by increased endometrial volume and qualitative differences with normal cycling endometrium. There is a balanced proliferation of both glands and stroma. The glands may exhibit marked variation in size and shape (Figures 7.2 and 7.3); most are round and tubular, but others are tortuous and cystically dilated (so-called cystic or Swiss-cheese hyperplasia). They may exhibit irregular outlines and limited epithelial budding. The epithelial lining is pseudostratified, with the cells being similar to those seen in the mid to late proliferative-phase endometrium (Figure 7.3), and secretory changes are rarely present. Tubal metaplasia with ciliated cells is frequently seen. The epithelial cells display oval nuclei with evenly dispersed chromatin and inconspicuous nucleoli. Mitotic figures and apoptotic bodies are frequently noted. The stroma is abundant and cellular, as is seen in the mid to late proliferative phase. The blood vessels are dilated and are frequently thrombosed. Finally, although occasional irregular glandular outpouchings can occur in isolated glands, if the outpouchings are numerous enough to produce a complex or "back-to-back" glandular pattern, the diagnosis of complex hyperplasia without atypia is justified.

Complex Hyperplasia without Atypia (CH) is characterized by increased gland crowding in comparison to SH with a shift in the gland-to-stroma ratio in favor of the glandular component (Figure 7.4). The glands have irregular profiles and show outpouchings and papillary intraluminal infoldings. Cell stratification and cellular polarity are generally maintained and the

cytologic features are similar to SH without significant nuclear atypia. Mitotic figures and apoptotic bodies are frequent. Varied metaplastic changes, including squamous, ciliated, and clear cell, may be present. The intervening stroma is cellular and compact. This lesion may be localized and restricted to a few fragments in an endometrial biopsy that otherwise shows a background of SH or disordered proliferative-phase endometrium.

Simple Hyperplasia with Atypia (SHA) is a rare type of hyperplasia characterized by the presence of architectural features of SH associated with cytologic atypia (see below).

Complex Hyperplasia with Atypia (CAH) is characterized by the presence of architectural features of CH, with the epithelial cells showing definite but variable degrees of cytologic atypia.

Atypical endometrial hyperplasia (SAH and CAH) is characterized by the presence of nuclear atypia in the cells lining the glands. The nuclear atypia may be either diffuse or focal (Figure 7.5). There is an increased nuclear-to-cytoplasmic ratio and loss of axial polarity, with the nuclei usually being large and round, in contrast to the elongated nuclei that are characteristic of endometrial hyperplasia without atypia. Nuclear pleomorphism, anisonucleosis, and nuclear hyperchromasia are also commonly seen. Nucleoli are enlarged and the chromatin may be either evenly or irregularly dispersed. Mitoses and apoptotic bodies are frequently found.

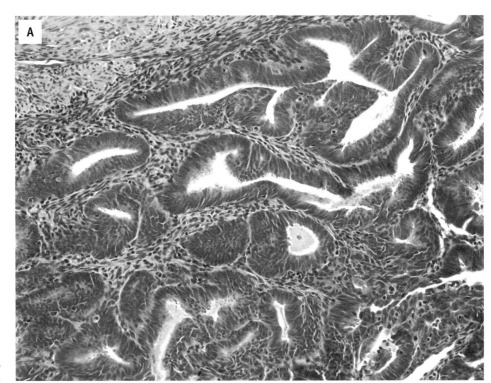

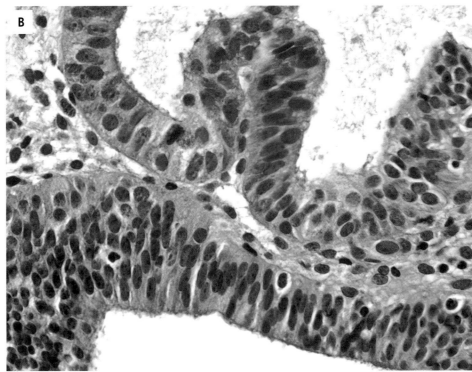

FIGURE 7.5

Complex hyperplasia with atypia. There is an increase in the glandular/ stromal ratio and the glands have a complex architecture (A). At high power, the cells show eosinophilic cytoplasm, loss of nuclear polarity, and round nuclei with nucleoli (B).

The Endometrial Intraepithelial Neoplasia System

The EIN system has been proposed as an alternative to the WHO classification of endometrial proliferative lesions. The rationale for the development of this alternative scheme comes from the poor reproducibility attributed to the WHO classification in several studies.

The EIN system is based on integrated morphologic, morphometric, molecular, and prognostic parameters.

According to this approach, true precancerous lesions are monoclonal proliferations that derive from polyclonal, normal cycling endometrial glands by mutations that confer small increases in growth advantage. Although genetically abnormal, these lesions may exhibit a benign growth pattern. Accumulation of sufficient genetic damage allows malignant transformation, a stage at which hormonal support is no longer required for survival. Morphometric analyses have sug-

BOX 7.2

PATHOLOGIC CATEGORIES ACCORDING TO THE ENDOMETRIAL INTRAEPITHELIAL NEOPLASIA APPROACH

1. Benign hyperplasia
2. Endometrial intraepithelial neoplasia (EIN)
3. Carcinoma

gested that the architecture of these lesions (glandular crowding) may be as important a diagnostic feature as nuclear atypia. In this system, three different categories are recognized: (1) endometrial hyperplasia related to benign architectural changes secondary to unopposed estrogen (benign hyperplasia sequence); (2) EIN; and (3) adenocarcinoma (Box 7.2).

Endometrial intraepithelial neoplasia is defined as the histopathological presentation of premalignant endometrial disease as identified by integrated clinical, histomorphometric, molecular, and genetic data. The fundamental aspect of EIN is the correlation of morphology with the so-called morphometric endometrial D-score, which quantifies architectural gland changes (volume percentage stroma and outer surface density of glands) and nuclear size variation (standard deviation of the shortest nuclear axis).

From the molecular point of view, EIN is defined as a proliferative lesion that is typically monoclonal and exhibits molecular alterations similar to those seen in EC (PTEN mutations and microsatellite instability). One of the key factor in defining EIN is the inactivation of the PTEN tumor suppressor gene, which is hormonally regulated in the normal endometrium and mutated in EIN. As the abnormal glands clonally proliferate, they generate cohesive radiating clusters of PTEN-negative glands that can be diagnosed as focal lesions by their altered cytology and architecture. Although PTEN immunohistochemistry can identify many of these lesions, it is not employed for routine clinical use, due to poor sensitivity and specificity.

The diagnostic criteria of EIN are:
1. Maximum linear dimension exceeding 1 mm in size, a scale that usually encompasses > 5–10 glands.
2. Gland area exceeding that of stroma (volume percentage stroma < 55 %).
3. Cytologic features that differ between the architecturally crowded focus and the background endometrial glands.

Benign mimics (basal endometrium, hypersecretory endometrium, endometrial polyps, and regenerative endometrium) as well as adenocarcinoma should be excluded. Most EIN cases correspond to lesions classified as complex atypical hyperplasia by the 2003 WHO classification (79 %). In contrast, only 2 % of SH and 44 % of CH belong to the diagnostic category of EIN. The risk of confusion when using the word *neoplasia* in a preneoplastic lesion is one of the main disadvantages of the EIN approach. Moreover, additional follow-up studies are required to validate this schema fully.

ENDOMETRIAL INTRAEPITHELIAL CARCINOMA

Endometrial intraepithelial carcinoma (EIC) is the precursor lesion of serous adenocarcinoma of the endometrium. It typically occurs in postmenopausal women, in the setting of an atrophic endometrium, and may be restricted to a small area of an otherwise typical endometrial polyp. It is characterized by highly malignant cells resembling those of invasive serous carcinoma, which replace the endometrial surface and glands without evidence of stromal invasion. The tumor cells show prominent pleomorphism, lack of polarity, large and atypical nuclei with prominent nucleoli, and frequent mitotic figures, many of them abnormal (Figure 7.6). The cells show increased Ki-67 (MIB-1) immunostaining, and strong p53 immunoreactivity. Even though EIC does not show stromal invasion, it may be associated with extrauterine tumor spread as typically seen in serous carcinoma; thus, the use of the term "intraepithelial" does not reflect its potential aggressive nature.

DIFFERENTIAL DIAGNOSIS

ENDOMETRIAL HYPERPLASIA VERSUS NONNEOPLASTIC ENDOMETRIAL LESIONS

Endometrial hyperplasias are frequently overdiagnosed. The most commonly overdiagnosed lesions include variations of the normal cycling endometrium (artifacts), anovulatory cycles, disordered proliferative-phase endometrium, cystic atrophy, polyps, metaplasias, and chronic endometritis. Of note, endometrial hyperplasia usually generates abundant material in endometrial samples, whereas the tissue obtained in other lesions is typically scant. Hyperplasia is usually a diffuse process, whereas polyps as well as metaplasias and artifact have a focal distribution. As mentioned earlier, even though CH may be focal, it is usually found in a background of diffuse SH. The diagnosis of *endometrial polyp* is aided by the presence of collagenous or densely cellular stroma, thick-walled vessels, and glands arranged in parallel to surface endometrial epithelium. However, the distinction between SH and an endometrial polyp is sometimes difficult, as hyperplasia may occur in polyps. The diagnosis of endometrial hyperplasia arising in polyps should be made with caution in premenopausal women, as some degree of proliferation is allowed in this setting. The distinction between SH and *disordered proliferative endometrium* is often difficult, since one may arise from the other, and mixed lesions are frequent. Transition from disordered proliferative-phase endometrium (with subtle architectural alterations) to SH (with irregularly shaped, cystically dilated glands) may be seen. *Cystic atrophy* may be confused with SH (cystic hyperplasia); however, the glands in cystic atrophy are usually lined by a single nonstratified layer of low cuboidal to columnar cells with no mitotic activity in a background of dense and compact (blue) or densely collagenous (pink) stroma, in contrast to glands lined by cells with pseudostratified nuclei and mitotic

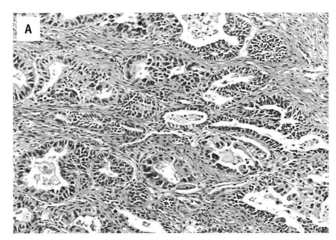

FIGURE 7.6

Endometrial intraepithelial carcinoma. Highly atypical cells lining
endometrial glands, without evidence of stromal invasion (A). The
cells show positivity for p53 (B)
and Ki-67 (C).

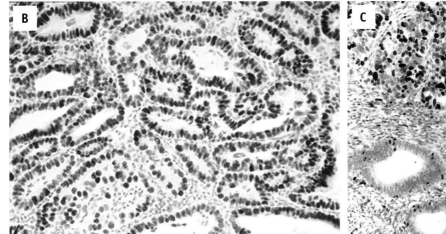

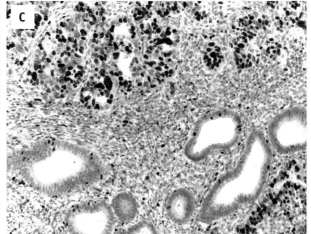

figures associated with mitotically active stroma seen in SH.

Metaplastic changes (ciliated, squamous, eosinophilic, mucinous) may be seen in endometrial hyperplasia, but they can also be present in normal endometrium. Attention should be paid to the architectural arrangement of the glands. If the low-power pattern shows abundant glands with striking variation in size and shape with budding or complexity and cell stratification, the diagnosis of endometrial hyperplasia should be made, regardless of the presence of any metaplasia. Finally, plasma cells, granulomas, and spindling of the endometrial stroma, features of *chronic endometritis*, are absent in endometrial hyperplasia.

COMPLEX ATYPICAL HYPERPLASIA VERSUS WELL-DIFFERENTIATED (GRADE 1) ENDOMETRIOID ADENOCARCINOMA

The distinction between CAH and well-differentiated carcinoma may be very difficult, especially in endometrial biopsies where the material is scant, because some of the required diagnostic criteria of carcinoma may be absent. Kurman and Norris first elaborated histologic criteria to aid in this differential diagnosis. As the main criterion for establishing the diagnosis of adenocarcinoma, they used the presence or absence of stromal invasion, defined by the finding of at least one

of the following features: (1) desmoplastic stromal response in the vicinity of infiltrating glands; (2) confluent or cribriform glandular growth; (3) extensive papillary pattern; and (4) replacement of stroma by squamous epithelium. To qualify as invasion, the last three findings were required to occupy at least half (2.1 mm) of a low-power field (4.2 mm).

Using these criteria, when stromal invasion was absent in the endometrial curettage, invasive endometrioid adenocarcinoma was present in the hysterectomy specimen in only 17 % of cases. These carcinomas were well differentiated and confined to the endometrium or had invaded the myometrium only superficially. In contrast, when stromal invasion was present in the curettage specimen, residual carcinoma was identified in the uterus in 50 % of cases, with one-third being moderately or poorly differentiated and one-quarter deeply invading the myometrium.

The most useful feature to distinguish CAH from well-differentiated endometrioid adenocarcinoma is the absence of stroma between adjacent glands due to confluent, back-to-back, villoglandular, or cribriform glandular growths. Additional important findings include the presence of stromal desmoplasia, tumor cell necrosis, and marked nuclear atypia. However, it is important to emphasize that some well-differentiated endometrioid adenocarcinomas may show significantly less cytologic atypia than CAH, and that approximately 25 % of patients with CAH in curettage specimens are found to have coexisting adenocarcinoma in hysterectomy specimens. Finally, the presence of mucinous differentiation has also been regarded as an indirect indicator for invasive adenocarcinoma.

In peri- and postmenopausal patients, the distinction between CAH and well-differentiated adenocarcinoma may not be critical, as both lesions are treated by hysterectomy. In contrast, in premenopausal women evaluation should be made with great care, as in young patients with CAH conservative therapy has yielded a 25% risk of concurrent carcinoma.

PROGNOSIS AND THERAPY

It has been difficult to determine the malignant potential of the various types of endometrial hyperplasia, due to problems in terminology and lack of follow-up data. When following the WHO classification, it appears that 1–10% of SH or CH and > 25% of CAH progress to carcinoma after 1–20 years. There are insufficient follow-up data in the literature on SHA to indicate that it is in fact a precancerous lesion. It is important to emphasize that when CAH is diagnosed in a biopsy specimen, a well-differentiated adenocarcinoma is discovered in the hysterectomy specimen in 25% of the cases, and that CAH will eventually evolve to carcinoma in approximately 30% of patients. Kurman and colleagues reported that the progression rate to carcinoma was significantly higher among premenopausal patients with CAH (23%) than in those who had endometrial hyperplasia without atypia (1.6%). Thus, hyperplasia without atypia appears to be a highly reversible lesion (80%), whereas CAH seems to be the immediate precursor of endometrioid adenocarcinoma and is not infrequently found in its proximity. Finally, of note, the premalignant potential of hyperplasias is also influenced by age, as 80% of SH occurring in women younger than 31 years will most likely regress.

Endometrial hyperplasia may be treated with progestins, and response rates vary from < 40 to 100%. Endometrial hyperplasia with atypia is less likely to respond to hormonal therapy, and for that reason, peri- and postmenopausal women with CAH are usually treated with hysterectomy. The treatment of choice in premenopausal women with CAH is controversial.

It is not possible from microscopic examination alone to predict which individual examples of EIN will progress to carcinoma, but overall the risk is high. If an immediate hysterectomy is performed, one third of the women with biopsy proven EIN will be found to have adenocarcinoma elsewhere in the endometrium. In addition to this high rate of occult concurrent carcinoma, women with EIN have a 45-fold increased risk of developing cancer compared to their EIN-free counterparts. The average progression interval from EIN to carcinoma is approximately 4 years. If the EIN scheme is used in the diagnosis of endometrial proliferations, the therapeutic decision recommended for benign endometrial hyperplasia (D-score > 1) consists of short-term

ablative progesterone followed by ultrasonographic and clinical surveillance, while either hormonal ablation or hysterectomy is recommended for EIN.

ENDOMETRIAL CARCINOMA

CLINICAL FEATURES

This is the most common malignant tumor of the female genital tract in western countries, accounting for 10–20 per 100 000 cases per year. EC typically occurs in peri- and postmenopausal women, although it may also be seen in premenopausal women, particularly in the setting of hyperestrogenism. The median age at the time of diagnosis is approximately 60 years. Several etiologi-

---

ENDOMETRIAL CARCINOMA – FACT SHEET

Definition
▸ Malignant epithelial tumor of the endometrium

Incidence
▸ Most common malignant tumor of the female genital tract (10–20 per 100,000 women per year in western countries)

Morbidity and Mortality
▸ Endometrioid carcinoma and its variants (type I): 5-year survival rate 85–90%
▸ Nonendometrioid carcinomas (type II): 5-year survival rate between 30–70%

Race and Age Distribution
▸ Higher incidence among Caucasian women
▸ Typically in perimenopausal women (type I), but it may also occur in postmenopausal patients (type II)

Clinical Features
▸ Abnormal vaginal bleeding

Prognosis and Treatment
▸ Poor prognostic indicators:
  1. Histologic type (serous and clear cell carcinoma)
  2. Histological grade
  3. Stage
  4. Depth of myometrial invasion
  5. Lymphovascular invasion
  6. Serosal and adnexal involvement
  7. Lymph node metastases
▸ Hysterectomy with bilateral salpingo-oophorectomy treatment of choice
▸ Pelvic and para-aortic lymphadenectomy in patients with poor prognostic indicators
▸ Omentectomy in serous carcinoma
▸ Radiation therapy added according to extent of disease at surgery
▸ Progestins and/or chemotherapy may be added in advanced stages

ENDOMETRIAL CARCINOMA – PATHOLOGIC FEATURES

Gross Findings

▸ Friable mass or irregular thickening involving the endometrium with or without invasion of the uterine wall

Microscopic Findings

▸ Endometrioid adenocarcinoma: variable resemblance to normal endometrial glands depending on degree of differentiation
  - Grade I: ≤ 5% solid growth
  - Grade II: 5–50% solid growth
  - Grade III: > 50% solid growth
  - Assessment based on solid glandular but not squamous component
▸ Endometrioid adenocarcinoma variants:
  ▸ With squamous differentiation
  ▸ Villoglandular
  ▸ Secretory
  ▸ Ciliated
  ▸ Other
▸ Mucinous adenocarcinoma: > 50% of cells with intracytoplasmic mucin
▸ Serous carcinoma: irregular, branching papillae with budding and prominent stratification of pleomorphic cells. Rarely, glandular architecture
▸ Clear cell carcinoma: cells arranged in tubulocystic, papillary, and solid patterns, frequently with clear and hobnail cells
▸ Mixed adenocarcinoma: composed of different types of carcinoma representing > 10% each
▸ Squamous cell carcinoma: exclusively composed of squamous cells
▸ Transitional cell carcinoma: similar morphology to tumors of the urinary tract
▸ Small cell carcinoma: similar to small cell carcinoma of the lung
▸ Undifferentiated carcinoma: lacks any recognizable type of cell differentiation

Differential Diagnosis

▸ Atypical polypoid adenomyoma (vs endometrioid carcinoma)
▸ Endocervical carcinoma (vs endometrioid carcinoma)
▸ Endometrial mucinous epithelial proliferations (vs endometrioid and mucinous carcinoma)
▸ Endometrioid carcinoma (vs serous carcinoma)
▸ Radiation changes (vs serous carcinoma)
▸ Secretory endometrioid carcinoma (vs clear cell carcinoma)
▸ Arias Stella effect (vs clear cell carcinoma)
▸ Malignant mixed müllerian tumor (vs poorly differentiated endometrioid EC)
▸ Metastatic tumors
▸ Trophoblastic lesions (vs poorly differentiated endometrioid EC and squamous cell carcinoma)

TABLE 7.1

Clinicopathologic types of endometrial carcinoma

	Type I	Type II
Age	Pre- and perimenopausal	Postmenopausal
Unopposed estrogen	Present	Absent
Hyperplasia precursor	Present	Absent
Grade	Low	High
Myometrial invasion	Minimal	Deep
Histologic types	Endometrioid carcinoma and variants, mucinous carcinoma	Serous, clear cell, squamous cell, and undifferentiated carcinoma
Behavior	Stable	Progressive
Molecular abnormalities	Microsatellite instability, PTEN and k-RAS mutations, and beta-catenin nuclear accumulation	p53 alterations, and loss of heterozygosity (LOH) at different loci

From the clinical point of view, EC has been divided into two main groups, type I and type II (Table 7.1). However, it is important to note that, in a given case, these two categories may overlap.

TYPE I ENDOMETRIAL CARCINOMA

These tumors usually develop in perimenopausal women in the setting of hyperestrogenism. They frequently coexist with, or are preceded by, CAH (EIN). They are typically low-grade tumors without deep myometrial invasion. Endometrioid carcinoma and its variants, as well as mucinous carcinoma, are the prototypes of type I EC. Microsatellite instability, mutations of PTEN and K-ras, and nuclear accumulation of β-catenin are the most characteristic molecular alterations associated with these tumors.

TYPE II ENDOMETRIAL CARCINOMA

These are very aggressive neoplasms unrelated to estrogen stimulation that usually occur in postmenopausal, elderly women. Type II ECs are high-grade and deeply invasive, and they are not preceded by, or associated with, CAH (EIN). From the pathologic viewpoint, they encompass the nonendometrioid carcinomas, including papillary serous, clear cell, squamous cell, and undifferentiated carcinoma. The molecular alterations associated with type II ECs are different from type I, and include abnormalities in p53, loss of heterozygosity at numerous loci, and alterations in genes involved in the regulation of cell division.

cal factors have been proposed in the pathogenesis of EC, such as unopposed estrogenic stimulation (anovulatory cycles, estrogen administration), conversion of androgens to estrone in adipose tissue in obese women or in patients with polycystic ovarian syndrome, and/or insulin resistance. The increasing use of tamoxifen (a nonsteroidal estrogen agonist and antagonist) for the treatment of breast carcinoma has been associated with increased risk of EC, although there is no absolute agreement among different studies. Abnormal bleeding is the most frequent presentation, yet a significant percentage of patients are asymptomatic.

PATHOLOGIC FEATURES

GROSS FINDINGS

The uterus may be enlarged, but also normal in size, or even small. The uterine cavity may be distended, containing large irregular masses of gray-white tissue that protrude into the endometrial cavity (Figure 7.7). In some cases, the tumor produces a diffuse thickening of the endometrium. Necrosis and hemorrhage may be present. Although the tumor may develop in any region of the uterus, it is more frequently located in the posterior wall, but in younger women, the lower uterine segment is more frequently involved. Myometrial invasion is usually present as poorly demarcated masses

with either a pushing or infiltrative border. However, sometimes, the myometrium may show diffuse thickening or deep myometrial invasion may not be evident on gross examination. Squamous cell carcinoma may be grossly similar to conventional EC, although occasionally it may have a condylomatous appearance, and may occur in association with pyometra.

MICROSCOPIC FINDINGS

The most recent WHO classification of EC is based primarily on cell type (Box 7.3), as follows:

ENDOMETRIOID ADENOCARCINOMA

This is the most common histological type, accounting for almost 80 % of all ECs. Endometrioid carcinoma encompasses a spectrum of neoplasms with variable histologic differentiation that ranges from well-differentiated to solid, poorly differentiated carcinomas (Figures 7.8–7.10). Well-differentiated adenocarcinomas are composed of glands that resemble those of the normal endometrium, some of them small, but others large or cystically dilated. The glands may be round to oval, but also may show irregular or angulated profiles. Marked complexity with back-to-back or cribriform growth, gland fusion, or solid areas are also seen as the tumor becomes less differentiated. Grading of the tumor is based on the amount of solid growth of the glandular (not squamous) component (grade I < 5 %; grade II 5–50 %; grade III > 50 %). The cells are larger than those of the proliferative-phase endometrium, they show round nuclei with variable nuclear pleomorphism (usually mild to moderate), and nucleoli may be prominent. Mitotic figures and apoptotic bodies are present. Although some tumors show intraluminal mucin, intracellular mucin is not a typical finding. Focal or confluent necrosis is seen, and necrotic debris may sometimes be found in the gland lumens. The stroma is usually des-

BOX 7.3

HISTOLOGIC CLASSIFICATION OF ENDOMETRIAL CARCINOMA (WORLD HEALTH ORGANIZATION, 2003)

1. Endometrioid carcinoma
2. Endometrioid carcinoma variants:
   (a) With squamous differentiation
   (b) Villoglandular
   (c) Secretory
   (d) Ciliated
   (e) Other
3. Mucinous adenocarcinoma
4. Serous adenocarcinoma
5. Clear cell adenocarcinoma
6. Mixed adenocarcinoma
7. Squamous cell carcinoma
8. Transitional cell carcinoma
9. Small cell carcinoma
10. Undifferentiated carcinoma

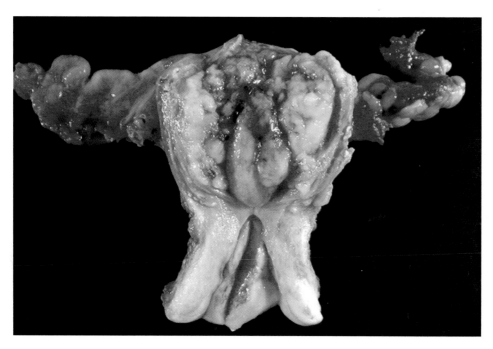

FIGURE 7.7
Endometrioid endometrial carcinoma. A large polypoid mass fills the endometrial cavity and superficially infiltrates the myometrial wall.

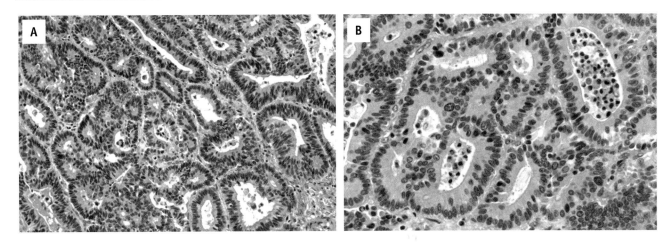

FIGURE 7.8
Endometrioid adenocarcinoma, grade I. The tumor forms well-defined glands (A) and only shows mild cytologic atypia (B).

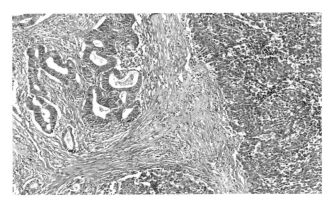

FIGURE 7.9
Endometrioid adenocarcinoma, grade II. A solid non-squamous growth is present (right); however, well-formed glands are still seen (left).

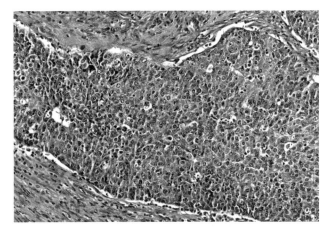

FIGURE 7.10
Endometrioid adenocarcinoma, grade III. The tumor cells have a predominant solid growth.

moplastic and contains variable numbers of inflammatory cells. Foamy cells are seen in the stroma in approximately 20 % of tumors, typically in the well-differentiated carcinomas.

Assessment of myometrial invasion is easy in the majority of cases, because the infiltrative border of the tumor usually contains irregular glands associated with desmoplastic stroma and an inflammatory response. However, it may occasionally be difficult, particularly when there is an irregular endomyometrial junction or in some myoinvasive tumors with an expansile border that may simulate a normal endomyometrial junction. Another caveat in the evaluation of myometrial invasion is involvement of foci of adenomyosis by adenocarcinoma, which occurs in approximately 25 % of cases. This phenomenon is important to distinguish from invasive adenocarcinoma, as it is not associated with an adverse prognosis. Useful features in the recognition of involvement of adenomyotic foci by adenocarcinoma and its distinction from true myometrial invasion include: (1) smooth, rounded contours of the myome-

trial tumor deposits; (2) presence of nonneoplastic endometrial glands or endometrial stroma; (3) absence of desmoplastic or inflammatory response; and (4) presence of adjacent uninvolved adenomyotic foci. CD-10 (a marker of endometrial stroma) is not a useful tool for evaluating tumor extension into adenomyosis, since the spindled cells that surround foci of myoinvasive carcinoma may express this marker. Finally, there are rare endometrioid carcinomas that diffusely infiltrate the myometrium in a deceptive manner, with the individual infiltrating glands associated with minimal or no stromal response. These tumors are typically low-grade and have been designated "adenoma malignum" because of the analogous microscopic appearance to that seen in minimal deviation adenocarcinomas of the cervix.

Endometrioid adenocarcinoma may show a variety of morphological features, including squamous differentiation, villoglandular growth, secretory change, and ciliated cells. When prominent in a particular tumor, the neoplasm should be classified as a specific variant of endometrioid carcinoma.

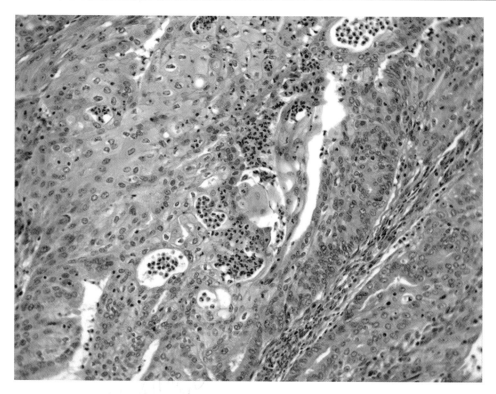

FIGURE 7.11

Endometrioid adenocarcinoma with squamous differentiation. Cytologically bland squamous cells are associated with the neoplastic glandular component.

ENDOMETRIOID CARCINOMA VARIANTS

Endometrioid Adenocarcinoma with Squamous Differentiation. This type of differentiation may be seen in up to 50% of all endometrioid adenocarcinomas. These tumors were formerly classified as adenoacanthomas or adenosquamous carcinomas, according to the degree of differentiation of the squamous component (Figure 7.11). Well-differentiated adenocarcinomas show rounded intraluminal aggregates of squamous cells (squamous morules) that may be confluent, and show central necrosis or keratinization. In contrast, in high-grade endometrioid carcinomas, the squamous component appears as large irregular masses of poorly differentiated cells with occasional intercellular bridges, well-defined cytoplasmic borders, and eosinophilic or, less frequently, clear cytoplasm.

It is important to emphasize that the squamous component of the tumor should not be taken into consideration when grading an endometrioid adenocarcinoma (see below). According to the 2003 WHO classification, criteria for establishing the presence of squamous differentiation include: (1) keratinization identified by standard staining techniques; (2) intercellular bridges; and/or (3) three or more of the following four criteria:
1. Sheet-like growth without gland formation or palisading.
2. Sharp cell margins.
3. Eosinophilic and thick or glassy cytoplasm.
4. Decreased nuclear-to-cytoplasmic ratio as compared with foci elsewhere in the same tumor.

Finally, some endometrioid adenocarcinomas with squamous differentiation are associated with the presence of keratin granulomas involving the peritoneum or ovarian surfaces. The granulomas are composed of aggregates of keratin surrounded by histiocytes, including foreign-body giant cells sometimes associated with ghost squamous cells; however, no viable epithelial tumor cells are seen. The presence of these keratin granulomas has no prognostic significance; however, it is important to sample these lesions thoroughly in order to exclude any viable tumor, as this finding would change tumor stage.

Villoglandular Variant. This is the second most common variant, accounting for 15–30% of all endometrioid adenocarcinomas. These are usually low-grade tumors, characterized by long, slender papillae with delicate fibrovascular cores lined by pseudostratified columnar cells oriented perpendicular to the basement membrane and morphologically similar to those of conventional endometrioid carcinoma (Figure 7.12). These tumors often show areas of conventional endometrioid carcinoma, which is more frequently seen in the myoinvasive component of the tumor; conversely, the villous architecture tends to be most noticeable in the superficial component of the tumor. Overall, the behavior of this variant is similar to that of conventional endometrioid carcinoma. However, villoglandular morphology in the invasive component may be associated with a higher frequency of lymphovascular invasion and lymph node metastases when compared to carcinomas having no villoglandular morphology in the invasive component.

Secretory Variant. This type of endometrioid carcinoma, also known as secretory carcinoma, is very rare. It is characterized by the presence of large glycogen vacuoles in the cell cytoplasm (more commonly sub-

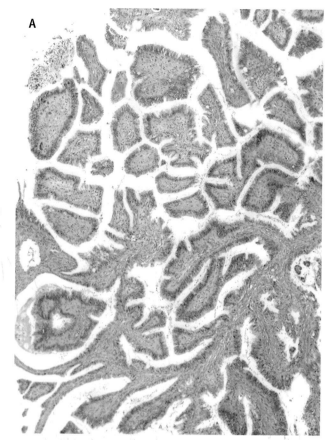

FIGURE 7.12

Villoglandular endometrioid adenocarcinoma. Slender and delicate papillae are lined by low-grade columnar epithelium (A). Neoplastic endometrial glands with prominent intrapapillary growth infiltrate the myometrium (B).

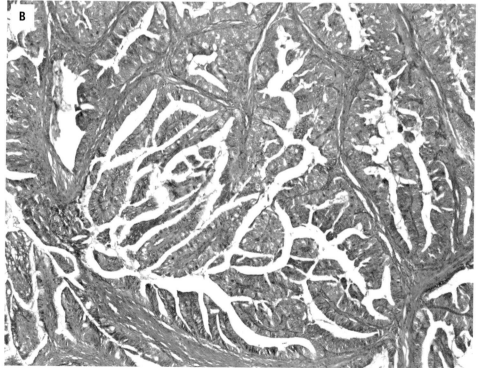

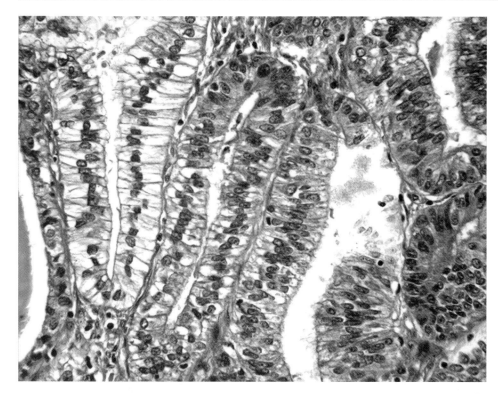

FIGURE 7.13
Secretory endometrioid adenocarcinoma. The neoplastic glands contain large subnuclear vacuoles imparting a "piano-key" appearance.

nuclear) (Figure 7.13) resembling early secretory-phase endometrium. Even though this morphologic feature is typically associated with progesterone stimulation, most patients do not have a known excess of progesterone. The tumors are usually well differentiated and behave similarly to well-differentiated endometrioid carcinomas.

Ciliated Variant. This is an uncommon variant of endometrioid adenocarcinoma, in which the neoplastic glands are lined by ciliated cells. It has the same biological behavior as conventional endometrioid adenocarcinoma.

In addition to the four variants included in the 2003 WHO classification, several authors have described small series of endometrioid adenocarcinomas that show specific morphological features:

Endometrioid Adenocarcinoma in the Setting of the Hereditary Nonpolyposis Colon Cancer Syndrome.
This is one of the most frequent tumors in patients with hereditary nonpolyposis colon cancer (HNPCC) syndrome (Lynch syndrome). It usually occurs in young premenopausal patients, and it is more frequent than colon cancer in female patients with this syndrome. The molecular basis for HNPCC is a defect in DNA mismatch repair genes, usually a germline mutation in MLH-1 or MSH-2. Several microscopic features have been found to be characteristic of tumors arising in this setting, including: (1) poor differentiation; (2) Crohn-like lymphoid reaction; (3) presence of tumor-infiltrating lymphocytes; and (4) lymphatic permeation. In these cases, immunostaining for MLH-1, MSH-2, or MSH-6 may be helpful in identification of the mutated gene and selection of patients for further counseling.

Endometrioid Adenocarcinoma with Small Nonvillous Papillae. This variant accounts for 8% of endometrioid adenocarcinomas and may be confused with serous papillary adenocarcinoma. In these tumors, small papillae lacking fibrovascular cores are present in endometrioid glands or in the villous projections of a villoglandular endometrioid adenocarcinoma. The papillae are composed of buds of cells with abundant eosinophilic cytoplasm and low-grade nuclear features (Figure 7.14). Half of these tumors also show squamous differentiation, and it is likely that the eosinophilic cells from the small buds represent, in many cases, abortive squamous differentiation. The behavior of this variant is identical to that of conventional endometrioid adenocarcinoma.

Endometrioid Adenocarcinoma with Microglandular Pattern. This variant is characterized by a conspicuous microglandular growth associated with luminal eosinophilic secretions, and numerous neutrophils (Figure 7.15). The microscopic appearance simulates microglandular hyperplasia of the cervix; however, the degree of cytologic atypia and mitotic activity exceeds that seen in microglandular hyperplasia.

Sertoliform Endometrioid Adenocarcinomas. This variant has a focal or predominant sertoliform appearance resembling the patterns of ovarian Sertoli cell tumors. The tumors are usually low-grade and are composed of hollow or solid tubules and/or compact thin cords of cells that have moderate amounts of eosinophilic or sometimes clear cytoplasm. This component usually coexists with areas of conventional endometrioid adenocarcinoma.

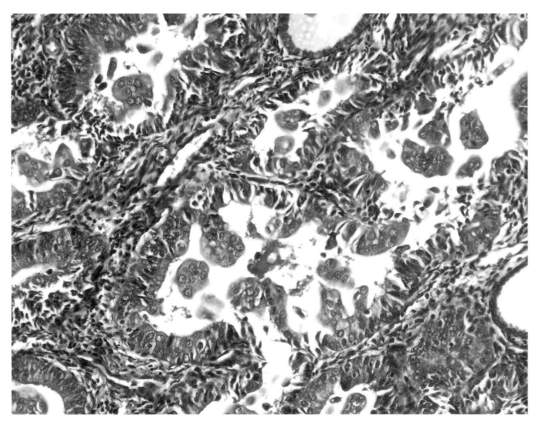

FIGURE 7.14
Endometrioid adenocarcinoma with small nonvillous papillae. Single cells and groups of cells with abundant cytoplasm and without a fibrovascular core are budding into the lumens of the neoplastic glands.

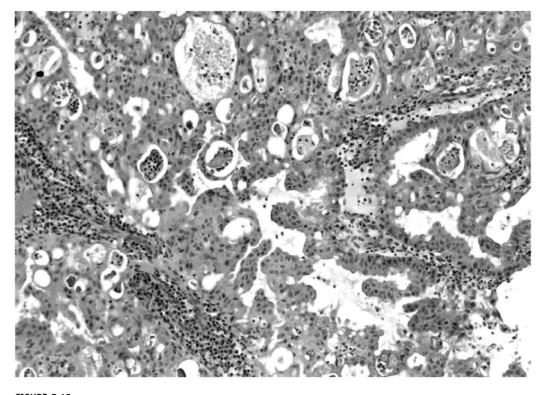

FIGURE 7.15
Endometrioid adenocarcinoma with microglandular-like features. Notice the abundant mucin, focal squamous differentiation, and bland cytologic features mimicking microglandular hyperplasia.

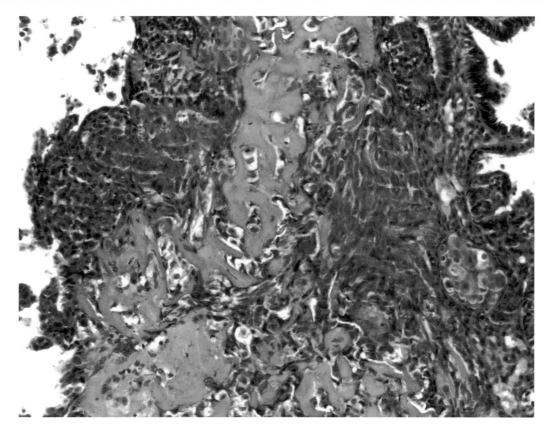

FIGURE 7.16
Endometrioid adenocarcinoma with spindle cell component. Neoplastic endometrial glands merge with spindle cells showing low-grade cytologic features.

Endometrioid Adenocarcinoma with Metaplastic Changes or Rare Patterns. A wide range of metaplastic changes (seen in up to 50%), including glycogen-rich, oxyphilic, and surface changes may be seen in endometrioid adenocarcinoma. On occasion, spindled epithelial cells or benign heterologous elements (more often mature bone) may be present (Figure 7.16). The presence of spindled cells (either glandular or squamous) in endometrioid adenocarcinomas, especially when prominent, may be misinterpreted as the sarcomatous component of a malignant mixed müllerian tumor (MMMT); however, the cells show much less cytologic atypia and the characteristic biphasic growth of the MMMT is lacking.

Endometrioid adenocarcinomas that have been treated with radiation or progesterone may show altered morphologic features. These include extensive necrosis, enlarged cell size, bizarre nuclei, pyknosis, karyorrhexis, or enlarged nucleoli. In some cases, radiation therapy may induce tumor cell maturation. Progestins may also induce tumor cell maturation or atrophy, and is frequently associated with decidual change of the endometrial stroma.

Rarely endometrioid adenocarcinomas contain signet-ring cells, trophoblastic differentiation, hepatoid differentiation, or a giant cell component. These findings are considered to represent a poorly differentiated component of the neoplasm.

MUCINOUS ADENOCARCINOMA

This is a rare subtype, accounting for < 10% of all EC. It is defined by the presence of intracytoplasmic mucin in at least 50% of tumor cells (Figure 7.17). Intraluminal mucin, which can be found in endometrioid adenocarcinomas, is not diagnostic of mucinous adenocarcinoma. These tumors are usually low-grade; however, myometrial invasion occurs in approximately 50% of them. The tumor cells are morphologically similar to mucinous cells of endocervical type, and they are frequently associated with a neutrophilic infiltrate. Areas of conventional endometrioid adenocarcinoma commonly coexist with mucinous areas, and it is not uncommon for endometrioid adenocarcinomas to have a minor mucinous surface component.

SEROUS ADENOCARCINOMA

This tumor accounts for 5–10% of ECs, frequently presents at an advanced stage, and represents the prototype of type II EC. It is not uncommon to find synchronous involvement of other areas of the female genital tract, such as the ovary, fallopian tube, or peritoneum. On microscopic examination, it shows a complex papillary pattern with irregular thick papillae associated with prominent cellular stratification and cellular budding (Figures 7.18 and 7.19). The tumor

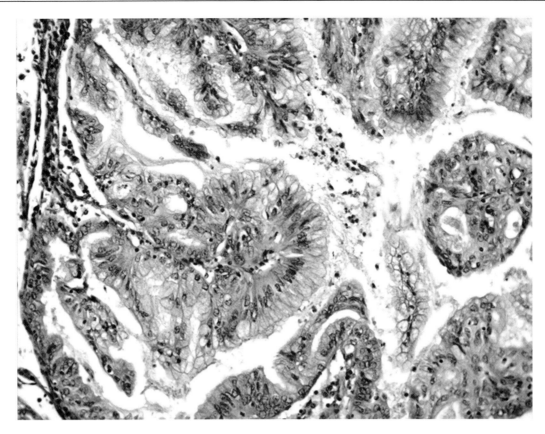

FIGURE 7.17
Mucinous adenocarcinoma. Abundant mucin is filling the cytoplasm of the neoplastic cells and is also present in luminal spaces associated with acute inflammatory cells.

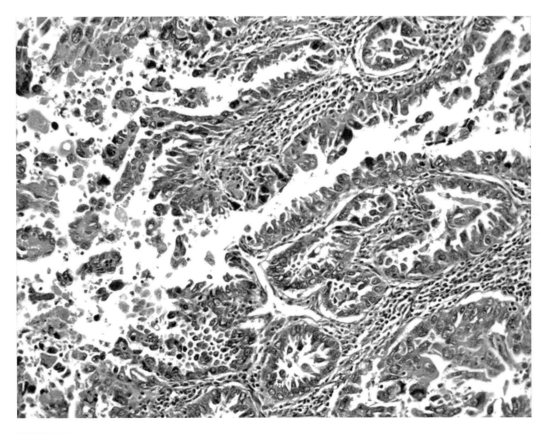

FIGURE 7.18
Papillary serous adenocarcinoma. Irregular thick papillae and glands are lined by highly pleomorphic cells.

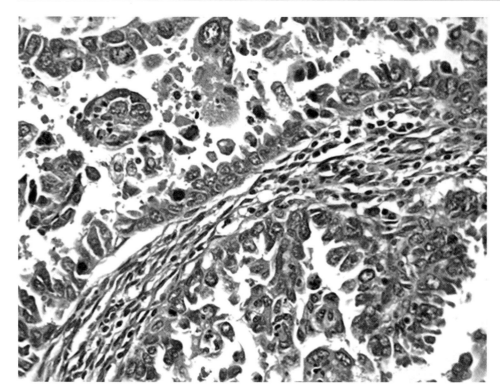

FIGURE 7.19

Papillary serous adenocarcinoma. The neoplastic cells show high nuclear-to-cytoplasmic ratio, atypical and hyperchromatic nuclei, and frequent mitotic figures.

may also show a solid growth pattern, slit-like irregular spaces, or less frequently, a glandular growth mimicking at low power an endometrioid adenocarcinoma (Figure 7.20). The cells display brightly eosinophilic cytoplasm and highly malignant nuclear features, with marked pleomorphism, hyperchromasia, and prominent nucleoli (Figure 7.19). Mitoses are frequent, and many of them are abnormal. Psammoma bodies are present in up to 30% of tumors, may be abundant, and sometimes are the initial finding in a routine cervicovaginal Pap smear.

Serous adenocarcinoma is usually associated with deep myometrial invasion and extensive lymphovascular permeation. Even in tumors with minimal or no myometrial invasion, such as those confined to an endometrial polyp, there is significant risk of extrauterine spread at the time of diagnosis. Although serous adenocarcinoma usually occurs in pure form, one-third of these tumors may coexist with conventional endometrioid adenocarcinoma or clear cell adenocarcinoma. It has been suggested that the serous component may arise as a result of progression of the endometrioid component.

The precursor lesion of serous adenocarcinoma is the so-called EIC (discussed earlier), which frequently involves pre-existing endometrial glands adjacent to the serous adenocarcinoma. Both lesions typically develop in the setting of atrophic endometrium. p53, a frequent molecular abnormality involved in the development and progression of this tumor, is usually strongly and diffusely positive in EIC and serous adenocarcinoma.

CLEAR CELL ADENOCARCINOMA

Clear cell adenocarcinoma is also a prototype of type II EC and comprises about 5% of all ECs. These tumors are characterized by a variety of patterns, including papillary, tubulocystic, and solid, which frequently coexist (Figure 7.21). The papillary pattern is the most common; the papillae are often small and rounded and frequently show hyalinized fibrovascular cores. The tumor cells may exhibit prominent clear cytoplasm due to abundant glycogen (Figure 7.21A), or may display oxyphilic cytoplasm. Typical hobnail cells, which frequently line papillae and tubules, are characterized by a nucleus that bulges into the lumen (Figure 7.21B). Cells lining cysts are commonly flattened or cuboidal. Intracytoplasmic hyaline bodies are very frequent and characteristic of this type of tumor. Mucin may be seen in the lumens of tubules and cysts but not in the cytoplasm; however, eosinophilic hyaline mucin droplets seen as intracytoplasmic vacuoles ("targetoid cells") are a characteristic feature. The nuclei are pleomorphic, with prominent nucleoli, and mitotic figures are frequent. Rarely, psammoma bodies may be found.

Clear cell adenocarcinomas may occasionally coexist with conventional endometrioid adenocarcinomas; however, recent studies show that they are more closely related to serous adenocarcinomas as they are typically high-grade tumors negative for ER and PR. However, in contrast to serous adenocarcinomas, they are frequently p53 negative.

MIXED ADENOCARCINOMA

Mixed adenocarcinomas are composed of an admixture of "type I" endometrioid adenocarcinomas or their variants (including mucinous adenocarcinoma), and "type II" (serous or clear cell) adenocarcinomas. The minor component should comprise at least 10% of the neoplasm. The prognosis depends on the proportion of the most aggressive component. However, the presence of any type II component should be stated in the pathol-

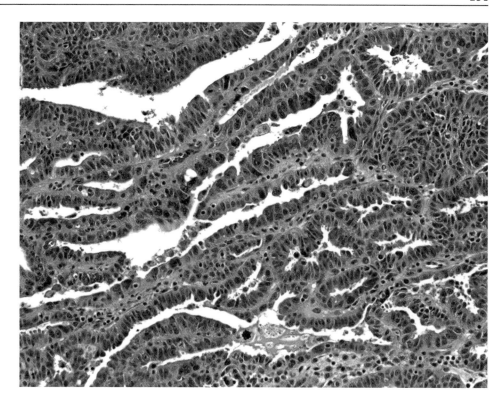

FIGURE 7.20
Serous adenocarcinoma. The tumor shows a prominent glandular architecture; however, note the marked cytologic atypia.

ogy report, as its significance is not yet well established.

SQUAMOUS CELL CARCINOMA

This is a very uncommon tumor, accounting for < 0.5 % of all ECs. It is exclusively composed of squamous cells with varying degrees of differentiation. Before establishing this diagnosis, one should exclude the presence of endometrioid glandular elements (endometrioid adenocarcinoma with extensive squamous differentiation) or the possibility of a primary squamous cell carcinoma of the cervix. This type of EC is sometimes associated with benign squamous metaplasia of the endometrium (ichthyosis uteri), and with cervical stenosis and pyometra.

TRANSITIONAL CELL CARCINOMA

This is an extremely infrequent variant of EC that morphologically resembles grade 2 or 3 papillary transitional cell carcinoma of the urinary tract (Figure 7.22). To establish the diagnosis of transitional cell carcinoma, this morphology should comprise > 90 % of the tumor. It is more common to see transitional areas admixed with other subtypes of EC, most frequently squamous, but also endometrioid or serous adenocarcinomas (Figure 7.22). The immunohistochemical profile of these tumors supports a müllerian derivation (CK7+/CK20–), and HPV type 16 has been detected in rare cases.

SMALL CELL CARCINOMA

This is an extremely infrequent tumor that resembles small cell carcinoma of the lung. These tumors fre-

quently coexist with a component of typical endometrioid adenocarcinoma.

UNDIFFERENTIATED CARCINOMA

Carcinomas that lack any evidence of differentiation after extensive sampling are classified as undifferentiated carcinoma. They are frequently composed of large pleomorphic cells with prominent nuclear atypia.

DIFFERENTIAL DIAGNOSIS

ATYPICAL POLYPOID ADENOMYOMA (APA) VERSUS ENDOMETRIOID ADENOCARCINOMA

This lesion was first described by Mazur as a benign polypoid lesion of the uterus that could be misinterpreted as endometrioid adenocarcinoma or endometrial hyperplasia. In contrast to endometrioid adenocarcinoma, APA usually occurs in premenopausal women, forms a well-circumscribed mass, and is typically located in the isthmus or lower uterine segment. The microscopic appearance is also quite distinctive, being characterized by a lobular proliferation of endometrial glands with variable degrees of architectural and cytologic atypia up to carcinoma in situ, separated by intersecting fascicles of mature smooth muscle. Cribriforming and squamous morular metaplasia (which occasionally shows central necrosis) are frequent findings. In small biopsies or curettages, the microscopic appearance may mimic a well-differentiated endometrial adenocarcinoma infiltrating the myometrium. However, the stroma in an APA lacks desmoplasia or inflammatory response

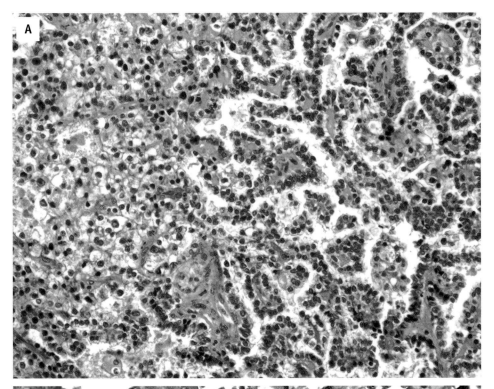

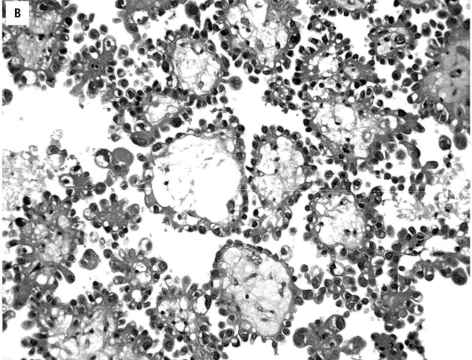

FIGURE 7.21

Clear cell adenocarcinoma. The tumor shows papillary and solid growth (A). On higher power, the clear cells lining the papillae show the typical "hobnail" morphology (B).

typically associated with myometrial invasion. Furthermore, it is very uncommon to see large fragments of smooth muscle invaded by carcinoma in a curettage or biopsy specimen.

Recently, some authors have subclassified APA into two categories: (1) atypical polypoid adenomyofibromas; and (2) atypical polypoid adenomyofibromas of low malignant potential, characterized by markedly complex glandular architecture indistinguishable from low-grade EC. The latter group was associated with a

higher risk of recurrence and myometrial invasion. Interestingly, APA is sometimes associated with complex endometrial hyperplasia in the adjacent endometrium. Some studies have reported APA coexisting with or preceding endometrial adenocarcinomas, which has led to the suggestion that APA may represent an unusual preneoplastic endometrial proliferation. Moreover, the same molecular abnormalities detected in endometrioid adenocarcinoma (MLH-1 promoter methylation, microsatellite instability, and beta-catenin nuclear accumula-

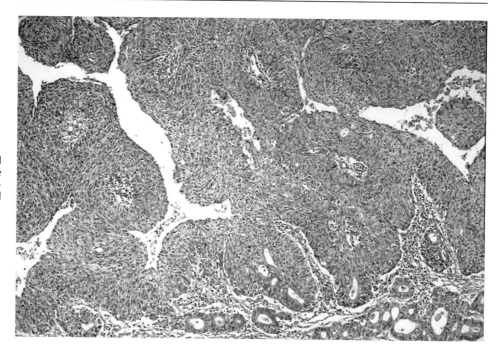

FIGURE 7.22

Transitional cell carcinoma. Broad papillae lined by transitional-type epithelium are present next to a component of conventional endometrioid carcinoma.

tion) have been identified in APAs, findings that support this hypothesis.

ENDOCERVICAL VS ENDOMETRIAL ADENOCARCINOMA

The distinction between endocervical and endometrial adenocarcinoma in small biopsies and curettage specimens may be very difficult. Even in hysterectomy specimens, determining the primary site of a uterine adenocarcinoma may be challenging when tumors involve both the lower uterine segment and endocervix. Endometrioid adenocarcinomas of the endometrium may contain a minor mucinous component, while some endocervical adenocarcinomas display endometrioid differentiation. The identification of a precursor lesion such as endometrial hyperplasia or in situ endocervical adenocarcinoma may provide support for an origin in the endometrium or the endocervix respectively, but these findings are often not seen. Marked desmoplasia has been regarded as a finding in favor of an endocervical origin, while the presence of stromal foamy histiocytes (present in 20% of endometrioid adenocarcinomas of the uterine corpus) would favor an endometrial origin. Immunohistochemical stains have been used to aid in this differential diagnosis. Coexpression of vimentin and cytokeratins, as well as strong nuclear positivity for ER, is more frequently seen in EC (Figure 7.23). In contrast, CEA positivity is more frequent in endocervical adenocarcinoma. However, in the differential diagnosis between endometrial (including mucinous) and endocervical adenocarcinoma it is best to use a panel that combines vimentin, ER, and CEA, always interpreting the results in the appropriate context. Finally, assessment of HPV may aid in this differential diagnosis, since most endocervical adenocarcinomas contain HPV DNA. HPV can be detected either by in situ hybridization or more recently by p16 immunostaining, a surrogate marker of HPV. p16 is an inhibitor of cyclin-

dependent kinases, which is involved in normal cell cycle control, and it is overexpressed in high-risk HPV-infected cells. A diffuse, moderate to strong p16 immunostaining is seen more frequently in endocervical tumors; however, this marker can show variable positivity in endometrioid adenocarcinoma and often diffuse positivity in serous adenocarcinoma.

The distinction between endometrial and endocervical adenocarcinoma is significant, since definitive therapy depends on the correct diagnosis. For an endocervical adenocarcinoma, the patient will undergo radical hysterectomy and pelvic lymphadenectomy or radiation therapy. In contrast, if the diagnosis is EC, a hysterectomy with para-aortic lymph node sampling is indicated.

ENDOMETRIAL MUCINOUS EPITHELIAL PROLIFERATIONS VERSUS MUCINOUS ADENOCARINOMA

The differential diagnosis between mucinous metaplasia of the endometrium and a well-differentiated mucinous adenocarcinoma may be very difficult, as mucinous metaplasia may occur in the setting of endometrial hyperplasia or endometrioid adenocarcinoma, and mucinous adenocarcinoma may exhibit a deceptively benign appearance. Some authors have divided mucinous endometrial metaplasias into three different categories according to the degree of architectural complexity and cytologic atypia. Type A includes mucin-containing epithelial cells, which are present singly or in small tufts within architecturally benign glands. Type B consists of mucin-containing epithelial cells that form small pseudoglands with rigid, punched-out spaces without supporting stroma. Type C is characterized by cytologic atypia or complex architecture including extensive glandular budding, cribriforming, and villous growth. Follow-up endometrial specimens demonstrated EC in 0%, 64.7%, and 100% of lesions classified as

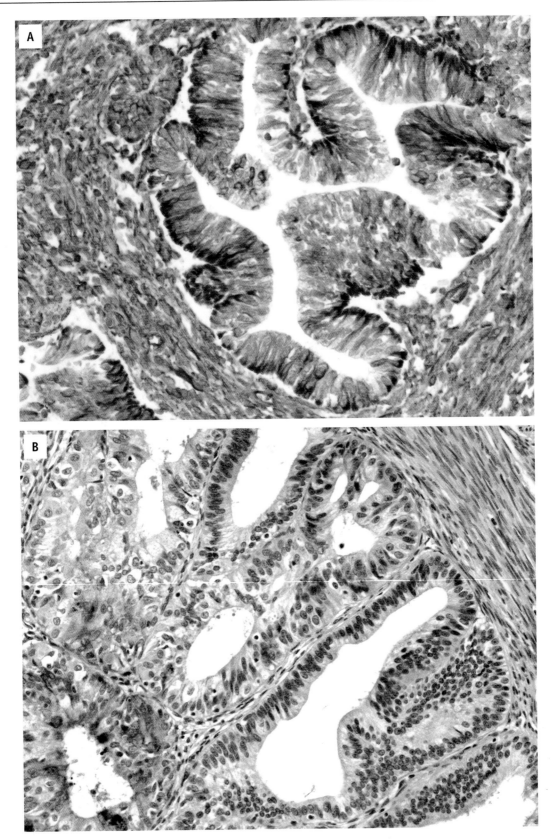

FIGURE 7.23
Endometrioid adenocarcinoma. The tumor cells are diffusely positive for vimentin (A) and ER (B).

types A, B, and C, respectively. From a practical viewpoint, the presence of mucinous metaplasia in an endometrial biopsy from a peri- and postmenopausal patient, outside the context of an endometrial polyp, should be interpreted with caution, especially when showing any degree of architectural complexity or cytologic atypia.

ENDOMETRIOID VERSUS SEROUS ADENOCARCINOMA

Villoglandular and non-villous papillary variants of endometrioid adenocarcinoma may be confused with serous adenocarcinoma because of the presence of papillae and cellular budding respectively. However, the papillae of villoglandular adenocarcinoma are slender and uniform, and the cytologic atypia is much less prominent (grade 1–2) than in serous adenocarcinoma (grade 3). The small non-villous papillae in some endometrioid adenocarcinomas frequently represent abortive squamous differentiation, with the cells having appreciable eosinophilic cytoplasm and minimal to absent cytologic atypia. The glandular variant of serous adenocarcinoma may mimic endometrioid adenocarcinoma; however, the prominent degree of cytologic atypia does not parallel the low-grade architecture (relatively well-formed glands) that one would expect in a well differentiated endometrioid adenocarcinoma.

PSEUDONEOPLASTIC CHANGES

Important non-neoplastic lesions that should not be confused with EC include radiation changes (serous adenocarcinoma) and Arias-Stella reaction (clear cell adenocarcinoma). Although radiation changes may simulate serous adenocarcinoma at high-power magnification, helpful distinguishing features include preserved nuclear-to-cytoplasmic ratio (enlarged nucleus and increased cytoplasm) and smudgy appearance of the nuclei without prominent nucleoli or mitotic activity. Arias-Stella reaction mimics clear cell adenocarcinoma because it contains clear and/or hobnail cells with enlarged nuclei. However, the normal architecture of the endometrial glands is preserved, frequently there is only partial gland involvement, the nuclei show degenerative changes with common pseudonuclear inclusions, and mitoses are absent.

ENDOMETRIOID VERSUS CLEAR CELL ADENOCARCINOMA

Even though endometrioid adenocarcinoma may show clear cells secondary to secretory change or squamous differentiation raising the possibility of clear cell adenocarcinoma, the overall architecture of these tumors differs from that seen in clear cell adenocarcinoma, usually showing low-grade cytologic features. Furthermore, in the secretory variant of endometrioid adenocarcinoma, there is a more uniform appearance of the clear vacuoles, and in squamous metaplasia, these cells commonly transition to more characteristic areas.

MALIGNANT MIXED MÜLLERIAN TUMOR

The differential diagnosis between MMMT and poorly differentiated carcinoma may be difficult, as EC may contain epithelial elements with a spindle cell morphology or sheets of poorly differentiated cells that may closely mimic the biphasic pattern of a MMMT. However, the spindle cells (either glandular or squamous) are almost always less atypical than the sarcomatous component of a MMMT, and there is usually transition to better-differentiated epithelial elements. Recognition of a biphasic pattern, with an obvious sarcomatous component, is the most important criterion for the diagnosis of MMMT. The finding of malignant heterologous elements (cartilage, skeletal muscle) is also very helpful.

CARCINOMAS METASTATIC TO THE ENDOMETRIUM

Metastatic carcinoma to the endometrium is infrequent and usually associated with disseminated disease. The most common carcinomas that metastasize to the endometrium are breast and colon. Screening programs for early diagnosis of endometrial disease in patients with breast cancer under tamoxifen treatment have led to the diagnosis of metastatic breast carcinoma in endometrial biopsies in a number of cases. The tumor (typically lobular carcinoma) frequently shows the distinctive morphologic features, including single-file and/or intracytoplasmic vacuoles, that help to establish the correct diagnosis in the vast majority of cases (Figure 7.24). As breast carcinoma expresses CK7, ER, and PR, similarly to endometrioid adenocarcinoma, GCDFP-15, if present, is most helpful. Colonic adenocarcinoma may involve the uterus either by direct extension or metastases. The tumor shows an architecture that may overlap with that seen in endometrioid carcinoma, but it is frequently associated with dirty necrosis, deeply eosinophilic cytoplasm, and goblet cells. CK7/CK20 are useful in the differential diagnosis, as metastatic colon adenocarcinoma is typically diffusely positive for CK20 but negative for CK7 and the opposite profile is seen in endometrioid adenocarcinoma.

TROPHOBLASTIC LESIONS

Trophoblastic proliferations may pose problems in the differential diagnosis with high-grade endometrioid carcinoma, squamous cell carcinoma, and ECs containing trophoblast cells. Placental site trophoblastic tumor is composed of intermediate trophoblast cells characterized by medium to large-sized mononuclear or, rarely, multinucleated cells showing enlarged nuclei, and prominent nucleoli. Helpful features include the finding of neoplastic cells replacing the vascular walls associated with fibrinoid necrosis and splitting of the muscle fibers by the tumor cells. Keratin and EMA are not helpful in the differential diagnosis between EC and placental site trophoblastic tumor. However, the latter is also positive for alpha-inhibin, hPL, CD146, and, focally, hCG. Finally, these patients have elevated serum levels of hCG in approximately 50% of cases.

The other trophoblastic proliferation that may be confused with a poorly differentiated endometrioid EC or a squamous cell carcinoma is the epithelioid trophoblastic tumor. This neoplasm is characterized by a proliferation of intermediate trophoblastic cells that

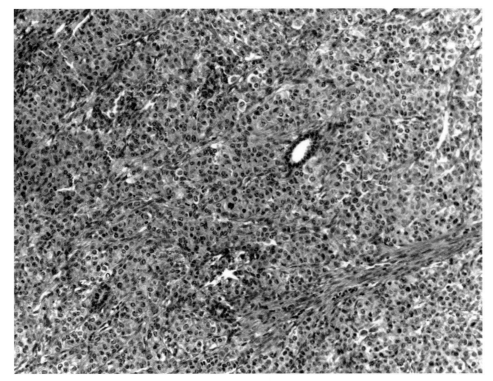

FIGURE 7.24

Lobular carcinoma metastatic to the endometrium. The tumor cells diffusely permeate the endometrium and have a monotonous appearance.

originate from the chorionic trophoblast, in which nests of mononuclear cells with clear to eosinophilic cytoplasm are frequently distributed around blood vessels without invading the vessel walls. Distinctive morphologic features include extensive hyaline-like necrosis with a geographic distribution and well-defined margins. Keratin and EMA are not helpful in the differential diagnosis between epithelioid trophoblastic tumor and EC. However, epithelioid trophoblastic tumor is also positive for alpha-inhibin and p63, and is focally positive for hPL, hCG, and CD116.

Choriocarcinoma is usually easy to distinguish from EC as it typically shows a biphasic growth, with mononuclear cells surrounded by syncytiotrophoblast cells. However, of note, choriocarcinoma may be seen in association with an endometrioid EC.

PROGNOSIS AND THERAPY

Several prognostic factors have been implicated in EC, and include:

STAGE

The 1988 International Federation of Gynecologists and Obstetricians (FIGO) staging system has been found stage to be the single strongest prognostic parameter for patients with EC. This is a surgical-pathologic staging system that divides EC into four stages and requires hysterectomy as well as assessment of any suspicious extrauterine lesions, pelvic as well as para-aortic lymph nodes, adnexae, and peritoneal fluid cytologic examination (Box 7.4).

BOX 7.4

STAGING OF ENDOMETRIAL CARCINOMA (INTERNATIONAL FEDERATION OF GYNECOLOGISTS AND OBSTETRICIANS, 1988)

I: Tumor confined to the uterus
    Ia: Tumor confined to the endometrium
    Ib: Tumor invades < 50% of the myometrial wall
    Ic: Tumor invades ≥ 50% of the myometrial wall
II: Tumor extends to the uterine cervix
    IIa: Tumor extends to the endocervical epithelial surface or glands
    IIb: Tumor infiltrates the cervical stroma
III: Tumor extends outside the uterus
    IIIa: Tumor involves serosa, and/or adnexa, and/or positive ascites, or peritoneal washings
    IIIb: Direct extension or metastasis to the vagina
    IIIc: Pelvic and/or para-aortic lymph node metastases
IV:
    IVa: Tumor invades bladder mucosa and/or bowel mucosa
    IVb: Distant metastases (excluding metastases to vagina, pelvic serosa, or adnexa)

The 5-year disease-free survival is 90% for stage I, 83% for stage II, and 43% for stage III tumors. When stratifying stage I tumors, a univariate analysis revealed 5-year survival rates of 93.8% for stage IA, 95.4% for stage IB, and 75% for stage IC EC.

HISTOLOGIC TYPE

Histologic type has been recognized as an important prognostic factor in EC. Low-grade endometrioid adenocarcinoma and its variants (with squamous differentiation, villoglandular, secretory, and ciliated) and mucinous adenocarcinoma (type I carcinomas) are associated with a favorable prognosis (5-year survival rate 85–90%). In contrast, serous, clear cell, high-grade endometrioid, and undifferentiated carcinoma (type II carcinomas) are associated with an unfavorable outcome, with overall 5-year survival rates ranging from 30 to 70%. In mixed carcinomas, the presence of > 25% of a serous, clear cell, or undifferentiated component has been shown to be an indicator of poor prognosis. However, the presence of any such component should be stated in the report as it may affect prognosis.

HISTOLOGIC GRADE

The prognostic importance of grading endometrioid adenocarcinomas has been recognized for many years. In contrast, nonendometrioid adenocarcinomas (serous and clear cell) are, by definition, considered high-grade. The 1988 FIGO/ISGP grading system of endometrioid adenocarcinomas is based primarily on architectural features (Table 7.2). Tumors with < 5% solid component are grade 1, those with 5–50% solid areas are grade 2, whereas tumors with > 50% solid areas are grade 3. Assessment of the solid growth is based only on the nonsquamous (glandular) component of the tumor. However, the presence of grade 3 nuclear features (marked nuclear pleomorphism, coarse chromatin, or prominent nuclei) in grade 1 or 2 carcinomas (based on architecture) increases their grade by 1. By using these criteria, the vast majority of endometrioid adenocarcinomas are grade 1. Assessment of nuclear features is more subjective, with poorer reproducibility.

The prognostic value of the FIGO grading system has been demonstrated in one univariate study of more than 600 patients with clinical stage I and/or occult stage II endometrioid adenocarcinoma. The 5-year relative survival for the patients with grade 1 tumors was 94%, while it decreased to 84 and 72% for those patients with grade 2 and 3 tumors respectively.

Recently, Lax and colleagues have proposed a binary architectural grading system of endometrial endometrioid carcinoma. In this scheme, the tumor is high-grade if at least two of the following three criteria are present: (1) > 50% solid growth (without distinction between squamous and glandular); (2) diffusely infiltrative rather than expansile growth pattern; and (3) tumor cell necrosis. This system stratifies patients into three prognostic and therapeutic groups: (1) patients with low-stage (Ia or Ib) low-grade tumors with a 100% 5-year survival rate; (2) patients with higher-stage (Ic and II–IV) low-grade tumors, and those with high-grade tumors confined to the myometrium (stages Ib and Ic) with a 5-year survival rate of 67–76%; and (3) patients with advanced-stage, high-grade tumors with 26% 5-year survival rate. The authors claim that this system has greater reproducibility in comparison to the FIGO scheme. However, these modifications of the FIGO grading system have not been adopted.

MYOMETRIAL INVASION

Myometrial invasion is an independent predictor of outcome in low-stage ECs. It correlates with the risk of extrauterine extension and with metastases to pelvic and para-aortic lymph nodes. However, identification of myometrial invasion may be difficult, especially when there is an irregular endomyometrial junction (Figure 7.25) or tumor extends into adenomyotic foci. In fact, myometrial invasion is overdiagnosed in 25% of cases.

The current FIGO staging system uses three subdivisions when evaluating depth of myometrial invasion: (1) tumor limited to the endometrium; (2) invasion < than one-half of myometrial wall; and (3) invasion ≥ one-half of myometrial wall without involvement of the uterine serosa. However, several other methods have been proposed, including division of myometrial thickness by thirds, depth of tumor invasion (in millimeters), and distance between the tumor and the uterine serosa (in millimeters).

CERVICAL INVOLVEMENT

Involvement of the cervix by EC may result from direct extension or lymphatic spread. In about 5%, implantation of EC in the denuded endocervix occurs after fractional dilatation and curettage. In stage IIa neoplasms, tumor cells are confined to the endocervical epithelial surface or glands, whereas in stage IIb, tumor cells infiltrate the cervical stroma. However, the prognostic value of this distinction has been questioned.

A peculiar pattern of cervical involvement has been recently described as "burrowing pattern." It occurs in low-grade endometrial endometrioid carcinoma, in which indolent-looking neoplastic glands may infiltrate the endocervical stroma deeply without any significant stromal reaction. This particular pattern of infiltration may raise the possibility of an independent cervical adenocarcinoma. However, thorough sampling shows continuity of the EC with the neoplastic endocervical proliferation.

TABLE 7.2

Histologic grading system for endometrioid carcinoma (International Federation of Gynecologists and Obstetricians, 1988)

Grade 1	< 5% of solid component
Grade 2	5–50% of solid component
Grade 3	> 50% of solid component

- High-grade nuclear features in architecturally grade 1 or 2 carcinomas increase their grade by one.
- Squamous elements should not be considered when assessing the solid component.

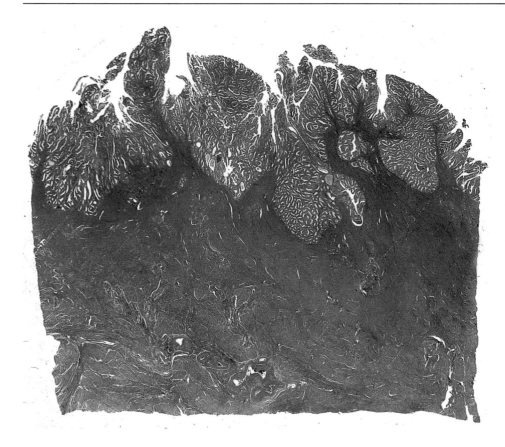

FIGURE 7.25

Endometrioid carcinoma confined to the endometrium. Notice the irregular endomyometrial junction that may be misinterpreted as myometrial invasion.

ADNEXAL INVOLVEMENT

Assessment of adnexal involvement can be difficult as it may reflect the existence of two simultaneous independent primaries (ovary and endometrium) rather than a primary EC with ovarian metastasis. Several clinicopathologic features can be used in this differential diagnosis, including tumor size, bilaterality and pattern of ovarian involvement, histologic type and grade of the tumors, presence and extent of lymphovascular invasion, myometrial and tubal invasion, coexistent endometrial hyperplasia or ovarian endometriosis, and follow-up. In difficult cases, a number of immunohistochemical, DNA flow cytometric, and molecular parameters have been proposed to aid in this differential diagnosis.

LYMPHOVASCULAR INVASION

Evidence of tumor cells within endothelial-lined spaces is an independent predictor of tumor recurrence and outcome. It is also associated with increased risk of lymph node metastasis. Lymphovascular space invasion is uncommon in endometrioid adenocarcinoma, but very frequent in serous adenocarcinoma. It should be distinguished from invasive tumor associated with retraction artifact, frequently seen at the infiltrative border with the myometrium.

LYMPH NODE INVOLVEMENT

The finding of pelvic and/or para-aortic lymph node metastases is classified as stage IIIc. The frequency of lymph node metastases in clinical stage I patients is related to the depth of myometrial invasion. One-third of patients with metastasis to pelvic lymph nodes also have positive para-aortic lymph nodes. Prognosis of EC with positive pelvic lymph nodes is better than that of those with positive para-aortic lymph nodes.

POSITIVE PERITONEAL CYTOLOGY

Positive peritoneal cytology has been associated with high histologic grade, deep myometrial invasion, and extrauterine spread.

OTHER PROGNOSTIC FACTORS

DNA ploidy has been shown to be a relatively useful prognostic factor. In stage I ECs, diploidy is associated with higher disease-free survival in comparison with aneuploid tumors. Approximately 67% of endometrioid adenocarcinomas are diploid, whereas diploid DNA is detected in only 45% of nonendometrioid adenocarcinomas.

Immunohistochemical staining for ER, bcl-2, c-erb B2, p53, and Ki-67 (MIB-1) has been suggested as important parameters in assessing prognosis in EC. However, further studies are required to confirm the independent prognostic value of these markers. Finally, a number of molecular alterations have also been proposed as putative prognostic factors of EC, including assessment of microsatellite instability and alterations in PTEN and CTNB-1 (β-catenin).

Hysterectomy with bilateral salpingo-oophorectomy is the primary treatment for over 90% of women with

EC accompanied by peritoneal cytologic sampling, as well as abdominal exploration with palpation and biopsy of any suspicious lymph nodes or lesions. Pelvic and para-aortic lymphadenectomy is appropriate when there is evidence of poor prognostic indicators (high grade, nonendometrioid morphology, deep myometrial invasion, or extension to the cervix or adnexa). Omentectomy is recommended for serous adenocarcinoma. After primary surgical treatment, the extent of disease can be determined and the field for adjuvant radiation therapy can be more appropriately tailored to treat the pelvis and para-aortic region, or the whole abdomen. For women with disseminated disease, systemic therapy with progestational hormones or cytotoxic chemotherapy may be considered.

SUGGESTED READING

Ambros RA, Sherman ME, Zahn ChM, et al. Endometrial intraepithelial carcinoma: a distinctive lesion specifically associated with tumors displaying serous differentiation. Hum Pathol 1995;26:1260–1267.

Baak JP, Mutter GL, Robboy S et al. The molecular genetics and morphometry-based endometrial neoplasia classification system predicts disease progression in endometrial hyperplasia more accurately than the 1994 World Health Organization classification system. Cancer 2005;103:2304–2312.

Bokhman JV. Two pathogenetic types of endometrial carcinoma. Gynecol Oncol 1983;15:10–17.

Clement PhB, Young RH. Endometrioid carcinoma of the uterus: a review of its pathology with emphasis on recent advances and problematic aspects. Adv Anat Pathol 2002;3:145–184.

Goff BA, Kata D, Schmidt RA. Uterine papillary serous carcinoma: patterns of metastatic spread. Gynecol Oncol 1994;54:264–268.

Hendrickson MR, Ross J, Eifel P, et al. Uterine papillary serous carcinoma: a highly malignant form of endometrial adenocarcinoma. Am J Surg Pathol 1982;6:93–108.

Kurman RJ, Norris HJ. Evaluation of criteria for distinguishing atypical endometrial hyperplasia from well differentiated carcinoma. Cancer 1982;49:2547–2559.

Kurman RJ, Kaminski PF, Norris HJ. The behavior of endometrial hyperplasia. A long term study of "untreated" endometrial hyperplasia in 170 patients. Cancer 1985;56:403–412.

Lax SF, Kurman RJ, Pizer ES, et al. A binary architectural grading system for uterine endometrial endometrioid carcinoma has superior reproducibility compared with FIGO grading and identifies subsets of advance-stage tumors with favorable and unfavorable prognosis. Am J Surg Pathol 2000;24:1201–1208.

Lee KR, Scully RE. Complex endometrial hyperplasia and carcinoma in adolescents and young women 15 to 20 years of age. Int J Gynecol Pathol 1989;8:201–213.

Longacre T, Chung MH, Jensen DN, et al. Proposed criteria for the diagnosis of well-differentiated endometrial carcinoma. A diagnostic test for myoinvasion. Am J Surg Pathol 1995;19:371–406.

Mazur MT. Atypical polypoid adenomyomas of the endometrium. Am J Surg Pathol 1981;5:473–482.

Mutter GL, Baak JPA, Crum CP, et al. Endometrial precancer diagnosis by histopathology, clonal analysis, and computerized morphometry. J Pathol 2000;190:462–469.

Mutter GL, Kandeser J, Baak JPA, et al. Biopsy histomorphometry predicts uterine myoinvasion by endometrial carcinoma. A Gynecologic Oncology Group Study. Hum Pathol 2008;39:866–874.

Mutter GL, Zaino RJ, Baak JP, et al. Benign endometrial hyperplasia sequence and endometrial intraepithelial neoplasia. Int J Gynecol Pathol 2007;26:103–114.

Prat J. Prognostic parameters of endometrial carcinoma. Hum Pathol 2004;35:649–662.

Sherman ME, Bitterman P, Rosenshein NB, et al. Uterine serous carcinoma: a morphologically diverse neoplasm with unifying clinicopathologic features. Am J Surg Pathol 1992;16:600–610.

Soslow RA, Bissonnette JP, Wetton A, et al. Clinicopathologic analysis of 187 high-grade endometrial carcinomas of different histologic subtypes: similar outcome belie distinctive biologic differences. Am J Surg Pathol 2007;31:979–987.

Tavasoli FA, Devilee P. Pathology and Genetics of Tumours of the Breast and Female Organs. WHO Classification of Tumours. Lyon: IARC Press: 2003.

Welch WR, Scully RE. Precancerous lesions of the endometrium. Hum Pathol 1977;8:503–512.

Wheeler DT, Bristow RE, Kurman RJ. Histologic alterations in endometrial hyperplasia and well-differentiated carcinoma treated with progestins. Am J Surg Pathol 2007;31:988–998.

8

Pure Mesenchymal and Mixed Müllerian Tumors of the Uterus

Esther Oliva

Pure mesenchymal tumors of the uterus consist mainly of smooth muscle and endometrial stromal tumors, leiomyomas being by far the most common. As benign smooth muscle tumors have a wide spectrum of microscopic appearances as well as unusual growth patterns, distinction from their malignant counterparts as well as from endometrial stromal tumors may become challenging in routine practice. Mixed müllerian tumors of the uterus represent the other main category of tumors with an important mesenchymal component. It encompasses a wide spectrum of tumors, with low-grade müllerian adenosarcoma, malignant mixed müllerian tumor, and adenomyoma being the best known. Malignant mixed müllerian tumors are the most common in this category, at the same time being associated with a worse prognosis. Even though they are discussed in this chapter, it is well known that these tumors are closely related to endometrial carcinomas and as such, behave as carcinomas, not as sarcomas. Accurate classification of the different categories of tumors is crucial for both prognostic and therapeutic purposes and morphology remains the cornerstone in the classification of all these tumors. This chapter reviews the salient diagnostic features of the main categories of pure mesenchymal and mixed müllerian tumors with emphasis on newly described variants, diagnostic criteria, problems in differential diagnosis, and the utility of adjunct immunohistochemistry as well as other techniques in establishing the correct diagnosis.

LEIOMYOMA AND LEIOMYOMA VARIANTS

This is the most common solid tumor in women and the most frequent among smooth muscle tumors, with an estimated incidence of 70% in hysterectomy specimens for noncancer-related conditions. Fibroids are also a common reason for hysterectomy, accounting for at least 200,000 such procedures annually in the US. They are present in 20–30% of women over 30 years of age, rising to > 40% in women older than 40 years. The prevalence of uterine leiomyomas varies among ethnic groups; black women tend to have leiomyomas at a younger age that are more often multiple and typically larger than those in white women, indicating the presence of a genetic predisposition or other influences.

CLINICAL FEATURES

Most patients with uterine leiomyomas are asymptomatic. When symptoms occur, they usually correlate with the location of the leiomyomas, their size, or associated degenerative changes. Abnormal uterine bleeding is the most common presenting symptom, either in the form of menorrhagia or hypermenorrhea, which may lead to severe anemia. Abdominal pain secondary to acute hemorrhage may occur, especially in apoplectic leiomyomas and those that undergo torsion or protrude through the cervical canal. Patients may have a history of infertility, increased rates of spontaneous abortion, and pregnancy-related problems when there is a submucosal myoma or a markedly distorted endometrial cavity that interferes with normal implantation. Rarely, the myoma is large and the patient may present with a pelvic mass and secondary gastrointestinal or urinary symptoms due to compression. Leiomyomas may rapidly enlarge and cause concern for malignant transformation; however, it is important to remember that a rapidly enlarging uterine mass in a premenopausal woman is still most likely to represent a leiomyoma, as the risk of malignant transformation remains very low. Some leiomyoma variants are seen more frequently in pregnant women or those taking oral contraceptives. Patients can present during pregnancy or the puerperium with acute abdominal signs secondary to rupture of the tumor into the peritoneal cavity. Patients with intravenous leiomyomatosis may occasionally present with cardiac manifestations due to tumor extension into the inferior vena cava and right heart. Other much less frequent signs and symptoms seen in leiomyomas include secondary erythrocytosis, infection, and ascites (pseudo-Meigs' syndrome). Uterine leiomyomas may be associated with rare genetic syndromes such as hereditary leiomyomatosis and renal cell carcinoma.

LEIOMYOMA, LEOIMYOMA VARIANTS, AND SMOOTH MUSCLE TUMORS WITH UNUSUAL GROWTH PATTERNS – FACT SHEET

Definition
▸ Benign smooth muscle tumors of the uterus with variable gross and microscopic appearances

Incidence
▸ Most common uterine neoplasm
▸ Present in 70% of hysterectomy specimens removed for noncancer-related conditions

Race and Age Distribution
▸ Higher incidence in black women
▸ Present in 20–30% of women over 30 years of age and > 40% in women > 40 years

Clinical Features
▸ Asymptomatic in 40–60% of cases
▸ Abnormal uterine bleeding (menorrhagia or hypermenorrhea)
▸ Abdominal pain due to acute hemorrhage (apoplectic leiomyoma)
▸ Infertility, frequent spontaneous abortions, and pregnancy-related problems
▸ Pelvic mass, rupture into peritoneal cavity, or rapid enlargement (risk of misinterpretation as leiomyosarcoma)
▸ Cardiac manifestations in intravenous leiomyomatosis
▸ Rarely erythrocytosis, infection, or ascites (pseudo-Meigs' syndrome)

Radiologic Features
▸ Hypoechoic or heterogeneous mass (transvaginal ultrasonography)
▸ Low signal intensity on T2 and thin hyperintense rim due to compression of adjacent muscle (MRI)
▸ High signal intensity on T1 in acute infarction

Prognosis and Treatment
▸ Excellent outcome for typical leiomyoma, leiomyoma variants, and most of the unusual growth patterns
▸ Pelvic or cardiac recurrences up to 15 years later in intravenous leiomyomatosis
▸ Association with benign smooth muscle nodules in lungs (benign metastasizing leiomyoma) in typical leiomyoma, leiomyoma with vascular invasion, and intravenous leiomyomatosis
▸ Myomectomy, hysterectomy, hormone therapy (gonadotropin-releasing hormone agonists: GnRHa), or uterine artery embolization based on symptoms and risk factors
▸ Hysterectomy, excision of extrauterine tumor, bilateral adnexectomy, and GnRHa in intravenous leiomyomatosis
▸ 5-year recurrence rate as high as 60% for myomectomy
▸ Transient effect with hormone therapy

RADIOLOGIC FEATURES

Transvaginal ultrasound with or without sonohysterography is used for standard assessment of leiomyomas. It typically shows a hypoechoic or heterogeneous mass. The sonographic texture depends on the relative ratio of fibrous tissue to smooth muscle and on the presence and type of degeneration. Hysterosalpingography is

useful for submucosal leiomyomas that show characteristic filling defects. The most common computed tomography findings include uterine enlargement or contour deformity with a range of enhancement. Although calcification is seen in < 10% of cases, it is the most specific finding. MRI is the most accurate imaging modality for the diagnosis, mapping, and characterization of leiomyomas. Nondegenerated leiomyomas characteristically display a low signal intensity on T2-weighted pulse sequences, and in approximately 30% of leiomyomas, there is compression of the surrounding myometrium which translates into a thin hyperintense rim resulting in a very clear demarcation in signal intensity between the leiomyoma and the surrounding tissues. Cystic degeneration and myxoid change are seen as areas of high signal intensity while the presence of fat in a leiomyoma can be selectively detected with fat suppression sequences. Necrosis displays variable signal intensities but acutely infarcted myomas have a high signal intensity on T1-weighted images.

PATHOLOGIC FEATURES

GROSS FINDINGS

Leiomyomas occur more commonly in the uterine fundus and they are often multiple. They are typically intramural, less frequently submucosal or subserosal, and rarely, they are found in the lower uterine segment or cervix. Subserosal leiomyomas can become pedunculated and may undergo torsion with secondary necrosis of the pedicle, losing its connection to the uterus, and on some occasions becoming attached to adjacent pelvic structures (parasitic leiomyoma). Leiomyomas are sharply circumscribed and easily shell out from the surrounding myometrium. They have a bulging white to slightly pink, firm and whorled cut surface (Figure 8.1), and areas of discrete hemorrhage may be seen. Degenerative changes are frequent and include ulceration (mainly in submucosal leiomyoma), edema, cyst formation and, less frequently, calcification or ossification. Red degeneration is characteristic of pregnancy or postpartum, but may occasionally be observed in nonpregnant patients (such as those on oral contraceptives) (Figure 8.2).

The following leiomyoma variants (Box 8.1) may display a different gross appearance:

Highly cellular leiomyoma often has a tan to yellow and soft cut surface (Figure 8.3).

Mitotically active leiomyoma often displays soft, fleshy or cystic areas and visible hemorrhage.

Apoplectic or hemorrhagic leiomyoma shows as a cardinal feature prominent stellate hemorrhage that may be accompanied by cystic change.

Leiomyoma with diffuse perinodular hydropic change may show a multinodular growth within the main mass, the nodules being separated by edematous tissue. In some cases, watery fluid may exude from the cut section of the tumor (Figure 8.4).

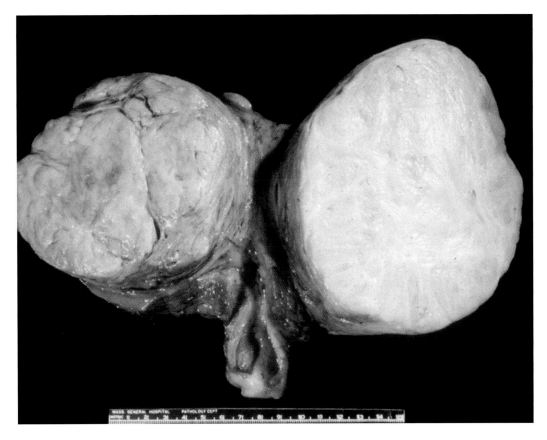

FIGURE 8.1
Uterus with two large intramyometrial leiomyomas. A white, whorled homogeneous cut surface characteristic of a typical leiomyoma is seen in the largest leiomyoma (right).

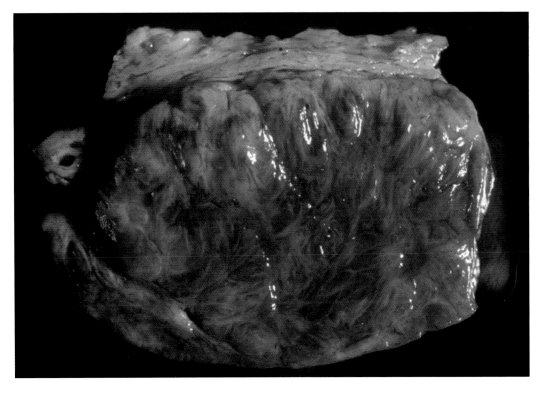

FIGURE 8.2
Leiomyoma with red degeneration. The tumor shows a diffusely hemorrhagic cut surface.

LEIOMYOMA, LEIOMYOMA VARIANTS, AND SMOOTH MUSCLE TUMORS WITH UNUSUAL GROWTH PATTERNS – PATHOLOGIC FEATURES

Gross Findings

▶ Intramural, submucosal, or subserosal in order of frequency
▶ Fundus most common location
▶ Often multiple; wide range of sizes
▶ Pedunculated if subserosal; torsion with secondary necrosis of its pedicle with loss of connection to the uterus (parasitic leiomyoma)
▶ Sharply circumscribed and easily shells out
▶ Bulging white to slightly pink, firm and whorled cut surface
▶ Degenerative changes include ulceration, edema, cystic change, calcification, or ossification
▶ Red degeneration characteristic of pregnancy, postpartum, and oral contraceptives

Leiomyoma Variants

▶ Highly cellular leiomyoma: often tan to yellow soft cut surface
▶ Mitotically active leiomyoma: frequently soft and fleshy; may have cystic areas and visible hemorrhage
▶ Apoplectic or hemorrhagic leiomyoma: prominent stellate hemorrhage ± cystic change
▶ Leiomyoma with hydropic change including diffuse perinodular: multinodular growth present within the main mass with edematous tissue separating nodules; watery fluid on sectioning
▶ Epithelioid leiomyoma: frequently soft and tan to pink cut surface; if ≤ 1 cm: "plexiform tumorlet"
▶ Myxoid leiomyoma: soft, gray, jelly-like cut surface
▶ Lipoleiomyoma: soft yellow areas admixed with firm white areas

Unusual Growth Patterns

▶ Dissecting leiomyoma including cotyledonoid leiomyoma ("Sternberg tumor"): irregular indistinct margins dissecting the myometrium with associated extrauterine exophytic extension as multiple bulbous red nodules attached to each other by thin adhesions resembling placental tissue
▶ Diffuse leiomyomatosis: diffuse and symmetrical thickening of the myometrium due to innumerable poorly circumscribed nodules typically < 1 cm
▶ Diffuse leiomyomatosis peritonealis: multiple small (typically < 2 cm) nodules with a white firm cut surface present in pelvic peritoneum and omentum
▶ Intravenous leiomyomatosis: multiple well-demarcated masses and sometimes visible coiled worm-like plugs of white tissue filling and distending myometrial and/or parametrial vessels outside the confines of, or in the absence of, a leiomyoma
▶ Benign metastasizing leiomyoma: small white and firm nodule(s) in lungs (more frequent), retroperitoneal and mediastinal lymph nodes, soft tissues, and bone (less frequent)

Microscopic Findings

▶ Well circumscribed
▶ Intersecting fascicles of spindled cells intermixed with variable amounts of collagen
▶ Abundant large blood vessels (when very numerous, vascular leiomyoma or angiomyoma)
▶ Abundant eosinophilic cytoplasm (when transversely cut, paranuclear vacuole) and elongated "cigar"-shaped nuclei
▶ Nuclear palisading may be seen
▶ Mild to absent cytologic atypia and mitoses
▶ Infarct-type necrosis: "mummified" and homogeneous appearance, area of transition between necrotic and viable tumor composed of granulation tissue or fibrous or hyalinized tissue
▶ Other findings: skeletal-like or rhabdoid cells, extramedullary hematopoiesis, collections of lymphocytes, mast cells, eosinophils, numerous histiocytes, acute inflammatory cells (pyomyoma)

Leiomyoma Variants

Cellular Leiomyoma

▶ Significantly more cellular than normal myometrium

Highly Cellular Leiomyoma

▶ Fascicles and sheets of cells with cellularity similar to that seen in endometrial stromal tumors
▶ Small cells with oval to spindle nuclei and scant cytoplasm
▶ Large and thick blood vessels as well as cleft-like spaces
▶ Imperceptibly merges with surrounding myometrium

Leiomyoma with Bizarre Nuclei ("Symplastic," "Atypical," or "Bizarre")

▶ Multinucleated or mononucleated cells
▶ "Spotty" distribution of cells with bizarre nuclei, although on occasion uniformly throughout the tumor
▶ Atypical nuclei and abundant eosinophilic cytoplasm
▶ Prominent nucleoli, coarse chromatin, and average mitotic count of 1–2/10 HPFs; but may reach 7/10 HPFs by highest count
▶ Other nuclear features: pseudoinclusions, pyknotic nuclei with dense smudged chromatin (may simulate abnormal mitoses)
▶ Uniform and bland cytologic features of spindled cells in areas uninvolved by bizarre cells

Mitotically Active Leiomyoma

▶ Spindled cells with bland nuclear features
▶ Increased mitotic activity (5–15/HPFs)
▶ No tumor cell necrosis
▶ Frequent hemorrhage or degenerative changes

Leiomyoma with Hormone-Related Changes ("Apoplectic Leiomyoma" or "Hemorrhagic Cellular Leiomyoma")

▶ Stellate hemorrhagic areas
▶ Edema and/or myxoid change around hemorrhage
▶ Hypercellularity surrounding hemorrhagic areas
▶ Mild to moderate nuclear atypia and up to 9 mitoses/10 HPFs
▶ Decreased cellularity and mitoses away from hemorrhage (zonation phenomenon) and no nuclear atypia
▶ Abnormal arteries with intimal thickening, fibrosis, and myxoid degeneration

Treated Leiomyomas with:

▶ Gonadotropin-releasing hormone agonists
  ▶ Reduced tumor size
  ▶ Increased hyalinization
  ▶ Smaller cell size, nuclear crowding, and increased apoptosis
  ▶ Infarct-type necrosis and lymphocytic infiltrate
  ▶ Vascular changes with fewer vessels, decreased vessel diameter, thickening and fibrosis, myxoid and fibrinoid changes, luminal narrowing, and thrombosis
▶ Uterine artery embolization
  ▶ Infarct-type necrosis
  ▶ Aggregates of embolized material in necrotic leiomyomas and myometrium
  ▶ Foreign body-type giant cells and macrophages

Leiomyoma with Diffuse Perinodular Hydropic Change

▶ Poorly defined areas of edematous connective tissue alternating with conventional areas of smooth muscle neoplasia
▶ Perinodular appearance or extensive effacement of architecture if prominent
▶ Occasional fibroblasts, sparse collagen fibers and vessels

LEIOMYOMA, LEIOMYOMA VARIANTS, AND SMOOTH MUSCLE TUMORS WITH UNUSUAL GROWTH PATTERNS – PATHOLOGIC FEATURES—cont'd

Epithelioid Leiomyoma
▸ At least 50% of the tumor cells are epithelioid
▸ Sheets, nests, cords, and trabeculae
▸ Polygonal or round cells
▸ Eosinophilic, granular, or clear cytoplasm
▸ Mild cytologic atypia, < 3 mitoses/10 HPFs
▸ No tumor cell necrosis

Myxoid Leiomyoma
▸ Hypocellular with abundant acellular myxoid matrix (positive for alcian blue or colloidal iron)
▸ May coexist with areas of conventional leiomyoma
▸ Oval to elongated or stellate cells
▸ Bland cytology with < 2 mitoses/10 HPFs
▸ No tumor cell necrosis

Leiomyoma with Heterologous Elements
▸ Adipose tissue: "lipoleiomyoma"
▸ Skeletal muscle
▸ Osseous or cartilaginous differentiation

Leiomyomas with Unusual Growth Patterns

Dissecting Leiomyoma Including Cotyledonoid Leiomyoma ("Sternberg Tumor")
▸ Fascicles of disorganized smooth muscle with a swirled growth
▸ Marked vascularity and extensive hydropic degeneration
▸ Large number of large muscular vessels in delicate fibrous matrix separating smooth muscle nodules

Diffuse Leiomyomatosis
▸ Multiple closely packed small nodules that tend to merge imperceptibly with each other
▸ Variable cellularity, but frequently cellular
▸ Perivascular arrangement of spindled cells
▸ Mature, mitotically inactive smooth-muscle cells

Diffuse Leiomyomatosis Peritonealis
▸ Multiple small to 10 cm (majority < 2 cm) nodules
▸ Spindled cells with minimal cytologic atypia and mitoses
▸ Decidual cells frequently admixed with smooth muscle cells
▸ Rarely, malignant transformation

Leiomyoma with Vascular Invasion
▸ Microscopic intravascular growth of benign-appearing smooth muscle cells within the tumor

Intravenous Leiomyomatosis
▸ Endothelium covered protrusions of smooth muscle
▸ Intersecting fascicles or appearance of a leiomyoma variant
▸ Clefted or lobulated contour, extensive hyalinization or hydropic change, and numerous thick-walled vessels
▸ Benign cytologic features and rare mitoses, except in cellular intravenous leiomyomatosis (up to 4/10 HPFs)
▸ Occasionally subendothelial proliferation of benign smooth muscle

Benign Metastasizing Leiomyoma
▸ Fascicles of smooth muscle cells
▸ Cells with no cytologic atypia or mitotic activity
▸ In the lung, alveolar spaces may be entrapped at the periphery

Immunohistochemical Features
▸ Actin, desmin, smooth-muscle myosin, HDCA8, h-caldesmon and oxytocin positive
▸ ER and PR positive
▸ Keratin and EMA frequently positive
▸ Variable CD10 expression (more commonly in highly cellular leiomyoma)
▸ Androgen receptor positive in 30% of cases
▸ Low MIB-1 expression, except in mitotically active leiomyoma
▸ Minimal p53 expression

Cytogenetic Features
▸ Simple karyotypic abnormalities in 40% of typical leiomyomas
▸ t(12;14)(q15;q24)

Differential Diagnosis
▸ Endometrial stromal tumor (vs highly cellular leiomyoma and intravenous leiomyomatosis)
▸ Spinded leiomyosarcoma (vs mitotically active leiomyoma and leiomyoma with bizarre nuclei)
▸ Myxoid leiomyosarcoma (vs hydropic leiomyoma and myxoid leiomyoma)
▸ Epithelioid leiomyosarcoma (vs epithelioid leiomyoma)
▸ Perivascular epithelioid cell tumor (vs epithelioid leiomyoma)
▸ Lymphangiomyomatosis (vs diffuse leiomyomatosis)
▸ Metastatic leiomyosarcoma (vs benign metastasizing leiomyoma)

BOX 8.1

LEIOMYOMA VARIANTS

1. Cellular and highly cellular
2. Mitotically active
3. With hormonal changes, including hemorrhagic or apoplectic leiomyoma
4. With hydropic change
5. Epithelioid
6. Myxoid

Epithelioid leiomyoma frequently has a soft and tan to pink cut surface.

Myxoid leiomyoma is characterized by a homogeneous, soft, gray, jelly-like cut surface.

Lipoleiomyoma appears as soft yellow areas randomly admixed with firm white areas (Figure 8.5).

Some leiomyomas are characterized by an unusual growth pattern (Box 8.2):

Dissecting leiomyoma, including cotyledonoid leiomyoma ("Sternberg tumor"), appears as multiple bulbous red nodules attached to each other by thin adhesions. They typically show irregular indistinct margins, dissect through the myometrium, and are associated

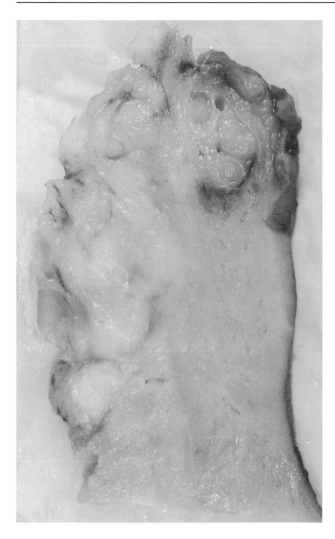

FIGURE 8.3

Highly cellular leiomyoma. The tumor has a homogeneous tan to yellow cut surface. Notice its association with multiple worm-like plugs of tumor distending the myometrial vessels outside the confines of the leiomyoma (intravenous leiomyomatosis component).

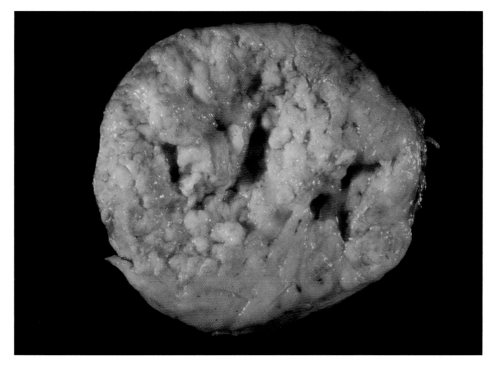

FIGURE 8.4

Leiomyoma with hydropic change. A well-circumscribed mass containing multiple nodules separated by empty spaces initially filled with watery fluid.

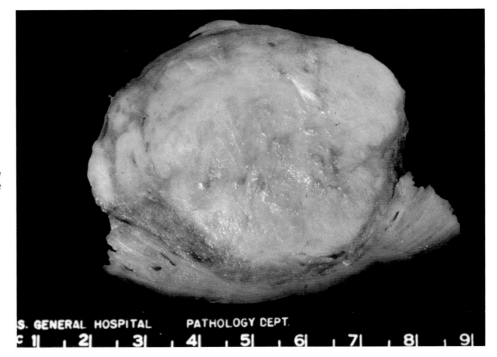

FIGURE 8.5

Lipoleiomyoma. Peripheral yellow areas are juxtaposed with white central areas.

BOX 8.2

UNUSUAL GROWTH PATTERNS IN BENIGN SMOOTH MUSCLE TUMORS

1. Dissecting leiomyoma, including cotyledonoid leiomyoma
2. Diffuse leiomyomatosis
3. Diffuse leiomyomatosis peritonealis
4. Leiomyoma with vascular invasion
5. Intravenous leiomyomatosis
6. Benign metastasizing leiomyoma

---

with extrauterine exophytic extension resembling placental tissue (Figure 8.6).

Diffuse leiomyomatosis shows a diffusely thickened myometrium almost completely replaced by innumerable nodules typically < 1 cm, imparting a symmetrical thickening of the myometrium. The nodules are poorly circumscribed and blend into the surrounding myometrium or adjacent nodules.

Diffuse leiomyomatosis peritonealis is characterized by multiple nodules scattered over the pelvic peritoneum, including the uterine serosa and omentum (Figure 8.7). The nodules are typically small (< 2 cm) but they may reach up to 10 cm and they have a white firm cut surface.

Intravenous leiomyomatosis displays multiple well-demarcated firm masses, typically intramyometrial. In some cases, it is possible to identify tumor within vascular spaces as convoluted or coiled worm-like plugs of white tissue that fills and distends the myometrial and sometimes parametrial vessels outside the confines of, or in the absence of, a leiomyoma (Figure 8.3).

Benign metastasizing leiomyoma is characterized by the presence of one or more extrauterine small (rarely up to 10 cm) white, firm nodules which occur most frequently in the lungs in women who have had typical uterine leiomyomas, leiomyomas with vascular invasion, or intravenous leiomyomatosis. Other sites that may be affected include retroperitoneal and mediastinal lymph nodes, soft tissues, and bone.

It is important to remember that the gross appearance of the tumor is critical, thus serial sections at every centimeter should be performed and areas with unusual appearances should be sampled more generously. On the other hand, grossly typical leiomyomas do not need excessive sampling and the rule of one section per centimeter may not necessarily apply.

MICROSCOPIC FINDINGS

On low-power examination, classic leiomyomas are typically well circumscribed. They are composed of intersecting fascicles of cells with relatively abundant eosinophilic cytoplasm and elongated "cigar"-shaped nuclei with mild to absent cytologic atypia and low mitotic activity (Figure 8.8). If cells are cut transversely the nuclei appear round with an associated paranuclear vacuole. Some leiomyomas may contain skeletal-like or rhabdoid cells with abundant eosinophilic cytoplasm. Sometimes, there is palisading of the nuclei, as is more commonly seen in benign nerve sheath tumors. Variable amounts of collagen may be seen in between the spindled cells and large blood vessels are interspersed throughout the tumor. When numerous muscular-walled blood vessels are present, the term "vascular

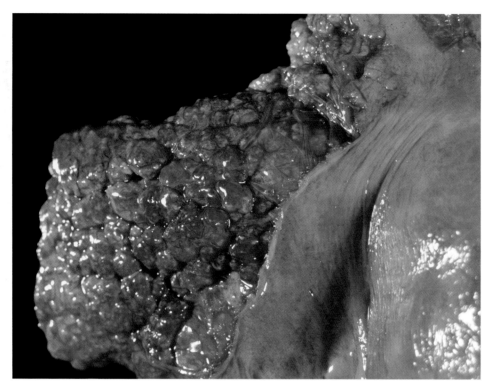

FIGURE 8.6

Dissecting cotyledonoid leiomyoma ("Sternberg tumor"). Multiple congested placenta-like masses are present dissecting through the myometrium into the parametrium.

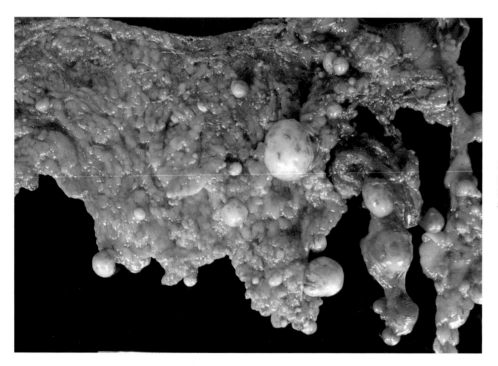

FIGURE 8.7

Diffuse leiomyomatosis peritonealis. Multiple well-defined white nodules are present in fat.

leiomyoma" or "angiomyoma" may be used. Leiomyomas may undergo ulcerative necrosis secondary to trauma (especially submucosal leiomyomas) and infarct-type necrosis. The latter is characterized by the finding of necrotic tissue with a "mummified" and homogeneous appearance, where the tumor cells as well as the vessels appear dead (Figure 8.9). There is an area of transition between the necrotic and the viable tumor that is composed of granulation tissue, fibrous or

hyalinized tissue depending on the age of the infarct, and may be associated with areas of recent hemorrhage (Figure 8.10). There is no perivascular growth of tumor cells or a dirty necrotic background, in contrast to tumor cell necrosis. Infarct-type necrosis may be seen in leiomyomas and leiomyosarcomas. Typical leiomyomas may contain foci of extramedullary hematopoiesis, striking collections of lymphocytes, mast cells, eosinophils, or numerous histiocytes, the latter especially in patients

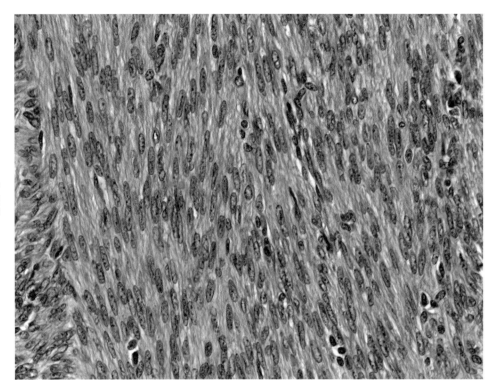

FIGURE 8.8

Typical leiomyoma. Long fascicles of spindle-shaped cells with elongated "cigar-shaped" nuclei, eosinophilic cytoplasm, and no cytologic atypia.

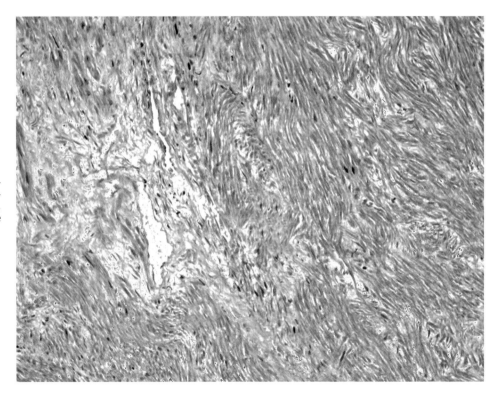

FIGURE 8.9

Infarct-type necrosis. Uniform mummified appearance of the non-viable smooth muscle cells; however, the cell outlines may still be appreciated.

taking gonadotropin-releasing hormone agonists (GnRHa). Some leiomyomas may become infected, showing large amounts of acute inflammatory cells which may form abscesses (pyomyoma).

It is important to recognize the different leiomyoma variants (Box 8.1). They may cause problems in diagnosis as they share one or more histologic features with leiomyosarcoma, such as high cellularity, striking cyto-logic atypia, and increased mitotic activity. Leiomyoma variants include the following:

Cellular and highly cellular leiomyoma. The World Health Organization (WHO) defines a cellular leiomyoma as an otherwise typical leiomyoma that is "significantly" more cellular than the normal myometrium (Figure 8.11). In contrast, a highly cellular leiomyoma is defined as a leiomyoma with a cellularity comparable

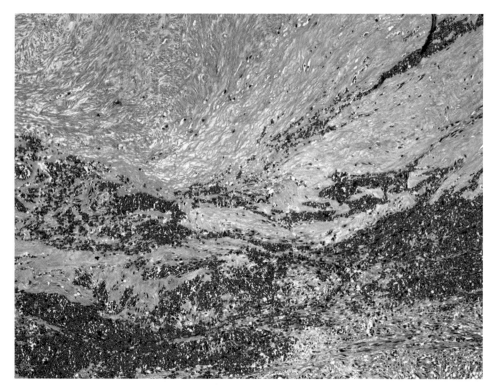

FIGURE 8.10

Infarct-type necrosis. An area of hyalinization associated with recent hemorrhage separates viable from nonviable tumor.

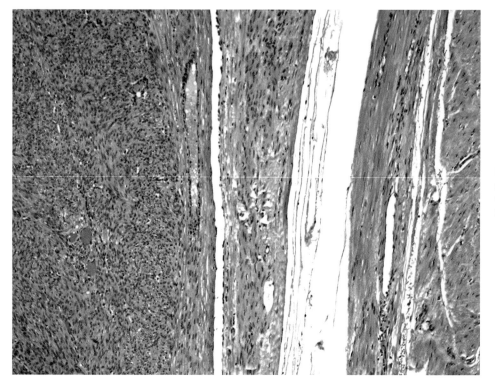

FIGURE 8.11

Cellular leiomyoma. Tumor cellularity is increased in relation to the surrounding myometrium.

to that encountered in endometrial stromal tumors, thus the cells have small oval to spindled nuclei with very scant cytoplasm (Figure 8.12). The cells often form fascicles and are associated with large and thick blood vessels as well as cleft-like spaces either representing compressed vessels or retraction artifact. At the periphery of the tumor, the neoplastic cells merge imperceptibly with the surrounding myometrium. Both tumors

typically have very low mitotic rates and are cytologically bland, but they may on occasion be mitotically active and then they should be labeled as cellular or highly cellular mitotically active leiomyoma.

Leiomyoma with bizarre nuclei ("symplastic," "atypical," or "bizarre" leiomyoma). The cardinal and defining feature of these tumors is the presence of cells with atypical pleomorphic nuclei, frequently

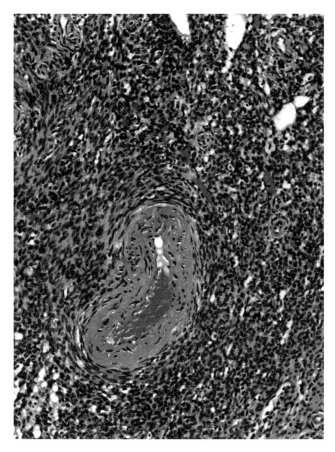

FIGURE 8.12
Highly cellular leiomyoma. Small cells with oval nuclei and scant cytoplasm focally form fascicles and are associated with a large and thick blood vessel.

multinucleated but sometimes mononucleated, associated with abundant eosinophilic cytoplasm which may sometimes form eosinophilic globules (Figure 8.13). Typically, the "bizarre cells" have a "spotty" distribution within the tumor, although on occasion, the cells may be seen uniformly throughout. The nuclei may show prominent nuclear pseudoinclusions or may be pyknotic with dense smudged chromatin. They frequently show prominent nucleoli and coarse chromatin and mitotic counts may be as high as 7/10 HPFs by the highest count method, although the average mitotic count is typically 1–2 mitoses/10 HPFs. Karyorrhectic nuclei simulating abnormal mitotic figures may be seen. Interspersed between the cells with bizarre nuclei, there are spindled cells with variable degrees of nuclear atypia; however, in areas of tumor uninvolved by bizarre cells, the spindled cells have uniform and bland cytologic features. It has been shown that excess of global DNA methylation associated with DNA inactivation may be one of the molecular mechanisms underlying the benign nature of this leiomyoma variant. The striking atypia most likely represents presence of abundant heterochromatin, which is known to be associated with inactivated DNA.

Mitotically active leiomyoma. This leiomyoma variant shows increased mitotic activity that ranges from 5 to 15 mitoses/HPFs. However, the single most important criterion to establish the diagnosis of mitotically active leiomyoma is the absence of cytologic atypia. Furthermore, tumor cell necrosis should be absent. Some smooth muscle tumors may have mitotic counts > 15 mitoses/10 HPFs and even though they could still be considered in this category, they are better classified

FIGURE 8.13
Leiomyoma with bizarre nuclei. Mono- or multinucleated cells in a patchy distribution show large nuclei with smudged chromatin and multiple nuclear pseudoinclusions.

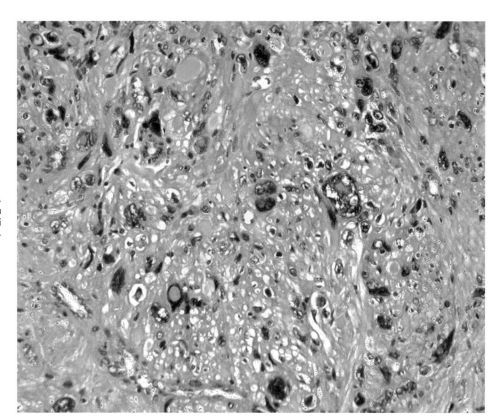

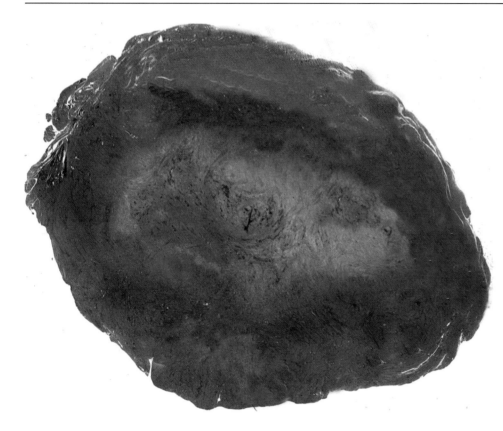

FIGURE 8.14

Apoplectic leiomyoma. A central area of hemorrhage is surrounded by a cellular rim of smooth muscle cells. The tumor away from the infarcted area is less cellular ("zonation" phenomenon).

as leiomyomas with increased mitotic index or smooth-muscle tumors of uncertain malignant behavior as experience with these tumors is very limited. These neoplasms are not infrequently associated with areas of hemorrhage or show degenerative changes. It seems that increased mitotic activity in these tumors may be related to the mitogenic effect of progesterone in the myometrium during the menstrual cycle, thus these tumors are seen in women of reproductive age but not postmenopausal women.

Leiomyoma with hormonal-related changes. Microscopic changes related to pregnancy or progestin include hemorrhage, edema, myxoid change, focal hypercellularity, nuclear pleomorphism, and increased mitotic activity. Among leiomyomas with hormonal-related changes, *apoplectic leiomyoma* or *hemorrhagic cellular leiomyoma* is characterized by the finding of stellate areas of recent hemorrhage surrounded by smooth muscle with markedly increased cellularity that may be focally associated with a myxoid background. The cells show slightly enlarged nuclei associated with prominent nucleoli and increased mitotic activity that may be as high as 8–9 mitoses/10 HPFs. Away from these areas, both cellularity and mitotic activity decrease. This zonation phenomenon is very characteristic and helps in establishing the diagnosis (Figure 8.14). Abnormal arteries characterized by thickening and fibrosis of the intima associated with myxoid accumulation are present in many of these tumors, as seen in patients taking oral contraceptives. It is likely that the apoplectic changes are secondary to vascular events, although the precise pathogenesis is unknown.

Treated leiomyoma. Histologic changes associated with GnRHa have not been consistent and some studies have not found differences between patients treated with GnRHa and untreated controls. The most common reported findings include: reduced tumor size, nuclear crowding, increased hyalinization, lymphocytic infiltrate, infarct-type necrosis, smaller cell size, vascular changes (fewer vessels, decreased vessel diameter, mural thickening, myxoid change, fibrinoid change, intimal or medial fibrosis, luminal narrowing, thrombosis), and increased apoptotic index. Surprisingly, no study has demonstrated any difference in the mitotic rate between leiomyomas removed during treatment and those from untreated women. In contrast, leiomyomas removed several weeks after withdrawal of GnRHa treatment can have increased mitotic activity. Rare GnRHa-treated smooth muscle tumors are unexpectedly found to be a leiomyosarcoma. Changes in leiomyomas can also be seen following uterine artery embolization with polyvinyl alcohol (PVA) particles or, more recently, trisacryl gelatin microspheres (TGM). Aggregates of PVA or TGM are seen within the necrotic leiomyomas and throughout the myometrium (Figure 8.15). Both are associated with infarct-type necrosis of the leiomyomas; however PVA may also be associated with infarction of the remainder of the uterus, including the cervix. Foreign body-type giant cells and mononuclear macrophages may be seen in association with the foreign material.

Leiomyoma with diffuse perinodular hydropic change. Hydropic degeneration is defined by the finding of well to poorly circumscribed zones of edematous con-

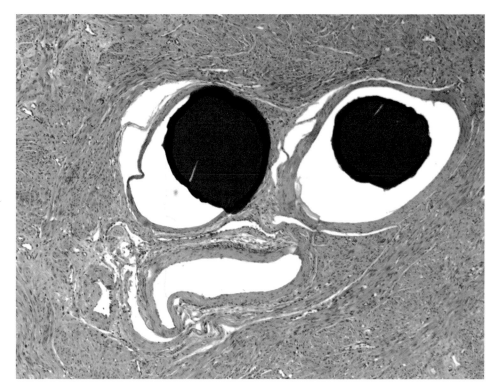

FIGURE 8.15

Treated leiomyoma. Blue polyvinyl alcohol particles fill the arteries.

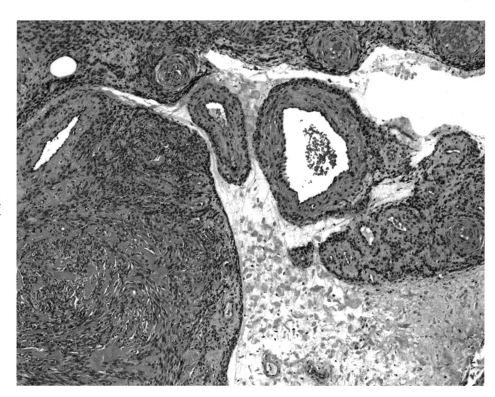

FIGURE 8.16

Leiomyoma with hydropic change. Extensive edema dissects the muscle fibers, imparting a false nodular appearance.

nective tissue alternating with neoplastic smooth muscle cells. This is a not uncommon focal finding in leiomyomas, but when it becomes prominent, a characteristic perinodular appearance or extensive effacement of the architecture of the leiomyoma may be seen (Figure 8.16). The hydropic areas show occasional fibroblasts and a sparse framework of collagen fibers admixed with vessels. These areas are negative for alcian blue or colloidal iron.

These changes are frequently associated with hyalinization in other areas.

Epithelioid leiomyoma. The WHO defines an epithelioid smooth muscle tumor as a neoplasm composed of cells resembling epithelial cells. As a general rule, the diagnosis of epithelioid smooth muscle tumor should be made when at least 50% of the tumor cells have an epithelioid morphology. In the past, these tumors were

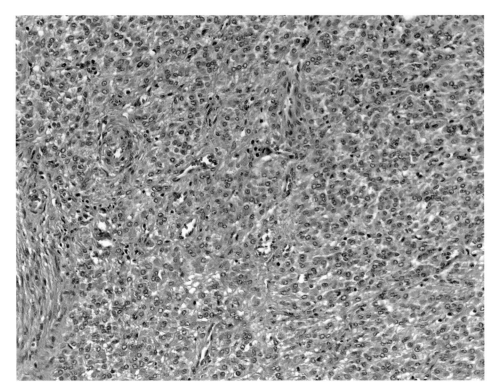

FIGURE 8.17
Benign epithelioid smooth muscle tumor. Diffuse growth of tumor cells with abundant eosinophilic cytoplasm. No cytologic atypia or mitoses are seen.

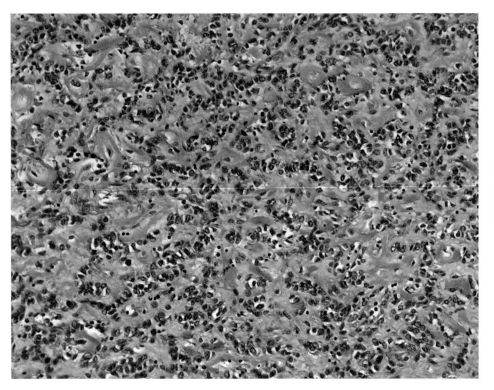

FIGURE 8.18
Benign epithelioid smooth muscle tumor. Anastomosing cords of tumor cells are separated by hypocellular stroma.

classified as leiomyoblastoma, clear cell, and plexiform subtypes based on their morphologic appearance (solid growth, clear cells, or presence of anastomosing cords and trabeculae respectively). At present, all these tumors are best designated as epithelioid smooth muscle tumors, with the exception of tumors with a plexiform architecture measuring < 1 cm, which are classified as "plexiform tumorlets." On low power, the most common

growth is solid (Figure 8.17), followed by nests, cords, and trabeculae (Figure 8.18), and rarely, pseudoglandular spaces, with more than one pattern frequently coexisting in a given tumor. The cells typically have abundant eosinophilic cytoplasm, but in some cases, may have clear cytoplasm (Figure 8.19). To establish the diagnosis of benign epithelioid smooth muscle tumor, the cells should show at most mild cytologic atypia, < 3 mitoses/

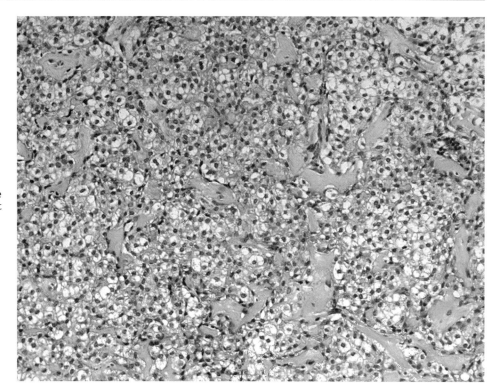

FIGURE 8.19
Benign epithelioid smooth muscle tumor. The tumor cells have abundant clear cytoplasm.

10 HPFs, and no tumor cell necrosis. It is important to keep in mind that the term "epithelioid" should not be loosely applied to smooth muscle tumors in which epithelial-like aggregation of cells results from hyalinization, hydropic, or other stromal changes.

Myxoid leiomyoma. Myxoid degeneration in leiomyomas has been reported to range from 3 to 13% among different series. Myxoid leiomyoma is characterized by the finding of abundant acellular myxoid matrix rich in acid mucins (positive for alcian blue or colloidal iron stains). The neoplastic cells are oval to elongated or stellate, and they show bland cytologic features, low mitotic rate (< 2 mitoses/10 HPFs), and no tumor cell necrosis. Myxoid change may occur focally in a conventional leiomyoma. This is important to note in order to avoid the potential misdiagnosis of leiomyosarcoma in a leiomyoma showing myxoid and nonmyxoid areas, imparting a pseudoinfiltrative appearance.

Leiomyoma with heterologous elements. Adipose tissue is the most common heterologous component in benign smooth muscle tumors. These tumors are classified as "lipoleiomyoma." Rarely leiomyomas may show skeletal muscle, osseous, or cartilaginous differentiation.

Leiomyomas can also cause problems in diagnosis due to unusual growth patterns (see Box 8.2). These include:

Dissecting leiomyoma including cotyledonoid leiomyoma ("Sternberg tumor"). As the name implies, these tumors are characterized by fascicles of disorganized smooth muscle with a swirled rather than a fascicular growth associated with marked vascularity and extensive hydropic degeneration. They are typically associated with a large number of large muscular vessels which cluster predominantly in the delicate fibrous matrix which separates the smooth muscle nodules (Figure 8.20).

Diffuse leiomyomatosis of the uterus. This condition is composed of multiple closely packed small nodules of cytologically mature, mitotically inactive smooth muscle cells within the myometrium that tend to merge imperceptibly with each other. They vary in cellularity but tend to be cellular and not infrequently the spindled cells have at least focally a perivascular arrangement. They are not associated with degenerative changes other than hyalinization.

Diffuse leiomyomatosis peritonealis. This condition is typically seen in pregnant or postpartum women. The nodules may range up to 10 cm, although the majority are < 2 cm in size. The nodules are composed of benign-appearing smooth muscle cells with minimal mitotic activity. Decidual cells are frequently admixed with the smooth muscle cells. Rarely, one of the nodules may undergo malignant transformation. This process is considered to originate from metaplastic transformation of submesothelial mesenchymal cells into smooth muscle cells.

Leiomyoma with vascular invasion. This is defined as a typical leiomyoma or leiomyoma variant with microscopic intravascular growth within the tumor.

Intravenous leiomyomatosis. The cardinal feature of this condition is the presence of endothelium-covered protrusions of smooth muscle resembling either a typical leiomyoma with spindle cells arranged in intersecting fascicles or the appearance of any leiomyoma variant (Figure 8.21). Features that are helpful in establishing

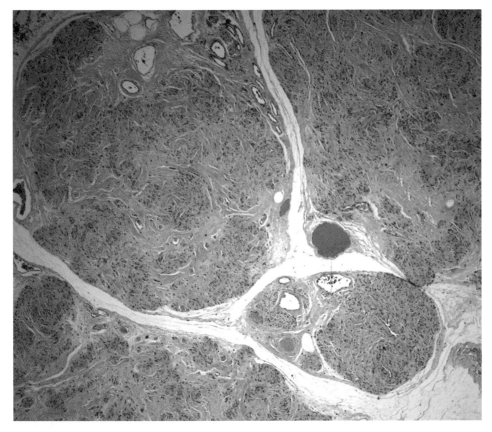

FIGURE 8.20
Dissecting cotyledonoid leiomyoma ("Sternberg tumor"). Swirling fascicles of disorganized smooth muscle are associated with marked vascularity.

the smooth muscle nature of the lesion include a clefted or lobulated contour, extensive hyalinization or hydropic change, and numerous thick-walled vessels. Mitotic figures are usually rare, but cellular intravenous leiomyomatosis may have up to 4 mitoses/10 HPFs. In some cases, a subendothelial proliferation of benign smooth muscle may merge with the intravascular tumor if this is attached to the vessel wall.

Benign metastasizing leiomyoma. It is composed of fascicles of cytologically benign smooth muscle cells. When involving the lung, it may entrap alveolar spaces at the periphery (Figure 8.22). The diagnosis of benign metastasizing leiomyoma should only be rendered when the uterine tumor has been thoroughly sampled to exclude the possibility of leiomyosarcoma.

ANCILLARY STUDIES

IMMUNOHISTOCHEMISTRY

Leiomyomas are typically positive for smooth muscle markers, including smooth muscle actin, desmin, smooth muscle myosin, HDCA8 and h-caldesmon. They are also positive for oxytocin and frequently express keratin and EMA (more often the epithelioid variant) whereas CD10 shows variable positivity. Estrogen and progesterone receptors are expressed in nearly 100% of uterine leiomyomas whereas androgen receptors (AR) are posi-

tive in approximately 30% of cases. MIB-1 expression is typically low except in mitotically active leiomyomas, whereas p53 staining is typically minimal to absent.

CYTOGENETICS

Approximately 40% of leiomyomas have cytogenetic alterations, typically described as simple karyotypic abnormalities. At least six cytogenetic subgroups have been identified within leiomyomas, but the best studied chromosomal aberration is t(12;14)(q15;q24).

DIFFERENTIAL DIAGNOSIS

Usual leiomyomas are straightforward; however several leiomyoma variants can be confused with a leiomyosarcoma or even with other less frequent types of uterine tumors because of their unusual macroscopic or microscopic features.

Highly cellular leiomyoma may be confused with an endometrial stromal tumor, either an endometrial stromal nodule or a low-grade endometrial stromal sarcoma, as they frequently appear tan to yellow on gross examination, they are very cellular, the cells have very scant cytoplasm and may grow in sheets instead of fascicles, they are associated with prominent vascularization, and may display at first glance a "tongue-like" growth into the surrounding myometrium. Helpful findings include, as highlighted earlier, the finding of large

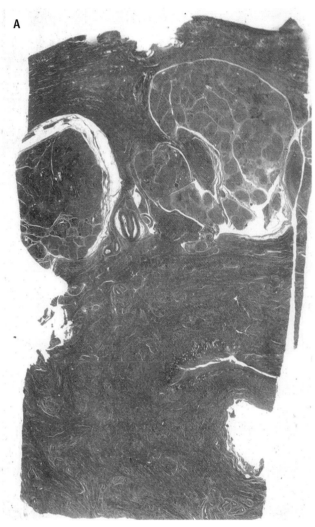

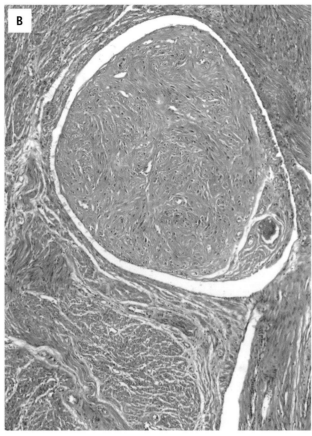

FIGURE 8.21

Intravenous leiomyomatosis. Multiple well-defined nodules of smooth muscle are present within the myometrium in the absence of a leiomyoma (A). At high magnification, one nodule is present within a distended myometrial vessel (B).

FIGURE 8.22

Benign metastasizing leiomyoma. A bland smooth muscle proliferation entraps and compresses respiratory epithelium.

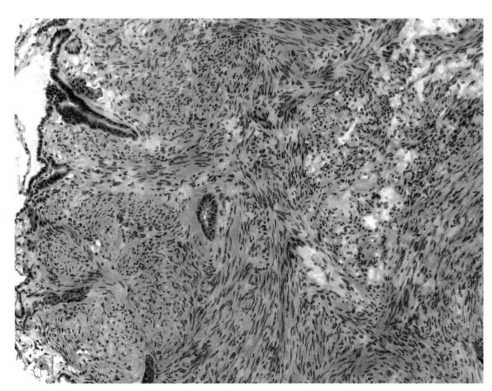

thick muscular walled blood vessels, in contrast to the arterioles seen in endometrial stromal tumors, cleft-like spaces, and focal merging of the highly cellular areas with typical areas of smooth-muscle neoplasia or with the surrounding myometrium. Finally, strong and multifocal or diffuse immunoreactivity for smooth muscle markers including desmin and h-caldesmon will confirm the smooth muscle nature of the tumor.

Mitotically active leiomyoma should not be confused with a leiomyosarcoma. It is important to remember that to establish the diagnosis of leiomyosarcoma, the finding of 10 mitoses/10 HPFs, as well as diffuse moderate to severe cytologic atypia and/or tumor cell necrosis should be present in the tumor.

Leiomyomas with bizarre nuclei can be distinguished from leiomyosarcoma by the absence of tumor cell necrosis and mitotic counts of < 10 mitoses/10 HPFs. Furthermore, the combination of aneuploidy, high MIB-1 activity, and p53 expression is rare in leiomyomas with bizarre nuclei, and this diagnosis should be made with caution when these features are seen.

Leiomyoma with hydropic change may lead to the erroneous consideration of intravenous leiomyomatosis because, on gross examination, the multinodular architecture may simulate intravascular growth. However, on microscopic examination, the nodules of smooth muscle are identified in a background of edema but not within vessels. In some cases, the hydropic change may be difficult to distinguish from myxoid background, this being an important distinction in order to rule out a myxoid leiomyosarcoma. Histochemical stains for alcian blue and/or colloidal iron are helpful in this distinction.

Epithelioid leiomyoma should be distinguished from an epithelioid leiomyosarcoma. The finding of moderate to severe cytologic atypia, ≥ 5 mitoses/10 HPFs, or tumor cell necrosis is diagnostic of epithelioid leiomyosarcoma. Other important entities in the differential diagnosis include perivascular epithelioid cell tumor (PEComa), trophoblastic tumors (placental site trophoblastic tumor (PSTT) and epithelioid trophoblastic tumor (ETT)), and a uterine tumor resembling an ovarian sex cord tumor (discussed in epithelioid leiomyosarcoma section, below).

Myxoid leiomyoma should be distinguished from myxoid leiomyosarcoma but this distinction may be difficult in curettage or biopsy specimens. A benign myxoid smooth muscle tumor can be favored if the tumor is well circumscribed and it lacks tumor cell necrosis or moderate to severe cytologic atypia. In the absence of these features, a mitotic index of < 2 mitoses/10 HPFs supports the diagnosis of a benign myxoid smooth muscle tumor.

Diffuse leiomyomatosis should be separated from the rare examples of uterine involvement by lymphangioleiomyomatosis, usually in patients with tuberous sclerosis. In such cases, the myometrium is usually grossly unremarkable, but shows numerous microscopic ill-defined nodules of smooth muscle surrounding lymphatics which protrude into their lumens. The smooth muscle cells of lymphangiomyomatosis are immunoreactive for HMB-45 and Melan-A.

Intravenous leiomyomatosis should not be confused with typical leiomyomas partially surrounded by compressed vascular spaces or leiomyomas with artifactual retraction from the surrounding myometrium. Stains for endothelial antigens may be useful in problematic cases. Leiomyoma with vascular invasion shares with intravenous leiomyomatosis the finding of smooth muscle within vascular spaces; however, in contrast to intravenous leiomyomatosis, the intravascular growth is seen within the confines of the leiomyoma. The differential diagnosis of intravenous leiomyomatosis and a low-grade endometrial stromal sarcoma may be challenging as both grow in vascular spaces, both have prominent vascularity, and intravenous leiomyomatosis may be cellular. In contrast to cellular intravenous leiomyomatosis, low-grade endometrial stromal sarcoma usually lacks thick-walled vessels, lobulation, and hydropic degeneration in its intravascular component, and is typically present in the endometrium as well as the myometrium.

Benign metastasizing leiomyoma should be distinguished from metastatic leiomyosarcoma, primary pulmonary smooth muscle tumors, pulmonary hamartomas with a prominent smooth muscle component, and lymphangioleiomyomatosis. The latter is a diffuse process seen exclusively in females that can exhibit a rapidly progressive and fatal course. Distinguishing pathologic features include cystic spaces and smooth muscle proliferation around endothelial spaces without the formation of gross nodules, as is typically seen in benign metastasizing leiomyoma. Additionally, the smooth muscle cells in lymphangioleiomyomatosis are HMB-45-positive. Pulmonary hamartomas typically show other histologic components and malignant smooth muscle tumors, either primary or metastatic, will show cytologic atypia as well as increased mitotic activity.

PROGNOSIS AND TREATMENT

Conventional leiomyomas are benign tumors that may be treated by myomectomy or hysterectomy depending on the symptoms and patient's associated risk factors. Myomectomy is associated with a higher morbidity than hysterectomy and some studies have shown that the 5-year recurrence rate for fibroids treated with local excision may be as high as 60%; the risk is lower in patients with a single fibroid, a smaller total uterine size, and those who subsequently had a successful pregnancy. Leiomyomas can also be treated with hormone therapy, more commonly GnRHa; however, the effects are transient, and within several cycles of discontinuing administration, myomas tend to return to their pre-therapy size. Uterine artery embolization is an emerging form of conservative treatment in women who are not candidates for surgery or who do not wish to accept the risks of surgery.

Leiomyoma variants are also associated with a benign outcome. For example, leiomyomas with a diffuse distribution of the bizarre nuclei treated with myomectomy and long follow-up (mean 15 years) have shown an unremarkable clinical course.

Among the unusual growth patterns seen in leiomyomas, intravenous leiomyomatosis is probably the only one that requires hysterectomy, excision of any extrauterine tumor if technically feasible, and bilateral adnexectomy, as the lesion is estrogen-dependent. The intravascular growth is probably inconsequential in most cases, especially if not extensive. In one study with 16 patients with a mean follow-up of 7.5 years, all had a favorable outcome. However, some patients develop pelvic or cardiac recurrences, up to 15 years after hysterectomy. Thus, as a preventive measure, postoperative imaging studies may be helpful in detecting and monitoring growth of residual intravascular tumor in these patients. GnRH agonists may be useful to control the growth of nonresectable tumor. Intravenous leiomyomatosis as well as conventional leiomyomas and leiomyomas with vascular invasion may occasionally be associated with benign smooth muscle nodules in the lungs as a secondary complication (benign metastasizing leiomyoma). The nodules typically appear years after the initial treatment; however, most cases still pursue a benign clinical outcome. After surgical removal of the nodules, additional treatment primarily consists of hormonal manipulation as the lung lesions are generally responsive to sex hormones, as evidenced by regression of lung nodules during pregnancy or after menopause.

LEIOMYOSARCOMA

Uterine leiomyosarcoma is an uncommon smooth muscle tumor with an annual incidence of 0.64/100,000 women. It is the most common uterine sarcoma among young women and it represents approximately 40% of all uterine sarcomas, but only 1% of all uterine malignancies. It is the malignant counterpart of uterine leiomyoma; however, the incidence of malignant transformation of leiomyomas has been reported to be very low, ranging between 0.13 and 0.80, while the incidence ratio between leiomyomas and leiomyosarcomas has been estimated to be 800:1. There seems to be an increased incidence of leiomyosarcoma among black women, although not as pronounced as with leiomyomas.

CLINICAL FEATURES

These tumors affect women with a mean age of 50 years, about 10 years older than in women with a leiomyoma; however, they may be seen in either pre- or postmenopausal women. These tumors are not known to be related to the risk factors described for endometrial carcinoma. Patients typically present with abnormal vaginal bleeding, pain, pelvic mass, or combination thereof. Although rapid enlargement of a myometrial

LEIOMYOSARCOMA – FACT SHEET

Definition
▶ Malignant smooth muscle tumor of the uterus. It is the malignant counterpart of uterine leiomyoma

Incidence
▶ 0.64/100,000 women
▶ 1% of all uterine malignancies
▶ Approximately 40% of all uterine sarcomas
▶ 800:1 incidence ratio between leiomyoma and leiomyosarcoma
▶ 0.13 and 0.80 incidence of malignant transformation of leiomyoma

Race and Age Distribution
▶ Increased incidence among black women
▶ Most common uterine sarcoma in young women (mean 50 years)

Clinical Features
▶ Abnormal vaginal bleeding
▶ Pain or pelvic mass
▶ Rapid enlargement of a presumed "fibroid" in postmenopausal women and patients on GnRHa treatment
▶ Occasionally hypercalcemia and eosinophilia
▶ Rarely, prior history of radiation therapy or tamoxifen treatment

Radiologic Features
▶ High signal on T2 or any small high-signal areas on T1 on MRI

Prognosis and Treatment
▶ 5-year survival rate of 12–40% for all stages
▶ 5-year survival rate of 50–70% for stage I tumors
▶ Recurrence rate of 71% for stages I and II and almost 100% for stages III and IV
▶ Median time to recurrence of 8–16 months for spindled type; up to 10 years for myxoid and epithelioid types
▶ Lungs and liver most common sites of metastasis
▶ Total abdominal hysterectomy and debulking of other tumor
▶ Removal of ovaries and lymph node dissection is controversial
▶ Staging based on a modified 1988 International Federation of Gynecologists and Obstetricians classification for endometrial cancer
▶ Uncertain benefit of adjuvant therapy on survival
▶ Tumor stage and grade most accurate predictive factors

tumor should raise the suspicion of leiomyosarcoma, this phenomenon occurs much more frequently in leiomyomas and it is not a reliable sign of malignancy. However, in postmenopausal women with an enlarging fibroid and in patients with presumed "fibroids" that continue to grow on treatment with GnRH agonists, concern for leiomyosarcoma should be raised. Less frequently, the presenting manifestations are related to tumor rupture and secondary hemoperitoneum, extrauterine extension, or metastases. Finally, in rare patients, symptoms are related to secretion of parathyroid hormone-related protein with secondary hypercalcemia and eosinophilia with secondary amyloidosis. Some patients may have a prior history of radiation therapy or tamoxifen treatment. On physical examination, the uterus is typically enlarged. More than 50% of patients have stage I or II tumors at the time of diagnosis.

RADIOLOGIC FEATURES

The diagnostic imaging criteria to separate leiomyosarcoma and leiomyoma are ill defined. MRI has become the imaging technique of choice for evaluation of uterine leiomyosarcomas because it can demonstrate the number, size, exact location, and extent of degeneration of the lesions. Smooth muscle tumors with poorly defined margins, with > 50% of the tumor with high signal on T2-weighted images or any small high-signal areas present on T1-weighted images are findings suggestive of leiomyosarcoma. The combined use of dynamic MRI and serum lactate dehydrogenase seems to be a useful tool in distinguishing leiomyosarcoma from leiomyoma.

PATHOLOGIC FEATURES

GROSS FINDINGS

These tumors are typically a large solitary mass or the largest tumor in a uterus, with multiple fibroids in up to 95% of cases. They have a mean diameter of approximately 10 cm. Most leiomyosarcomas are intramyometrial or submucosal, much less frequently subserosal, and 5% arise in the cervix. They are often poorly circumscribed and cannot be shelled out from the adjacent myometrium, in contrast to leiomyomas. The cut surface is soft and fleshy with frequently associated areas of necrosis and hemorrhage (Figure 8.23). Epithelioid leiomyosarcomas have a gross appearance similar to spindled leiomyosarcomas, whereas myxoid leiomyosarcomas typically show a gelatinous cut surface and not infrequently a deceptively well-circumscribed border. Even though leiomyosarcomas are frequently seen in uteri with leiomyomas, bona fide examples of leiomyosarcoma arising in a leiomyoma are rare. Some tumors may display a prominent intravascular growth that may be seen on gross examination (Figure 8.24).

MICROSCOPIC FINDINGS

Spindled leiomyosarcoma. At low power scrutiny, these tumors frequently show an infiltrative growth with destruction of the surrounding myometrium. They are composed of long intersecting fascicles of spindled cells with eosinophilic fibrillary cytoplasm and elongated blunt-ended nuclei. These tumors are frequently, although not always, hypercellular. They typically exhibit diffuse moderate to marked nuclear atypia with hyperchromatic pleomorphic nuclei and multinucleated giant cells (Figure 8.25). Leiomyosarcomas typically display > 10 mitoses/10 HPFs and atypical mitoses are not uncommon (Figure 8.26). Although the finding of atypical mitoses is worrisome for malignancy, they may

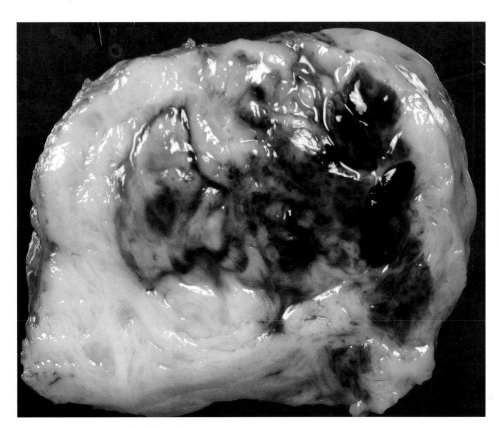

FIGURE 8.23
Uterine leiomyosarcoma. Heterogeneous cut surface with fleshy areas juxtaposed with extensive necrosis and hemorrhage.

LEIOMYOSARCOMA – PATHOLOGIC FEATURES

Gross Findings

▶ Large solitary mass or largest mass (mean 10 cm)
▶ Intramyometrial (most common), submucosal, or subserosal
▶ 5% arise in the cervix
▶ Poorly circumscribed; cannot be shelled out from adjacent myometrium
▶ Soft and fleshy cut surface
▶ Frequent necrosis and hemorrhage
▶ Gelatinous cut surface and deceptively well-circumscribed border in myxoid leiomyosarcomas
▶ Rarely, prominent intravascular growth

Microscopic Findings

Spindled Leiomyosarcoma

▶ Infiltrative growth
▶ Frequently hypercellular but may be hypocellular
▶ Long intersecting fascicles of spindled cells
▶ Cells with eosinophilic fibrillary cytoplasm and elongated blunt-ended nuclei
▶ Frequently diffuse moderate to marked nuclear atypia, including multinucleated giant cells
▶ Typically ≥ 10 mitoses/10 HPFs, including atypical forms
▶ Frequent tumor cell necrosis; may also show infarct-type necrosis
▶ Diagnosis based on combination of two of the following features:
  ▶ Diffuse moderate to severe cytologic atypia
  ▶ > 10 mitoses/10 HPFs
  ▶ Tumor cell necrosis
▶ Vascular invasion in 20% of cases

Epithelioid Leiomyosarcoma

▶ > 50% of the cells with an "epithelial-like" appearance
▶ Sheets, nests, cords, or rarely, pseudoglandular spaces
▶ Common hyalinization if cords and nests (plexiform growth)
▶ Cells with eosinophilic granular or clear cytoplasm and round or angular nucleus
▶ Diagnosis based on combination of ≥ 5 mitoses/10 HPFs, diffuse moderate to severe cytologic atypia, or tumor cell necrosis

Myxoid Leiomyosarcoma

▶ Infiltrative growth
▶ Typically hypocellular with abundant extracellular myxoid matrix
▶ Loose or thin fascicles or no particular pattern
▶ Cells with stellate, spindle, or abundant cytoplasm with marked degree of cytologic atypia
▶ Not infrequently cells with scant cytoplasm, minimal cytologic atypia and rare mitoses (< 5/10 HPFs)
▶ Diagnosis based on finding moderate to severe cytologic atypia or tumor cell necrosis, and in their absence finding ≥ 2 mitoses/10 HPFs

Other

▶ Osteoclastic-type giant cells
▶ "Xanthoma cells"
▶ Rhabdomyoblastic differentiation
▶ Liposarcoma component

Immunohistochemical Features

▶ Desmin, h-caldesmon, smooth muscle myosin, HDCA8 and other smooth muscle markers positive in conventional type; in epithelioid or myxoid types, less extensive positivity
▶ CD10, keratin, and EMA frequently positive (even more so in epithelioid variant)
▶ Estrogen, progesterone, and androgen receptor positive in approximately 30–40% of cases
▶ CD117 (c-kit) may be positive
▶ High MIB-1 and strong p53 positivity

Ultrastructual Features

▶ Syncytial arrangement of spindled cells in a matrix of collagen
▶ Basal lamina surrounding cells
▶ Thin microfilaments and dense bodies of microfilaments within processes (may be the only findings in epithelioid type)
▶ Abundant intracytoplasmic mitochondria in epithelioid type

Ploidy

▶ Frequently aneuploid but can be diploid

Cytogenetics

▶ Complex karyotypes
▶ Frequent gains and losses of several chromosomal regions

Differential Diagnosis

Spindled Leiomyosarcoma

▶ Leiomyoma variants
▶ Spindled rhabdomyosarcoma
▶ Undifferentiated endometrial sarcoma

Epithelioid Leiomyosarcoma

▶ Poorly differentiated carcinoma
▶ Metastatic and primary malignant melanoma
▶ Placental site trophoblastic tumor/epithelioid trophoblastic tumor
▶ Uterine tumor resembling ovarian sex cord tumor
▶ Perivascular epithelioid cell tumor

Myxoid Leiomyosarcoma

▶ Myxoid leiomyoma
▶ Intravenous leiomyomatosis with myxoid change
▶ Leiomyoma with prominent hydropic change

---

occasionally be encountered in leiomyomas. Tumor cell necrosis is a feature only seen in malignant smooth muscle tumors. It is characterized by an abrupt transition from viable tumor cells to necrotic cells without an interposed zone of granulation or fibrous tissue. Preserved nuclei with marked pleomorphism and hyperchromasia as well as apoptotic cells may still be seen within the necrotic foci. Often there is a perivascular growth of the viable tumor cells (Figure 8.27). Even though special emphasis has been given to tumor cell

necrosis in establishing the malignant nature of a smooth muscle tumor, this feature is rarely seen in isolation and, when present, high mitotic activity and marked cytologic atypia are also present in the tumor. The combination of any two of the following three features: (1) diffuse moderate to severe atypia; (2) > 10 mitoses/10 HPFs; and (3) tumor cell necrosis, establishes the diagnosis of spindle cell leiomyosarcoma. Infarct-type necrosis may be seen in benign and malignant smooth muscle tumors and thus is not helpful in establishing

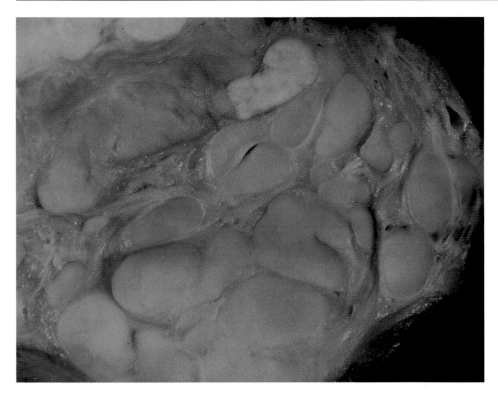

FIGURE 8.24

Uterine leiomyosarcoma. Prominent worm-like plugs of fleshy tumor distend myometrial vessels.

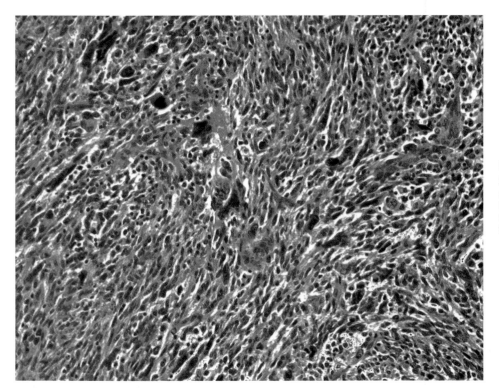

FIGURE 8.25

Spindle cell leiomyosarcoma. Highly atypical spindled cells, some of them multinucleated, with eosinophilic cytoplasm and elongated nuclei, form long intersecting fascicles.

the diagnosis of malignancy. In some cases, the distinction between early infarct-type necrosis and tumor cell necrosis may be extremely difficult. Vascular invasion is detected in approximately 20% of leiomyosarcomas but some tumors may have a prominent intravascular growth, simulating intravenous leiomyomatosis.

Leiomyosarcoma variants are uncommon: epithelioid and myxoid leiomyosarcomas are the most common subtypes (Box 8.3).

Epithelioid leiomyosarcoma. As mentioned earlier (see epithelioid leiomyoma section), the unifying term "epithelioid" is preferred for the classification of these

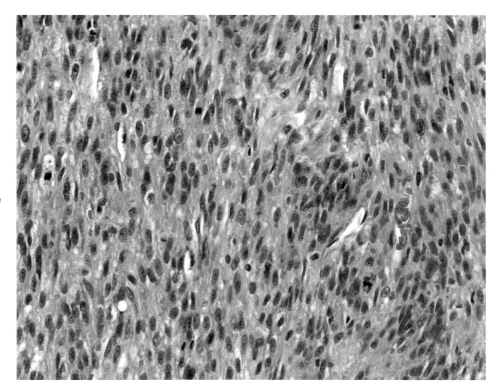

FIGURE 8.26

Spindle cell leiomyosarcoma. Note brisk mitotic activity.

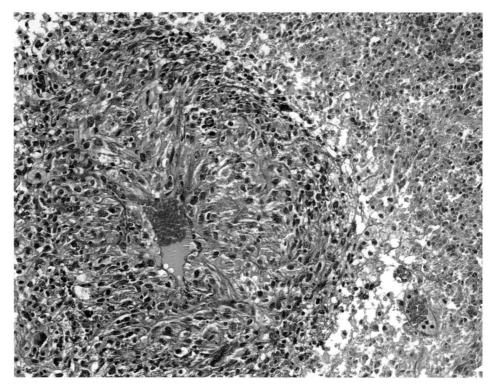

FIGURE 8.27

Tumor cell necrosis. Abrupt transition from viable to nonviable tumor cells. The viable tumor cells grow in a perivascular distribution and show marked cytologic atypia.

tumors regardless of the architectural or cytoplasmic characteristics that they may display. A leiomyosarcoma is classified as epithelioid when > 50 % of the cells have an "epithelial-like" appearance. On low-power examination, these tumors most frequently show a diffuse growth, but nests, cords, or occasionally pseudoglandular spaces may be seen and not infrequently these different patterns coexist (Figure 8.28). Hyalinization is commonly seen, particularly in association with a plexi-

form growth. The cytoplasm is usually eosinophilic and granular, but may be clear, and in about 25 % of cases the entire tumor is composed of clear cells (clear cell leiomyosarcoma). The round or angular nucleus is typically central but may be eccentric, occasionally mimicking signet-ring cells or lipoblasts, and even more so if the cytoplasm appears vacuolated. Because of the rarity of these tumors, criteria predictive of malignancy are less well established than for spindle cell leiomyosarcomas. However, as a general rule the finding of ≥ 5 mitoses/10 HPFs (Figure 8.29), diffuse moderate to severe cytologic atypia, or tumor cell necrosis warrants the diagnosis of epithelioid leiomyosarcoma.

Myxoid leiomyosarcoma. On low power, these tumors show an infiltrative growth which contrasts with the relative circumscription observed on gross examination (Figure 8.30). They are typically hypocellular due to abundant extracellular myxoid matrix, which is strongly positive for alcian blue and colloidal iron histochemical stains. The tumor cells may be arranged in loose or thin fascicles or may be distributed throughout the myxoid stroma without a particular pattern (Figure 8.31). They have stellate, spindle, or abundant cytoplasm with a marked degree of cytologic atypia, but in some instances the cells are small with scant cytoplasm, oval or spindle nuclei, and inconspicuous nucleoli associated with low mitotic activity (frequently < 5 mitoses/10 HPFs) (Figure 8.32). In these cases, the diagnosis of leiomyosarcoma may be challenging. The finding of an infiltra-

tive growth as well as areas of spindled leiomyosarcoma may facilitate the diagnosis. It is now recommended that, in the absence of tumor cell necrosis and severe cytologic atypia, the finding of ≥ 2 mitoses/10 HPFs in a myxoid smooth muscle tumor establishes the diagnosis of myxoid leiomyosarcoma. Thus, extensive sampling is crucial.

Rare leiomyosarcomas have a prominent component of *osteoclastic-type giant cells* that may be more conspicuous in areas of hemorrhage or have cells with abundant cytoplasm, lipid vacuoles, and multiple or multilobulated nuclei sometimes disposed in a wreath-like arrangement – *xanthomatous leiomyosarcoma*. Rarely, spindled leiomyosarcomas may show *rhabdomyoblastic differentiation* or may display a small component of *clear cells* or a component of *liposarcoma*.

ANCILLARY STUDIES

IMMUNOHISTOCHEMISTRY

Leiomyosarcomas express desmin, h-caldesmon (Figure 8.33), smooth muscle myosin, HDCA8 and other smooth muscle markers; however, epithelioid and myxoid subtypes may show less extensive positivity for these markers. Leiomyosarcomas are also frequently positive for CD10 (Figure 8.34) and epithelial markers, including keratin (Figure 8.35) and EMA (more frequent in the epithelioid variant). These tumors express ER, PR, and AR in approximately 30–40% of cases. It has been shown that leiomyosarcomas may variably stain for CD117 (c-kit),

---

BOX 8.3

LEIOMYOSARCOMA VARIANTS

1. Conventional (spindled)
2. Epithelioid
3. Myxoid
4. With prominent intravascular growth
5. With osteoclast-type cells
6. With clear cells
7. With xanthoma-type cells

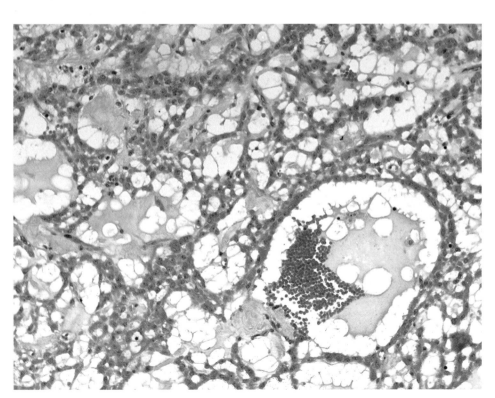

FIGURE 8.28

Epithelioid leiomyosarcoma. Anastomosing cords and trabeculae with pseudoglandular formation.

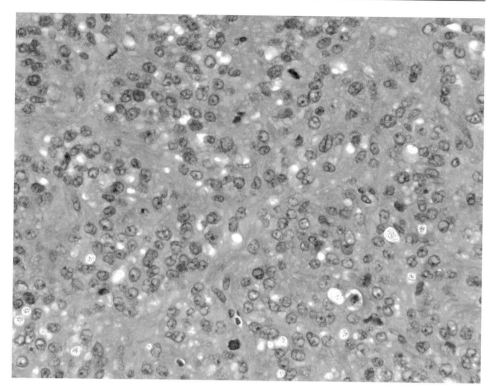

FIGURE 8.29

Epithelioid leiomyosarcoma. Diffuse growth of tumor cells with noticeable mitotic activity in the absence of marked cytologic atypia.

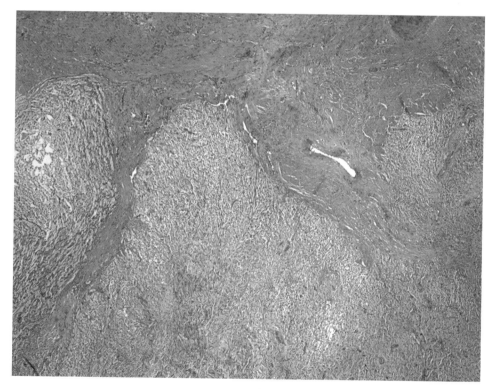

FIGURE 8.30

Myxoid leiomyosarcoma. Prominent irregular myometrial invasion.

although c-kit mutations have not been detected. Leiomyosarcomas frequently display high MIB-1 as well as strong p53 positivity.

ULTRASTRUCTURAL EXAMINATION

Diagnostic criteria for leiomyosarcoma include: (1) syncytial arrangement of spindle cells in a matrix of collagen; (2) basal lamina surrounding cells; and (3) thin microfilaments and dense bodies of microfilaments within processes. The diagnosis of an epithelioid smooth muscle tumor depends on the finding of thin filaments and dense bodies as other features may be missing. They may have abundant intracytoplasmic mitochondria. Smooth muscle cells in epithelioid smooth muscle tumors have been described as being immature and mimic mesenchymal cells of fetal uterus during 14–26 weeks of gestation.

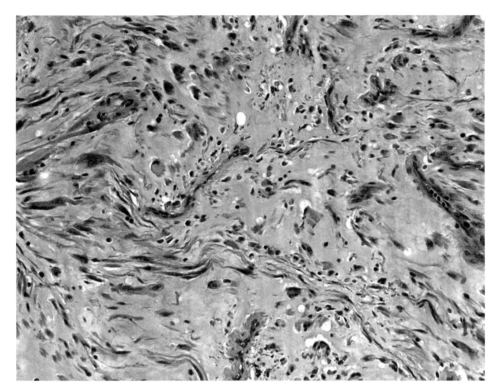

FIGURE 8.31
Myxoid leiomyosarcoma. Atypical spindled cells are present in a hypocellular myxoid background.

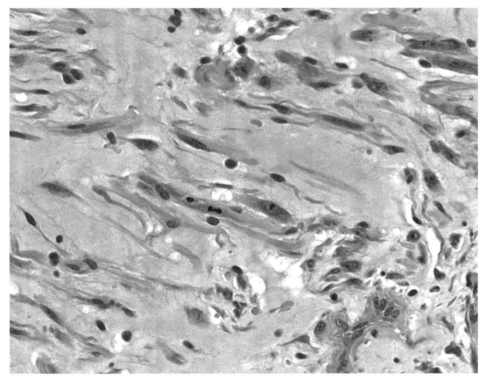

FIGURE 8.32
Myxoid leiomyosarcoma. Elongated cells with enlarged nuclei, prominent nucleoli, as well as one mitotic figure.

PLOIDY

Leiomyosarcomas may be diploid but frequently they are aneuploid, although this finding has not been consistently correlated with prognosis.

CYTOGENETICS

Numerical or structural cytogenetic abnormalities have been detected in > 60% of uterine leiomyosarcomas and, although the vast majority of reported karyo-

types are complex, consistent abnormalities have not been identified. A high frequency of gains or losses of several chromosomal regions has been reported.

DIFFERENTIAL DIAGNOSIS

Uterine leiomyosarcoma should be distinguished from *leiomyoma variants*, more commonly leiomyoma with

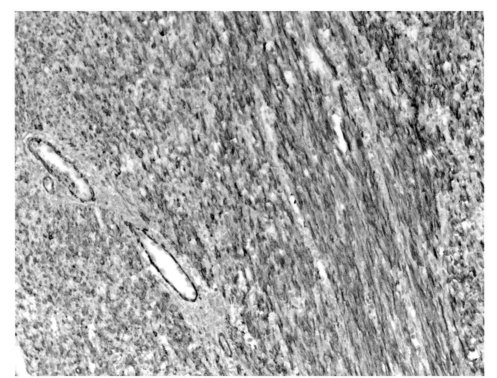

FIGURE 8.33

Spindle cell leiomyosarcoma. Diffuse staining of the tumor cells for h-caldesmon.

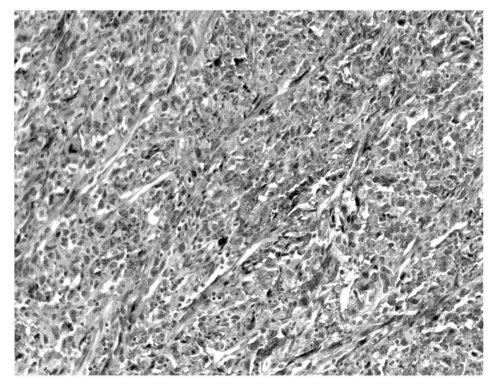

FIGURE 8.34

Spindle cell leiomyosarcoma. The tumor cells are diffusely positive for CD10.

bizarre nuclei and mitotically active leiomyoma (previously discussed). It should also be distinguished from spindle cell rhabdomyosarcoma and undifferentiated endometrial sarcoma. *Uterine rhabdomyosarcoma* is rare, with pleomorphic rhabdomyosarcoma being the most common subtype in the corpus. In the spindle cell variant, the cells are predominantly spindled and have elongated nuclei, a microscopic appearance that closely overlaps with that observed in spindled leiomyosarcoma. The finding of occasional cells with eosinophilic cytoplasm, cytoplasmic cross-striations, and positivity for skeletal muscle markers such as sarcomeric actin,

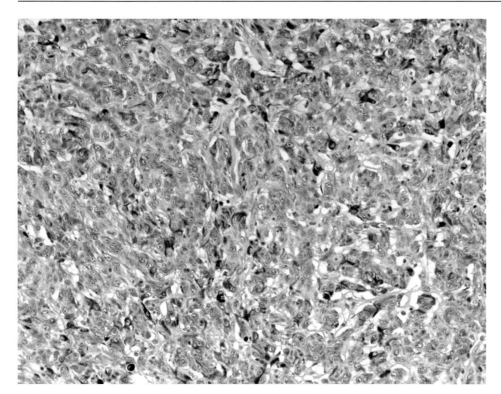

FIGURE 8.35
Epithelioid leiomyosarcoma. The malignant cells show extensive positivity for keratin.

myoglobin, and myoD1 is helpful in this differential diagnosis. Finally, as its name implies *undifferentiated endometrial sarcoma* is a high-grade sarcoma with no specific differentiation. Thus, the diagnosis should be made after excluding an undifferentiated carcinoma, malignant mixed müllerian tumor, and high-grade leiomyosarcoma.

Epithelioid leiomyosarcoma should be distinguished from *poorly differentiated carcinoma,* especially when composed of eosinophilic or clear cells. Many such carcinomas, however, exhibit, at least focally, overt glandular or squamous differentiation. In some cases, immunohistochemical or ultrastructural studies may be needed to facilitate the diagnosis. The use of a panel of antibodies is recommended as epithelioid smooth muscle tumors are frequently positive for keratin and EMA. *Metastatic and, less commonly, primary malignant melanoma* can be excluded by their immunoreactivity for S-100 and HMB-45 and lack of reactivity for smooth muscle markers. *PSTT* and *ETT* also enter in the differential diagnosis as they may grow in sheets and their cells typically have abundant eosinophilic or clear cytoplasm. Features favoring a diagnosis of a trophoblastic tumor include a history of recent pregnancy, an elevated serum HCG level, an infiltrative growth pattern with tumor cells dissecting pre-existing smooth muscle bundles (PSTT), prominent vascular involvement (PSTT), fibrinoid change in vessel walls (PSTT), well-circumscribed margins (ETT), nested growth around vessels (ETT), extensive areas of geographical necrosis (ETT), and immunoreactivity for CK18, inhibin and HPL (both), and p63 (ETT). A *uterine tumor resembling*

an ovarian sex cord tumor (UTROSCT) may cause confusion with an epithelioid tumor as it also shows prominent "epithelial-like" differentiation and furthermore, frequently expresses smooth muscle and epithelial markers. However, in most cases the degree of epithelial differentiation is more pronounced and some of these tumors may also express inhibin, CD99, and calretinin. *PEComa* enters in the differential diagnosis as the tumor cells have abundant clear or eosinophilic cytoplasm with oval to round nuclei, they are disposed in sheets or small solid nests, and they may express smooth muscle markers. However, in contrast to smooth muscle tumors, PEComas are characteristically positive for HMB-45, Melan-A, and other melanocytic markers. Finally, it is important to be aware that epithelioid leiomyosarcomas with variable amounts of clear cells may be focally positive for HMB-45.

Myxoid leiomyosarcoma should be primarily distinguished from its benign counterpart, the *myxoid leiomyoma.* The presence of cytologic atypia, tumor cell necrosis, or $\geq$ 2 mitoses/10 HPFs will point towards malignancy. *Intravenous leiomyomatosis with myxoid change* may rarely enter into the differential diagnosis because of the intravascular growth pattern. The finding of any degree of cytologic atypia or mitotic activity will favor the diagnosis of leiomyosarcoma. Finally, *leiomyoma with prominent hydropic change* may enter into this differential diagnosis if the edematous background is confused with myxoid matrix, or if the hydropic change extends beyond the confines of the leiomyoma mimicking infiltrative growth. This distinction is crucial and can be achieved with alcian blue or colloidal iron stains which are negative in leiomyomas with hydropic change.

PROGNOSIS AND TREATMENT

Leiomyosarcomas are aggressive tumors with an overall poor prognosis. The 5-year survival rate ranges from 12% to 40% for all stages and is approximately 50–70% for tumors confined to the uterus. This wide range mirrors the differences in defining criteria used in the diagnosis of these tumors until recently. In a large Gynecology Oncology Group (GOG) study of early-stage leiomyosarcomas (stages I and II), the recurrence rate was 71% whereas the 3-year progression-free interval was 31%. Up to 70% of patients with leiomyosarcomas confined to the uterus and nearly all with extrauterine disease at initial diagnosis will eventually recur with a median time to recurrence of 8–16 months. Leiomyosarcomas spread hematogenously and lungs are the most common site of recurrence, followed by the liver. In the GOG study, lung recurrences occurred in 40%, whereas pelvic recurrences occur in only 13%.

The treatment of choice is total abdominal hysterectomy and debulking of tumor if present outside the uterus. Removal of the ovaries and lymph node dissection remains controversial as metastasis occurs in only a small percentage of patients and it is frequently associated with the presence of extrauterine disease. Patients are staged based on a modified 1988 staging system of the International Federation of Gynecology and Obstetrics (FIGO) for endometrial cancer. Adjuvant therapy has an uncertain benefit in survival, although radiotherapy may be useful in controlling local recurrences, and chemotherapy with doxorubicin or placlitaxel is used for advanced or recurrent disease, with response rates ranging from 19% to 30%. It has been shown that time to recurrence of > 12 months and optimal surgical resection of the recurrent tumor appear to increase survival. Hormonal status does not influence overall survival when corrected for stage; however, some patients may respond to hormonal treatment. No consistent correlation has been shown between survival and clinical or pathologic parameters in multiple studies. However, in a very recent study of 208 uterine leiomyosarcomas, tumor grade and stage emerged as the most accurate predictive parameters in these tumors. Other parameters, including patient age > 51 years, tumor size > 5 cm, and menopausal status, also seemed to be associated with reduced overall survival, at least by univariate analysis. Parameters including p53, DNA ploidy, and Bcl-2 may have a role in predicting outcome in leiomyosarcomas, but it is not clear that these factors act independently of stage. Stage is still the most powerful prognostic factor in these tumors.

Myxoid leiomyosarcomas are also aggressive tumors, but in contrast to spindled leiomyosarcoma, the post-operative interval to recurrence or metastases may be as long as 10 years. Awareness of the major discrepancy between the relatively innocuous appearance of myxoid leiomyosarcomas and their obvious malignant course should always prompt caution with this type of smooth muscle neoplasm. Patients with epithelioid leiomyosarcomas may die from tumor, often after multiple recurrences, > 5 or even > 10 years after hysterectomy. Finally, it is important to point out that experience with cervical smooth muscle tumors is very limited and that these tumors may have a lower threshold for metastases when compared to leiomyosarcomas occurring in the uterine corpus.

SMOOTH MUSCLE TUMORS OF LOW OR UNCERTAIN MALIGNANT POTENTIAL (STUMP)

Uterine smooth-muscle tumors that show some worrisome histologic features but do not fulfill the diagnostic criteria of leiomyosarcoma fall into this category. They include: (1) banal leiomyoma with tumor cell necrosis; (2) necrosis of uncertain type with ≥ 10 mitoses/10 HPFs; (3) marked diffuse atypia and borderline mitotic counts; (4) tumors with cytologic atypia where it is difficult to be sure about mitotic counts; and (5) tumors with early necrosis that is difficult to classify. The term "smooth muscle tumor of low malignant potential" should not be abused and every effort should be made to classify a smooth muscle tumor into a specific category when possible (Figure 8.36).

PECOMA

PEComa is a relatively newly described low-grade mesenchymal tumor first reported in the uterus by Pea and colleagues in 1996. It belongs to the family of lesions which includes the clear cell "sugar" tumors of the lung and pancreas, some forms of angiomyolipoma, the clear cell myelomelanocytic tumor of ligamentum teres/falciform ligament, and others. In the female gynecologic tract, the uterus is the most common location. This tumor shows a particular association with lymphangioleiomyomatosis and tuberous sclerosis. All these tumors originate from the perivascular epithelioid cell (PEC), a cell defined by the presence of abundant clear to eosinophilic granular cytoplasm and positive staining for HMB-45, as well as frequent expression of muscle markers.

CLINICAL FEATURES

The tumors are typically seen in reproductive-age or postmenopausal patients who most commonly present with uterine bleeding.

PECOMA – FACT SHEET

Definition
- Tumor composed of "perivascular epithelioid cells" (PEC), a cell defined by abundant clear to eosinophilic granular cytoplasm and HMB-45 positivity
- Belongs to the family of lesions which includes clear cell "sugar" tumors of the lung and pancreas, some forms of angiomyolipoma, clear cell myelomelanocytic tumor of ligamentum teres, and others

Incidence
- Rare

Age Distribution
- Reproductive-age and postmenopausal women

Clinical Features
- Uterine bleeding
- Association with lymphangioleiomyomatosis and tuberous sclerosis

Prognosis and Treatment
- Survival rate of 95% for stage I tumors and 75% for advanced tumors
- Long term prognosis not well established
- Aggressive behavior if > 5 cm, infiltrative growth pattern, high-grade cytologic atypia, necrosis, and mitotic activity > 1/50 HPFs

---

PATHOLOGIC FEATURES

GROSS FINDINGS

The majority of these tumors present as solitary lesions ranging from 0.6 to 12 cm. They can have either a well-circumscribed white, whorled cut surface resembling a leiomyoma or poorly defined margins with a fleshy, soft cut surface which is gray-white to tan or yellow resembling the gross appearance of an endometrial stromal tumor. In most cases, the tumors are confined to the uterus at the time of diagnosis.

MICROSCOPIC FINDINGS

On low-power examination, some tumors have a tongue-like infiltrative growth, while in others the interface between the tumor and the surrounding tissue is smooth. The tumor cells typically grow in sheets with scant amounts of intervening stroma (Figure 8.37), the presence of which may result focally in a nested growth pattern. However, extensive areas of stromal hyalinization may be seen. Not infrequently, focal fascicular growth is present. In some tumors, a prominent lymphangioleiomyomatous growth is most prominent. The cells usually have well-defined borders, abundant clear to eosinophilic and granular cytoplasm, and oval to round nuclei, imparting an epithelioid pattern (Figure

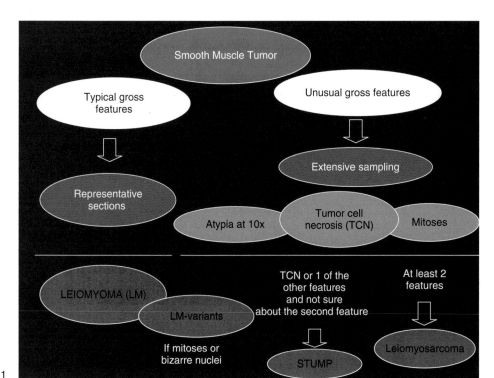

FIGURE 8.36

Proposed flow chart showing a practical approach to smooth muscle tumors of the uterus.

PECOMA – PATHOLOGIC FEATURES

Gross Findings

▸ Solitary mass ranging from 0.6 to 12 cm
▸ Either well-circumscribed or with poorly defined margins
▸ Gray-white, whorled or fleshy and soft cut-surface

Microscopic Findings

▸ Smooth and regular interface or tongue-like infiltration
▸ Sheets or nests of cells with scant amounts of intervening stroma
▸ Focal fascicular growth
▸ Prominent lymphangioleiomyomatous growth in some cases
▸ Occasionally extensive areas of stromal hyalinization
▸ Two cell types:
  ▸ Cells with well-defined borders, abundant clear to eosinophilic cytoplasm, and oval to round nuclei
  ▸ Spindled cells
▸ Cells may be tightly arranged around blood vessels
▸ Variable degree of nuclear atypia (more commonly absent)
▸ Low mitotic rate in most cases
▸ Necrosis in high-grade tumors

Immunohistochemical Features

▸ HMB-45, Melan-A and MiTF positive
▸ Variable positivity for smooth muscle markers and CD10
▸ Cytokeratin, inhibin, and S-100 negative

Cytogenetic Features

▸ 16p deletion in the TSC2 locus

Differential Diagnosis

▸ Low-grade endometrial stromal sarcoma (at low power)
▸ Epithelioid smooth muscle tumor
▸ Metastatic or primary melanoma
▸ Endometrial carcinoma

8.38). Sometimes the cells may be tightly arranged around blood vessels. The spindled areas have cells with elongated nuclei, an appearance that closely resembles that seen in smooth muscle tumors. Nuclear atypia is typically absent but may be moderate, whereas mitotic rates are low in most cases. High-grade tumors may show associated necrosis.

ANCILLARY STUDIES

IMMUNOHISTOCHEMISTRY

The tumors are characteristically positive for HMB-45 (Figure 8.39) and Melan-A, and in most cases negative for S-100. They are frequently positive for microphthalmia transcription factor (MiTF) and muscle markers, including smooth muscle actin and desmin. Coexpression of HMB-45 and muscle markers is highly specific. These tumors may be positive for CD10, but are negative for inhibin and keratin.

CYTOGENETICS

Some PEComas have a 16p deletion in the TSC2 locus, an abnormality detected in some angiomyolipomas. This may indicate an oncogenetic relationship between PEComa and angiomyolipoma as a TSC2-linked neoplasm.

DIFFERENTIAL DIAGNOSIS

This tumor needs to be distinguished from *low-grade endometrial stromal sarcoma*, as at low power, a tongue-

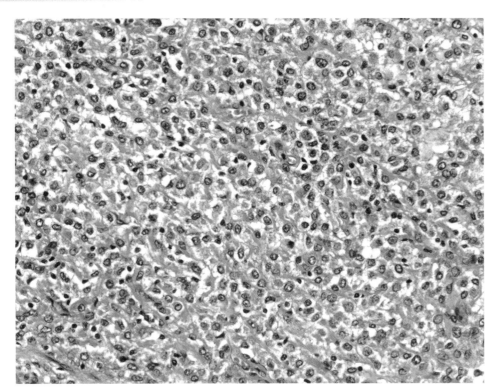

FIGURE 8.37
Perivascular epithelioid cell tumor (PEComa). Diffuse to vaguely nested growth of tumor cells is present.

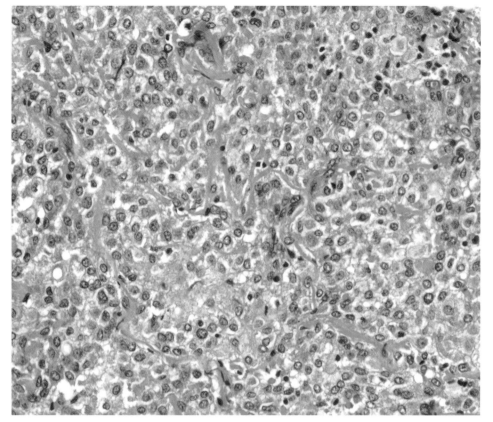

FIGURE 8.38

Perivascular epithelioid cell tumor (PEComa). The neoplastic cells display abundant clear cytoplasm, round nuclei, and minimal cytologic atypia.

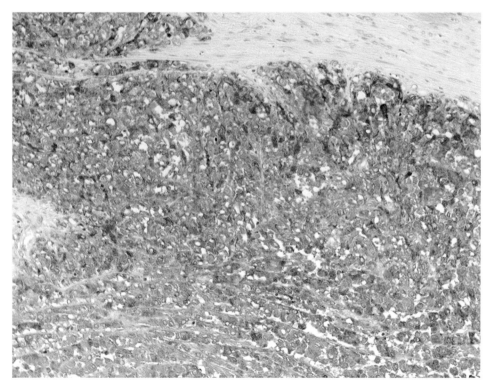

FIGURE 8.39

Perivascular epithelioid cell tumor (PEComa). Diffuse and strong HMB-45 positivity.

like pattern of infiltration and a diffuse growth may be seen in both tumors. Clear cells have rarely been described in endometrial stromal tumors; however, the latter are also characterized by focal areas resembling proliferative endometrial stroma with associated arterioles. Endometrial stromal tumors may be positive for smooth muscle markers but they do not express HMB-45 or Melan-A. *Epithelioid smooth muscle tumors* frequently share with PEComas a diffuse or nested growth, stromal hyalinization, and cells with eosinophilic or clear cytoplasm; it is not infrequent to see a spindle cell component as well. Furthermore, PEComas are positive for muscle markers (although to a lesser extent when compared to spindled smooth muscle tumors). In contrast to PEComas, epithelioid smooth muscle tumors are frequently positive for keratins and negative for HMB-45, although experience with this antibody is limited. It is important to note the reported HMB-45 positivity in smooth muscle tumors including epithelioid leiomyosarcomas with a variable number of clear cells. *Primary or metastatic malignant melanomas* are typically S-100 positive and lack reactivity for smooth-muscle markers. *Primary endometrial carcinoma* may rarely enter into the differential diagnosis; however, it usually exhibits, at least focally, overt epithelial differentiation. Keratin may aid in difficult cases as it is typically negative in PEComa.

PROGNOSIS AND TREATMENT

The long-term prognosis of these tumors is not well established as experience is very limited. At least 13 of the uterine PEComas reported in the literature have behaved in an aggressive fashion. A significant correlation with subsequent aggressive behavior has been observed in tumors > 5 cm, those with an infiltrative growth pattern, high cytologic atypia, necrosis, and mitotic activity > 1/50 HPFs in a combined statistical analysis of all previously reported cases, mostly in soft tissues and uterine corpus and cervix.

ENDOMETRIAL STROMAL TUMORS

Endometrial stromal tumors of the uterus are the second most common mesenchymal tumor of the uterus, even though they account for < 10% of all such tumors. In the latest WHO classification, endometrial stromal tumors are divided into: (1) endometrial stromal nodule (ESN); (2) low-grade endometrial stromal sarcoma; and (3) undifferentiated endometrial sarcoma.

ENDOMETRIAL STROMAL NODULE

This tumor is very rare. It is composed of cells that are reminiscent of proliferative-phase endometrial stroma. It represents the benign end of the spectrum within the category of endometrial stromal tumors.

ENDOMETRIAL STROMAL TUMORS – FACT SHEET

Definition

Endometrial Stromal Nodule

▸ Well-circumscribed noninvasive endometrial stromal tumor composed of cells that are reminiscent of proliferative-phase endometrial stroma

Low-Grade Endometrial Stromal Sarcoma

▸ Low-grade malignant endometrial stromal tumor composed of cells reminiscent of proliferative-phase endometrial stroma characterized by myometrial and vascular invasion and late recurrences

Incidence

Endometrial Stromal Nodule

▸ Very rare

Low-Grade Endometrial Stromal Sarcoma

▸ 0.2% of all uterine malignancies
▸ 10–15% of malignant tumors of the uterus with a mesenchymal component

Age Distribution

Endometrial Stromal Nodule

▸ Any age (median 47 years)
▸ One-third postmenopausal

Low-Grade Endometrial Stromal Sarcoma

▸ Mean age 45 years

Clinical Features

▸ Abnormal uterine bleeding
▸ Pelvic or abdominal pain

Prognosis and Treatment

Endometrial Stromal Nodule

▸ Excellent prognosis with no recurrences if completely excised
▸ Hysterectomy and, on rare occasions, excision of lesion only if complete examination of margins possible

Low-Grade Endometrial Stromal Sarcoma

▸ 5-year survival rate of approximately 60–80%
▸ Low malignant potential with late recurrences
▸ Recurrences in one-third or more of patients with stage I tumors
▸ Pelvic recurrences (occurring in up to one-half of the patients up to 20 years later), abdominal, and less frequently, vaginal recurrences or lung metastases (up to 27 years later)
▸ Total abdominal hysterectomy and bilateral salpingo-oophorectomy and debulking of any visible tumor
▸ Radiation or hormonal treatment (progestational agents or aromatase inhibitors) as adjuvant treatment or for recurrent or metastatic tumor
▸ Endometrial stromal tumors with unusual types of differentiation should be reported as endometrial stromal nodule or low-grade endometrial stromal sarcoma based on the margins of the tumor, as this is the discriminating prognostic factor

ENDOMETRIAL STROMAL TUMORS – PATHOLOGIC FEATURES

Gross Findings

Endometrial Stromal Nodule

▶ Solitary well-circumscribed mass
▶ Variable size (0.5–22 cm; mean 7 cm)
▶ Uniform soft, tan to yellow cut surface
▶ Occasional cyst formation, hemorrhage and/or necrosis

Low-Grade Endometrial Stromal Sarcoma

▶ Solid nodules or diffuse growth involving myometrium with/without endometrial involvement
▶ Frequent worm-like plugs of tumor in myometrial or parametrial veins
▶ Some tumors deceptively well circumscribed with minimal or absent vascular permeation
▶ Soft, fleshy, bulging with tan to yellow cut surface
▶ Occasional hemorrhage, necrosis, and cyst formation

Microscopic Findings

Endometrial Stromal Nodule (Diagnostic Criteria)

▶ Smooth interface (most important)
▶ Sometimes focal irregularities such as lobulated or finger-like projections into adjacent myometrium < 3 mm and ≤ 3 in number
▶ No vascular invasion

Low-Grade Endometrial Stromal Sarcoma (Diagnostic Criteria)

▶ Irregular tongues and/or islands of tumor extensively permeating the myometrium; frequent growth within myometrial veins and lymphatics with extrauterine extension

Endometrial Stromal Nodule and Low-Grade Endometrial Stromal Sarcoma (Shared Features)

▶ Typically hypercellular stroma, rarely hypocellular
▶ Collagen bands, histiocytes, or extensive hyalinization variably present
▶ Typically thin-walled vessels (arterioles) that may become hyalinized; however, vasculature not always striking
▶ Sheets of small blue cells closely resembling proliferative-phase endometrial stroma
▶ Cells with scant cytoplasm, oval to round nuclei, and inconspicuous nucleoli. Occasionally, abundant eosinophilic cytoplasm

▶ Bland cytologic features and low mitotic activity (1–5 mitoses/ 10 HPFs), but higher mitotic rate does not exclude either diagnosis
▶ Infarct-type necrosis associated with cholesterol clefts
▶ Other findings:
  ▶ Smooth ("starburst") and skeletal muscle differentiation
  ▶ Fibrous or myxoid background
  ▶ Sex cord-like differentiation
  ▶ Glandular differentiation (endometrioid-type benign or atypical glands)
  ▶ Rhabdoid differentiation
  ▶ Clear/epithelioid cells
  ▶ Bizarre stromal cells
  ▶ Fatty metaplasia

Immunohistochemical Features

▶ CD10 and vimentin typically positive
▶ Keratin, muscle-specific, smooth-muscle actin frequently positive
▶ ER and PR frequently positive
▶ Desmin, h-caldesmon, myosin, and HDCA8 rarely positive in stromal component but typically positive in smooth muscle areas
▶ Inhibin, calretinin, CD99, WT-1, and Melan-A may be positive in areas of sex cord-like differentiation

Cytogenetic Features

▶ t(7;17) common aberration in conventional endometrial stromal tumors and variants

Differential Diagnosis

▶ Highly cellular leiomyoma (vs endometrial stromal nodule and low-grade endometrial stromal sarcoma)
▶ Highly cellular intravenous leiomyomatosis (vs low-grade endometrial stromal sarcoma)
▶ Cellular endometrial polyp (vs endometrial stromal nodule and low-grade endometrial stromal sarcoma)
▶ Adenomyosis (vs low-grade endometrial stromal sarcoma)
▶ Low-grade müllerian adenosarcoma (vs low-grade endometrial stromal sarcoma)
▶ Uterine tumor resembling sex cord-stromal tumor (vs endometrial stromal nodule and low-grade endometrial stromal sarcoma)

CLINICAL FEATURES

These tumors occur in women of any age (median 47 years), with approximately one-third being postmenopausal. Patients usually present with abnormal uterine bleeding and pelvic or abdominal pain.

PATHOLOGIC FEATURES

GROSS FINDINGS

Endometrial stromal nodules are typically well-circumscribed but not encapsulated tumors ranging in size from 0.5 to 22 (mean 7) cm. If centered in the endometrium, they are frequently polypoid; however, they may be intramyometrial or subserosal. They have a uniform soft, tan to yellow cut surface (Figure 8.40) which may be associated with cyst formation as well as hemorrhage and/or necrosis.

MICROSCOPIC FINDINGS

On low-power examination, these tumors are well demarcated from the adjacent myometrium. This is the most important microscopic feature to differentiate ESN from low-grade endometrial stromal sarcoma, as both share the same high-power microscopic appearance. Focal irregularities in the form of lobulated or finger-like projections into the adjacent myometrium may occur but they should not exceed 3 mm and should be ≤ 3 in number. No vascular invasion should be seen. On high-power examination, the tumors are typically hypercellular but may be hypocellular secondary to a fibrous

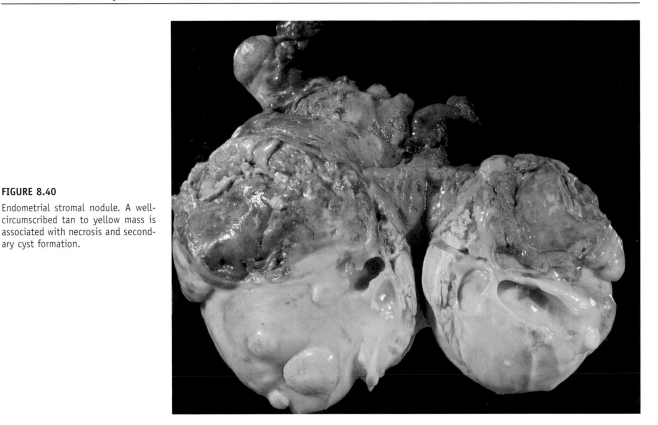

FIGURE 8.40

Endometrial stromal nodule. A well-circumscribed tan to yellow mass is associated with necrosis and secondary cyst formation.

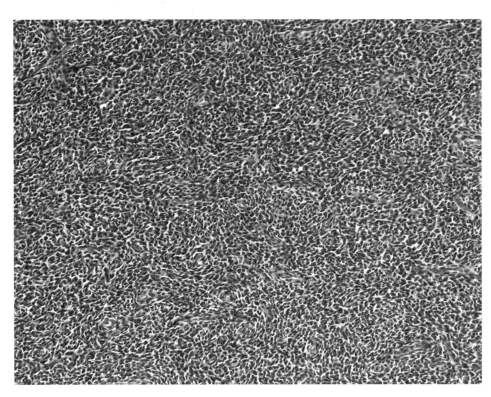

FIGURE 8.41

Endometrial stromal tumor. Diffuse growth of homogeneous small cells with scant cytoplasm and oval to slightly elongated nuclei.

or myxoid background. They are composed of sheets of small blue cells closely resembling proliferative-phase endometrial stroma (Figure 8.41). The cells have scant cytoplasm and oval to round nuclei with inconspicuous nucleoli, but occasionally, they have abundant eosinophilic cytoplasm imparting an epithelioid appearance.

Mitotic activity typically ranges from 1 to 5 mitoses/10 HPFs. The cells often whorl around arterioles which typically have thin walls (Figure 8.42) but may become hyalinized. This characteristic arborizing vasculature, however, is not always striking. Large thick-walled blood vessels, if present, are typically close to the tumor–myo-

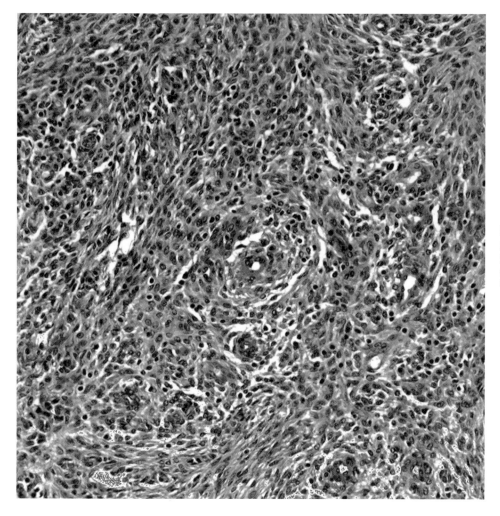

FIGURE 8.42

Endometrial stromal tumor. The small blue tumor cells whorl around delicate and thin blood vessels reminiscent of endometrial arterioles.

metrium interface. Sex cord-like differentiation may be present and represent up to 70% of the tumor. It is seen in the form of sertoliform or retiform tubules, anastomosing cords, trabeculae, nests, or diffuse sheets reminiscent of an adult granulosa cell tumor (Figure 8.43). Smooth and skeletal muscle differentiation, fibrous or myxoid change, glandular differentiation (as benign or malignant endometrioid-type glands), and rhabdoid cells may also be seen (see low-grade endometrial stromal sarcoma, below). Other microscopic findings include irregular bands of collagen, extensive areas of hyalinization, foamy histiocytes, either isolated or in small groups (Figure 8.44), and cysts with cholesterol clefts associated with infarct-type necrosis.

ANCILLARY STUDIES

The immunohistochemical profile as well as cytogenetic findings are similar to those encountered in low-grade endometrial stromal sarcoma (see ancillary studies in low-grade endometrial stromal sarcoma section, below).

DIFFERENTIAL DIAGNOSIS

The differentiation of ESN from *low-grade endometrial stromal sarcoma* is not possible in a curettage specimen, except in the rare case where the lesion is so small that it can be completely removed and the pathologist can evaluate the margins, since their distinction is based on the presence of infiltrative margins or vascular permeation. The finding of one of these two features establishes the diagnosis of a low-grade endometrial stromal sarcoma. Some tumors may not fulfill the criteria for an ESN but still do not have the typical permeative growth of an endometrial stromal sarcoma. These tumors have been descriptively referred to as "endometrial stromal tumors with limited infiltration" until more information is known regarding their prognosis.

A *highly cellular leiomyoma* closely resembles the gross appearance of an ESN because it is soft with a yellow or yellow-tan cut surface. On microscopic examination, it is as cellular and may have prominent vascularity similar to that of an ESN. Helpful clues to the correct diagnosis include focal merging of the highly

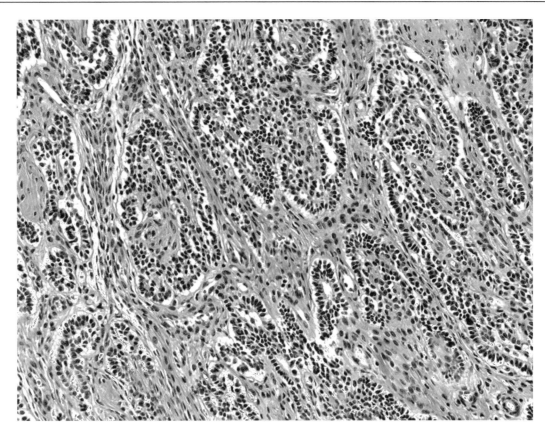

FIGURE 8.43
Endometrial stromal nodule with sex cord-like differentiation. Irregular nests of epithelial-like cells with peripheral palisading are present in a background of endometrial stromal neoplasia.

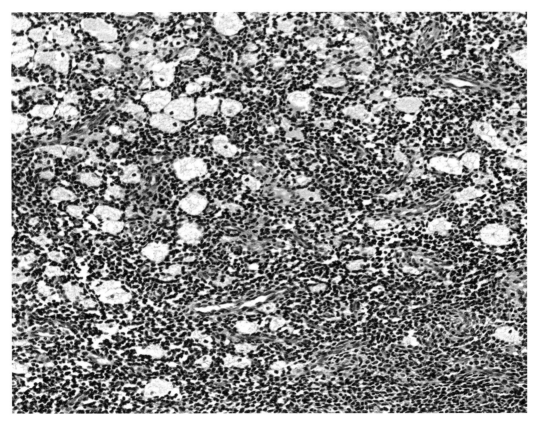

FIGURE 8.44
Endometrial stromal tumor. Histiocytes are intimately admixed with the neoplastic endometrial stromal cells.

cellular component with typical fascicular areas of smooth muscle neoplasia, large thick-walled blood vessels, and the presence of cleft-like spaces. Strong and extensive immunoreactivity for smooth muscle markers is also helpful. A *uterine tumor resembling a sex cord-stromal tumor* may enter in the differential diagnosis, especially in curettage specimens if the endometrial stromal component is not evident. Immunohistochemical stains are not helpful in this differential diagnosis and in these cases the final report should convey that the possibility of an endometrial stromal tumor cannot be excluded.

PROGNOSIS AND TREATMENT

Endometrial stromal nodules have an excellent prognosis and patients are cured by hysterectomy. Conservative treatment with excision of the mass is only performed when complete examination of the margins can be done, which only occurs in rare instances.

LOW-GRADE ENDOMETRIAL STROMAL SARCOMA

Low-grade endometrial stromal sarcoma accounts for approximately 0.2% of all malignant uterine tumors and 10–15% of uterine malignancies with a mesenchymal component, being much less common than carcinosarcoma and leiomyosarcoma.

CLINICAL FEATURES

These tumors frequently occur in women between 40 and 55 years of age, although they may be seen in younger or older women. Some of them have been reported in association with ovarian polycystic disease, estrogen use, or tamoxifen therapy. The patients commonly present with abnormal uterine bleeding, pelvic pain, and dysmenorrhea, but as many as 25% of patients are asymptomatic. Extrauterine pelvic extension at the time of presentation is found in up to one-third of patients and, rarely, patients present with manifestations at the metastatic site. Physical examination is nonspecific, often revealing uterine enlargement, and endometrial sampling provides a diagnosis in only 30% of cases.

RADIOLOGIC FEATURES

The MRI appearance is similar to that of other pelvic masses. The tumor is isointense relative to the myometrium on T1-weighted images, is hyperintense on T2-weighted images, and demonstrates heterogeneous enhancement on contrast-enhanced images.

PATHOLOGIC FEATURES

GROSS FINDINGS

Most low-grade endometrial stromal sarcomas are centered in the myometrium, but some may arise in the endometrium and form one or multiple polypoid masses. The tumors range in size from less than < 4 cm to > 15 cm. They typically grow in solid nodules or diffusely into the myometrium, and they are frequently associated with worm-like plugs of tumor in myometrial or parametrial veins (Figure 8.45), with extension to the serosa in approximately 50% of cases. However, some tumors may be deceptively well circumscribed with minimal or absent vascular permeation. The cut surface is soft, fleshy, bulging, and tan to yellow. Areas of hemorrhage, necrosis, and cyst formation may also be identified.

MICROSCOPIC FINDINGS

On low-power examination, these tumors form irregularly shaped tongues and/or islands that are densely cellular, extensively permeate the myometrium (Figure 8.46), and frequently grow within myometrial veins and lymphatics with extrauterine extension (Figure 8.45). They are composed of a uniform proliferation of oval to spindle-shaped cells with scant cytoplasm and oval to round nuclei without significant cytologic atypia. The overall appearance is highly reminiscent of proliferative-phase endometrial stroma and similar to ESNs. The cells in some tumors may appear decidualized with relatively abundant eosinophilic cytoplasm and round nuclei; some tumors may contain bizarre nuclei. Mitotic activity is usually < 3/10 HPFs, but may be higher. Even in cases with brisk mitotic activity, the diagnosis of low-grade endometrial stromal sarcoma is still valid if the architectural and cytologic features of the tumor are reminiscent of endometrial stroma. Foam cells can be identified, singly or in small clusters, and may be associated with areas of necrosis and cholesterol clefts. Collagen bands, extensive areas of hyalinization, or edema may also be encountered.

Low-grade endometrial stromal sarcomas may show sex cord-like differentiation, glandular differentiation (typically endometrioid-like, either benign or atypical) (Figure 8.47), smooth muscle and skeletal muscle differentiation, fibrous and/or myxoid change (Figure 8.48), and, very rarely, cells with an epithelioid, clear, or rhabdoid phenotype similar to that described in ESNs. Fatty metaplasia has been described in one case (Box 8.4). Sex cord-like areas with patterns resembling those seen in sex cord-stromal tumors of the ovary, including cords, trabeculae, solid or hollow tubules, or even a retiform pattern, may be found. Smooth muscle differentiation may be seen as irregular discrete epithe-

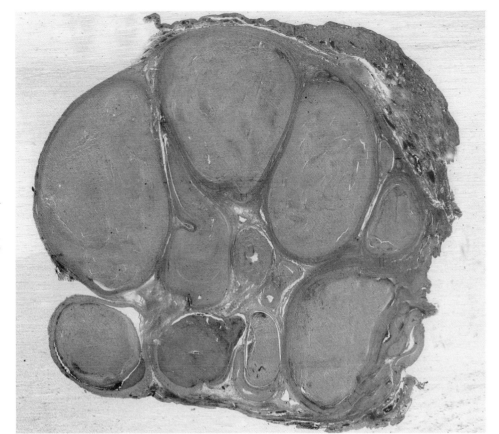

FIGURE 8.45

Low-grade endometrial stromal sarcoma. Plugs of densely packed blue tumor cells are filling and distending the parametrial vessels in a tumor that was centered in the uterus.

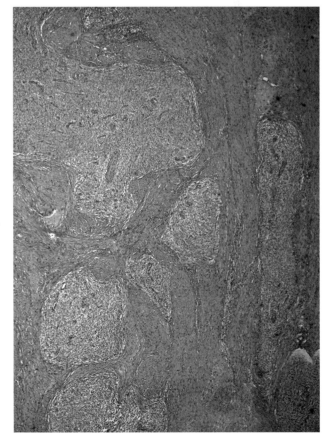

FIGURE 8.46

Low-grade endometrial stromal sarcoma. Irregular islands of small blue cells are diffusely permeating the myometrium.

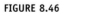

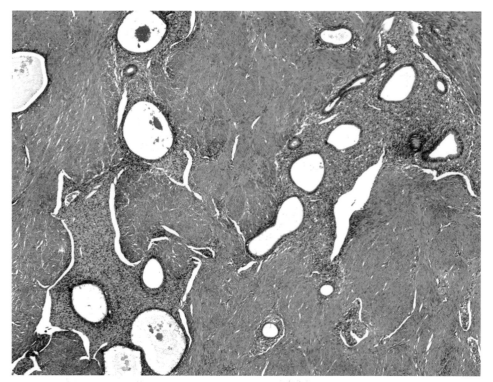

FIGURE 8.47

Low-grade endometrial stromal sarcoma with glandular differentiation. Benign endometrial-type glands are intimately admixed with the neoplastic endometrial stroma and diffusely permeate the myometrium.

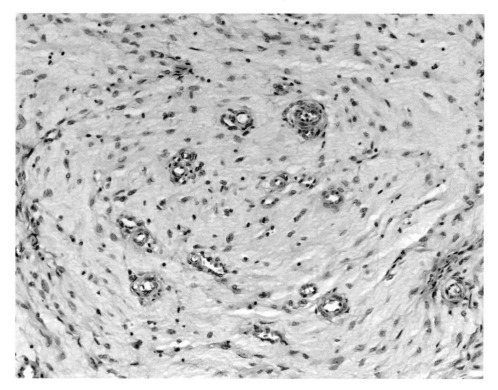

FIGURE 8.48

Low-grade endometrial stromal tumor with myxoid change. Prominent arteriole-like vessels are seen in a striking hypocellular myxoid background.

lioid islands in a background of endometrial stromal neoplasia, or more characteristically as nodules with prominent central hyalinization (so-called "starburst" pattern) with collagen bands radiating towards the periphery where plump round cells are embedded (Figure 8.49). These nodules may be juxtaposed with small and disorganized bundles of immature muscle or adjacent to more organized and mature bundles of muscle. The smooth muscle component almost always has benign cytologic features. Smooth muscle may be identified grossly in some cases as firm, white areas alternating with tan to yellow soft areas. Smooth muscle differentiation should account for at least 30% of the tumor based on hematoxylin-eosin examination to be included in the report. A common pitfall in the evaluation of these tumors is posed by the irregular interdigitation of the two components, particularly when the smooth muscle is mature and relatively well organized, as it may be misconstrued as myometrium, and thus a well-circumscribed tumor may be misinterpreted as an invasive low-grade endometrial stromal sarcoma. In such cases, it is crucial to appreciate the existence of regions with divergent differentiation within the mass, rather than invasion into the myometrium. Endometrial stromal tumors with unusual types of differentiation should be reported as ESN or low-grade endometrial stromal sarcoma based on the margins of the tumors, as this is the discriminating prognostic factor in these tumors.

BOX 8.4

ENDOMETRIAL STROMAL TUMOR VARIANTS

1. Smooth muscle
2. Fibrous or myxoid
3. Endometrioid-type glands
4. Sex cord-like
5. Skeletal muscle
6. Epithelioid and/or eosinophilic
7. Clear cells
8. Rhabdoid
9. With bizarre nuclei
10. Fat

ANCILLARY STUDIES

IMMUNOHISTOCHEMISTRY

Endometrial stromal tumors are typically immunoreactive for vimentin, muscle specific actin, smooth muscle actin, and frequently keratin. Most endometrial stromal tumors as well as normal endometrial stromal cells stain for CD10. However, it is important to point out that smooth muscle tumors, mixed müllerian tumors (including low-grade müllerian adenosarcoma and malignant mixed müllerian tumor), or even rhabdomyosarcomas may be CD10-positive. Thus, this antibody should not be used in isolation when evaluating the cell of origin in a mesenchymal tumor of the uterus. Desmin staining in endometrial stromal tumors varies among studies and it should not be used in isolation to differentiate these tumors from smooth muscle tumors. Other muscle markers, including h-caldesmon, myosin, and HDCA8, are also helpful in this differential diagnosis. Areas of smooth muscle differentiation are positive for all smooth muscle markers as well as for CD10. Areas of sex cord-like differentiation may be positive for inhibin, calretinin, CD99, WT-1, and Melan-A. Finally, endometrial stromal tumors frequently contain ER and PR, although the presence of these receptors is not specific.

CYTOGENETICS

Conventional endometrial stromal tumors as well as endometrial stromal tumors with smooth muscle differentiation and those with fibrous or myxoid change

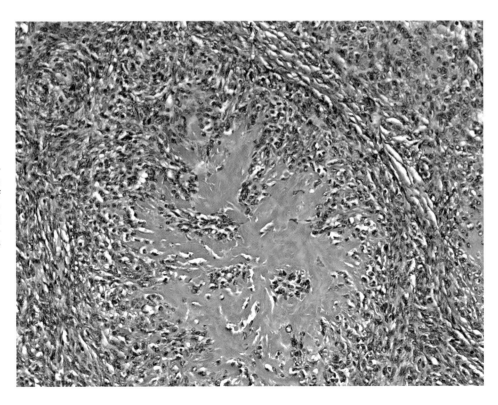

FIGURE 8.49

Low-grade endometrial stromal tumor with smooth-muscle differentiation (starburst pattern). A central area of hyalinization is associated with radiating bands of collagen embedding round neoplastic cells at the periphery which merge with short fascicles of spindled cells.

show as most common translocation t(7;17) with involvement of two zinc finger genes, *JAZF1* and *JJAZ1*.

DIFFERENTIAL DIAGNOSIS

Highly cellular leiomyoma is the lesion that most frequently causes problems in the differential diagnosis with a low-grade endometrial stromal sarcoma, as both tumors share dense cellularity, prominent vascularity, and an irregular margin with the surrounding myometrium. However, highly cellular leiomyoma has fascicular growth at the periphery of the lesion, tumor cells merge with the surrounding myometrium, and vessels are typically thick and large, in contrast to the delicate arteriolar network present in endometrial stromal tumors. *Intravenous leiomyomatosis* may cause confusion with low-grade endometrial stromal sarcoma because both show prominent intravascular growth and on occasion intravenous leiomyomatosis may be as cellular as a low-grade endometrial stromal sarcoma. The findings of a clefted contour, focal fascicular growth, thick-walled vessels and hydropic change, as seen in conventional leiomyoma, are helpful in this differential diagnosis. The finding of tumor cells "colonizing" the walls of veins also supports the diagnosis of intravenous leiomyomatosis.

Among benign lesions, an *endometrial polyp* may not infrequently be fragmented in a curettage specimen and some of the fragments may consist of cellular stroma, raising concern for an endometrial stromal tumor. Features helpful in separating these entities include a compact, atrophic appearance of the endometrial stroma of the polyp in which vessels, if prominent, tend to be large, thick-walled, and irregularly distributed. In contrast, an endometrial stromal tumor (either a nodule or a low-grade endometrial stromal sarcoma) has an expansile appearance with active growth of the endometrial stroma (typical vascular network, plump cells, and some mitotic activity). *Adenomyosis* enters into the differential diagnosis with low-grade endometrial stromal sarcoma, as it may show a scant glandular component or the gland-poor adenomyotic foci may be seen within vascular spaces. However, adenomyosis is typically an incidental finding, which even in florid cases produces only an ill-defined nodularity or asymmetric thickening of the uterine wall. Furthermore, there is an atrophic appearance of the stromal cells which lack mitotic activity, in contrast to the expansile growth of the stromal nests and proliferative appearance of the cells in low-grade endometrial stromal sarcoma. Typical areas of adenomyosis are usually present in close vicinity, whereas other typical features of low-grade endometrial stromal sarcoma are lacking. On the other hand, low-grade endometrial stromal sarcoma may have glands and mimic adenomyosis; however, the former has an expansile growth of the stromal component with an active proliferative appearance. Low-grade endometrial stromal sarcoma with gland differentiation should also

be distinguished from *low-grade müllerian adenosarcoma* as both show endometrial-type stroma admixed with müllerian-type glands. However, intraluminal polypoid projections of stroma as well as hypercellular collaring around the glands are lacking in low-grade endometrial stromal sarcoma.

Uterine tumor resembling an ovarian sex cord tumor (UTROSCT) may enter in this differential diagnosis as low-grade endometrial stromal sarcoma may have extensive sex cord-like differentiation. As mentioned earlier, if no evident endometrial stromal component is seen in the curettage specimen, the final diagnosis can only be established with a hysterectomy specimen.

A low-grade endometrial stromal sarcoma at metastatic sites may have a different morphologic appearance than the primary tumor, and in these cases, the differential diagnosis may include primary tumors at those specific locations. For example, an endometrial stromal sarcoma metastatic to the ovary may simulate a *sex cord-stromal tumor*, while in the lung it may simulate a *solitary fibrous tumor*, and in the gastrointestinal tract the differential diagnosis may include a *gastrointestinal stromal tumor*. CD34 and ER may be helpful in the differential diagnosis of endometrial stromal sarcoma and solitary fibrous tumor as the latter is ER negative and CD34 positive, while the opposite profile is seen in low-grade endometrial stromal sarcoma. Gastrointestinal stromal tumors are positive for c-kit and CD34, markers typically not expressed in low-grade endometrial stromal sarcoma.

PROGNOSIS AND TREATMENT

Patients with low-grade endometrial stromal sarcoma have a 5-year survival rate of approximately 60–80%. These tumors have a low malignant potential and are characterized by late recurrences, even in patients with stage I disease, as one-third or more of them develop recurrences. The most common sites of recurrence include pelvis (occurring in up to one-half of the patients up to 20 years later), abdomen and vagina, and less frequently, lung (up to 27 years later). Standard initial surgical treatment encompasses total abdominal hysterectomy accompanied by bilateral salpingo-oophorectomy because these tumors are often hormone-sensitive and it has been shown that patients retaining their ovaries have a much higher risk of recurrence (up to 100%). Patients with tumors extending outside the uterus usually undergo debulking of any visible tumor. Lymph node dissection does not seem to have a role in treatment. Patients may also receive adjuvant radiation or hormonal treatment with progestational agents (as these tumors are frequently PR positive) or alternatively they can be treated with aromatase inhibitors. The same treatment may be used for recurrent or metastatic tumor. Postoperative radiation therapy may improve local control of the disease but it does not improve the frequency of distal recurrences or overall survival.

UTERINE TUMORS RESEMBLING OVARIAN SEX CORD TUMORS

These tumors constitute an unusual group of neoplasms defined by the presence of pure or prominent microscopic patterns closely overlapping with those seen in sex cord-stromal tumors of the ovary without an associated conspicuous endometrial stromal component. Even though most investigators classify these tumors as a variant of endometrial stromal tumors, the most recent WHO classification of tumors of the uterine corpus placed them in the miscellaneous category and designated them as "sex cord-like tumors."

CLINICAL FEATURES

These tumors may be seen in either reproductive- or postmenopausal-age patients. They frequently present with abnormal vaginal bleeding or uterine enlargement, but patients may be asymptomatic.

PATHOLOGIC FEATURES

GROSS FINDINGS

Most tumors are centered in the uterine corpus, either myometrium or endometrium, but they have rarely been reported in the cervix. They are typically well circumscribed and polypoid if endometrial-based, with a mean diameter of 6 cm. On sectioning, they frequently show a homogeneous yellow to tan cut surface.

MICROSCOPIC FINDINGS

On low-power examination, most tumors are well circumscribed, but some may infiltrate in between the muscle fibers of the surrounding myometrium. They typically recapitulate the different growth patterns seen in sex cord-stromal tumors of the ovary. These include diffuse sheets, tight nests, thin cords, broad interconnecting trabeculae (Figure 8.50), irregular islands, hollow or solid tubules (Figure 8.51), and rarely a retiform architecture separated by variable amounts of fibrous stroma that may be hyalinized. The cells vary from small with scant cytoplasm to large with abundant eosinophilic, clear, or foamy cytoplasm reminiscent of Sertoli or granulosa cells. No Leydig cell differentiation has been reported in these tumors, although some cases have been described to contain luteinized-like cells. The nuclei range from small to medium-sized, they are round to oval, and rarely grooved, with inconspicuous nucleoli and typically low mitotic rates are present. Importantly, no neoplastic endometrial stroma should be identified within the tumor.

UTERINE TUMOR RESEMBLING OVARIAN SEX CORD-STROMAL TUMOR – FACT SHEET

Definition
▸ Tumors with pure or prominent microscopic patterns that closely overlap with those seen in sex cord-stromal tumors of the ovary without an associated conspicuous endometrial stromal component

Incidence
▸ Rare

Age Distribution
▸ Typically reproductive-age and postmenopausal women

Clinical Features
▸ Abnormal vaginal bleeding
▸ Enlarged uterus
▸ May be asymptomatic

Prognosis and Treatment
▸ Excellent prognosis, only rare recurrences
▸ Excision or simple hysterectomy

UTERINE TUMOR RESEMBLING OVARIAN SEX CORD-STROMAL TUMOR – PATHOLOGIC FEATURES

Gross Findings
▸ Well circumscribed
▸ Polypoid if endometrial-based
▸ Variable size (mean 6 cm)
▸ Homogeneous yellow to tan cut surface

Microscopic Findings
▸ Well circumscribed but rarely may infiltrate between neighboring muscle fibers
▸ Sheets, tight nests, thin cords, broad interconnecting trabeculae, irregular islands, hollow or solid tubules, and rarely retiform
▸ Variable amounts of fibrous stroma ± hyalinization
▸ Cells with scant to abundant eosinophilic, clear, or foamy cytoplasm reminiscent of Sertoli or granulosa cells
▸ Bland cytologic features with rare mitoses in most cases
▸ No areas of endometrial stromal neoplasia

Immunohistochemical Features
▸ Smooth muscle markers, WT-1 and CD10 frequently positive
▸ Inhibin, calretinin, CD99, Melan-A and epithelial markers variably positive
▸ ER and PR positive

Differential Diagnosis
▸ Endometrial stromal nodule or low-grade endometrial stromal sarcoma with extensive sex cord-like differentiation
▸ Epithelioid smooth muscle tumor
▸ Endometrial carcinoma with a sex cord arrangement

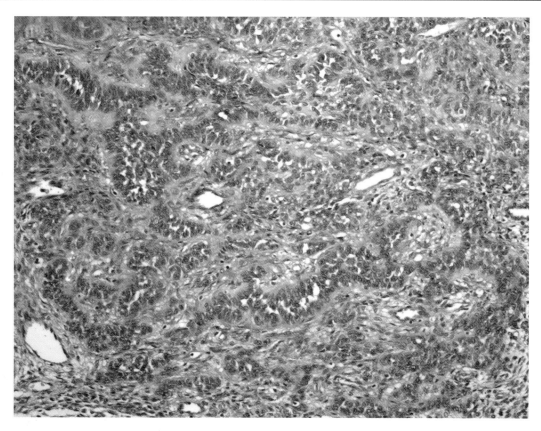

FIGURE 8.50
Uterine tumor resembling ovarian sex cord tumor. Anastomosing cords and trabeculae are seen in a relatively hyalinized background.

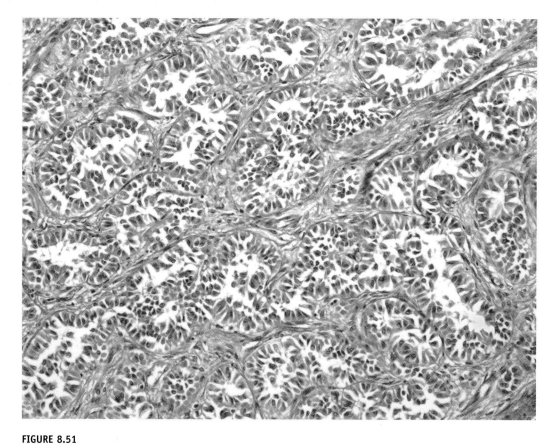

FIGURE 8.51
Uterine tumor resembling ovarian sex cord tumor. Relatively well-developed tubules are lined by cells with abundant eosinophilic cytoplasm.

ANCILLARY STUDIES

IMMUNOHISTOCHEMISTRY

The tumor cells are frequently positive for smooth muscle markers and variably positive for epithelial markers, inhibin, calretinin, CD99, Melan-A, WT-1, and CD10. This immunohistochemical profile is indistinguishable from sex cord areas in endometrial stromal tumors. The tumors also express ER and PR.

ULTRASTRUCTURAL EXAMINATION

Ultrastructural studies of UTROSCT have yielded different interpretations regarding its differentiation, including epithelial, smooth muscle, and sex cord. The finding of cells resting in a basal lamina and the presence of desmosomes favor epithelial differentiation. On the other hand, the finding of external lamina, abundant intermediate filaments, and subplasmalemmal densities in some tumors is consistent with smooth muscle differentiation. However, the absence of cytoplasmic dense bodies with associated actin-like filaments argues against it. The background stroma shows evidence of fibroblastic and myofibroblastic differentiation.

DIFFERENTIAL DIAGNOSIS

Endometrial stromal tumors with extensive sex cord-like differentiation, either an ESN or a low-grade endometrial stromal sarcoma, should be considered before establishing the diagnosis of UTROSCT. Endometrial stromal tumors will display well-defined areas of pure endometrial stromal neoplasia. However, the distinction may be difficult in curettage specimens. In such cases, the best approach includes a descriptive diagnosis of stromal tumor with sex cord-like differentiation, stating in a note that the tumor could either represent an endometrial stromal tumor with massive sex cord-like elements or a UTROSCT, and thus, a hysterectomy is needed to further categorize the tumor. Immunohistochemical stains are not helpful in this differential diagnosis.

Epithelioid smooth muscle tumors are the other main category of tumors in the differential diagnosis. These tumors are composed of epithelial-like cells that may be arranged in cords, trabeculae, and nests, closely mimicking the microscopic patterns of UTROSCTs. Furthermore, the immunohistochemical profile shows overlap, as both tumors are positive for muscle markers and can be positive for epithelial markers, WT-1 and CD10. Smooth muscle tumors are typically negative for inhibin and calretinin. The distinction is important as most UTROSCTs behave in a benign fashion, whereas epithelioid smooth muscle tumors frequently recur or metastasize, particularly when associated with some degree of mitotic activity. Finally, *endometrial carcinomas with a sex cord arrangement* may superficially mimic a UTROSCT. However, conventional areas of obvious glandular differentiation, higher degree of cytologic atypia, as well as absence of immunoreactivity for smooth muscle or sex cord markers will support the diagnosis of carcinoma.

PROGNOSIS AND TREATMENT

Most of these tumors behave in a benign fashion, in part because they are small or well circumscribed and can be treated by hysterectomy or excision, especially in women of reproductive age. Recurrences or metastases are rare and, in general, only close follow-up is advised.

UNDIFFERENTIATED ENDOMETRIAL SARCOMA

The lack of specific evidence of endometrial stromal cell origin in most cases precludes their placement in the endometrial stromal group of uterine tumors (Figure 8.52). Destructive myometrial invasion is common, but, the intravascular worm-like plugs of tumor characteristic of low-grade endometrial stromal sarcoma are typically absent. These tumors have marked cellular pleomorphism and brisk mitotic activity, and carry a very poor prognosis. The diagnosis of undifferentiated endometrial sarcoma should only be made after extensive sampling has excluded smooth or skeletal muscle differentiation or even small foci of carcinoma (the latter finding would result in a diagnosis of malignant mixed müllerian tumor). Occasional tumors have a component of low-grade endometrial stromal sarcoma, indicating that, in these cases, the high-grade component is presumably of endometrial stromal derivation.

MIXED MÜLLERIAN TUMORS

These tumors are divided into six main categories by the WHO (Box 8.5): (1) müllerian adenofibroma; (2) low-grade müllerian adenosarcoma; (3) malignant mixed müllerian tumor; (4) carcinofibroma; (5) carcinomesenchymoma; and (6) adenomyoma. Only the three most common subtypes will be discussed here, including low-grade müllerian adenosarcoma, malignant mixed müllerian tumor, and adenomyomas.

LOW-GRADE MÜLLERIAN ADENOSARCOMA

This is a rare variant in the category of mixed müllerian tumors characterized by an admixture of a benign (or sometimes atypical) epithelial component with a low-

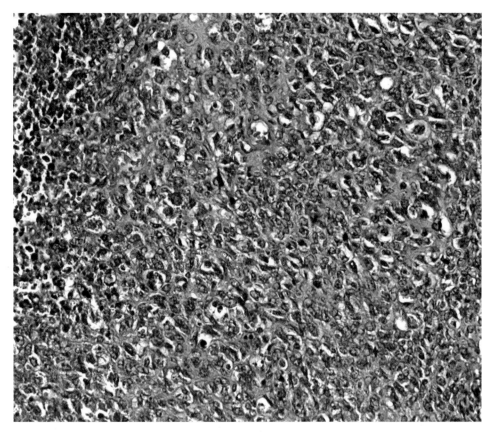

FIGURE 8.52
Undifferentiated endometrial sarcoma. Highly malignant poorly differentiated mesenchymal cells are associated with focal necrosis.

BOX 8.5

MIXED MÜLLERIAN TUMORS OF THE UTERUS

Müllerian adenofibroma
Low-grade Müllerian adenosarcoma
   Homologous
   Heterologous
Malignant mixed müllerian tumor
   Homologous
   Heterologous
Müllerian carcinofibroma and carcinomesenchymoma
Müllerian adenomyoma
   Endometrioid-type
   Endocervical-type
   Atypical polypoid adenomyoma

---

grade malignant stromal component. It represents approximately 8% of uterine sarcomas.

CLINICAL FEATURES

Low-grade müllerian adenosarcoma typically occurs in postmenopausal women (median age 58 years), but 30% are found in premenopausal patients, while those arising in the cervix tend to occur at a younger age. Frequently, they present with abnormal vaginal bleeding, often accompanied by pelvic pain and an enlarged uterus. In one-half of cases, tumor protrudes through the external os. Occasionally, the diagnosis is made in retrospect in patients who have a history of recurrent endometrial or endocervical polyps. Associated risk factors include hyperestrinism (e.g. tamoxifen therapy) and prior radiation therapy.

RADIOLOGIC FEATURES

The tumors are frequently seen on MRI imaging as a large multiseptated cystic mass with multiple heterogeneous solid components that fill the endometrial cavity. The solid component has low signal intensity on T2-weighted MRI images and enhances on contrast-enhanced T1-weighted images.

PATHOLOGIC FEATURES

GROSS FINDINGS

Most low-grade müllerian adenosarcomas arise in the endometrium but they may originate in the cervix (9%) or be centered within the myometrium (4%). They may be solitary, sessile, or pedunculated, polypoid to papillary intraluminal tumors with a mean size of 5 (range 1–20) cm (Figure 8.53A). The cut surface varies from firm to soft and spongy secondary to variably sized cysts, but it can also be clefted, reminiscent of a phyllodes tumor (Figure 8.53B). Myometrial invasion is only rarely appreciated.

MICROSCOPIC FINDINGS

On low-power scrutiny, the tumors show a biphasic growth of benign glands and low-grade malignant stroma. The glands are often dilated or show a papillary or leaf-like configuration with frequent polypoid intraluminal projections of the stroma (Figures 8.54 and 8.55). The stromal component shows condensation around the glands, a phenomenon described as "periglandular collaring" (Figure 8.56). On high power, the glands are frequently lined by endometrioid-type epithelium, but also may contain mucinous, squamous, ciliated, or hobnail-type cells. The lining epithelium is typically benign but occasionally may be atypical. The stromal component is a low-grade sarcoma in 80% of cases, resembling a low-grade endometrial stromal sarcoma, fibrosarcoma, or combinations thereof. This stroma is typically more cellular around the glands and

in these areas, the cells show higher nuclear-to-cytoplasmic ratio with enlarged nuclei and prominent nucleoli (Figure 8.57). In areas away from the glands, the stroma is typically less cellular or even hypocellular and may be myxoid or hyalinized. The cells are smaller and cyto-

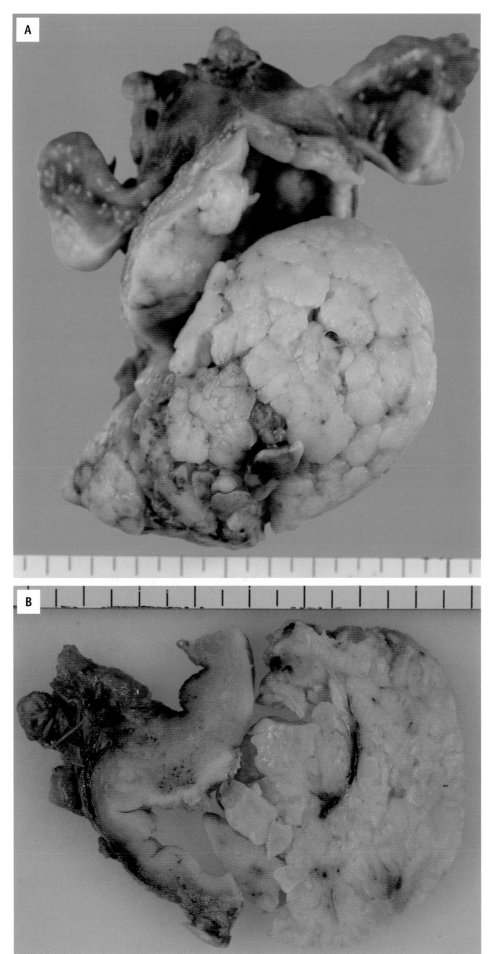

FIGURE 8.53

Low-grade müllerian adenosarcoma. A large polypoid mass distends the endometrial cavity (A), and a prominent leaf-like outline is seen on cut surface (B).

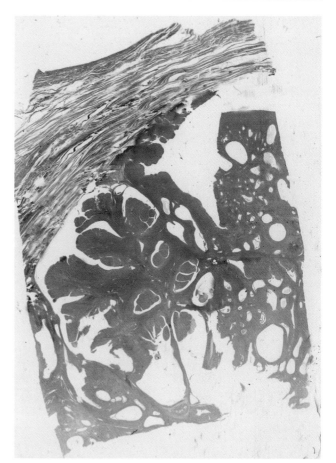

FIGURE 8.54

Low-grade müllerian adenosarcoma. The tumor has a pushing margin into the myometrium and contains multiple cysts, some of them with a complex papillary architecture.

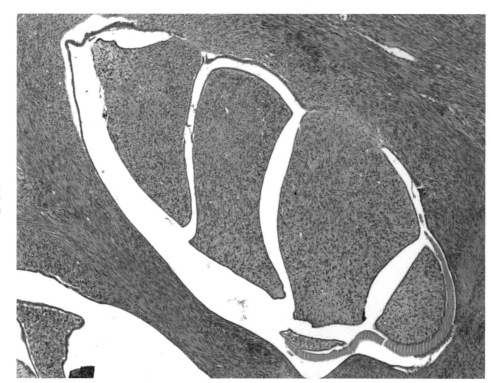

FIGURE 8.55

Low-grade müllerian adenosarcoma. Multiple stromal intraluminal polypoid projections are seen, imparting a "phyllodes" appearance.

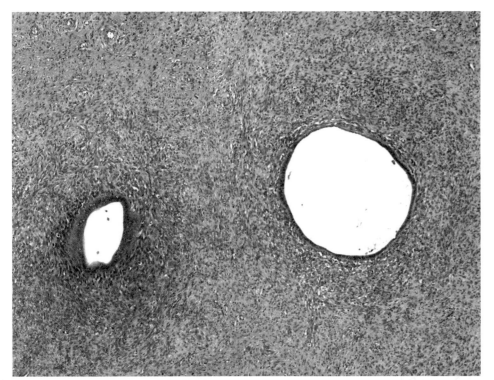

FIGURE 8.56

Low-grade müllerian adenosarcoma. Condensation of the malignant stromal cells around the epithelial elements is seen ("periglandular collaring").

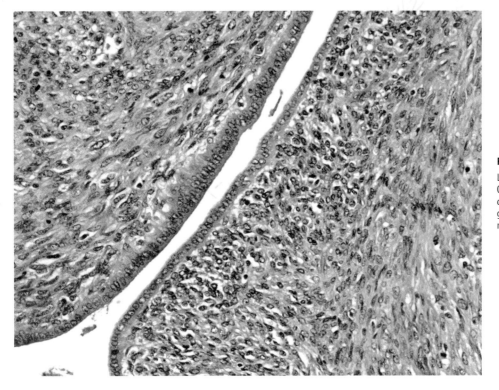

FIGURE 8.57

Low-grade müllerian adenosarcoma. Collaring of malignant mesenchymal cells around the endometrial-type gland showing cytologic atypia and mitotic activity.

logically less atypical. Mitotic activity of the stromal component is higher but still variable around the glands (mean 9/10 HPFs). A cut-off ≥ 4 mitoses/10 HPFs has been used to establish the diagnosis of adenosarcoma, as over two-thirds of tumors have been reported to have such counts; however, of note, some cases with lower mitotic counts have behaved in an aggressive fashion. It is important to search diligently for mitoses in the hypercellular areas, as some tumors may be underdiagnosed. Useful criteria in diagnosing low-grade müllerian adenosarcoma include the finding of ≥ 2 mitoses/

10 HPFs in the stromal component, marked stromal cellularity, or significant cytologic atypia of the stromal component. Myometrial invasion is found in one-sixth of tumors and is superficial in most cases. Vascular invasion is rarely seen.

Sarcomatous overgrowth ("müllerian adenosarcoma with sarcomatous overgrowth", MASO) occurs in 10 % of tumors. To establish the diagnosis of MASO, the area of pure sarcoma should occupy at least 25 % of the tumor volume or 1 low-power field in one slide. The sarcoma in most cases is high-grade with a destructive

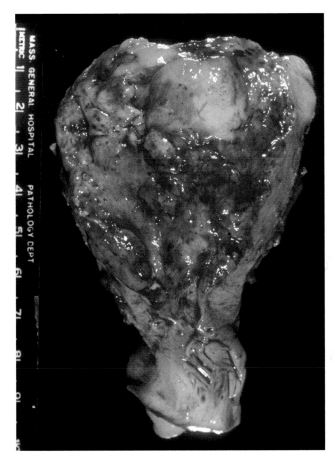

FIGURE 8.58

Low-grade müllerian adenosarcoma with sarcomatous overgrowth. Multiple fleshy nodules are diffusely present in the endometrium and focally infiltrate deeply into the myometrium.

growth, but it can have a similar appearance to the low-grade sarcoma of conventional adenosarcoma (Figures 8.58 and 8.59). Tumors with stromal overgrowth invade the myometrium more often and deeply than those without overgrowth.

Heterologous elements are seen in approximately 20–25% of low-grade müllerian adenosarcomas, varying from minor foci of fat, cartilage, or rhabdomyoblasts to embryonal rhabdomyosarcoma occupying most or all of the stroma. Cases containing nodules of fetal-type cartilage are typically seen in the cervix. Sex cord-like elements are seen in up to 7% of tumors and may occupy up to 50% of the tumor. They are present within the stromal component and are composed of benign-appearing epithelial-type cells arranged in nests, trabeculae, cords, and solid or hollow tubules. The cells have eosinophilic or foamy, lipid-rich cytoplasm and round to oval nuclei with inconspicuous nucleoli. Smooth muscle differentiation can be extensive. Multinucleated giant cells, as seen in the lower female genital tract and in endometrial polyps, typically have enlarged atypical nuclei with smudgy chromatin but no mitotic activity. Abundant xanthoma cells with a histiocytic appearance may occupy large areas of the tumor.

ANCILLARY STUDIES

IMMUNOHISTOCHEMISTRY

The stromal component of a low-grade müllerian adenosarcoma is typically positive for vimentin, WT1, CD10, ER and PR with variable expression of cytokeratin, muscle actin, and AR, an immunohistochemical

FIGURE 8.59

Low-grade müllerian adenosarcoma with sarcomatous overgrowth. Spindled cells with cytologic atypia and brisk mitotic activity are present in the absence of an epithelial component.

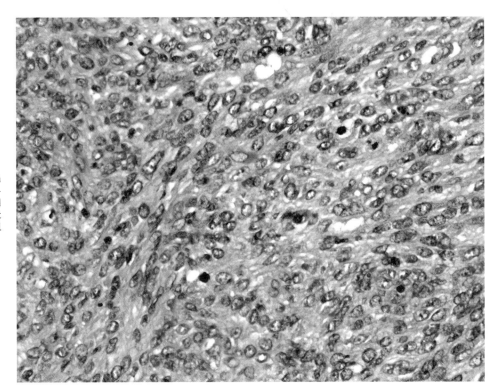

profile that overlaps with that of endometrial stromal neoplasms. Areas of MASO are frequently CD10, ER, and PR negative.

HISTOGENESIS

Low-grade müllerian adenosarcomas have an uncertain origin. It appears that 9–15% of carcinosarcomas have an adenosarcoma-like component and it is hypothesized that these tumors have a common origin. However, the majority of malignant mixed müllerian tumors are felt to represent dedifferentiated carcinomas, as shown by immunohistochemical, ultrastructural, and genetic data, findings not reported in müllerian adenosarcomas. It is also hypothesized that these tumors may originate from endometrial stromal cells and have a common origin with endometrial stromal tumors.

DIFFERENTIAL DIAGNOSIS

Cellular endometrial polyps may be confused at low power with a low-grade müllerian adenosarcoma. However, the stroma is homogeneously cellular with no periglandular cuffing. Cytologic atypia and mitotic activity are absent in the stromal component. It is important to keep in mind that adenosarcomas may arise in endometrial/endocervical polyps and that endometrial polyps may also contain cells with bizarre nuclei, as has been reported in low-grade müllerian adenosarcomas.

Müllerian adenofibromas are extremely rare, accounting for < 5% of tumors in the category of mixed müllerian tumors. They have benign epithelial and stromal components. The features of the epithelial elements overlap with those seen in adenosarcomas. In contrast to müllerian adenosarcomas, the stromal component is hypocellular, does not condense around the glands, lacks cytologic atypia, and shows only rare mitoses (< 2/10 HPFs).

Atypical polypoid adenomyoma, like low-grade müllerian adenosarcoma, is a biphasic tumor containing smooth muscle. However, in atypical polypoid adenomyoma, smooth muscle is the predominant mesenchymal component that is typically seen intimately admixed with a glandular component frequently associated with squamous morules. There is no periglandular cuffing, intraluminal polypoid projections, and no heterologous components. Furthermore, at low-power examination, atypical polypoid adenomyoma shows a vague nodular arrangement of the glandular and mesenchymal components, a feature not seen in adenosarcoma.

Malignant mixed müllerian tumor is the most common tumor in the category of mixed müllerian tumors, but in contrast to adenosarcoma, the carcinomatous and mesenchymal components are typically high-grade. Moreover, the phyllodes-type glands and the periglandular stromal condensation of adenosarcoma are lacking.

Endometrial stromal sarcoma with glandular or sex cord-like differentiation may enter into the differential diagnosis. However, low-grade endometrial stromal sarcoma shows the typical lymphovascular invasion and tongue-like infiltrative growth pattern but not the destructive myometrial invasion seen in adenosarcoma. Furthermore, epithelial elements are typically scant without the typical appearance of an adenosarcoma.

Low-grade müllerian adenosarcoma with sarcomatous overgrowth should be distinguished from a *pure high-grade sarcoma* or a *malignant mixed müllerian tumor*, which may be difficult in small samples. Additional sampling is required in these cases, as immunohistochemical stains may not be helpful in arriving at the correct diagnosis.

In the cervix, the most important and difficult differential diagnosis is that of an *embryonal rhabdomyosarcoma*, as both tumors present as polypoid masses, show condensation of stroma around the glands and beneath the surface epithelium, display heterologous elements such as cartilage (rhabdomyosarcoma in 50% and adenosarcoma in 25% of cases respectively), and low-grade müllerian adenosarcoma may uncommonly show rhabdomyoblastic differentiation. Distinguishing features include a more edematous/myxoid background, a sparse glandular component (which is largely entrapped), and absence of leaf-like or cystic glands in embryonal rhabdomyosarcoma.

PROGNOSIS AND TREATMENT

This tumor has low malignant potential, characterized predominantly by late local recurrences (primarily vaginal or pelvic) in approximately 25–40% of patients. Long-term follow-up is required. Distant metastases and death occur in < 5% and between 10% and 20% of patients respectively. Hematogenous spread occurs in < 10% of patients, all of whom have purely sarcomatous tumors. The histology of the recurrent tumor is a pure sarcoma (70%), less frequently an adenocarcinoma (30%), and rarely a carcinosarcoma. The only morphologic features that have been associated with a high rate of recurrence are deep myometrial invasion and the presence of MASO. The latter is associated with a greater frequency of deep myometrial invasion (60% versus 25% in conventional adenosarcomas), recurrences, hematogenous metastases, and death from tumor (70%, 40%, and 60% of patients respectively, even in patients with stage I MASO). Some studies have reported that the prognosis for MASO is even worse than that of malignant mixed müllerian tumor. It is not clear whether the presence of heterologous elements in the stromal component is of prognostic significance; however, rhabdomyosarcomatous differentiation has been associated with a worse prognosis in some studies. Surgical therapy consisting of total abdominal hysterectomy and bilateral salpingo-oophorectomy is the cornerstone of treatment. Patients with stage I or II MASO may undergo lymph node sampling and receive whole pelvis radiation, whereas intraperitoneal disease may be treated with whole abdomen radiation or chemotherapy. However, there is no consensus regarding adjuvant therapy, as experience with MASO is limited.

CARCINOSARCOMA (MALIGNANT MIXED MÜLLERIAN TUMOR)

These tumors represent the most common subtype of mixed müllerian tumors, accounting for almost half of all uterine sarcomas but < 5 % of all malignant tumors of the uterus. They are defined as tumors composed of an admixture of malignant epithelial and mesenchymal components. They are currently designated as "carcinosarcomas" by the WHO classification, although the term "malignant mixed müllerian tumor" is more often utilized.

CLINICAL FEATURES

Carcinosarcomas tumors typically occur in postmenopausal women (mean age 65 years), but may be seen in younger patients (< 5 % in patients ≤ 50 years), and seem to affect black women more commonly. The typical presenting signs and symptoms include postmenopausal bleeding followed by an enlarged uterus and/or pelvic pain. Up to two-thirds of patients present at an advanced stage with tumor extending outside the uterus (stage III–IV). It has been shown that carcinosarcoma and endometrioid endometrial adenocarcinoma share similar risk factors. Both tumors are associated with obesity, use of exogenous estrogens, tamoxifen therapy, and nulliparity. In contrast, oral contraceptive use protects against both. Finally, up to 37 % of women with carcinosarcoma have a history of previous radiation; these women develop tumor at a younger age. Patients with tumors arising in the cervix present with vaginal bleeding and are found to have a polypoid mass protruding from the cervical os. Tumors in the cervix have been related to HPV infection, as occurs with the majority of primary epithelial cervical lesions. Serum CEA level is elevated in the majority of patients.

RADIOLOGIC FEATURES

These tumors may show findings similar to endometrial carcinomas but tend to manifest as a larger, more heterogeneous mass, with the polypoid portion of the tumor showing intense enhancement, with frequent hemorrhage, necrosis, and myometrial invasion.

PATHOLOGIC FEATURES

GROSS FINDINGS

Carcinosarcomas appear typically as large, bulky polypoid masses, filling the uterine cavity and prolapsing through the endocervical canal. The cut surface is

---

MALIGNANT MIXED MÜLLERIAN TUMOR – FACT SHEET

Definition
▸ Tumor composed of malignant epithelial and mesenchymal elements, commonly admixed

Incidence
▸ Approximately half of all uterine sarcomas
▸ < 5% of malignant tumors of the uterus

Race and Age Distribution
▸ Higher incidence in black women
▸ Postmenopausal women (mean age 65 years)
▸ < 5% in patients ≤50 years

Clinical Features
▸ Postmenopausal bleeding
▸ Enlarged uterus and/or pelvic pain
▸ Risk factors similar to those associated with endometrial cancer (obesity, exogenous estrogens, tamoxifen therapy, nulliparity)
▸ History of previous radiation in up to 37% of women (younger age at presentation)
▸ Vaginal bleeding and polypoid mass through os in cervical tumors
▸ HPV linkage in cervical tumors
▸ Elevated serum CEA level

Radiologic Features
▸ Large, heterogeneous mass
▸ Intense enhancement of polypoid portion with frequent hemorrhage, necrosis, and myometrial invasion

Prognosis and Treatment
▸ 5-year survival rate from 5 to 35% for all stages (median survival around 2 years for all stages)
▸ 5-year survival rate from 40 to 60% for stage I–II tumors
▸ Tumor extends outside the uterus (stages III–IV) at time of diagnosis in up to two-thirds
▸ Overall recurrence rate of 55%; ovaries, fallopian tubes, and omentum most common sites
▸ Carcinoma, infrequently carcinosarcoma, and rarely sarcoma seen in recurrences or metastases
▸ Tumor stage most important prognostic factor
▸ Higher incidence of metastases if serous and clear cell components
▸ Heterologous sarcomatous component may influence prognosis
▸ More extensive disease at time of diagnosis if radiation-induced
▸ Total abdominal hysterectomy with bilateral salpingo-oophorectomy, removal of pelvic and aortic lymph nodes, omentectomy, and peritoneal cytology
▸ Cisplatin-based chemotherapy for metastatic tumor and radiation for local disease

---

usually fleshy and often shows areas of hemorrhage and necrosis with secondary cyst formation (Figure 8.60). Myometrial invasion is frequently seen. Tumors uncommonly arise in the cervix, accounting for < 3 % of all uterine malignant mixed müllerian tumors.

MALIGNANT MIXED MÜLLERIAN TUMOR – PATHOLOGIC FEATURES

Gross Findings

▶ Large, bulky polypoid masses, filling uterine cavity and prolapsing through endocervical canal
▶ < 3% arise in cervix
▶ Fleshy cut surface
▶ Frequent hemorrhage and necrosis with secondary cyst formation
▶ Myometrial invasion common

Microscopic Findings

▶ Typically intimate but haphazard admixture of high-grade malignant epithelial and mesenchymal components; rarely, one or both components may be low-grade
▶ High-grade endometrioid carcinoma (more common), serous, clear cell, mucinous, squamous, or undifferentiated carcinoma (including small cell carcinoma)
▶ Endometrial hyperplasia, endometrial intraepithelial carcinoma, or frank carcinoma in adjacent endometrium in up to 50% of cases
▶ Squamous cell or adenoid cystic carcinoma (much less frequent) in cervical tumors with associated high-grade squamous intraepithelial neoplasia
▶ Homologous or heterologous (50%) sarcomatous component
▶ Homologous sarcomatous component resembles endometrial stromal sarcoma, leiomyosarcoma, malignant fibrous histiocytoma, or undifferentiated sarcoma
▶ Rhabdomyosarcoma, benign-appearing cartilage or chondrosarcoma, and less frequently osteosarcoma or liposarcoma as heterologous elements
▶ In cervical tumors, homologous sarcomatous elements present in a myxoid background
▶ Eosinophilic hyaline droplets are common but not indicative of rhabdomyoblastic differentiation

Immunohistochemical Features

▶ Cytokeratin, EMA, and vimentin positive in epithelial component and frequently in mesenchymal component
▶ Neuroendocrine markers (synaptophysin, neuron-specific enolase, and Leu-7) may be positive in epithelial component
▶ Vimentin and smooth muscle actin positive in mesenchymal component
▶ CD10 and CD34 may be positive in mesenchymal component
▶ Myoglobin, myogenin, MyoD1 positive in rhabdomyosarcoma component
▶ p53 positive in both components

Ultrastructural Features

▶ Epithelial cells surrounded by basal lamina
▶ "Hybrid" epithelial/stromal-appearing cells have prominent rough endoplasmic reticulum, cytoplasmic projections, poorly formed intercellular junctions, and incomplete basal lamina

Cytogenetic and Molecular Features

▶ Monoclonal nature of epithelial and mesenchymal components (identical patterns of X-chromosome inactivation, mutations of p53 and K-ras, and loss of heterozygosity for identical alleles)
▶ Multiple and complex chromosomal abnormalities

Differential Diagnosis

▶ Sarcomatoid endometrioid carcinoma
▶ Endometrioid carcinoma with heterologous elements
▶ Undifferentiated endometrial sarcoma, pure heterologous sarcoma
▶ Adenosarcoma with sarcomatous overgrowth

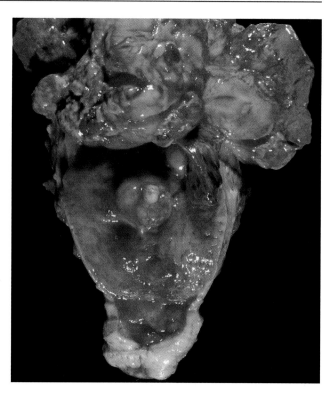

FIGURE 8.60

Malignant mixed müllerian tumor. Large and fleshy polypoid masses are associated with hemorrhage and necrosis.

MICROSCOPIC FINDINGS

Typically, there is an intimate but haphazard admixture of high-grade malignant epithelial and mesenchymal components, although in rare instances, one or both components may be low-grade and the proportion of each element is variable within each tumor. Thus, any uterine neoplasm composed of a high-grade sarcoma or carcinoma should be extensively sampled to exclude the possibility of malignant mixed müllerian tumor. The carcinomatous component is more frequently a high-grade endometrioid carcinoma with or without squamous differentiation (Figure 8.61), but it can also be represented by a serous carcinoma (Figure 8.62) and less frequently clear cell, mucinous, squamous, or undifferentiated carcinoma (including small cell carcinoma), or an admixture thereof. Spindle cell areas initially misinterpreted as sarcoma may be identified but when seen merging with solid epithelial clusters, a diagnosis of spindle cell carcinoma is more appropriate. Endometrial hyperplasia, endometrial intraepithelial carcinoma, or frank carcinoma (endometrioid or serous) in the adjacent endometrium is identified in up to 50% of cases. Cervical malignant mixed müllerian tumors typically contain a keratinizing, nonkeratinizing, or basaloid squamous cell carcinoma, and less frequently have an adenoid cystic carcinoma. High-grade squamous intraepithelial neoplasia is often seen overlying the tumor.

The sarcomatous component may be homologous or heterologous. The homologous sarcomatous component resembles endometrial stromal sarcoma, leiomyosar-

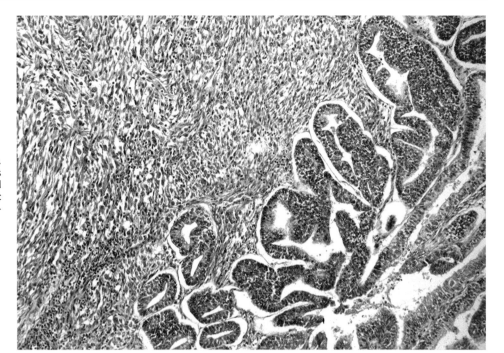

FIGURE 8.61

Malignant mixed müllerian tumor. Malignant endometrioid-type glands are juxtaposed to malignant spindled cells with abundant eosinophilic cytoplasm (rhabdomyosarcoma component).

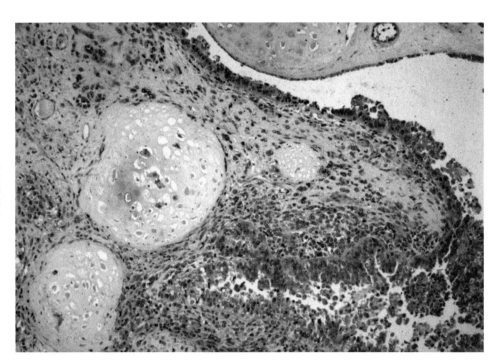

FIGURE 8.62

Malignant mixed müllerian tumor. Malignant epithelial cells forming small papillae (serous carcinoma) are admixed with malignant mesenchyme that focally shows cartilaginous differentiation.

coma, malignant fibrous histiocytoma, undifferentiated sarcoma, or any combination thereof. When heterologous elements are present (in approximately 50% of tumors), the most common include rhabdomyosarcoma (Figure 8.61), benign-appearing cartilage (Figure 8.62), or chondrosarcoma, and, less frequently, osteosarcoma or liposarcoma. Rarely, neuroectodermal, melanocytic, yolk sac, and rhabdoid differentiation may be seen. The heterologous elements typically merge with the homologous sarcoma. Eosinophilic hyaline droplets are a common finding, but their presence does not indicate rhabdomyoblastic differentiation. Tumors arising in the uterine cervix usually show homologous sarcomatous

elements that may be present in a myxoid background.

ANCILLARY STUDIES

IMMUNOHISTOCHEMISTRY

The carcinomatous elements are typically positive for epithelial markers (cytokeratin, EMA) and vimentin as seen in endometrial carcinoma. The sarcomatous elements are typically positive for vimentin and frequently for smooth muscle actin. They also frequently express epithelial markers, reflecting a common origin of these tumors. The sarcomatous component can also express CD10 and CD34. The rhabdomyosarcomatous component stains for myoglobin, myogenin, MyoD1, and CD34. The carcinomatous and sarcomatous elements may show positivity for neuroendocrine markers, including synaptophysin, neuron-specific enolase, and Leu-7. In most instances, immunohistochemical stains are not needed to establish the diagnosis of malignant mixed müllerian tumor, as this diagnosis is typically made on morphological basis. However, it may be helpful in delineating the two components of the tumor. p53 staining has been found in both the epithelial and mesenchymal components.

ULTRASTRUCTURAL EXAMINATION

At the ultrastructural level, epithelial cells are usually surrounded by basal lamina. Cells with a "hybrid" epithelial/mesenchymal appearance show prominent rough endoplasmic reticulum, cytoplasmic projections, poorly formed intercellular junctions, and incomplete basal lamina.

CYTOGENETICS AND MOLECULAR STUDIES

Identical patterns of X-chromosome inactivation as well as identical mutations of p53 and K-ras and loss of heterozygosity for identical alleles have been demonstrated in the epithelial and mesenchymal components of most carcinosarcomas. Although very limited data are available, most malignant mixed müllerian tumors have shown multiple and complex but not consistent chromosomal abnormalities. The findings support a monoclonal origin for most uterine carcinosarcomas.

HISTOGENESIS

Four main theories have been postulated to explain the histogenesis of malignant mixed müllerian tumors. The "composition" theory interpreted the spindle cell component as a pseudosarcomatous mesenchymal reaction to the carcinoma; however, it has been shown that the mesenchymal component of the tumor is also malignant, and this theory has been dismissed. The "collision" theory hypothesizes that two independent tumors collide, the epithelial and sarcomatous components appear distinct rather than admixed, and this theory may explain the origin of a small number of tumors. The "combination" theory hypothesizes that the two components arise from a common pluripotential cell; and finally in the "conversion" theory, the sarcomatous component evolves from the carcinomatous component by a metaplastic process or dedifferentiation. The "combination" and "conversion" theories are currently widely accepted as the modes of development of most malignant mixed müllerian tumors. Molecular data have shown that most tumors are monoclonal in origin, based on patterns of X-chromosome inactivation, loss of

heterozygosity, and p53 mutations. Furthermore, tissue culture studies have shown the conversion of carcinoma cells to sarcoma cells with transitional forms showing biphasic morphologic and immunohistochemical features. Finally, some malignant mixed müllerian tumors arising in the cervix have been shown to contain HPV DNA, with integrated HPV 16 being present in the carcinomatous and sarcomatous components.

DIFFERENTIAL DIAGNOSIS

Sarcomatoid endometrioid carcinoma, an uncommon type of endometrial carcinoma, can be distinguished from malignant mixed müllerian tumor because it shows transition from typical carcinomatous areas to spindled areas but lacks heterologous components. Another unusual variant of endometrial adenocarcinoma that may be confused with a malignant mixed müllerian tumor is the *endometrioid carcinoma with heterologous elements*; however, these tumors are characterized by otherwise typical endometrial carcinoma associated with minor foci of benign cartilage, fat, or bone. Finally, *undifferentiated endometrial sarcomas, pure heterologous sarcomas,* and *low-grade müllerian adenosarcomas with sarcomatous overgrowth* may cause problems if the carcinomatous component of the malignant mixed müllerian tumor is minor and therefore difficult to identify. In these cases, extensive sampling as well as immunohistochemistry may be needed to exclude the presence of an epithelial component.

PROGNOSIS AND TREATMENT

The 5-year survival rate ranges from 5 to 35% for patients with tumors of all stages, and 40 to 60% for stage I and II tumors, with a median survival around 2 years for all stages. Some studies have reported that the behavior of malignant mixed müllerian tumors is akin to high-grade endometrial carcinomas stage for stage, whereas other studies have shown that malignant mixed müllerian tumors behave more aggressively than both high-grade and high-risk endometrial carcinomas. Tumor stage is the most important independent prognostic factor, but recurrences may be encountered even in cases lacking myometrial invasion. Other important prognostic factors include depth of myometrial invasion, advanced age (> 70 years), and amount of residual tumor. Deep myometrial invasion is seen in 40% of tumors. Metastatic and recurrent tumor is more often composed of carcinoma, infrequently shows both components, and rarely consists of only sarcoma. The overall recurrence rate is 55% and the most common metastatic sites include ovaries, fallopian tubes, and omentum. Pulmonary metastases appear late in the course of the disease, as occurs with endometrial carcinoma. Within the carcinomatous component, serous and clear cell components are associated with a higher incidence of metastases, deep myometrial invasion, lymphatic or vascular invasion, and cervical extension – all parameters indicative of aggressive behavior. In contrast, within the sarcomatous component, only the presence of heterologous elements may affect prognosis. Radiation-induced tumors have more extensive disease at the time of diagnosis.

Appropriate treatment includes total abdominal hysterectomy with bilateral salpingo-oophorectomy, removal of pelvic and aortic lymph nodes, omentectomy, and peritoneal cytology. The role of adjuvant therapy is not clear but some studies have demonstrated the advantage of radiotherapy to disease-specific survival in early-stage tumors as well as local control in advanced-stage tumors. As malignant mixed müllerian tumors are associated with a high rate of distant metastases, chemotherapy is used, although the agents administered have traditionally been the same as those for uterine sarcomas. Modern cisplatin-based chemotherapy may lead to increased survival in patients with metastatic malignant mixed müllerian tumors.

MÜLLERIAN ADENOMYOMAS

ADENOMYOMA, ENDOCERVICAL-TYPE

This is a rare variant of adenomyoma composed of benign endocervical-type glands and smooth muscle typically arising within the cervix.

CLINICAL FEATURES

The tumors may occur in women at any age, but more typically in women of reproductive age. Most patients are asymptomatic but they may present with abnormal vaginal bleeding, mucoid vaginal discharge, or with an "endocervical polyp." On physical examination, a prolapsing mass may be visible at the external os.

PATHOLOGIC FEATURES

GROSS FINDINGS

The tumors are well circumscribed and range from 1 to 23 cm in greatest dimension. On sectioning they display a firm and gray or tawny cut surface. Grossly apparent cysts containing gelatinous material and areas of hemorrhage may be seen.

MICROSCOPIC FINDINGS

On low-power examination, the tumors have a biphasic growth with mesenchymal and epithelial components

(Figures 8.63 and 8.64). The mesenchymal component shows predominantly smooth muscle admixed with varying amounts of fibrous tissue. The smooth muscle merges imperceptibly with the surrounding cervical smooth muscle outside the lesion, resulting in poorly defined borders. The glandular component consists of glands and cysts lined by a single layer of endocervical-type mucinous epithelium (Figure 8.63). The glands

---

ENDOCERVICAL-TYPE ADENOMYOMA – FACT SHEET

Definition
▶ Rare subtype of adenomyoma composed of benign endocervical-type glands and smooth muscle

Incidence
▶ Rare

Age Distribution
▶ Women of reproductive age

Clinical Features
▶ Mostly asymptomatic
▶ Abnormal vaginal bleeding
▶ Mucoid vaginal discharge or "endocervical polyp"
▶ Prolapsing mass

Prognosis and Treatment
▶ Excellent prognosis
▶ Complete excision or hysterectomy
▶ May recur if not completely excised

ENDOCERVICAL-TYPE ADENOMYOMA – PATHOLOGIC FEATURES

Gross Findings
▶ Well circumscribed
▶ Variable size (1–23 cm)
▶ Firm and gray or tawny cut surface with apparent cysts containing gelatinous material
▶ Rarely hemorrhage

Microscopic Findings
▶ Poorly defined borders
▶ Biphasic growth with mesenchymal and epithelial components intimately admixed; no associated stromal reaction
▶ Benign smooth muscle (predominant) admixed to variable extent with fibrous tissue
▶ Glands with lobular architecture (large irregular gland surrounded by smaller glands and cysts) or complex papillary architecture
▶ Glands lined by single layer of benign endocervical-type mucinous epithelium; tubal or endometrioid-type very minor component

Immunohistochemical Features
▶ Apical CEA positivity in endocervical glands
▶ Smooth muscle markers positive in smooth muscle (desmin, h-caldesmon, others)

Differential Diagnosis
▶ Adenoma malignum

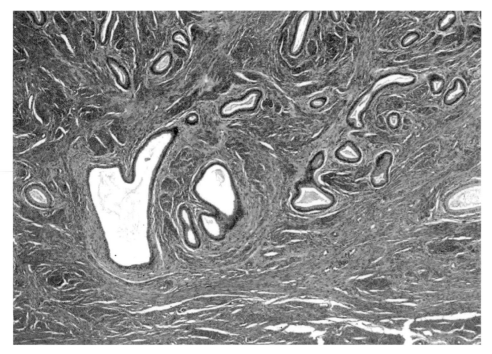

FIGURE 8.63

Adenomyoma, endocervical-type. Intimate admixture of endocervical-type glands and smooth muscle. Note that the smooth muscle component merges imperceptibly with the non-neoplastic cervical smooth muscle.

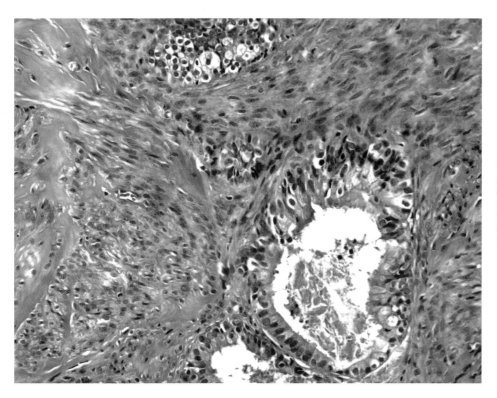

FIGURE 8.64

Adenomyoma, endocervical-type. The endocervical-type glands show abundant mucin and focally pseudostratified nuclei. There is no cytologic atypia in the glandular or smooth muscle cells.

frequently have a lobular architecture with large irregular glands surrounded by smaller glands. Some of the glands may have a more complex papillary architecture with prominent infolding of the epithelium. Tubal or endometrioid-type epithelium may also be seen but typically represents a very minor component. The glandular and mesenchymal components are intimately admixed with no associated stromal reaction, and both cell types are uniformly bland with ≤ 1 mitoses/10 HPFs.

ANCILLARY STUDIES

IMMUNOHISTOCHEMISTRY

The endocervical glands show apical positivity for CEA whereas the smooth muscle component is positive for smooth muscle markers, including desmin and h-caldesmon.

DIFFERENTIAL DIAGNOSIS

The main differential diagnosis, especially in small biopsies or fragmented specimens, is with *adenoma malignum* because of the finding of bland-appearing endocervical glands admixed with smooth muscle. The clinical impression of a diffuse thickening of the uterine cervix (adenoma malignum) versus the finding of a well-defined mass (adenomyoma) may be of help. In a hysterectomy specimen, the circumscription of the adenomyoma and the polypoid appearance (at least in some cases) are helpful gross features that support the benign nature of the lesion. On microscopic examination, the frequent lobular arrangement of the glands, their bland appearance and the lack of a desmoplastic stromal reaction are also helpful. CEA should be used with caution in the final interpretation of a cervical glandular lesion as some cases of adenoma malignum are CEA-negative or only show focal CEA positivity. Rarely, cytoplasmic CEA positivity has been reported in cervical adenomyomas.

PROGNOSIS AND TREATMENT

These are benign tumors but if excision is incomplete they may recur.

ADENOMYOMA, ENDOMETRIOID-TYPE

This is an uncommon subtype of adenomyoma, defined by the presence of endometrioid-type glands (that lack any degree of cytologic atypia) admixed with benign smooth muscle.

ENDOMETRIOID-TYPE ADENOMYOMA – FACT SHEET

Definition
▶ Biphasic uterine tumor composed of smooth muscle and cytologically bland endometrioid-type epithelium

Incidence
▶ Rare

Age Distribution
▶ 26 to 64 years

Clinical Features
▶ Abnormal vaginal bleeding
▶ May mimic a prolapsed endometrial polyp or leiomyoma
▶ Incidental finding

Prognosis and Treatment
▶ Excellent prognosis
▶ Excision or simple hysterectomy

CLINICAL FEATURES

Patients range in age from 26 to 64 years and frequently present with abnormal vaginal bleeding. On physical examination, the lesion may mimic a prolapsed endometrial polyp or leiomyoma. In some cases, the tumor may be an incidental finding.

PATHOLOGIC FEATURES

GROSS FINDINGS

The tumors are typically centered in the uterine corpus, more commonly being submucosal, but they may be centered in the myometrium, subserosa, or cervix. They range from 1 to 17 cm in largest dimension, are well circumscribed, and when submucosal or subserosal they are frequently pedunculated. The cut surface shows firm white-gray areas reminiscent of a leiomyoma with frequent cysts containing mucin or hemorrhagic fluid (Figure 8.65).

ENDOMETRIOID-TYPE ADENOMYOMA – PATHOLOGIC FEATURES

Gross Findings
▶ Submucosal (more common), myometrial, subserosal, or cervical
▶ Frequently pedunculated if submucosal or subserosal
▶ Variable size (1–17 cm)
▶ Well circumscribed
▶ Firm white-gray cut surface with frequent cysts containing mucin or hemorrhagic fluid

Microscopic Findings
▶ Well demarcated
▶ Proliferative endometrioid-type glands vary in number and shape; other types of müllerian epithelium may be seen
▶ Endometrial-type stroma and smooth muscle (which may display same changes as seen in benign smooth muscle tumors)
▶ Glands surrounded by a rim of benign endometrial-type stroma (minor component), in turn surrounded by smooth muscle (most prominent component)
▶ No cytologic atypia and only scattered mitoses

Differential Diagnosis
▶ Endometrial polyp with smooth muscle metaplasia
▶ Leiomyoma with entrapped endometrial glands
▶ Atypical polypoid adenomyoma
▶ Low-grade müllerian adenosarcoma with smooth muscle differentiation
▶ Endometrial stromal tumor with smooth muscle differentiation

---

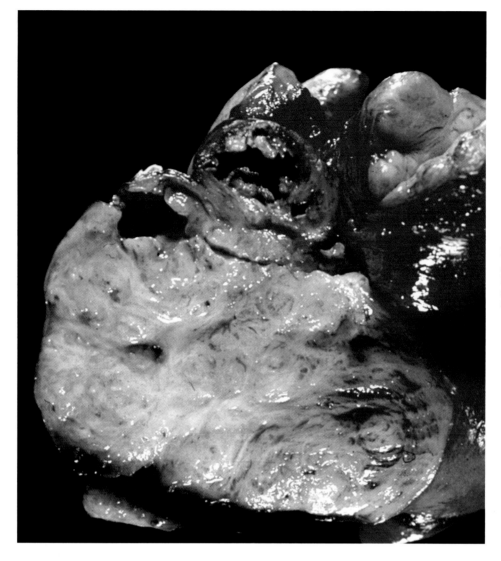

FIGURE 8.65
Adenomyoma, endometrioid-type. A lobulated, fairly well-defined mass shows admixed white and yellow areas and focal cyst formation.

MICROSCOPIC FINDINGS

On low-power examination, the tumors are well demarcated from the myometrium or adjacent cervical stroma. The glands, which vary in number and shape, are irregular and range from small to large with cyst formation. They are typically lined by proliferative endometrioid-type epithelium, but other types of müllerian epithelium may be seen. Cytologic atypia is absent, and only scattered mitotic figures are present. The mesenchymal component consists of a rim of endometrial-type stroma and smooth muscle (Figure 8.66). The endometrial-type stroma surrounds the glands and frequently represents a minor portion of the tumor. Smooth muscle surrounds the endometrial stroma, and typically is most prominent. The endometrial stromal component is characterized by small oval to spindle cells with scant cytoplasm and benign nuclear features which may show sex cord-like differentiation. The smooth muscle forms hyper- or hypocellular fascicles and may display the same changes seen in benign smooth muscle tumors. Mitotic activity is sparse, but if present is more often seen in the endometrial stromal than in the smooth muscle component.

DIFFERENTIAL DIAGNOSIS

In most cases, the diagnosis of endometrioid-type adenomyoma is straightforward. Occasionally, the differential diagnosis may include an *endometrial polyp with smooth-muscle metaplasia*; however, the smooth muscle component tends to be centrally located within the polyp, with the glands being near the surface. The stroma around the glands is typically fibrous and the spatial arrangement of endometrial stroma and muscle as seen in adenomyoma is lacking. In *leiomyoma with entrapped endometrial glands*, the glands are usually seen at the periphery and are not surrounded by endometrial stroma. Another entity that may be included in the differential diagnosis is *atypical polypoid adenomyoma*. In contrast to the typical endometrioid-type adenomyoma, atypical polypoid adenomyoma is characterized by a nodular growth with variably crowded endometrioid glands showing variable degrees of cytologic atypia and, in the majority of cases, squamous morules. The glands are embedded in a cellular, sometimes mitotically active stroma composed, in large part, of smooth muscle. *Low-grade müllerian adenosarcoma with smooth*

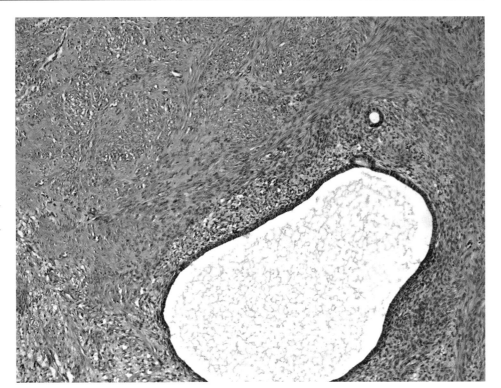

FIGURE 8.66

Endometrioid-type adenomyoma. Long fascicles of benign smooth muscle are juxtaposed to a rim of endometrial stroma which in turn surrounds a cystically dilated benign endometrial gland.

muscle differentiation may bear a vague resemblance to adenomyoma because of its biphasic growth. However, the characteristic low-power appearance of dilated or leaf-like glands with periglandular condensation and malignant cytologic appearance of the stroma (albeit low-grade) are absent in the endometrioid-type adenomyoma. Finally, *endometrial stromal tumors with smooth muscle differentiation* may enter in the differential diagnosis if the adenomyoma has a very minor glandular component. Extensive sampling may be helpful, as well as the finding of typical areas of smooth muscle metaplasia with the characteristic "starburst" appearance.

PROGNOSIS AND TREATMENT

These are benign tumors with no recurrence or spread reported to date.

ATYPICAL POLYPOID ADENOMYOMA

These are unusual biphasic tumors of the uterus, initially reported by Mazur in 1981. This term reflects the polypoid nature of the lesion and emphasizes the complex proliferation of endometrial glands with variable cytologic atypia admixed with a cellular smooth muscle component, which could be confused with an endometrial adenocarcinoma.

ATYPICAL POLYPOID ADENOMYOMA – FACT SHEET

Definition
▶ Unusual biphasic polypoid tumor of the uterus occurring in young women characterized by a complex proliferation of endometrial glands with variable cytologic atypia and cellular smooth muscle

Incidence
▶ Rare

Age Distribution
▶ Reproductive-age women (mean, 39 years)
▶ Occasionally postmenopausal women

Clinical Features
▶ Abnormal vaginal bleeding
▶ Polypoid mass protruding from external os
▶ Rare association with long-term estrogen therapy

Prognosis and Treatment
▶ Excellent prognosis
▶ Curettage or excision with follow-up or simple hysterectomy
▶ Recurrence rate of 45% if treated conservatively; and in those cases rare progression to adenocarcinoma
▶ Recurrence rate of 60% if foci resembling well-differentiated carcinoma; however, no overt malignant behavior
▶ Important to search for endometrial hyperplasia in areas not involved by atypical polypoid adenomyoma if lesion only curetted

CLINICAL FEATURES

Most of these tumors occur in women of reproductive age (mean, 39 years), but occasional tumors occur in postmenopausal women. Rare cases are associated with long-term estrogen therapy. Patients typically present with abnormal vaginal bleeding. Pelvic examination is usually unremarkable, but in some cases a polypoid mass protrudes from the external os.

PATHOLOGIC FEATURES

GROSS FINDINGS

These tumors frequently involve the lower uterine segment, but they may arise in the corpus or cervix. They are typically solitary and well circumscribed, frequently

---

ATYPICAL POLYPOID ADENOMYOMA – PATHOLOGIC FEATURES

Gross Findings

▶ Lower uterine segment (more frequent), corpus or cervix
▶ Solitary and well circumscribed, frequently pedunculated or sessile
▶ Variable size (mean 2 cm)
▶ Bulging, lobulated, or bosselated, solid and firm or rubbery, and yellow-tan to gray or white cut surface

Microscopic Findings

▶ Well-demarcated boundaries with vague lobulated architecture
▶ Juxtaposition of epithelial and mesenchymal components
▶ Endometrioid-type glands with squamous morules (90%), ± central necrosis; other types of müllerian epithelium less common
▶ Glands with varying degrees of architectural complexity, cytologic atypia, and mitotic activity
▶ Rarely, cribriforming, severe cytologic atypia, or foci resembling well-differentiated adenocarcinoma
▶ Interlacing bundles of cellular smooth muscle with a variable admixture of myofibroblasts
▶ At most mild to moderate cytologic atypia and ≤ 2–3 mitoses/ 10 HPFs in mesenchymal cells
▶ Superficial infiltration of myometrium may occur, especially with foci resembling well-differentiated carcinoma

Immunohistochemical Features

▶ Smooth muscle actin positive in mesenchymal component
▶ Desmin and other smooth-muscle markers frequently positive in mesenchymal component
▶ CD34 variably positive in mesenchymal component
▶ AE1-3, CAM 5.2, ER and PR positive in epithelial component

Molecular Studies

▶ Overlapping molecular alterations with endometrial hyperplasia
▶ MLH-1 promoter hypermethylation and focal lack of MLH-1

Differential Diagnosis

▶ Invasive endometrial adenocarcinoma
▶ Endometrioid-type adenomyoma
▶ Low-grade müllerian adenosarcoma

---

pedunculated or sessile, and range from 0.7 to 5 cm, with a mean diameter of approximately 2 cm. The sectioned surface is bulging, lobulated or bosselated, solid and firm or rubbery, and yellow-tan to gray or white.

MICROSCOPIC FINDINGS

On low-power examination, the lesion has a vague lobulated architecture with epithelial and mesenchymal components (Figure 8.67). If the curetting contains adjacent endometrium or myometrium, the boundaries between the atypical polypoid adenomyoma and the surrounding tissues appear well demarcated. The epithelial component has endometrioid-type glands with varying degrees of architectural complexity ranging from widely spaced to closely packed and markedly complex with prominent branching (in at least half) (Figures 8.68 and 8.69). The lining cells frequently show a moderate degree of cytologic atypia and mitotic activity. Squamous morules, seen in 90 % of cases, obliterate the glandular lumens (Figure 8.70) and may show central necrosis. Other types of müllerian-type epithelium may be seen. Rarely, a cribriform pattern, severe cytologic atypia, or even foci resembling well-differentiated adenocarcinoma may be seen, and in fact, some atypical polypoid adenomyomas are contiguous with, and appear to be the origin of, a well-differentiated adenocarcinoma. The mesenchymal component contains interlacing bundles of cellular smooth muscle with a variable admixture of myofibroblasts (Figures 8.67 and 8.68) which is juxtaposed to the glands but it is not condensed around them. The mesenchymal cells exhibit at most mild to moderate atypia and ≤ 2–3 mitoses/ 10 HPFs. Atypical polypoid adenomyomas are typically noninvasive, with a well-circumscribed border in hysterectomy specimens, although some may infiltrate the superficial myometrium. In one study, only rare atypical polypoid adenomyomas associated with foci resembling well-differentiated adenocarcinoma superficially invaded the myometrium.

ANCILLARY STUDIES

IMMUNOHISTOCHEMISTRY

The mesenchymal cells typically stain for smooth muscle actin, and frequently for desmin or other smooth muscle markers, and may show some degree of positivity for CD34. As expected, the endometrioid-type glands are positive for cytokeratin (AE1-3 and CAM5.2), ER, and PR.

MOLECULAR STUDIES

These lesions share some of the molecular alterations seen in endometrial hyperplasia as some of them exhibit MLH-1 promoter hypermethylation with focal lack of MLH-1 immunostaining, a molecular abnormality

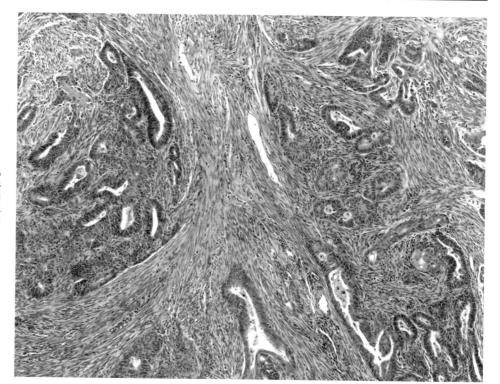

FIGURE 8.67

Atypical polypoid adenomyoma. A striking lobulated architecture is seen. Endometrioid-type glands with variable degrees of architectural complexity are admixed with long smooth muscle fascicles.

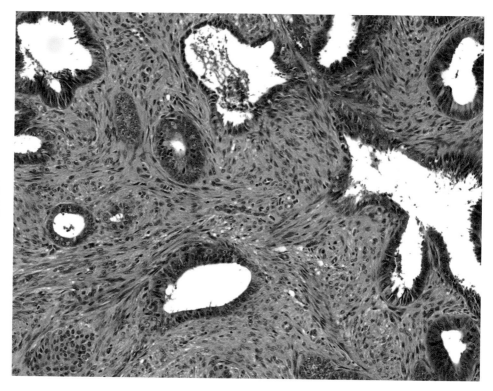

FIGURE 8.68

Atypical polypoid adenomyoma. Simple endometrioid-type glands are surrounded by benign-appearing smooth muscle and myofibroblastic cells.

involved in the transition from complex atypical hyperplasia to endometrioid adenocarcinoma.

DIFFERENTIAL DIAGNOSIS

Invasive endometrial adenocarcinoma may enter in the differential diagnosis, especially in a curettage specimen due to the glandular complexity, presence of squamous metaplasia, and the intimate admixture of endometrial glands and smooth muscle. Features favoring adenocarcinoma include postmenopausal age of the patient, presence of glands with overt malignant features as well as, at least in some areas, the finding of desmoplastic stroma. Typical *endometrioid-type adenomyoma* is also composed of endometrioid-type glands and smooth muscle. In contrast to atypical polypoid adenomyoma, the tumors

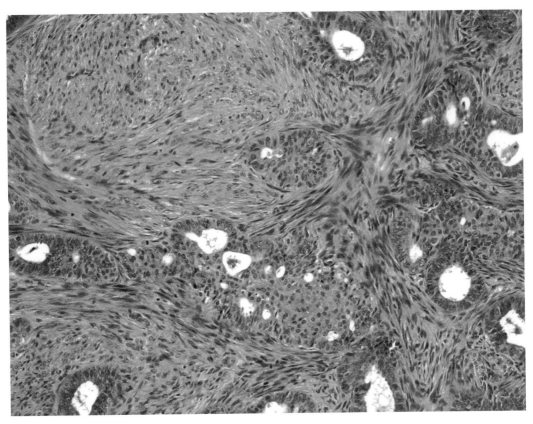

FIGURE 8.69
Atypical polypoid adenomyoma. Endometrioid-type glands show cribriforming and focal morular formation.

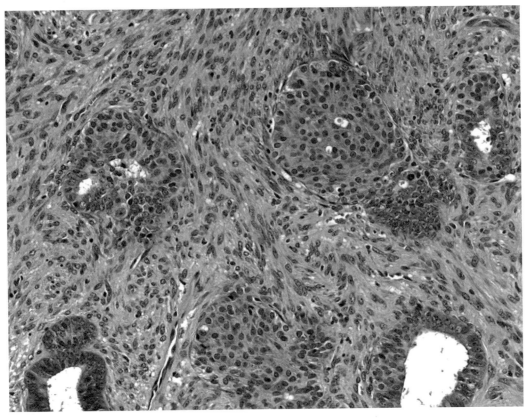

FIGURE 8.70
Atypical polypoid adenomyoma. Several immature squamous morules fill the endometrial glands.

also have a rim of endometrial stroma between the glands and the smooth muscle, and the glandular component does not show cytologic atypia or architectural complexity. *Low-grade müllerian adenosarcoma* may show prominent smooth muscle metaplasia; however, the finding of periglandular condensation of the stromal component around the glands as well as intraluminal polypoid projections will help in this distinction.

PROGNOSIS AND TREATMENT

These tumors have an excellent prognosis. The treatment may consist of curettage or excision with follow-up, or simple hysterectomy. However, there is a recurrence rate of 45% in patients treated conservatively and those treated in this manner may rarely progress to adenocarcinoma. Atypical polypoid adenomyomas with foci resembling well-differentiated carcinomas have a higher recurrence rate, and for that reason they have been designated "atypical polypoid adenomyoma of low malignant potential," since they are capable of locally aggressive but not overt malignant behavior (60% versus 33%). Finally, if the lesion has only been curetted, it is important to search for endometrial hyperplasia in areas not involved by atypical polypoid adenomyoma, which is not an infrequent finding.

RHABDOMYOSARCOMA

There are three main types of rhabdomyosarcoma: (1) embryonal; (2) pleomorphic; and (3) alveolar. They are all rare, the most common of which is embryonal rhabdomyosarcoma.

EMBRYONAL RHABDOMYOSARCOMA (SARCOMA BOTRYOIDES)

CLINICAL FEATURES

The tumors typically occur in the cervix of young women (mean 18 years). Patients usually present with abnormal vaginal bleeding, discharge, or a mass protruding from the cervix.

PATHOLOGIC FEATURES

GROSS FINDINGS

The tumors are frequently polypoid (Figure 8.71) with a myxoid cut surface and a mean size of 3–4 cm.

FIGURE 8.71
Embryonal rhabdomyosarcoma. A large broad-based polypoid tumor with a heterogeneous surface is arising from the cervical canal.

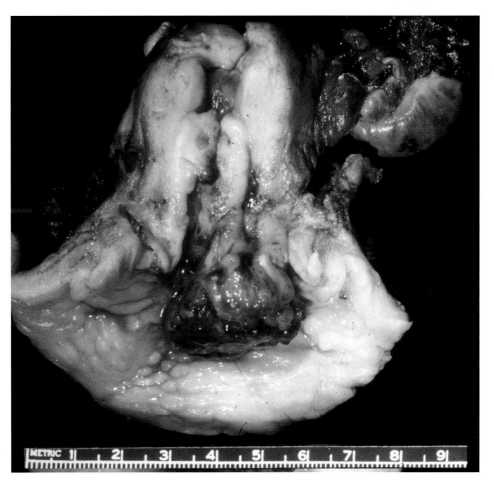

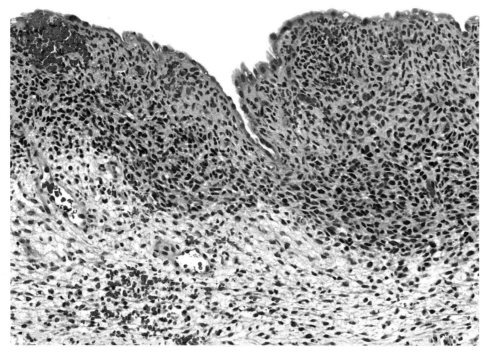

FIGURE 8.72

Embryonal rhabdomyosarcoma. Condensation of small blue cells directly beneath the glandular epithelium ("cambium layer"). In addition, there are alternating zones of cellularity.

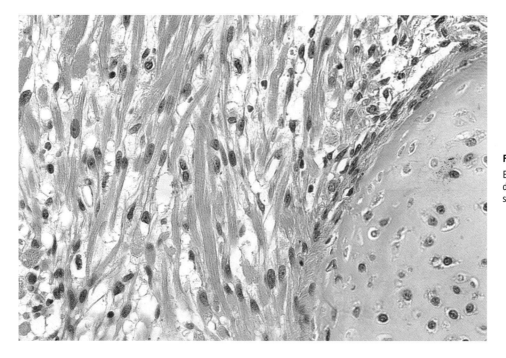

FIGURE 8.73

Embryonal rhabdomyosarcoma. Rhabdomyoblasts with cross-striations are seen next to fetal-type cartilage.

MICROSCOPIC FINDINGS

They are characterized by the typical finding of a superficial hypercellular zone, known as the "cambium layer," composed of small, mitotically active cells beneath the surface epithelium (Figure 8.72). The tumor shows alternating cellular and less cellular myxoid/edematous areas that contain similar small cells and cells with abundant eosinophilic cytoplasm, some with cross striations (rhabdomyoblasts). Nodules of hyaline

cartilage are seen in approximately 50% of tumors (Figure 8.73).

DIFFERENTIAL DIAGNOSIS

The differential diagnosis includes *fibroepithelial polyp*, particularly those containing bizarre stromal cells with abundant eosinophilic cytoplasm. *Cervical müllerian adenosarcoma* may exhibit skeletal muscle or cartilaginous differentiation, and on the other hand, nonneoplastic endocervical glands may be entrapped within a rhabdomyosarcoma, mimicking the appearance of the neoplastic glands of an adenosarcoma. However, adenosarcoma typically exhibits periglandular condensation of stroma and has more widely distributed glands within the tumor. Nevertheless, in rare instances, the distinction between these two tumors may be exceedingly difficult.

PROGNOSIS AND TREATMENT

After surgery and adjuvant chemotherapy, the prognosis is favorable in most cases, with an 80% survival rate for patients with cervical tumors; and up to 90% survival rate in early-stage tumors. The main adverse prognostic factor is the presence of deep invasion. Tumors with superficial invasion may occasionally be cured by conservative local excision.

PLEOMORPHIC RHABDOMYOSARCOMA

These tumors occur in an older age group (35–87 years; mean 64.6 years). They are usually polypoid endometrial masses but may be intramyometrial or located in the cervix. They range in size up to 15 cm in greatest dimension. These tumors are very pleomorphic with many bizarre cells, plentiful rhabdomyoblasts, and numerous mitoses; there is no cambium layer.

The differential diagnosis with other *high-grade sarcomas* is dependent on the finding of definite skeletal muscle differentiation. The one benign tumor with skeletal muscle differentiation, *rhabdomyoma*, lacks the atypia seen in pleomorphic rhabdomyosarcoma. Prognosis is dismal, and most patients die within 15 months of initial presentation, despite aggressive chemotherapy.

SUGGESTED READING

Smooth Muscle Tumors

General

Bell SW, Kempson RL, Hendrickson MR. Problematic uterine smooth muscle neoplasms. A clinicopathologic study of 213 cases. Am J Surg Pathol 1994;18:535–558.

Longrace TA, Hendrickson MR, Kempson RL. Predicting clinical outcome for uterine smooth muscle neoplasms with a reasonable degree of certainty. Adv Anat Pathol 1997;4:95–104.

Oliva E, Clement PB, Young RY. Mesenchymal tumors of the uterus: selected topics emphasizing diagnostic pitfalls. Curr Diagn Pathol 2002;8:268–282.

Tavassoli F, Devilee P (eds) Pathology and genetics of tumours of the breast and female genital organs. In: Kleihues P, Sobin LH (eds) World Health Organization Classification of Tumours, vol. 5. Lyon: IARC Press, 2003:233–249.

Wilkinson N, Rollason TP. Recent advances in the pathology of smooth muscle tumours of the uterus. Histopathology 2001;39:331–341.

Leiomyoma

Canzonieri V, D'Amore ES, Bartoloni G, et al. Leiomyomatosis with vascular invasion. A unified pathogenesis regarding leiomyoma with vascular microinvasion, benign metastasizing leiomyoma and intravenous leiomyomatosis. Virchows Arch 1994;425:541–545.

Clement PB, Young RH. Diffuse leiomyomatosis of the uterus: a report of four cases. Int J Gynecol Pathol 1987;6:322–330.

Clement PB, Young RH, Scully RE. Intravenous leiomyomatosis of the uterus: a clinicopathologic analysis of 16 cases with unusual histologic features. Am J Surg Pathol 1988;12:932–945.

Clement PB, Young RH, Scully RE. Diffuse, perinodular, and other patterns hydropic degeneration within and adjacent to uterine leiomyomas. Problems in differential diagnosis. Am J Surg Pathol 1992;16:26–32.

Downes KA, Hart WR. Bizarre leiomyomas of the uterus: a comprehensive pathologic study of 24 cases with long term follow-up. Am J Surg Pathol 1997;21:1261–1270.

Gal AA, Brooks JS, Pietra GG. Leiomyomatous neoplasms of the lung: a clinical, histologic, and immunohistochemical study. Mod Pathol 1989;2:209–216.

Mulvany NJ, Ostor AG, Ross I. Diffuse leiomyomatosis of the uterus. Histopathology 1995;27:175–179.

O'Connor DM, Norris HJ. Mitotically active leiomyomas of the uterus. Hum Pathol 1990;21:223–227.

Oliva E, Young RH, Clement PB, et al. Cellular benign mesenchymal tumors of the uterus. A comparative morphologic and immunohistochemical analysis of 33 highly cellular leiomyomas and six endometrial stromal nodules, two frequently confused tumors. Am J Surg Pathol 1995;19:757–768.

Prayson RA, Hart WR. Mitotically active leiomyomas of the uterus. Am J Clin Pathol 1992;97:14–20.

Roth LM, Reed RJ. Dissecting leiomyomas of the uterus other than cotyledonoid dissecting leiomyomas: a report of eight cases. Am J Surg Pathol 1999;23:1032–1039.

Roth LM, Reed RJ, Sternberg WH. Cotyledonoid dissecting leiomyoma of the uterus. The Sternberg tumor. Am J Surg Pathol 1996;20:1455–1461.

Sreenan JJ, Prayson RA, Biscotti CV, et al. Histopathologic findings in 107 uterine leiomyomas treated with leuprolide acetate compared with 126 controls. Am J Surg Pathol 1996;20:427–432.

Walach EE, Vlahos NF. Uterine myomas: an overview of development, clinical features, and management. Obstet Gynecol 2004;104:393–406.

Wang X, Kumar D, Seidman JD. Uterine lipoleiomyomas: a clinicopathologic study of 50 cases. Int J Gynecol Pathol 2006;25:239–242.

Leiomyosarcoma

Bodner K, Bodner-Adler B, Kimberger O, et al. Evaluating prognostic parameters in women with uterine leiomyosarcoma. A clinicopathologic study. J Reprod Med 2003;48:95–100.

Dinh TA, Oliva E, Fuller AF, et al. The treatment of uterine leiomyosarcoma. Results from a 10-year experience (1990–1999) at the Massachusetts General Hospital. Gynecol Oncol 2004;92:648–652.

Giuntoli RL, Metzinger DS, DiMarco CS, et al. Retrospective review of 208 patients with leiomyosarcoma of the uterus: prognostic indicators, surgical management, and adjuvant therapy. Gynecol Oncol 2003;89:460–469.

Jones MW, Norris HJ. Clinicopathologic study of 28 uterine leiomyosarcomas with metastasis. Int J Gynecol Pathol 1995;14:243–249.

Larson B, Silfversward C, Nilsson B, et al. Prognostic factors in uterine leiomyosarcoma. A clinical and histopathological study of 143 cases. The Radiumhemmet series 1936–1981. Acta Oncol 1990;29:185–191.

Leiato MM, Sonoda Y, Brennan MF, et al. Incidence of lymph node metastases in leiomyosarcoma of the uterus. Gynecol Oncol 2003;91:209–212.

Major FJ, Blessing JA, Silverberg SG, et al. Prognostic factors in early-stage uterine sarcoma. A Gynecologic Oncology Group study. Cancer 1993;71:1702–1709.

Myxoid Leiomyosarcoma

King ME, Dickersin GR, Scully RE. Myxoid leiomyosarcoma of the uterus. A report of six cases. Am J Surg Pathol 1982;6:589–598.

Pounder DJ, Iyer PV. Uterine leiomyosarcoma with myxoid stroma. Arch Pathol Lab Med 1985;109:762–764.

Schneider D, Halperin R, Segal M, et al. Myxoid leiomyosarcoma of the uterus with unusual malignant histologic pattern: a case report. Gynecol Oncol 1995;59:156–158.

Epithelioid Smooth Muscle Tumors

Kaminski PF, Tavassoli FA. Plexiform tumorlet: a clinical and pathologic study of 15 cases with ultrastructural observations. Int J Gynecol Pathol 1984;3:124–134.

Kurman RJ, Norris HJ. Mesenchymal tumors of the uterus. VI. Epithelioid smooth-muscle tumors including leiomyoblastoma and clear-cell leiomyoma. A clinical and pathological analysis of 26 cases. Cancer 1976;37:1853–1865.

Prayson RA, Goldblum JR, Hart WR. Epithelioid smooth-muscle tumors of the uterus: a clinicopathologic study of 18 patients. Am J Surg Pathol 1997;21:383–391.

Silva EG, Tornos C, Ordonez NG, et al. Uterine leiomyosarcoma with clear cell areas. Int J Gynecol Pathol 1995;14:174–178.

PEComa

Bosincu L, Rocca P, Martignoni G, et al. Perivascular epithelioid cell (PEC) tumors of the uterus: a clinicopathologic study of two cases with aggressive features. Mod Pathol 2005;18:1336–1342.

Folpe A, Mentzel T, Lehr HA, et al. Perivascular epithelioid cell neoplasms of soft tissue and gynecologic origin: a clinicopathologic study of 26 cases and review of the literature. Am J Surg Pathol 2005;29:1558–1575.

Hornick JL, Fletcher CD. PEComa: what do we know so far? Histopathology 2006;48:75–82.

Pan CC, Jong YJ, Chai CY, et al. Comparative genomic hybridization study of perivascular epithelioid cell tumor: molecular genetic evidence of perivascular epithelioid cell tumor as a distinctive neoplasm. Hum Pathol 2006;37:606–612.

Silva EG, Deavers MT, Bodurka D, et al. Uterine epithelioid leiomyosarcomas with clear cells. Reactivity with HMB-45 and the concept of PEComa. Am J Surg Pathol 2004;28:244–249.

Simpson KW, Albores-Saavedra J. HMB-45 reactivity in conventional uterine leiomyosarcomas. Am J Surg Pathol 2007;31:95–8.

Vang R, Kempson RL. Perivascular epithelioid cell tumor (PEComa) of the uterus: a subset of HMB-45-positive epithelioid mesenchymal neoplasms with an uncertain relationship to pure smooth-muscle tumors. Am J Surg Pathol 2002;26:1–13.

Endometrial Stromal Tumors

Baker PM, Moch H, Oliva E. Unusual morphologic features of endometrial stromal tumors: a report of 2 cases. Am J Surg Pathol 2005;29:1394–1398.

Chang KL, Crabtree GS, Lim-Tan SK, et al. Primary uterine endometrial stromal neoplasms. A clinicopathologic study of 117 cases. Am J Surg Pathol 1990;14:415–438.

Clement PB, Scully RE. Endometrial stromal sarcomas of the uterus with extensive endometrioid glandular differentiation: a report of three cases that caused problems in differential diagnosis. Int J Gynecol Pathol 1992;11:163–173.

Dionigi A, Oliva E, Clement P, et al. Endometrial stromal nodules and endometrial stromal tumors with limited infiltration: a clinicopathologic analysis of 50 cases. Am J Surg Pathol 2002;26:567–581.

Huang HY, Ladanyi M, Sostow RA. Molecular detection of JAZF1-JJAZ1 gene fusion in endometrial stromal neoplasms with classic and variant histology: evidence for genetic heterogeneity. Am J Surg Pathol 2002;26:1142–50.

Kempson RL, Hendrickson MR. Smooth muscle, endometrial stromal, and mixed müllerian tumors of the uterus. Mod Pathol 2000;13:328–342.

Koontz JI, Soreng AL, Nucci M, et al. Frequent fusion of the JAZF1 and JJAZ1 genes in endometrial stromal tumors. Proc Natl Acad Sci USA 2001;98:6348–6353.

Levine PH, Abou-Nassar S, Mittal K. Extauterine low-grade endometrial stromal sarcoma with florid endometrioid glandular differentiation. Int J Gynecol Pathol 2001;20:395–398.

Nucci MR, Harburger D, Dal Cin P, Koontz J, Sklar J. Molecular Analysis of the JAZF1/JJAZ1 Gene Fusion by RT-PCR and Fluorescence in situ Hybridization in Endometrial Stromal Neoplasms Am J Surg Pathol 2007;31:65–70.

Oliva E, Clement PB, Young RH, et al. Mixed endometrial stromal and smooth-muscle tumors of the uterus: a clinicopathologic study of 15 cases. Am J Surg Pathol 1998;22:997–1005.

Oliva E, Clement PB, Young RH, et al. Myxoid and fibrous endometrial stromal tumors of the uterus: a report of ten cases. Int J Gynecol Pathol 1999;18:310–319.

Oliva E, Clement PB, Young RH. Endometrial stromal tumors: an update on a group of tumors with a protean phenotype. Adv Anat Pathol 2000;7:257–281.

Oliva E, de Leval L, Soslow RA et al. High frequency of JAZF1-JJAZ1 gene fusion in endometrial stromal tumor with smooth muscle differentiation by interphase FISH detection. Am J Surg Pathol 2007;31:1277–84.

Tavassoli FA, Norris HJ. Mesenchymal tumors of the uterus. VII. A clinicopathological study of 60 endometrial stromal nodules. Histopathology 1981;5:1–10.

Yilmaz A, Rush DS, Soslow RA. Endometrial stromal sarcomas with unusual histologic features. A report of 24 primary and metastatic tumors emphasizing fibroblastic and smooth muscle differentiation. Am J Surg Pathol 2002;26:1142–1150.

Uterine Tumors Resembling Ovarian Sex Cord-Stromal Tumors

Baker RJ, Hildebrandt RH, Rouse RV, et al. Inhibin and CD99 (MIC2) expression in uterine stromal neoplasms with sex-cord-like elements. Hum Pathol 1999;30:671–679.

Clement PB, Scully RE: Uterine tumors resembling ovarian sex-cord tumors. A clinicopathologic analysis of fourteen cases. Am J Clin Pathol 1976;66:512–525.

Irving JA, Carinelli S, Prat J. Uterine tumors resembling ovarian sex cord tumors are polyphenotypic neoplasms with true sex cord differentiation. Mod Pathol 2006;19:17–24.

Krishnamurthy S, Jungbluth AA, Busam KJ, et al. Uterine tumors resembling ovarian sex-cord tumors have an immunophenotype consistent with true sex-cord differentiation. Am J Surg Pathol 1998;22:1078–1082.

Low-Grade Müllerian Adenosarcoma

Clement PB. Müllerian adenosarcomas of the uterus with sarcomatous overgrowth. A clinicopathological analysis of 10 cases. Am J Surg Pathol 1989;13:28–38.

Clement PB, Scully RE. Müllerian adenosarcomas of the uterus with sex cord-like elements. A clinicopathologic analysis of eight cases. Am J Clin Pathol 1989;91:664–672.

Clement PB, Scully RE. Müllerian adenosarcoma of the uterus: a clinicopathologic analysis of 100 cases with a review of the literature. Hum Pathol 1990;21:363–381.

Clement PB, Oliva E, Young RH. Müllerian adenosarcoma of the uterine corpus associated with tamoxifen therapy; a report of six cases and review of the tamoxifen-associated endometrial lesions. Int J Gynecol Pathol 1996;15:222–229.

Jessop FA, Roberts PF. Müllerian adenosarcoma of the uterus in association with tamoxifen therapy. Histopathology 2000;36:91–92.

Kaku T, Silverberg SG, Major FJ, et al. Adenosarcoma of the uterus: a Gynecologic Oncology Group clinicopathologic study of 31 cases. Int J Gynecol Pathol 1992;11:75–88.

Kaku T, Ogawa S, Ariyoshi K, et al. Adenosarcoma of the uterus with sarcomatous overgrowth. Pathol Case Rev 2000;11:168–172.

Miller KN, McClure SP. Papillary adenofibroma of the uterus. Report of a case involved by adenocarcinoma and review of the literature. Am J Clin Pathol 1992;97:806–809.

Ramos P, Ruiz A, Carabias E, et al. Müllerian adenosarcoma of the cervix with heterologous elements: report of a case and review of the literature. Gynecol Oncol 2002;84:161–166.

Tai LH, Tavassoli FA. Endometrial polyps with atypical (bizarre) stromal cells. Am J Surg Pathol 2002;26:505–509.

Malignant Mixed Müllerian Tumors

Clement PB, Scully RE. Uterine tumors with mixed epithelial and mesenchymal elements. Semin Diagn Pathol 1988;5:199–222.

Clement PB, Zubovits JT, Young RH, et al. Malignant müllerian mixed tumors of the uterine cervix: a report of 9 cases of a neoplasm with morphology often different from its counterpart in the corpus. Int J Gynecol Pathol 1998;17:211–222.

Gagne E, Tetu B, Blondeau L, et al. Morphologic prognostic factors of malignant mixed müllerian tumor of the uterus: a clinicopathologic study of 58 cases. Mod Pathol 1989;2:433–438.

George E, Manivel JC, Dehner LP, et al. Malignant mixed müllerian tumors: an immunohistochemical study of 47 cases, with histogenetic considerations and clinical correlation. Hum Pathol 1991;22:215–223.

Grayson W, Taylor LF, Cooper K. Carcinosarcoma of the uterine cervix. A report of 8 cases with immunohistochemical analysis and evaluation of human papillomavirus status. Am J Surg Pathol 2001;25:338–347.

Inthasorn P, Carter J, Valmadre S, et al. Analysis of clinicopathologic factors in malignant mixed müllerian tumors of the uterine corpus. Int J Gynecol Cancer 2002;12:348–353.

Iwasa Y, Haga H, Konishi I, et al. Prognostic factors in uterine carcinosarcoma: a clinicopathologic study of 25 patients. Cancer 1998;82:512–519.

McCluggage WG. Malignant biphasic uterine tumors: carcinosarcomas or metaplastic carcinomas? J Clin Pathol 2002;55:321–325.

Meis JM, Lawrence WD. The immunohistochemical profile of malignant mixed müllerian tumor. Overlap with endometrial adenocarcinoma. Am J Clin Pathol 1990;94:1–7.

Nordal RR, Kristensen GB, Stenwig AE, et al. An evaluation of prognostic factors in uterine carcinosarcoma. Gynecol Oncol 1997;67:316–321.

Silverberg SG, Major FJ, Blessing JA, et al. Carcinosarcoma (malignant mixed mesodermal tumor) of the uterus. A Gynecologic Oncology Group pathologic study of 203 cases. Int J Gynecol Pathol 1990;9:1–19.

Wada H, Enomoto T, Fujita M, et al. Molecular evidence that most but not all carcinosarcomas of the uterus are combination tumors. Cancer Res 1997;57:5379–5385.

Adenomyomas

Gilks CB, Young RH, Clement PB, et al. Benign endocervical adenomyomas and adenoma malignum. Modern Pathol 1996;9:220–224.

Gilks CB, Clement PB, Hart WR, et al. Uterine adenomyomas excluding atypical polypoid adenomyomas and adenomyomas of endocervical type: a clinicopathologic study of 30 cases of an underemphasized lesion that may cause diagnostic problems with brief consideration of adenomyomas of other female genital tract sites. Int J Gynecol Pathol 2000;19:195–205.

Longacre MH, Chung MH, Rouse RV, et al. Atypical polypoid adenomyofibromas (atypical polypoid adenomyomas) of the uterus. A clinicopathologic study of 55 cases. Am J Surg Pathol 1996;20:1–20.

Mazur MT. Atypical polypoid adenomyomas of the endometrium. Am J Surg Pathol 1981;5:473–482.

Ota S, Catasus L, Matias-Guiu X, et al. Molecular pathology of atypical polypoid adenomyoma of the uterus. Hum Pathol 2003;34:784–788.

Soslow RA, Chung MH, Rouse RV, et al. Atypical polypoid adenomyofibroma (APA) versus well-differentiated endometrial carcinoma with prominent stromal matrix: an immunohistochemical study. Int J Gynecol Pathol 1996;15:209–216.

Young RH, Treger T, Scully RE. Atypical polypoid adenomyoma of the uterus. A report of 27 cases. Am J Clin Pathol 1986;86:139–145.

Rhabdomyosarcoma

Bernal KL, Fahmy L, Remmenga S, et al. Embryonal rhabdomyosarcoma (sarcoma botryoides) of the cervix presenting as a cervical polyp treated with fertility-sparing surgery and adjuvant chemotherapy. Gynecol Oncol 2004;95:243–246.

Brand E, Berek JS, Nieberg RK, et al. Rhabdomyosarcoma of the uterine cervix. Sarcoma botryoides. Cancer 1987;60:1552–1560.

Caruso RA, Napoli P, Villari D, et al. Anaplastic (pleomorphic) subtype embryonal rhabdomyosarcoma of the cervix. Arch Gynecol Obstet 2004;270:278–280.

Daya DA, Scully RE. Sarcoma botrioides of the uterine cervix in young women; a clinicopathologic study of 13 cases. Gynecol Oncol 1988;29:290–304.

McCluggage WG, Lioe TF, McClelland HR, et al. Rhabdomyosarcoma of the uterus: report of two cases, including one of the spindle cell variant. Int J Gynecol Cancer 2002;12:128–32.

Ordi J, Stamatakos MD, Tavassoli FA. Pure pleomorphic rhabdomyosarcomas of the uterus. Int J Gynecol Pathol 1997;16:369–377.

Immunohistochemistry

Chu PG, Arber DA, Weiss LM, et al. Utility of CD10 in distinguishing between endometrial stromal sarcoma and uterine smooth-muscle tumors: an immunohistochemical comparison of 34 cases. Mod Pathol 2001;14:465–471.

De Leval L, Waltregny D, Boniver J, et al. Use of histone deacetylase 8 (HDAC8), a new marker of smooth muscle differentiation, in the classification of mesenchymal tumors of the uterus. Am J Surg Pathol 2006;30:319–327.

Klein WM, Kurman RJ. The lack of expression of c-kit protein (CD117) in mesenchymal tumors of the uterus and ovary. Int Gynecol Pathol 2003;22:181–184.

Leitao MM, Soslow RA, Nonaka D, et al. Tissue microarray immunohistochemical expression of estrogen, progesterone, and androgen receptors in uterine leiomyomata and leiomyosarcoma. Cancer 2004;101:1455–1462.

Leunen M, Breugelmans M, De Sutter P, et al. Low-grade endometrial stromal sarcoma treated with the aromatase inhibitor letrozole. Gynecol Oncol 2004;95:769–771.

Loddenkemper C, Mechsner S, Fos HD, et al. Use of oxytocin receptor expression in distinguishing between uterine smooth-muscle tumors and endometrial stromal sarcoma. Am J Surg Pathol 2003;27:1458–1462.

McGlugage WG. Immunohistochemical and functional biomarkers of value in female genital tract lesions. Int J Gynecol Pathol 2006;25:101–120.

McCluggage WG, Sumathi VP, Maxwell P. CD10 is a sensitive and diagnostically useful immunohistochemical marker of normal endometrial stroma and of endometrial stromal neoplasms. Histopathology 2001;39:273–278.

Nucci MR, O'Connell JT, Cviko A, et al. h-Caldesmon expression distinguishes endometrial stromal neoplasms from smooth-muscle tumors. Am J Surg Pathol 2001;25:445–463.

Oliva E. CD10 expression in the female genital tract: does it have useful diagnostic applications? Adv Anat Pathol 2004;11:310–315.

Oliva E, Young RH, Amin MB, et al. Immunohistochemical analysis of endometrial stromal and smooth-muscle tumors of the uterus. A study of 54 cases emphasizing the importance of using a panel because of overlap in immunoreactivity for individual antibodies. Am J Surg Pathol 2002;26:403–412.

Rush DS, Tan J, Baergen RN, et al. h-Caldesmon, a novel smooth muscle-specific antibody, distinguishes between cellular leiomyoma and endometrial stromal sarcoma. Am J Surg Pathol 2001;25:253–258.

Winter WE, Seidman JD, Krivac TC, et al. Clinicopathological analysis of c-kit expression in carcinosarcomas and leiomyosarcomas of the uterine corpus. Gynecol Oncol 2003;91:3–8.

9 Pathology of the Fallopian Tube and Broad Ligament

Isabel Alvarado-Cabrero

The fallopian tube extends from the cornu of the uterus to the median pole of the ovary and it plays a crucial role in reproduction. Malformations, infections, and inflammation may severely affect its function and are responsible for over 20% of cases of infertility in women, most of them having no cure. The fallopian tube is an organ of müllerian derivation and as such

it is susceptible to the same spectrum of metaplastic changes and neoplasms seen in the uterus and ovary, though with a much lower frequency. The broad ligament runs parallel to the fallopian tube enclosing the mesonephric remnants, and associated abnormalities are even rarer than those reported in the fallopian tube.

Fallopian Tube

TUMOR-LIKE LESIONS

METAPLASIAS

CLINICAL FEATURES

Metaplasia, defined as a change from one differentiated tissue to a different type of differentiated tissue, is very common in the müllerian system, although the fallopian tube is the least affected site. Nevertheless, it may undergo a variety of metaplastic changes, the most common being decidual change, which may occur in 5–12% of intrauterine pregnancies and in up to 80% of ectopic pregnancies. Ectopic decidual change of the tubal mucosa is also a common finding in peripartum tubal ligation specimens. Occasionally, similar changes have been documented in tubal specimens removed following hormonal therapy.

Mucinous metaplasia is less common but important to recognize because of its association with mucinous tumors of the female genital tract (cervix and ovary) and with the Peutz–Jeghers syndrome. Transitional and squamous cell metaplasias are even rarer and typically represent an incidental finding.

PATHOLOGIC FEATURES

GROSS FINDINGS

Decidual change is usually an incidental finding on microscopic examination; however, in florid examples, multiple small white nodules or plaques may be visible lining peritoneal surfaces.

Mucinous metaplasia is also typically an incidental finding but it may be associated with visible luminal mucin.

MICROSCOPIC FINDINGS

Decidual change is characterized by collections of polygonal cells with abundant pale eosinophilic to amphophilic cytoplasm with well-defined membrane borders and bland ovoid to round nuclei (Figure 9.1). It typically involves the stromal cells of the lamina propria and submesothelial cells.

Mucinous metaplasia typically appears as an abrupt transition from ciliated-type epithelium to a single layer of mucinous epithelium with preservation of the normal architecture of the fallopian tube. The mucinous cells have tall cytoplasm with a basally placed small nucleus that may appear hyperchromatic secondary to compression. Mucinous metaplasia rarely may be associated

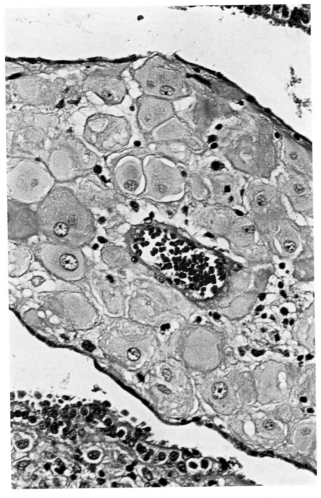

FIGURE 9.1
Stromal decidual reaction. A compact collection of cells within the lamina propria have bland ovoid nuclei and abundant eosinophilic cytoplasm.

with extravasated mucin and hyperplastic changes, as well as malignant transformation.

DIFFERENTIAL DIAGNOSIS

Florid decidual change may mimic a disseminated neoplasm at the time of surgery. Histologically, the differential diagnosis includes epithelioid neoplasms with abundant eosinophilic cytoplasm such as malignant mesothelioma (deciduoid type) and metastatic carcinoma (particularly breast carcinoma), especially in biopsy specimens. Decidual change is readily distinguished from *malignant mesothelioma and metastatic breast carcinoma* by the lack of tissue invasion, significant nuclear pleomorphism, and paucity or absence of mitotic activity. Furthermore, malignant mesothelioma is positive for keratin 5/6 and calretinin while breast carcinoma is positive for keratin and, in some cases, GCDFP 15. In contrast, decidual cells are positive for vimentin and desmin, but negative for keratins.

Mucinous metaplasia should be distinguished from a *primary mucinous tumor of borderline malignancy,* or *primary or metastatic mucinous carcinomas.* The latter may colonize the fallopian tube lining epithelium in a very deceptive manner. However, in most cases of carcinoma, effacement of the pre-existing fallopian tube architecture, cytologic atypia, and destructive invasion are seen.

Transitional and squamous metaplasia typically represent a focal finding, are associated with bland cytologic features, and do not pose problems in differential diagnosis. However, transitional cell metaplasia has been suggested as a potential precursor lesion of transitional cell carcinoma that can rarely occur in the fallopian tube.

PROGNOSIS AND THERAPY

Decidual change typically regresses following pregnancy or cessation of hormonal therapy. The finding of mucinous metaplasia should raise the possibility of multifocal mucinous neoplasia and Peutz–Jeghers syndrome.

WALTHARD NESTS

CLINICAL FEATURES

Walthard nests/cysts are typically incidental findings of no clinical significance. However, they may sometimes resemble granulomas at the time of surgery.

PATHOLOGIC FEATURES

GROSS FINDINGS

Walthard nests appear as white/yellow nodules or cysts up to 2 mm on the serosal and subserosal aspects of the fallopian tube, mesosalpinx, and mesovarian soft tissues.

MICROSCOPIC FINDINGS

Histologically, they form well-circumscribed, small, solid nests (Figure 9.2) or cysts (Figure 9.3) composed of flat or cuboidal transitional cells with pink cytoplasm and elongated nuclei, often displaying prominent nuclear grooves, one or two small nucleoli but no cytologic atypia.

DIFFERENTIAL DIAGNOSIS

Walthard nests may be clinically confused with granulomatous salpingitis or deposits of metastatic tumor,

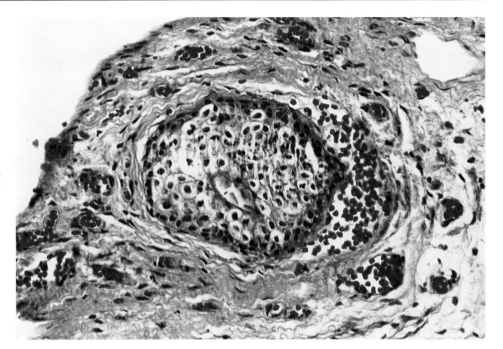

FIGURE 9.2
Walthard nest. The cells have pale eosinophilic cytoplasm and elongated nuclei without atypia.

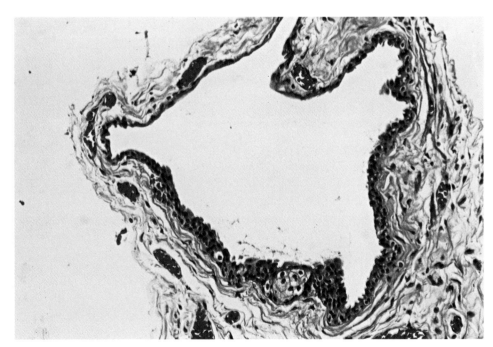

FIGURE 9.3
Cystic Walthard nest. A unilocular cyst is lined by attenuated epithelium. More than one cell layer is focally present.

but can be easily distinguished on microscopic examination.

PROGNOSIS AND THERAPY

Walthard nests are benign, usually incidental microscopic findings and no further therapy is necessary.

PSEUDOCARCINOMATOUS HYPERPLASIA

CLINICAL FEATURES

Tubal epithelial hyperplasia has been reported in association with exogenous or endogenous estrogenic stimulation, including tamoxifen administration (18%), ovarian tumors, some of which are estrogenic (69 %), salpingitis (48.5 %), BRCA1 mutations, and serous borderline tumors of the ovary, although it may occur without any known predisposing condition. Pseudocarcinomatous changes typically occur in young patients between 17 and 40 (mean 28.6) years and are usually secondary to pelvic inflammatory disease (PID), with the most atypical forms associated with both tuberculous and nontuberculous salpingitis. The lesions usually represent an incidental finding at the time of surgery for other causes (e.g., uterine leiomyomas, pelvic endometriosis).

PSEUDOCARCINOMATOUS HYPERPLASIA – FACT SHEET

Definition
‣ Reactive florid hyperplasia that mimics carcinoma

Incidence
‣ Associated with estrogenic stimulation in 18% of cases, with ovarian tumors in 69%, and salpingitis in 18.5%

Morbidity and Mortality
‣ A correct diagnosis may avoid radical treatment
‣ Related to underlying process

Age Distribution
‣ 27 to 40 (mean 28.6) years

Clinical Features
‣ Incidental finding at the time of surgery for another gynecologic disorder
‣ Usually secondary to pelvic inflammatory disease

Prognosis and Treatment
‣ Treatment and prognosis depends on predisposing disease

PATHOLOGIC FEATURES

GROSS FINDINGS

The fallopian tubes may be grossly unremarkable or enlarged, and show thickened walls; pyosalpinx or hydrosalpinx can also be observed. The gross abnormalities are typically related to the underlying disease.

MICROSCOPIC FINDINGS

This lesion is characterized by florid epithelial hyperplasia. The plicae are often fused, resulting in a back-to-back pseudoglandular pattern frequently associated with a cribriform architecture and pseudoinfiltrative growth. The tubal epithelium shows mild to moderate nuclear atypia, occasional mitotic figures, and usually dense chronic inflammation (Figure 9.4).

PSEUDOCARCINOMATOUS HYPERPLASIA – PATHOLOGIC FEATURES

Gross Findings
‣ Enlarged fallopian tube with thickened wall
‣ No evidence of tumor

Microscopic Findings
‣ Epithelial hyperplasia with cribriform and pseudoinfiltrative growths
‣ Adjacent plicae often fuse resulting in a pseudoglandular pattern
‣ Epithelium with mild to moderate atypia but rare mitoses
‣ Frequent dense chronic inflammation

Differential Diagnosis
‣ Carcinoma

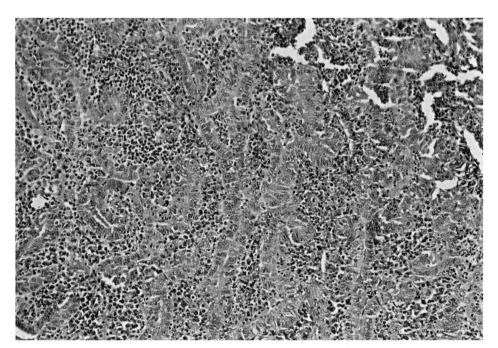

FIGURE 9.4
Pseudocarcinomatous hyperplasia. The tubal epithelium froms pseudoglands and shows reactive cytologic changes. Note the associated florid acute inflammation.

DIFFERENTIAL DIAGNOSIS

The most important differential diagnosis of pseudocarcinomatous hyperplasia is *carcinoma*. The young age of the patient, absence of a visible mass, presence of severe chronic inflammation, lack of desmoplastic reaction, absence of overt nuclear atypia, and paucity of mitotic figures favor the diagnosis of pseudocarcinomatous hyperplasia.

PROGNOSIS AND THERAPY

In these cases it is most important to treat the predisposing disease.

TORSION

CLINICAL FEATURES

Torsion of the fallopian tube is uncommon, but when it occurs, it is usually associated with torsion of the ipsilateral ovary. It may occur at any age; however, it most often affects reproductive-aged women. Patients often present with severe acute low abdominal pain which may become a surgical emergency. Other presenting symptoms include gastrointestinal manifestations and urinary frequency. Predisposing factors include tubal enlargement secondary to hydrosalpinx, pyosalpinx, or previous sterilization.

PATHOLOGIC FEATURES

GROSS FINDINGS

Depending on the duration of the disruption of blood flow, the affected fallopian tube may appear normal but more commonly is edematous, hyperemic, and often contains serous or bloody fluid. In severe cases, the fallopian tube and surrounding tissues, including the ovary, may undergo hemorrhagic infarction.

MICROSCOPIC FINDINGS

The wall of the fallopian tube shows variable amounts of edema, inflammatory infiltrate, vascular congestion, and, if severe, massive hemorrhage.

DIFFERENTIAL DIAGNOSIS

Clinically and pathologically, the main differential diagnostic consideration is a *malignant neoplasm* of the fallopian tube, which can also cause tubal enlargement and undergo secondary torsion with similar clinical presentation. In most instances, this distinction is readily made upon microscopic examination.

FALLOPIAN/TUBE TORSION – FACT SHEET
Definition
▶ Twisted fallopian tube
Incidence and Location
▶ Rare
▶ Involves the fallopian tube and/or ipsilateral ovary
Morbidity and Mortality
▶ Tubo-ovarian autoamputation rare complication
Race and Age Distribution
▶ Racial distribution unknown
▶ All ages
Clinical Features
▶ Acute and severe low abdominal pain
▶ Gastrointestinal symptoms
▶ Urinary frequency
▶ Often surgical emergency
Prognosis and Treatment
▶ Surgery preferred treatment

FALLOPIAN/TUBE TORSION – PATHOLOGIC FEATURES
Gross Findings
▶ Normal or swollen fallopian tube
▶ Serous or bloody fluid may be present in lumen
Microscopic Findings
▶ Acute inflammation, edema, and vascular congestion
▶ Secondary infarction and necrosis
Differential Diagnosis
▶ Carcinoma with secondary infarction

PROGNOSIS AND THERAPY

If surgical intervention is prompt, the fallopian tube may be preserved. A rare complication of torsion is tubo-ovarian autoamputation.

SALPINGITIS ISTHMICA NODOSA

CLINICAL FEATURES

Salpingitis isthmica nodosa (SIN) or "adenomyosis" of the fallopian tube consists of one or more outpouchings or diverticula of tubal epithelium into the muscular wall

SALPINGITIS ISTHMICA NODOSA – FACT SHEET

Definition
▶ Nodular thickening of the fallopian tube of uncertain nature

Incidence and Location
▶ 0.6–11% in healthy women
▶ Higher frequency in the setting of ectopic pregnancy
▶ Proximal portion of the fallopian tube (isthmus)

Morbidity
▶ Higher rate of primary infertility and ectopic pregnancy

Race and Age Distribution
▶ No racial predilection
▶ 25 to 60 (average 30) years

Clinical Features
▶ Incidental finding

Radiologic Features
▶ Multiple small diverticular collections protruding from the lumen into the wall of the isthmus by hysterosalpingography

Prognosis and Treatment
▶ Microtubal surgery may be definitive treatment for qualified woman

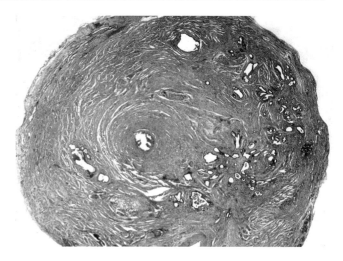

FIGURE 9.5
Salpingitis isthmica nodosa. Small to medium-sized glands, some with irregular outlines, penetrate the wall of the fallopian tube.

SALPINGITIS ISTHMICA NODOSA – PATHOLOGIC FEATURES

Gross Findings
▶ Frequently bilateral
▶ One or more yellow-white nodules up to 2 cm

Microscopic Findings
▶ Pseudoinfiltrative epithelial growth typically associated with hyperplasia of the muscular wall
▶ Glands communicate with the tubal lumen in serial sections
▶ Tubal epithelium with bland cytologic features

Differential Diagnosis
▶ Chronic follicular salpingitis
▶ Endometriosis
▶ Invasive carcinoma

typically in the isthmic region. It most commonly occurs in women between 25 and 60 (average age at diagnosis is 30) years. The incidence of SIN in healthy, fertile women ranges from 0.6% to 11%; however, it is significantly more common in the setting of ectopic pregnancy and infertility. Salpingitis isthmica nodosa predisposes to a higher rate of primary infertility by interfering with upward sperm migration and ectopic pregnancy by trapping the fertilized ovum within the fallopian tube.

RADIOLOGIC FEATURES

Hysterosalpingography may demonstrate multiple small diverticular collections of contrast protruding from the lumen into the wall of the isthmic portion of the fallopian tube.

PATHOLOGIC FEATURES

GROSS FINDINGS

Salpingitis isthmica nodosa frequently involves both fallopian tubes. It typically consists of one or more yellow-white nodules up to 2 cm in diameter, which on cut section may disclose small diverticula.

MICROSCOPIC FINDINGS

On low-power examination, there is a nodular growth of discrete but irregular glandular structures lined by bland tubal-type epithelium showing a pseudoinfiltrative growth into the underlying muscular wall which appears disorganized and hyperplastic (Figure 9.5). Serial sectioning demonstrates that the glands are diverticula that communicate with the fallopian tube lumen. This appearance has led some to prefer to use the term "diverticulosis" in describing this process. The diverticula may closely approach, but do not usually connect with, the serosal surface.

DIFFERENTIAL DIAGNOSIS

The main differential diagnostic considerations include chronic follicular salpingitis, endometriosis, and carcinoma. *Follicular salpingitis* consists of small glandular spaces separated by fibrous tissue, but not smooth muscle, associated with prominent lymphoid inflammation. A diagnosis of *endometriosis* requires the presence of endometrial-type stroma surrounding endometrioid glands, a feature typically absent in SIN. Finally, *tubal carcinoma* shows an irregular distribution of the glands, and it is frequently associated with significant cytologic atypia and a desmoplastic stromal response.

PROGNOSIS AND THERAPY

As infertility is a common complication, microsurgical excision/treatment may benefit patients who wish to become pregnant.

TUBAL PREGNANCY

CLINICAL FEATURES

More than 95% of ectopic pregnancies, defined as a pregnancy that occurs outside the uterus or in an abnormal site within the uterus, arise in the fallopian tube. The vast majority (~80%) occur in the ampulla, with the isthmus (~10%) and infundibulum (~5%) being less common sites. Ectopic pregnancies are usually associated with conditions that interfere with the passage of the fertilized egg into the uterus, and more commonly include prior salpingitis, pelvic inflammatory disease, endometriosis, tubal surgery, and structural (acquired or congenital) abnormalities of the fallopian tube. Ectopic pregnancy is usually diagnosed within the first 2 months of pregnancy and symptoms include missed period, abnormal vaginal bleeding, and lower abdomen or pelvic pain. Even though in the past ectopic pregnancies were associated with significant morbidity and mortality, the maternal death rate from ectopic pregnancy in the US has decreased to < 0.1% in the last 30 years.

RADIOLOGIC FEATURES

Transvaginal ultrasound is utilized to identify whether or not a gestational sac is present within the uterus or if there is evidence of an adnexal mass, which may indicate an ectopic gestation. In some instances, an embryo with a visible heart beat may be evident within

---

TUBAL PREGNANCY – FACT SHEET

Definition
▶ Pregnancy occurring in fallopian tube

Incidence and Location
▶ 80% occur in ampulla, 10% in isthmus, and 5% in infundibulum

Morbidity and Mortality
▶ Internal bleeding or hemorrhage due to organ rupture may lead to shock and/or death

Race and Age Distribution
▶ No race predilection
▶ 15–24 years (sexually active woman)

Clinical Features
▶ Missed period or abdominal vaginal bleeding
▶ Lower abdomen or pelvic pain
▶ History of salpingitis or pelvic inflammatory disease in up to 50% of women

Radiologic Features
▶ Ultrasound demonstrates if gestational sac is in uterus or fallopian tube

Prognosis and Treatment
▶ About 85% of women are later able to achieve a normal pregnancy
▶ Salpingectomy treatment of choice

---

the adnexal mass. Radiologic guided culdocentesis may indicate a ruptured fallopian tube if there is blood in the pelvic cavity.

PATHOLOGIC FEATURES

GROSS FINDINGS

The fallopian tube is usually dilated in the ampullary region, typically resulting in a "sausage-shaped" appearance with distention and attenuation of the muscular wall by intraluminal hemorrhage. The cut surface reveals abundant luminal blood, and sometimes admixed placental tissue. Occasionally, an embryo is present (Figure 9.6). Not infrequently, rupture may occur, which can be evidenced by blood clot or placental tissue protruding through the wall of the fallopian tube.

MICROSCOPIC FINDINGS

Abundant intraluminal blood admixed with chorionic villi and extravillous trophoblast is frequently seen

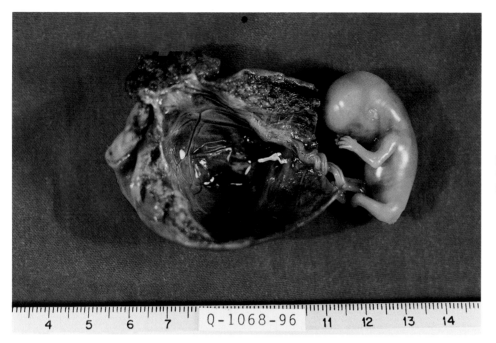

FIGURE 9.6
Tubal ectopic pregnancy. Placental tissue and an embryo are present.

TUBAL PREGNANCY – PATHOLOGIC FEATURES

Gross Findings
- "Sausage-shaped" appearance
- Luminal blood mixed with placental tissue on cut section

Microscopic Findings
- Intraluminal chorionic villi and extravillous trophoblast
- Rarely fetal/embryonic tissue
- Decidual change

Differential Diagnosis
- Gestational trophoblastic disease including choriocarcinoma

---

on low-power examination. Implantation may occur in the wall of the fallopian tube although chorionic villi and extravillous intermediate trophoblast can grow predominantly intraluminally. Microscopic evidence of an underlying predisposing disorder such as chronic salpingitis or endometriosis may be present.

DIFFERENTIAL DIAGNOSIS

The distended blood-filled fallopian tube may clinically and grossly simulate a tumor, fallopian tube torsion with hemorrhagic infarction, or an endometriotic mass, all of which are readily diagnosed on microscopic examination. In some occasions, submission of the entire specimen may be required to confirm the ectopic gesta-

tion. *Gestational trophoblastic disease* involving the fallopian tube is uncommon, with an incidence of approximately 1.5 per 1,000,000 births. Criteria for distinction from a normally developing pregnancy are the same as those used for intrauterine gestations (Chapter 16).

PROGNOSIS AND THERAPY

Rupture of an ectopic pregnancy is life-threatening because of the risk of bleeding. The treatment of tubal pregnancy may be surgical (salpingectomy with preservation of the ovary if feasible), or medically managed with administration of methotrexate. Approximately 85 % of women who have experienced one ectopic pregnancy are later able to achieve a normal pregnancy.

ENDOMETRIOSIS

CLINICAL FEATURES

Endometriosis, classically defined as the presence of endometrial-type glands and stroma in an extrauterine location, is almost exclusively a disease of women of reproductive age and most commonly results in dysmenorrhea, pelvic pain, and infertility. Tubal endometriosis is identified in approximately 10 % of tubal specimens and, when present, most commonly involves

---

TUBAL ENDOMETRIOSIS – FACT SHEET

Definition
▸ Presence of endometrial-type glands and stroma in mucosa, muscular wall, or serosa of fallopian tube

Incidence and Location
▸ 10% frequency
▸ Often distal end of fallopian tube

Race and Age Distribution
▸ No racial differences
▸ Reproductive years

Morbidity and Mortality
▸ Large intraluminal nodules may produce complete blockage resulting in infertility
▸ Increased risk for developing carcinoma

Clinical Features
▸ Dysmenorrhea
▸ Pelvic pain
▸ Infertility

Prognosis and Treatment
▸ Hormonal suppressive treatment
▸ Surgery an option in refractory cases

TUBAL ENDOMETRIOSIS – PATHOLOGIC FEATURES

Gross Findings
▸ Small dark blue/brown intraluminal/subserosal nodules
▸ May form polyps or fill the lumen

Microscopic Findings
▸ Endometrial-type glands and stroma +/− hemorrhage
▸ Decidual or Arias–Stella reaction (as response to pregnancy)

Differential Diagnosis
▸ Salpingitis isthmica nodosa
▸ Endosalpingiosis
▸ Endometrioid adenocarcinoma
▸ Low-grade müllerian adenosarcoma

---

the distal end. This distribution, along with the common occurrence of endometriosis in the posterior cul de sac, has suggested that retrograde flow of blood and cellular material during menses from the uterus through the fallopian tube into the pelvis may be an important cause of endometriosis.

PATHOLOGIC FEATURES

GROSS FINDINGS

Endometriosis commonly appears as dark blue/brown nodules or as raised patches or cysts involving the lumen or serosa. Lesions usually range from a few millimeters to 1–2 cm in diameter, but they may form visible polyps ("polypoid endometriosis") or occlude the fallopian tube lumen.

MICROSCOPIC FINDINGS

Endometriosis most commonly involves the subserosa or mesosalpinx, but may also replace the tubal mucosa (so-called "endometrialization"), more commonly involving the interstitial and isthmic portions (considered a variation of normal morphology), and on occasion may fill the tubal lumen. In classic examples, endometrial-type glands are surrounded by abundant endometrial-type stroma containing small vessels associated with recent hemorrhage. Hemosiderin deposition is often present, but in isolation is not sufficient for the diagnosis of endometriosis. Similar to eutopic endometrium, endometriosis may undergo decidual change or Arias–Stella reaction as a response to intrauterine or ectopic pregnancy. In older lesions, the stroma may be scanty and fibrotic, making its recognition more difficult.

DIFFERENTIAL DIAGNOSIS

Endometriosis should be distinguished from SIN, endosalpingiosis, well-differentiated endometrioid adenocarcinoma, and low-grade müllerian adenosarcoma. When endometriosis involves the wall of the fallopian tube it may simulate *SIN*; however, the latter is characterized by glands lined by tubal-type epithelium set within a nodular myomatous proliferation, analogous to uterine adenomyoma and lacks endometrial-type stroma. Endometriosis should also be distinguished from *endosalpingiosis*, which is also composed of glands lined by benign tubal-type epithelium but not associated with endometrial-type stroma. This distinction may be very difficult in postmenopausal women due to absence (involution) of endometrial-type stroma in endometriosis. A spectrum ranging from *hyperplastic changes to adenocarcinoma* similar to those occurring in the endometrium have been described in endometriosis involving the fallopian tube. Criteria used to distinguish hyperplasia from well-differentiated endometrioid adenocarcinoma are identical to those applied in the endometrium (Chapter 7). Finally, endometriosis can be distinguished from *low-grade müllerian adenosarcoma* since the latter typically forms a mass that on microscopic examination exhibits periglandular stromal cuffing, intraluminal stromal protrusions, and some cytologic atypia of the stromal component.

PROGNOSIS AND THERAPY

In younger women, the main impact of tubal endometriosis is on fertility, with the rate of successful pregnancy diminished depending on the extent of tubal occlusion. Similar to its natural history at other sites, patients with endometriosis have an increased risk for subsequent malignancy. Hormonal suppressive therapy is the treatment of choice. In refractory cases, surgery may be indicated.

INFLAMMATORY PROCESSES

ACUTE INFECTIOUS SALPINGITIS

CLINICAL FEATURES

The incidence of acute infectious salpingitis, which correlates clinically with pelvic inflammatory disease, is highest in sexually active women aged 15–24 years. Risk factors are related to sexual behavior and include age at first intercourse, number of sexual partners, and history of a sexually transmitted disease. Other potential causes of pelvic inflammatory disease include prior instrumentation and the use of an intrauterine device. The most common organisms associated with pelvic inflammatory disease are *Neisseria gonorrhoeae, Chlamydia trachomatis, Mycoplasma,* and anaerobic bacteria. The microorganisms may reach the fallopian tubes via lymphatic or blood vessels (especially after abortion or pregnancy) or may spread directly from the lower to the upper genital tract via the cervical canal and endometrial cavity.

Acute infectious salpingitis may be manifested clinically by fever, pelvic pain, nausea, vomiting, menstrual abnormalities, and peritonitis; however, subclinical infection, particularly with *C. trachomatis,* is not uncommon, particularly in infertile patients. Repeated infections result in recurrent symptoms as well as anatomic changes of chronic salpingitis. Complications of acute salpingitis include peritonitis, abscess formation (pyosalpinx, tubo-ovarian or cul de sac abscess) with adnexal destruction and subsequent infertility.

RADIOLOGIC FEATURES

Advances in transvaginal sonography of the female reproductive tract have resulted in identifying characteristic markers for acute and chronic pelvic inflammatory disease. In particular, incomplete septation of the tubal wall (so-called "cogwheel sign") is a marker for acute salpingitis.

PATHOLOGIC FEATURES

GROSS FINDINGS

In established cases, there is redness and edema of the fallopian tube and ovary which is frequently associated with fibrinopurulent serosal exudate and adhesions. Cross-section of the fallopian tube typically reveals a thick edematous wall with congested mucosal plicae. In addition, the lumen often contains serous fluid or purulent exudate.

MICROSCOPIC FINDINGS

The plicae of the fallopian tube are edematous and densely infiltrated by neutrophils (Figure 9.7). When

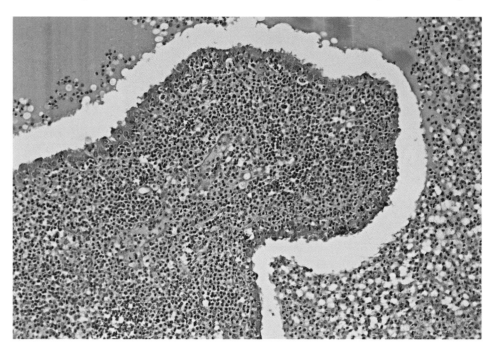

FIGURE 9.7

Acute salpingitis. A plica is distended and filled with a dense neutrophilic infiltrate.

the inflammation is severe, the mucosa may be ulcerated and the lumen filled with acute inflammatory cells. The entrapped epithelium is often hyperplastic, and in severe cases may show a complex glandular architecture (see pseudocarcinomatous hyperplasia) as well as significant cytologic atypia (Figure 9.4). The glandular proliferation may extend through the muscular wall, closely mimicking an invasive carcinoma.

DIFFERENTIAL DIAGNOSIS

Florid reactive epithelial changes associated with inflammation should be distinguished from *in situ and invasive carcinoma*. Young age of the patient, evidence of pelvic inflammatory disease, absence of a grossly visible mass, along with the presence of pronounced inflammation (which is typically absent or scant in carcinomas), and absence of severe cytologic atypia are helpful to establish the diagnosis of reactive changes associated with either acute or chronic salpingitis.

PROGNOSIS AND THERAPY

The most important prognostic factor in women with pelvic infection is timely clinical diagnosis. The mortality rate, directly related to acute infectious salpingitis and pelvic inflammatory disease, has been estimated at 9–29 per 1,000,000 cases for patients aged between 15 and 44 years with most fatalities resulting from rupture of a tubo-ovarian abscess. Treatment consists of antibiotics, analgesics, and bed rest, and removal of intrauterine device (if present).

ACUTE AND CHRONIC SALPINGITIS – FACT SHEET

Definition
▸ Inflammation of the fallopian tube nearly always infectious in origin

Incidence
▸ Worldwide frequency difficult to estimate
▸ World Health Organization (1995): 31 million cases of gonorrhea infection

Morbidity and Mortality
▸ Infertility and ectopic pregnancy most common and serious sequelae
▸ Mortality rate: 9–29 patients per 1,00,000 cases for patients aged 15–44 years

Race and Age Distribution
▸ Higher incidence among women in developing areas (sub-Saharan Africa and Southeast Asia)
▸ 15 to 44 years

Clinical Features
▸ Fever, pelvic pain, peritonitis
▸ Infertility

Radiologic Features
▸ Acute salpingitis: incomplete septation of the tubal wall ("cogwheel sign") by ultrasound
▸ Chronic salpingitis: thin tubal wall ("beaded string") by ultrasound

Prognosis and Treatment
▸ Most deaths result from rupture of tubo-ovarian abscess
▸ Antibiotics and intrauterine device removal (if present) treatment of choice

---

CHRONIC SALPINGITIS

CLINICAL FEATURES

Chronic salpingitis typically occurs following one or more episodes of acute salpingitis and may be manifested clinically by pelvic pain or infertility.

RADIOLOGIC FEATURES

Transabdominal ultrasound is unable to differentiate between pyosalpinx, hydrosalpinx or salpingitis; however, transvaginal sonography of the fallopian tube may show a thin wall (the "beading string" sign).

PATHOLOGIC FEATURES

GROSS FINDINGS

The fallopian tube is enlarged and distorted with multiple adhesions to surrounding paratubal and paraovarian soft tissues. The serosa appears rough with alternating red and white patches, the latter secondary to scarring. On sectioning, the wall may be thickened or very thin and the lumen dilated, often with secondary hydrosalpinx or pyosalpinx (Figures 9.8 and 9.9).

MICROSCOPIC FINDINGS

The tubal wall and plicae are densely infiltrated by plasma cells, lymphocytes, and histiocytes and associated with fibrosis and effacement of the mucosal folds.

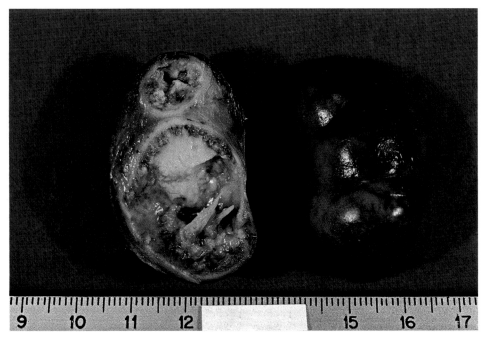

FIGURE 9.8
Pyosalpinx. The fallopian tube is markedly distended. The lumen is septated and contains yellow material.

ACUTE AND CHRONIC SALPINGITIS – PATHOLOGIC FEATURES

Gross Findings

Acute Salpingitis
▸ Redness and edema
▸ Fibrinopurulent serosal and luminal exudate
▸ Often adherent to adjacent tissues

Chronic Salpingitis
▸ Enlarged distorted tube adherent to ovary
▸ May be associated with hydrosalpinx or pyosalpinx

Microscopic Findings

Acute Salpingitis
▸ Prominent edema with dense neutrophilic infiltrate
▸ Mucosal ulceration
▸ Reactive epithelial changes which may be striking (pseudocarcinomatous hyperplasia)

Chronic Salpingitis
▸ Blunted, shortened plicae, associated with chronic inflammation and fibroris

Differential Diagnosis

▸ Carcinoma

The plicae are shortened and blunted with secondary fusion forming dilated gland-like spaces.

DIFFERENTIAL DIAGNOSIS

See acute infectious salpingitis.

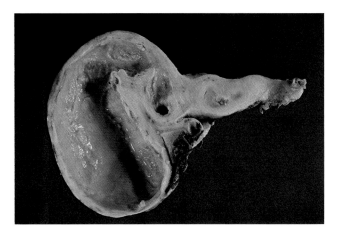

FIGURE 9.9
Pyosalpinx. The fallopian tube lumen is distended and filled with pus.

PROGNOSIS AND THERAPY

See acute infectious salpingitis.

TUBERCULOUS SALPINGITIS

Granulomatous salpingitides comprise a group of disorders characterized by the presence of granulomas in the mucosa or wall of the fallopian tube. Their symptoms overlap with those described in chronic salpingitis. Identification of granulomas requires further studies to determine the precise etiology as both infectious and noninfectious processes may cause granulomatous salpingitis. Among the infectious causes, tuberculosis is the most common, but other infectious agents such as actinomycosis and parasites (schistosomiasis and *Enterobius vermicularis*) may produce a similar granulomatous host response. Granulomatous salpingitis may also be seen as a part of a systemic, noninfectious process, such as sarcoidosis and Crohn disease, or as part of a reaction to a foreign body introduced into the fallopian tube.

CLINICAL FEATURES

Tuberculous salpingitis can affect women of any age but occurs most frequently in adolescents with an overall incidence of approximately 5%. In occurs more commonly secondary to hematogenous spread from a primary lung infection. If the infection spreads to the gynecologic tract, up to 90% of women will have bilateral tubal involvement. Genital tuberculosis may remain latent for long periods or may manifest itself with pain and bleeding, and in some countries, two-thirds of all women with genital tuberculosis are infertile.

TUBERCULOUS SALPINGITIS – FACT SHEET

Definition
▸ Granulomatous salpingitis caused by *Mycobacterium tuberculosis* or *M. bovis*

Incidence
▸ Endemic in less developed areas of the world
▸ Overall 5% incidence in patients with tuberculosis

Race and Age Distribution
▸ Vast majority in developing world; rare in US
▸ All ages, more frequent in adolescence

Morbidity and Mortality
▸ Infertility in two-thirds of all women with pelvic tuberculosis

Radiologic Features
▸ Saccular diverticula extending from the ampulla by hysterosalpingography ("cluster of currants")

Prognosis and Treatment
▸ Good prognosis
▸ Antituberculous medication

RADIOLOGIC FEATURES

Hysterosalpingography may show saccular diverticula extending from the ampulla (giving the impression of clusters of currants), which is a characteristic finding of granulomatous salpingitis.

PATHOLOGIC FEATURES

GROSS FINDINGS

Tuberculosis is nearly always bilateral. In 50% of cases, the fallopian tubes are enlarged; however, they may appear normal, only slightly edematous or may show patchy involvement. Serosal soft and grayish tubercles are visible in about 20% of cases. The fimbriated end of the fallopian tube is usually patent and the lumen contains caseous debris (Figure 9.10) or serosanguineous fluid. The wall is generally thickened and mural caseation may be seen.

TUBERCULOUS SALPINGITIS – PATHOLOGIC FEATURES

Gross Findings
▸ Frequent bilateral involvement
▸ Visible serosal tubercles in about 20%
▸ Luminal caseous debris on sectioning
▸ Less frequently normal appearance

Microscopic Findings
▸ Caseating granulomas within mucosa
▸ Chronic inflammation and fibrosis in muscularis propria
▸ Schaumann bodies often present

Differential Diagnosis
▸ Lipoid salpingitis
▸ Parasitic infections
▸ Necrotic pseudoxanthomatous nodules
▸ Carcinoma

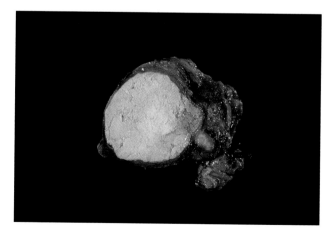

FIGURE 9.10
Tuberculous salpingitis. The wall of the fallopian tube is distended and the lumen contains caseous debris.

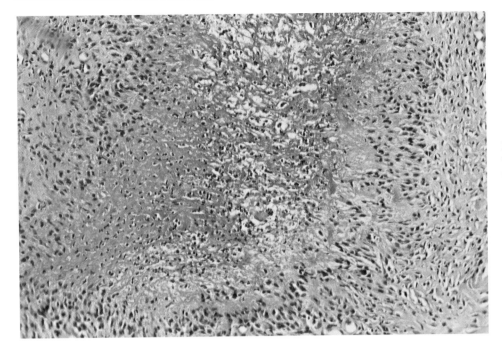

FIGURE 9.11
Tuberculous salpingitis. Caseous necrosis is surrounded by palisading histiocytes (granulomatous inflammation).

MICROSCOPIC FINDINGS

The presence within the mucosa of tuberculous granulomas, which are usually caseating and may be single or confluent (Figure 9.11), is the most characteristic histologic feature. An associated dense lymphocytic infiltrate involving both the lamina propria and the muscular wall is common. The epithelium often exhibits marked reactive epithelial hyperplasia that may be misinterpreted as carcinoma. Identification of acid-fast bacilli on tissue sections or preferably isolation of the organism in cultures is necessary to establish a definitive diagnosis of tuberculous salpingitis.

DIFFERENTIAL DIAGNOSIS

Lipoidal salpingitis, parasitic infections, necrotic pseudoxanthomatous nodules associated with endometriosis, and carcinoma are the entities most commonly considered in the differential diagnosis. *Lipoidal salpingitis* is a granulomatous reaction secondary to lipoidal contrast agents, which when introduced into the fallopian tube may result in variably sized, discrete, round to ovoid spaces within the lamina propria (corresponding to lipid droplets that dissipate during routine processing) surrounded by histiocytes and foreign-body giant cells. *Infection by* Enterobius vermicularis *(pinworm)* typically shows abundant eosinophilic inflammation associated with fragments of the worms or their ova, surrounded by necrotic debris, foreign-body giant cells, granulation tissue, and fibrosis. Classically, the ova are 25 × 30 μm, covered by a thick shell, and have an asymmetric configuration with one flattened side. *Schistosoma infection* also elicits a granulomatous response; however, in most cases, identification of the characteristic ova allows its recognition. In cases

of granulomatous salpingitis in which a diagnosis of schistosomiasis is considered, sodium hydroxide digestion of the remaining tubal tissue may reveal ova. *Necrotic pseudoxanthomatous nodules* represent end-stage endometriosis typically showing a necrotic center surrounded by palisading pseudoxanthoma cells and minimal or absent inflammation. Distinction of reactive/reparative changes of the epithelium from *carcinoma* may be difficult; however, the usual young age of the patient, the associated granulomatous inflammatory response, and the lack of overt malignant cytologic features (with preservation of a normal nuclear-to-cytoplasmic ratio) help to classify the process as reactive.

PROGNOSIS AND THERAPY

Granulomatous salpingitis is not life-threatening if the appropriate treatment is promptly instituted. However, many patients become infertile as a result of infection. The treatment of pelvic tuberculosis is similar to that of pulmonary tuberculosis. Current regimens last 6–9 months and may include isoniazid, rifampin, ethambutol, and pyrazinamide.

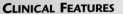

ACTINOMYCOTIC SALPINGITIS

CLINICAL FEATURES

Actinomycosis is a rare, chronic suppurative and granulomatous infection that produces pyogenic lesions associ-

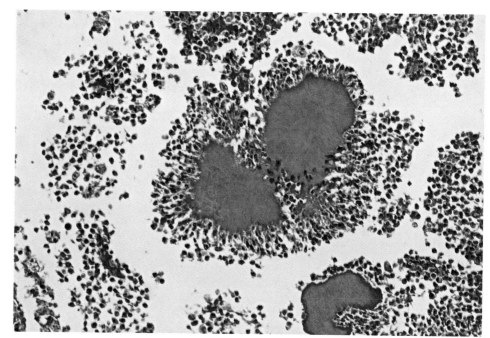

FIGURE 9.12

Actinomyces israelii. A sulfur granule is surrounded by polymorphonuclear leukocytes.

TUBAL ACTINOMYCOSIS – FACT SHEET

Definition

▶ Chronic suppurative and granulomatous infection caused by Gram-positive, anaerobic to microaerophilic bacteria

Incidence

▶ 1.6–36% among intrauterine device users

Morbidity and Mortality

▶ Availability of antibiotics has greatly reduced morbidity for all forms of actinomycosis
▶ High frequency of secondary sinus tracts

Race and Age Distribution

▶ No race predilection
▶ Young to middle-aged (20–50 years)

Clinical Features

▶ Pelvic or abdominal pain

Prognosis and Treatment

▶ Simple regimen of antibiotics can be curative
▶ Aggressive surgical management in advanced cases

TUBAL ACTINOMYCOSIS – PATHOLOGIC FEATURES

Gross Findings

▶ Large firm mass often also involving the ovary
▶ Yellow sulfur granules in tissue (specific finding)
▶ Frequent fistulous tracts (bowel, bladder, or skin)

Microscopic Findings

▶ Numerous histiocytes, plasma cells, and lymphocytes with abscess formation
▶ Purulent exudate with sulfur granules (bacteria)

Differential Diagnosis

▶ Carcinoma
▶ Inflammatory bowel disease
▶ Diverticulitis

PATHOLOGIC FEATURES

GROSS FINDINGS

A large irregular mass is found often encasing the fallopian tube and ovary. Fistulous tracts involving the bowel, urinary bladder, or skin may also be present. The only specific finding is the presence of yellow granules up to 1 mm ("sulfur granules") within the exudate.

MICROSCOPIC FINDINGS

Numerous histiocytes, plasma cells, lymphocytes, and neutrophils are present admixed with the sulfur granules (composed of filamentous bacteria) forming abscesses (Figure 9.12). Gram and methenamine-silver

ated with prominent sinus tracts. The infection is caused by filamentous, Gram-positive, anaerobic to microaerophilic non acid-fast bacteria. Actinomycosis of the abdomen and pelvis accounts for 10–20% of reported cases; it can affect women of all ages, but the majority are seen in young to middle-aged adults (20–50 years) with an increased incidence among users of intrauterine devices (up to 36%). In most cases, the diagnosis is made postoperatively because of its non-specific clinical presentation (pelvic or abdominal pain).

stains may be used to confirm the diagnosis of actinomycosis.

DIFFERENTIAL DIAGNOSIS

Pelvic actinomycosis may clinically mimic malignancy, inflammatory bowel disease, or diverticulitis; however, its diagnosis is readily apparent on microscopic examination.

PROGNOSIS AND THERAPY

If pelvic actinomycosis is recognized preoperatively, a simple regimen of antibiotics can be curative. However, aggressive surgical management in advanced cases with multiorgan involvement seems to have reemerged in recent years.

BENIGN TUMORS

ADENOMATOID TUMOR

CLINICAL FEATURES

Adenomatoid tumor is derived from mesothelial cells and represents the most frequent benign neoplasm of the fallopian tube, although it is also commonly found in the uterus. It is usually an incidental finding in middle-aged or elderly women.

ADENOMATOID TUMOR – FACT SHEET

Definition
▸ Benign tumor derived from mesothelial cells

Incidence and Location
▸ Most frequent benign tumor of fallopian tube
▸ Beneath the serosa

Age Distribution
▸ Middle-aged or elderly woman

Clinical Features
▸ Usually an incidental finding

Prognosis and Treatment
▸ Excellent prognosis
▸ It can be treated successfully by surgery alone

PATHOLOGIC FEATURES

GROSS FINDINGS

These tumors are often located under the serosa, although may be present in the mucosa or lamina propria. They form well-circumscribed but unencapsulated, round to oval, gray to yellowish nodules, which are typically small (≤ 2 cm) (Figure 9.13).

MICROSCOPIC FINDINGS

On low-power examination, adenomatoid tumors are poorly circumscribed. They may show a variety of architectural patterns, but tubular and angiomatoid growths are most frequent and extensive. They are characterized by anastomosing gland-like spaces that may show cribriforming and/or slit-like, ovoid to round spaces reminiscent of vascular structures (Figures 9.14 and 9.15). Cysts, signet ring-like cells and, less frequently, papillae or solid growth are also seen (Figure 9.15). The lining cells are cuboidal to flat with bland cytologic features and minimal to absent mitotic activity. The spaces may contain basophilic secretions. The pseudoglandular spaces intermingle with bands of connective tissue or less frequently with hyperplastic smooth muscle (the latter being a feature more characteristic of adenomatoid tumors of the uterus). A sprinkling of lymphocytes may be present in the stroma, and on occasion may form lymphoid aggregates.

ANCILLARY STUDIES

IMMUNOHISTOCHEMISTRY

The tumor cells are diffusely and strongly positive for low-molecular-weight keratin, calretinin, and WT1

ADENOMATOID TUMOR – PATHOLOGIC FEATURES

Gross Findings
▸ Most commonly subserosal
▸ Well circumscribed but unencapsulated
▸ Round or oval, gray to yellow nodule
▸ Typically ≤ 2 cm

Microscopic Findings
▸ Gland-like and slit-like spaces
▸ Single signet ring-like cells and cysts less common
▸ Cuboidal to flat cells with bland cytologic features
▸ Sprinkling of lymphocytes

Immunohistochemical Features
▸ Low-molecular-weight keratin, calretinin and WT1 positive
▸ Negative for CEA, factor VIII, CD15, TAG-72

Differential Diagnosis
▸ Adenocarcinoma (frozen section)
▸ Lymphangioma
▸ Leiomyoma

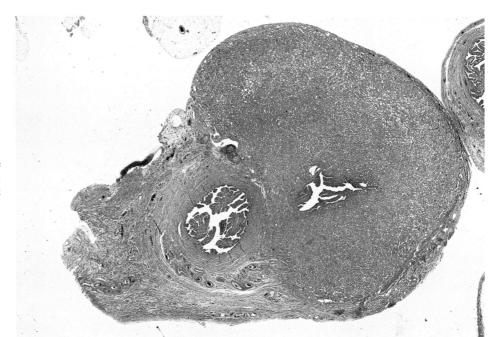

FIGURE 9.13

Adenomatoid tumor. The wall of the fallopian tube is expanded by a subserosal circumscribed but uncapsulated tumor.

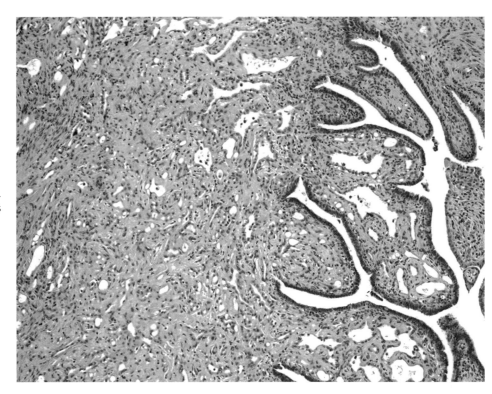

FIGURE 9.14

Adenomatoid tumor. Irregular gland-like spaces and stromal lymphocytes are present.

(in keeping with their mesothelial origin), and negative for CEA, factor VIII, CD15 and TAG-72.

DIFFERENTIAL DIAGNOSIS

On frozen section, the most important distinction is from *adenocarcinoma*, including signet-ring cell carcinoma, as both tumors share an infiltrative growth, irregularly shaped spaces, signet ring cells, and luminal basophilic secretions. The well-circumscribed gross appearance,

bland cytology, and lack of mitotic activity support a benign diagnosis. Adenomatoid tumor should also be distinguished from other benign tumors such as lymphangioma and leiomyoma. In difficult cases, CD34 and *Ulex europaeus* are needed to support the endothelial nature of *lymphangioma*. The stroma of an adenomatoid tumor may contain prominent smooth muscle, suggesting the diagnosis of *leiomyoma*. However, in contrast with an adenomatoid tumor, leiomyoma is typically easily enucleated from the surrounding tissues, is whiter and firmer on gross examination, and lacks the characteristic spaces of an adenomatoid tumor.

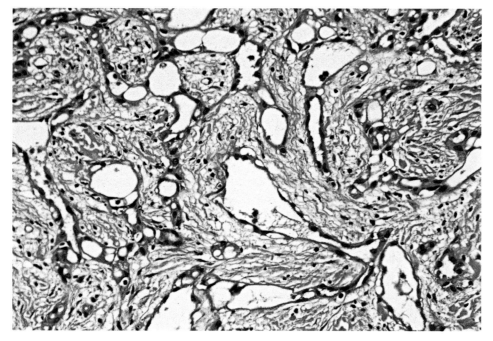

FIGURE 9.15
Adenomatoid tumor. The tumor shows numerous slit-like spaces. Note also the presence of signet ring-like cells.

METAPLASTIC PAPILLARY TUMOR

CLINICAL FEATURES

Metaplastic papillary tumor is an uncommon but distinctive intraluminal papillary epithelial proliferation that only occurs in the fallopian tube. This lesion is almost exclusively detected in pregnant and postpartum women (27–33 years).

**METAPLASTIC PAPILLARY TUMOR –
FACT SHEET**

Definition
▶ Intraluminal papillary epithelial proliferation of the fallopian tube seen during pregnancy or postpartum

Incidence and Location
▶ Rare
▶ No predilection for a specific location

Race and Age Distribution
▶ Racial distribution unknown
▶ 27–33 years (pregnant or postpartum women)

Clinical Features
▶ Incidental microscopic finding

Prognosis
▶ Benign

PATHOLOGIC FEATURES

GROSS FINDINGS

This lesion is an incidental microscopic finding in a grossly normal fallopian tube.

MICROSCOPIC FINDINGS

On low-power examination, metaplastic papillary tumor involves only part of the lumen. It has a papillary configuration and the cores are thin, but sometimes edematous and rounded (Figure 9.16A). The lining epithelium is composed of columnar, nonciliated cells arranged either as a single layer with basal and bland nuclei, or as pseudostratified epithelium (Figure 9.16B). The majority of the cells have abundant bright eosino-

---

METAPLASTIC PAPILLARY TUMOR – PATHOLOGIC FEATURES

Gross Findings
▶ Unremarkable fallopian tube

Microscopic Findings
▶ Luminal papillary proliferation
▶ Pseudostratified or single layer of columnar, nonciliated cells
▶ Cells with abundant eosinophilic cytoplasm and bland cytologic features

Differential Diagnosis
▶ Borderline (serous/mucinous endocervical) tumors
▶ Carcinoma

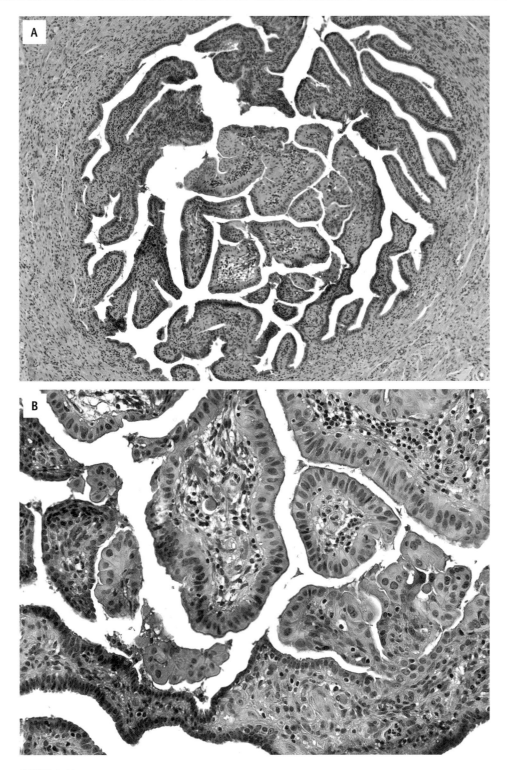

FIGURE 9.16

Papillary metaplastic tumor. A limited papillary proliferation occupies the center of the lumen of the fallopian tube (A). The lining cells have abundant eosinophilic cytoplasm and bland nuclei (B).

philic cytoplasm, and sparsely interspersed among these cells are cells containing intracytoplasmic mucin.

ANCILLARY STUDIES

IMMUNOHISTOCHEMISTRY

The lesional cells are positive for keratin and EMA, but negative for CEA.

DIFFERENTIAL DIAGNOSIS

The metaplastic papillary tumor is grossly and histologically distinct from primary tubal borderline (serous/ mucinous endocervical) tumors. *Borderline tumors* are not typically associated with pregnancy; in most cases they are grossly visible, have hierarchical branching of papillae with prominent budding, and most cells typically have less abundant eosinophilic cytoplasm (if serous) or are associated with a prominent inflammatory infiltrate (if mucinous endocervical). *Fallopian tube carcinoma*, unlike metaplastic papillary tumor, is frequently associated with fusiform enlargement of the fallopian tube. Even when incidentally found, the tumor cells show high nuclear-to-cytoplasmic ratio, moderate to severe cytologic atypia with brisk mitotic activity, and are frequently associated with stromal invasion.

PROGNOSIS AND THERAPY

No treatment is necessary as it is a benign incidental lesion that is completely removed when performing surgery for other reasons.

TUMORS OF BORDERLINE MALIGNANCY AND MALIGNANT TUMORS

SEROUS BORDERLINE TUMORS

CLINICAL FEATURES

In general, borderline tumors of the fallopian tube are rare, in contrast to their ovarian counterparts. They typically occur in reproductive-aged women and are usually incidental findings at the time of surgery for another gynecologic disorder.

SEROUS BORDERLINE TUMORS OF THE FALLOPIAN TUBE – FACT SHEET

Definition
▸ Tumors of low-grade malignancy with a generally favorable outcome

Incidence
▸ Rare

Race and Age Distribution
▸ Similar incidence among racial groups
▸ 31 to 73 (average 39.7) years

Morbidity and Mortality
▸ Related to extension outside fallopian tube

Clinical Features
▸ Usually incidental finding

Prognosis and Treatment
▸ Favorable outcome
▸ Treatment can be conservative

SEROUS BORDERLINE TUMORS OF THE FALLOPIAN TUBE – PATHOLOGIC FEATURES

Gross Findings
▸ Soft, tan, delicate papillary fronds
▸ From 2.6 to 6 (mean 1.8) cm

Microscopic Findings
▸ Overlapping features with its ovarian counterpart

Differential Diagnosis
▸ Metaplastic papillary tumor
▸ Papilloma
▸ Carcinoma

PATHOLOGIC FEATURES

GROSS FINDINGS

The tumors are usually < 6 cm in largest diameter (mean size 1.8 cm), and their gross appearance is similar to their ovarian counterparts, being composed of soft, tan, usually numerous and sometimes coalescing, delicate papillary fronds.

MICROSCOPIC FINDINGS

Serous borderline tumors of the fallopian tube closely resemble their ovarian counterparts. On low-power examination, they are characterized by hierarchical branching of the papillae, epithelial pseudostratification, and detached cell clusters. The tumor cells are usually ciliated, resembling nonneoplastic fallopian tube epithelium. Often cells with abundant eosinophilic cytoplasm are interspersed, as are cells that are cuboidal or have a hobnail appearance. The tumor cell nuclei may show mild to focal moderate degrees of nuclear pleomorphism with slightly irregular nuclear contours and hyperchromasia; nucleoli may be prominent but mitoses are infrequent.

DIFFERENTIAL DIAGNOSIS

Borderline tumors originating in the fallopian tube should be distinguished from the rare *metaplastic papillary tumor*. The latter is a microscopic incidental papillary proliferation in segments of fallopian tube removed during the postpartum period that lack hierarchical branching. *Papillomas* show delicate branching stromal stalks lined by a single layer of nonciliated columnar or oncocytic cells with uniform nuclei. *Fallopian tube carcinoma* shows complex papillae or slit-like spaces lined by multiple layers of cells with enlarged pleomorphic hyperchromatic nuclei containing abnormal mitotic figures, and it is frequently associated with stromal invasion.

PROGNOSIS AND THERAPY

Overall, prognosis is favorable, and treatment can be conservative.

TUBAL INTRAEPITHELIAL CARCINOMA

CLINICAL FEATURES

This tumor occurs more frequently in the fallopian tubes of women with proven BRCA-1 or BRCA-2 mutations.

PATHOLOGIC FEATURES

GROSS FINDINGS

Tubal intraepithelial carcinoma is not grossly identifiable but may be present adjacent to a gross tumor involving the fallopian tube.

MICROSCOPIC FINDINGS

Pseudostratified epithelium, nuclear enlargement, varying degrees of nuclear atypia, mitotic activity, and

prominent nucleoli (Figure 9.17) are characteristic features of this lesion. Tubal intraepithelial carcinoma may also be seen adjacent to invasive carcinoma, supporting the concept that it represents a precursor lesion. Because these lesions may be focal and more frequently involve the fimbriated end of the fallopian tube, the entire fallopian tube should be examined, with particular attention to the fimbriated end, in all patients with known or suspected BRCA mutations.

ANCILLARY STUDIES

Tubal intraepithelial carcinoma displays diffuse and strong p53 and MIB-1 positivity, similar to the immunohistochemical profile seen in serous adenocarcinoma.

DIFFERENTIAL DIAGNOSIS

Entities in the differential diagnosis include reactive atypia and thermal artifact. Hyperplastic changes associated with *reactive cytologic atypia* of the tubal epithelium may occur in response to salpingitis and may closely simulate carcinoma in situ; however, severe nuclear atypia and prominent mitotic activity are absent. *Thermal artifact* can also simulate carcinoma because it causes marked nuclear pseudostratification, elongation, and hyperchromatism. However, the distorted appearance of the epithelium can be readily identifiable in most cases.

PROGNOSIS AND THERAPY

When tubal intraepithelial carcinoma is seen in association with a carcinoma, the treatment is based on the stage of the invasive carcinoma. When discovered as an isolated finding, adjunctive therapy, particularly chemotherapy, may be considered since shedding tumor cells put the peritoneal cavity at risk.

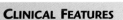

FALLOPIAN TUBE CARCINOMA

CLINICAL FEATURES

Fallopian tube carcinoma is a rare malignancy, accounting for only 0.3–1.1% of all malignant tumors of the female reproductive tract. The age of the patients ranges from 26 to 85 (average 58) years. The most common presenting complaints are abnormal vaginal bleeding and abdominal-pelvic pain; patients may also have a palpable pelvic mass. The clinical complex designated

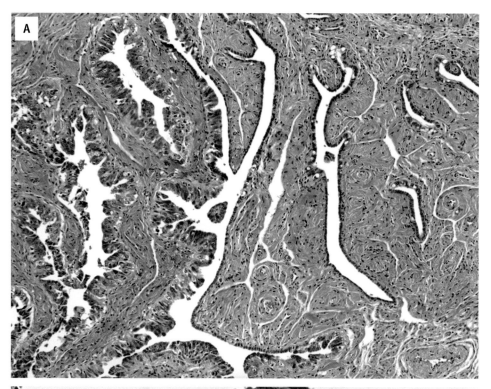

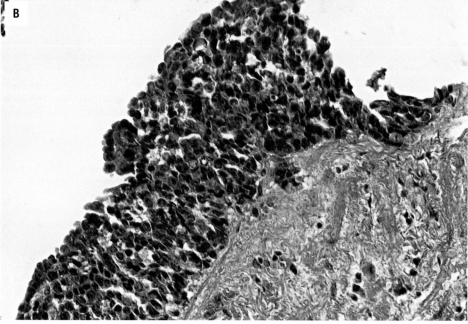

FIGURE 9.17

Tubal intraepithelial carcinoma. Partial involvement of the fallopian tube mucosa by pseudostratified and hyperchromatic cells (A). Marked pseudostratification is associated with striking nuclear pleomorphism and mitotic activity (B).

"hydrops tubae profluens" (pelvic pain, copious watery discharge, and adnexal mass), although thought to be fairly specific for tubal carcinoma, occurs in < 5% of patients.

The finding of fallopian tube carcinoma in members of families with BRCA1/BRCA2 germline mutations has suggested an etiologic role of these mutations in the development of fallopian tube carcinoma and the possibility that this type of carcinoma may be part of hereditary breast–ovarian cancer syndrome. It is important to consider the risk of fallopian tube carcinoma when a prophylactic oophorectomy is performed in high-risk women. In one study of 26 women with BRCA1/BRCA2 mutations who had undergone prophylactic oophorectomy with salpingectomy, two atypical hyperplasias and two "in situ" carcinomas of the tube were discovered.

The diagnosis of fallopian tube carcinoma is rarely made prior to surgery. The majority of tubal cancers are misdiagnosed preoperatively as hydrosalpinx, pyosalpinx or an ovarian malignancy. When postmenopausal bleeding persists after negative endometrial curettage, the possibility of tubal cancer should be a consideration.

FALLOPIAN TUBE CARCINOMA – FACT SHEET

Definition
▶ Malignant epithelial tumor of müllerian derivation

Incidence
▶ Rare (0.3–1.1% of all malignant tumors of the female genital tract)

Morbidity and Mortality
▶ 50% 5-year survival rate if outside the pelvis

Race and Age Distribution
▶ Similar incidence among different racial groups
▶ 26 to 85 years

Clinical Features
▶ Abnormal vaginal bleeding
▶ Pelvic pain
▶ Palpable pelvic mass
▶ Hydrops tubae profluens (pelvic pain, watery discharge, and adnexal mass)

Prognosis and Treatment
▶ Adverse prognostic factors include high stage, high grade, and large volume of residual tumor after initial surgery
▶ Hysterectomy and bilateral salpingo-oophorectomy with debulking and adjuvant therapy

---

FALLOPIAN TUBE CARCINOMA – PATHOLOGIC FEATURES

Gross Findings
▶ Middle to outer third more common locations
▶ Distended fallopian tube simulating hydro- or pyosalpinx
▶ Closed fimbriated end in 50% of cases
▶ Friable, gray to white solid or nodular masses
▶ 0.2–14 (mean 7) cm

Microscopic Findings
▶ Close resemblance to ovarian carcinomas of all cell types
▶ Grade 3 serous carcinomas represent vast majority
▶ Giant cells are more often seen than in their serous ovarian counterparts
▶ Endometrioid and transitional carcinomas less common subtypes
▶ Mucinous, clear cell, and squamous cell carcinomas rare subtypes

Differential Diagnosis
Serous Carcinoma
▶ Tuberculous or nontuberculous salpingitis
▶ Pseudocarcinomatous hyperplasia

Endometrioid Carcinoma
▶ Female adnexal tumor of probable wolffian origin

Pap smear, although abnormal in 10–20% of patients, is usually not diagnostic, and ancillary diagnostic procedures are of limited value.

PATHOLOGIC FEATURES

GROSS FINDINGS

Most primary fallopian tube carcinomas are unilateral (< 3% bilateral) and are located in the middle and outer thirds of the fallopian tube. The fimbriated end of the fallopian was involved in 8% of the cases in one large study. Tubal carcinoma often simulates a hydro- or pyosalpinx, particularly if advanced, where the tumor has undergone extensive necrosis and the contents are largely composed of thick fluid or debris. When the tubal wall is not infiltrated by tumor and the fimbriated end is patent, the serosa is usually smooth; but, it may be granular (Figure 9.18). The fimbriated end of the tube is occluded in approximately 50% of cases. Sectioning reveals single or multiple solid, soft, gray to white friable nodules or papillary/polypoid growths (Figure 9.19) with tumor size ranging from 0.2 to 14 (mean 7) cm. Extensive associated necrosis and hemorrhage are often seen.

MICROSCOPIC FINDINGS

Serous carcinoma is the most common subtype of fallopian tube carcinoma, accounting for approximately 50% of malignant neoplasms in this organ. It is histologically similar to its ovarian counterpart. Grade 1 tumors represent < 10% of serous carcinomas; they show well-formed papillae with slender and delicate fibrovascular branching cores (Figure 9.20) lined by cuboidal cells with mild to focally moderate cytologic atypia and variable mitotic activity (Figure 9.21). Grade 2 tumors exhibit a more complex papillary architecture as well as irregular glands forming slit-like and alveolar spaces and moderate cytologic atypia. Poorly differentiated (grade 3) carcinomas comprise the vast majority of serous carcinomas. They may show a complex papillary growth, slit-like spaces, or solid sheets, and more frequently a combination thereof. The tumor cells display marked nuclear pleomorphism and have a high mitotic rate. Scattered to large numbers of tumor giant cells are more often seen in serous fallopian tube carcinomas than in their ovarian counterparts (Figure 9.22). Psammoma bodies may also be seen. Prominent necrosis as well as wall and vascular invasion are common findings.

Endometrioid carcinoma represents approximately 25% of fallopian tube carcinomas. The tumors may resemble an endometrioid carcinoma of the uterus and ovary (Figure 9.23) or may have an appearance similar to the female adnexal tumor of probable wolffian origin (FATWO) showing closely packed small to cystically dilated glands with banal cytologic features. Oxyphilic and spindled subtypes may also occur. Endometrioid

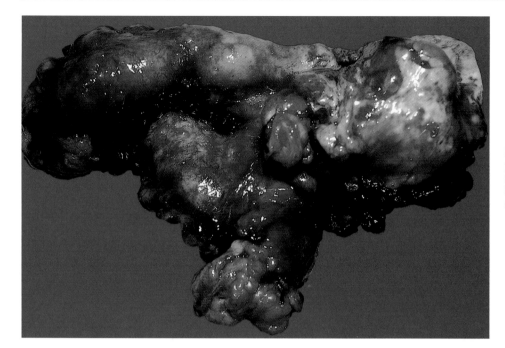

FIGURE 9.18

Fallopian tube carcinoma. The tube is uniformly enlarged and has a nodular and hemorrhagic appearance.

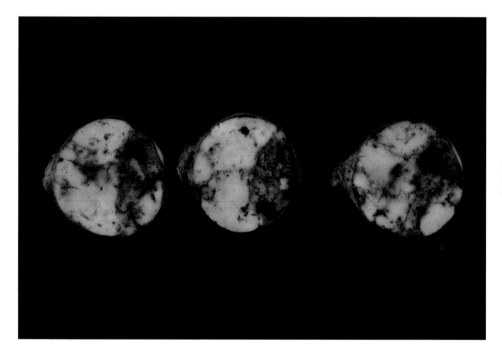

FIGURE 9.19

Fallopian tube carcinoma. A friable gray tumor fills the lumen.

adenocarcinomas of the fallopian tube are commonly confined to the mucosa or lamina propria.

Transitional cell carcinoma is the third most common histologic type of carcinoma found in the fallopian tube. The tumors may have an exophytic papillary (Figure 9.24), endophytic, or solid growth, or a combination thereof. They are typically high-grade and the cells have scant to moderate eosinophilic cytoplasm, pleomorphic nuclei, and brisk mitotic activity. However, some of the nuclei may show nuclear grooves. These tumors are typically associated with extensive necrosis. They are not infrequently seen in combination with a component of serous carcinoma.

Mucinous carcinoma is extremely rare but of interest because of its association with other mucinous lesions of the female genital tract and with Peutz–Jeghers syndrome. In one large series of tubal carcinoma, mucinous carcinoma accounted for 5% of cases. The histologic appearance of mucinous fallopian tube carcinomas is similar to that of their ovarian counterparts.

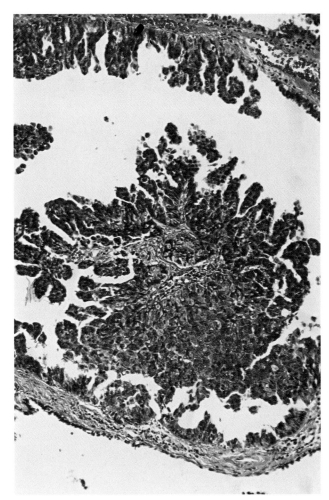

FIGURE 9.20

Low-grade papillary serous carcinoma. Complex branching papillae fill the fallopian tube lumen. Note the absence of invasion into the wall (stage IA-0).

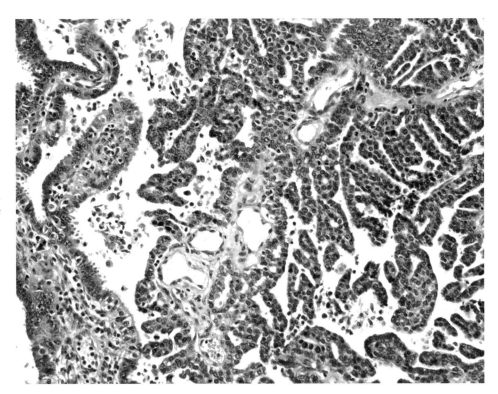

FIGURE 9.21

Low-grade papillary serous carcinoma. Cells with mild to moderate cytologic atypia line slender papillae.

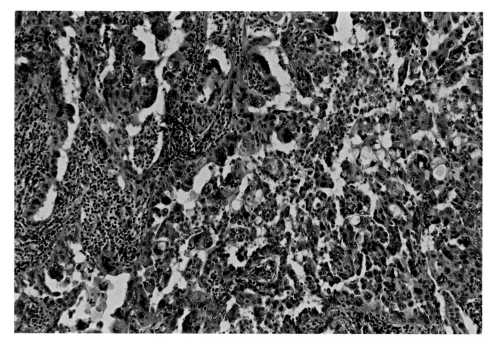

FIGURE 9.22
High-grade serous carcinoma. Numerous tumor giant cells are present.

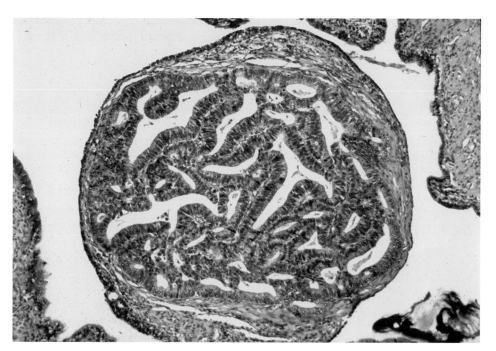

FIGURE 9.23
Endometrioid carcinoma. Back-to-back glands form an intraluminal nodule (stage IA-0).

Clear cell carcinoma is also rare; with a frequency ranging from 2–5% of all tubal carcinomas. These tumors show an admixture of different architectural patterns, including solid, papillary, and tubulocystic, similar to those seen in the uterus and ovary. They are high-grade and may show prominent hobnail and clear cells.

Squamous and adenosquamous carcinomas of the fallopian tube are very rare. Adenosquamous carcinoma is composed of large cells with distinct cell membranes, amphophilic cytoplasm, often with a ground-glass finely granular appearance, and large nuclei with prominent nucleoli. The stroma is infiltrated by numerous plasma cells, lymphocytes, and some eosinophils.

INTERNATIONAL FEDERATION OF GYNECOLOGISTS AND OBSTETRICIANS (FIGO) STAGING SYSTEM

There is no FIGO staging classification for fallopian tube carcinoma and the current clinical staging system is too simple (Table I). In 1999, modifications to the FIGO system were suggested in order to accommodate noninvasive carcinomas and those confined to the fimbriae. Stage IA-0 was proposed for intraluminal or intramucosal tumors without invasion into the lamina propria; stage IA-1 for tumors with extension into lamina propria, but without extension into the muscularis propria; and stage IA-2 for tumors with extension

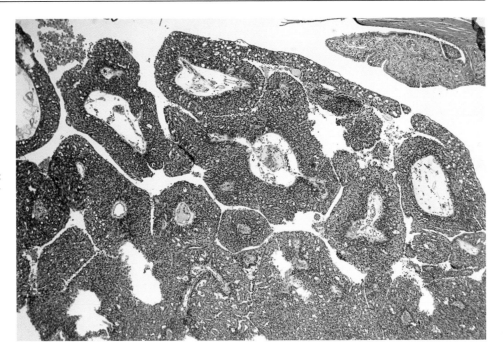

FIGURE 9.24

Transitional cell carcinoma. Exophytic growth with a striking papillary configuration is seen.

TABLE I

Carcinomas of the fallopian tube: TNM and FIGO staging

TNM	FIGO	
Tis	0	Carcinoma in situ (preinvasive carcinoma)
T1	I	Tumor confined to fallopian tube(s)
T1a	IA	Tumor limited to one tube, without penetrating the serosal surface
T1b	IB	Tumor limited to both tubes, without penetrating the serosal surface
T1c	IC	Tumor limited to one or both tube(s) with extension onto or through the tubal serosa, or with malignant cells in ascites or peritoneal washings
T2	II	Tumor involves one or both fallopian tube(s) with pelvic extension
T2a	IIA	Extension and/or metastasis to uterus and/or ovaries
T2b	IIB	Extension to other pelvic structures
T2c	IIC	Pelvic extension with malignant cells in ascites or peritoneal washings
T3 and/or N1	III	Tumor involves one or both fallopian tube(s) with peritoneal implants outside the pelvis and/or positive regional lymph nodes
T3a	IIIA	Microscopic peritoneal metastasis outside pelvis
T3b	IIIB	Microscopic peritoneal metastasis outside pelvis ≤ 2 cm in greatest dimension
T3c	IIIC	Peritoneal metastasis > 2 cm in greatest dimension and/or positive regional lymph nodes

into the muscularis propria. This modification of the FIGO staging system enhances the prognostic significance of staging in patients with fallopian tube carcinoma, as there are statistically significant differences in survival rates between patients with stage IA-0 or 1 and those with stage IA-2 tumors. Finally, carcinomas confined to the fimbriae are classified as stage I(F).

DIFFERENTIAL DIAGNOSIS

Once a fallopian tube origin has been established, the most important entity in the differential diagnosis is *pseudocarcinomatous hyperplasia* which can closely simulate invasive carcinoma, more commonly serous carcinoma. However, the degree of cytologic atypia is limited, mitotic activity is low to absent, without atypical forms, and this lesion is frequently associated with salpingitis.

Endometrioid carcinoma should be distinguished from *female adnexal tumor of probable wolffian origin* (FATWO). On gross examination, *FATWO* typically involves the outer aspect of the fallopian tube, and it has a homogeneous rubbery, white to tan to yellow cut surface, in contrast to the more friable and heterogeneous appearance of an endometrioid carcinoma. On microscopic examination, FATWO lacks glands with true luminal borders, luminal mucin, as well as squamous differentiation. Immunohistochemical stains may be helpful in this differential diagnosis as endometrioid carcinomas are typically EMA positive and most FATWOs are negative for this marker.

Finally, although rare, *tumors derived from intermediate trophoblast*, including placental site nodule, placental-site trophoblastic tumor, and epithelioid trophoblastic

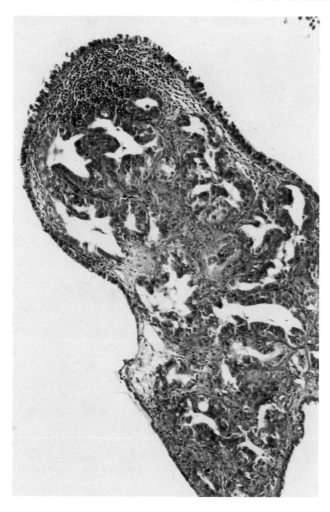

FIGURE 9.25
Papillary serous adenocarcinoma. The tumor is limited to the fimbriated end of the fallopian tube.

tumor have been described to arise in the fallopian tube. These tumors are composed of cells with abundant eosinophilic cytoplasm and may mimic a squamous cell carcinoma, as is more often the case in the cervix (Chapter 16). A previous history of an ectopic pregnancy can be discovered in some cases.

PROGNOSIS AND THERAPY

Fallopian tube carcinoma usually presents at advanced stage and has a poor prognosis. When the disease has extended beyond the fallopian tube, but is confined to the pelvis, the 5-year survival rate is close to 50%. Adverse prognostic factors include high stage, high grade, large volume of residual tumor after initial surgery, absence of closure of the fimbriated end, and fimbrial location (Figure 9.25). Treatment strategies are similar to those for carcinoma of the ovary.

CYSTS OF THE BROAD LIGAMENT – FACT SHEET

Definition
▶ Cysts lined by mesothelial, müllerian, or mesonephric epithelium

Incidence and Location
▶ 10% of all adnexal masses
▶ Near the fimbriated end of the fallopian tube or within the leaves of the broad ligament

Morbidity and Mortality
▶ Secondary torsion and/or rupture

Race and Age Distribution
▶ Racial distribution unknown
▶ Mean age 42.1 years

Clinical Features
▶ Incidental microscopic finding most common
▶ If symptomatic lower abdominal pain

Prognosis and Treatment
▶ Benign
▶ Surgery alone preferred treatment

CYSTS OF THE BROAD LIGAMENT – PATHOLOGIC FEATURES

Gross Findings
▶ Typically round unilocular cyst
▶ Mesothelial cysts may be uni- or multilocular
▶ From few millimeters to 20 cm

Microscopic Findings
▶ Müllerian cyst (hydatid of Morgagni): ciliated cells
▶ Mesothelial cyst: cuboidal to transitional cells
▶ Mesonephric cyst: cuboidal nonciliated cells

Differential Diagnosis
▶ Physiologic ovarian cyst
▶ Unilocular ovarian cystadenoma

METASTATIC TUMORS

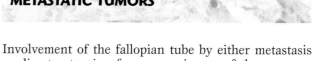

Involvement of the fallopian tube by either metastasis or direct extension from a carcinoma of the ovary or endometrium accounts for the majority of tubal malignancies. When both fallopian tube and ovary are intimately involved by tumor, the assumption of an ovarian origin may not always be correct. Metastases to the fallopian tube from extragenital carcinomas are uncommon; they are often seen within lymphovascular spaces, but they can also infiltrate the fallopian tube (Figure 9.26).

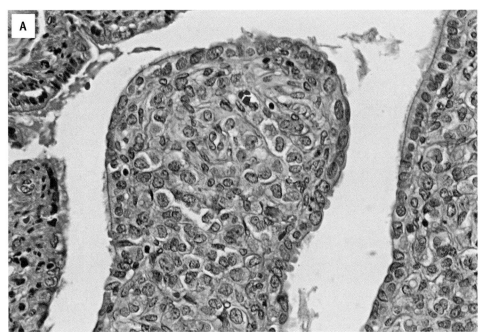

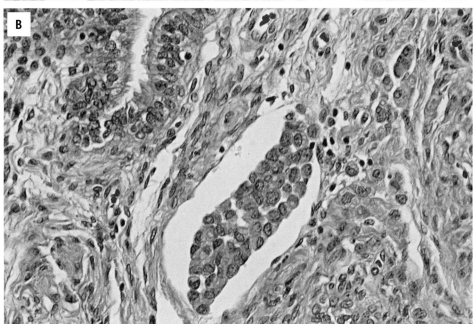

FIGURE 9.26
Metastatic breast carcinoma. Neoplastic cells expand the tubal plicae (A). A nest of neoplastic cells are present in a lymphovascular space (B).

BROAD LIGAMENT

CYSTS

CLINICAL FEATURES

Paraovarian cysts, which account for approximately 10% of all adnexal masses, may arise from the mesothelium as well as from müllerian or mesonephric (wolffian) rests. When large, the cysts become symptomatic due to pressure effect, with the most common presentation being lower abdominal pain. On imaging studies (radiology or ultrasonography), cysts of the broad ligament may be misclassified as primary lesions of the ovary, fallopian tubes, or uterus.

PATHOLOGIC FEATURES

GROSS FINDINGS

The cysts vary in size from a few millimeters to ≥ 20 cm. They are often round, unilocular cysts with a smooth inner surface.

MICROSCOPIC FINDINGS

Cysts are classified based upon their epithelial lining. *Hydatids of Morgagni* are the most common (müllerian cysts), and they are lined by ciliated epithelium similar to that of the fallopian tube. Mesothelial and transitional cell-lined cysts (cystic change of Walthard nests) are also common. Finally, mesonephric cysts arise from mesonephric remnants; they are lined by cuboidal nonciliated cells, and may be surrounded by smooth muscle fibers.

DIFFERENTIAL DIAGNOSIS

Clinically, paraovarian cysts should be included in the differential diagnosis of large *physiologic ovarian cysts* and *unilocular ovarian cystadenomas*. Microscopically, the distinction is not difficult; however, if the cyst is large and the cells become flattened it may not be possible to determine its origin, and a diagnosis of a simple cyst will suffice.

PROGNOSIS AND THERAPY

Paraovarian cysts and cysts of the broad ligament are benign but they may undergo torsion and rupture. Surgical excision is the preferred treatment.

FEMALE ADNEXAL TUMOR OF PROBABLE WOLFFIAN ORIGIN

CLINICAL FEATURES

This is a rare tumor, which is believed to originate from mesonephric (wolffian) remnants on the basis of their shared location in the broad ligament. Even though it was originally described in the broad ligament, it may also be seen in the ovary and retroperitoneum. These tumors occur in patients with a mean age of 46 (range 15–72) years. Symptoms at presentation include abdominal pain and/or a palpable mass and, in some cases, the tumor may be incidentally discovered.

PATHOLOGIC FEATURES

GROSS FINDINGS

This tumor is typically a well-circumscribed, solid mass with a bosselated external surface arising in the leaves of the broad ligament or a pedunculated mass arising from the fallopian tube serosa (Figure 9.27). They average approximately 8 cm in diameter. On sectioning, they frequently show a firm or rubbery, white

---

FEMALE ADNEXAL TUMOR OF PROBABLE WOLFFIAN ORIGIN – FACT SHEET

Definition
▸ Tumor believed to originate from mesonephric (wolffian) remnants

Incidence and Location
▸ Rare
▸ More common in broad ligament but can also be present in ovary

Morbidity and Mortality
▸ Very low morbidity

Race and Age Distribution
▸ Similar incidence for all racial groups
▸ 15 to 72 years

Clinical Features
▸ Abdominal pain
▸ Palpable mass
▸ Sometimes incidental finding

Prognosis and Treatment
▸ Most tumors behave in a benign fashion
▸ Rarely malignant with multiple recurrences and/or metastases
▸ Excision treatment of choice

FEMALE ADNEXAL TUMOR OF PROBABLE WOLFFIAN ORIGIN – PATHOLOGIC FEATURES

Gross Findings
▸ Solid tumor involving the broad ligament or paratubal soft tissues
▸ Average 8 cm
▸ Rounded with bosselated external surface
▸ Mostly solid and rubbery white to tan to yellow
▸ May have small cysts

Microscopic Findings
▸ Diffuse, tubular, or cystic (sieve-like) patterns
▸ Oval to spindled cells with minimal pale cytoplasm and small, round/oval nuclei

Immunohistochemical Features
▸ AE1/AE3, CAM 5.2, keratin 7, CD10, calretinin, vimentin positive
▸ Inhibin only focally positive
▸ EMA, CEA, S100, B72.3 typically negative

Ultrastructural Features
▸ Thick peritubular basal lamina, no/minimal cilia
▸ Golgi apparatus, secretory granules, and glycogen

Differential Diagnosis
▸ Endometrioid carcinoma

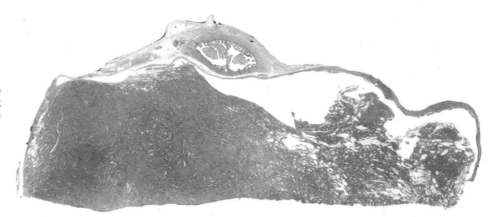

FIGURE 9.27
Female adnexal tumor of probable wolffian origin. A well-defined but unencapsulated tumor is centered in the paratubal tissues.

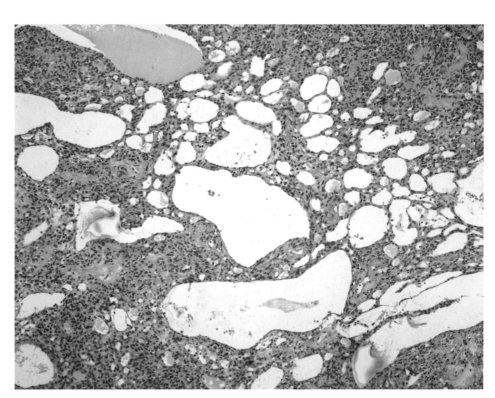

FIGURE 9.28
Female adnexal tumor of probable wolffian origin. The tumor shows a prominent cystic pattern.

to tan to yellow, homogeneous cut surface; small cysts and calcifications may also be present.

MICROSCOPIC FINDINGS

On low-power examination, these tumors often show an intimate and variable admixture of solid, tubular, and cystic growth (Figures 9.28 and 9.29). A sieve-like pattern secondary to a prominent cystic component and reminiscent of an adenomatoid tumor may be seen. The tubules are closely apposed but do not have a true luminal border whereas the solid component has a vaguely spindled appearance. The tumor cells have scant pale eosinophilic cytoplasm and oval to slightly elongated nuclei. Cytologic atypia is minimal and mitotic rate is very low in most cases (Figure 9.30).

ANCILLARY STUDIES

IMMUNOHISTOCHEMISTRY

Female adnexal tumors of probably wolffian origin are immunoreactive for pancytokeratin, CAM 5.2, cytokeratin 7, cytokeratin 903, ER, PR, AR, inhibin (albeit focal and faint), calretinin, CD10, and vimentin. Most tumors are negative for EMA.

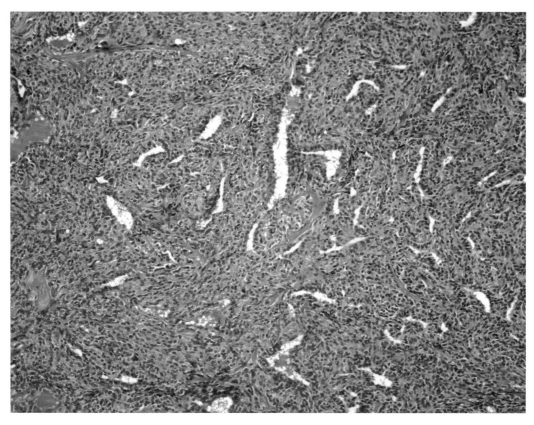

FIGURE 9.29
Female adnexal tumor of probable wolffian origin. Pseudotubules and solid areas are intimately admixed.

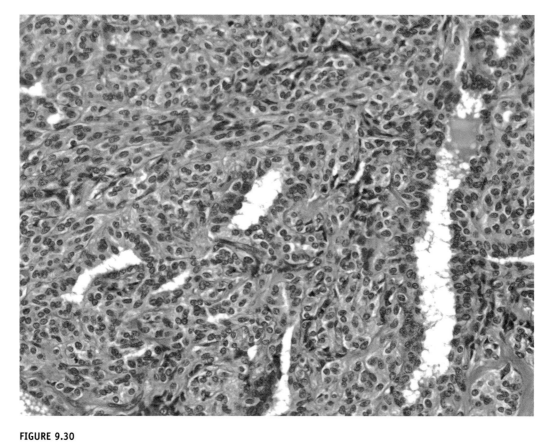

FIGURE 9.30
Female adnexal tumor of probable wolffian origin. The tumor cells are ovoid to slightly spindled with scant pale cytoplasm, have oval nuclei, and show bland cytologic features.

ULTRASTRUCTURAL EXAMINATION

The tumor cells show thick peritubular basal lamina and an absence or paucity of cilia, Golgi complexes, secretory granules, and glycogen.

DIFFERENTIAL DIAGNOSIS

Endometrioid adenocarcinoma of the fallopian tube is the main consideration in the differential diagnosis as it may closely resemble a FATWO. Microscopically, *endometrioid adenocarcinomas* may have spindle cells with a sieve-like architecture. However, unlike FATWO, they exhibit true glands, focal squamous differentiation, intraluminal mucin, and they are typically centered in the luminal aspect of the fallopian tube.

PROGNOSIS AND THERAPY

Most of these tumors behave in a benign fashion. Rare FATWOs exhibit a malignant behavior with multiple local recurrences and metastasis. No histologic features have been linked with malignant behavior. While most patients are treated with surgery, malignant tumors have been treated with multiple chemotherapy regimens.

PAPILLARY SEROUS CYSTADENOMA OF BORDERLINE MALIGNANCY

CLINICAL FEATURES

Papillary serous cystadenoma of borderline malignancy arising in the broad ligament is extremely rare. Patients range in age from 19 to 67 (average 32) years. The most common symptoms at presentation are lower abdominal and pelvic pain; however, some cases are discovered on routine gynecologic examination.

PATHOLOGIC FEATURES

GROSS FINDINGS

These tumors have a smooth outer surface and contain watery fluid. The inner surface has single or multiple 0.3–2.5-cm excrescences.

MICROSCOPIC FINDINGS

Simple to pseudostratified cuboidal to columnar, and focally ciliated epithelium lines the cyst wall and their papillary structures. The stroma resembles ovarian stroma but lacks follicles.

DIFFERENTIAL DIAGNOSIS

Distinction of a borderline tumor from a *serous carcinoma* is based on the absence of frank stromal invasion and marked nuclear atypia.

PROGNOSIS AND THERAPY

Patients have an excellent prognosis and local excision is curative.

EPENDYMOMA OF THE BROAD LIGAMENT

CLINICAL FEATURES

Ependymoma of the broad ligament is an extremely rare tumor that occurs in patients with a mean age of 38 (range 13–48) years who typically present with a pelvic mass or acute abdominal pain.

EPENDYMOMA – FACT SHEET

Definition
▶ Tumors showing ependymal differentiation akin to neoplasms of the central nervous system

Incidence
▶ Very rare

Morbidity and Mortality
▶ Related to recurrences and metastases

Race and Age Distribution
▶ Racial distribution unknown
▶ 13–48 years

Clinical Features
▶ Pelvic mass
▶ Acute lower abdominal pain

Prognosis and Treatment
▶ May metastasize
▶ No data available regarding treatment

PATHOLOGIC FEATURES

GROSS FINDINGS

Ependymomas may be solid, multicystic, multilobulated tumors of varying sizes with a soft friable consistency, frequently showing patchy hemorrhage and necrosis.

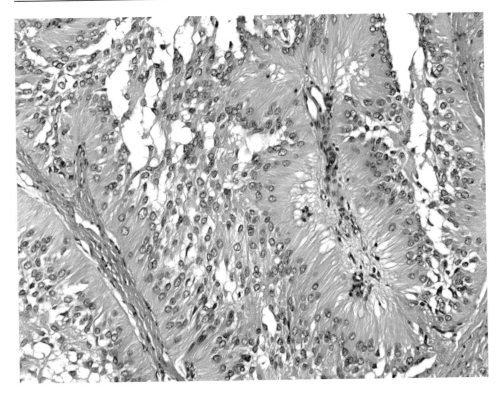

FIGURE 9.31

Ependymoma. Elongated cells with abundant pink cytoplasm and elongated processes show a perivascular arrangement.

EPENDYMOMA – PATHOLOGIC FEATURES

Gross Findings
▶ Solid, multicystic and multilobulated
▶ Soft friable consistency

Microscopic Findings
▶ Papillae, closely packed tubules, and solid growth
▶ Cells with abundant eosinophilic cytoplasm and long cilia
▶ True perivascular rosettes
▶ Psammoma bodies

Immunohistochemical Features
▶ Glial fibrillary acidic protein positive

Differential Diagnosis
▶ Papillary serous carcinoma

MICROSCOPIC FINDINGS

These tumors are similar in appearance to their counterparts in the central nervous system. They are composed of papillae, closely packed tubules, and solid growth. The papillae and tubules are lined by flat to columnar ciliated cells with central to apical, round to elongated nuclei. True perivascular rosettes (Figure 9.31), psammoma bodies, and small nodules of mature cartilage may be present.

DIFFERENTIAL DIAGNOSIS

These tumors are easily confused with *papillary serous carcinoma* because both exhibit papillary architecture

and may contain psammoma bodies. However, ependymal differentiation is evidenced by the presence of perivascular rosettes and positive reaction for glial fibrillary acidic protein.

PROGNOSIS AND THERAPY

Due to its rarity, information regarding outcome and therapeutic options is limited. Some tumors may be metastatic at the time of presentation. Recurrences, sometimes over decades, may also occur.

SUGGESTED READING

Metaplasias

Bramsilver BR, Ferenczy A, Richart RM. Brenner tumors and Walthard cell nests. Arch Pathol 1974;98:76–86.
Egan AJM, Russell P. Transitional cell metaplasia of the fallopian tube mucosa: morphologic assessment of three cases. Int J Gynecol Pathol 1996;15:72–76.
Hunt JL, Lynn AA. Histologic features of surgically removed fallopian tubes. Arch Pathol Lab Med 2002;126:951–955.
Seidman JD. Mucinous lesions of the fallopian tube: a report of seven cases. Am J Surg Pathol 1994;18:1205–1212.

Pseudocarcinomatous Hyperplasia

Cheung AN, Young RH, Scully RE. Pseudocarcinomatous hyperplasia of the fallopian tube associated with salpingitis. A report of 14 cases. Am J Surg Pathol 1994;18:1125–1130.
Dougherty CM, Cotten NM. Proliferative epithelial lesions of the uterine tube. I. Adenomatous hyperplasia. Obstet Gynecol 1964;24:849–854.
Moore SW, Enterline HT. Significance of proliferative epithelial lesions of the uterine tube. Obstet Gynecol 1975;45:385–390.
Pauerstein CJ, Woodruff JD. Cellular patterns in pyroliferative and anaplastic disease of the fallopian tube. Am J Obstet Gynecol 1966;96:486–492.

Roboy SS, Silva EG. Epithelial hyperplasia of the fallopian tube. Its association with serous borderline tumors of the ovary. Int J Gynecol Pathol 1989;8:214–220.

Torsion

Bernardus RE, Van der Slikke JW, Roex AJM, et al. Torsion of the fallopian tube: some considerations on its etiology. Obstet Gynecol 1984; 64:675.

Breen JL. A 21 year survey of 654 ectopic pregnancies. Am J Obstet Gynecol 1970;106:1004–1019.

Chambers JT, Thiagarajah S, Kitchin JD III. Torsion of the normal fallopian tube in pregnancy. Obstet Gynecol 1979;54:487–489.

Gold MA, Schmidt RR, Parks N, et al. Bilateral absence of the ovaries and distal fallopian tubes. A case report. J Reprod Med 1997;42:375–377.

Hibbard LT. Adnexal torsion. Am J Obstet Gynecol 1985;152:456–461.

Salpingitis Isthmica Nodosa

Honoré LH. Salpingitis isthmica nodosa in female infertility and ectopic tubal pregnancy. Fertil Steril 1978;29:164–168.

Jenkins CS, Williams RS, Schmidt GE. Salpingitis isthmica nodosa- a review of the literature, discussion of clinical significance, and consideration of patient management. Fertil Steril 1993;60:599–607.

Mc Comb PF, Rowe TC. Salpingitis isthmica nodosa: evidence it is a progressive disease. Fertil Steril 1989;51:542–545.

Persaud V. Etiology of tubal pregnancy. Obstet Gynecol 1970; 36:257–263.

Punnonen R, Soderstrom KO. Inflammatory etiology of salpingitis isthmica nodosa: a clinical, histological and ultrastructural study. Acta Eur Fertil 1986;17:199–203.

Tubal Pregnancy

Bickell NA, Bodian C, Anderson RM, et al. Time and the risk of ruptured tubal pregnancy. Obstet Gynecol 2004;104:789–794.

Budowick M, Johnson TR, Genadry R, et al. The histopathology of the developing tubal ectopic pregnancy. Fertil Steril 1980;34:169–171.

Giannopoulus T, Katesmark M. Ruptured tubal ectopic pregnancy with secondary implantation in the pouch of Douglas. J Obstet Gynaecol 2004;24:199–200.

Jacques SM, Qureshi F, Ramirez NC, et al. Retained trophoblastic tissue in fallopian tubes: a consequence of unsuspected ectopic pregnancies. Int J Gynecol Pathol 1997;16:219–224.

Pauerstein CJ, Croxatto HB, Eddy CA, et al. Anatomy and pathology of tubal pregnancy. Obstet Gynecol 1986;67:301–308.

Endometriosis

Clement PB. Pathology of endometriosis. Pathol Annu 1990;25:245–295.

Donnez J, Casanas-Roux F, Ferin J, et al. Tubal polyps, epithelial inclusions, and endometriosis after tubal sterilization. Fertil Steril 1984;41: 564–568.

Kuzela DC, Speers WC. Heterotopic endometrium of the fallopian tube. Fertil Steril 1985;44:552–553.

Rock JA, Parmley TH, King TM, et al. Endometriosis and the development of tuboperitoneal fistulas after tubal ligation. Fertil Steril 1981;35: 16–20.

Stock RJ. Postsalpingectomy endometriosis: a reassessment. Obstet Gynecol 1982;60:560–570.

Acute Infectious Salpingitis

Keith LG, Berger GS, Edelman DA. On the causation of pelvic inflammatory disease. Am J Obstet Gynecol 1984;149:215–224.

Mardh PA. Tubal factor infertility with special regard to chlamydial salpingitis. Curr Opin Infect Dis 2004;17:49–52.

Mc Cormack WM. Pelvic inflammatory disease. N Engl J Med 1994;330:115–119.

Soper DE, Brockwell NJ, Dalton HP, et al. Observations concerning the microbial etiology of acute salpingitis. Am J Obstet Gynecol 1994;170:1008–1017.

Thompson SE, Hager WD, Wong KH. The microbiology and therapy of acute pelvic inflammatory disease in hospitalized patients. Am J Obstet Gynecol 1980;136:179–186.

Chronic Salpingitis

Ault KA, Faro S. Pelvic inflammatory disease. Current diagnostic and treatment guidelines. Postgrad Med 1993;93:85–86.

Cohen MA, Lindheim SR, Sauer MV. Hydrosalpinges adversely affect implantation in donor oocyte cycles. Hum Reprod 1999; 14:1087–1089.

Parsons AK. Regarding the best approach to the pyosalpinx. Ultrasound Obstet Gynecol 1996;7:398–400.

Vasquez G, Boeckx W, Brosens I. Prospective study of tubal mucosa lesions and fertility in hydrosalpinges. Hum Reprod 1995;10:1075–1078.

Westrom L, Wolnerhanssen P. Pathogenesis of pelvic inflammatory disease. Genitourin Med 1993;69:9–17.

Tuberculous Salpingitis

Hallo HC. Female genital tuberculosis. Bull Int Union Tuberc 1968; 41:99–101.

Nogales-Ortíz F, Tarancon II, Nogales FF. The pathology of female genital tuberculosis. Obstet Gynecol 1979;53:422–428.

Parikh FR, Nadkarni SG, Kamat SA, et al. Genital tuberculosis – a major pelvis factor causing infertility in Indian women. Fertil Steril 1997;67:497–500.

Punnonen R, Kiilholma P, Meurman L. Female genital tuberculosis and consequent infertility. Int J Fertil 1983;28:235–238.

Schaefer G. Tuberculosis of the female genital tract. Clin Obstet Gynecol 1970;13:965–998.

Actinomycosis

Braby HH, Dougerty CM, Mikal A. Actinomycosis of the female genital tract. Obstet Gynecol 1964;23:580–583.

Dische FE, Burt JM, Davison NJH, et al. Tuboovarian actinomycosis associated with intrauterine contraceptive devices. J Obstet Gynaecol Br Commonw 1974;81:724–729.

Goodman HM, Tuomala RE, Leavitt T Jr. Actinomycotic pelvic inflammatory disease simulating malignancy. J Reprod Med 1986;31:625–628.

Persson E, Holmberg K. A longitudinal study of actinomyces israelii in the female genital tract. Acta Obstet Gynecol Scand 1984;63:207–216.

Yoonesi M, Crickard K, Cellini IS, et al. Association of actinomyces and intrauterine contraceptive devices. J Reprod Med 1985;30:48–52.

Adenomatoid Tumor

Bolton RN, Hunter WC. Adenomatoid tumors of the uterus and adnexa. Report of eleven cases. Am J Obstet Gynecol 1958;76:647–652.

Pauerstein CJ, Woodruff JD, Quinton SW. Developmental patterns in "adenomatoid lesions" of the fallopian tube. Am J Obstet Gynecol 1968;100:1000–1007.

Schwartz EJ, Longacre TA. Adenomatoid tumors of the female and male genital tracts express WT1. Int J Gynecol Pathol 2004;23:123–8.

Stephenson TJ, Mills PM. Adenomatoid tumors: an immunohistochemical and ultrastructural appraisal of their histogenesis. J Pathol 1986; 148:327–335.

Metaplastic Papillary Tumor

Bartnik J, Powell WS, Moriber-Katz S, et al. Metaplastic papillary tumor of the fallopian tube. Case report, immunohistochemical features, and review of the literature. Arch Pathol Lab Med 1989;113:545–547.

Keeney GL, Thrasher TV. Metaplastic papillary tumor of the fallopian tube: a case report with ultrastructure. Int J Gynecol Pathol 1988;7:86–92.

Pang LC. Hydrosalpinx due to asymptomatic bilateral tubal pregnancies associated with metaplastic papillary tumor of the fallopian tube. South Med J 1999;92:725–727.

Saffos RO, Rhatigan RM, Scully RE. Metaplastic papillary tumor of the fallopian tube—a distinctive lesion of pregnancy. Am J Clin Pathol 1980;74:232–236.

Borderline Epithelial Tumors of the Fallopian Tube

Alvarado-Cabrero I, Navani SS, Young RH, et al. Tumors of the fimbriated end of the fallopian tube. A clinicopathological analysis of 20 cases, including nine carcinomas. Int J Gynecol Pathol 1997;16:189–196.

Casasola SV, Mindan JP. Cystadenofibroma of fallopian tube. Appl Pathol 1989;7:256–259.

Kayaalp E, Heller DS, Majmudar B. Serous tumor of low malignant potencial of the fallopian tube. Int J Gynecol Pathol 2000;19:398–400.

Mc Carthy JH, Aga R. A fallopian tube lesion of borderline malignancy associated with pseudomyxoma peritonei. Histopathology 1998;13:223–225.

Zheng W, Wolf S, Kramer EE, et al. Borderline papillary serous tumor of the fallopian tube. Am J Surg Pathol 1996;20:30–35.

Intraepithelial Carcinoma

Agoff SN, Garcia RL, Goff B, et al. Follow-up of in situ and early stage fallopian tube carcinoma in patients undergoing prophylactic surgery for proven or suspected BRCA-1 or BRCA-2 mutations. Am J Surg Pathol 2004;28:1112–1114.

Bannatyne P, Russell P. Early adenocarcinoma of the fallopian tubes. A case for multifocal tumorigenesis. Diagn Gynecol Obstet 1981;3:49–60.

Colgan TJ. Challenges in the early diagnosis and staging of fallopian tube carcinomas associated with BRCA mutations. Int J Gynecol Pathol 2003;22:109–20.

Colgan TJ, Murphy J, Cole DE, et al. Occult carcinoma in prophylactic oophorectomy specimens: prevalence and association with BRCA germline mutation status. Am J Surg Pathol 2001;25:1283–9.

Lee Y, Medeiros F, Kindelberger D, et al. Advances in the recognition of tubal intraepithelial carcinoma: applications to cancer screening and the pathogenesis of ovarian cancer. Adv Anat Pathol 2006;13:1–7.

Medeiros F, Muto MG, Lee Y, et al. The tubal fimbria is a preferred site for early adenocarcinoma in women with familial ovarian cancer syndrome. Am J Surg Pathol 2006;30:230–236.

Sonnendecker HE, Cooper K, Kalian KN. Primary fallopian tube adenocarcinoma in situ associated with adjuvant tamoxifen therapy for breast carcinoma. Gynecol Oncol 1994;52:402–407.

Fallopian Tube Carcinoma

Alvarado-Cabrero I, Young RH, Vamvakas EC, et al. Carcinoma of the fallopian tube: a clinicopathological study of 105 cases with observations on staging and prognostic factors. Gynecol Oncol 1999;72:367–379.

Aziz S, Kuperstein G, Rosen B, et al. A genetic epidemiological study of carcinoma of the fallopian tube. Gynecol Oncol 2001;80:341–345.

Baekelandt M, Jorunn NA, Kristensen GB, et al. Carcinoma of the fallopian tube. Cancer 2000;89:2076–2084.

Finch A, Shaw P, Rosen B, et al. Clinical and pathologic findings of prophylactic salpingo-oophorectomies in 159 BRCA1 and BRCA2 carriers. Gynecol Oncol 2006;100:58–64.

Hellström AC, Frankendal B, Nilsson B, et al. Primary fallopian tube carcinoma: the prognostic impact of stage, histopathology and biologic parameters. Int J Gynecol Cancer 1996;6:456–462.

Rosen AC, Ausch CH, Hafner E, et al. A 15 year overview of management and prognosis in primary fallopian tube carcinoma. Eur J Cancer 1998;34:1725–1729.

Cysts of the Broad Ligament

Chudeka-Glaz A, Menkiszak J, Rzepka-Gorska I. Paraovarian cysts – not always benign. Gynekol Pol 2002;73:1078–1083.

Genadry R, Parmley T, Woodruff JD. The origin and clinical behavior of the paraovarian tumor. Am J Obstet Gynecol 1977;129:873–880.

Kishimoto K, Ito K, Awaya H, et al. Paraovarian cysts: MR imaging features. Abdom Imaging 2002;27:685–689.

Stock RJ. Large intraligamentous cysts. Technique of surgical removal and correlation of surgical observations and histologic findings pertaining to origin. J Reprod Med 1987;32:347–352.

Varras M, Akrivis CH, Polyzos D, et al. A voluminous twisted paraovarian cyst in a 74 year old patient: case report and review of the literature. Clin Exp Obstet Gynecol 2003;30:253–256.

Female Adnexal Tumor of Probable Wolffian Origin

Daya D. Malignant female adnexal tumor of probable wolffian origin with review of the literature. Arch Pathol Lab Med 1994;118:310–312.

Demopoulus RI, Sitelman A, Flotte T, et al. Ultrastructural study of a female adnexal tumor of probable wolffian origin. Cancer 1980;46:2273–2280.

Devouassoux-Shisheboran M, Silver SA, Tavassoli FA. Wolffian adnexal tumor, so called female adnexal tumor of probable wolffian origin. (FATWO): immunohistochemical evidence in support of a wolffian origin. Hum Pathol 1999;30:856–863.

Kariminejad MH, Scully RE. Female adnexal tumor of probable wolffian origin. A distinctive pathology entity. Cancer 1973;31:671–677.

Rahilly MA, William AR, Krausz T, et al. Female adnexal tumor of probable wolffian origin. A clinicopathological and immunohistochemical study of three cases. Histopathology 1995;26:69–74.

Borderline Tumors of the Broad Ligament

Aslani M, Ahn GH, Scully RE. Broad ligament mucinous and serous cystadenoma of borderline malignancy. Acta Obstet Gynecol Scand 1989;68:663–667.

Däblaing G, Klatt EC, Dirocco G, et al. Broad ligament serous tumor of low malignant potential. Int J Gynecol Pathol 1983;2:93–99.

Jensen ML, Nielsen MN. Broad ligament mucinous and serous cystadenomas of borderline malignancy. Acta Obstet Gynecol Scand 1989;68:663–667.

Jensen ML, Nielsen MN. Broad ligament mucinous cystadenoma of borderline malignancy. Histopathology 1990;16:89–91.

Loverro G, Cormio G, Renzulli G, et al. Serous papillary cystadenoma of borderline malignancy of the broad ligament. Eur J Obstet Gynecol Reprod Biol 1997;74:211–213.

Ependymoma of the Broad Ligament

Bell DA, Woodruff JM, Scully RE. Ependymoma of the broad ligament. A report of two cases. Am J Surg Pathol 1984;8:203–209.

Duggan MA, Hugh J, Nation JG, et al. Ependymoma of the uterosacral ligament. Cancer 1989;64:2565–2571.

Grody WW, Nieberg RK, Bhuta S. Ependymoma-like tumor of the mesoovarium. Arch Pathol Lab Med 1985;109:291–293.

10 Nonneoplastic Lesions of the Ovary

Teri A Longacre · C Blake Gilks

Nonneoplastic lesions of the ovary may be entirely asymptomatic incidental findings identified on gross or microscopic examination of the ovary, or they may be associated with a pelvic mass, pain, or manifestations of abnormal hormonal regulation. Many occur during the reproductive years and may be associated with infertility.

CYSTS OF FOLLICULAR ORIGIN

Solitary ovarian cysts of follicular origin are regularly encountered in women of reproductive age, where they can be a transient finding. They can also occur in neonates and children, and be associated with endocrine manifestations. Multiple follicular cysts, associated with sclerosis of the superficial cortical stroma (sclerocystic ovaries), are seen in association with chronic anovulation. Multiple follicular cysts secondary to excess of gonadotropins (hyperreactio luteinalis or ovarian hyperstimulation syndrome) are discussed later in this chapter, under the heading "Pregnancy-associated changes."

CLINICAL FEATURES

Solitary follicular cysts or corpora lutea cysts are usually an incidental finding in patients of reproductive age. When persistent, they may cause symptoms secondary to a pelvic mass, and occasional cases are associated with manifestations of excess estrogen production (isosexual pseudoprecocity in children, or irregular menses and/or endometrial hyperplasia in women of reproductive age). Follicular cysts or corpora lutea cysts may also rupture, leading to hemoperitoneum. Multiple follicular cysts are part of the spectrum of abnormalities seen in polycystic ovarian syndrome (PCOS), a common disorder, characterized by hyperandrogenism of ovarian origin, resulting in virilization, infertility, obesity, and insulin resistance (Stein–Leventhal syndrome). Up to 10 % of women with PCOS may have clinical manifestations. A family history is frequent but genetic factors in PCOS are poorly understood. The histopathologic find-

ings of multiple ovarian cysts associated with cortical sclerosis, although part of the spectrum of PCOS, is not specific, and can be seen in other causes of chronic anovulation; therefore, clinical and biochemical assessment is required for a diagnosis of PCOS. Solitary and multiple follicular cysts may also occur in association with McCune–Albright syndrome (polyostotic fibrous dysplasia, cutaneous melanin pigmentation, and endocrine organ hyperactivity) and in prepubertal patients with hypothyroidism.

CYSTS OF FOLLICULAR ORIGIN – FACT SHEET

Definition
- Physiologic (functional) follicle cyst or corpus luteum cyst measuring > 3 cm in diameter

Incidence and Location
- Common, especially during prepubertal and reproductive years

Morbidity and Mortality
- Often self-limited condition, but may cause acute abdominal pain secondary to rupture and hemoperitoneum, or torsion
- Persistence requires intervention in order to exclude a borderline or malignant surface epithelial tumor

Race and Age Distribution
- Prepubertal and reproductive-age women
- Rarely in neonates

Clinical Features
- Menstrual irregularities, occasionally amenorrhea
- Precocious pseudopuberty in prepubertal patients
- Sudden onset of abdominal pain if cyst ruptures with consequent hemoperitoneum

Radiologic Features
- Unilocular cyst > 3 cm

Prognosis and Treatment
- Benign
- Most solitary cysts resolve spontaneously
- Cystectomy if persistence or rupture

RADIOLOGIC FEATURES

Transvaginal ultrasound of follicular or corpora lutea cysts will show simple thin-walled cysts. With intracystic hemorrhage, the appearance can mimic a complex adnexal mass and may suggest a neoplasm. Small cysts can be followed with ultrasound; their disappearance over a period of weeks allows a presumptive benign diagnosis. The ultrasound appearance of multiple cysts in the cortex, associated with PCOS, is characteristic but, as noted previously, not specific for PCOS and correlation with other clinical findings is required for its diagnosis.

PATHOLOGIC FEATURES

GROSS FINDINGS

Solitary follicular cysts (Figure 10.1A) are thin-walled and > 3 cm in diameter (but usually < 10 cm). By definition, cysts < 3 cm are referred to as cystic follicles, and are considered to be within the range of normal follicular development. A corpus luteum cyst, also > 3 cm in diameter, more commonly contains intracystic hemorrhage and exhibits a yellow rim of variable thickness (Figure 10.2). Sclerocystic ovaries show bilateral ovarian enlargement with numerous cortical cysts, most measuring < 3 cm, and a band of white firm tissue that replaces the superficial cortex overlying the cysts (Figure 10.3).

MICROSCOPIC FINDINGS

Follicular cysts, whether solitary or multiple, are lined by granulosa cells with a surrounding layer of theca cells (Figure 10.1). Both layers may show luteinization. They are characterized by cells with abundant eosinophilic or clear cytoplasm and a round nucleus with a central nucleolus. Corpora lutea cysts show prominent luteinization of both granulosa and theca cell layers and undulating contours (Figure 10.2). In sclerocystic ovaries there is prominent sclerosis of the superficial ovarian cortex, visible as a pale rim of heavily collagenized ovarian stroma underlying the surface epithelium associated with multiple follicle cysts. Evidence of prior ovulation (e.g., corpora albicantia or lutea) is sparse (Figure 10.4).

CYSTS OF FOLLICUCAR ORIGIN – PATHOLOGIC FEATURES

Gross Findings

▸ Solitary, fluid-filled cyst measuring > 3 cm in diameter

Microscopic Findings

▸ Follicular cyst is lined by granulosa cells, with a surrounding layer of theca cells; both layers may show luteinization
▸ Corpus luteum cyst is composed of a thick undulating layer of granulosa and theca cells with prominent luteinization

Immunohistochemical Features

▸ Granulosa and theca cells are positive for inhibin and calretinin

Differential Diagnosis

▸ Cystic granulosa cell tumor
▸ Surface epithelial cystadenoma

POLYCYSTIC OVARIAN DISEASE – FACT SHEET

Definition

▸ Clinicopathologic syndrome characterized by anovulation, menstrual dysfunction, hyperandrogenism, and enlarged polycystic ovaries (Stein–Leventhal syndrome). Heterogeneous etiology, more commonly insulin resistance of peripheral tissue and/or an abnormality of the hypothalamic–pituitary–ovarian axis

Incidence and Location

▸ Very common, affecting up to 10% of reproductive-age women
▸ Increased incidence among first-degree relatives suggesting autosomal-dominant mode of inheritance in some cases

Morbidity and Mortality

▸ Infertility, insulin resistance (when present), and sequelae of increased peripheral conversion of androgenic to estrogenic compounds (e.g., endometrial hyperplasia, well-differentiated endometrial adenocarcinoma)

Age Distribution

▸ Age of onset typically perimenarchal

Clinical Features

▸ Anovulation, infertility, menstrual disturbances
▸ Obesity
▸ Hirsutism, acne, male-pattern baldness (some patients)

Radiologic Features

▸ Enlarged, multicystic ovaries with cystic follicles (typically ≥ 10) lining up at the periphery of the ovaries on ultrasound

Prognosis and Treatment

▸ Ovulation induction, weight loss, hormonal therapy (oral contraceptives or progestins), treatment of underlying insulin resistance, medical treatment for hirsutism

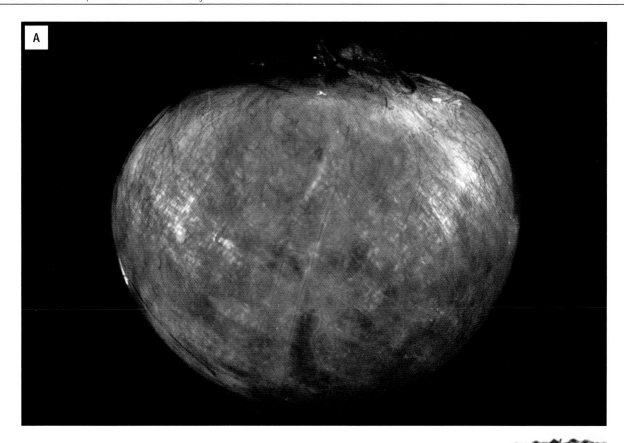

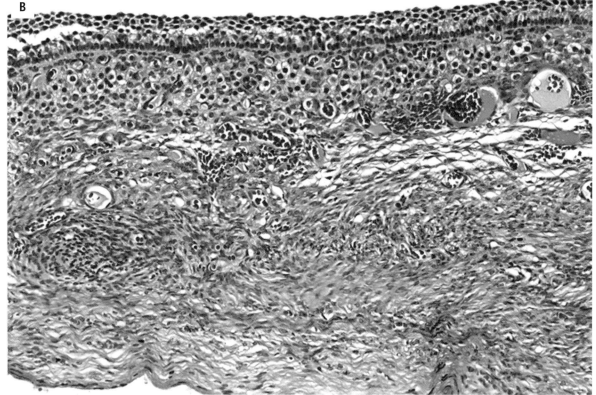

FIGURE 10.1

Follicular cyst. Unilocular thin-walled cyst with a smooth external surface measuring < 8 cm (A). The cyst is lined by several layers of granulosa cells and luteinized theca cells (B).

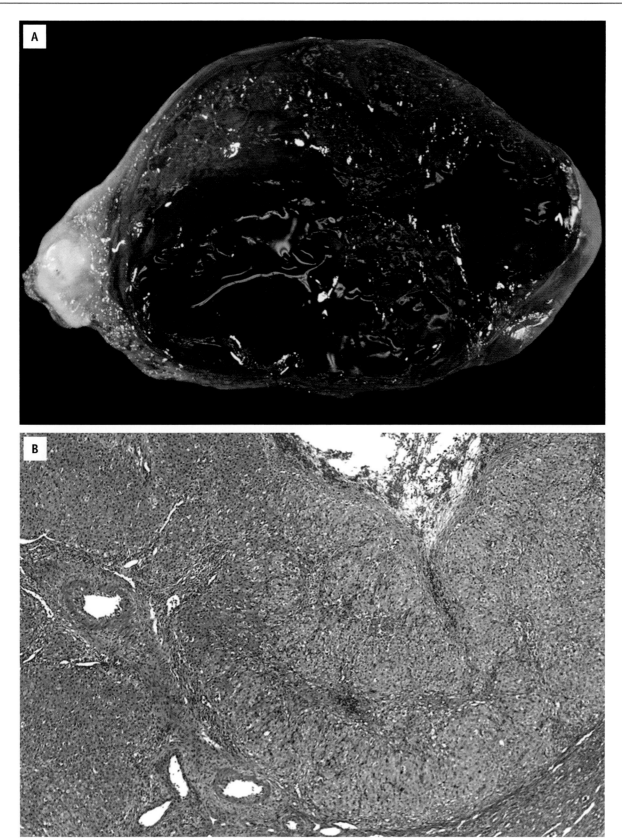

FIGURE 10.2

Corpus luteum cyst. Orange-brown cut surface with central hemorrhage (A). A corpus luteum cyst is distinguished from a follicular cyst by its undulating contour and marked luteinization of the granulosa cells (B).

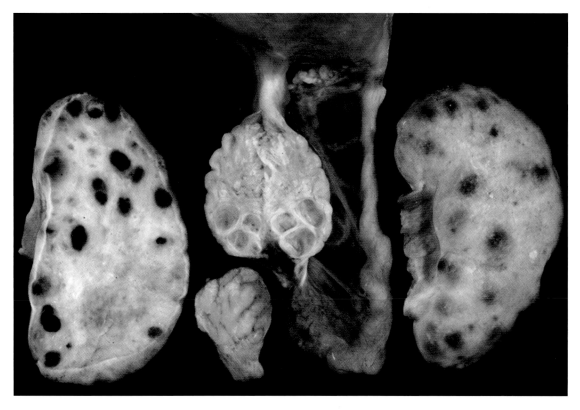

FIGURE 10.3

Polycystic ovarian syndrome. The ovaries are enlarged bilaterally due to multiple follicle cysts and expanded stroma. Note normal-sized ovaries in the middle for comparison (Courtesy of Dr. Michael Hendrickson).

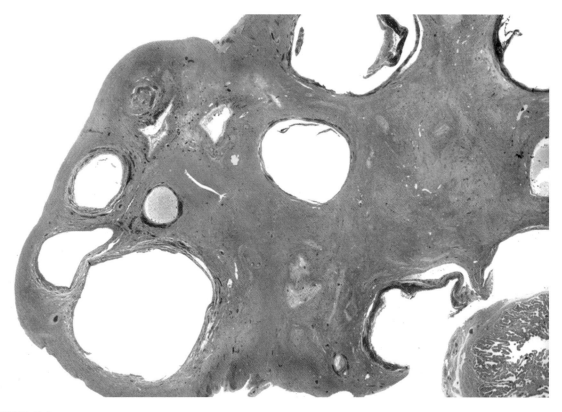

FIGURE 10.4

Polycystic ovarian syndrome. The follicular cysts are mainly distributed beneath the superficial sclerotic cortex.

ANCILLARY STUDIES

IMMUNOHISTOCHEMISTRY

The granulosa and theca cells stain positively for inhibin and calretinin.

CYTOLOGY

Aspiration of cyst fluid shows clusters of granulosa cells, distinguished cytologically from epithelial cells by their scant cytoplasm and indistinct cell margins.

DIFFERENTIAL DIAGNOSIS

The chief differential diagnosis is with *epithelial cysts* of surface epithelial stromal origin. There is generally no problem in differentiating between epithelial lining and granulosa cells; the former are typically monolayered and may contain cilia. Immunohistochemistry can be used in difficult cases as epithelial cells are negative for inhibin and calretinin. Solitary follicular cysts must also be distinguished from *unilocular cystic granulosa cell tumors*, which are usually larger and do not exhibit the well-organized granulosa cell-theca cell layers of follicular cysts, but rather have granulosa cell proliferations in the cyst wall, scattered Call-Exner bodies, and cells with less abundant cytoplasm.

PROGNOSIS AND THERAPY

Solitary follicular and corpora lutea cysts will usually resolve spontaneously. Management of PCOS depends on the clinical manifestations and whether pregnancy is desired. Since PCOS is considered to be an endocrinologic abnormality as opposed to a purely ovarian

---

POLYCYSTIC OVARIAN DISEASE – PATHOLOGIC FEATURES

Gross Findings
▸ Bilaterally enlarged ovaries with multiple, often uniformly sized follicular cysts
▸ Thickened superficial cortex

Microscopic Findings
▸ Multiple follicular cysts with prominent theca interna layer distributed beneath a collagenized hypocellular zone in superficial cortex, immediately underlying ovarian surface

Differential Diagnosis
▸ Normal variant in prepubertal ovaries
▸ McCune–Albright syndrome
▸ Multiple follicular cysts secondary to hypothyroidism
▸ Congenital adrenal hyperplasia

---

abnormality, current treatment is not directed at the ovarian changes per se as these may be encountered as an incidental finding in women without other features of PCOS.

STROMAL HYPERPLASIA AND HYPERTHECOSIS

Stromal hyperplasia is characterized by a nonneoplastic proliferation of ovarian stromal cells, whereas stromal hyperthecosis is characterized by stromal cell luteinization in a background of stromal hyperplasia.

CLINICAL FEATURES

Stromal hyperplasia and hyperthecosis are most common in the sixth to seventh decades, occurring in more than

---

STROMAL HYPERPLASIA AND HYPERTHECOSIS – FACT SHEET

Definition
▸ Stromal hyperplasia: Non-neoplastic cellular proliferation of non-luteinized ovarian stromal cells
▸ Stromal hyperthecosis: Luteinized stromal cells present in a background of stromal hyperplasia

Incidence and Location
▸ Common
▸ Bilateral

Morbidity and Mortality
▸ Secondary to hormonal manifestations

Age Distribution
▸ More common in sixth to seventh decades
▸ Less common in reproductive-age except in PCOS

Clinical Features
▸ Often asymptomatic
▸ Estrogenic manifestations (endometrial hyperplasia/carcinoma)
▸ Androgenic manifestations (virilization, acne)
▸ Obesity, hypertension, glucose intolerance
▸ Rarely HAIR-AN syndrome (hyperandrogenism, insulin resistance, and acanthosis nigricans)

Radiologic Features
▸ Bilateral ovarian enlargement with or without hypoechogenicity on ultrasound

Prognosis and Treatment
▸ GnRH agonists or oral contraceptives if hyperandrogenic manifestations
▸ Complete resolution of androgenic symptoms with bilateral oophorectomy; insulin resistance in HAIR-AN syndrome usually persists

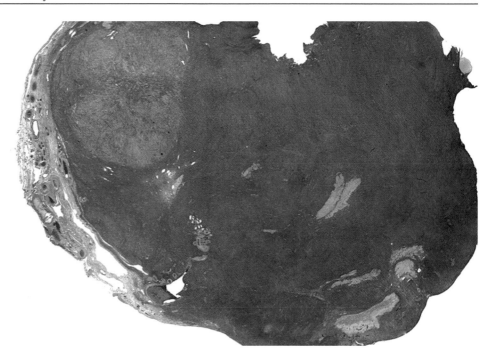

FIGURE 10.5

Stromal hyperplasia. Nodular and diffuse hyperplastic proliferation of cellular stroma is typically bilateral and found during menopause.

one-third of women in this age group. Many patients are asymptomatic, but androgen hypersecretion may be present, particularly in younger, reproductive-aged women with stromal hyperthecosis. These patients are characteristically virilized, obese, hypertensive, and hyperinsulinemic. A small percentage of patients with hyperthecosis have HAIR-AN syndrome, which consists of hyperandrogenism (HA), insulin resistance (IR), and acanthosis nigricans (AN). Some patients with hyperthecosis have estrogenic manifestations, such as endometrial hyperplasia or even well-differentiated adenocarcinoma.

RADIOLOGIC FEATURES

The ovaries may be normal or slightly enlarged. Variation in echogenicity may be present on ultrasound.

PATHOLOGIC FEATURES

GROSS FINDINGS

Stromal hyperplasia and stromal hyperthecosis are typically bilateral and may be associated with normal-sized or enlarged (up to 7.0 cm) ovaries, which have a diffuse or nodular firm, white to yellow cut surface.

MICROSCOPIC FINDINGS

In stromal hyperplasia, there is a nodular and/or diffuse, bilateral cortical and medullary proliferation of mitotically inactive stromal cells with ovoid nuclei and indistinct nucleoli, present more frequently in the med-

---

**STROMAL HYPERPLASIA AND HYPERTHECOSIS –
PATHOLOGIC FEATURES**

Gross Findings

▶ Bilateral normal or enlarged ovaries (up to 7 cm) with diffuse or nodular firm, white or yellow parenchyma

Microscopic Findings

▶ *Stromal hyperplasia*
  ▶ Diffuse or nodular proliferation
  ▶ Oval to spindled cells with scant cytoplasm
  ▶ May be associated with Leydig cell hyperplasia
▶ *Stromal hyperthecosis*
  ▶ Single cells or aggregates of large rounded cells with abundant eosinophilic or vacuolated cytoplasm and central, round nuclei with small nucleoli
  ▶ Typical background of stromal hyperplasia
  ▶ May be associated with Leydig cell hyperplasia

Immunohistochemical Features

▶ Luteinized cells are positive for inhibin and calretinin

Differential Diagnosis

▶ Leydig cell hyperplasia
▶ Stromal luteoma
▶ Luteinized thecoma
▶ Steroid cell tumor

---

ullary region (Figure 10.5). In stromal hyperthecosis, there are aggregates of luteinized cells, which have abundant eosinophilic or vacuolated cytoplasm and central, round nuclei with small nucleoli, typically present in a background of stromal hyperplasia (Figure 10.6).

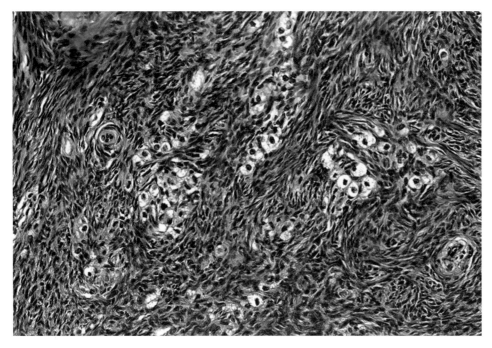

FIGURE 10.6
Stromal hyperthecosis. Nests of eosinophilic and vacuolated luteinized cells are dispersed throughout the hyperplastic ovarian stroma.

DIFFERENTIAL DIAGNOSIS

Stromal hyperplasia/hyperthecosis should be distinguished from other processes characterized by lipid-laden cells such as Leydig cell hyperplasia, stromal luteoma, luteinized thecoma, and steroid cell tumors. *Leydig cell hyperplasia* may accompany stromal hyperplasia and hyperthecosis, but it is typically seen at the hilus of the ovary. Like stromal hyperthecosis, Leydig cell hyperplasia may be asymptomatic or manifest as androgenic disturbances; however, it is associated with some degree of nuclear pleomorphism and multinucleation. Reinke crystals may also be present. *Stromal luteoma* is defined as a tumor composed of lutein cells ≥ 0.5 cm in size. It typically arises in a background of stromal hyperthecosis. *Luteinized thecoma* and *steroid cell tumor* form a distinct mass or nodule on macroscopic examination and are almost always unilateral.

PROGNOSIS AND THERAPY

Patients with hyperandrogenic manifestations may respond to gonadotropin-releasing hormone (GnRH) agonists or oral contraceptives. Bilateral oophorectomy results in complete resolution of the androgenic symptoms, but the insulin resistance in HAIR-AN syndrome usually persists.

LEYDIG CELL HYPERPLASIA

This is a nodular or diffuse benign proliferation of Leydig cells that may occur within the ovarian hilus,

where they normally exist (hilar Leydig cell hyperplasia), or much less frequently within the ovarian stroma (stromal Leydig cell hyperplasia), in the wall of the fallopian tube or adjacent to an ovarian tumor.

CLINICAL FEATURES

Leydig cell hyperplasia typically occurs in postmenopausal women in association with stromal hyperplasia or stromal hyperthecosis. Mild hyperplasia is most common and is not usually associated with relevant clinical endocrine disturbances. More pronounced degrees of Leydig cell hyperplasia may be associated with virilization and most frequently occur in younger women, occasionally during pregnancy.

RADIOLOGIC FEATURES

There are no specific radiologic features associated with Leydig cell hyperplasia.

PATHOLOGIC FEATURES

GROSS FINDINGS

Leydig cell hyperplasia, in the absence of associated stromal hyperplasia or stromal hyperthecosis, does not have any specific gross ovarian findings. Most affected ovaries are grossly unremarkable.

MICROSCOPIC FINDINGS

Leydig cell hyperplasia results in small aggregates, nests, clusters or, less commonly, diffuse sheets of polygonal cells with abundant eosinophilic cytoplasm and rounded, hyperchromatic nuclei, typically in the hilus of the ovary (hilus cell hyperplasia) (Figure 10.7). Mitotic figures may be present and there may be significant cellular and nuclear pleomorphism. Intracytoplasmic elongated, eosinophilic Reinke crystals, when present, are considered to be specific for Leydig cells.

ANCILLARY STUDIES

IMMUNOHISTOCHEMISTRY

The hyperplastic Leydig cells, like normal Leydig cells, will stain for inhibin or calretinin.

ULTRASTRUCTURAL EXAMINATION

Crystals of Reinke in Leydig cells form needle-shaped structures when cut in longitudinal section and hexagonal microtubular units when cut in cross-section.

DIFFERENTIAL DIAGNOSIS

Leydig cell hyperplasia is distinguished from *luteinized stromal cells* primarily on the basis of its hilar location (for the hilar variant) and the presence of Reinke crystals (for the rare stromal variant). *Leydig cell tumors* are larger, discrete, solid masses and are more frequently associated with virilization.

PROGNOSIS AND THERAPY

Leydig cell hyperplasia is often an incidental finding in ovaries removed for an unrelated gynecologic disorder. Patients with associated virilization exhibit complete resolution of androgenic symptoms following oophorectomy.

PREGNANCY-ASSOCIATED CHANGES

The ovaries can undergo changes in pregnancy that can mimic a neoplasm, both grossly and microscopically. Specific entities include: pregnancy luteoma, large solitary luteinized follicle cyst of pregnancy and puerperium, hyperreactio luteinalis, decidual reaction of the ovarian stroma, and granulosa cell proliferations. Prior to diagnosing an ovarian neoplasm during pregnancy, exclusion of these nonneoplastic pregnancy-associated entities that are either specific for pregnancy, or seen most commonly during pregnancy is essential.

CLINICAL FEATURES

Knowledge of the clinical setting (i.e., pregnancy) is important and, regrettably, may not always be indicated on the specimen requisition. If there is any question of a pregnancy-associated condition, consultation with the primary care physician or the patient record should take place early in the diagnostic work-up. Pregnancy luteoma, unlike the large solitary luteinized follicle cyst of pregnancy and hyperreactio luteinalis, occurs more frequently in black women. Virilization is the presenting manifestation of pregnancy luteoma in 25 % of cases, and both pregnancy luteoma and solitary luteinized follicle cyst of pregnancy and puerperium may present as a palpable adnexal mass. These pregnancy-associated changes are otherwise asymptomatic and discovered

---

PREGNANCY LUTEOMA – FACT SHEET

Definition
▶ Nonneoplastic ovarian tumor-like lesion composed of luteinized cells occurring during pregnancy

Incidence and Location
▶ Uncommon
▶ 30% bilateral and 50% multiple

Morbidity and Mortality
▶ Secondary to hormonal manifestations

Race and Age Distribution
▶ More common in black women
▶ Reproductive age

Clinical Features
▶ Typically in second half of pregnancy
▶ Incidental finding at cesarean section
▶ Hirsutism or virilization in mother (25%) or female infants (70%)

Radiologic Features
▶ Solid mass(es) on ultrasound; may exhibit cystic area(s)

Prognosis and Treatment
▶ Benign, regresses following delivery

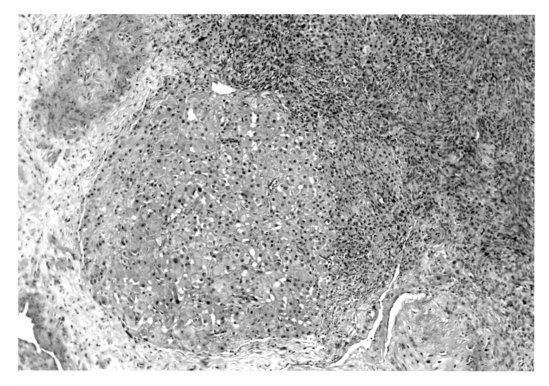

FIGURE 10.7
Leydig cell hyperplasia (hilus cell hyperplasia). A nodule of Leydig cells is present in the hilus of the ovary.

PREGNANCY LUTEOMA – PATHOLOGIC FEATURES

Gross Findings
▶ One or multiple (more common), red to brown fleshy mass(es)

Microscopic Findings
▶ Well circumscribed
▶ Luteinized cells with abundant eosinophilic cytoplasm, central round and regular nuclei, and prominent nucleoli
▶ Mitoses (up to 7/10 HPFs)
▶ Necrosis and degenerative changes may be seen

Immunohistochemical Features
▶ Positive for inhibin and calretinin

Differential Diagnosis
▶ Steroid cell tumor
▶ Leydig cell tumor
▶ Thecoma

LARGE SOLITARY LUTEINIZED FOLLICLE CYST OF PREGNANCY AND PUERPERIUM – FACT SHEET

Definition
▶ Nonneoplastic large luteinized cyst occurring during pregnancy

Incidence and Location
▶ Rare
▶ Unilateral

Morbidity and Mortality
▶ Primarily associated with excessive surgery to exclude neoplastic condition(s)

Age Distribution
▶ Reproductive age

Clinical Features
▶ Asymptomatic
▶ Palpable adnexal mass discovered during pregnancy or cesarean section

Radiologic Features
▶ Unilateral, large unilocular cyst

Prognosis and Treatment
▶ Benign
▶ Limited resection curative

---

incidentally (usually at the time of cesarean section). Hyperreactio luteinalis or ovarian hyperstimulation syndrome occurs as a result of an excess of either endogenous or exogenous gonadotrophins respectively, and is associated with virilization in 15 % of women. Ovarian hyperstimulation syndrome can be associated with massive edema, ascites, and hydrothorax, findings not encountered in patients with non-iatrogenic hyperreactio luteinalis.

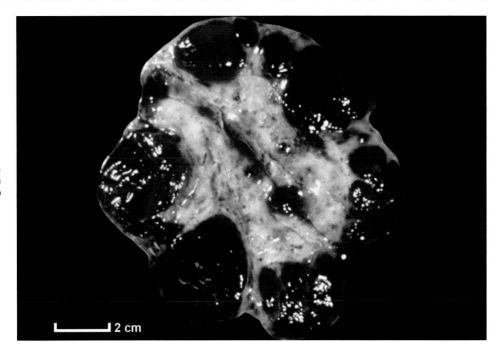

FIGURE 10.8
Pregnancy luteoma. Multiple circum-scribed nodules show a red-brown cut surface (Courtesy of Dr. Philip Clement).

RADIOLOGIC FEATURES

Findings on imaging are not specific. Pregnancy luteoma can appear as a solid mass, but may exhibit cystic areas secondary to necrosis. Solitary luteinized follicle cyst of pregnancy and puerperium appears as a large (median 25 cm) thin-walled unilocular cyst. Hyperreactio luteinalis can appear as symmetric ovarian enlargement with multiple peripheral uniformly sized cysts.

PATHOLOGIC FEATURES

GROSS FINDINGS

Pregnancy luteomas are bilateral in one-third of cases and are often multinodular. Red, brown, or gray solid and fleshy, sometimes hemorrhagic nodules, replace the ovarian parenchyma (Figure 10.8). Large solitary luteinized follicle cyst of pregnancy and puerperium is invariably unilateral and appears as a thin-walled cyst with a smooth lining. The gross appearance of hyperreactio luteinalis or ovarian hyperstimulation syndrome is that of variable, but sometimes massive, ovarian enlargement secondary to numerous thin-walled cysts which may be hemorrhagic. Decidual reaction may be visible as soft red fleshy foci on the ovarian surface or peritoneum, or may be an incidental microscopic finding. Granulosa cell proliferations of pregnancy are invariably incidental microscopic findings.

LARGE SOLITARY LUTEINIZED FOLLICLE CYST OF PREGNANCY AND PUERPERIUM – PATHOLOGIC FEATURES

Gross Findings

▶ Large (8–36 cm; median 25 cm) unilocular, thin-walled cyst containing serous fluid

Microscopic Findings

▶ Luteinized granulosa and theca cells (the latter inconspicuous) with ample cytoplasm lining the cyst wall
▶ Nuclear hyperchromasia and focal marked nuclear pleomorphism but no mitoses

Immunohistochemical Features

▶ Granulosa and theca cells positive for inhibin

Differential Diagnosis

▶ Unilocular cystic granulosa cell tumor
▶ Surface epithelial cystadenoma

MICROSCOPIC FINDINGS

Pregnancy luteomas are composed of sharply circumscribed nodules of polygonal cells with abundant eosinophilic cytoplasm, central nuclei and prominent nucleoli, typical of steroid-producing cells (Figure 10.9); occasional mitotic figures may be seen. Large solitary luteinized follicle cyst of pregnancy and puerperium is lined by large cells with abundant cytoplasm with focal pleomorphic and hyperchromatic nuclei (Figure 10.10). The

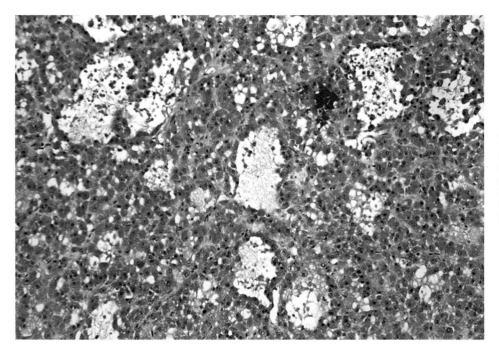

FIGURE 10.9
Pregnancy luteoma. Large polygonal cells contain abundant eosinophilic cytoplasm and regular, round centrally positioned nuclei with small nucleoli, and focally form pseudoglandular spaces.

HYPERREACTIO LUTEINALIS – FACT SHEET

Definition
▶ Bilateral ovarian enlargement secondary to development of multiple luteinized cysts that can occur during pregnancy, in association with beta-HCG-producing tumors, or during ovulation induction (ovarian hyperstimulation syndrome)

Incidence and Location
▶ Rare in normal pregnancy
▶ May occur in 10–40% of women with gestational trophoblastic disease and in women undergoing ovulation induction (especially those with pre-existing polycystic ovaries)

Morbidity and Mortality
▶ Potential cyst rupture and intraabdominal hemorrhage

Age Distribution
▶ Reproductive age

Clinical Features
▶ Typically asymptomatic; usually discovered during pregnancy, delivery, puerperium, or following ovulation induction
▶ Abdominal pain secondary to hemorrhage
▶ Virilization (15%)

Radiologic Features
▶ Symmetrical and bilateral ovarian enlargement with multiple peripheral uniform cysts (1–3 cm in diameter)
▶ Ascites or pleural effusions may occur in ovarian hyperstimulation syndrome

Prognosis and Treatment
▶ Regression, especially following delivery or treatment of underlying gestational trophoblastic disease, but complete regression may take 4–6 months
▶ Ovarian hyperstimulation syndrome treated by cyst aspiration under ultrasound guidance or surgical excision if complicated by infarction, hemorrhage, or persistence

---

HYPERREACTIO LUTEINALIS – PATHOLOGIC FEATURES

Gross Findings
▶ Moderately to markedly enlarged ovaries (> 5 cm) with multiple thin-walled cysts containing serous or serosanguineous fluid

Microscopic Findings
▶ Multiple follicle cysts lined by luteinized theca interna cells (more prominent) and granulosa cells, the latter showing occasional cytologic alypia
▶ Marked edema in surrounding ovarian stroma

Immunohistochemical Features
▶ Granulosa and luteinized theca cells positive for inhibin

Differential Diagnosis
▶ Surface epithelial neoplasm/metastases (macroscopically)
▶ Large solitary luteinized follicle cyst of pregnancy and puerperium

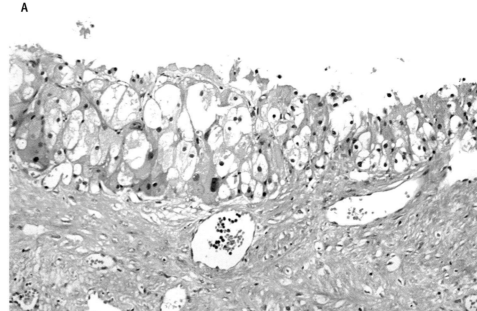

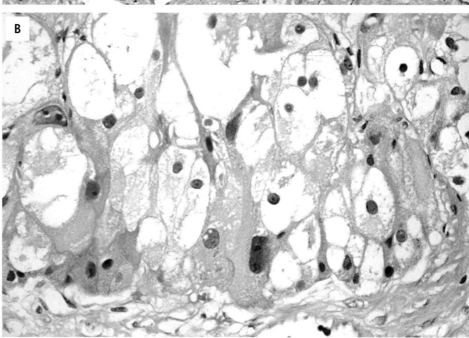

FIGURE 10.10

Large solitary luteinized cyst of pregnancy and puerperium. The cyst wall is lined by luteinized granulosa and theca cells with ample cytoplasm which appear indistinguishable (A). Nuclear hyperchromasia and focal marked nuclear pleomorphism are seen (B).

atypia is thought to be of degenerative type. Unlike usual follicular cysts, a distinct theca layer is not identifiable. The cysts in hyperreactio luteinalis are lined by hyperplastic and luteinized granulosa and theca interna cells (the latter being more conspicuous) (Figure 10.11). Decidual reaction consists of cells indistinguishable from decidualized endometrial stromal cells, and are thought to arise by metaplasia of ovarian stroma. They range in size from a few cells to sheets of cells, forming excrescences on the ovarian surface (Figure 10.12). Granulosa cell proliferations of pregnancy consist of uniform non-luteinized granulosa cells arranged in sheets, trabeculae, insulae or microfollicles, they occur within atretic follicles, typically < 5 mm in size.

ANCILLARY STUDIES

IMMUNOHISTOCHEMISTRY

The sex cord nature of the cells of pregnancy luteoma, large solitary luteinized follicle cyst of pregnancy and puerperium, and granulosa cell proliferations can be

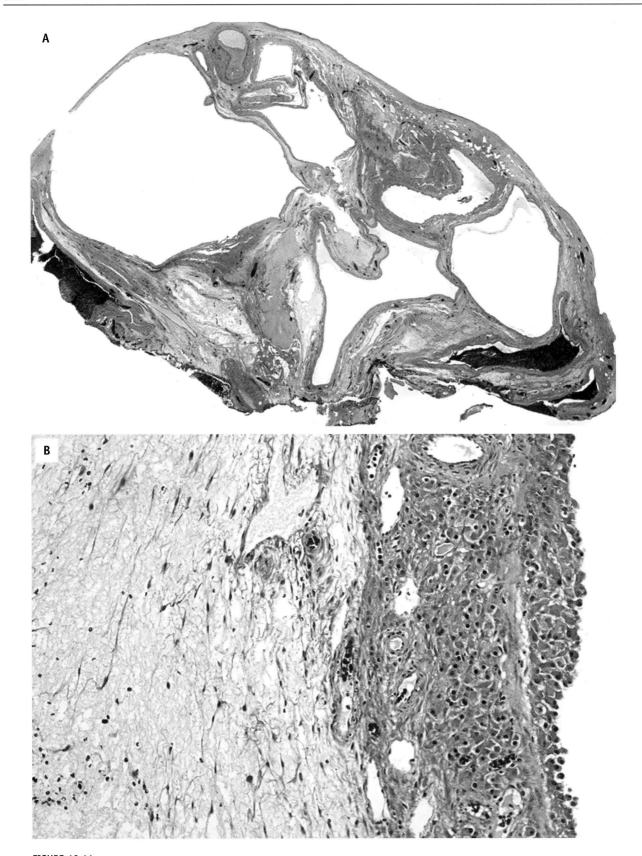

FIGURE 10.11

Hyperreactio luteinalis. Multiple enlarged thin-walled cysts replace the ovarian parenchyma (A). The theca interna layer appears more prominent than the granulosa layer and striking edema is present outside the cyst wall (B).

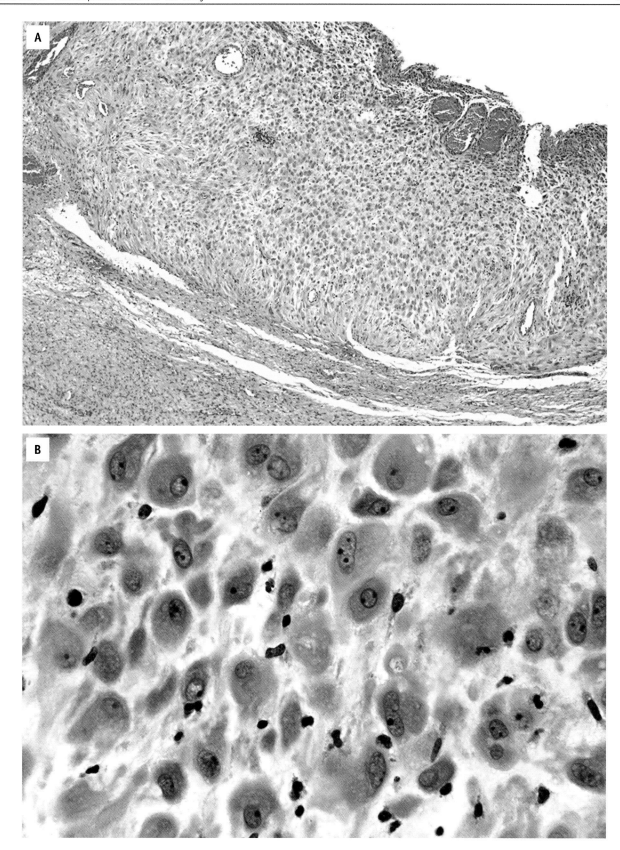

FIGURE 10.12

Ectopic decidua. A nodule (A) composed of polygonal cells with eosinophilic and vacuolated cytoplasm and central, pale, vesicular nuclei (B) is present within the ovarian cortex.

confirmed with staining for inhibin or other sex-cord stromal markers. The decidualized stromal cells of ectopic decidua are negative for keratin.

DIFFERENTIAL DIAGNOSIS

The differential diagnosis of pregnancy luteoma mainly includes *sex cord stromal tumors composed of luteinized cells* (particularly steroid cell tumor, Leydig cell tumor, and thecoma). The distinctive gross appearance of pregnancy luteoma and the clinical setting are key in reaching a correct diagnosis. In cases where a firm diagnosis is not possible based on a biopsy specimen, a conservative approach is recommended, with the diagnosis of pregnancy luteoma confirmed on clinical follow-up when there is prompt regression of the mass after delivery. Large solitary luteinized follicle cyst of pregnancy and puerperium must be distinguished from a *cystadenoma of surface epithelial stromal origin* or a *cystic granulosa cell tumor*. If there is doubt about the origin of the cells lining the cyst, immunohistochemistry can be used to differentiate between granulosa cells and epithelial cells. With respect to the differential diagnosis with cystic granulosa cell tumor, the intramural proliferations of granulosa cells characteristic of cystic granulosa cell tumor are not seen in large solitary luteinized follicle cyst of pregnancy and puerperium. Rarely, *hyperrectio luteinalis* can be grossly confused with a primary or metastatic neoplasm, but on microscopic examination the correct diagnosis is easily established. Hyperreactio luteinalis can be separated from a large, solitary, luteinized follicle cyst of pregnancy because it is typically bilateral, multiple, and may be associated with a pregnancy luteoma. Decidual reaction must be distinguished from *metastatic carcinoma*; immunohistochemistry can be of help in problematic cases, although it is not usually required since decidual reaction lacks the atypia and mitotic activity commonly seen in metastatic carcinoma. Granulosa cell proliferations of pregnancy can mimic small granulosa cell tumors. The clinical setting (pregnancy) and their microscopic size are features which allow for a correct diagnosis.

PROGNOSIS AND TREATMENT

Pregnancy luteoma should be treated conservatively, with preservation of the ovaries. Biopsy and frozen section can be done to confirm the diagnosis. Pregnancy luteoma will start to regress within days after delivery, involuting completely within weeks. Large solitary luteinized follicle cysts are typically removed surgically because of their large size; no further therapy is required. Hyperreactio luteinalis typically resolves weeks to months following removal of the precipitating cause of gonadotropin excess (e.g., pregnancy or gestational tro-

phoblastic disease). Ovarian hyperstimulation syndrome similarly regresses upon cessation of ovulation induction. Decidual reaction and granulosa cell proliferations regress postpartum. Decidual reaction can occur unrelated to pregnancy, where it is seen as an incidental finding and no treatment is required.

OVARIAN TORSION

Ovarian torsion is the fifth most common cause of a gynecologic surgical emergency. In these cases, the ovary and often the ipsilateral fallopian tube twist with the vascular pedicle, resulting in vascular compromise. Unrelieved torsion leads to hemorrhagic infarction. It is commonly associated with an underlying ovarian cystic lesion, mass, or other abnormality, although torsion of a normal ovary may occur, especially in infants and children.

CLINICAL FEATURES

Most women with ovarian torsion are young (mean 26 years). Approximately 20% of cases occur in pregnant women. Patients present with sudden onset or episodic acute abdominal pain. Occasionally, an adnexal mass can be palpated on pelvic examination.

RADIOLOGIC FEATURES

Ovarian torsion is seen as an uniformly echogenic mass on ultrasonography. Computed tomography (CT) and MRI may also be useful diagnostic tools. Common CT and MRI features of adnexal torsion include fallopian tube thickening, smooth wall thickening of the twisted adnexal cystic mass, and ascites.

PATHOLOGIC FEATURES

GROSS FINDINGS

The torsed ovary is enlarged, edematous, often engorged with blood, and may be infarcted.

MICROSCOPIC FINDINGS

Ovarian torsion shows massive edema and hemorrhage separating normal ovarian structures, which may be preserved or infarcted. An underlying nonneoplastic cyst, abscess, or neoplasm should be excluded. When

383

there is an underlying neoplasm, it may not be possible to make a histopathological diagnosis because of massive necrosis; however, the large majority of such tumors, although there is uncertainty about their precise classification, will follow a benign course.

ANCILLARY STUDIES

CYTOLOGIC EXAMINATION

Culdocentesis may yield blood, but this is not a specific finding.

DIFFERENTIAL DIAGNOSIS

Ovarian hemorrhage secondary to rupture of a corpus luteum in a patient receiving anticoagulant therapy may mimic ovarian torsion and is distinguished from the latter by the clinical history. *Ovarian vein thrombosis* may also simulate ovarian torsion, but it is much less common, and occurs postpartum, following pelvic surgery or trauma, or as a complication of pelvic inflammatory disease. *Ovarian abscess* and *endometrioma* are distinguished from torsion by the finding of more prominent acute and chronic inflammation in the former and the presence, at least focally, of ectopic endometrial glands and stroma in the latter.

PROGNOSIS AND THERAPY

Early diagnosis and intervention may permit conservative management and ovarian-sparing treatment. Late or delayed diagnosis usually results in oophorectomy or salpingo-oophorectomy.

MASSIVE OVARIAN EDEMA
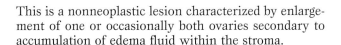

This is a nonneoplastic lesion characterized by enlargement of one or occasionally both ovaries secondary to accumulation of edema fluid within the stroma.

CLINICAL FEATURES

Massive ovarian edema is an unusual cause of ovarian enlargement occurring in children, adolescents, and young women (mean 21 years). Venous and lymphatic obstruction with resultant edema, which may occur secondary to partial or intermittent ovarian torsion, is

---

MASSIVE OVARIAN EDEMA – FACT SHEET

Definition
▶ Ovarian enlargement due to edema fluid

Incidence and Location
▶ Almost always unilateral; right > left (7:3)

Morbidity and Mortality
▶ Potential torsion

Age Distribution
▶ Children, adolescents, young women (mean 21 years)

Clinical Features
▶ Abdominal pain or torsion
▶ Virilism, hirsutism, and rarely, precocious pseudopuberty

Radiologic Features
▶ Solid or solid and cystic enlarged ovary

Prognosis and Treatment
▶ Biopsy with frozen section to exclude a neoplasm, followed by ovarian suspension and fixation
▶ Advanced cases may require excision

---

thought to be the underlying etiology in most cases. For unclear reasons, the right ovary is more commonly affected. Patients typically present with abdominal pain, distension, and menstrual irregularities. Hormonal symptoms include virilism, hirsutism, and rarely, precocious pseudopuberty. Serum CA-125 is not usually elevated.

RADIOLOGIC FEATURES

Ultrasound shows ovarian enlargement with solid or solid and cystic changes. The demonstration of multiple ovarian follicles situated in the peripheral cortex of the enlarged ovary on ultrasound or MRI is considered to be a relatively specific diagnostic feature.

MASSIVE OVARIAN EDEMA – PATHOLOGIC FEATURES

Gross Findings
▶ Enlarged ovary: 5.5–35 (mean 11.5) cm
▶ Watery cut surface and thickened capsule

Microscopic Findings
▶ Stromal edema and entrapped follicles
▶ Aggregates of luteinized cells (40%) in stroma

Differential Diagnosis
▶ Fibroma with marked edema
▶ Sclerosing stromal tumor

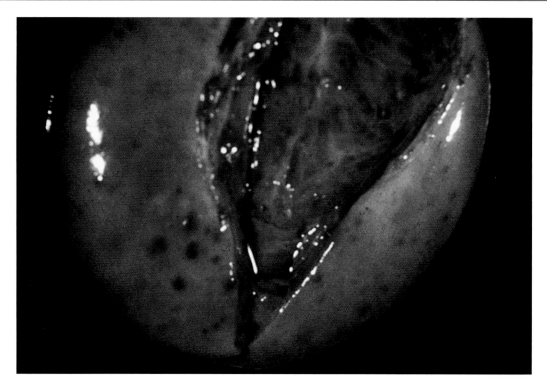

FIGURE 10.13
Massive ovarian edema. The ovary is enlarged and distended by accumulation of edema fluid.

PATHOLOGIC FEATURES

GROSS FINDINGS

There is enlargement of the ovary(s), ranging from 5.5 to 35 (mean 11.5) cm with a smooth pale outer surface and solid, glistering interior that exudes watery fluid (Figure 10.13). The ipsilateral fallopian tube may also be edematous.

MICROSCOPIC FINDINGS

Diffuse edema is present throughout the ovarian parenchyma, separating and sometimes entrapping preexisting follicular structures (Figure 10.14). Small foci of luteinized cells are present in 40% of cases. The stroma may also contain extravasated red blood cells, but extensive hemorrhage is not characteristic. Ovarian fibromatosis is closely related to massive ovarian edema in that it also is characterized by diffuse enlargement of one or both ovaries; however, it is histologically characterized by diffuse fibromatous background.

DIFFERENTIAL DIAGNOSIS

Ovarian fibroma with marked edema and *sclerosing stromal tumor* either replace or push aside normal ovarian follicular structures, whereas massive edema diffusely entraps follicles and their derivatives.

PROGNOSIS AND THERAPY

Uncomplicated massive ovarian edema is a benign, surgically correctable condition. Since conservative treatment with suspension and preservation of the ovary is often possible, it is important to consider the possibility of ovarian edema in a young patient with a complex but nonspecific ovarian mass. Clinical and ultrasonographic features may not be completely diagnostic and definitive diagnosis may require histologic examination. A laparoscopic diagnostic wedge resection with subsequent frozen section may be performed. Rare cases have been secondary to lymphatic or venous obstruction due to metastatic adenocarcinoma; in these cases, the prognosis is determined by the underlying malignancy.

SURFACE EPITHELIAL INCLUSION CYSTS

Surface epithelial inclusion cysts are cortical inclusions of ovarian surface epithelium. They are thought to form as a consequence of entrapment of ovarian surface epithelium within the cortex as part of the healing reaction after follicular rupture. They are differentiated from cystadenomas based on size; surface epithelial inclusion cysts are < 1 cm in diameter, whereas larger epithelial-lined cysts are arbitrarily designated cystadenomas. Because of their small size, they are never symptomatic, and their importance lies primarily in their

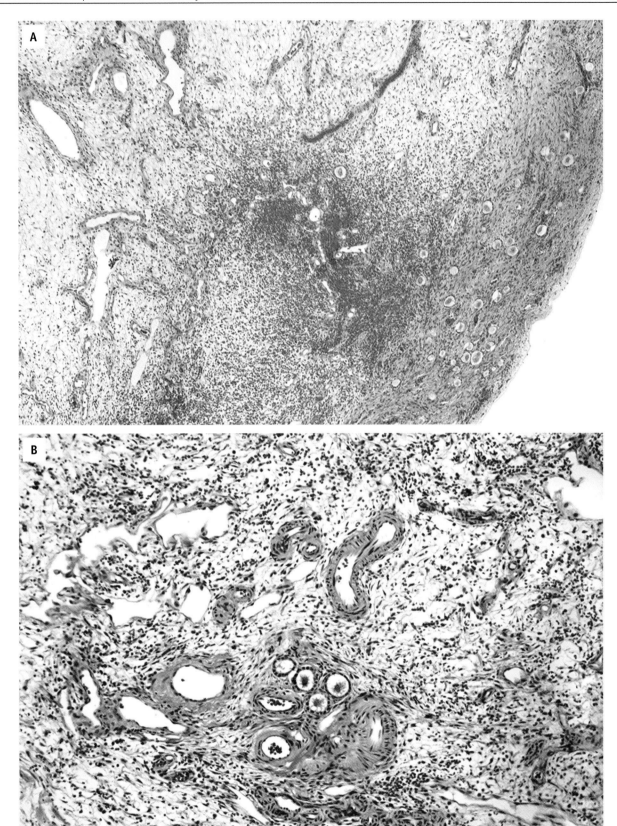

FIGURE 10.14

Massive ovarian edema. The ovarian parenchyma is expanded by striking edema associated with extravasated erythrocytes (A). Note the presence of entrapped primordial follicles (B).

seen in children and women of reproductive age. They are never symptomatic.

PATHOLOGIC FEATURES

GROSS FINDINGS

They are not usually appreciated on gross examination, as they measure < 1 cm.

MICROSCOPIC FINDINGS

Surface epithelial inclusion cysts are present in the ovarian cortex and are lined by a single layer of epithelium which is most commonly of ciliated, serous type

being the possible origin of development of surface epithelial neoplasms.

CLINICAL FEATURES

Surface epithelial inclusion cysts are most commonly encountered in postmenopausal women but can also be

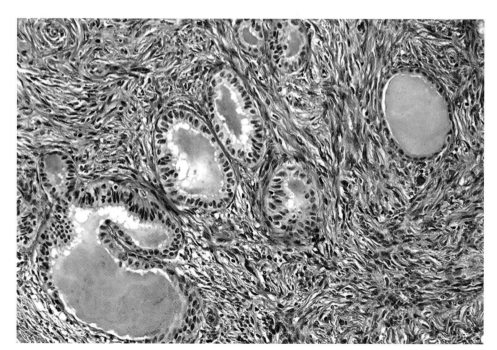

FIGURE 10.15

Surface epithelial inclusion cysts. Cuboidal or columnar serous (tubal-type) epithelium lines the glands and cysts.

(Figure 10.15). Less commonly, the lining cells are of endometrioid or endocervical type. Psammoma bodies may be present.

DIFFERENTIAL DIAGNOSIS

Distinction between a surface epithelial inclusion cyst and *cystadenoma* is based on size. *Walthard rests* or *cysts* lined by transitional epithelium are more commonly found adjacent to the fallopian tube but may occur in the ovary. Finally, follicular cysts are lined by more than one layer of granulosa and theca cells.

PROGNOSIS AND TREATMENT

Surface epithelial inclusion cysts are incidental findings and do not require treatment.

ENDOMETRIOSIS

Ovarian endometriosis is characterized by the presence of ectopic endometrial glands and stroma. Endometriotic cysts (endometriomas) of the ovaries are common, often bilateral, and usually present during the reproductive years.

CLINICAL FEATURES

The majority of patients are reproductive age women who present with abdominal pain, symptoms referable to a mass lesion, dysmenorrhea, infertility, or irregular vaginal bleeding. Up to 10% of patients with endometriosis are adolescents, whereas 5% present during the postmenopausal years without a preceding premenopausal diagnosis. A significant proportion of patients are asymptomatic and the diagnosis is established during evaluation of another pelvic process. Serum CA-125 is often elevated, but typically to a lesser degree than is seen with serous carcinoma of the ovary.

RADIOLOGIC FEATURES

Endometriomas often form a characteristic homogeneous hypoechoic cystic mass with echogenic mural foci on ultrasound. Ovarian endometriomas that are multilocular and septated with areas of diffuse wall thickening and/or mural nodularity on ultrasound may be difficult to distinguish from a malignant process. In these cases, the identification of a hyperintense image with shading on MRI may be helpful in excluding a neoplasm.

ENDOMETRIOSIS – FACT SHEET

Definition
▶ Presence of ectopic endometrial tissue in the ovary, usually consisting of endometrial glands and stroma

Incidence and Location
▶ Common (10% reproductive-aged women)
▶ Ovary most common site

Morbidity and Mortality
▶ Infertility, adhesions, and pain depending on extent of disease
▶ Secondary malignant tumors in < 1%

Race and Age Distribution
▶ More frequent in Caucasian women
▶ Young women

Clinical Features
▶ Symptoms vary depending on extent of disease
▶ Often asymptomatic if microscopic
▶ Often symptomatic if macroscopic: dysmenorrhea, infertility, pain, hemoperitoneum with acute pain secondary to cyst rupture

Radiologic Features
▶ Homogeneous hypoechoic cystic mass with echogenic wall foci
▶ Multilocular and septated lesions with areas of diffuse wall thickening and/or mural nodularity on ultrasound may be distinguished from a malignant process by a hyperintense image with shading on MRI

Prognosis and Treatment
▶ Treatment depends on extent of disease and symptoms, i.e., conservative therapy with analgesics for limited disease; androgens, progestins, GnRH agonists, and aromatase inhibitors for extensive disease; and laparoscopic laser ablation and microsurgical excision for severe disease
▶ Severe, intractable symptoms and mass lesions may require surgical excision of ovaries
▶ Simple cystectomy is usually curative for uncomplicated endometriomas
▶ Secondary neoplasms can develop, including benign and borderline endometrioid tumors, carcinoma (endometrioid and clear cell), müllerian mucinous borderline tumor, endometrial stromal sarcoma, low-grade müllerian adenosarcoma, and carcinosarcoma (malignant mixed müllerian tumor)

PATHOLOGIC FEATURES

GROSS FINDINGS

Ovarian endometriosis may be a microscopic finding or may form large cystic masses (usually not exceeding 15 cm) with intracystic inspissated brown chocolate-colored material (so-called "chocolate cyst") (Figure 10.16). In these cases, the cyst wall is often thickened and the ovarian surface is covered by dense fibrous adhesions. Complete replacement of the ovary may occur.

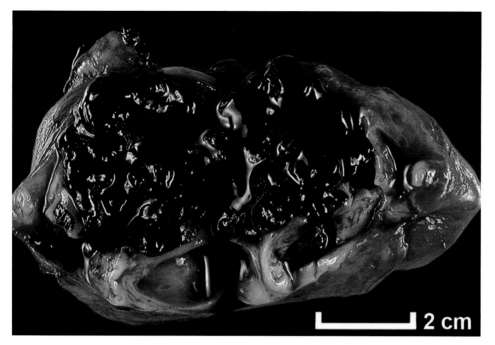

FIGURE 10.16
Endometriosis. Large and small blood-filled ("chocolate") cysts are seen.

_____

ENDOMETRIOSIS – PATHOLOGIC FEATURES

Gross Findings

▸ Frequently bilateral
▸ Red, brown, or white areas on ovarian surface
▸ Enlarged, thick-walled cyst containing dark "chocolate" fluid associated with surface adhesions

Microscopic Findings

▸ Endometrial-type glands and stroma with associated fibrosis, hemosiderin deposition, and histocytes
▸ Epithelium may be cytologically atypical (hyperchromatic nuclei with smudgy chromatin)
▸ Decidualization of the stroma and gestational changes may occur (Arias–Stella reaction)

Immunohistochemical Features

▸ ER, PR (epithelium and stroma) and CD10 (stroma) positive

Differential Diagnosis

▸ Solitary follicle or corpus luteum cyst
▸ Tubo-ovarian abscess
▸ Surface epithelial cyst/cystadenoma
▸ Unilocular cystic granulosa cell tumor
▸ Secondary neoplasm (most commonly clear cell or endometrioid carcinoma)

MICROSCOPIC FINDINGS

The microscopic appearance of ovarian endometriosis varies depending on the duration, extent of associated inflammation and fibrosis, and degree to which the ectopic foci exhibit morphologic response to the fluctu-ating hormonal milieu of the menstrual cycle. Most cases exhibit, at least focally, endometrial glands surrounded by a cuff of endometrial stroma (Figure 10.17). The individual glands and stroma may be inactive or demonstrate proliferative, secretory, or atrophic changes. Many endometriomas feature an extremely attenuated epithelial/stromal lining and recognition of endometriosis depends on a constellation of findings including granulation tissue, hemosiderin deposition, pseudoxanthoma cells, and islands of residual cuboidal glandular epithelium or endometrial stroma.

Occasionally, the ectopic glandular epithelium exhibits abundant eosinophilic cytoplasm and nuclear enlargement with marked atypia (sometimes referred to as "atypical endometriosis") (Figure 10.17). Cells with these features may merge with areas of clear cell carcinoma and cysts bearing such atypical foci should be carefully examined to exclude malignant transformation.

ANCILLARY STUDIES

IMMUNOHISTOCHEMISTRY

Endometriotic glands exhibit an immunohistochemical phenotype that is similar to that of eutopic endometrium. Expression of ER and PR in the epithelium is common, but may be decreased relative to normal cycling endometrial tissue. The endometrial stroma is also typically positive for ER, PR and CD10.

CYTOLOGY

Examination of peritoneal fluid typically shows marked reactive mesothelial changes and recent or old

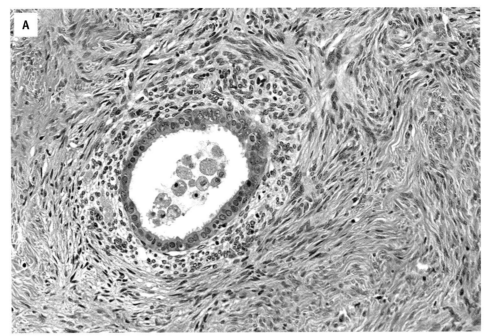

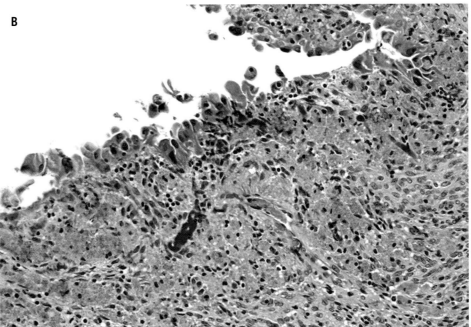

FIGURE 10.17

Endometriosis. An endometrioid gland is surrounded by endometrial-type stroma (A). Abundant hemosiderin-laden macrophages and associated endometrioid epithelium is diagnostic of endometriosis. Note the degenerative type epithelial atypia (B).

hemorrhage (hemosiderin). With rupture of an endometriotic cyst, endometrial glands and stroma may be present in the fluid.

DIFFERENTIAL DIAGNOSIS

Benign hemorrhagic cysts of follicular origin exhibit a granulosa-theca cell lining, which may or may not be luteinized. Blood breakdown products may be present, but are not usually as prominent as in endometriosis.

Chronic tubo-ovarian abscesses may exhibit similar inflammatory changes associated with foamy histiocytes, but do not have endometrial-type glands and stroma. *Cystadenomas* lack endometrial-type stroma and are uncommonly associated with hemosiderin deposition. *Unilocular granulosa cell tumors* are multilayered, resembling a typical granulosa cell tumor with Call-Exner bodies and grooved nuclei, at least focally. Since carcinoma may develop within an endometrioma, any thickened areas or solid nodules within the wall of an endometriotic cyst should be sectioned and evaluated to exclude a malignant tumor, most often endometrioid or clear cell carcinoma.

PROGNOSIS AND THERAPY

Uncomplicated endometriomas are clinically benign and simple excision is curative; however, a range of benign, borderline, and malignant epithelial, stromal, and mixed müllerian tumors can arise from ovarian endometriosis. Malignant tumors, most often endometrioid or clear cell adenocarcinoma, arise in up to 1% of cases. Although severe cytologic atypia in endometriosis may be a precursor of carcinoma, such atypia alone does not warrant any treatment beyond surgical removal, and recurrences as carcinoma have not been recorded.

OOPHORITIS

Inflammatory conditions primarily involving the ovary, without fallopian tube involvement or systemic disease, are rare. Oophoritis may be secondary to bacterial infection (e.g., pelvic inflammatory disease with tubo-ovarian abscess formation) or may be autoimmune. Oophoritis secondary to viral, fungal or parasitic infection is rarely encountered.

CLINICAL FEATURES

The clinical manifestations of oophoritis are determined by the underlying etiology. For most cases of infectious oophoritis, the presenting symptoms are those of pelvic inflammatory disease and consist primarily of pelvic pain, with fever and/or vaginal discharge being variably present. On physical examination, there is tenderness of the cervix. In advanced disease, unilateral or bilateral adnexal masses may develop. Chronic pelvic inflammatory disease may be insidious in onset and only recognized when scarring of the fallopian tube and ovarian surface is identified during investigation for infertility. Oophoritis unrelated to fallopian tube disease may be secondary to fistula formation from the gastrointestinal tract (most commonly associated with diverticulitis, appendicitis, or Crohn disease). Autoimmune oophoritis results in premature ovarian failure with early onset of menopause, usually preceded by a variable period of oligomenorrhea; there may be other autoimmune manifestations such as Hashimoto's thyroiditis, Graves disease, or Addison disease.

RADIOLOGIC FEATURES

Ultrasound of a tubo-ovarian abscess may show complex solid and cystic masses that are indistinguishable from malignancy.

PATHOLOGIC FEATURES

GROSS FINDINGS

In cases of tubo-ovarian abscess, there is congestion, fibrinous exudate, and adhesions involving the surface of ovary and fallopian tube. Bilateral involvement is common (Figure 10.18). The severe inflammatory process obscures the normal anatomic landmarks and recognition of normal fallopian tube or ovary may not be possible. On sectioning, unilocular or multilocular thick-walled cysts are characteristically present. (This represents selection bias towards more severe cases of pelvic inflammatory disease, as most patients are treated with antibiotics and no surgical pathology specimen is received). After resolution of the acute phase, the gross findings include dilation of the fallopian tube (hydrosalpinx) with adherence to the ovary. Although there are no specific gross findings associated with autoimmune oophoritis, patients may have bilateral ovarian enlargement with multiple follicle cysts at the time of presentation.

MICROSCOPIC FINDINGS

The findings in tubo-ovarian abscess are typical of pyogenic inflammation, with edema, hemorrhage, marked acute and chronic inflammation, and abscess formation. If granulomatous inflammation is present, stains for mycobacteria and fungi should be performed. So-called "sulfur granules," consisting of colonies of filamentous Gram-positive bacilli, are seen in cases of tubo-ovarian abscess secondary to *Actinomyces* (typically in patients who have the same intrauterine device in place for years). The histological findings in autoimmune oophoritis are characterized by a lymphoplasmacytic and histiocytic infiltration of developing follicles, with sparing of primordial follicles. Occasional eosinophils or granulomas can be seen. The infiltrate is typically most severe in the theca layers, and becomes more intense with progressive maturation of the follicle. As the disease progresses there are diminishing numbers of follicles in the ovary.

ANCILLARY STUDIES

CYTOLOGY

Culdocentesis from patients with tubo-ovarian abscess shows acute inflammatory cells and reactive mesothelial cells. With rupture of the abscess, pus is identified.

MICROBIOLOGIC EXAMINATION

The fluid from most tubo-ovarian abscesses grows mixed anaerobic bacteria.

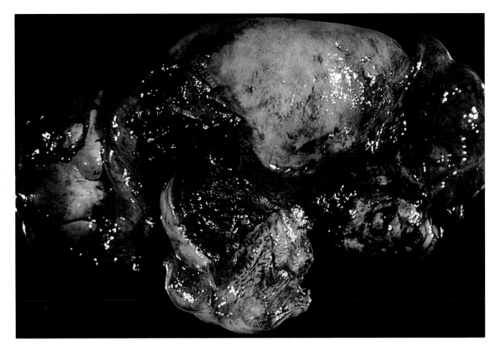

FIGURE 10.18
Bilateral tubo-ovarian abscess. Note adhesions of the tubal fimbriae to ovarian surface.

SEROLOGIC EXAMINATION

Most patients with autoimmune oophoritis will have antibodies to steroid cell antigens in their serum.

DIFFERENTIAL DIAGNOSIS

The clinical differential diagnosis of tubo-ovarian abscess includes an ovarian neoplasm; however this is not a diagnostic issue microscopically. The microscopic differential diagnosis does include *endometriosis*, however, absence of endometrial-type stroma and glands and more prominent inflammatory infiltrate are distinguishing features. In end stage cases of *autoimmune oophoritis* or in small biopsies, the findings may be equivocal and correlation with clinical findings is necessary for diagnosis.

PROGNOSIS AND THERAPY

Treatment of tubo-ovarian abscess requires identification of the etiologic agent and specific antimicrobial therapy. Surgery is not indicated in most patients but will occasionally be required if ruptured, disease not responding completely to antibiotic therapy, or there is chronic pelvic pain. The most common sequelae are infertility or ectopic pregnancy. The frequency of infertility after medical treatment of tubo-ovarian abscess is high, and related to chronic scarring of the fallopian tube and ovary. An unusual complication of surgery for tubo-ovarian abscess is the ovarian remnant syndrome. After salpingo-oophorectomy, some ovarian tissue is left in the pelvic sidewall, presumably because of ovarian surface adhesions, and the patient subsequently develops a cystic pelvic mass that is seen histologically to be a follicular cyst arising in the residual ovarian tissue. Autoimmune oophoritis ultimately results in premature ovarian failure. Although immunosuppressive therapy can be used empirically, it has shown variable results.

SUGGESTED READING

Clement PB. Histology of the ovary. In: Sternberg S (ed.) Histology for Pathologists, 2nd edn. Philadelphia: Lippincott-Raven, 1997:929–959.

Clement PB. Nonneoplastic lesions of the ovary. In: Kurman RJ (ed.) Blaustein's Pathology of the Female Genital Tract. New York: Springer Verlag, 2002:675–727.

Scully RE, Young RH, Clement PB. Atlas of Tumor Pathology. Tumors of the Ovary, Maldeveloped Gonads, Fallopian Tube, and Broad Ligament, 3rd edn. Washington, DC: AFIP, 1998.

Surface Epithelial Stromal Tumors of the Ovary

Teri A Longacre · C Blake Gilks

Surface epithelial stromal tumors, the most common neoplasms of the ovary, encompass five distinct subtypes. Differentiation into these epithelial cell types is under the control of the same genes that determine different epithelial lineages in the female reproductive tract during embryonic development (e.g., mucinous epithelium in the endocervix, endometrioid epithelium in the endometrium, serous or tubal epithelium in the fallopian tube). Surface epithelial stromal tumors are further subclassified into benign, borderline (low malignant potential, atypical proliferating), or malignant on the basis of their histologic features. Benign, borderline, and malignant subclasses account for 60%, 5%, and 35% of all the surface epithelial stromal tumors, respectively. They have been historically considered to arise from the surface epithelium of the ovary or its derivatives, but they may also arise from the fallopian tube epithelium or endometriosis.

The division of the various epithelial subtypes into benign, borderline, and malignant forms is based on the premise that tumors with architectural and cytologic features that are intermediate between those of clinically benign and malignant tumors of the same epithelial cell type have a significantly better prognosis, stage for stage, than their malignant counterpart. By definition, borderline tumors lack destructive stromal invasion, but have other histologic features of malignancy (e.g., nuclear atypia, cellular stratification, mitotic activity). For the most part, the clinical behavior of these histologically intermediate or borderline tumors is benign, with the exception of serous borderline surface epithelial stromal tumors, which are frequently associated with extraovarian disease and exhibit a clinical behavior intermediate between benign serous tumors and invasive serous carcinomas.

The overtly malignant surface epithelial tumors (carcinomas) comprise 85% of all malignant ovarian neoplasms and are the fourth most common cause of cancer death in women in the US. Approximately 1 in 70 women in industrialized countries develops ovarian cancer and 1 in 100 dies of it. The incidence is lower in nonindustrialized nations; decreased dietary fat intake is a possible factor. Risk factors include nulliparity, infertility, late child-bearing and delayed menopause, whereas oral contraceptive use, breast-feeding and tubal ligation are protective. A personal or family history of endometrial, breast, or colon cancer is also associated with increased risk, as is inherited germline mutations in the autosomal-dominant cancer susceptibility genes

BRCA1/BRCA2 or in one of the DNA base mismatch repair genes, the most frequent of which are MLH1 and MSH2 (hereditary nonpolyposis colon carcinoma).

The most important factor in determining the prognosis of patients with surface epithelial carcinomas is tumor stage. The widely used International Federation of Gynecologists and Obstetricians (FIGO) staging system is shown in Table 11.1. Stage can only be assigned after completion of a proper surgical staging procedure. Prognosis for patients with low-grade, stage IA tumors (i.e., tumor confined to one ovary, without ovarian surface involvement or extraovarian spread) is excellent, with > 90% being disease-free at 5 years. Unfortunately, most patients with ovarian cancer present with advanced-stage disease, and in these patients the most important prognostic factor is whether or not the extraovarian disease is resectable; if all macroscopic disease can be surgically removed, there is > 40% 5-year disease-free survival compared to < 20% 5-year disease-free survival for patients with macroscopic residual disease after maximal surgical debulking. Current screening modalities for the early detection of ovarian cancer (including ultrasound and serum tumor marker assays) have been not nearly as effective as those for cervical, breast, or colon cancer. The development of an adequate screening program for early ovarian cancer is especially challenging due to the apparent absence of a long latent or in situ phase; the most common forms of surface epithelial carcinoma give rise to early and often extensive spread to extraovarian sites, resulting in the rapid development of nonresectable disease.

Tumor grade has consistently been shown to be of prognostic significance, although it is not as important as stage. Grading can be done according to a number of different systems, most of which are dependent on tumor cell type, and the grading criteria for each cell type will be discussed subsequently. Within the past 5 years a grading system has been proposed for ovarian carcinoma that is universally applicable to all cell types and recapitulates the Nottingham Grading System used for breast carcinoma, in that architecture, nuclear atypia, and mitotic activity are independently assessed. Details of this grading system, commonly referred to as the Silverberg grading system, are shown in Table 11.2. Architecture refers to the predominant tumor growth pattern. For assessment of cytologic atypia, the most atypical area occupying at least one-half of a low-power field (4× objective, 10× ocular) is assessed. Score 1 atypia

TABLE 11.1

International Federation of Gynecologists and Obstetricians (FIGO) 1988 staging of ovarian carcinomas

Stage	Description
Stage I	Growth limited to the ovaries
Stage IA	Growth limited to one ovary; no ascites. No tumor on the external surface; capsule intact
Stage IB	Growth limited to both ovaries; no ascites. No tumor on the external surface; capsules intact
Stage IC*	Tumor either stage IA or IB but with tumor on the surface of one or both ovaries, or with capsule ruptured, or with ascites containing malignant cells, or with positive peritoneal washings
Stage II	Growth involving one or both ovaries with pelvic extension
Stage IIA	Extension and/or metastases to the uterus and/or tubes
Stage IIB	Extension to other pelvic tissues
Stage IIC	Tumor either stage IIA or IIB but with tumor on the surface of one or both ovaries with capsule(s) ruptured, or with ascites containing malignant cells, or with positive peritoneal washings
Stage III	Tumor involving one or both ovaries with peritoneal implants outside the pelvis and/or positive retroperitoneal or inguinal nodes. Superficial liver metastasis equals stage III. Tumor is limited to the true pelvis but with histologically verified malignant extension to small bowel or omentum
Stage IIIA	Tumor grossly limited to the true pelvis with negative nodes but with histologically confirmed microscopic seeding of abdominal peritoneal surfaces
Stage IIIB	Tumor of one or both ovaries with histologically confirmed implants of abdominal peritoneal surfaces, ≤ 2 cm in diameter; nodes negative
Stage IIIC	Abdominal implants > 2 cm in diameter and/or positive retroperitoneal or inguinal nodes
Stage IV	Growth involving one or both ovaries with distant metastasis. If pleural effusion is present, there must be positive cytologic test results to allot a case to stage IV. Parenchymal liver metastasis equals stage IV

*In order to evaluate the impact on prognosis of the different criteria for allotting cases to stage IC or IIC, it would be of value to know if rupture of the capsule was (1) spontaneous or (2) caused by the surgeon, and if the source of malignant cells detected was (1) peritoneal washings or (2) ascites.

TABLE 11.2

A proposed universal grading system for ovarian carcinoma

Score	Architecture	Cytologic atypia	Mitoses/10 HPFs*
1	Glandular	Slight	0–9
2	Papillary	Moderate	10–24
3	Solid	Marked	≥25

Total score 3–5 = grade 1, 6–7 = grade 2, and 8–9 = grade 3.
*Mitotic figures are counted in the most active area, field area = 0.345 mm².

is present when the tumor cell nuclei are regular and uniform, with no more than twofold variation in nuclear diameter, and there is no chromatin clumping or prominent nucleoli. Score 2 is assigned when there is greater variation in nuclear size (up to fourfold); there may be small nucleoli present and some clumping of nuclear chromatin. For score 3, there is marked variation in nuclear size (> fourfold) and shape, with a high nuclear-to-cytoplasmic ratio and prominent nucleoli. Mitotic counts are assessed in the most mitotically active area, typically at the periphery of the tumor, and a minimum of 30 fields should be counted. This grading system has

not gained wide acceptance and its prognostic value and reproducibility remain to be determined. One exception to the potential universal applicability of this grading system is clear cell carcinoma, where grading does not appear to be prognostically significant.

Although ovarian surface epithelial carcinomas are subclassified according to cell type, and tumors of different cell types have different prognoses and show different rates of response to adjuvant chemotherapy, current treatment is predominantly based on tumor stage and grade, and does not take into account tumor cell type. Most patients with surface epithelial carcinomas are

TABLE 11.3
Histologic classification of surface epithelial stromal tumors*

Histologic type	Total (%)
Serous	46
Mucinous	36
Endometrioid	8
Clear	3
Transitional	2
Undifferentiated	2
Mixed	3

*Tumors with squamous differentiation have also historically been included among the surface epithelial stromal tumors, but pure squamous tumors are rare, as most arise in a teratoma.

TABLE 11.4
Classification of serous surface epithelial stromal tumors (modified from World Health Organization)

Benign (cystadenoma, cystadenofibroma, adenofibroma)	50%
Variant, with focal proliferation	
Borderline (low malignant potential)	15%
Variant, with micropapillary features	
Variant, with stromal microinvasion	
Variant, with intraepithelial carcinoma	
Malignant (adenocarcinoma, cystadenocarcinoma, malignant adenofibroma)	35%

CLINICAL FEATURES

Benign serous tumors occur over a wide age range, but are most common in the reproductive age group. They are often bilateral. Women may present with abdominal

treated by surgery followed by adjuvant chemotherapy. The surgical management usually consists of abdominal hysterectomy, bilateral salpingo-oophorectomy, omentectomy, and removal of as much tumor as technically feasible. First-line chemotherapy typically consists of combination of platinum and taxane. Chemotherapy is not routinely given to patients with borderline tumors. The relative frequency of the main histologic subtypes of surface epithelial stromal tumors, including the undifferentiated and mixed tumors, is provided in Table 11.3.

SEROUS SURFACE EPITHELIAL STROMAL TUMORS

Tumors with serous differentiation, representing 46% of all surface epithelial stromal ovarian neoplasms, are characterized by epithelial cells resembling those of the fallopian tube and encompass a group of three biologically distinct entities, including serous cystadenoma/adenofibroma, serous borderline tumor (tumor of low malignant potential), and serous carcinoma (Table 11.4). Serous borderline tumors have the capacity for extraovarian spread, recurrence, and death, even though the tempo of disease progression is significantly more indolent when compared to serous carcinoma.

SEROUS CYSTADENOMA (SEROUS CYSTADENOFIBROMA, SEROUS ADENOFIBROMA)

Benign serous tumors comprise 50% of all serous ovarian neoplasms. They are almost always confined to the ovary.

SEROUS CYSTADENOMA (ADENOFIBROMA, CYSTADENOFIBROMA) – FACT SHEET

Definition
- Benign ovarian tumor composed of tubal-type epithelium and varying amounts of stroma
- If predominantly cystic: cystadenoma
- If prominent stromal component without grossly visible cysts: adenofibroma
- If prominent stromal component with grossly visible cysts: cystadenofibroma

Incidence and Location
- Most common benign surface epithelial tumor
- Bilateral (20%)

Morbidity and Mortality
- No significant morbidity or mortality unless torsion, rupture, or infection

Age Distribution
- Wide age range including premenarchal to postmenopausal women, but predominantly reproductive age

Clinical Features
- Often asymptomatic, incidental finding during routine examination or evaluation for unrelated condition

Radiologic Features
- Simple, smooth-walled unilocular or multilocular cystic mass (often < 4 cm) on ultrasound

Prognosis and Treatment
- Benign tumors
- Simple excision (cystectomy or adnexectomy) is curative

enlargement, pain, or vaginal bleeding, but most benign tumors are asymptomatic and discovered incidentally.

RADIOLOGIC FEATURES

Benign serous tumors tend to form simple, smooth-walled unilocular or multilocular cystic masses on pelvic ultrasound. They are typically smaller (< 4 cm) than their borderline and malignant counterparts, and are distinguished by the lack of intracystic internal complexity.

PATHOLOGIC FEATURES

GROSS FINDINGS

Benign serous tumors, frequently bilateral and meta-chronous (especially in older women), are composed of varying amounts of fibrous stroma (when predominant, serous adenofibroma) and cysts (when > 1 cm, serous cystadenoma or cystadenofibroma), and range in size from 1 to 10 cm (rarely up to 30 cm). Surface papillomas are not uncommon. The cysts are unilocular or multilocular and may contain papillary projections (Figure 11.1).

SEROUS CYSTADENOMA (ADENOFIBROMA, CYSTADENOFIBROMA) – PATHOLOGIC FEATURES

Gross Findings

▸ Simple, smooth-walled unilocular or multilocular cyst with varying amounts of fibromatous stroma (often < 4 cm)
▸ Solid areas may be present (fibromatous component) and are firm
▸ Necrosis absent, unless complicated by torsion, infection, or infarction

Microscopic Findings

▸ Simple architecture; non-branching papillae (if present) with rare to absent tufting
▸ Single, orderly layer of nonstratified, cuboidal to columnar epithelium, often ciliated
▸ Nuclear atypia minimal or absent, and rare mitoses

Immunohistochemical Findings

▸ CK7, EMA, and WT1 positive
▸ CK20 negative

Differential Diagnosis

▸ Epithelial inclusion cyst
▸ Rete cyst
▸ Endometriotic cyst
▸ Struma ovarii
▸ Serous tumor with focal proliferation
▸ Serous borderline tumor (low malignant potential)
▸ Mucinous cystadenoma

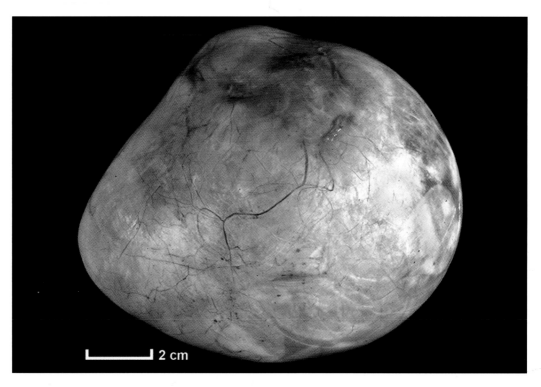

FIGURE 11.1
Serous cystadenoma. Thin-walled cyst is smooth and glistening without surface excrescences.

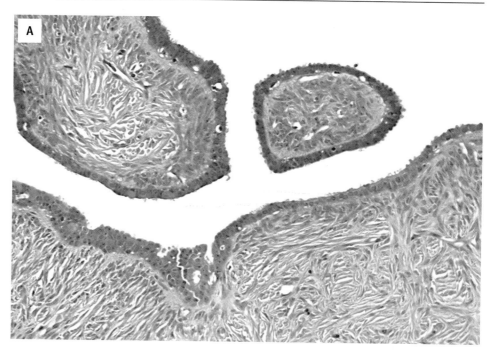

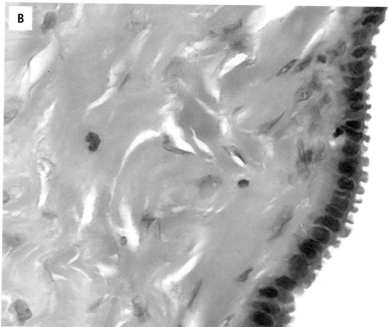

FIGURE 11.2

Serous cystadenoma. The cyst is lined by ciliated epithelium with minimal nuclear atypia (A). Note resemblance to fallopian tube lining epithelium (B).

MICROSCOPIC FINDINGS

Benign serous tumors are lined by epithelium that closely recapitulates the ciliated and secretory cells of the fallopian tube (Figure 11.2). Varying amounts of stroma (adenofibroma, cystadenofibroma) and cystic change (cystadenofibroma) are present.

ANCILLARY STUDIES

IMMUNOHISTOCHEMISTRY

Benign serous tumors express an immunohistochemical profile that is similar to borderline and malignant serous tumors. Like many other surface epithelial stromal tumors, they show a CK7 positive, CK20 negative phenotype. In addition, serous tumors express WT1, BerEP4, and CD15 (Leu-M1).

DIFFERENTIAL DIAGNOSIS

Serous cystadenomas are distinguished from *serous epithelial inclusion cysts* on the basis of size (> 1 cm) and from *rete cysts* on the basis of location (rete cysts are hilar), presence of prominent cilia, absence of a smooth muscle layer and hyperplastic hilar cells. An *endometriotic cyst*, especially in postmenopausal women, can closely mimic a serous cystadenoma. The presence of endometrial-type stroma, at least focally, helps in this distinction. If cystic, *struma ovarii* may resemble a serous cystadenoma, but the constituent cysts of struma contain colloid and are immunoreactive for thyroglobulin. The chief differential diagnosis is between benign and borderline serous tumors. *Borderline tumors* have a hierarchical papillary architecture, epithelial stratification, tufting with detached epithelial cell clusters, cytologic atypia, and occasional mitotic figures. By definition, serous tumors with focal borderline change (< 10 % of the tumor epithelium) in an otherwise benign tumor are designated serous cystadenoma (or cystadenofibroma) with "focal proliferation" or "focal atypia". Occasionally, serous tumors can secrete watery material resembling mucin, and thus, resemble a *mucinous cystadenoma*, but its constituent cells do not contain intracytoplasmic mucin (PAS-diastase or mucicarmine negative).

PROGNOSIS AND THERAPY

Serous cystadenomas, adenofibromas, and cystadenofibromas are clinically benign. Complete excision (cystectomy or oophorectomy) is curative. To minimize surgical morbidity, laparoscopic removal is often performed. Occasionally, similar tumors in extraovarian sites accompany benign serous ovarian tumors.

SEROUS BORDERLINE TUMOR (SEROUS TUMOR OF LOW MALIGNANT POTENTIAL)

Serous borderline tumors are an enigmatic and controversial group of surface epithelial ovarian neoplasms. They comprise approximately 15 % of all ovarian serous tumors and account for the vast majority of all borderline surface epithelial stromal neoplasms.

CLINICAL FEATURES

Serous borderline tumors are more often bilateral and larger than benign serous tumors. They occur at a slightly younger age than serous carcinoma (mean 45 versus 60 years), and may present with disease beyond the confines of the ovary. Patients are often asymptomatic, but may have abdominal enlargement or pain. Younger women often present with infertility. A signifi-

cant minority of women are pregnant at the time of diagnosis.

RADIOLOGIC FEATURES

Serous borderline tumors tend to form bilateral cystic adnexal masses with profuse papillary projections. No areas of necrosis or solid mural nodules are seen on ultrasound.

PATHOLOGIC FEATURES

GROSS FINDINGS

Serous neoplasms in the borderline or low malignant potential group are predominantly cystic with variable amounts of papillary epithelial projections (Figure 11.3), or solid with surface papillary excrescences (or combination thereof).

MICROSCOPIC FINDINGS

Serous borderline tumors are composed of complex hierarchical branching papillae associated with detached cellular buds; destructive invasion of the ovarian stroma is not seen. The lining cells are tall to columnar and may or may not display cilia. The nuclei are uniform, mildly to moderately atypical and mitotic activity is low. Psammoma bodies may be present, but are not diagnostic (Figure 11.4).

Approximately 5–10% of all serous borderline tumors contain foci of significant micropapillary architecture (Figure 11.5), defined as either nonhierarchical branching of slender, elongated papillae that are at least five times as long as they are wide, or a sieve-like cribriform pattern, occupying a continuous 5-mm extent. This tumor is designated as the micropapillary variant of serous borderline tumor, which is more frequently associated with bilaterality, ovarian surface involvement, and the presence of extraovarian implants, a higher proportion of which may be invasive.

Foci of stromal microinvasion (Figure 11.6), defined as individual eosinophilic cells, small cell clusters or papillae (more frequently small) lying within stromal spaces ≤ 5 mm in linear extent or 10 mm^2 in area, may be found in 10–15% of serous borderline tumors (Box 11.1); stromal microinvasion is more often seen in pregnant women. Although it may be associated with increased long-term risk of disease recurrence, the presence of stromal microinvasion does not warrant a diagnosis of carcinoma.

Approximately 30–40% of serous tumors in the borderline group are associated with similar-appearing lesions in the pelvis and intra-abdominal sites, including lymph nodes (high-stage disease) (Figure 11.7). These lesions, termed implants, may be microscopic or macroscopic and are subclassified into noninvasive (Figures 11.8 A and B) and invasive types (Figures 11.9 and 10), based on the presence of destructive infiltration into underlying normal tissue (Table 11.5). Noninvasive epithelial implants are exclusively composed of glands or cysts with variable degree of papillary formation present on the peritoneal surfaces. The interface between the implant and surrounding tissue is typically smooth. Noninvasive desmoplastic-type implants may occur over the ovarian surface or between exophytic surface papillae (autoimplants) as well as in the peritoneum. They form plaques or nodules without associated invasion of underlying organs/tissues, and thus, are easily removed. They are characterized by prominent desmoplastic reaction and inflammation surrounding single cells or irregular nests of tumor cells which typically represent a minor component of the lesion. In both types of non-invasive implants, the cytologic features should be similar to those seen in the primary ovarian serous borderline tumor. Invasive implants may also be

---

SEROUS BORDERLINE TUMOR (SEROUS TUMOR OF LOW MALIGNANT POTENTIAL) – PATHOLOGIC FEATURES

Gross Findings

▸ Large cystic or solid and cystic mass with soft papillary projections and/or surface papillary excrescences

Microscopic Findings

▸ Numerous papillae, often broad and edematous, with complex, typically hierarchical branching
▸ Cuboidal to columnar epithelium, often ciliated with interspersed eosinophilic (pink) cells with cellular stratification and tufting
▸ Mild to focally moderate nuclear atypia, and sparse mitoses
▸ Psammoma bodies
▸ Micropapillary variant: elongated papillae with nonhierarchical branching (at least five times long as they are wide and at least 5 mm in continuous linear extent)
▸ Stromal microinvasion (≤ 5 mm in linear extent or 10 mm^2 in area) may be present (10%)
▸ Extraovarian peritoneal and lymph node implants may be present

Immunohistochemical Findings

▸ CK7, EMA, WT1, BerEP4, CA125, CD15 positive
▸ CK20 negative

Molecular Studies

▸ K-RAS and BRAF mutations
▸ No association with germline or somatic *BRCA1/BRCA2* mutations

Differential Diagnosis

▸ Benign serous tumor with focal proliferation
▸ Serous adenocarcinoma
▸ Well-differentiated papillary mesothelioma
▸ Mucinous borderline tumor, endocervical-like
▸ Struma ovarii
▸ Retiform Sertoli–Leydig cell tumor

BOX 11.1

DIAGNOSTIC CRITERIA FOR STROMAL MICROINVASION IN SEROUS BORDERLINE (LOW MALIGNANT POTENTIAL) TUMORS*

– Individual cells or small, irregular clusters of cells with abundant eosinophilic cytoplasm within the stromal stalks of serous papillae, commonly surrounded by a tissue space or cleft. The pink cells often have enlarged nuclei with distinct nucleoli.
– Small aggregates of simple and branching papillae, often composed of eosinophilic cells surrounded by a tissue space or cleft often coexist with microinvasion by individual eosinophilic cells.
– Micropapillae, macropapillae, or cribriform glands lined by serous borderline epithelium surrounded by a cleft. This is an uncommon form of microinvasion.

---

*Individual foci of microinvasion must not exceed 5 mm in linear extent or 10 mm^2 in area.

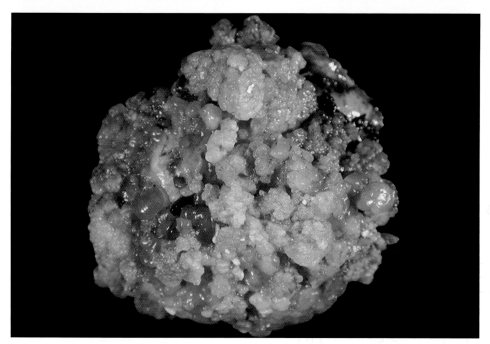

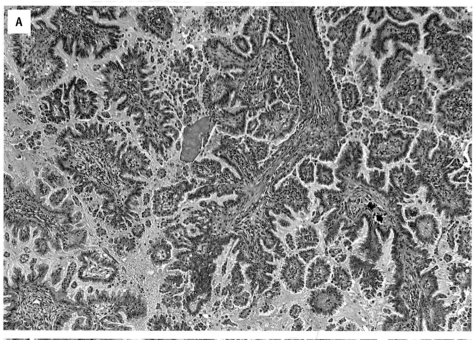

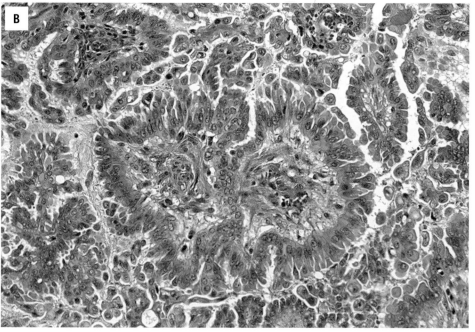

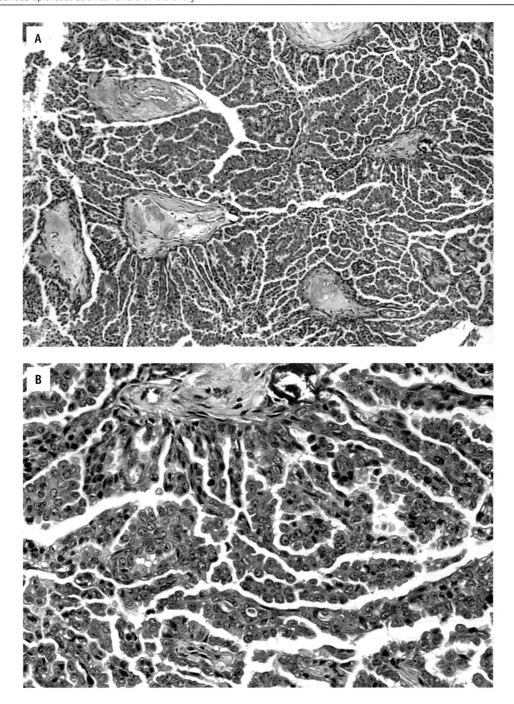

FIGURE 11.5

Serous borderline tumor (serous tumor of low malignant potential) with micropapillary features. Complex elongated papillae with nonhierarchical branching are at least five times as long as they are wide and involve at least one confluent area measuring ≥ 5 mm in one dimension (A). The cytologic appearance is uniform with moderate atypia (B).

associated with a desmoplastic response but typically show destructive invasion of underlying tissue, and often the cells show cytologic features of low-grade carcinoma. Borderline tumors with invasive implants are associated with an increased risk of recurrence and often a more aggressive clinical course. Since both types of implants may feature a prominent stromal connective tissue response, occasional implants may be especially difficult to subclassify; in these instances, the implants should probably be classified as indeterminate. The

presence of a micropapillary morphology is considered by some investigators as evidence of invasion in an implant (Figure 11.10A). Rarely, extraovarian invasion by single cells with abundant eosinophilic cytoplasm may be seen (Figure 11.10B). Foci of endosalpingiosis involving extraovarian peritoneum and lymph nodes are common in women with serous borderline tumors. These foci, characterized by simple glands lined by tubal-type epithelium, should be distinguished from extraovarian borderline implants, since the presence of

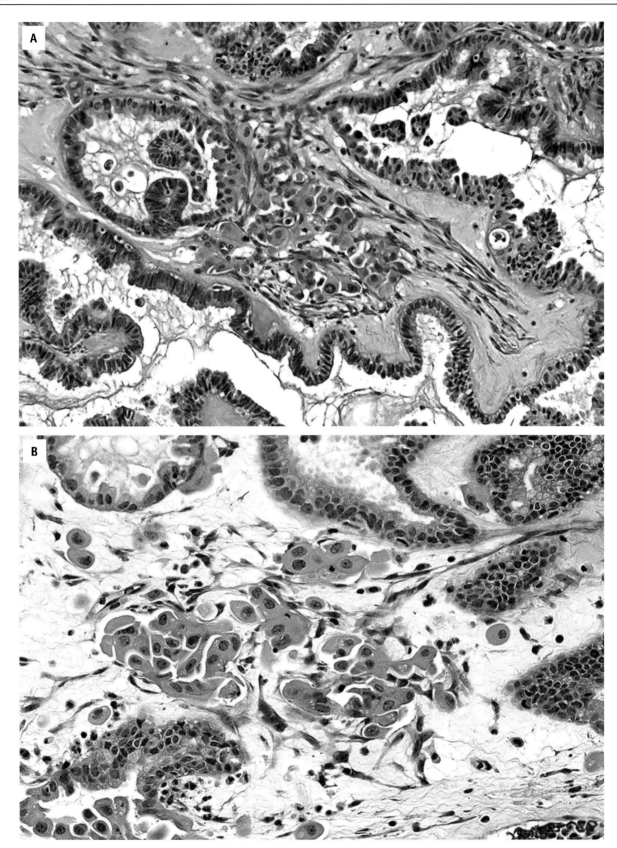

FIGURE 11.6

Serous borderline tumor (serous tumor of low malignant potential) with microinvasion. Noncohesive individual cells and small cell clusters are dispersed throughout the stroma (A). Most of the cells have abundant eosinophilic cytoplasm and are similar in appearance to overlying pink cells lining the glands and papillae (B).

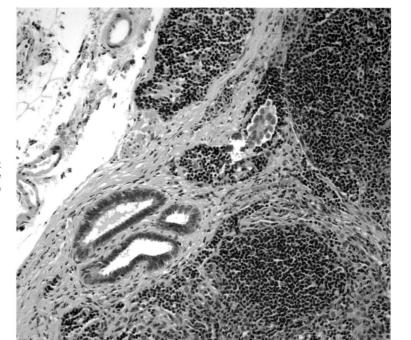

FIGURE 11.7

Serous borderline tumor (serous tumor of low malignant potential) involving a lymph node. A single small papillary cluster of tumor cells is present in a subcapsular sinus. Also notice the presence of endosalpingiosis.

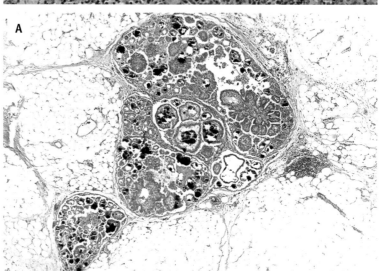

FIGURE 11.8

Noninvasive implants. Cysts containing multiple papillae are present in omental septa. The interface between the implant and adjacent fat is smooth and no desmoplastic reaction is seen (epithelial, non-invasive implant) (A). Small papillae and single cells are embedded in abundant edematous, inflamed, and/or desmoplastic tissue. Note the well demarcated interface between the implant and adjacent fat (desmoplastic, non-invasive implant) (B).

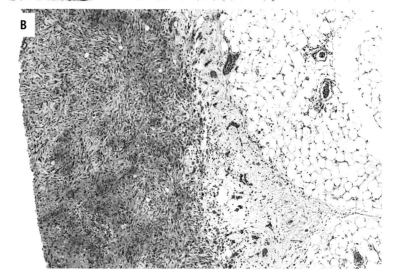

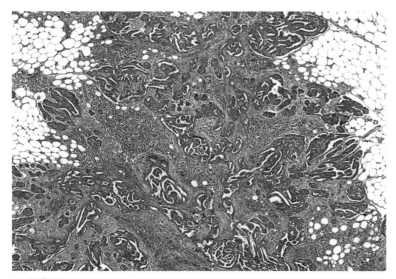

FIGURE 11.9

Invasive implant. Complex glands and branching papillae irregularly invade into adjacent normal omental tissue effacing the preexisting architecture. Epithelial predominance is characteristic of this type of implant.

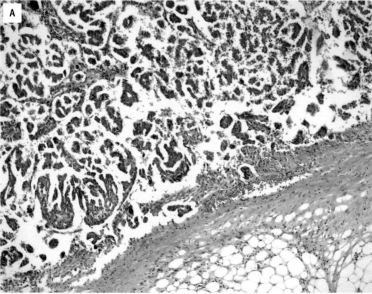

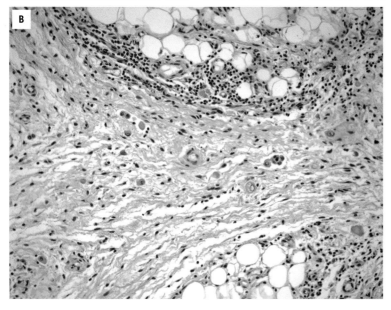

FIGURE 11.10

Invasive implants. Complex micropapillary morphology is present (A). Single cells with abundant eosinophilic cytoplasm are seen within the fibrous septa (B).

TABLE 11.5

Classification of extraovarian serous implants (modified from World Health Organization)*

	Diagnostic features
Endosalpingiosis	Small, ciliated tubular glands, may have simple papillary infoldings, no atypia, smooth epithelial–stromal interface
Noninvasive implants	
Epithelial implants	Branching papillae, glands with complex papillary infoldings, single cell and small cell clusters, mild to moderate atypia, smooth interface with underlying/surrounding normal tissue
Desmoplastic implants	Branching papillae, glands with complex papillary infoldings, single cell and small cell clusters, mild to moderate atypia, desmoplastic fasciitis-like stroma, smooth interface with underlying/surrounding normal tissue
Invasive implants†	Branching papillae, glands with complex papillary and micropapillary infoldings, single cell and small cell clusters, with abundant epithelial component, moderate to carcinomatous atypia, jagged and irregular interface with underlying/surrounding normal tissue

*Implants should be distinguished from endosalpingiosis (which is a benign process and does not warrant upstaging of an accompanying ovarian serous borderline tumor) and are classified as invasive or noninvasive on the basis of the interface between the implant and normal tissue. Implants with no attached normal tissue (so-called detached implants) are classified as noninvasive (either epithelial or desmoplastic) provided the atypia is moderate at most (e.g., no marked cytologic atypia) and the architecture is not overtly complex. When marked cytologic and architectural atypia is present, the implant should probably be classified as invasive or, alternatively, as indeterminate since there is no evaluable interface. Implants in which it is difficult to determine whether the interface is smooth and expansile or focally irregular and infiltrative should also be classified as indeterminate.
†Fewer than 15% of extraovarian implants are invasive.

endosalpingiosis does not warrant upstaging of an accompanying ovarian serous borderline tumor (Figure 11.11).

ANCILLARY STUDIES

IMMUNOHISTOCHEMISTRY

Serous borderline tumors express an immunohistochemical profile that is similar to benign and malignant serous tumors. They are usually CK7 positive, CK20 negative, and in addition, express WT1, BerEP4, and CD15 (Leu-M1).

MOLECULAR STUDIES

The profile of mRNA expression patterns is significantly different for serous borderline tumors and serous carcinomas, as is the pattern of genetic alterations, e.g., the presence of point mutations in *BRAF* or *KRAS* is more frequently associated with borderline tumors, whereas p53 mutation and somatic or germline abnormalities of *BRCA1* and/or *BRCA2* are more frequently associated with carcinoma.

CYTOLOGY

Positive peritoneal cytologic preparations are characterized by papillary aggregates and/or tight clusters of cells with minimal nuclear atypia and can be difficult to distinguish from benign serous epithelium (endosalpingiosis), reactive mesothelial proliferations, and

well-differentiated serous adenocarcinomas. Psammoma bodies may be present, but are not diagnostic. Fine-needle aspiration is only indicated for confirmation of suspected recurrent disease.

DIFFERENTIAL DIAGNOSIS

Borderline serous tumors are distinguished from *benign serous tumors* on the basis of epithelial proliferation. By definition, serous tumors featuring ≤ 10 % proliferation of borderline type are designated as serous tumors with "focal proliferation" or "focal atypia". *Serous carcinoma* is distinguished from serous borderline tumor by the presence of destructive stromal invasion ($> 10 \, \text{mm}^2$) or by cytologically malignant cells lining the papillae, in the cyst wall or stromal component of a predominantly fibromatous tumor. *Well-differentiated papillary mesothelioma* may mimic a surface ovarian (or extraovarian) serous borderline tumor and is distinguished by less hierarchical branching of the papillae, prominent papillary connective tissue cores lined by cuboidal cells with less pseudostratification, strong calretinin staining, and lack of staining for BerEP4 and CD 15. *Mucinous borderline tumors of endocervical-like type* (also referred to as seromucinous type) are distinguished from serous borderline tumors by the presence of both serous and mucinous endocervical-like epithelial cells, abundant neutrophils in large edematous papillae, and their more frequent association with endometriosis. *Struma ovarii* with cystic and papillary architecture may resemble a serous borderline tumor, but

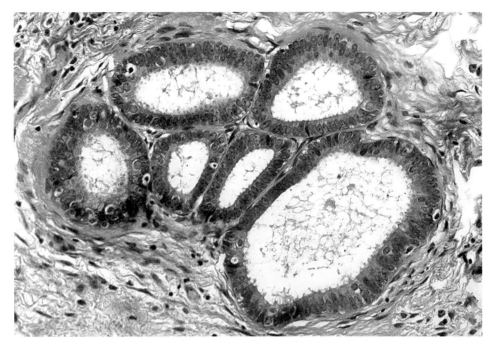

FIGURE 11.11

Endosalpingiosis. Simple glands are lined by ciliated cuboidal to columnar epithelium with minimal cytologic atypia. Note the absence of papillary infolding.

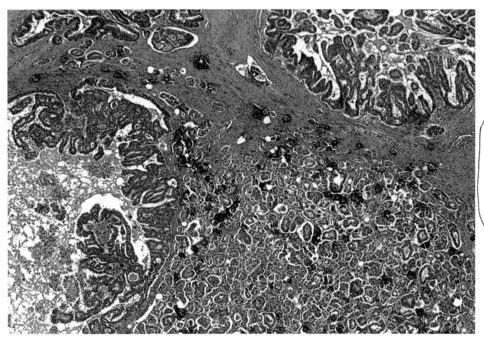

FIGURE 11.12

Serous borderline tumor (serous tumor of low malignant potential) with transformation to low-grade carcinoma. Borderline tumor (upper right) is present juxtaposed to confluent invasion within the stroma.

more classical areas with thyroid follicles and immunoreactivity for thyroglobulin are helpful in this differential diagnosis. *Retiform Sertoli–Leydig cell tumor* may simulate a serous borderline tumor; however, the papillae are typically edematous and lack branching and cell budding. Moreover, this tumor typically has distinctive features of sex cord stromal differentiation elsewhere provided there is adequate tumor sampling.

PROGNOSIS AND THERAPY

Serous borderline tumors offer the potential for ovarian uterine conservative surgery, especially in young, repro-

ductive-aged women, although initial staging surgery is often performed in order to accurately determine stage and exclude the presence of invasive implants. Even in high-stage tumors, the disease tempo in women with serous borderline tumors is characteristically indolent and protracted. Prolonged periods of dormancy and even spontaneous regression may occur. Patients with invasive implants have an increased risk of disease recurrence and progression, except those with single cell infiltration. Transformation to low-grade serous carcinoma (Figure 11.12) occurs in up to 7% of women, occasionally decades after initial diagnosis, and is associated with increased tempo of disease and a significantly more aggressive disease course. Stromal microinvasion and lymph node involvement appear not to be associated with risk of recurrence or progression. In a meta-analysis of studies of serous borderline tumors, disease-specific survival was > 95 % for patients with low-stage (stage I) tumors and approximately 65 % for patients with high-stage (stage II–IV) tumors. Since late recurrences do occur, and follow-up is limited in many of the studies analyzed, these are conservative estimates of risk of recurrence. Whether or not all patients with serous borderline tumors need to undergo complete surgical staging is controversial. Currently, there is no indication for adjuvant chemotherapy or radiation therapy for women with serous borderline tumors who have disease confined to the ovary or noninvasive extraovarian implants only. Patients with invasive implants have been treated with aggressive chemotherapy, but the efficacy of such treatment in this subset of patients has not been determined.

SEROUS ADENOCARCINOMA (SEROUS CYSTADENOCARCINOMA)

Serous carcinomas account for 35 % of all serous ovarian neoplasms and approximately 75 % of ovarian surface epithelial stromal carcinomas. Ovarian tumors that occur in women with germline *BRCA1/BRCA2* mutations are usually serous carcinomas, which may also arise in the fallopian tube in most cases.

CLINICAL FEATURES

Serous carcinoma is very uncommon in women < 20 years, but the incidence progressively increases with age, peaking in the sixth to seventh decades (mean 56 years). Most women present with advanced-stage disease. Symptoms are often vague and nonspecific and include dyspepsia, bloating, early satiety, backache or urinary symptoms. The most common finding is an adnexal, pelvic, or abdominal mass on pelvic examination or imaging studies. A subset of patients present with sudden onset of severe abdominal pain, due to torsion of the ovarian mass. A variety of paraneoplastic syndromes have been reported in association with serous carcinoma, but these are rarely the presenting sign or symptom. Elevated serum CA-125, although nonspecific, is present in > 80 % of patients.

RADIOLOGIC FEATURES

Carcinomas tend to form large, complex, solid and cystic masses on pelvic ultrasound. Irregular, thick cyst walls with septations, necrosis, and solid mural nodules on

---

SEROUS ADENOCARCINOMA – FACT SHEET

Definition
▸ Malignant surface epithelial ovarian tumor composed of serous (tubal-type) epithelium

Incidence and Location
▸ Most common histologic subtype of surface epithelial ovarian carcinoma
▸ Bilateral (60%)

Morbidity and Mortality
▸ Advanced stage (> 80%) with Transabdominal spread to involve peritoneum (with omental caking) and abdominal lymph nodes
▸ Lungs, liver, and pleura common sites of distant metastases

Geographic, and Age Distribution
▸ More common in western hemisphere
▸ Rare in first two decades, but steady increase thereafter (mean age 56 years)

Clinical Features
▸ Pelvic or abdominal enlargement, vague pain, urinary or gastrointestinal symptoms
▸ Ascites
▸ Elevated serum CA125

Radiologic Features
▸ Complex, solid and cystic mass with irregular, thick cyst walls, septations, necrosis, and solid mural nodules
▸ Ascites
▸ Psammomatous calcifications on X-ray

Prognosis and Treatment
▸ Most patients present with extraovarian disease
▸ Overall 5-year survival 30–40%, dependent on stage
▸ Treatment similar to that of other ovarian surface epithelial stromal carcinomas

---

contrast-enhanced CT and MRI are characteristic of ovarian carcinoma. Massive ascites and the presence of diffuse multilocular cystic peritoneal implants are also often present in patients with advanced-stage disease. Psammomatous calcifications may be visible as small granular opacities on plain (X-ray) films of the pelvis and abdomen, especially in women with psammocarcinoma.

PATHOLOGIC FEATURES

GROSS FINDINGS

Serous carcinomas are solid and cystic tumors that frequently show areas of necrosis and hemorrhage. The solid areas are often composed of coalescent friable tissue. Two-thirds are bilateral (Figure 11.13) and in the vast majority, there is spread beyond the ovary at the time of diagnosis.

MICROSCOPIC FINDINGS

Grading of serous carcinomas according to the World Health Organization (WHO) is based on assessment of architectural features and nuclear atypia (without specific criteria) and assignment of a grade from 1 (low-grade) to 3 (high-grade). As expected, it is subject to significant interobserver variability, and the previously described universal grading system of Silverberg (Table 11.2) may be more reproducible. A two-tiered grading scheme based on nuclear atypia (< 3:1 or ≥ 3:1 variation in nuclear size and shape) and if needed, mitotic index (≤ 12/10 HPFs or > 12/10 HPFs) has also been proposed.

High-grade serous carcinomas are characterized by complex, branching papillae and glands forming narrow, slit-like spaces with destructive stromal invasion, which is recognized by confluent growth of malignant cells or irregularly arranged glands, papillae and/or nests of

tumor cells in a desmoplastic stroma. Poorly differentiated tumors often demonstrate large areas of solid epithelial proliferation. Psammoma bodies are frequent but not diagnostic. Nuclear atypia is often pronounced, with bizarre cells present. Mitotic activity is usually brisk and abnormal figures are common. Low-grade serous carcinomas (Figure 11.14) are much less common (< 10%) than high-grade tumors (Figure 11.15) and are commonly associated with a component of serous borderline tumor. They tend to have a more uniform architecture, mostly being composed of small nests and papillae showing slight nuclear enlargement and relatively uniform nucleoli. Serous psammocarcinoma, a very rare variant of low-grade serous carcinoma that uncommonly occurs in the ovary, is defined by the presence of massive psammomatous calcification (at least 75% of the tumor cell nests containing psammoma bodies) (Figure 11.16).

ANCILLARY STUDIES

IMMUNOHISTOCHEMISTRY

Serous carcinomas express an immunohistochemical profile that is similar to benign and borderline serous tumors, i.e., positive for CK7, WT1, Ber-EP4, and CD15 (Leu-M1), but negative for CK20.

MOLECULAR STUDIES

High-grade serous carcinoma usually exhibits *p53* mutations and somatic or germline abnormalities of *BRCA1* and/or *BRCA2*. Marked genomic instability, with complex karyotypic abnormalities and aneuploidy, is the norm. Low-grade (grade 1) serous carcinomas, in contrast, show genetic abnormalities similar to those seen in serous borderline tumors (e.g., *BRAF or K-RAS* mutations).

CYTOLOGY

Cytologic examination of ascitic fluid or abdominal/pelvic peritoneal washings is part of the formal staging of ovarian-surface carcinoma. Positive peritoneal cytologic preparations (seen in up to 95% of cases) are characterized by loose papillary aggregates and/or tight clusters of cells with cytoplasmic vacuolization and hyperchromatic and/or pleomorphic nuclei (Figure 11.17). Psammoma bodies may be present, but are not diagnostic. Fine-needle aspiration is only indicated for the diagnosis of an inoperable cancer or confirmation of suspected recurrent disease.

DIFFERENTIAL DIAGNOSIS

Serous carcinoma should be distinguished from *endometrioid carcinoma* which features more elongated villous

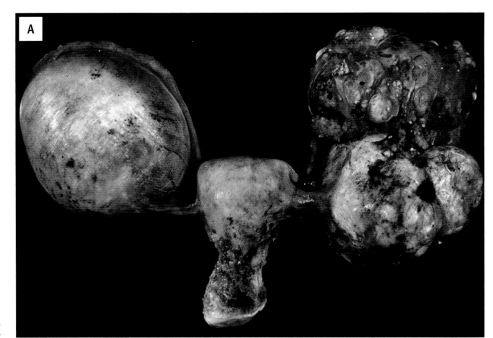

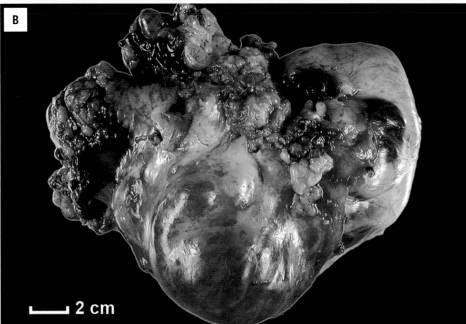

FIGURE 11.13

Serous adenocarcinoma. Predominantly solid and focally necrotic tumors replace both ovaries (A). Surface excrescences are present (B).

FIGURE 11.14

Serous adenocarcinoma, low-grade. Closely packed papillae and small nests of cells are surrounded by stromal clefts. The degree of cytologic atypia is beyond that seen in serous borderline tumor.

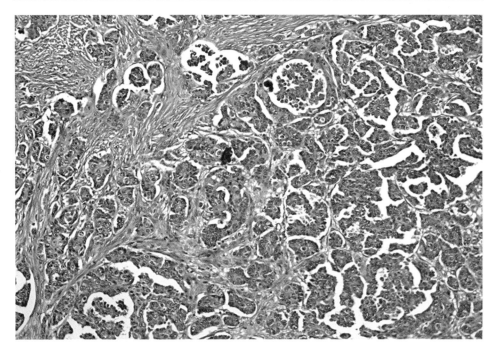

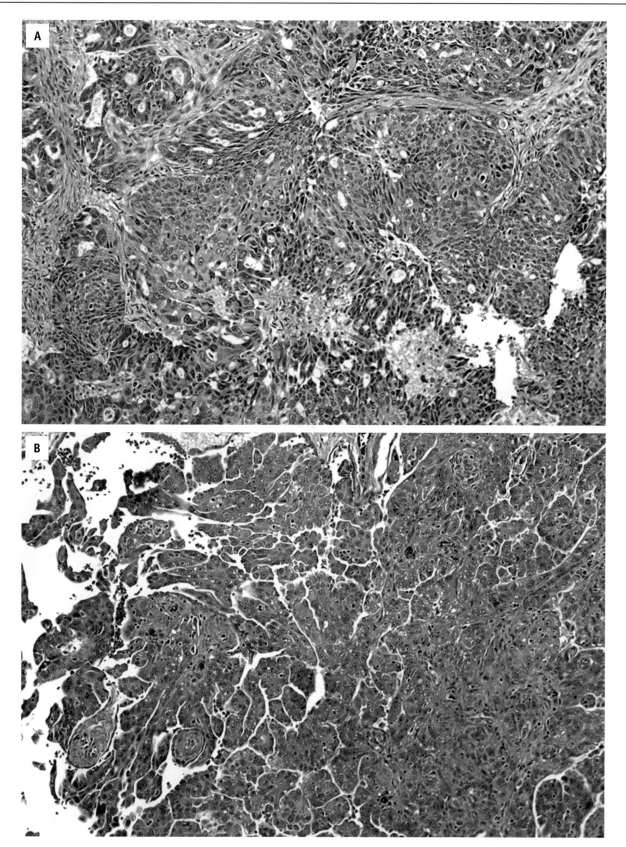

FIGURE 11.15

Serous adenocarcinoma, high-grade. The tumor cells grow in sheets and also form pseudoglandular spaces and papillae (A, B). The epithelial cells are pleomorphic with prominent nucleoli (B).

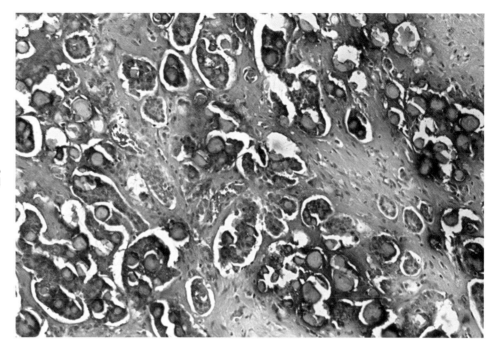

FIGURE 11.16

Psammocarcinoma. Greater than 75% of the tumor cell nests are associated with psammoma bodies.

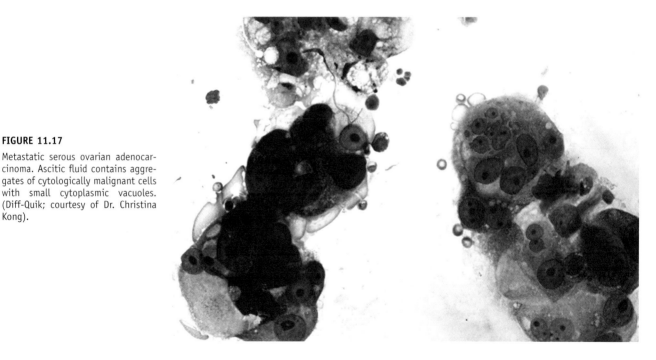

FIGURE 11.17

Metastatic serous ovarian adenocarcinoma. Ascitic fluid contains aggregates of cytologically malignant cells with small cytoplasmic vacuoles. (Diff-Quik; courtesy of Dr. Christina Kong).

papillae, glands with more rounded luminal contours and nuclear polarity, and (often) foci of squamous (or morular) metaplasia. Finally, endometrioid carcinomas are rarely positive for WT1 in contrast to serous carcinomas. *Clear cell carcinoma* frequently has papillae, but are distinguished from serous carcinoma by their small round appearance, more prominent hyalinized cores and less epithelial stratification in the lining cells which may be hobnailing or show clear cytoplasm. *Transitional cell*

carcinoma exhibits significant morphologic overlap with serous carcinoma, but is distinguished by the presence of prominent papillary architecture, with highly atypical multilayered epithelium lining the papillae, similar to that seen in urothelial transitional cell carcinoma. However, not infrequently, serous and transitional cell carcinomas coexist or merge with one another. When a *serous carcinoma involves the ovary and the uterus*, available evidence suggests that these tumors are clonal (i.e., not independent primaries) and primary in the endometrium in most if not all cases, even if there is little or no myometrial invasion by the uterine tumor.

By definition (Gynecologic Oncology Group criteria), serous carcinoma of the ovary is distinguished from *serous carcinoma of the peritoneum* with secondary ovarian involvement by the presence of at least 5 mm of ovarian parenchymal involvement. *Retiform Sertoli–Leydig cell tumors* may simulate a low-grade serous carcinoma, but the former tumors occur at a younger age and typically demonstrate other areas with distinctive features of sex cord stromal differentiation. *Malignant papillary mesothelioma* is distinguished from low-grade serous carcinoma on the basis of prominent tubulopapillary architecture and cuboidal cells as well as the presence of strong staining for calretinin and absence of staining for epithelial markers. *Metastatic breast carcinoma* is recognized on the basis of the clinical history and strong, diffuse staining for GCDFP-15, and absent WT-1 staining. However, negative BRST-2 staining does not exclude the diagnosis of metastatic breast carcinoma.

PROGNOSIS AND THERAPY

The treatment of serous carcinoma does not differ from that of other ovarian surface epithelial stromal carcinomas. As high-grade serous carcinoma accounts for most advanced-stage ovarian carcinomas, the grim survival statistics largely reflect the prognosis of patients with this subtype of ovarian carcinoma. Although most high-grade serous carcinomas initially respond to chemotherapy, responses are not durable and most patients die of their disease. Low-grade serous carcinoma is much less likely to respond to chemotherapy, but has a more favorable prognosis than high-grade carcinoma because of its indolent growth.

MUCINOUS SURFACE EPITHELIAL STROMAL TUMORS

Surface epithelial tumors with mucinous differentiation account for 12–15% of all ovarian neoplasms in the US and Europe. In Japan, where other subtypes of ovarian surface epithelial tumors are less common, mucinous tumors account for a higher percentage. These tumors are characterized by epithelial cells resembling those of the endocervix (endocervical-like) or gastrointestinal tract (intestinal-type) and encompass a group of three biologically distinct entities: (1) mucinous cystadenoma/adenofibroma; (2) mucinous borderline tumor (tumor of low malignant potential); and (3) mucinous carcinoma. While all surface epithelial stromal tumors may exhibit some degree of intratumoral heterogeneity, mucinous surface epithelial tumors are notorious for containing foci of benign, borderline, and malignant

TABLE 11.6

Classification of mucinous surface epithelial stromal tumors (modified from World Health Organization)

Benign (cystadenoma, adenofibroma, cystadenofibroma)	80%
Variant, with focal proliferation	
Borderline (low malignant potential)	15%
Intestinal type	(85%)
Variant, with stromal microinvasion	
Variant, with microinvasive carcinoma	
Variant, with intraepithelial carcinoma	
Endocervical-like	(15%)
Variant, with stromal microinvasion	
Variant, with microinvasive carcinoma	
Variant, with intraepithelial carcinoma	
Malignant (adenocarcinoma, malignant adenofibroma)	5%
Mucinous cystic tumor with mural nodules	
Sarcoma-like	
Anaplastic carcinoma	
Sarcoma	
Mixed	
Mucinous cystic tumor with pseudomyxoma peritonei	

cytoarchitecture intermingled within the same neoplasm, making careful gross examination and histologic sampling particularly important. Tumors indistinguishable from ovarian mucinous tumors (cystadenoma, borderline tumor, and carcinoma) can also occur at extraovarian sites, most commonly in the retroperitoneum, but also in the pancreas, biliary tract, and inguinal region, in the absence of a primary tumor in the ovary. Mucinous epithelial tumors may coexist with Brenner tumors (transitional cell adenofibromas), carcinoids, Sertoli–Leydig cell tumors, or mature cystic teratomas in up to 5% of cases. Rarely, intestinal-type mucinous tumors are admixed with a high-grade neuroendocrine carcinoma (nonsmall cell type). The full classification of mucinous surface epithelial stromal tumors is given in Table 11.6.

BENIGN MUCINOUS TUMORS

Benign mucinous tumors comprise 80% of all mucinous ovarian neoplasms.

CLINICAL FEATURES

Benign mucinous tumors occur over a wide age range, but are most commonly diagnosed in the reproductive age group. They are infrequently bilateral and women typically present with abdominal enlargement or pain.

MUCINOUS CYSTADENOMA (ADENOFIBROMA, CYSTADENOFIBROMA) – FACT SHEET

Definition
▸ Benign surface epithelial tumor composed of endocervical-like (müllerian) or intestinal-type mucinous epithelium

Incidence and Location
▸ Most common mucinous ovarian tumor (80%)
▸ Unilateral

Morbidity and Mortality
▸ Benign

Age Distribution
▸ Wide age range, but most common during reproductive years

Clinical Features
▸ Often asymptomatic
▸ Abdominal enlargement or pain

Radiologic Features
▸ Simple smooth-walled unilocular or multilocular cystic mass
▸ Larger and more frequently unilateral than serous cystadenomas

Prognosis and Treatment
▸ Complete excision is curative

RADIOLOGIC FEATURES

These tumors tend to form simple, smooth-walled unilocular or multilocular cystic masses on pelvic ultrasound. They are typically large and are distinguished from borderline or malignant mucinous tumors by the lack of intracystic complexity.

PATHOLOGIC FEATURES

GROSS FINDINGS

Benign mucinous tumors can reach very large size and range from 1 to ≥ 30 cm (Figure 11.18A). They are

composed of unilocular or multilocular smooth lined cystic spaces often filled with thick and tenacious fluid, although the cysts contents are not reliable in determining the type of lining epithelium. A prominent stromal component (mucinous adenofibroma) may be seen.

MICROSCOPIC FINDINGS

The lining epithelium resembles that of the endocervix or upper gastrointestinal type (most commonly foveolar cells), typically composed of columnar cells with abundant, pale-staining intracellular mucin (Figure 11.18B) and small, bland, basally located nuclei. Goblet cells are rare in contrast to mucinous tumors of low malignant potential or mucinous carcinomas.

MUCINOUS CYSTADENOMA (ADENOFIBROMA, CYSTADENOFIBROMA) – PATHOLOGIC FEATURES

Gross Findings
▸ Unilocular or multilocular, predominantly cystic mass
▸ Often very large (> 30 cm)
▸ Smooth capsule and cyst lining

Microscopic Findings
▸ Columnar, pale-staining mucinous epithelium resembling endocervix or upper gastrointestinal tract
▸ Minimal or absent epithelial stratification
▸ Minimal or absent atypia

Differential Diagnosis
▸ Serous cystadenoma
▸ Mucinous borderline tumor

DIFFERENTIAL DIAGNOSIS

Mucinous cystadenoma is distinguished from other benign cysts based on the type of lining epithelium. The chief differential diagnosis rests between benign mucinous cystadenoma and mucinous borderline tumor (either endocervical-like or intestinal type). *Mucinous borderline tumor of intestinal type* features epithelial stratification and atypia, numerous goblet cells, and occasional mitotic figures. *Endocervical-like mucinous borderline tumor* (also referred to as müllerian mucinous borderline tumor or seromucinous borderline tumor) is characterized by papillae covered by stratified ciliated and mucinous epithelium with abundant neutrophils within the edematous papillae. By definition, mucinous tumors that are otherwise benign but show focal epithelial proliferation, with stratification and atypia (accounting for < 10% of the epithelium), are designated mucinous cystadenoma with "focal proliferation" or

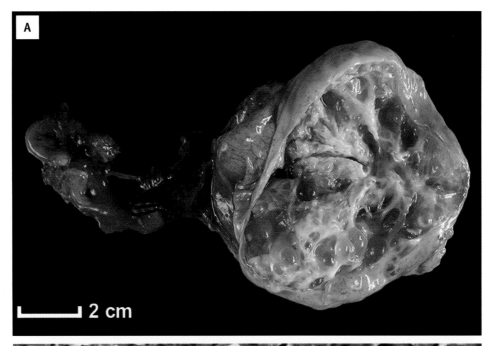

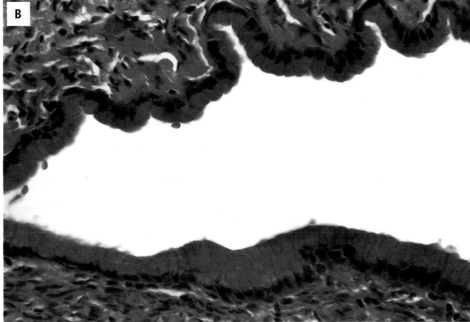

FIGURE 11.18
Mucinous cystadenoma. The bisected surface shows a multiloculated cystic tumor with smooth cyst walls (A). The cyst shows nonstratified columnar mucinous epithelium with small, basal nuclei (B).

"focal atypia" (either endocervical-like or intestinal type).

PROGNOSIS AND THERAPY

Mucinous cystadenomas and cystadenofibromas are clinically benign. Complete excision (cystectomy or oophorectomy) is curative. To minimize surgical morbidity, laparoscopic removal may be performed, although many tumors are too large to be removed by this method.

MUCINOUS BORDERLINE TUMOR (MUCINOUS TUMOR OF LOW MALIGNANT POTENTIAL), INTESTINAL-TYPE

Mucinous borderline tumors comprise approximately 15% of all ovarian mucinous neoplasms and can be subdivided into intestinal-type and endocervical-like subsets. In North America they are less common than serous borderline tumors, whereas in Japan, serous and mucinous borderline tumors are encountered with approximately equal frequency. The following discussion refers only to the mucinous borderline tumors of intestinal type, which are far more common. The endocervical-like mucinous borderline tumors are discussed separately.

CLINICAL FEATURES

Mucinous borderline tumor of intestinal type occurs at a similar age as mucinous carcinoma (mean 45 years). Patients are often asymptomatic, or present with abdominal enlargement or pain. Unlike serous borderline tumors, which have a distinctive, indolent, and often prolonged natural history, mucinous borderline tumors, in the absence of intraepithelial carcinoma or frank carcinoma, appear to follow an invariably benign clinical course. Thus, the proposed terminology of "atypically proliferating mucinous tumor" is arguably more

accurate, since it describes the histologic features without suggesting potential malignant behavior.

RADIOLOGIC FEATURES

Mucinous borderline tumors tend to form unilateral cystic adnexal masses. Bilaterality is sufficiently uncommon and, if present, should prompt consideration of a metastasis. No areas of necrosis are seen on imaging studies, with the exception of those tumors that have undergone torsion and/or infarction.

PATHOLOGIC FEATURES

GROSS FINDINGS

Mucinous neoplasms in the borderline or low-malignant-potential group are unilateral and often larger than benign mucinous tumors (can reach > 30 cm). They have a smooth surface and are predominantly cystic, with frequent multiple locules (Figure 11.19). Distinction from a benign or malignant mucinous tumor cannot be made based solely on gross examination; therefore,

---

MUCINOUS BORDERLINE TUMOR (MUCINOUS TUMOR OF LOW MALIGNANT POTENTIAL), INTESTINAL-TYPE – FACT SHEET

Definition
▸ Surface epithelial tumor composed of intestinal-type mucinous epithelium with limited epithelial stratification and cytologic atypia and no stromal invasion

Incidence and Location
▸ Most common mucinous borderline tumor (85%)
▸ Unilateral

Morbidity and Mortality
▸ Invariably benign unless associated with invasive adenocarcinoma

Geographic and Age Distribution
▸ Comparatively more common in Japan
▸ Predominantly reproductive-age women (mean 45 years)

Clinical Features
▸ Often asymptomatic
▸ Abdominal enlargement, pain, change in bowel or bladder function

Radiologic Features
▸ Large, multilocular cystic mass
▸ Almost always unilateral
▸ Necrosis absent, unless torsion or infarction

Prognosis and Treatment
▸ Cystectomy or oophorectomy curative in most cases, provided adequate sampling and exclusion of extraovarian disease
▸ Surgical staging should be considered for intraepithelial carcinoma and invasive adenocarcinoma
▸ No indication for adjuvant radiation therapy or chemotherapy

---

MUCINOUS BORDERLINE TUMOR (MUCINOUS TUMOR OF LOW MALIGNANT POTENTIAL), INTESTINAL-TYPE – PATHOLOGIC FEATURES

Gross Findings
▸ Large (often > 30 cm), predominantly cystic mass with multiple locules

Microscopic Findings
▸ Stratification of intestinal-type (often gastric-type) epithelium into 2–3 cell layers with arborizing villous architecture
▸ Mild to moderate cytologic atypia with maturation at the tips of villous structures, and scattered mitoses
▸ Goblet cells common; Paneth cells and neuroendocrine cells may be present
▸ Limited stromal invasion may occur (≤ 5 mm in linear extent or 10 mm² in area)
▸ Intraepithelial carcinoma: Cellular stratification with loss of maturation, severe cytologic atypia, and frequent mitoses

Immunohistochemical Features
▸ CK7, CK20, CEA positive

Molecular Studies
▸ K-RAS mutations
▸ No association with germline or somatic BRCA1/BRCA2 mutations

Differential Diagnosis
▸ Mucinous cystadenoma with focal proliferation
▸ Mucinous adenocarcinoma
▸ Metastatic adenocarcinoma (e.g., appendix, colon, stomach, pancreaticobiliary tract, cervix or lung)

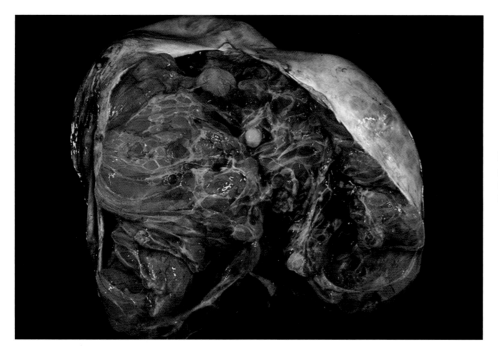

FIGURE 11.19

Borderline mucinous tumor, intestinal type. Multiloculated cysts contain mucoid material.

extensive sampling is required (*at least* one section per centimeter), particularly directed to more complex microcystic or solid areas.

MICROSCOPIC FINDINGS

Mucinous borderline tumors of intestinal type show stratification of the epithelial cells into ≤ 3 layers. Assessment of stratification can be difficult in areas of tangential sectioning, but it is invariably accompanied by some degree of cytologic atypia. Unlike the flat lining of benign mucinous tumors, the epithelium in borderline tumors is often thrown into variably complex papillary folds (Figure 11.20). The individual cells show mild to moderate cytologic atypia, with an increased nuclear-to-cytoplasmic ratio and variability in nuclear size and shape. Mitotic figures are usually present but are not striking. The amount of intracytoplasmic mucin is variable, but overall, it appears to be more abundant towards the surface indicating "maturation" as seen in the gastrointestinal tract epithelium. Goblet cells are present and Paneth and neuroendocrine cells may also be found. The lower limit for diagnosis of a mucinous borderline tumor of intestinal type is not well defined, and in equivocal cases it is preferable to make a diagnosis of benign mucinous cystadenoma, provided the tumor has been well sampled. When a borderline component is unequivocally present but accounts for < 10% of the tumor, the preferred diagnostic terminology is benign mucinous cystadenoma with "focal proliferation" or "focal atypia". The upper limit of cytologic atypia accepted for a mucinous borderline tumor of intestinal type (versus mucinous borderline tumor with intraepithelial carcinoma) is similarly ill-defined. The presence of marked or severe nuclear atypia involving the full thickness of stratified epithelium with or without brisk mitotic activity (i.e., not limited to the crypts) warrants a diagnosis of mucinous borderline tumor of intestinal type with intraepithelial carcinoma (Figure 11.21).

Two patterns of microinvasion are recognized in mucinous borderline tumors of intestinal type. The first pattern consists of infiltration of stroma by individual cells or small nests of cells that are cytologically similar to the cells elsewhere in the borderline tumor. Such foci must not exceed 5 mm in linear extent or 10 mm^2 in area. This is an uncommon finding in mucinous borderline tumors (in comparison to the frequency of microinvasion in serous borderline tumors) and, although it should be noted, it does not warrant a diagnosis of carcinoma. The second pattern of microinvasion consists of one or more small foci (≤ 5 mm in linear extent or 10 mm^2 in area) of nests, individual cells, and glands exhibiting cytologic features of high-grade carcinoma. The term "mucinous borderline tumor of intestinal type with microinvasive carcinoma" has been proposed and it is the most common pattern of stromal microinvasion in these tumors. When these foci are small, they are of uncertain prognostic significance, but their presence should prompt a search for frank invasive carcinoma.

ANCILLARY STUDIES

IMMUNOHISTOCHEMISTRY

Mucinous borderline tumors of intestinal type, because of their intestinal differentiation, express an immunohistochemical profile that is somewhat different from serous tumors, with similarities to tumors of the gastrointestinal tract. For example, most mucinous borderline tumors of intestinal type are CEA positive and CA125 negative.

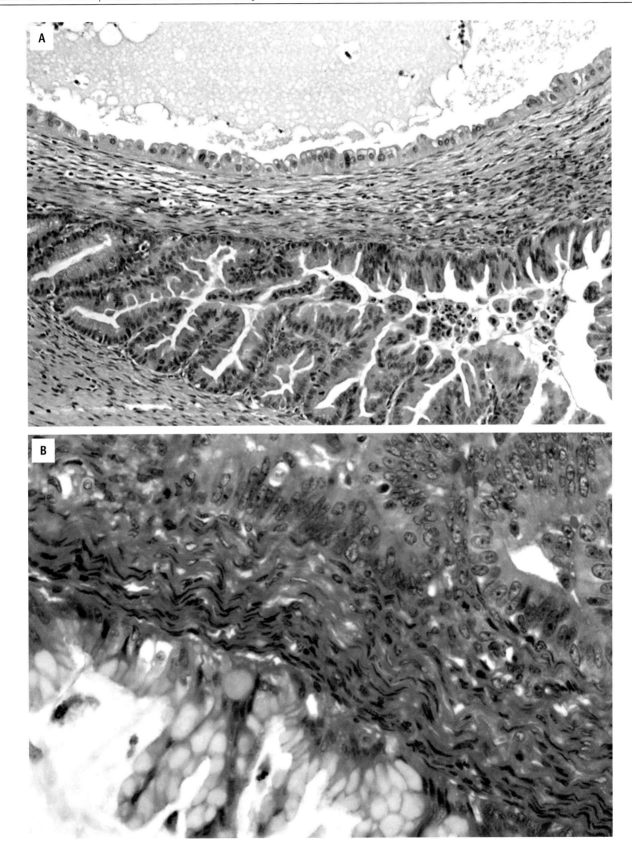

FIGURE 11.20

Borderline mucinous tumor, intestinal type. A complex villous architecture resembles a villous polyp of the colorectum (A). The cells have enlarged nuclei with visible nucleoli (upper right) which contrast with the banal nuclear appearance in the coexisting benign appearing areas (B).

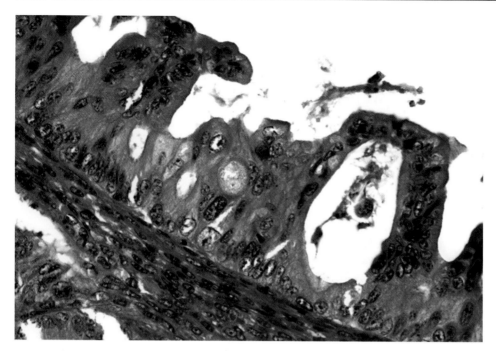

FIGURE 11.21

Mucinous borderline tumor with intraepithelial carcinoma. Cellular stratification with loss of maturation, nuclear hyperchromasia, and marked nuclear pleomorphism are present.

Additionally, they are usually CK7 positive and stain for CK20 in the majority of cases, although positivity is frequently patchy. CDX2 staining is also common but is typically less diffuse and intense than in intestinal tumors. Although some qualitative differences in staining pattern have been observed between mucinous borderline tumors of intestinal type and mucinous tumors primary at other sites which can metastasize to the ovary and mimic a primary mucinous tumor, there is sufficient overlap that these stains may be less than completely discriminatory in individual cases.

MOLECULAR STUDIES

Mucinous borderline tumors of intestinal type frequently show *KRAS* mutations. They are not associated with somatic or germline abnormalities of *BRCA1* and/ or *BRCA2*.

DIFFERENTIAL DIAGNOSIS

Mucinous borderline tumors should be distinguished from *mucinous cystadenomas with focal proliferation*. In such cases, most of the tumor (> 90 %) is composed of a flat lining of cells with no nuclear pseudostratification or atypia. *Mucinous adenocarcinomas* typically show a more complex architecture with cribriform, back to back, or less commonly, irregularly infiltrative glands associated with marked cytologic atypia. However, not infrequently, the chief concern in the differential diagnosis is a *metastasis* from the gastrointestinal tract, pancreaticobiliary system, uterine cervix, or lung, as these tumors may have coexisting benign, borderline, and

malignant areas. The clinical setting is most helpful in alerting the pathologist to the possibility of metastases. Metastatic tumors are frequently bilateral, multinodular and show ovarian surface involvement, although absence of these features do not exclude a metastasis. Bilaterality, nodularity and ovarian surface involvement are rare in primary mucinous borderline tumors of intestinal type. Even though the latter are typically larger than metastases, this is not a reliable feature as ovarian metastases are frequently much larger than the primary extraovarian tumor (e.g., of vermiform appendix, cervix, or pancreas). A history of a previous extraovarian primary is of course helpful, although the adnexal mass may be the presenting manifestation of a primary extraovarian tumor. Finally, the presence of pseudomyxoma peritonei or extraovarian implants is very uncommon in primary ovarian mucinous tumors and should suggest the possibility of metastasis. Often, review of the histologic features of the extraovarian primary tumor and comparison with the ovarian tumor, with or without immunohistochemical studies, will be sufficient to determine whether or not a tumor is a metastasis.

PROGNOSIS AND THERAPY

Mucinous borderline tumors of intestinal type with no evidence of intraepithelial carcinoma or invasive carcinoma, if confined to the ovary, are invariably benign provided careful histopathologic examination has been performed. Occasional old reports of stage I mucinous borderline tumors of intestinal type followed a malignant course, but most likely these tumors were not well sampled. Thus, there is the potential for conservative surgery, especially in young, reproductive-aged women. Unilateral salpingo-oophorectomy, with careful examination for extraovarian disease, is sufficient treatment. There is no indication for adjuvant chemotherapy or radiation therapy.

Mucinous borderline tumors of intestinal type with stromal microinvasion are probably not associated with an increased risk of recurrence, but relatively few cases have been reported. Occasional mucinous borderline tumors of intestinal type with intraepithelial carcinoma have recurred (< 5 %) as high-grade carcinoma, within 5 years of initial diagnosis. These tumors have been associated with a rapidly progressive course, frequently with distant metastases. Finally, most if not all, advanced-stage mucinous borderline tumors of intestinal type reported are now thought to most likely represent metastases.

MUCINOUS BORDERLINE TUMOR (MUCINOUS TUMOR OF LOW MALIGNANT POTENTIAL), ENDOCERVICAL-LIKE

These tumors account for 5–15 % of mucinous borderline tumors. Endocervical-like mucinous borderline tumors are also known as müllerian mucinous papillary cystadenomas of borderline malignancy and seromucinous borderline tumors. The latter accurately conveys the striking clinical and pathologic similarity to serous borderline tumors, as well as the fact that these tumors are often admixed with a component of serous borderline tumor, in contrast to mucinous borderline tumors of intestinal type, which are typically purely mucinous.

CLINICAL FEATURES

Patients with endocervical-like mucinous borderline tumors range in age between 19 and 59 (mean 35) years; up to 40 % are bilateral and 20 % have extraovarian disease at presentation. There is a strong association with endometriosis (present in up to 50 % of cases).

PATHOLOGIC FEATURES

GROSS FINDINGS

Mucinous borderline tumors with endocervical-like differentiation are generally smaller than those of intestinal type (mean diameter 8–10 cm). They are unilocular or multilocular, and often exhibit papillary excrescences along the inner cyst wall similar to serous borderline tumors. Foci of endometriosis may be grossly apparent.

MICROSCOPIC FINDINGS

Endocervical-like mucinous borderline tumors are composed of variably complex papillae, architecturally similar to those of serous borderline tumors. They are lined by cuboidal to columnar mucin-secreting epithelium, ciliated epithelium, and eosinophilic "pink" cells that frequently exfoliate from the tips of the papillae (Figure 11.22); goblet cells are absent. Nuclear atypia is mild to moderate and mitotic figures may be present, but are usually infrequent. A prominent neutrophilic infiltrate is typically seen in the stroma of the papillae (which are frequently edematous) and in the luminal contents. Stromal microinvasion, and extraovarian implants similar to that in serous borderline tumors, may be present, but are not associated with poorer prognosis.

DIFFERENTIAL DIAGNOSIS

The presence of intracellular mucin and a prominent neutrophilic infiltrate distinguishes these tumors from their serous counterpart, while the absence of definitive intestinal-type differentiation (e.g., goblet cells) and

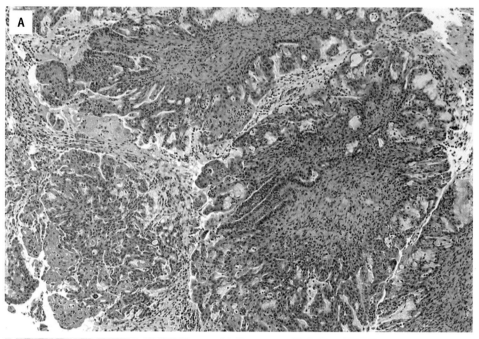

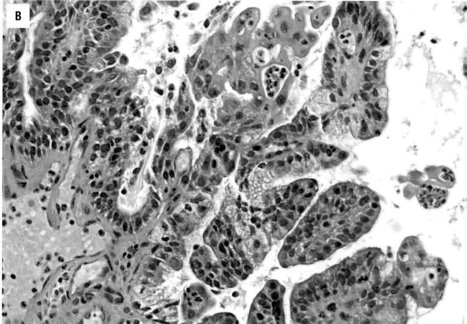

FIGURE 11.22
Borderline mucinous tumor, endocervical-like (müllerian mucinous borderline tumor). Large edematous papillae are associated with prominent acute inflammation and cellular tufting (A). Endocervical-like, ciliated, and pink cells are seen (B).

MUCINOUS BORDERLINE TUMOR (MUCINOUS TUMOR OF LOW MALIGNANT POTENTIAL), ENDOCERVICAL-LIKE – PATHOLOGIC FEATURES

Gross Findings

▶ Unilocular or multilocular cyst with papillary excrescences along inner cyst wall similar to serous borderline tumor
▶ Foci of endometriosis may be apparent

Microscopic Findings

▶ Variably complex papillae, frequently edematous, lined by a mixture of mucin-secreting columnar endocervical-like cells, ciliated cells, and eosinophilic "pink" cells
▶ Neutrophilic infiltrate in papillary cores and cyst contents
▶ Low-grade nuclear atypia and infrequent mitoses

▶ Stromal microinvasion may occur
▶ Endometriosis often present

Immunohistochemical Features

▶ CK7 positive
▶ CK20 negative

Differential Diagnosis

▶ Serous borderline tumor
▶ Mucinous borderline tumor, intestinal type

papillary rather than villous architecture distinguishes them from mucinous borderline tumor of intestinal type.

PROGNOSIS AND THERAPY

The natural history of endocervical-like borderline tumors appears to be similar to that of serous borderline tumors. Although no deaths have been attributed to endocervical-like mucinous borderline tumors, relatively few cases with long-term follow-up have been reported. Women with stage I tumors can be conservatively treated with cystectomy or adnexectomy, but follow-up is recommended as recurrences may occur. Chemotherapy is not indicated, even for patients with high-stage disease.

MUCINOUS ADENOCARCINOMA (MUCINOUS CYSTADENOCARCINOMA)

Mucinous adenocarcinomas account for < 15 % of all mucinous ovarian neoplasms and < 10 % of all ovarian surface epithelial stromal carcinomas.

CLINICAL FEATURES

The age at presentation is similar to that of patients with mucinous borderline tumors of intestinal type (mean 45 years). Patients are either asymptomatic or present with abdominal enlargement or pain, and less frequently, with changes in bowel or bladder function. In contrast to serous carcinomas, CA-125 may not be markedly elevated. Most mucinous adenocarcinomas are confined to the ovary at presentation.

RADIOLOGIC FEATURES

These tumors form large, complex, solid and cystic masses on pelvic ultrasound. Irregular, thick cyst walls with septations, necrosis, and solid mural nodules on contrast-enhanced CT and MRI are characteristic. Ascites may be present but is not common.

PATHOLOGIC FEATURES

GROSS FINDINGS

Mucinous adenocarcinomas are predominantly unilateral, solid and cystic and often large (> 10 cm) tumors. Surface ovarian involvement is not identifiable in most cases, although larger tumors may exhibit rupture and/ or adhesions.

MICROSCOPIC FINDINGS

Mucinous carcinomas are distinguished from mucinous borderline tumors of intestinal type by a combination of architectural and cytologic features. Typically, primary mucinous carcinoma demonstrates a continuum of architectural and cytologic atypia that includes borderline and frankly carcinomatous areas. Tumors with the architectural features of typical mucinous borderline tumors of intestinal type, containing foci of epithelial stratification and severe nuclear atypia, are classified as mucinous borderline tumor of intestinal type with intraepithelial carcinoma. Invasive carcinoma can be diagnosed based on two different patterns of invasion, which may coexist in a single tumor. The confluent glandular or expansile invasive pattern is recognized by marked glandular crowding with little intervening stroma, creating a labyrinthine appearance (Figure 11.23A); cribriforming may also be present (Figure 11.23B). The destructive stromal invasive pattern, which is less common, is recognized by irregular nests and single cells with malignant cytologic features infiltrating the stroma (Figure 11.24). The presence

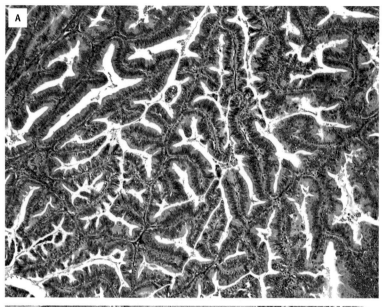

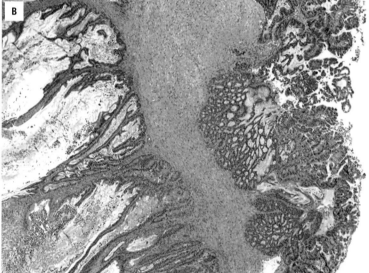

FIGURE 11.23

Mucinous adenocarcinoma. The tumor glands are back to back with minimal intervening stroma (expansile pattern) (A). A confluent cribriform architecture diagnostic of carcinoma (right) coexists with foci of mucinous borderline tumor (left) (B).

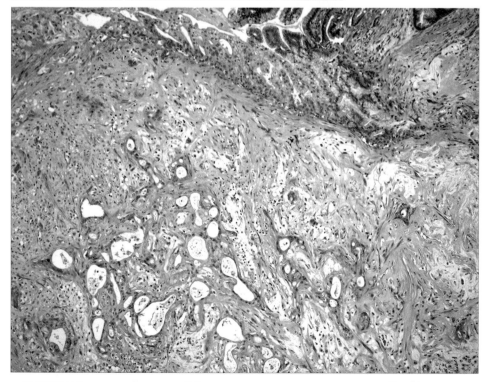

FIGURE 11.24

Mucinous adenocarcinoma with destructive stromal invasion (infiltrative pattern). Small glands and individual nests of cytologically malignant tumor cells infiltrate the stroma in a disorderly fashion.

MUCINOUS ADENOCARCINOMA (CYSTADENOCARCINOMA) – PATHOLOGIC FEATURES

Gross Findings

▸ Solid and cystic mass
▸ Surface involvement typically absent, but large tumors often exhibit rupture and/or adhesions
▸ May reach very large size (> 30 cm)

Microscopic Findings

▸ Cytoarchitectural features similar to, but more severe than, mucinous borderline tumors (intestinal type) with areas of invasive adenocarcinoma exceeding 5 mm in linear extent or 10 mm² in area
▸ Two patterns of invasion:
  – Destructive: malignant glands and individual cells irregularly infiltrating ovarian stroma
  – Expansile: Confluent glands forming labyrinthine or cribriform patterns
▸ Mitotic figures may be numerous with atypical forms
▸ Areas of benign, borderline, and invasive mucinous carcinoma may coexist in same tumor

Immunohistochemical Features

▸ CK7, CK20, CEA positive

Molecular Studies

▸ K-RAS mutations
▸ No association with germline or somatic BRCA1/BRCA2 mutations

Differential Diagnosis

▸ Metastatic adenocarcinoma (e.g., appendix, colon, stomach, pancreatobiliary tract)
▸ Mucinous borderline tumor, intestinal type

of stromal invasion, whether of destructive or confluent type, must exceed 5 mm in linear extent or 10 mm² in area in order to be classified as carcinoma; otherwise a diagnosis of microinvasion is warranted. Recognizable mucinous epithelium may give way to anaplastic carcinoma, especially in tumors showing destructive stromal invasion. Mitotic activity is often quite high and abnormal forms are frequently present. A very rare variant of mucinous carcinoma has been described which is endocervical-like, and is considered the malignant counterpart of endocervical-like mucinous borderline tumor, but this subgroup of tumors is not well characterized at present.

ANCILLARY STUDIES

IMMUNOHISTOCHEMISTRY

Mucinous adenocarcinomas show intestinal differentiation and are positive for CEA, CK7, CK20, and CDX2, but negative for CA125. As with mucinous borderline tumors of intestinal type, there are some qualitative differences in immunostaining between primary and metastatic adenomucinous carcinomas, but there is sufficient overlap to make these stains less than completely discriminatory in some cases.

MOLECULAR STUDIES

Mucinous carcinomas commonly show *KRAS* mutations. These tumors are unique amongst subtypes of surface epithelial carcinomas in not being associated with somatic or germline abnormalities of *BRCA1* and/or *BRCA2*.

DIFFERENTIAL DIAGNOSIS

The chief differential diagnosis is with *metastatic mucinous adenocarcinoma*, which should always be strongly considered when evaluating an ovarian mucinous carcinoma. Features suggestive of metastatic carcinoma include history of a primary mucinous carcinoma at another site, bilaterality, multinodularity, ovarian surface involvement, destructive stromal invasion, hilar lymphovascular invasion, and extraovarian disease. The presence of a benign or borderline component is not a useful distinguishing feature, since metastatic mucinous carcinomas are as likely as primary ovarian mucinous carcinomas to exhibit this appearance.

PROGNOSIS AND THERAPY

Stage is the most important prognostic indicator in patients with mucinous adenocarcinoma. Most tumors are stage I at presentation and these patients have an excellent prognosis. Fewer than 5% of patients with stage I mucinous borderline tumor of intestinal type with intraepithelial carcinoma, mucinous borderline tumor of intestinal type with stromal microinvasion or microinvasive carcinoma, or mucinous carcinoma with confluent glandular invasion (and no destructive stromal invasion) experience recurrences, accounting for a large majority of patients with mucinous carcinoma. Thus, for these patients no adjuvant therapy is warranted. Importantly, when these patients do experience a recurrence they tend to be early (within 3 years of diagnosis), do not appear to respond well to chemotherapy or radiotherapy, and lead to the death of the patient. Prognosis for patients with either destructive stromal invasion or extraovarian disease at presentation is less favorable. Fourteen to 25% of patients with stage I mucinous carcinomas with destructive stromal invasion experience recurrences, while most patients with extraovarian disease at presentation die of disease. Chemotherapy appears to be less effective against mucinous carcinoma than serous carcinoma.

MUCINOUS CYSTIC TUMOR WITH MURAL NODULES

The presence of one or more discrete nodules in the wall of a mucinous cystic neoplasm (benign, borderline, or malignant) is a well-described but uncommon occurrence. They are divided into: (1) sarcoma-like mural nodules which are composed of spindle cells, epulis-like

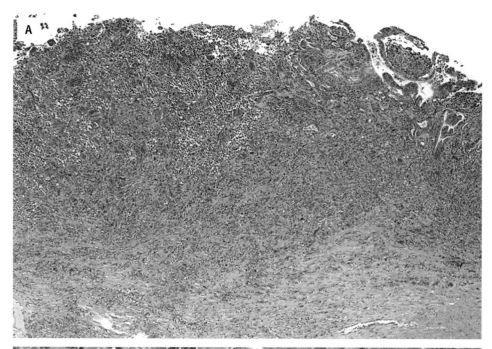

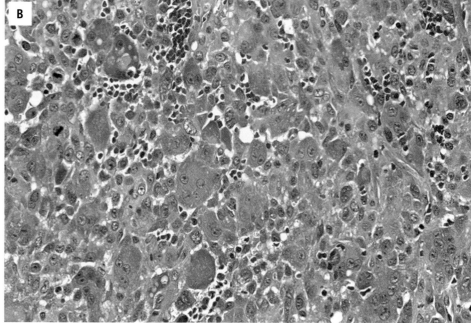

FIGURE 11.25

Sarcoma-like nodule in a mucinous borderline tumor. A large nodule is present in the wall (A). It is composed of mononuclear cells and osteoclast-like giant cells (B).

giant cells, and/or inflammatory cells; (2) anaplastic carcinoma; (3) sarcoma; and (4) mixed nodules. Not surprisingly, the presence of sarcoma-like nodules is not of prognostic significance, while nodules of anaplastic carcinoma, sarcoma, or any mixture thereof are associated with a poor outcome. Sarcoma-like nodules may occur in benign, borderline, or malignant mucinous tumors (Figure 11.25). They are often multiple, may be visualized on gross examination as red-brown nodules (0.6–6 cm in diameter), are frequently mitotically active (5–10/10 HPFs), stain strongly for histiocyte markers, and may show weak immunoreactivity for cytokeratin. Nodules of anaplastic carcinoma almost always occur in borderline or malignant mucinous tumors. They may be microscopic or macroscopic (up to 10 cm), single or mul-

tiple, with spindled or epithelioid cells, and stain strongly for cytokeratin (Figure 11.26). Sarcomatous nodules exhibit a variety of patterns, including fibrosarcoma, rhabdomyosarcoma, and undifferentiated sarcoma. Mixed nodules may feature carcinosarcoma or a mixed anaplastic carcinoma and sarcoma-like nodule.

MUCINOUS CYSTIC TUMOR WITH PSEUDOMYXOMA PERITONEI

Although mucinous tumors associated with pseudomyxoma peritonei are listed as a separate category by

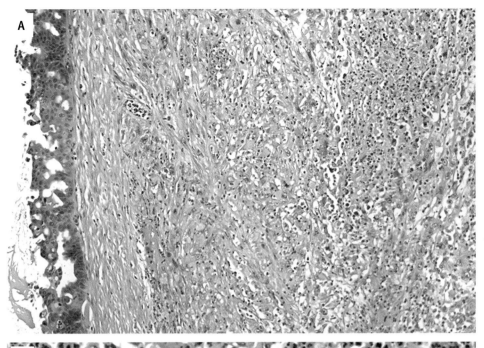

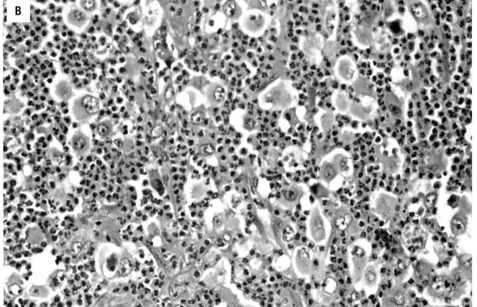

FIGURE 11.26

Anaplastic carcinoma in a mucinous cystic tumor. A mucinous borderline tumor (intestinal type) is juxtaposed to a mural nodule (A), which is composed of sheets of undifferentiated malignant cells with admixed inflammatory cells (B). The undifferentiated malignant cells are strongly positive for cytokeratin (C).

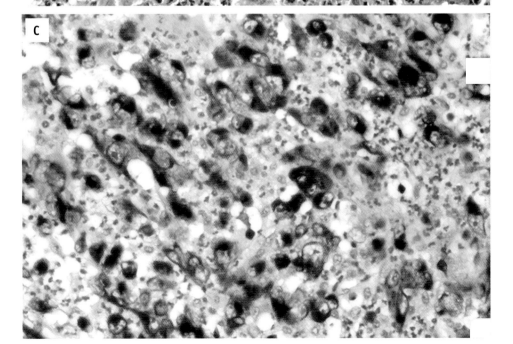

the WHO, it is now appreciated that most of these tumors are metastases from primary mucinous tumors of the vermiform appendix (Chapter 14). Rare examples of mucinous ovarian tumors associated with pseudomyxoma peritonei and a normal vermiform appendix do occur. The ovarian tumors typically show features of mucinous borderline tumor of intestinal type and some have an associated teratoma in the ovary, suggesting a germ cell origin for these tumors. As only few well-documented primary ovarian tumors associated with pseudomyxoma peritonei have been reported, their natural history is not well understood.

ENDOMETRIOID SURFACE EPITHELIAL STROMAL TUMORS

Surface epithelial tumors with endometrioid differentiation (benign, borderline (low malignant potential), or malignant) have glands and/or stroma resembling endometrial endometrial-type glands and stroma. Most endometrioid ovarian tumors are carcinomas (Table 11.7). The frequency with which endometrioid carcinoma is diagnosed varies widely, particularly when high-grade, because of its poor interobserver reproducibility and the fact that some represent high-grade serous carcinomas. Typical endometrioid adenocarcinomas account for 5–10% of ovarian surface epithelial carcinomas, and although classified as of surface epithelial stromal origin, many show a close association with endometriosis, suggesting that at least some of them arise directly from malignant transformation of endometriosis and not from the ovarian surface epithelium.

Endometrioid carcinomas are associated with synchronous low-grade endometrioid carcinomas of the endometrium in 15–20% of cases. Primary ovarian malignant mixed mesodermal tumor (carcinosarcoma), adenosarcoma, and (low-grade) endometrioid stromal sarcoma are rare.

TABLE 11.7

Classification of endometrioid surface epithelial stromal tumors (modified from World Health Organization)

Benign (cystadenoma, adenofibroma, cystadenofibroma)	5%
Borderline (low malignant potential) Variant, with intraepithelial carcinoma	20%
Malignant Adenocarcinoma (cystadenocarcinoma, malignant adenofibroma)	75%
Malignant mixed mesodermal tumor (carcinosarcoma)	
Mesodermal adenosarcoma	
Endometrioid stromal sarcoma, low-grade	

CLINICAL FEATURES

The majority of endometrioid surface epithelial tumors are malignant (endometrioid carcinoma) and, if diagnosed according to strict criteria, comprise about 5–10%

ENDOMETRIOID SURFACE EPITHELIAL STROMAL TUMORS – FACT SHEET

Definition
▸ Spectrum of surface epithelial stromal tumors composed of glands and/or stroma resembling endometrial-type glands and stroma showing variable degrees of cytologic atypia
▸ Common types:
– Benign (adenofibroma most common)
– Borderline (low malignant potential)
– Malignant (adenocarcinoma)
▸ Less common types:
– Mesodermal adenosarcoma
– Endometrioid stromal sarcoma
– Malignant mixed mesodermal tumor

Incidence and Location
▸ Endometrioid epithelial tumors: 8% of all epithelial stromal tumors; most malignant
▸ Unilateral (if benign)
▸ Unilateral (70%) or bilateral (30%) (if borderline or malignant)
▸ Mesodermal adenosarcoma, malignant mixed mesodermal tumor, and endometrioid stromal sarcoma rare

Morbidity and Mortality
▸ Endometrioid adenocarcinoma associated with synchronous primary endometrial adenocarcinoma (15–20%)
▸ If association with clear cell carcinoma more aggressive behavior

Age Distribution
▸ Wide age range, but predominant in fifth to seventh decades

Clinical Features
▸ Asymptomatic
▸ Pelvic or abdominal mass, pain, or vaginal bleeding
▸ Symptoms and signs related to endometriosis

Prognosis and Treatment
▸ Benign and borderline endometrioid tumors clinically benign
▸ Greater than 90% 5-year survival for low-grade, low-stage endometrioid adenocarcinomas (including those with synchronous low-grade endometrial primary cancer)
▸ High-grade and high-stage endometrioid adenocarcinoma similar clinical course to usual ovarian cancer
▸ Poorer prognosis for mesodermal adenosarcoma when compared to its uterine counterpart with frequent recurrences
▸ Endometrioid stromal sarcoma often indolent, even when high-stage
▸ Aggressive behavior associated with malignant mixed mesodermal tumor
▸ Benign and borderline tumors conservatively treated by simple excision
▸ High-grade and high-stage endometrioid adenocarcinoma surgically staged and treated similarly to other ovarian adenocarcinomas
▸ Mesodermal adenosarcoma, malignant mesodermal tumor, and endometrioid stromal sarcoma treated similarly to their uterine counterparts

of all ovarian carcinomas. Benign and borderline endometrioid tumors (almost all adenofibromas) are extremely rare and occur in the second to seventh decade of life, but most commonly in perimenopausal and postmenopausal women. Endometrioid carcinomas tend to occur in the fifth to seventh decade (10 % in fourth decade), often with symptoms of an enlarging abdominal mass, pelvic pain, and occasionally vaginal bleeding (particularly when associated with a concurrent endometrial adenocarcinoma). Serum CA-125 levels are commonly elevated. Many patients with endometrioid tumors have associated pelvic endometriosis (11–38 %) and/or endometriosis involving the ovary (40 %).

RADIOLOGIC FEATURES

Endometrioid adenocarcinomas often show a similar appearance to endometriomas, but frequently have a solid component within the cyst wall.

PATHOLOGIC FEATURES

GROSS FINDINGS

Benign endometrioid tumors are unilateral and solid with small cysts on sectioning, an appearance typical of adenofibroma. Borderline tumors and carcinomas may be uni- or bilateral, may have an adenofibromatous appearance, or be cystic with intracystic solid nodules. Finally, endometrioid carcinomas may be cystic and solid with areas of hemorrhage and necrosis, an appearance indistinguishable from other ovarian surface epithelial carcinomas (Figure 11.27). Ovarian mesodermal adenosarcoma typically shows a solid, or solid and cystic, fleshy cut surface, while endometrioid stromal tumors have a solid or solid and cystic, tan to yellow appearance, similar to that of their more common uterine counterparts. Malignant mixed mesodermal tumor is indistinguishable from high-grade surface epithelial carcinoma.

MICROSCOPIC FINDINGS

Endometrioid tumors are composed of glands and/or stroma resembling endometrial-type glands and stroma. Endometrioid adenofibroma/cystadenofibroma is composed of well-spaced glands that vary in number, size and shape and are embedded in a fibromatous stroma. The glands are lined by columnar to cuboidal cells with eosinophilic cytoplasm and oval, small, and uniform neclei without appreciable mitotic activity (Figure 11.28A). Metaplastic changes may be seen but are uncommon.

The WHO classification defines endometrioid borderline tumors as being "composed of atypical or histologically malignant endometrioid-type glands or cysts

---

ENDOMETRIOID SURFACE EPITHELIAL STROMAL TUMORS – PATHOLOGIC FEATURES

Gross Findings

▸ Solid with small cysts (adenofibroma)
▸ Solid or solid and cystic with intracystic solid projections and hemorrhage (borderline tumor, adenocarcinoma, and adenosarcoma)
▸ Solid and cystic, often fleshy and necrotic (malignant mesodermal tumor)
▸ Solid or solid and cystic, tan to yellow (endometrioid stromal sarcoma)

Microscopic Findings

▸ Endometrioid adenofibroma: Cuboidal to columnar cells lining simple glands present in a fibromatous stroma
▸ Endometrioid borderline tumor: Closely packed glands often with morular squamous metaplasia, showing a lobular architecture and set in a fibromatous stroma. Cytologic atypia mirrors that seen in atypical complex hyperplasia
▸ Endometrioid adenocarcinoma: glandular (round to elongated glands in contrast to slit-like spaces in serous tumors), villoglandular, cribriform, or solid architecture, +/– squamous or morular differentiation; grading similar to its uterine counterpart
▸ Endometrioid stromal neoplasms: Diffuse growth of uniform endometrial stromal cells with a prominent vascular pattern (small arterioles)
▸ Malignant mixed mesodermal tumor: malignant glands and stroma (homologous or heterologous)
▸ Mesodermal adenosarcoma: benign endometrioid and/or other müllerian-type glands and low-grade malignant stroma featuring prominent periglandular condensation and/or phyllodes-like architecture. Heterologous elements may be seen
▸ Endometriosis often present

Immunohistochemical Features

▸ CK7, ER, and PR positive (epithelial component)
▸ CK20 and inhibin typically negative (epithelial component)

Molecular Studies

▸ Somatic mutations in *beta-catenin* and *PTEN*
▸ Microsatellite instability
▸ Germline mutations in DNA mismatch repair genes in hereditary nonpolyposis colorectal cancer syndrome

Differential Diagnosis

▸ Serous adenocarcinoma (vs endometrioid carcinoma)
▸ Sex cord stromal tumors (vs endometrioid carcinoma)
▸ Carcinoid tumor (vs endometrioid carcinoma)
▸ Metastatic colorectal or endometrial adenocarcinoma (vs endometrioid carcinoma)
▸ Adenofibroma or polypoid endometriosis (vs mesodermal adenosarcoma)
▸ Fibroma or diffuse granulosa cell tumor (vs endometrioid stromal tumor)
▸ High-grade carcinoma (vs malignant mixed mesodermal tumor)

---

often set in a dense fibrous stroma with absence of stromal invasion." The appearance of borderline endometrioid tumors is analogous to that seen in complex atypical hyperplasia of the endometrium, in that there is both cytologic and architectural atypia (Figure 11.28B). These tumors often show a lobular architec-

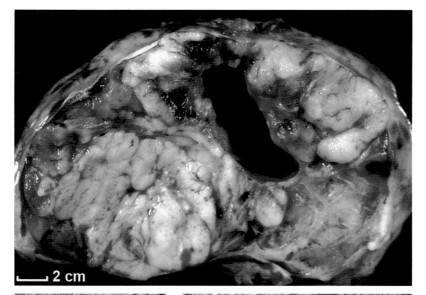

FIGURE 11.27

Endometrioid adenocarcinoma, low-grade. The tumor shows a solid and cystic cut surface with foci of hemorrhage.

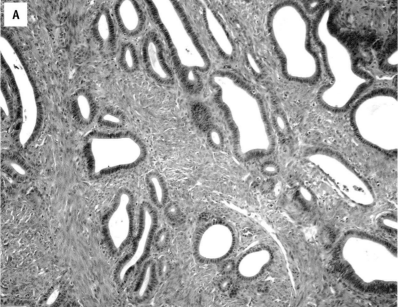

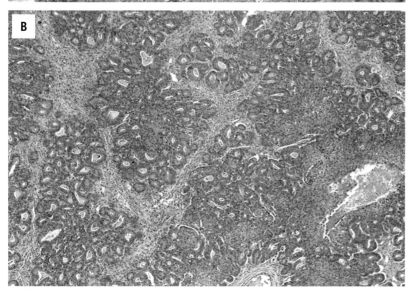

FIGURE 11.28

Endometrioid adenofibroma. Variably sized, banal appearing glands are embedded in a fibromatous stroma (A). Endometrioid borderline tumor (endometrioid tumor of low malignant potential). Endometrial-type glands with complex architecture and prominent immature squamous (morular) metaplasia showing occasional central necrosis are separated by fibromatous stroma (B).

ture, with the neoplastic glands being closely packed, and frequently associated with morular squamous differentiation.

The appearance of typical ovarian endometrioid adenocarcinoma is usually comparable to FIGO grade 1 or 2 endometrial adenocarcinoma of endometrioid type, although occasional tumors are grade 3 featuring a solid growth. Squamous metaplasia is very common and other metaplastic changes (secretory, ciliated cell, oxyphilic) may also be seen. A minor mucinous component similar to that occasionally seen in low-grade endometrial adenocarcinomas of endometrioid type, may also be encountered. Endometrioid carcinomas of the ovary are capable of exhibiting a wide array of morphologies, including tubular, insular, trabecular, microglandular, adenoid basal, adenoid cystic, and spindled (Figure 11.29). These less common patterns, when present, coexist with more typical endometrioid carcinoma in most cases, and not infrequently, there is a histologic spectrum from endometriosis, to borderline areas, to endometrioid carcinoma. Criteria for grading endometrioid carcinomas are the same as for their endometrial counterpart: < 5% solid growth – grade 1; 5–50% solid growth – grade 2; > 50% solid growth – grade 3. Areas with squamous and/or spindled differentiation are not included in the assessment of the percentage of the solid component, and marked nuclear atypia raises the grade by 1. Alternately, the previously described universal grading system (Table 11.2) can be used. With either system, the large majority of endometrioid carcinomas are grade 1 or 2.

Mesodermal adenosarcoma is composed of benign müllerian-type glands (more often endometrioid, but also other müllerian cell types) within a malignant, homologous stromal component, often resembling endometrial stroma (Figure 11.30). Periglandular cuffs or intraglandular protrusions of cellular stroma are typical features. The stromal component shows at least mild atypia and variable mitotic counts (sometimes > 40/10 HPFs). Heterologous mesenchymal components may be seen.

Endometrioid stromal sarcoma is composed of sheets of monomorphic small stromal cells with prominent delicate vessels, recapitulating the spiral arterioles of the proliferative-phase endometrial stroma (Figure 11.31). Mitotic activity may be brisk (> 10/10 HPFs). Almost 50% of these tumors are associated with endometriosis.

Malignant mixed mesodermal tumor has varying proportions of high-grade carcinoma and high-grade sarcoma of homologous or heterologous type (commonly chondrosarcoma, rhabdomyosarcoma, or both), similar to the much more common malignant mixed mullerian tumor of the uterus (Figure 11.32).

ANCILLARY STUDIES

IMMUNOHISTOCHEMISTRY

Endometrioid tumors express epithelial markers, including cytokeratin and EMA. Most exhibit a CK7 positive, CK20 negative profile. The tumor cells are also typically positive for B72.3, ER, and PR, but are negative for alpha-inhibin and calretinin.

MOLECULAR STUDIES

Most endometrioid adenocarcinomas of the ovary are sporadic, but a small subset occurs in patients with germline mutations in DNA mismatch repair genes in association with the hereditary nonpolyposis colorectal cancer syndrome. Somatic mutations of *beta-catenin* and *PTEN* are the most common genetic abnormalities in sporadic ovarian endometrioid carcinomas, followed by microsatellite instability due to MLH1 promoter methylation.

DIFFERENTIAL DIAGNOSIS

Endometrioid adenofibromas may be difficult to differentiate from adenofibromas of other cell types, particularly Brenner tumors. Such a distinction, even though not clinically important, should be done based on histologic examination of the lining epithelial cells. The distinction between benign and borderline endometrioid tumors is based on the degree of architectural and cytologic atypia of the epithelial component. Closely packed glands, cribriforming and presence of any degree of cytologic atypia favors a diagnosis of borderline tumor. The diagnosis of endometrioid carcinoma should be reserved for tumors clearly resembling endometrial adenocarcinomas of endometrioid type. High-grade endometrioid carcinomas may be confused with *high-grade serous carcinomas*, and in fact the latter is frequently misdiagnosed as high-grade endometrioid carcinoma. The finding of slit-like spaces, severe cytologic atypia and presence of psammoma bodies support the diagnosis of high-grade serous carcinoma. Endometrioid carcinomas exhibiting a prominent sex cord-like growth pattern are distinguished from *sex cord stromal tumors* on the basis of the older age of the patient, typical endometrioid adenocarcinoma elsewhere, squamous differentiation, intraluminal mucin, and adenofibromatous background. In difficult cases immunohistochemical stainings may be helpful, since endometrioid carcinomas stain for EMA, and hormone receptors, but not for alpha-inhibin. Similarly, *carcinoid tumor* is distinguished from endometrioid carcinoma by the finding of well-formed acini, "salt and pepper" chromatin, and on the basis of their strong and diffuse staining for chromogranin or synaptophysin. *Metastatic colon adenocarcinoma* can mimic endometrioid carcinoma. The presence of extensive "dirty cell" necrosis with abundant karyorrhectic debris associated with segmental necrosis of the neoplastic glands, a garland-like glandular pattern, and a characteristic CK7 negative, CK20 positive phenotype should prompt the search for an intestinal tumor, if no previous history is known. Mesodermal adenosarcoma is distinguished from *adenofibroma* and *polypoid endometriosis* on the basis of

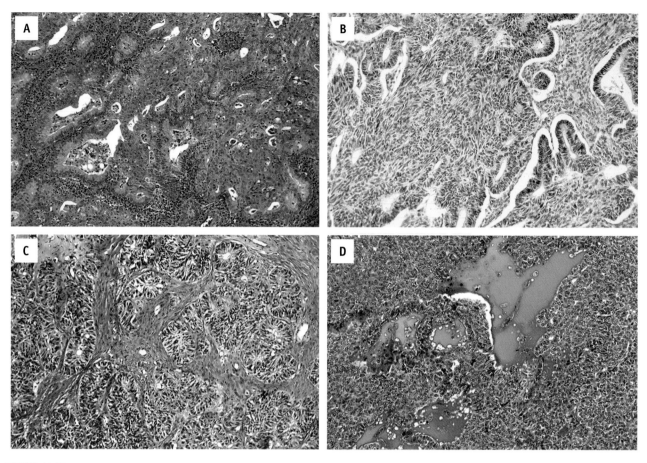

FIGURE 11.29

Endometrioid adenocarcinoma. The tumor frequently shows a confluent cribriform architecture (A); but may also have a prominent spindled growth (B); solid tubular pattern (simulating Sertoli cell tumor) (C); or follicular pattern (simulating granulosa cell tumor) (D).

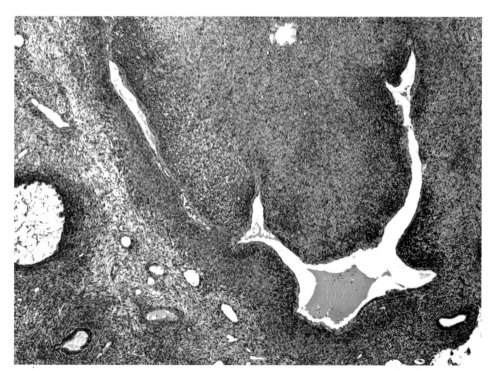

FIGURE 11.30

Mesodermal adenosarcoma. An endometrioid-type gland shows intraglandular polypoid projections and prominent periglandular cuffing by cellular stroma.

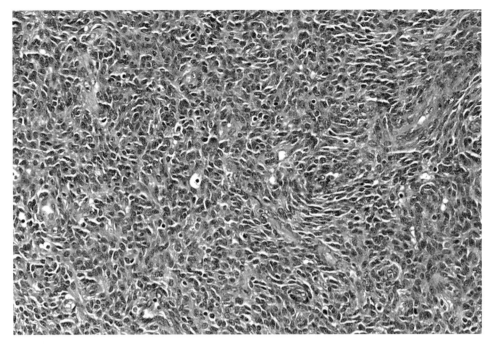

FIGURE 11.31

Endometrioid stromal sarcoma. The tumor is composed of a cellular pro-liferation of uniform small stromal cells with small oval nuclei. Note numerous delicate arterioles resem-bling spiral arteries of proliferative-phase endometrium.

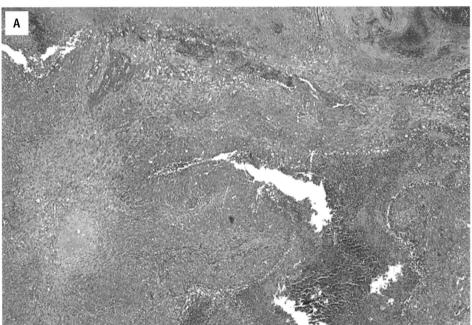

FIGURE 11.32

Malignant mixed mesodermal tumor with heterologous elements. Malig-nant glands are separated by cellular, sarcomatous stroma containing aty-pical, cellular cartilage (A). Note the distinct biphasic pattern (B).

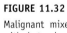

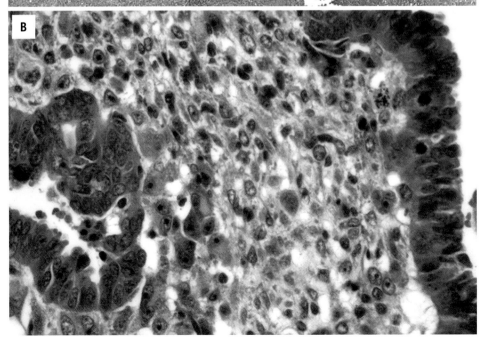

periglandular stromal hypercellularity, nuclear atypicality, and increased number of mitotic figures in the stromal component. Endometrioid stromal sarcoma may be confused with the diffuse pattern of *adult-type granulosa cell tumor* or a *cellular fibroma*; however, it has a distinctive vascular pattern, the cells lack nuclear grooves and are negative for alpha-inhibin if no sex cord-like elements are present. Finally, malignant mixed mesodermal tumor should be distinguished from *high-grade carcinoma*. The latter typically shows a transition from evident epithelial regions to spindled areas, while malignant mixed mesodermal tumor features an abrupt transition between the high grade epithelial and mesenchymal components.

PROGNOSIS AND THERAPY

Endometrioid adenofibromas and borderline tumors have a benign clinical course. Complete excision (unilateral oophorectomy or total hysterectomy and bilateral oophorectomy) is curative. Endometrioid adenocarcinomas are typically confined to the ovary, and patients have 5-year survival > 90 %. When there is extraovarian spread, the prognosis is guarded and adjuvant therapy is routinely offered. The surgical treatment for endometrioid adenocarcinoma is similar to that of other surface epithelial carcinomas. Malignant mixed mesodermal tumor is associated with a very poor prognosis, although survivors have been reported among patients with tumor confined to the ovary at presentation. The prognosis of patients with ovarian mesodermal adenosarcoma is much worse than that of uterine müllerian adenosarcoma, with recurrences occurring in two-thirds of patients (mean of 2.6 years after operation) even though most patients present with stage I tumors. Ovarian endometrioid stromal sarcomas are often high-stage at presentation (25 % bilateral; 30 % associated with a similar tumor in the uterus), but tend to pursue a comparatively indolent course, with fatalities occurring 10 or more years after initial diagnosis. Progestational agents have been used for residual or recurrent disease.

CLEAR CELL SURFACE EPITHELIAL STROMAL TUMORS

Surface epithelial tumors with clear cell differentiation (benign, low malignant potential (borderline), or malignant) are composed of epithelial cells containing glycogen-rich clear cytoplasm and hobnail cells (Table 11.8). Initially thought to be of mesonephric origin (hence the old term "mesonephroma"), clear cell surface epithelial tumors are now recognized as of müllerian derivation.

TABLE 11.8

Classification of clear cell surface epithelial stromal tumors (modified from World Health Organization)

Benign (cystadenoma, adenofibroma, cystadenofibroma)	<1%
Borderline (low malignant potential)	<1%
Malignant (adenocarcinoma, cystadenocarcinoma, malignant adenofibroma)	99%

CLEAR CELL SURFACE EPITHELIAL TUMORS – FACT SHEET

Definition

▸ Spectrum of ovarian surface epithelial tumors composed of cells with clear or eosinophilic cytoplasm and large nuclei with hobnail cells
▸ Three types:
  – Benign clear cell adenofibroma
  – Borderline clear cell tumor (tumor of low malignant potential)
  – Clear cell adenocarcinoma

Incidence and Location

▸ Clear cell carcinoma most common (6% of all surface epithelial carcinomas)
▸ Benign and borderline variants very rare (< 50 reported cases)
▸ Typically unilateral (benign, borderline and malignant)

Morbidity and Mortality

▸ Related to pelvic mass and/or abdominal disease

Geographic, Race, and Age Distribution

▸ Clear cell carcinoma more prevalent in Japan than in western countries
▸ Benign and borderline clear cell tumor: Second to seventh decades
▸ Clear cell carcinoma: Fifth to seventh decades (10% in fourth decade)

Clinical Features

▸ Benign and borderline tumor: Asymptomatic and present as incidental mass
▸ Clear cell carcinoma: Similar to usual surface epithelial carcinoma, but significant proportion present at younger age (fourth decade)
▸ Clear cell carcinoma frequently associated with pelvic endometriosis (50–70%); one-fourth arise in endometriotic cyst
▸ Two thirds of women with clear cell carcinoma are nulliparous
▸ Clear cell carcinoma associated with paraneoplastic hypercalcemia

Prognosis and Treatment

▸ Clear cell adenofibroma and borderline tumors clinically benign and treated by oophorectomy ± hysterectomy
▸ 30% 5-year mortality for women with stage I disease versus 85% with stage III clear cell carcinoma
▸ Stage for stage, clear cell carcinoma has a worse prognosis than other surface epithelial carcinomas
▸ Clear cell carcinoma treated like other surface epithelial tumors with optimal debulking and adjuvant chemotherapy, but common resistance to platinum-based chemotherapy

CLINICAL FEATURES

The vast majority of clear cell surface epithelial tumors are malignant (clear cell carcinoma) and comprise about 5% of all ovarian cancers in North America. There is an unexplained increased prevalence of clear cell carcinoma in Japan relative to western countries, even though the overall incidence of ovarian carcinoma in Japan is relatively low. Benign and borderline clear cell adenofibromatous tumors are extremely rare (< 50 reported in the English literature) and present in the second to seventh decade of life with a median age of 45 years for clear cell adenofibroma and 62 years for clear cell tumor of borderline malignancy. Clear cell carcinomas tend to occur in the fifth to seventh decades (10% in fourth decade); patients often presenting with symptoms related to an enlarging abdominal mass. Two-thirds of women with clear cell carcinoma are nulliparous. Many (50–70%) have associated pelvic endometriosis and/or endometriosis involving the ovary (25%). Paraneoplastic hypercalcemia and pelvic venous thromboses have been associated with clear cell carcinoma. Almost all benign and borderline clear cell tumors are unilateral, as are most clear cell carcinomas (80%), and approximately 40–60% of patients with clear cell carcinoma present with FIGO stage I disease.

RADIOLOGIC FEATURES

Clear cell carcinomas often show areas of hemorrhage and necrosis and are indistinguishable from other high-grade surface epithelial stromal carcinomas. Alternatively, they may show features similar to endometriomas, but with a solid component within the cyst wall.

PATHOLOGIC FEATURES

GROSS FINDINGS

Clear cell benign and borderline adenofibromatous tumors are unilateral neoplasms composed of firm tissue with small cysts containing clear, watery fluid. Size may vary, but tumors up to 23 cm have been reported (mean 12–15 cm). The external surface is smooth and lobulated, and the tumor may exhibit a fine honeycomb appearance on cut section. Hemorrhage, necrosis, and adhesions are absent. Clear cell carcinomas, although often unilateral, are usually distinguished from their benign counterparts by their unilocular, solid, and cystic appearance with foci of necrosis and hemorrhage. Clear cell carcinomas measure up to 30 cm (mean 15 cm). When occurring in association with an endometriotic cyst, it may form a soft, fleshy nodule along the cyst wall (Figure 11.33). Capsular adhesions may be present.

CLEAR CELL SURFACE EPITHELIAL STROMAL TUMORS – PATHOLOGIC FEATURES

Gross Findings

Adenofibroma and borderline tumor:
▶ Smooth, lobulated external surface
▶ Fine honeycomb cut surface

Carcinoma
▶ Thick-walled unilocular (less commonly, multilocular) cystic and solid mass with fleshy nodules
▶ hemorrhage and necrosis on inner cyst wall and adhesions over capsule
▶ May present as single fleshy nodule in an endometriotic cyst (25%)

Microscopic Findings
▶ Borderline adenofibromatous tumor: Variably sized glands/tubules lined by flat (usually one or two cell layers) or hobnail cells, present in a fibromatous stroma
▶ Clear cell carcinoma: Tubulocystic, papillary (with prominent hyalinized cores), and/or solid architecture
▶ Polyhedral or hobnail cells with abundant clear and/or eosinophilic granular cytoplasm (containing glycogen); signet ring-type or targetoid cells in clear cell carcinoma
▶ Eccentric, rounded or angular, hyperchromatic nuclei. Minimal, mild to moderate nuclear atypia (adenofibroma and borderline tumor respectively) to marked nuclear pleomorphism, at least focally (carcinoma)
▶ Mitoses absent to very rare in adenofibromatous and borderline tumors (< 1/10 HPFs), but present in carcinomas

Ultrastructural Features
▶ Epithelial cells with abundant glycogen granules and endoplasmic reticulum
▶ Stubby microvilli on apical surface

Immunohistochemical Features
▶ CK7, CK20, EMA and CD15 positive
▶ Clear cell carcinoma may express AFP
▶ ER and WT1 negative

Differential Diagnosis
▶ Yolk sac tumor
▶ Metastatic renal cell carcinoma
▶ Endometrioid adenocarcinoma, secretory variant or with clear squamous cell differentiation
▶ Serous adenocarcinoma
▶ Juvenile granulosa cell tumor

MICROSCOPIC FINDINGS

Clear cell tumors are characterized by polyhedral cells with abundant clear and/or eosinophilic granular cytoplasm, and hobnail cells with scant cytoplasm and enlarged, bulbous nuclei that protrude into the lumens of the cystic spaces. Cells can also be cuboidal or flat. The cytoplasm is glycogen-rich and PAS-positive. PAS-positive, diastase-resistant, and mucicarmine staining material may be present at the apical cell membranes and within gland lumens. Clear cell neoplasms often have a

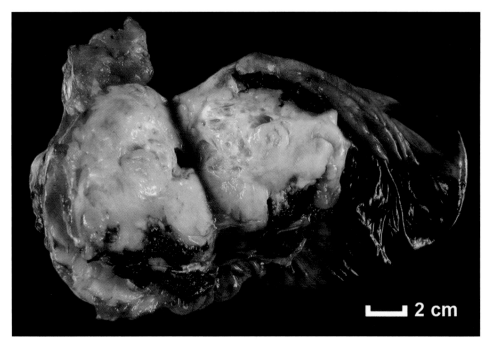

FIGURE 11.33
Clear cell carcinoma arising in an endometriotic cyst. A partially collapsed endometriotic cyst contains a solid and partially cystic mural nodule.

fibromatous component, which may be more cellular around the glands or tubules in borderline adenofibromatous tumors (Figure 11.34). The finding of confluent tubular growth in an adenofibromatous tumor should strongly suggest carcinoma. Furthermore, as clear cell carcinoma may contain foci of clear cell borderline adenofibroma, the diagnosis of the latter should only be made after thorough sampling of the tumor to exclude areas of clear cell carcinoma. Clear cell carcinoma often shows an admixture of tubulocystic, papillary and solid patterns (Figure 11.35). The papillae are typically small and round, and dense hyaline basement membrane material forms the cores of papillary stalks. The nuclei are rounded or angular, often eccentric and hyperchromatic without prominent nucleoli. Nuclear atypia is minimal or absent in clear cell adenofibromas, and mild to moderate in borderline variants. By definition, marked nuclear pleomorphism is only seen in clear cell carcinoma. Unlike other surface epithelial carcinomas, grading of clear cell carcinoma does not appear to correlate with prognosis and is not routinely performed, nevertheless, all clear cell carcinomas are considered high-grade. Mitotic figures are absent or exceedingly rare in clear cell adenofibromas and borderline tumors, and are relatively infrequent even in carcinomas (as compared to other surface epithelial carcinomas). Microcalcifications and psammoma bodies may be seen in carcinomas and up to 25% also contain eosinophilic hyaline bodies. The oxyphilic variant of clear cell carcinoma is composed of polygonal cells with granular eosinophilic cytoplasm; however, typical patterns of clear cell carcinoma are usually present. Mixed clear cell and endometrioid carcinoma occurs in 20–25% of cases.

ANCILLARY STUDIES

IMMUNOHISTOCHEMISTRY

Clear cell tumors express epithelial markers, including cytokeratin and EMA. Most exhibit a CK7 positive, CK20 negative profile. They may also express B72.3, CD15, (Leu-M1), CEA, CA125 and rarely, AFP.

ULTRASTRUCTURAL EXAMINATION

These tumors contain abundant cytoplasmic glycogen granules, packets of rough endoplasmic reticulum, and short, stubby microvilli along the apical surfaces. Intracellular mucin is rarely present.

MOLECULAR STUDIES

Similar genetic alterations have been described in endometrioid adenocarcinoma and some clear cell carcinomas, but overall, molecular abnormalities in clear cell carcinoma are still largely undetermined.

DIFFERENTIAL DIAGNOSIS

Clear cell carcinoma may be difficult to distinguish from yolk sac tumor, particularly when it occurs in younger women, although clear cell carcinoma is rare under 40 years of age. *Yolk sac tumor* is associated with elevated serum AFP levels, a reticular growth of primitive tumor cells within a loose background stroma, and in

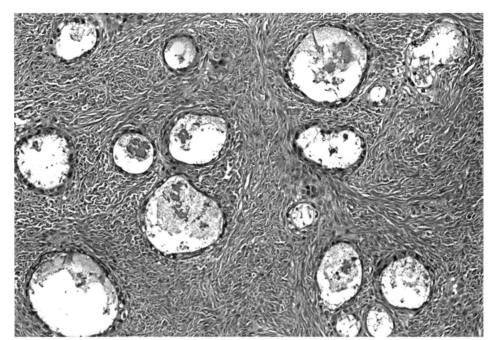

FIGURE 11.34
Borderline clear cell adenofibroma. Cystic glands, lined by flat and hobnail cells with clear or pale eosinophilic cytoplasm, are separated by abundant fibromatous stroma. Nuclear atypia is not striking and mitoses are absent.

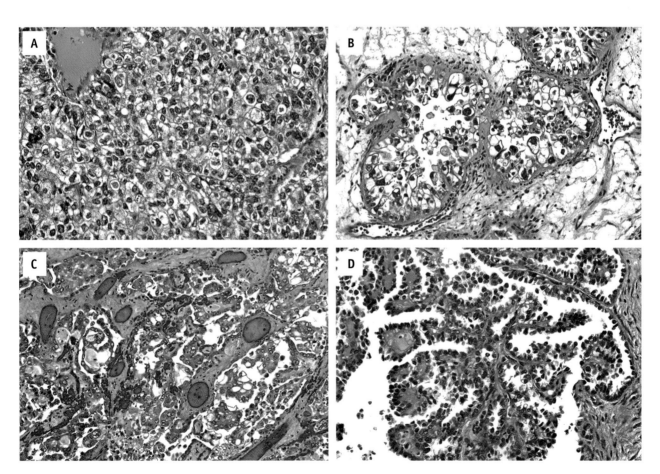

FIGURE 11.35
Clear cell carcinoma. Solid (A), tubulocystic (B), tubulopapillary (C), and papillary (D) patterns may be seen. Note the clear to pale eosinophilic cytoplasm and prominent hobnail cells (B and D). Intracytoplasmic eosinophilic material is present, occasionally resulting in a "targetoid pattern" (A).

some cases, the presence of Schiller-Duval bodies. Although clear cell carcinoma may rarely express AFP and yolk sac tumors may express CD15 (Leu-M1), the expression of CD15 in the absence of AFP staining supports the diagnosis of clear cell carcinoma. CK7 is also helpful in this differential diagnosis (positive in clear cell carcinoma). *Metastatic renal clear cell carcinoma* involving the ovary is uncommon, but may be initially misdiagnosed as an ovarian primary carcinoma. Renal cell carcinomas do not exhibit hobnail cells and are typically associated with a prominent sinusoidal vascular framework, not present in ovarian clear cell carcinoma. *Endometrioid adenocarcinoma* with *secretory change or squamous metaplasia with clear cytoplasm* is separated from clear cell carcinoma by the absence of the typical architectural patterns and lack of hobnail cells with high-grade nuclei. *Serous adenocarcinoma* is distinguished from clear cell carcinoma by the findings of irregular thick papillae, more prominent cellular stratification and budding, marked nuclear pleomorphism, and higher mitotic rates. In difficult cases, immunostains may aid in the diagnosis, as clear cell carcinomas are typically ER and WT1 negative. Occasionally, clear cell and endometrioid carcinoma coexist. *Juvenile granulosa cell tumor*, a sex cord stromal tumor occurring in younger women, is distinguished from clear cell carcinoma by the presence of large follicle-like cysts containing pale-staining, often basophilic fluid, positive staining for inhibin, and lack of EMA expression.

PROGNOSIS AND THERAPY

Clear cell adenofibromas and borderline tumors have a benign clinical course. Complete excision (unilateral oophorectomy or hysterectomy and bilateral oophorectomy) is almost always curative. Clear cell carcinoma is associated with 70% and 15% 5-year survival for women with stage I and stage III respectively. These survival rates are, in general, poorer than those for surface epithelial carcinomas of other cell types. The treatment for clear cell carcinoma, similar to that of other surface epithelial carcinomas, is surgical, as chemoresistance is common.

TRANSITIONAL CELL (BRENNER) SURFACE EPITHELIAL STROMAL NEOPLASMS

Ovarian surface epithelial neoplasms composed of transitional (urothelial)-type epithelial cells (benign, low malignant potential (borderline), or malignant (malignant Brenner, transitional cell carcinoma)) comprise approximately 2% of all primary surface epithelial neoplasms (Table 11.9). These tumors are thought to arise through metaplasia of the ovarian surface epithelium and are analogous to Walthard nests, which are transitional-type epithelial inclusions occurring beneath the serosa of the fallopian tubes and in the hilar region of the ovaries.

CLINICAL FEATURES

Most transitional cell tumors occurring within the ovaries are benign (Brenner tumors), and are typically incidental findings discovered at laparotomy for unrelated pelvic conditions in patients during the fourth to eighth decades (mean age 50 years). Proliferating or borderline transitional cell tumors are less common,

---

TRANSITIONAL CELL SURFACE EPITHELIAL STROMAL TUMORS – FACT SHEET

Definition
▸ Spectrum of surface epithelial neoplasms composed of transitional (urothelial)-type epithelium
▸ Types:
  – Benign Brenner (adenofibroma)
  – Borderline Brenner (low-malignant potential)
  – Malignant Brenner
  – Transitional cell carcinoma (no benign or borderline Brenner component)

Incidence and Location
▸ Benign Brenner tumor: Most common subtype of ovarian transitional tumor; usually unilateral (90–95%)
▸ Borderline and malignant Brenner tumors: Very uncommon (approximately 50–60 reported cases); usually unilateral
▸ Transitional cell carcinoma: Very rare and often unilateral (85%)

Morbidity and Mortality
▸ Rarely, synchronous or metachronous papillary urothelial carcinomas in the urinary bladder
▸ Related to metastatic disease

Age Distribution
▸ Benign Brenner tumor: Fourth to eighth decades (mean age 50 years)
▸ Borderline, malignant Brenner tumors, and transitional cell carcinomas: Second to seventh decades (mean age 60 years)

Clinical Features
▸ Benign Brenner tumor: Frequently asymptomatic, incidental finding. Occasionally, estrogenic or, less often, androgenic endocrine manifestations
▸ Borderline and malignant Brenner tumors: Commonly present as abdominal masses
▸ Transitional cell carcinoma: Similar presentation to other high-grade ovarian cancers

Prognosis and Treatment
▸ Benign and borderline Brenner tumors benign
▸ 10–20% of malignant Brenner tumors and 70–100% of transitional cell carcinomas high stage
▸ Benign and borderline Brenner tumors treated by oophorectomy ± hysterectomy
▸ Malignant Brenner tumor and transitional cell carcinoma treated like other surface epithelial tumors with optimal debulking and adjuvant chemotherapy
▸ Transitional cell carcinoma may have improved response to chemotherapy compared to other surface epithelial carcinomas

TABLE 11.9

Classification of transitional surface epithelial stromal tumors (modified from World Health Organization)

Benign (Brenner tumor)	99%
Borderline (proliferating Brenner tumor)	<1%
Malignant	<1%
Malignant Brenner tumor	
Transitional cell carcinoma (non-Brenner-type)	

occur at an older age (mean 60 years), and are larger, and more likely to present with symptoms referable to an enlarging abdominal mass than benign Brenner tumors. Even rarer are malignant transitional cell tumors, which have been subclassified into transitional cell carcinoma and malignant Brenner tumor. Malignant transitional cell tumors occur during the fifth and sixth decades (mean age 55 years). Approximately 80 % of malignant Brenner tumors are stage I, while greater than two-thirds of transitional cell carcinomas have spread to adjacent pelvic structures or abdomen at the time of diagnosis.

RADIOLOGIC FEATURES

Brenner tumors form small, mostly solid masses if benign or multilocular cystic masses with a solid component, the latter being mildly or moderately enhanced on CT-scan and exhibiting low signal intensity similar to that of a fibroma on T2-weighted MRI. Extensive amorphous calcification is often present within the solid component.

PATHOLOGIC FEATURES

GROSS FINDINGS

Benign Brenner tumors are typically solid and unilateral, with a smooth external surface and firm yellow or white cut section containing small cysts (occasionally large cysts are present) (Figure 11.36); they vary in size from < 2 to > 20 cm, but most are < 2 cm and up to one-third are microscopic. Brenner tumors may have a gritty consistency due to flecks of calcification. Borderline tumors, also unilateral, are usually larger (10–25 cm), solid and cystic (unilocular or multilocular) with soft, friable polypoid projections lining the cyst wall or surface. Both, benign and borderline Brenner tumous may be associated with a mucinous cystic tumor (Figure 11.37). Malignant Brenner

---

TRANSITIONAL CELL SURFACE EPITHELIAL STROMAL TUMORS – PATHOLOGIC FEATURES

Gross Findings

Benign Brenner tumor:
- Well circumscribed, solid with smooth external surface, from < 2 to > 20 cm
- Yellow or white tissue with small cysts (occasionally large cysts are present) and gritty on cut section

Borderline and malignant Brenner tumor:
- Unilateral, large (10–25 cm), cystic (may be unilocular or multilocular), and solid with soft, friable polypoid structures present on inner cyst wall and surface

Transitional cell carcinoma:
- Indistinguishable grossly from other high-grade ovarian carcinomas

Microscopic Findings

Benign Brenner tumor:
- Well-circumscribed solid and cystic nests of uniform transitional-type epithelium embedded in abundant, fibromatous stroma with hyalinization and spiculated dystrophic calcification (50%)
- Ovoid cells with small nuclei with discernible grooves and small, indistinct nucleoli
- Associated with mucinous cystadenoma, serous cystadenoma, or dermoid cyst in ≈ 25%. Frequent stromal luteinization

Borderline Brenner tumor:
- Large papillary structures with both exophytic and endophytic growth, similar to low-grade papillary urothelial carcinoma of the urinary bladder
- Benign transitional cell (Brenner) elements

Malignant Brenner tumor:
- Papillae with thick stalks projecting into cystic spaces similar to high-grade papillary urothelial carcinoma of the urinary bladder +/– stromal invasion

- Mucinous, squamous, or spindle cell differentiation
- Benign Brenner component

Transitional cell carcinoma:
- Cystic spaces with undulating macropapillae with smooth borders
- Extensive necrosis unusual
- Marked nuclear atypia
- No benign or borderline Brenner component

Immunohistochemical Features
- CK7, CA125, CEA, WT1 and EMA positive

Differential Diagnosis

Benign Brenner Tumor
- Endometrioid adenofibroma with squamous differentiation

Borderline Brenner Tumor
- Benign Brenner tumor
- Malignant Brenner tumor
- Metastatic papillary urothelial carcinoma

Malignant Brenner Tumor/Transitional cell carcinoma
- Metastatic papillary urothelial carcinoma
- Undifferentiated carcinoma
- Granulosa cell tumor (vs transitional cell carcinoma)
- Metastatic transitional cell carcinoma
- Serous carcinoma

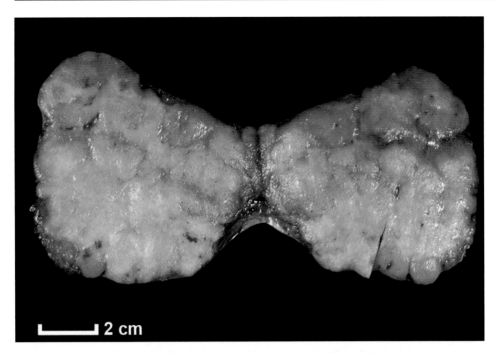

FIGURE 11.36

Benign Brenner tumor. The tumor has a firm, lobulated, yellow and white cut surface with scattered microcysts.

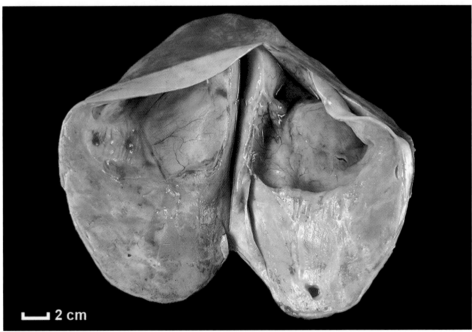

FIGURE 11.37

Benign Brenner tumor associated with a mucinous cystic tumor. A large cyst (top) coexists with a solid yellow nodule (bottom).

tumors appear similar to borderline tumors, but additionally feature areas of hemorrhage or necrosis and foci of gritty calcification (50%). Transitional cell carcinomas resemble other high-grade surface epithelial carcinomas, and they are usually unilateral (85%).

MICROSCOPIC FINDINGS

Transitional cell tumors of the ovary are composed of ovoid or polygonal cells that are histologically similar to urothelium, although the resemblance is closer for benign, borderline, and malignant Brenner tumors than it is for transitional cell carcinomas. Benign Brenner tumors are composed of well-demarcated nests of cyto-

logically bland transitional-type epithelium enmeshed in prominent fibromatous stroma (Figure 11.38), while borderline Brenner tumors feature coarse papillary fronds lined by multilayered epithelium reminiscent of low-grade transitional cell carcinoma of the urinary tract (Figure 11.39). The constituent cells often have longitudinal nuclear grooves, exhibiting the characteristic (but nonspecific) "coffee bean" nuclei. Mitotic figures are rare to absent in benign Brenner tumors, but may be present in borderline tumors (typically along the base of the papillary fronds). The cell nests often show central microcysts, which may contain eosinophilic material or be partially lined by metaplastic mucinous (endocervical-like) epithelium, squamous epithelium, or

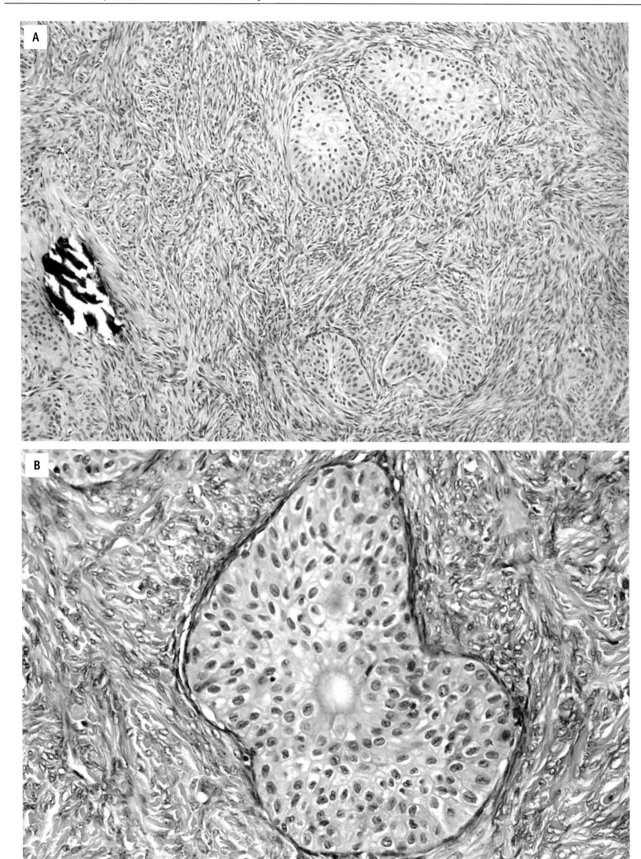

FIGURE 11.38

Brenner tumor. Solid epithelial nests are dispersed throughout fibromatous stroma associated with stromal calcification (A). The nests are composed of uniform cells with bland, often grooved nuclei, and may have central lumina containing eosinophilic material (B).

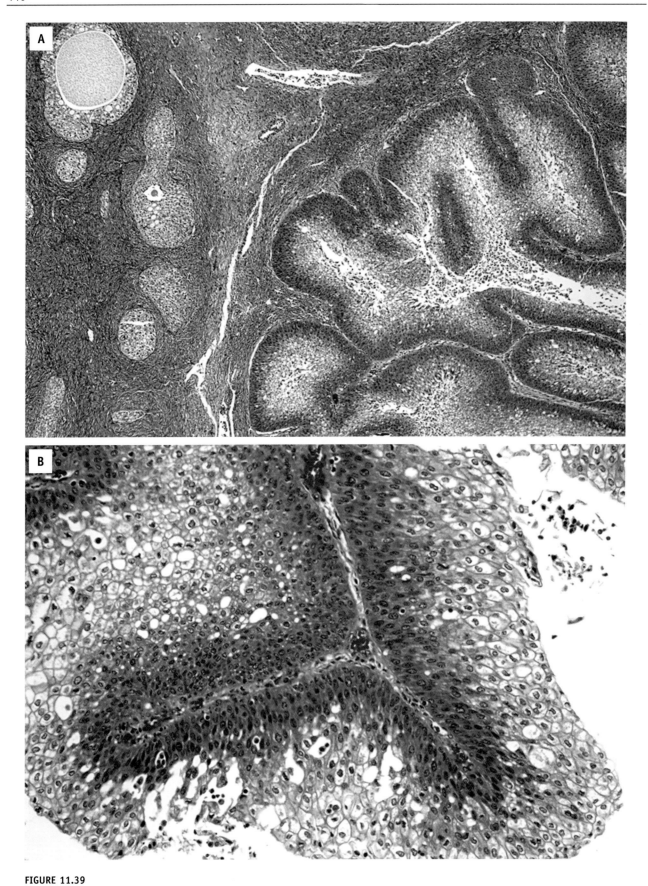

FIGURE 11.39
Borderline (low-malignant potential) Brenner tumor. Nests and papillae (A) are lined by stratified transitional-type epithelium with mild to moderate cytologic atypia, similar to that seen in low-grade papillary urothelial carcinoma (B).

ciliated cells. Stromal luteinization and dystrophic calcification (present in 50% of benign tumors) may be seen (Figure 11.38). Malignant transitional cell tumors feature stromal invasion and nuclear pleomorphism with hyperchromasia and numerous mitotic figures. Areas of necrosis are common but extensive necrosis is unusual. Malignant transitional cell tumors with benign or borderline transitional areas are designated as malignant Brenner tumor (Figure 11.40), whereas those without these elements are designated as transitional cell carcinoma (Figure 11.41).

ANCILLARY STUDIES

IMMUNOHISTOCHEMISTRY

Transitional cell tumors are positive for cytokeratin, EMA, and WT1. Most exhibit a CK7-positive, CK20-negative profile, similar to other primary ovarian-surface epithelial tumors, whereas transitional cell tumors of the urinary tract exhibit a CK7 and CK20-positive profile.

ULTRASTRUCTURAL EXAMINATION

The ultrastructural features of primary ovarian transitional cell tumors resemble those of transitional cell tumors of the urinary tract, i.e., ovoid, prominently grooved nuclei and villiform cytoplasmic processes.

DIFFERENTIAL DIAGNOSIS

Brenner tumor is distinguished from *endometrioid adenofibroma* by the presence of stratified epithelium, prominent nuclear grooves and frequent association with a mucinous component. Borderline Brenner tumors are distinguished from benign and malignant Brenner tumors by the presence of prominent papillary epithelial proliferation (benign Brenner) and absence of stromal invasion and marked cytologic atypia (malignant Brenner). Malignant Brenner tumor is distinguished from transitional cell carcinoma by the presence of benign or borderline Brenner elements in the former. Transitional cell carcinoma is distinguished from *serous adenocarcinoma* by the presence of prominent, thick papillae projecting into cystic spaces, although there is considerable histologic overlap among these entities and often transitional areas merge with typical serous carcinoma. *Undifferentiated carcinoma* also shows high-grade nuclear features, but the cells lack urothelial morphology, and the tumor often grows in sheets without a papillary architecture. *Metastatic urothelial carcinoma* is recognized on the basis of the clinical history of a prior or concurrent primary urothelial carcinoma, features typical of metastases, and positive CK20 and negative WT-1 staining; CK7 is not helpful in this differential diagnosis. *Granulosa cell tumors*, may show a papillary architecture and nuclear grooves similar to borderline Brenner tumors or transitional cell carcinomas; however, high-power examination discloses other typical features of these tumors.

PROGNOSIS AND THERAPY

Transitional cell adenofibroma (Brenner) and borderline tumors have a benign clinical course. Complete excision (unilateral oophorectomy or total hysterectomy and bilateral oophorectomy) is curative. Transitional cell carcinomas are more often advanced-stage (70–100%) and clinically more aggressive than malignant Brenner tumors (10–20%). Transitional cell carcinomas may exhibit an improved response to chemotherapy and more favorable prognosis compared to nontransitional cell carcinomas, but this is controversial.

UNDIFFERENTIATED SURFACE EPITHELIAL STROMAL TUMORS

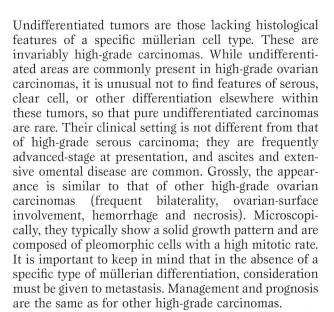

Undifferentiated tumors are those lacking histological features of a specific müllerian cell type. These are invariably high-grade carcinomas. While undifferentiated areas are commonly present in high-grade ovarian carcinomas, it is unusual not to find features of serous, clear cell, or other differentiation elsewhere within these tumors, so that pure undifferentiated carcinomas are rare. Their clinical setting is not different from that of high-grade serous carcinoma; they are frequently advanced-stage at presentation, and ascites and extensive omental disease are common. Grossly, the appearance is similar to that of other high-grade ovarian carcinomas (frequent bilaterality, ovarian-surface involvement, hemorrhage and necrosis). Microscopically, they typically show a solid growth pattern and are composed of pleomorphic cells with a high mitotic rate. It is important to keep in mind that in the absence of a specific type of müllerian differentiation, consideration must be given to metastasis. Management and prognosis are the same as for other high-grade carcinomas.

MIXED SURFACE EPITHELIAL STROMAL TUMORS

By definition, mixed tumors have at least a 10% component of one or more minor types of müllerian differentiation (Table 11.10). The frequency with which mixed tumors are diagnosed varies greatly, reflecting the avidity of individual observers for identification of subtle differences within tumors. The following are among the more common combinations encountered: mucinous cystadenoma and Brenner tumor, serous borderline tumor and endocervical-like mucinous borderline tumor, serous carcinoma and transitional carcinoma, and finally endometrioid carcinoma and clear cell carcinoma. Except for the last example, where a high-grade clear cell component and lower-grade endometrioid component coexist, there is little clinical significance associated with the minor component of mixed tumors.

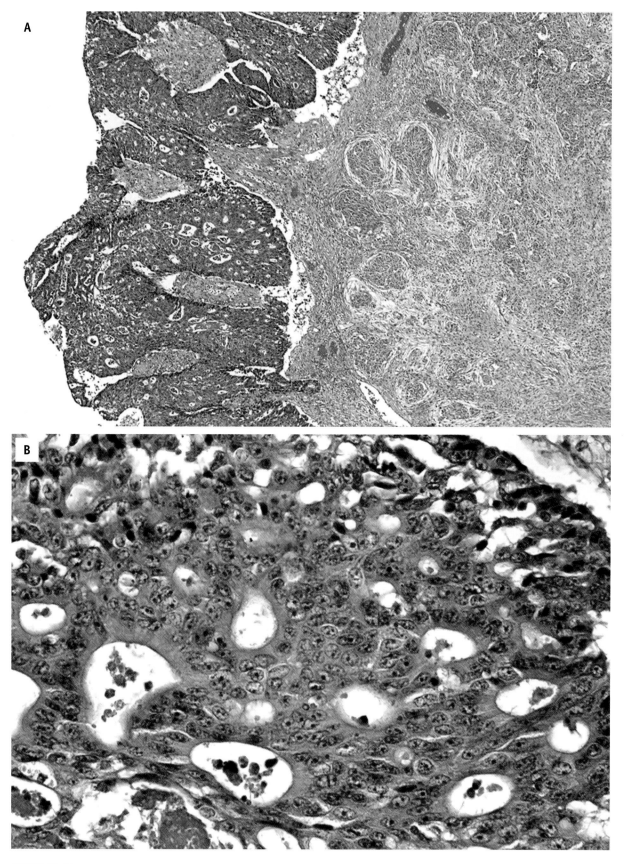

FIGURE 11.40

Malignant Brenner tumor. Cyst lined by solid and cribriform growths merges imperceptibly with areas of benign Brenner tumor (A). The transitional-type epithelium in the solid and cribriform areas is similar to high-grade papillary urothelial carcinoma with marked nuclear atypia and mitotic figures (B).

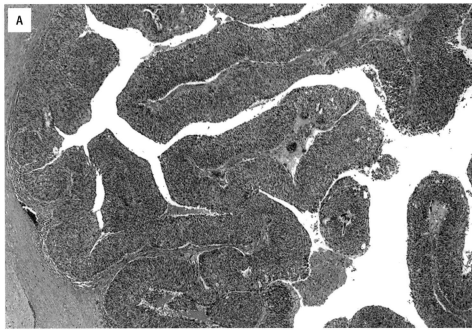

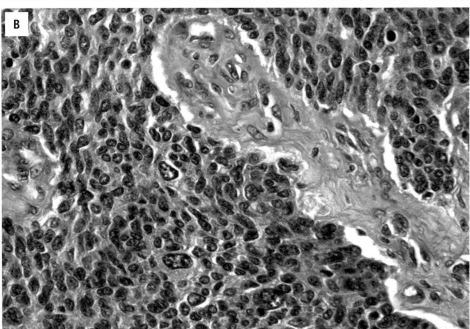

FIGURE 11.41

Transitional cell carcinoma. The tumor is composed of broad, undulating papillae projecting into cystic spaces with minimal necrosis (A). Cytologic atypia is comparable to that seen in high-grade papillary urothelial carcinoma (B).

TABLE 11.10

Classification of mixed surface epithelial stromal tumors (modified from World Health Organization)

Benign (cystadenoma, adenofibroma, cystadenofibroma)	<1%
Borderline (low malignant potential)	10%
Malignant (adenocarcinoma, cystadenocarcinoma, malignant adenofibroma)	90%

SUGGESTED READING

General

Cheng W, Liu J, Yoshida H, et al. Lineage infidelity of epithelial ovarian cancers is controlled by HOX genes that specify regional identity in the reproductive tract. Nat Med 2005;531–537.

Dubeau L. Ovarian cancer. In: Vogelstein B, Kinzler KW (eds) The Genetic Basis of Human Cancer, 2nd edn. New York: McGraw-Hill, 2002: 675–680.

Heintz AP, Odicino F, Maisonneuve P, et al. Carcinoma of the ovary. J Epidemiol Biostat 2001;6:107–138.

Hendrickson MR, Longacre TA. Classification of surface epithelial neoplasms of the ovary. Pathology (Phila) 1993;1:189–254.

Lee KR, Tavassoli FA, Prat J, et al. Tumours of the ovary and peritoneum. In: Tavassoli FA, Devillee P (eds) Tumours of the Breast and Female Genital Organs. Lyon: IARC Press, 2003:119–124.

Malpica A, Deavers MT, Lu K, et al. Grading ovarian serous carcinoma using a two-tier system. Am J Surg Pathol 2004;28:496–504.

Scully RE, Young RH, Clement PB. Atlas of Tumor Pathology. Tumors of the Ovary, Maldeveloped Gonads, Fallopian Tube, and Broad Ligament, 3rd edn. Washington, DC: AFIP, 1998.

Silverberg SG. Histopathologic grading of ovarian carcinoma: a review and proposal. Int J Gynecol Pathol 2000;19:7–15.

Werness BA, Ramus SJ, Whittemore AS, et al. Histopathology of familial ovarian tumors in women from families with and without germline BRCA1 mutations. Hum Pathol 2000;31:1420–1424.

Serous Surface Epithelial Stromal Tumors

Bell DA, Longacre TA, Prat J, et al. Serous borderline (low malignant potential, atypical proliferative) ovarian tumors workshop perspectives. Hum Pathol 2004;35:934–948.

Bell DA, Scully RE. Ovarian serous borderline tumors with stromal micro-invasion: a report of 21 cases. Hum Pathol 1990;21:397–403.

Burks RT, Sherman ME, Kurman RJ. Micropapillary serous carcinoma of the ovary. A distinctive low-grade carcinoma related to serous borderline tumors. Am J Surg Pathol 1996;20:1319–1330.

Crum CP, Drapkin R, Miron A, et al. The distal fallopian tube: a new model for pelvic serous carcinogenesis. Curr Opin Obstet Gynecol 2007;19:3–9.

Eichhorn JH, Bell DA, Young RH, et al. Ovarian serous borderline tumors with micropapillary and cribriform patterns: a study of 40 cases and comparison with 44 cases without these patterns. Am J Surg Pathol 1999;23:397–409.

Gilks CB, Bell DA, Scully RE. Serous psammocarcinoma of the ovary and peritoneum. Int J Gynecol Pathol 1990;9:110–121.

Gilks CB, Alkushi A, Yue JJ, et al. Advanced-stage serous borderline tumors of the ovary: a clinicopathological study of 49 cases. Int J Gynecol Pathol 2003;22:29–36.

Longacre TA, Kempson RL, Hendrickson MR. Well differentiated serous neoplasms of the ovary. In: Hendrickson MR (ed.) Surface Epithelial Neoplasms of the Ovary. Philadelphia: Hanley and Belfus, 1993: 255–306.

Longacre TA, McKenney JK, Tazelaar HD, et al. Ovarian serous tumors of low malignant potential (borderline tumors). Outcome-based study of 276 patients with long-term (> 5-year) follow-up. Am J Surg Pathol 2005;29:707–723.

Malpica A, Deavers MT, Lu K, et al. Grading ovarian serous carcinoma using a two-tiered system. Am J Surg Pathol 2004;28:496–504.

McKenney JK, Balzer BL, Longacre TA. Lymph node involvement in ovarian serous tumors of low malignant potential (borderline tumors): pathology, prognosis, and proposed classification. Am J Surg Pathol 2006;30:614–624.

Prat J, De Nictolis M. Serous borderline tumors of the ovary: a long-term follow-up study of 137 cases, including 18 with a micropapillary pattern and 20 with microinvasion. Am J Surg Pathol 2002;26:1111–1128.

Rollins SE, Young RH, Bell DA. Autoimplants in serous borderline tumors of the ovary: a clinicopathologic study of 30 cases of a process to be distinguished from serous adenocarcinoma. Am J Surg Pathol 2006;30:457–462.

Seidman JD, Kurman RJ. Ovarian serous borderline tumors: a critical review of the literature with emphasis on prognostic indicators. Hum Pathol 2000;31:539–557.

Singer G, Oldt R 3rd, Cohen Y, et al. Mutations in BRAF and KRAS characterize the development of low-grade ovarian serous carcinoma. J Natl Cancer Inst 2003;95:484–486.

Slomovitz BM, Caputo TA, Gretz HF 3rd, et al. A comparative analysis of 57 serous borderline tumors with and without a noninvasive micropapillary component. Am J Surg Pathol 2002;26:592–600.

Mucinous Surface Epithelial Stromal Tumors

Baergen RN, Rutgers JL. Mural nodules in common epithelial tumors of the ovary. Int J Gynecol Pathol 1994;13:62–72.

Bagué S, Rodríguez IM, Prat J. Sarcoma-like mural nodules in mucinous cystic tumors of the ovary revisited: a clinicopathologic analysis of 10 additional cases. Am J Surg Pathol 2002;26:1467–1476.

Hart WR. Mucinous tumors of the ovary: a review. Int J Gynecol Pathol 2005;24:4–25.

Lee KR, Nucci MR. Ovarian mucinous and mixed epithelial carcinomas of mullerian (endocervical-like) type: a clinicopathologic analysis of four cases of an uncommon variant associated with endometriosis. Int J Gynecol Pathol 2003;22:42–51.

Lee KR, Scully RE. Mucinous tumors of the ovary: a clinicopathologic study of 196 borderline tumors (of intestinal type) and carcinomas, including an evaluation of 11 cases with "pseudomyxoma peritonei". Am J Surg Pathol 2000;24:1447–1464.

Lee KR, Young RH. The distinction between primary and metastatic mucinous carcinomas of the ovary: gross and histologic findings in 50 cases. Am J Surg Pathol 2003;27:281–292.

Rodríguez IM, Prat J. Mucinous tumors of the ovary: a clinicopathologic analysis of 75 borderline tumors (of intestinal type) and carcinomas. Am J Surg Pathol 2002;26:139–152.

Rodriguez IM, Irving JA, Prat J. Endocervical-like mucinous borderline tumors of the ovary: a clinicopathologic analysis of 31 cases. Am J Surg Pathol 2004;28:1311–1318.

Ronnett BM, Kajdacsy-Balla A, Gilks CB, et al. Mucinous borderline ovarian tumors: points of general agreement and persistent controversies regarding nomenclature, diagnostic criteria, and behavior. Hum Pathol 2004;35:949–960.

Silverberg SG, Bell DA, Kurman RJ, et al. Borderline ovarian tumors: key points and workshop summary. Hum Pathol 2004;35:910–917.

Endometrioid, Clear Cell, Brenner, and Mixed Surface Epithelial Stromal Tumors

Bell KA, Kurman RJ. A clinicopathologic analysis of atypical proliferative (borderline) tumors and well-differentiated endometrioid adenocarcinomas of the ovary. Am J Surg Pathol 2000;24:1465–1479.

Bell DA, Scully RE. Atypical and borderline endometrioid adenofibromas of the ovary. A report of 27 cases. Am J Surg Pathol 1985;9:205–214.

Bell DA, Scully RE. Benign and borderline clear cell adenofibromas of the ovary. Cancer 1985;56:2922–2931.

Catasús L, Bussaglia E, Rodrguez I, et al. Molecular genetic alterations in endometrioid carcinomas of the ovary: similar frequency of beta-catenin abnormalities but lower rate of microsatellite instability and PTEN alterations than in uterine endometrioid carcinomas. Hum Pathol 2004;35:1360–1368.

Eichhorn JH, Scully RE. Endometrioid ciliated-cell tumors of the ovary: a report of five cases. Int J Gynecol Pathol 1996;15:248–256.

Eichhorn JH, Young RH. Transitional cell carcinoma of the ovary: a morphologic study of 100 cases with emphasis on differential diagnosis. Am J Surg Pathol 2004;28:453–463.

Eichhorn JH, Young RH, Clement PB, et al. Mesodermal (müllerian) adenosarcoma of the ovary: a clinicopathologic analysis of 40 cases and a review of the literature. Am J Surg Pathol 2002;26:1243–1258.

Kempson RL, Hendrickson MR. Miscellaneous types of surface epithelial neoplasms. The well-differentiated end of the morphologic spectrum of endometrioid, clear-cell, and Brenner tumors and mixed epithelioid tumors of low malignant potential of müllerian type. Pathol (Phila) 1993;1:335–365.

Logani S, Oliva E, Amin MB, et al. Immunoprofile of ovarian tumors with putative transitional cell (urothelial) differentiation using novel urothelial markers: histogenetic and diagnostic implications. Am J Surg Pathol 2003;27:1434–1441.

Oliva E, Sarrió D, Brachtel EF, et al. High frequency of beta-catenin mutations in borderline endometrioid tumours of the ovary. J Pathol 2006;208:708–713.

Ordi J, Schammel DP, Rasekh L, et al. Sertoliform endometrioid carcinomas of the ovary: a clinicopathologic and immunohistochemical study of 13 cases. Mod Pathol 1999;12:933–940.

Silva EG, Young RH. Endometrioid neoplasms with clear cells: a report of 21 cases in which the alteration is not of typical secretory type. Am J Surg Pathol 2007;31:1203–1208.

Tornos C, Silva EG, Ordoñez NG, et al. Endometrioid carcinoma of the ovary with a prominent spindle-cell component, a source of diagnostic confusion. A report of 14 cases. Am J Surg Pathol 1995;19:1343–1353.

Yamamoto S, Tsuda H, Yoshikawa T, et al. Clear cell adenocarcinoma associated with clear cell adenofibromatous components: a subgroup of ovarian clear cell adenocarcinoma with distinct clinicopathologic characteristics. Am J Surg Pathol 2007;31:999–1006.

Young RH, Prat J, Scully RE. Ovarian endometrioid carcinomas resembling sex cord-stromal tumors. A clinicopathological analysis of 13 cases. Am J Surg Pathol 1982;6:513–522.

12 Sex Cord-Stromal Tumors of the Ovary

Michael T Deavers · Esther Oliva · Marisa R Nucci

This category of ovarian tumors includes a diverse group of neoplasms with a wide morphologic spectrum composed of ovarian and testicular stromal-type cells. As a group, they represent 8% of all primary ovarian neoplasms. The WHO classification divides them into four main categories: (1) granulosa stromal cell tumors, composed of ovarian-type cells; (2) Sertoli stromal cell tumors, composed of testicular-type cells; (3) sex cord-stromal tumors of mixed or unclassified cell types and (4) steroid cell tumors (Box 12.1). By far, the most frequently encountered of these tumors are in the granulosa stromal cell group and include thecomas/fibromas and granulosa cell tumors.

GRANULOSA STROMAL CELL TUMORS

This group of tumors is composed of various combinations of granulosa cells, theca cells, and fibroblasts. The presence or absence of a granulosa cell component (10% of the tumor at minimum) is the basis for their classification into the fibroma/thecoma or granulosa cell category.

FIBROMA

This is the most common sex cord-stromal tumor, accounting for approximately 70% of ovarian tumors in this category, although they only represent < 10% of all ovarian tumors.

CLINICAL FEATURES

Fibromas may occur at any age, but are seen most commonly in middle-aged women, with an average age at presentation in the fifth decade. They are uncommon in women < 30 years, except for patients with the Gorlin syndrome (nevoid basal cell carcinoma syndrome), an autosomal-dominant disorder, characterized by congenital abnormalities (e.g., developmental defects of the skeletal system) and predisposition to multiple basal cell carcinomas, ovarian fibromas (which are frequently

bilateral, multinodular, and calcified), as well as other tumors, which gradually appear with increasing patient age. Most fibromas are incidental findings removed at the time of surgery for an unrelated condition; however, if symptomatic, patients most commonly present with abdominal pain, reported in approximately 40% of cases. Fibromas are rarely associated with evidence of

---

BOX 12.1

WORLD HEALTH ORGANIZATION CLASSIFICATION OF OVARIAN SEX CORD-STROMAL TUMORS

I. Granulosa stromal cell tumors
    A. Granulosa cell tumors
       1. Adult granulosa cell tumor
       2. Juvenile granulosa cell tumor
    B. Thecoma/fibroma
       1. Thecoma
          (a) Luteinized thecoma
       2. Fibroma
          (a) Cellular fibroma
       3. Fibrosarcoma
       4. Stromal tumor with minor sex cord elements
       5. Sclerosing stromal tumor
       6. Signet-ring stromal tumor
II. Sertoli stromal cell tumors
    A. Sertoli–Leydig cell tumors
       1. Well-differentiated
       2. Intermediate differentiation
          (a) With heterologous elements
       3. Poorly differentiated
          (a) With heterologous elements
       4. Retiform
          (a) With heterologous elements
    B. Sertoli cell tumor
    C. Stromal–Leydig cell tumor
III. Sex cord-stromal tumors of mixed or unclassified cell types
    A. Sex cord tumor with annular tubules
    B. Gynandroblastoma
    C. Sex cord-stromal tumor, not otherwise specified (unclassified)
IV. Steroid cell tumors
    A. Steroid cell tumor, not otherwise specified
    B. Stromal luteoma
    C. Leydig cell tumor
       1. Hilus cell tumor
       2. Leydig cell tumor, nonhilar type

FIBROMA – FACT SHEET

Definition
▸ Benign fibromatous tumor of varying cellularity composed of spindle, oval, or round collagen-producing cells

Incidence and Location
▸ < 10% of primary ovarian tumors
▸ Typically unilateral
▸ If associated with Gorlin syndrome, more commonly bilateral

Morbidity and Mortality
▸ Secondary torsion
▸ If cellular, may be associated with extraovarian adhesions

Age Distribution
▸ Average age fifth decade
▸ Younger age in patients with Gorlin syndrome

Clinical Features
▸ Pelvic mass, abdominal/pelvic pain, ascites, urinary frequency
▸ Increased CA-125 serum levels
▸ Meigs syndrome in 1% of patients (ascites and pleural effusion)
▸ Association with Gorlin syndrome (hereditary basal cell nevus syndrome)

Prognosis and Treatment
▸ Excellent prognosis
▸ Oophorectomy; complete surgical resection if adherent to other structures (e.g., pelvic wall, omentum)
▸ Adhesions and rupture may be associated with recurrence in cellular and/or mitotically active fibroma
▸ Long-term follow-up recommended for patients with cellular and/or mitotically active fibroma

FIBROMA – PATHOLOGIC FEATURES

Gross Findings
▸ 1–21.5 (average 6) cm
▸ Firm, white cut surface; may be lobulated
▸ Soft, white to yellow cut surface if cellular
▸ Pedunculated or polypoid growth in up to one-fifth
▸ Cystic change in approximately one-quarter
▸ Hemorrhage and necrosis, particularly with torsion
▸ Bilaterality, multinodularity, and calcification if associated with the basal cell nevus syndrome (Gorlin syndrome)

Microscopic Findings
▸ Intersecting fascicles or storiform pattern of spindle cells
▸ Variable degrees of collagen production with occasional hyaline plaques
▸ Variants:
  ▸ Cellular (cellularity similar to adult granulosa cell tumor)
  ▸ Mitotically active (4–19 (mean 6.7) mitoses/10 HPFs)
▸ Other features:
  ▸ Sex cord-like differentiation (< 10% of the tumor)
  ▸ Intracytoplasmic hyaline droplets
  ▸ Bizarre nuclei
  ▸ Verocay-like areas
  ▸ Prominent edema

Immunohistochemical Features
▸ Vimentin positive
▸ Smooth muscle actin often positive; desmin and CD10 negative
▸ Focal and weak positivity for calretinin and inhibin

Differential Diagnosis
Conventional Fibroma
▸ Stromal hyperplasia
▸ Massive ovarian edema/fibromatosis
▸ Thecoma

Cellular Mitotically Active Fibroma
▸ Fibrosarcoma
▸ Luteinized thecoma with sclerosing peritonitis
▸ Diffuse adult granulosa cell tumor

steroid hormone production, but they have been reported to be associated with elevated levels of CA-125, which not surprisingly raises clinical suspicion for ovarian carcinoma. Fibromas > 10 cm may also be associated with ascites in 10–15% of cases or with Meigs syndrome (ascites and pleural effusion) in a small percentage of patients, both typically disappearing after removal of the tumor.

PATHOLOGIC FEATURES

GROSS FINDINGS

Conventional fibromas are typically unilateral tumors (90%) and may range in size from microscopic to > 20 cm, with an average size of 6 cm. They have a smooth or lobulated surface and a homogeneous, firm, white cut section (Figure 12.1). Edema and cyst formation are frequent and calcification is seen in up to 10% of tumors. Fibromas associated with the Gorlin syndrome, however, are bilateral in approximately 75% and typically show multinodular growth and calcifications in almost all

cases. Fibromas that are histologically cellular tend to be larger, and may have a softer, white to yellow cut surface in comparison to conventional fibromas (Figure 12.2). It is not infrequent for cellular fibromas to be associated with ovarian surface adhesions, adhesions to surrounding structures, or rupture.

MICROSCOPIC FINDINGS

Fibromas are composed of fascicles of bland spindle cells that often display a striking storiform or whorled arrangement (Figure 12.3). The cells have scant cytoplasm and uniform oval to elongated wavy nuclei with pointy ends. There is minimal cytologic atypia and mitotic activity is rare. These tumors are variably cellular depending on the amounts of edema and collagenous stroma. Hyaline bands and calcified plaques may

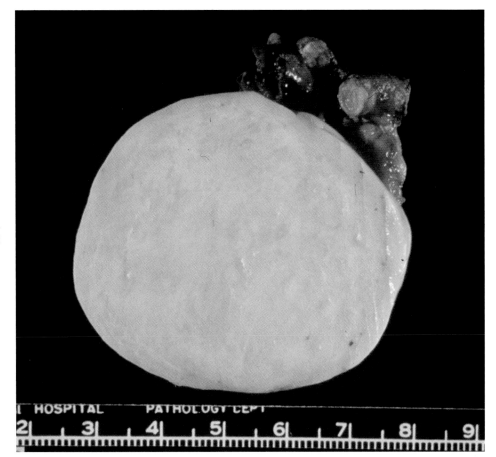

FIGURE 12.1

Fibroma. The tumor is well circum-scribed, has a smooth surface, and a homogeneous white cut section.

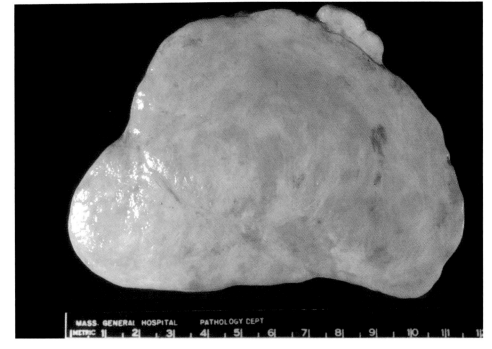

FIGURE 12.2

Cellular fibroma. The tumor is exten-sively tan to yellow, except in the lower left portion, where it shows the more conventional white appear-ance of a fibroma.

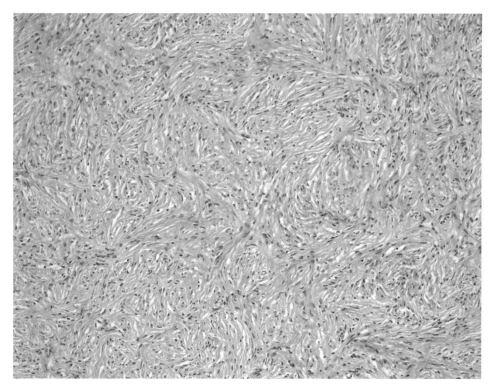

FIGURE 12.3

Fibroma. The tumor is composed of short fascicles of bland spindle cells displaying a striking storiform arrangement.

be seen, but they are not as common as seen in theco-mas. Unusual features include increased cellularity ("cellular fibroma"), increased mitotic activity (> 3/10 HPFs), sex cord-like differentiation (< 10% of the tumor; termed "fibroma with minor sex cord elements"), intracytoplasmic hyaline droplets, bizarre nuclei, and Verocay-like areas. More than one of these unusual features may be present in the same tumor. Small foci of hemorrhage may be seen, but necrosis is typically absent (except with infarction).

Fibromas with increased cellularity similar to that seen in diffuse adult granulosa cell tumors (AGCTs) are termed cellular fibroma. Tumors with this degree of cellularity are uncommon and represent approximately 10% of all ovarian fibromas. Cellular fibroma frequently has areas morphologically similar to conventional fibroma; however, in contrast to its typical counterpart, cellular fibroma is much less frequently associated with edema and hyaline bands. Importantly, these tumors show only minimal cytologic atypia, the most important feature to establish this diagnosis (Figure 12.4). In contrast, increased mitotic activity is not infrequent and it is not necessarily indicative of malignancy. A recent study has shown that cellular fibromas have a mean mitotic count of 1.5/10 HPFs (with a highest mitotic rate ranging from 0 to 3), whereas in mitotically active cellular fibromas, the mean mitotic rate was 6.7/10 HPFs (ranging from 4 to 19), with 15% of tumors having 10–19 mitoses/10 HPFs (Figure 12.5). In contrast to conventional fibromas, both cellular fibromas and mitotically active cellular fibromas may show necrosis that appears sharply demarcated from the surround-

ing viable tumor, the latter commonly present in a perivascular location, a morphologic appearance that overlaps with tumor cell necrosis in uterine smooth-muscle tumors.

ANCILLARY STUDIES

IMMUNOHISTOCHEMISTRY

Fibromas typically are diffusely positive for vimentin, frequently positive for smooth muscle actin, and rarely positive for CD34 and desmin. In some tumors, inhibin and calretinin may be focally and weakly positive. They are negative for CD10.

GENETICS

Patients with the Gorlin syndrome have mutations in the human homologue of *Drosophila* patched gene (PTCH). Some sporadic typical and cellular fibromas have shown loss of heterozygosity (LOH) at 19p13.3, with the highest frequency at microsatellite marker D9S15, which localizes proximal to the PTCH gene. In one study, LOH at 19p13.3 was seen in 50% of cellular fibromas and 25% of conventional fibromas, but not in fibrosarcomas. These results suggest that sporadic cellular fibromas and fibromas associated with Gorlin syndrome may arise through similar genetic pathways.

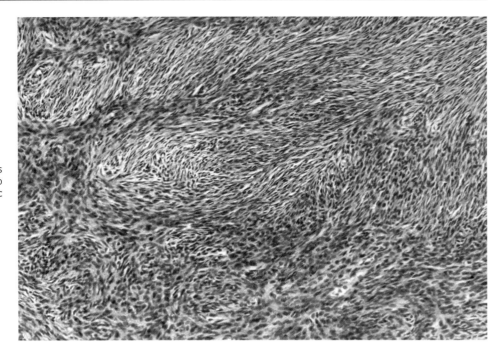

FIGURE 12.4

Cellular fibroma. The tumor shows increased cellularity with minimal to no collagen deposition. No cytologic atypia is present.

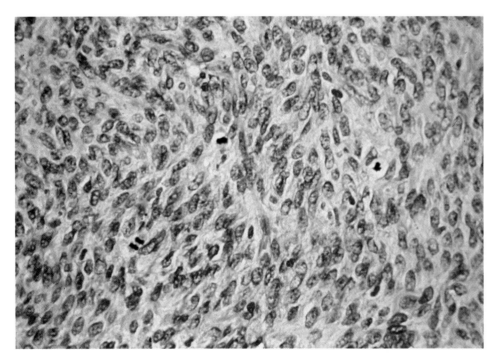

FIGURE 12.5

Mitotically active cellular fibroma. Increased mitotic activity is seen in the absence of cytologic atypia.

DIFFERENTIAL DIAGNOSIS

Conventional fibroma must be mainly distinguished from stromal hyperplasia, massive ovarian edema/fibromatosis, and thecoma. Cellular fibroma should be distinguished from fibrosarcoma, diffuse AGCT, and luteinized thecoma. In contrast to fibroma, *stromal hyperplasia* is typically a bilateral process characterized by a diffuse and cellular proliferation of ovarian stromal cells within the cortex and medulla of the ovary, which may exhibit variable nodularity and lacks collagenous stroma and hyaline plaques. *Massive ovarian edema/fibromatosis* and fibroma are usually unilateral and may be histologically quite similar; however, massive ovarian edema/fibromatosis does not displace normal ovarian structures (e.g., follicles, corpora lutea, and corpora albicantia). Fibroma and *thecoma* may show significant morphologic overlap (and hence the use of the term "fibrothecoma"); nevertheless, fibromas lack nodular growth, tumor cells with abundant pale or vacuolated cytoplasm, tend to show much less staining for inhibin and are negative for CD10 in comparison to thecoma.

Morphologic criteria for the distinction between cellular fibroma and *fibrosarcoma* have evolved over time. In contrast to the initial criteria proposed by Prat and Scully, a recent study found that only cytologic atypia plays a key role in the classification of cellular fibromatous neoplasms. Based on this study, a cellular tumor showing bland cytologic features should be classified as fibroma as it is associated with good outcome despite a high mitotic rate, while tumors with moderate to severe nuclear atypia and high mitotic activity should be classified as fibrosarcoma. On gross examination, fibrosarcoma tends to be larger, softer, and more commonly shows hemorrhage and necrosis. Furthermore, fibrosarcoma is rare, accounting for < 1 % of all primary ovarian tumors. Cellular fibroma and *luteinized thecoma with sclerosing peritonitis* may both be densely cellular, lack cytologic atypia, and have brisk mitotic activity; however, cellular fibromas are more homogeneously cellular, they lack luteinized cells, are typically unilateral, and are not associated with sclerosing peritonitis. Furthermore, hormonal manifestations are common in luteinized thecoma with sclerosing peritonitis but extremely unusual in cellular fibroma. Finally, *diffuse AGCTs*, which may sometimes have a striking fibromatous background, can be distinguished from cellular fibromas at higher magnification as the cells in the former often show grooved nuclei. Finding other areas with patterns characteristic of AGCT is also helpful.

PROGNOSIS AND THERAPY

Conventional fibromas are benign tumors and oophorectomy is adequate treatment. Cellular mitotically active fibromas also behave in a benign fashion even when associated with ovarian adhesions or extraovarian extension. Thus, these tumors should be treated conservatively with surgery. Long-term follow-up is particularly advised for those patients with tumor rupture or adhesions as they may recur locally.

THECOMA

CLINICAL FEATURES

Thecomas typically occur in postmenopausal women, most commonly in the sixth decade, but they may occur at any age, with some presenting in women ≤ 30 years (more often luteinized thecomas); however, they are rare before puberty. These tumors are commonly estrogenic and most women present with abnormal vaginal bleeding. Approximately 20 % of patients will also develop concurrent endometrial carcinoma. Of note,

---

THECOMA – FACT SHEET

Definition
▶ Stromal tumor composed of lipid-containing cells resembling theca cells with a variable fibromatous component

Incidence and Location
▶ Approximately one-third as common as granulosa cell tumors
▶ 95% unilateral

Morbidity and Mortality
▶ Association with endometrial neoplasia

Age Distribution
▶ Conventional thecoma: mostly postmenopausal women (mean age 59 years)
▶ Luteinized thecoma: 30% in patients ≤ 30 years

Clinical Features
▶ Pelvic mass or swelling
▶ Vaginal bleeding (both conventional and luteinized thecoma)
▶ Endometrial adenocarcinoma in one-fifth of patients (secondary to estrogen production)
▶ Virilization (more common in luteinized thecoma)

Prognosis and Treatment
▶ All but rare cases benign
▶ Unilateral salpingo-oophorectomy (unless associated with endometrial adenocarcinoma: hysterectomy and bilateral salpingo-oophorectomy)

---

luteinized thecomas are androgenic in approximately 10 % of cases.

PATHOLOGIC FEATURES

GROSS FINDINGS

The vast majority of thecomas are unilateral (~ 95 %) and can range in size from microscopic tumors to large masses; most being between 5 and 10 cm. These tumors are typically solid (but may occasionally be cystic) and have a tan-yellow, sometimes lobulated sectioned surface (Figure 12.6). On occasion, they may show areas of necrosis, hemorrhage, or calcification; the latter is more common in tumors occurring in younger women.

MICROSCOPIC FINDINGS

These tumors are composed of sheets or nodular aggregates of plump to spindle cells with pale or vacuolated cytoplasm (Figure 12.7). The plump cells resemble

THECOMA – PATHOLOGIC FEATURES

Gross Findings

▶ Unilateral (except luteinized thecomas with sclerosing peritonitis)
▶ < 1 to 15 cm; most between 5–10 cm
▶ Solid and yellow to gray-white and sometimes lobulated cut surface
▶ Occasional cystic change, focal calcification, hemorrhage, and necrosis
▶ Extensive calcification in young women

Microscopic Findings

▶ Aggregates of oval to round cells alternating with spindled cells (conventional thecoma) ± groups or single lutein cells (luteinized thecoma)
▶ Theca cells with abundant pale to vacuolated cytoplasm and round to oval nuclei
▶ Lutein cells with abundant eosinophilic cytoplasm and large round nuclei
▶ Minimal cytologic atypia and rare mitotic figures
▶ Hyaline plaques and, less frequently, calcification may be seen
▶ Unusual features:
  ▶ Minor sex cord elements
  ▶ Bizarre nuclei
  ▶ Fatty metaplasia

Immunohistochemical Features

▶ Inhibin, calretinin, CD10, and vimentin positive
▶ EMA and cytokeratin negative

Ultrastructural Features

▶ Cells with abundant intracytoplasmic lipid, granular endoplasmic reticulum, and mitochondria with tubular cristae
▶ Cells lack desmosomes and basal lamina and are separated by collagen

Differential Diagnosis

▶ Fibroma
▶ Granulosa cell tumor
▶ Sclerosing stromal tumor
▶ Pregnancy luteoma (vs luteinized thecoma)
▶ Steroid cell tumor (vs luteinized thecoma)

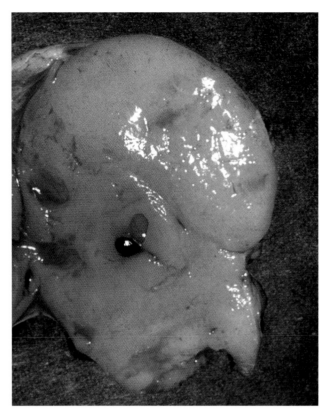

FIGURE 12.6
Thecoma. The tumor has a solid, tan to yellow cut surface.

ANCILLARY STUDIES

HISTOCHEMISTRY AND IMMUNOHISTOCHEMISTRY

Reticulin stain reveals a dense fibrillar network that surrounds individual tumor cells. Oil red O stain demonstrates intracytoplasmic lipid. Thecomas are typically positive for vimentin, inhibin, calretinin, and CD10, but are negative for cytokeratin and EMA.

ULTRASTRUCTURAL EXAMINATION

Electron microscopy reveals that thecomas are composed of cells with abundant intracytoplasmic lipid, granular endoplasmic reticulum, and mitochondria with tubular cristae. The tumor cells lack desmosomes and basal lamina, and are separated by collagen. A variable amount of admixed fibroblastic cells may also be present.

DIFFERENTIAL DIAGNOSIS

The principal differential diagnostic considerations include fibroma, AGCT (diffuse pattern), and sclerosing stromal tumor.

theca interna cells of a developing follicle. If the tumor is mainly composed of spindle cells (fibromatous background) or plump cells (thecomatous background) with single or variable-size clusters of lutein cells, the term "luteinized thecoma" is applied. The nuclei of the theca cells are round to oval with fine, dispersed chromatin with infrequent mitotic figures. The lutein cells have abundant eosinophilic cytoplasm, round nuclei, and prominent central nucleoli. Hyaline plaques are often present, and stromal calcification may occur and is sometimes prominent, particularly in tumors occurring in younger women. These tumors may have focal sex cord-like differentiation but, to be classified as a thecoma, the tumor must show < 10 % of such component. Rarely, fatty metaplasia and bizarre nuclei may be seen.

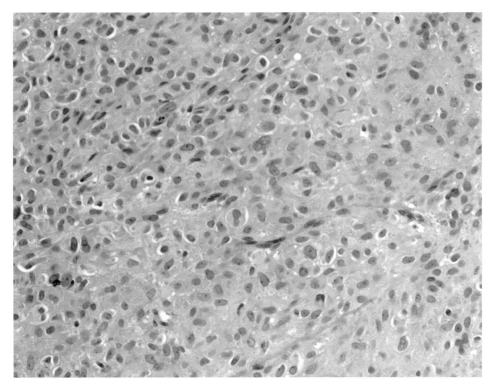

FIGURE 12.7
Thecoma. The tumor is composed of spindle to plump cells with pale to vacuolated cytoplasm.

Distinction between *fibroma* and thecoma can be problematic since these two entities have varying combinations of bland spindled cells and plumper cells with more abundant eosinophilic or clear cytoplasm. Because of this morphologic overlap, tumors with features of both fibroma and thecoma have been called "fibrothecoma." Nevertheless, the diagnosis of thecoma should be reserved for those tumors in which most of the tumor cells have abundant pale or vacuolated cytoplasm (lipid-rich cells). In addition, diffuse staining for inhibin supports the diagnosis of thecoma, as fibromas tend to show minimal to absent staining for this marker. The diffuse pattern of *granulosa cell tumor* may mimic a thecoma or may have a very prominent thecomatous component. It can be distinguished from thecoma by the presence of characteristic nuclear grooves (although this may require careful scrutiny of nuclear morphology) and lack of investment of individual cells by a dense fibrillar network, as highlighted by a reticulin stain. Thecoma may mimic a *sclerosing stromal tumor* as it may show a prominent nodular growth and cells with spindle and epithelioid appearance. However, sclerosing stromal tumor more commonly occurs in the first three decades of life and is less commonly associated with clinical manifestations. In addition, sclerosing stromal tumors are more vascular and contain numerous vessels with a hemangiopericytoma-like appearance. In pregnant women, thecomas may undergo extensive luteinization and may cause problems in the differential diagnosis with *pregnancy luteoma*. However, the latter are typically multiple and bilateral, do not have the fibromatous or thecomatous background, and the cells contain little

or no lipid. Finally *steroid cell tumors* typically have a diffuse growth of cells showing well defined borders and containing aboundant lipid vacuoles.

PROGNOSIS AND THERAPY

Thecoma is a benign tumor except for a very few exceptions, and unilateral salpingo-oophorectomy is considered adequate treatment. Because of their association with endometrial neoplasia, endometrial sampling should be performed. In cases associated with carcinoma, hysterectomy and bilateral salpingo-oophorectomy is the standard treatment.

LUTEINIZED THECOMA WITH SCLEROSING PERITONITIS

CLINICAL FEATURES

Luteinized thecoma with sclerosing peritonitis (LT with SP) is a variant of thecoma that typically affects women in their third and fourth decades. This is an enigmatic entity in which patients present with abdominal swelling, abdominal pain, ascites or, in some cases, pleural effusion or symptoms of bowel obstruction. On pelvic examination, they are found to have unilateral or more frequently bilateral pelvic masses.

LUTEINIZED THECOMA WITH SCLEROSING PERITONITIS – FACT SHEET

Definition

▸ Densely cellular tumor composed predominantly of spindle cells admixed with less prominent small lutein cells (steroid hormone-producing cells) typically associated with sclerosing peritonitis

Incidence and Location

▸ Rare
▸ Typically bilateral but can be unilateral

Morbidity and Mortality

▸ Bowel obstruction and enterocutaneous fistulae secondary to sclerosing peritonitis
▸ No recurrence or metastases
▸ Death secondary to surgical complications

Age Distribution

▸ Reproductive age (mean 25 years; frequently < 40 years)

Clinical Features

▸ Abdominal pain or swelling
▸ Symptoms secondary to bowel obstruction

Prognosis and Treatment

▸ Prognosis related to intestinal/peritoneal disease
▸ Bilateral oophorectomy and resection of adhesions
▸ Bowel obstruction managed by surgical intervention, conservative measures, or hormonal therapy
▸ Extensive and multiple surgeries if adhesions with increased risk of bowel obstruction

LUTEINIZED THECOMA WITH SCLEROSING PERITONITIS – PATHOLOGIC FEATURES

Gross Findings

▸ Typically bilateral
▸ Slightly enlarged to nodular ovaries or large masses (up to 31 cm)
▸ Cerebriform surface
▸ Solid and edematous cut surface

Microscopic Findings

▸ Frequent diffuse ovarian involvement
▸ Densely cellular with diffuse or loose fascicular architecture
▸ Predominant population of spindle cells admixed with small groups of lutein cells (smaller than usual luteinized cells)
▸ Absent to mild cytologic atypia
▸ Brisk mitotic activity in spindle cells (up to 80/10 HPFs)
▸ Not infrequently, edema with microcyst formation
▸ May entrap normal ovarian structures

Immunohistochemical Features

▸ Inhibin, calretinin and CD56 positive in luteinized cells
▸ Smooth muscle actin, desmin, calretinin, CD56, and AE1/3 focally positive
▸ Inhibin negative in spindle cells

Differential Diagnosis

▸ Stromal hyperthecosis
▸ Massive edema/fibromatosis
▸ Edematous cellular fibroma
▸ Sclerosing stromal tumor
▸ Fibrosarcoma

PATHOLOGIC FEATURES

GROSS FINDINGS

The ovarian lesions may form bilateral large masses (up to 31 cm) or result in only slightly enlarged ovaries (Figure 12.8A) replacing the entire ovary or less commonly involving the cortex in most cases. When they form a mass, the tumors typically have a prominent nodular or cerebriform surface and a solid, homogeneous, white to tan-pink and edematous sectioned surface (Figure 12.8B).

The sclerosing peritonitis, which can involve omentum, peritoneum, and intestinal serosa, appears as areas of thickening up to 2–3 mm, which is generally well demarcated from the underlying normal tissue.

MICROSCOPIC FINDINGS

The ovarian lesion is poorly demarcated and is composed of sheets or cellular/loose intersecting fascicles of spindle cells with scanty eosinophilic cytoplasm and round to spindled nuclei with small nucleoli that display minimal atypia (Figure 12.9). In some cases, discrete masses are not present but rather there is diffuse cortical spindle cell expansion resulting in nodular cortical thickening. Scattered throughout the lesion are small nests and clusters of small luteinized stromal cells (hence designation as luteinized thecoma) (Figure 12.10). Mitotic activity can be striking (up to 80 mitoses/10 HPFs), sometimes with markedly varied counts between the ovarian lesions on both sides (Figure 12.9). Marked edema may be seen with secondary microcyst formation (Figure 12.11). Residual ovarian follicles are often present within the lesion.

The associated sclerosing peritonitis is composed of a fascicular or, less commonly, storiform, variably cellular (but generally moderately cellular) proliferation of bland-appearing fibroblasts, collagen deposition, and inflammatory cells (Figure 12.12); surface fibrin and focal mesothelial hyperplasia may also be present. Extensive involvement of the omentum results in envelopment of individual lobules of adipose tissue by the fibroblastic proliferation, resulting in a dramatic accentuation of the normal lobular architecture.

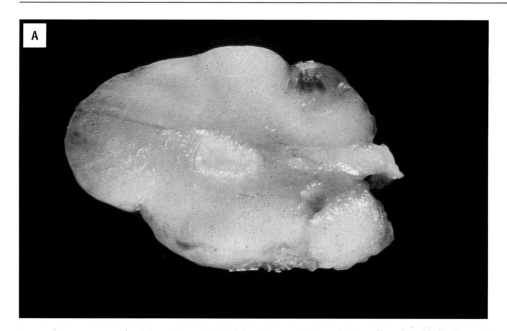

FIGURE 12.8

Luteinized thecoma with sclerosing peritonitis. The ovary can be slightly enlarged (A) or have a multinodular growth involving the cortex (B).

ANCILLARY STUDIES

IMMUNOHISTOCHEMISTRY

The luteinized cells are typically diffusely positive for inhibin, calretinin, and CD56. The spindle cell component is usually focally positive for smooth muscle actin and desmin and occasionally positive for cytokeratin AE1/AE3, calretinin, and CD56, but is negative for inhibin.

DIFFERENTIAL DIAGNOSIS

The ovarian lesion of LT with SP should be differentiated from stromal hyperthecosis, massive ovarian edema and fibromatosis, edematous cellular fibroma, sclerosing stromal tumor, and fibrosarcoma.

Stromal hyperthecosis falls into the differential diagnosis because it is almost always bilateral and characterized by the presence of nests of luteinized cells within

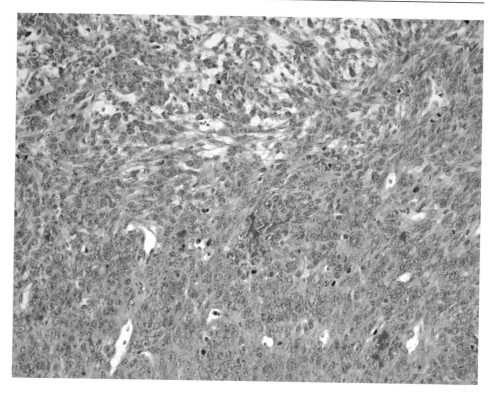

FIGURE 12.9

Luteinized thecoma with sclerosing peritonitis. The ovarian tumor is composed of dense short intersecting fascicles of spindle cells with scanty eosinophilic cytoplasm and round to spindled nuclei with small nucleoli, minimal cytologic atypia and brisk mitotic activity.

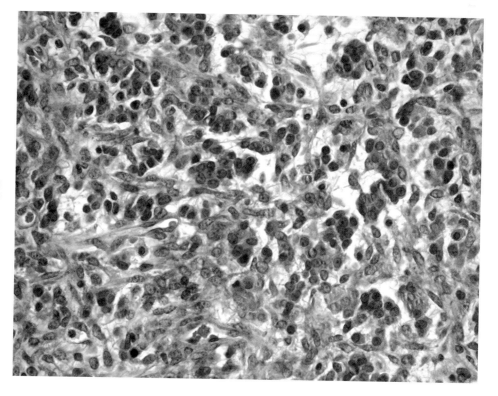

FIGURE 12.10

Luteinized thecoma with sclerosing peritonitis. Interspersed between the spindled cells there are nests and clusters of small luteinized cells.

hyperplastic stroma and, similarly to LT with SP, it can also entrap normal ovarian follicles; however, it is not accompanied by ascites, prominent ovarian enlargement, or obliteration of the ovarian architecture. In addition, the stromal cells in stromal hyperthecosis lack mitotic activity which is in stark contrast to most LT with SP. Although *massive ovarian edema/fibromatosis* may cause significant ovarian enlargement, occasionally may be bilateral, and contain rare foci of luteinized cells, they are typically hypocellular and associated with either diffuse marked edema or collagen deposition. *Edematous cellular fibroma* can be distinguished from LT with SP because it is typically unilateral, and although it may be associated with ascites, it is not associated with

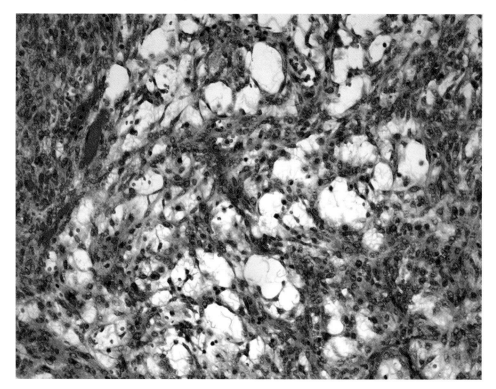

FIGURE 12.11

Luteinized thecoma with sclerosing peritonitis. Marked edema of the ovarian tumor produces microcyst formation.

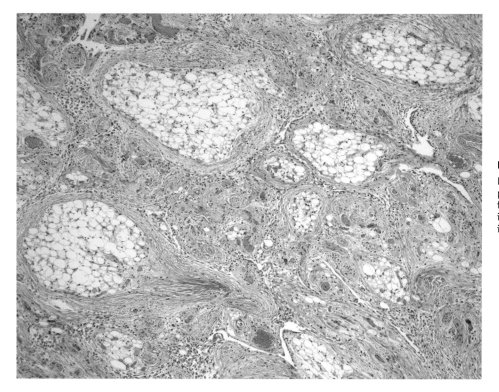

FIGURE 12.12

Luteinized thecoma with sclerosing peritonitis. A moderately cellular fibroblastic proliferation surrounds individual lobules of adipose tissue in the omentum.

sclerosing peritonitis. *Sclerosing stromal tumor* is also typically unilateral and differs morphologically from LT with SP in that it is composed of a biphasic population of mitotically inactive spindle-shaped and luteinized cells arranged in a characteristic pseudolobular arrange-

ment and admixed with a prominent hemangiopericy-toma-like vascular pattern. Even though *fibrosarcoma* can exhibit brisk mitotic activity, it is associated with tight fascicles of spindle cells with moderate to severe cytologic atypia, features not seen in LT with SP.

PROGNOSIS AND THERAPY

Treatment consists of removal of the ovarian lesion(s), as well as omentectomy, lysis of adhesions, and bowel resection when necessary, to relieve symptoms of obstruction. Rare patients have benefited from hormonal treatment. Although it appears that the ovarian lesions are benign, with no evidence of recurrence or metastases, a small number of patients have died of complications related to the sclerosing peritonitis.

SCLEROSING STROMAL TUMOR

Sclerosing stromal tumor is a rare benign neoplasm that accounts for 2–6% of ovarian stromal tumors.

SCLEROSING STROMAL TUMOR – FACT SHEET

Definition
▸ Benign stromal tumor with cellular areas composed of fibroblasts and lutein cells separated by hypocellular edematous or collagenized areas imparting a pseudolobular appearance

Incidence and Location
▸ 2–6% of ovarian stromal tumors
▸ < 1% of all primary ovarian tumors
▸ Unilateral

Morbidity and Mortality
▸ Rare torsion

Age Distribution
▸ 80% of women < 30 years of age

Clinical Features
▸ Pain, pelvic mass
▸ Very rarely, estrogenic or androgenic manifestations

Radiologic Features
▸ Solid mass with a pseudolobular pattern by CT scan and MRI
▸ Medium signal intensity of tumor periphery and high signal in center by nonenhancing MRI
▸ Initial enhancement of tumor periphery with centripetal progression of contrast by dynamic enhanced MRI

Prognosis and Treatment
▸ Excellent prognosis
▸ Unilateral oophorectomy

CLINICAL FEATURES

It is generally found in patients who are younger than those with either thecomas or fibromas, as 80% are < 30 years of age. Patients often present with menstrual irregularities or symptoms related to the presence of a pelvic mass. Evidence of hormone production, either estrogenic or androgenic, has been documented only rarely. Ascites, Meigs syndrome, or elevated serum levels of CA125 are infrequent.

RADIOLOGIC FEATURES

Imaging findings are reported to be typical and diagnostic of this type of ovarian tumor, particularly by dynamic contrast-enhanced CT and MRI. They show a well-defined, predominantly solid mass with a pseudo-lobular pattern. The nonenhancing MRI shows medium signal intensity of the tumor periphery and high signal in the center while by dynamic-enhanced MRI, there is initial enhancement of the periphery of the tumor with centripetal progression of the contrast.

PATHOLOGIC FEATURES

GROSS FINDINGS

The tumors are almost always unilateral and range from 1.5 to 20 cm in largest dimension. They have a well-defined border that, in some cases, has led to enucleation of the tumor at surgery. They are white to yellow and typically solid, or solid with multiple cystic spaces; occasional tumors may have a large central cyst (Figure 12.13).

MICROSCOPIC FINDINGS

Sclerosing stromal tumor is typically well circumscribed with a sharply demarcated thin rim of normal ovarian tissue at the periphery. At low magnification, the tumor has a pseudolobular appearance with cellular nodules alternating with hypocellular edematous or markedly collagenized connective tissue (Figure 12.14). The cellular areas contain a random and heterogeneous mixture of spindled cells and round lutein cells, and a characteristic vascular network composed of numerous thin-walled vessels, some of which can be dilated and branched, resembling those seen in hemangiopericytoma (Figure 12.14). The lutein cells have eosinophilic to clear vacuolated cytoplasm and round nuclei with vesicular chromatin and prominent nucleoli (Figure 12.15). These cells may form small clusters, and occasionaly, may have a signet-ring appearance. The spindle

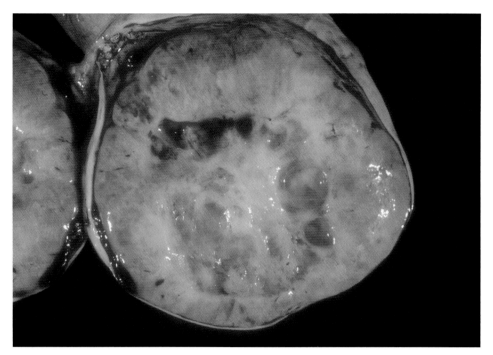

FIGURE 12.13
Sclerosing stromal tumor. A well circumscribed, tan to yellow solid cut surface with a central cyst is seen.

SCLEROSING STROMAL TUMOR – PATHOLOGIC FEATURES

Gross Findings

‣ 1.5–20 cm
‣ Well-defined border with normal ovarian tissue
‣ White to yellow and solid, or solid with multiple cystic spaces
‣ Occasionally large central cyst

Microscopic Findings

‣ Pseudolobular architecture
‣ Cellular nodules alternating with hypocellular edematous or collagenized areas
‣ Numerous thin-walled vessels, some branched and dilated (hemangiopericytoma-like vascular network)
‣ Cellular areas with heterogeneous admixture of spindle and round cells
‣ Round cells with vacuolated to eosinophilic cytoplasm and round nuclei with vesicular chromatin and prominent nucleoli
‣ Minimal cytologic atypia and low mitotic rate

Immunohistochemical Features

‣ Calretinin, ER, PR, vimentin and smooth muscle actin positive
‣ Variable inhibin and desmin expression
‣ Keratin and EMA negative

Ultrastructural Features

‣ Variegated appearance of cells
‣ Abundant membrane-bound lipid granules and rough endoplasmic reticulum
‣ No desmosomes
‣ Basal lamina adjacent to cell membranes

Differential Diagnosis

‣ Fibroma
‣ Luteinized thecoma
‣ Krukenberg tumor
‣ Carcinoid tumor

cells have scant pale cytoplasm and elongated nuclei. Cytologic atypia and mitoses are rare.

ANCILLARY STUDIES

IMMUNOHISTOCHEMISTRY

Sclerosing stromal tumors, particularly the lutein cells, are positive for calretinin and less frequently for inhibin (not universally expressed). Estrogen and progesterone receptors, vimentin, and smooth muscle actin are also positive. Keratin and EMA are negative, while there are conflicting reports regarding desmin expression.

ULTRASTRUCTURAL EXAMINATION

On electron microscopic examination, there is a wide spectrum of cells with a variegated appearance, including luteinized cells, spindle-shaped fibroblastic cells, and primitive mesenchymal cells. The nuclei range in appearance from oval to elongated and irregular with prominent nucleoli. The cytoplasm contains abundant membrane-bound lipid granules and rough endoplasmic reticulum. Basal lamina is present adjacent to the cytoplasmic membranes, but desmosomes are lacking.

DIFFERENTIAL DIAGNOSIS

Depending upon which component is most prominent in the tumor, the entities to be considered in the differential diagnosis can vary. If the spindle cells predomi-

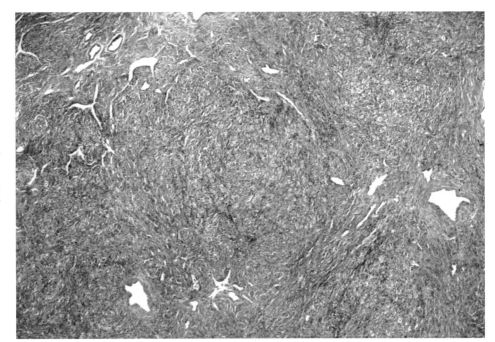

FIGURE 12.14

Sclerosing stromal tumor. The tumor shows a prominent lobulated architecture, has hypocellular and hypercellular areas, and a conspicuous hemangiopericytoma-like vascular pattern.

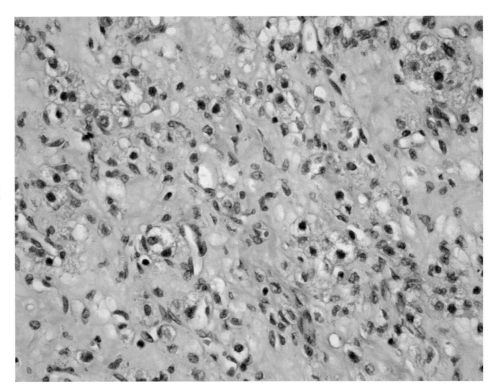

FIGURE 12.15

Sclerosing stromal tumor. The tumor is composed of an admixture of spindle cells and round luteinized cells.

nate, a sclerosing stromal tumor may be confused with a fibroma or luteinized thecoma. *Fibroma* tends to occur in older patients (average age is approximately 50 years and < 10% of these patients are under 30 years of age), and histologically they frequently show hyalinized plaques and lack the pseudolobulation, prominent vascularity, and cellular heterogeneity characteristic of

sclerosing stromal tumors. *Luteinized thecoma* and sclerosing stromal tumor share several clinical and pathologic features. Both occur in young patients more frequently than fibromas or thecomas (30% of patients with luteinized thecoma are 30 years of age or younger); both are stromal tumors containing spindled and lutein cells, and express inhibin and calretinin. However, the variegated appearance of sclerosing stromal tumor and its prominent thin-walled vessels are absent in luteinized thecoma. Because the lutein cells of sclerosing stromal tumors often have clear cytoplasm, and sometimes a signet-ring cell appearance, they can mimic *metastatic signet-ring cell carcinoma*. Krukenberg tumors, however, contain mucin and are positive for keratin and EMA while the vacuoles in the signet-ring-like cells of the sclerosing stromal tumor contain lipid. If the lutein cells are arranged in cords, they can mimic *metastatic breast carcinoma or carcinoid tumor*; however, both lack the prominent hemangiopericytoma-like vascular network seen in sclerosing stromal tumors. Negative keratin and EMA, and positive inhibin and calretinin staining should distinguish sclerosing stromal tumor from those two entities. It should be kept in mind that both sclerosing stromal tumor and metastatic breast carcinoma can be ER and PR positive.

PROGNOSIS AND THERAPY

As these tumors are typically benign, simple oophorectomy is adequate therapy.

ADULT GRANULOSA CELL TUMOR

This tumor is the most frequent among sex cord-stromal tumors with an annual incidence of 0.5–1.5 cases per 100,000 women and accounts for approximately 2–3 % of primary ovarian tumors.

CLINICAL FEATURES

Adult granulosa cell tumors can occur at any age, but are most common in peri- and postmenopausal women. They are the most common ovarian tumor associated with estrogenic manifestations. Because of estrogen production, patients frequently present with menometrorrhagia or postmenopausal bleeding, and they are at risk for concurrent endometrial hyperplasia (up to 50 %) and adenocarcinoma (up to 10 %). In prepubertal patients, the most common manifestation is isosexual pseudoprecocity. Other common presentations include abdominal pain and the presence of a pelvic mass. Less commonly, the tumor is androgenic and can be virilizing. Occasionally, AGCTs are diagnosed during pregnancy; in this setting, hormonal manifestations are less common and they are more often complicated by rupture and hemoperitoneum.

ADULT GRANULOSA CELL TUMOR – FACT SHEET

Definition

‣ Granulosa stromal cell tumor with at minimum a 10% component of granulosa cells, often in a fibrothecomatous background

Incidence and Location

‣ 2–3% of primary ovarian tumors
‣ > 95% unilateral

Morbidity and Mortality

‣ Propensity for late recurrences
‣ Association with endometrial neoplasia

Age Distribution

‣ First to tenth decade, with a median age of approximately 50 years

Clinical Features

‣ Abdominal mass or pain
‣ Estrogenic manifestations in one- to two-thirds:
  – Abnormal vaginal bleeding in reproductive or postmenopausal women
  – Isosexual pseudoprecocity in prepubertal girls
‣ Androgenic manifestations (10%)
‣ Hemoperitoneum secondary to rupture (10%)

Radiologic Features

‣ Varied patterns, including multilocular cystic, unilocular cystic, and homogeneously or heterogeneously solid by ultrasound and CT scan
‣ Frequently thickened endometrium by ultrasound

Prognosis and Treatment

‣ Stage strongest prognostic factor
‣ Tumor rupture, size, and mitotic activity may have prognostic significance
‣ 5-, 10-, and 20-year survival rates of 77–90%, 67–90% and 41–62%, respectively
‣ Surgical resection primary mode of therapy
‣ Combination chemotherapy for advanced-stage and recurrent tumors
‣ Secondary cytoreduction surgery, radiation therapy, or hormonal therapy if recurrence
‣ Serum inhibin levels to monitor tumor recurrence

RADIOLOGIC FEATURES

Adult granulosa cell tumors have varied radiologic appearances, from solid to multilocular or unilocular cysts. Intratumoral hemorrhage, necrosis, and fibrosis can add to the heterogeneity of the imaging findings. These tumors also have a complex pattern by ultrasonography, and a low-impedance Doppler flow pattern because of neovascularization. Ultrasound may detect a thickened endometrium in those patients with secondary endometrial hyperplasia or adenocarcinoma. However, there are no radiographic features that

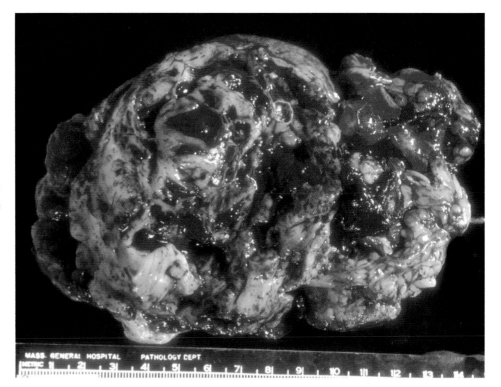

FIGURE 12.16

Adult granulosa cell tumor. The tumor is solid and cystic, with a tan to yellow cut surface and areas of hemorrhage.

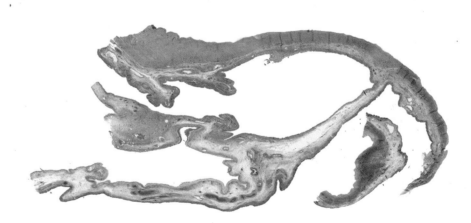

FIGURE 12.17

Adult granulosa cell tumor. This tumor is strikingly cystic.

specifically distinguish AGCTs from the more common category of epithelial ovarian tumors.

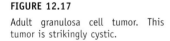
PATHOLOGIC FEATURES

GROSS FINDINGS

The vast majority of these tumors are unilateral (> 95 %). They range from microscopic incidental findings to 30 cm in maximum dimension, with an average size of 12 cm. The tumors are predominantly solid or solid and cystic with a yellow to white cut surface

(Figure 12.16). Occasional tumors consist of uni- or multilocular cysts (Figure 12.17) which tend to be smooth-walled and filled with serous to sanguineous fluid.

MICROSCOPIC FINDINGS

The neoplastic cells can be arranged in a number of different patterns and frequently there is a combination of patterns in the same tumor. A diffuse or solid growth of cells is most frequent, followed by trabecular (cords), microfollicular, macrofollicular, and insular patterns; gyriform and watered silk patterns are less common (Figure 12.18). Call–Exner bodies, the hallmark of the microfollicular pattern, are microcystic spaces that can

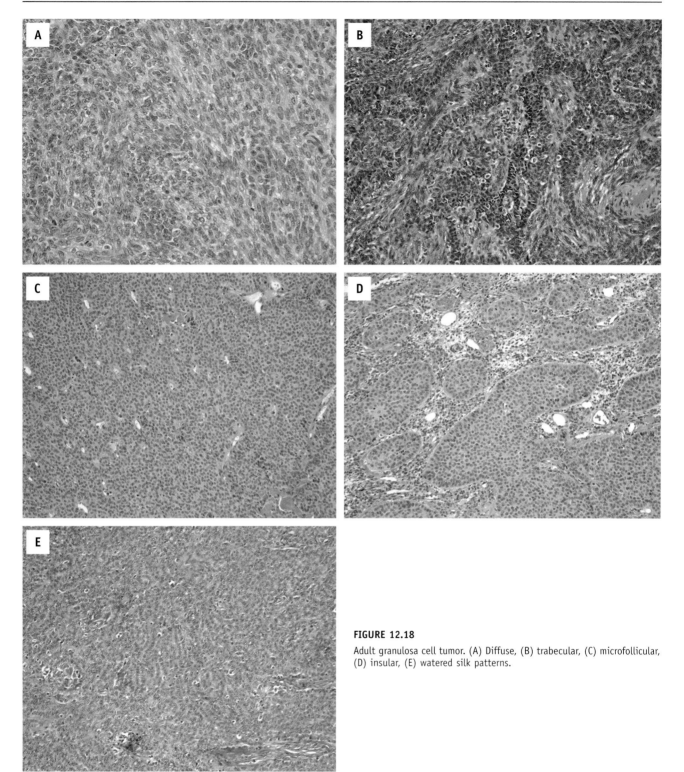

FIGURE 12.18
Adult granulosa cell tumor. (A) Diffuse, (B) trabecular, (C) microfollicular, (D) insular, (E) watered silk patterns.

ADULT GRANULOSA CELL TUMOR – PATHOLOGIC FEATURES

Gross Findings

▸ <1 to 30 (average 12) cm
▸ Predominantly solid or solid and cystic
▸ Rarely uni or multilocular cyst
▸ Yellow-white cut surface
▸ Frequent areas of hemorrhage

Microscopic Findings

▸ Proliferation of granulosa cells in a fibrothecomatous background
▸ Diffuse, trabecular, microfollicular (Call–Exner bodies), macrofollicular, insular, gyriform, and watered-silk growth patterns
▸ Cells with scant cytoplasm and round to oval nuclei with a longitudinal groove
▸ Minimal cytologic atypia and low mitotic rate (typically < 5/10 HPFs)
▸ Rarely:
  ▸ Bizarre nuclei
  ▸ Extensive luteinization (luteinized granulosa cell tumor)
  ▸ Hepatic differentiation

Histochemical and Immunohistochemical Features

▸ Reticulin surrounds groups of cells
▸ Inhibin, calretinin, CD99, CD56, and vimentin positive
▸ Keratin (CAM 5.2, AE1/AE3), CD10, S-100, WT-1, smooth-muscle actin, and desmin can be positive
▸ EMA and CK7 negative

Ultrastructural Features

▸ Deeply indented nuclei with uniformly dispersed chromatin
▸ Call–Exner bodies consist of basal lamina-lined spaces surrounded by tumor cells
▸ Variable numbers of immature desmosomes
▸ Basal lamina around groups of granulosa cells

Fine-Needle Aspiration Biopsy Findings

▸ Cellular smears with cell aggregates, rosette-like follicles, and Call–Exner bodies
▸ Call–Exner bodies have amorphous, metachromatic material on Diff-Quik stain
▸ Small cells with pale cytoplasm, uniform round to oval nuclei and vesicular chromatin
▸ Nuclear grooves not always prominent

Differential Diagnosis

▸ Endometrial stromal sarcoma (primary/metastatic)
▸ Undifferentiated carcinoma/transitional cell carcinoma
▸ Endometrioid adenocarcinoma with sex cord-like differentiation
▸ Carcinoid tumor
▸ Thecoma
▸ Sex cord-stromal tumor with annular tubules
▸ Metastatic breast carcinoma

---

contain deeply eosinophilic basal lamina material (Figure 12.19A). Although less commonly present, they are helpful in the diagnosis of the cystic variant of AGCT (Figure 12.19B). The granulosa cell proliferation frequently has a fibrothecomatous background (Figure 12.18B). The neoplastic granulosa cells generally have scant cytoplasm and round to oval or angular nuclei with a longitudinal groove (Figure 12.20). Nuclear grooves, however, are not limited to AGCT (also seen in Brenner tumors, some Sertoli cell tumors, cellular fibromas, and transitional cell carcinomas) and may be present only in scattered cells in some cases. Mitotic activity is variable, but typically < 5/10 HPFs in the majority of AGCTs. Rare findings include: (1) hyperchromatic, irregular, enlarged nuclei (bizarre nuclei), typically with a focal distribution in the tumor (Figure 12.21); (2) extensive luteinization of the cells (luteinized AGCT) characterized by abundant eosinophilic to vacuolated cytoplasm and oval to round nuclei lacking nuclear grooves (Figure 12.22); and (3) hepatic differentiation with cells arranged in acini, nests, and trabeculae.

ANCILLARY STUDIES

HISTOCHEMISTRY AND IMMUNOHISTOCHEMISTRY

Reticulin staining demonstrates well-defined fibers surrounding aggregates of tumor cells (Figure 12.23).

Inhibin and calretinin are sensitive markers of AGCT. While one or the other may be negative or sparsely expressed, it is unusual to find a tumor negative for both markers. Vimentin is universally expressed and WT1 and CD99 stain the majority of tumors, showing nuclear and membranous staining respectively. These tumors have also been reported to be CD56 positive. Cytokeratin AE1/3-Cam5.2 (punctate), smooth muscle actin, desmin, S100, ER, and PR also show variable positivity, but EMA and CK7 are typically negative. Areas of hepatic differentiation are CEA, EMA, Cam 5.2, and AFP positive but negative for inhibin and vimentin.

ULTRASTRUCTURAL EXAMINATION

The nuclei of the neoplastic cells are characteristically deeply indented and have dispersed chromatin. Call–Exner bodies, if present, consist of granulosa cells surrounding basal lamina-lined spaces. The granulosa cells are attached by immature desmosomes and groups of cells are surrounded by basal lamina.

FINE-NEEDLE ASPIRATION BIOPSY

Although primary ovarian tumors are not usually aspirated, recurrent AGCT may be diagnosed by fine-needle aspiration. The smears are cellular and contain irregular aggregates, rosette-like follicles, and Call–Exner bodies in some cases (Figure 12.24). With Diff-Quik staining, the Call–Exner bodies are readily identified by

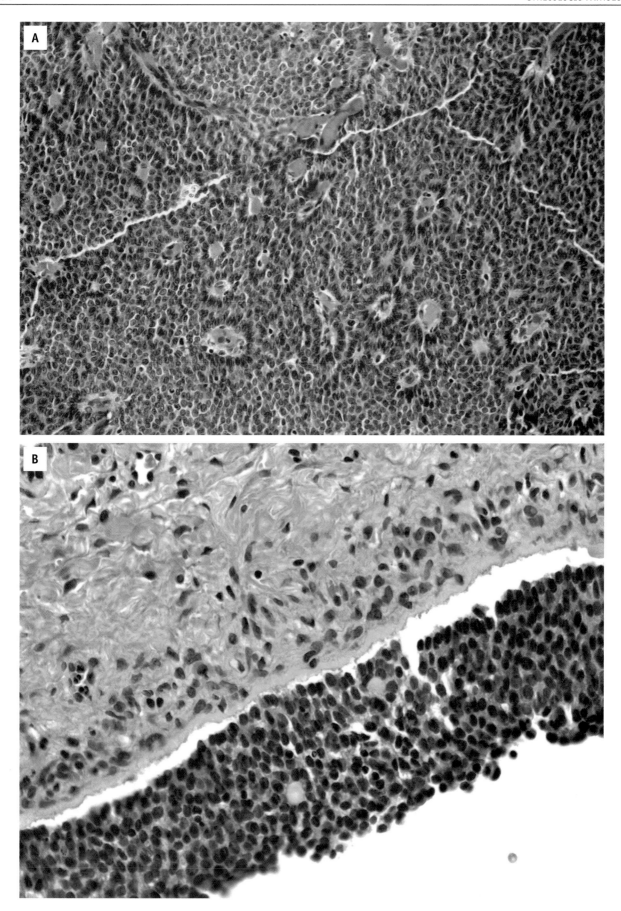

FIGURE 12.19

Adult granulosa cell tumor. Prominent Call–Exner bodies contain deeply eosinophilic basal lamina material (A). In the cystic variant, Call–Exner bodies are only focally seen (B).

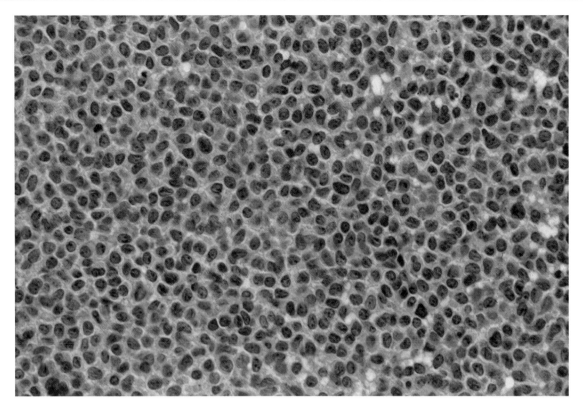

FIGURE 12.20
Adult granulosa cell tumor. Tumor cells characteristically show longitudinally grooved nuclei.

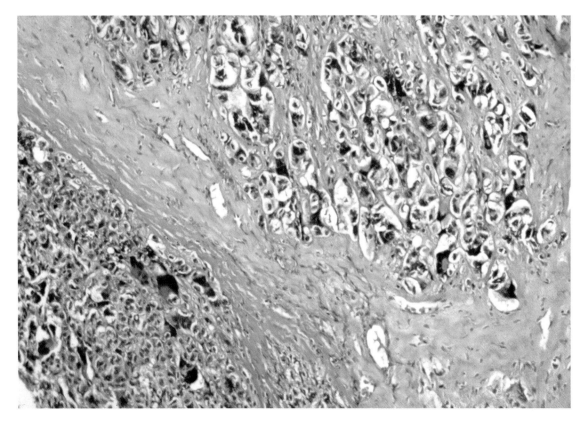

FIGURE 12.21
Adult granulosa cell tumor. Conspicuous enlarged, hyperchromatic (bizarre) nuclei are seen.

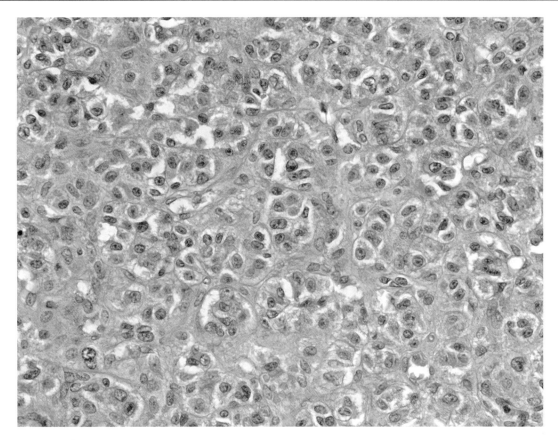

FIGURE 12.22
Luteinized adult granulosa cell tumor. Cells have abundant eosinophilic cytoplasm and lack grooved nuclei.

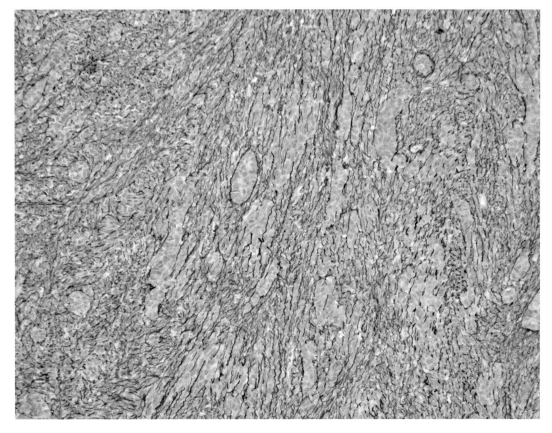

FIGURE 12.23
Adult granulosa cell tumor. Reticulin staining demonstrates well-defined fibers surrounding aggregates of tumor cells.

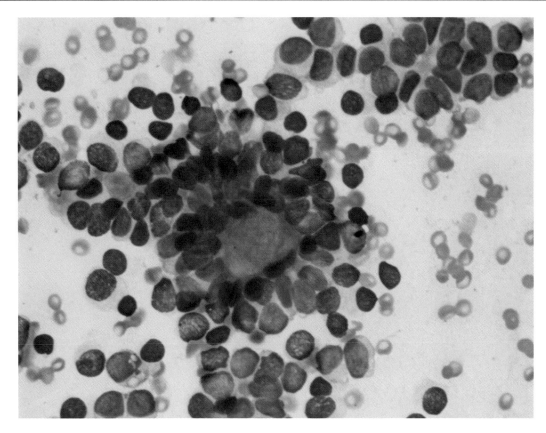

FIGURE 12.24
Adult granulosa cell tumor, fine-needle aspiration biopsy. A cellular smear contains a Call–Exner body.

the presence of metachromatic amorphous material. The cells tend to be small with scant cytoplasm, the nuclei are vesicular with small nucleoli, and nuclear grooves are characteristic but may not be prominent.

DIFFERENTIAL DIAGNOSIS

An AGCT with a diffuse pattern can mimic an endometrioid stromal sarcoma or an undifferentiated carcinoma. Even though *primary or metastatic endometrial stromal sarcomas* may focally show histologic patterns that closely overlap with those seen in a granulosa cell tumor, absence of the characteristic arteriolar vascular pattern, presence of nuclear grooves, and staining for inhibin are helpful findings in establishing the diagnosis of AGCT. Relatively uniform nuclei with grooves, a low mitotic rate, absence of EMA staining, and tumor limited to the ovary help to exclude an *undifferentiated carcinoma*. Rarely, at low-power examination, some cystic AGCT may mimic the papillary growth of a *transitional cell carcinoma* (Figure 12.25). Furthermore both tumors share the presence of nuclear grooves. However, at higher magnification, AGCT lacks uniform high-grade cytologic atypia, tumor necrosis, and high mitotic rate. AGCTs with trabecular, insular, and microfollicular patterns may resemble an endometrioid adenocarcinoma or a carcinoid tumor. Furthermore, *endometrioid adenocarcinomas* may also show grooved nuclei. Absence of squamous or mucinous differentiation, associated endometriosis, and negative EMA staining help to rule out an endometrioid adenocarcinoma. In *carcinoid tumors*, the cells frequently have granular cytoplasm, the nuclei show perpendicular orientation in relation to the main axis of the cords/trabeculae, and they have a "salt-and-pepper" appearance to the chromatin. Moreover, these tumors are positive for neuroendocrine markers. It is important to distinguish luteinized AGCTs from *thecomas*, because the latter are benign neoplasms. In contrast to the distinct reticulum fibers surrounding large groups of granulosa cells, *thecomas* have small fibers and "rootlets" surrounding many individual cells. The microfollicular pattern of an AGCT can also have a superficial resemblance to a *sex cord tumor with annular tubules (SCTAT)*. However, the tubules of SCTAT are either simple or complex, with the nuclei placed near the lumen and at the periphery of the tubules. In addition, there are deposits of dense hyalinized basement membrane material in the lumens. The gyriform or watered-silk patterns may suggest the possibility of *metastatic breast carcinoma*, but the nuclear features differ from those seen in an AGCT, and the presence of other histologic patterns as well as a positive inhibin and negative EMA staining rules out this possibility.

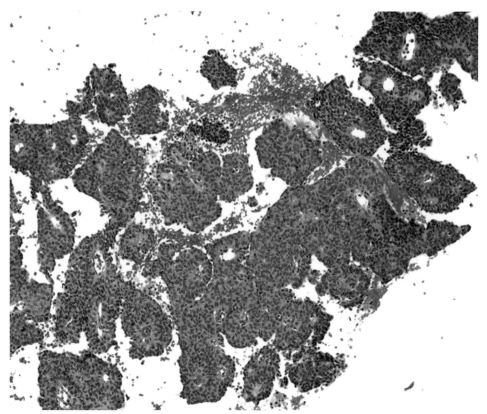

FIGURE 12.25
Adult granulosa cell tumor. A pseudopapillary architecture may mimic at low-power magnification the appearance of a transitional cell carcinoma.

PROGNOSIS AND THERAPY

The most important prognostic indicator in AGCT is tumor stage. Patients with stage I tumors have a 10-year survival rate of 84–87% compared to 38–60% for those with advanced-stage disease. These tumors have a propensity for late recurrences, with an average time to recurrence of 5 years (some developing up to 30 years after initial diagnosis). Pathologic factors such as size (> 5 cm), mitotic activity (> 5 mitoses/10 HPFs), and tumor rupture have been associated with a worse prognosis in some studies. Salpingo-oophorectomy with complete staging is the initial therapeutic approach; tumor-reductive surgery is performed in patients with advanced disease. These patients are also treated with combination chemotherapy. Those with recurrence may benefit from secondary cytoreductive surgery, chemotherapy, and hormonal therapy; radiation therapy can also be effective in some instances. Serum levels of inhibin may be used to monitor tumor recurrence.

JUVENILE GRANULOSA CELL TUMOR

Juvenile granulosa cell tumor (JGCT) comprises 5–15% of granulosa cell tumors and represents 10% of ovarian tumors in patients < 20 years of age.

CLINICAL FEATURES

A total of 97% of JGCTs present in patients < 30 years and approximately 40% under the age of 10 years, with an average age of 13 years at presentation. These tumors frequently produce estrogens and are typically associated with isosexual pseudoprecocity in most prepubertal patients. JGCTs presenting after puberty may be detected secondary to abdominal swelling, pain, pelvic mass, or menstrual irregularities. A few tumors have been found in association with Ollier disease (enchondromatosis) and Maffucci syndrome (multiple enchondromas, hemangiomas, and other mesenchymal tumors).

PATHOLOGIC FEATURES

GROSS FINDINGS

Approximately 98% of JGCTs are unilateral and range from 2.5 to 32 cm in maximum dimension, with an average of 12.5 cm. The gross appearance is similar to that of AGCT and ranges from solid and cystic (approximately 50%), to predominantly solid. The solid areas frequently have a nodular, rubbery, tan to yellow cut surface while the cysts contain serous or serosanguineous fluid (Figure 12.26). Hemorrhage and necrosis may be seen.

JUVENILE GRANULOSA CELL TUMOR – FACT SHEET

Definition
▸ Subtype of granulosa cell tumor almost always found during the first three decades of life, with histologic features that differ from the adult type and resemble the appearance of the granulosa cells of the developing follicle

Incidence and Location
▸ 10% of ovarian tumors in patients < 20 years
▸ 5–15% of all granulosa cell tumors
▸ 98% unilateral

Morbidity and Mortality
▸ High-stage tumors often fatal
▸ Most recurrences within 3 years of initial surgery

Age Distribution
▸ 97% before 30 years (average 13 years)
▸ 6% in children < 1 year
▸ 3% in adults > 30 years

Clinical Features
▸ In prepubertal girls: typically isosexual pseudoprecocity
▸ In reproductive-age women: abdominal swelling, pain, pelvic mass, and menstrual irregularities
▸ Rare manifestations: hemoperitoneum secondary to rupture, androgenic manifestations, association with Maffucci syndrome or Ollier disease

Prognosis and Treatment
▸ Stage strongest prognostic factor
▸ > 90% survival rate for patients with stage Ia tumors
▸ Unilateral salpingo-oophorectomy for stage Ia tumors
▸ Debulking surgery and/or combination chemotherapy for advanced-stage and recurrent tumors
▸ Serum inhibin levels to monitor recurrences

JUVENILE GRANULOSA CELL TUMOR – PATHOLOGIC FEATURES

Gross Findings
▸ 2.5–32 (mean 12.5) cm
▸ Solid and cystic most frequent
▸ Lobulated, gray-white to tan to yellow cut surface
▸ Occasional hemorrhage and necrosis

Microscopic Findings
▸ Diffuse or nodular, and less frequently follicular architecture
▸ Nodules may be completely hyalinized
▸ Myxomatous to edematous background
▸ Irregularly shaped and variable-sized follicles with basophilic or eosinophilic fluid
▸ Call–Exner bodies rare
▸ Granulosa cells with moderate to abundant eosinophilic to vacuolated cytoplasm and round, hyperchromatic nuclei lacking grooves
▸ Variable nuclear atypia (marked in up to 5%) and mitotic rate (up to 32/10 HPFs)
▸ Theca cells surround nodules and follicles, or intermix with granulosa cells if solid growth
▸ Unusual features:
  ▸ bizarre nuclei
  ▸ hyaline globules
  ▸ small foci of adult granulosa cell tumors

Immunohistochemical Features
▸ Inhibin and calretinin positive
▸ Keratin, WT-1, CD10, S100, CD56, and smooth muscle actin frequently positive
▸ EMA focally positive in 25–50% of tumors, in contrast to other sex cord-stromal tumors

Ultrastructural Features
▸ Oval to polygonal cells with abundant rough endoplasmic reticulum, mitochondria, variable amounts of lipid, microfilaments, and irregular nuclei
▸ Groups of cells are surrounded by basal lamina and attached by desmosomes

Differential Diagnosis
▸ Adult granulosa cell tumor
▸ Thecoma
▸ Yolk sac tumor
▸ Small cell carcinoma of hypercalcemic type
▸ Clear cell carcinoma
▸ Metastatic and primary melanoma

MICROSCOPIC FINDINGS

These tumors are composed of a diffuse or nodular proliferation of granulosa cells set in a myxoid (rich in hyaluronic acid) or edematous background (Figure 12.27A). The nodules may become completely hyalinized (Figure 12.27B). Characteristic follicular spaces are found within the nodules or scattered in the solid areas. They vary in shape from round to irregular, and in size from very large to small (Figure 12.28), but Call–Exner bodies are rare. Their content may be either eosinophilic or basophilic. The granulosa cells are generally larger than those seen in AGCT and often have moderate to abundant, pale or eosinophilic cytoplasm. The nuclei are round or oval and hyperchromatic, and grooves are rarely present (Figure 12.29). In some instances, cells lining the cysts have bulbous hyperchromatic nuclei that partially mimic the hobnail cells seen in clear cell carcinoma. Cytologic atypia varies from mild to severe and mitotic activity ranges from 1 to 32/10 HPFs (median of 6–8/10 HPFs). Atypical mitoses may be seen. Theca cells can be seen in JGCTs surrounding nodules of granulosa cells, intermixed with the granulosa cells in solid areas and, much less frequently, surrounding the granulosa cells lining the follicles. They are typically more spindle-shaped than the granulosa cells. Other features seen in these tumors include bizarre nuclei, hyaline globules or rarely, hyaline bands and not infrequently, minor areas of AGCT may

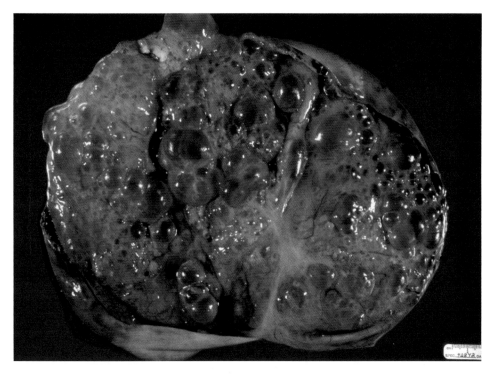

FIGURE 12.26
Juvenile granulosa cell tumor. Solid and cystic tumor with a tan to yellow cut surface.

be encountered in an otherwise typical JGCT. During pregnancy, the tumor cells may have a more disordered arrangement lacking recognizable differentiation, being associated with prominent edema and increased number of lutein cells.

ANCILLARY STUDIES

HISTOCHEMISTRY AND IMMUNOHISTOCHEMISTRY

Reticulin stain demonstrates fibers around groups of granulosa cells, while surrounding individual theca cells. The fluid in the follicular spaces is mucicarmine-positive in two-thirds of cases. These tumors are characteristically positive for inhibin and/or calretinin. Vimentin and keratin are positive in most cases, and WT-1, CD56, and S-100 are also frequently expressed. It should be kept in mind that, in contrast to other sex cord-stromal tumors, focal staining for EMA (< 25 % of tumor cells in most cases) can be seen in 25–50 % of JGCTs. Most tumors are positive for smooth muscle actin, but negative for desmin.

ULTRASTRUCTURAL EXAMINATION

The cells are oval to polygonal with variable amounts of cytoplasm that contains abundant rough endoplasmic reticulum, free ribosomes, and microfilaments. The quantity of cytoplasmic lipid varies from cell to cell. The nuclei are oval or angular, with dispersed chromatin and distinct nucleoli. Basal lamina surrounds groups of cells and poorly formed intercellular junctions and desmosomes interconnect the neoplastic cells.

DIFFERENTIAL DIAGNOSIS

The finding of diffuse and nodular patterns with irregular follicular spaces, cells with round to oval hyperchromatic nuclei lacking grooves embedded in a myxoid background, and frequent luteinized cells distinguish JGCT from *AGCT*. Because of luteinization, JGCT may be mistaken for a thecoma. *Thecomas*, however, lack the follicular spaces and generally the mitotic activity seen in JGCTs. Furthermore, the reticulin fiber pattern is also different in these tumors, typically surrounding individual cells. Because of the young age of most patients with JGCT, a germ cell tumor, specifically a *yolk sac tumor*, may be considered in the differential diagnosis. Both tumors may display a myxomatous background, microcystic architecture, and brisk mitotic activity. However, yolk sac tumors typically form anastomosing channels, have cells with large and primitive nuclei, may contain Schiller–Duval bodies, and may be associated with other germ cell components (commonly a mature cystic teratoma); while follicular spaces, admixture with theca cells, and inhibin expression are absent. *Small cell carcinoma of the hypercalcemic type* also characteristically occurs in young patients; it has follicle-like spaces and the cells are hyperchromatic with brisk mitotic activity. The distinction between these two entities is extremely important as the tumors are associated with very different outcomes. Small cell car-

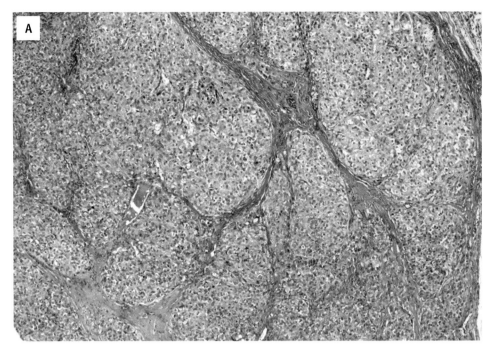

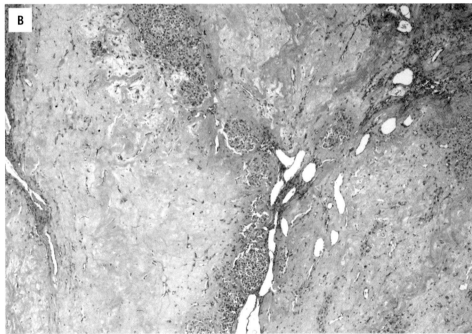

FIGURE 12.27

Juvenile granulosa cell tumor. Prominent nodular growth of granulosa cells (A). The tumor nodules are extensively hyalinized (B).

cinoma of the hypercalcemic type occurs more frequently in women > 20 years, is frequently associated with hypercalcemia, and lacks estrogenic manifestations. In contrast to JGCTs, at the time of diagnosis, these tumors frequently show extraovarian spread and are associated with a poor outcome. From the microscopic point of view, small cell carcinoma of the hypercalcemic type typically grows in sheets but lacks a nodular pattern and has fewer follicles. The cells lining the follicles are not surrounded by theca cells, and inhibin expression is negative. Rarely, as mentioned

earlier, the cells lining the cysts in some JGCTs may have a hobnail configuration and/or the luteinized cells may have abundant pale to clear cytoplasm resembling a *clear cell carcinoma*. However, the latter typically occurs in older patients, it is frequently associated with endometriosis or an adenofibromatous background, shows an admixture of tubulocystic, papillary, and/or solid growths, is positive for EMA and CK7, but negative for inhibin. Either *primary or metastatic melanoma* can involve ovaries of young patients (< 30 years), may have follicle-like spaces, and cells with abundant eosino-

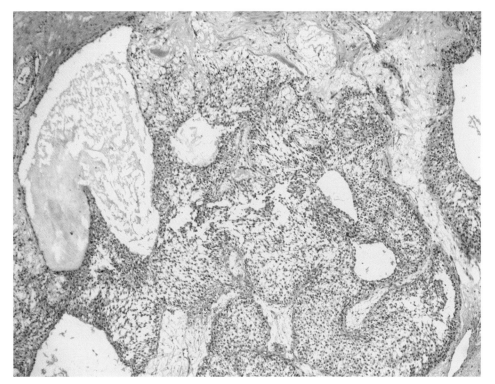

FIGURE 12.28

Juvenile granulosa cell tumor. Follicle-like spaces characteristically vary in size and shape, in contrast to adult granulosa cell tumor.

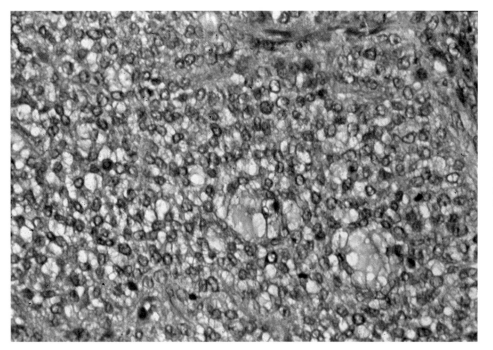

FIGURE 12.29

Juvenile granulosa cell tumor. The cells have round to oval and hyperchromatic nuclei, and they are present within a myxoid matrix.

philic cytoplasm. In cases of metastatic melanoma, the tumors are frequently bilateral and there is often a previous clinical history, while primary ovarian melanomas are frequently associated with a mature cystic teratoma or monodermal teratoma. Both metastatic and primary melanomas are also frequently composed of spindle cells, contain melanin pigment, and react with melanocytic markers. It should be cautioned that focal inhibin expression has been noted in some melanomas involving the ovary.

PROGNOSIS AND THERAPY

Stage is the most important prognostic parameter in these tumors. Nearly all patients with stage Ia tumors remain free of disease, whereas the few patients who present with advanced-stage tumors generally die of disease. Nuclear atypia and mitotic activity have not been found to correlate with prognosis in stage I tumors. In contrast to the late recurrences of AGCTs, recurrences of JGCTs most frequently occur within 3 years of presentation.

As the majority of patients with JGCT are young and 98% have unilateral disease, conservative surgery (unilateral salpingo-oophorectomy and complete staging) with preservation of fertility is the preferred treatment. In advanced-stage disease, total abdominal hysterectomy with bilateral salpingo-oophorectomy and tumor debulking is indicated. Combination chemotherapy is used to treat patients with tumors beyond stage Ia and those with recurrences. Serum inhibin levels may be useful to monitor tumor recurrence.

SERTOLI STROMAL CELL TUMORS

Sertoli stromal cell tumors are composed of Sertoli cells, cells morphologically similar to rete epithelial cells, cells resembling fibroblasts, and Leydig cells either in pure form, or in varying combinations and with variable degrees of differentiation. Included within this category are Sertoli–Leydig cell tumors (SLCTs) and Sertoli cell tumors (SCTs).

SERTOLI–LEYDIG CELL TUMOR

CLINICAL FEATURES

These are uncommon tumors, accounting for < 1% of ovarian neoplasms. SLCTs typically occur in reproductive-age women (average 25 years); however, the retiform variant usually occurs at a younger age (average 15 years) whereas well-differentiated SLCTs occur more commonly at an average age of 35 years. Approximately half of patients have nonspecific symptoms, including abdominal swelling and pain. One-third of patients present with signs of virilization (except for retiform SLCTs, which are less commonly androgenic), and only occasionally, these tumors may be estrogenic or result in elevation AFP.

PATHOLOGIC FEATURES

GROSS FINDINGS

The vast majority of SLCTs are unilateral, with only 2% being bilateral. The average size of most SLCTs is

---

SERTOLI–LEYDIG CELL TUMOR – FACT SHEET

Definition
▶ Tumors composed of Sertoli cells showing varying degrees of differentiation admixed with variable numbers of Leydig cells

Incidence and Location
▶ < 1% of ovarian neoplasms
▶ Most common neoplasm in the category of Sertoli stromal cell tumors
▶ Most unilateral

Morbidity and Mortality
▶ Approximately 12% clinically malignant

Age Distribution
▶ Average age 25 years
▶ Well-differentiated, older age at presentation (average 35 years)
▶ Retiform variant, younger age at presentation (average 15 years)

Clinical Features
▶ Commonly nonspecific symptoms, including abdominal swelling and pain
▶ One-third androgenic manifestations (less frequently in retiform Sertoli–Leydig cell tumors)
▶ Occasionally estrogenic or associated with increased AFP levels

Prognosis and Treatment
▶ 80% of tumors stage Ia
▶ Prognosis related to stage, degree of differentiation of the tumor, and presence of heterologous elements or retiform component
▶ Almost all malignant tumors are poorly differentiated, retiform, or contain heterologous mesenchymal elements
▶ Salpingo-oophorectomy for well-differentiated stage I tumors
▶ Chemotherapy for poorly differentiated tumors, unusual variants, and ruptured intermediate differentiated tumors
▶ Early recurrences, more often confined to pelvis and abdomen

---

approximately 15 cm, although poorly differentiated tumors tend to be larger. They typically have a solid yellow to yellow-tan cut surface with focal cyst formation (Figure 12.30), except retiform SLCTs and SLCTs with heterologous elements, which are more commonly cystic. In the former, the cut surface may be soft and "spongy" or when the cysts are prominent, they may contain multiple edematous to gelatinous polypoid/papillary excrescences, which may simulate the gross appearance of the vesicles of a hydatidiform mole or a serous borderline tumor of the ovary. Poorly differentiated tumors more often contain areas of necrosis and hemorrhage.

MICROSCOPIC FINDINGS

Sertoli-Leydig cell tumors are classified into five major histologic categories due to important clinical

SERTOLI–LEYDIG CELL TUMOR – PATHOLOGIC FEATURES

Gross Findings

▶ 15 cm average size
▶ Solid, lobulated, yellow cut surface
▶ Retiform variant and those with heterologous elements more commonly soft and "spongy" or cystic with intracystic papillae and polypoid excrescences

Microscopic Findings

Well Differentiated

▶ Lobules separated by fibromatous tissue
▶ Lobules composed of solid or hollow tubules
▶ Tubules may resemble endometrioid-type glands
▶ Sertoli cells with abundant eosinophilic or pale and vacuolated cytoplasm and round nuclei with small nucleoli
▶ Minimal cytologic atypia and absent mitotic activity
▶ Leydig cells in between lobules

Intermediate Differentiated

▶ Cellular "blue" lobules separated by hypocellular edematous stroma
▶ Lobules composed of Sertoli cells with diffuse or tubular (poorly developed), nested or cord-like arrangements
▶ Microcystic pattern reminiscent of thyroid tissue
▶ Immature Sertoli cells with scant cytoplasm and small round to oval nuclei
▶ Leydig cells either admixed with Sertoli cells or more frequently at the periphery of lobules

Poorly differentiated

▶ Diffuse or sarcomatoid growth of poorly differentiated Sertoli cells
▶ Rarely, small areas of poorly formed tubules
▶ Sparse to absent Leydig cells

Retiform Variant

▶ Frequently associated with moderately to poorly differentiated Sertoli–Leydig cell tumors
▶ Often slit-like tubules and cysts with short and rounded or blunt papillae
▶ Cysts may resemble thyroid tissue due to luminal eosinophilic secretion
▶ Papillary cores often hyalinized
▶ Tubules, papillae, and cysts lined by a single layer of cuboidal cells with round to oval nuclei
▶ Variable mitotic rate
▶ Cellular and fibromatous or immature mesenchymal intervening stroma

With Heterologous Elements

▶ In ~20% of Sertoli–Leydig cell tumors, typically in intermediate and poorly differentiated tumors
▶ Gastrointestinal-type mucinous epithelium most common
▶ Carcinoid tumor
▶ Immature cartilage or skeletal muscle
▶ Very rarely, hepatoid and neuroblastoma foci

Immunohistochemical Features

Sertoli Cells

▶ Vimentin, cytokeratin, inhibin, calretinin and CD56-positive
▶ CD99, WT-1, CD10, smooth muscle actin variably positive
▶ EMA negative

Leydig Cells

▶ Vimentin, inhibin, and calretinin positive
▶ Melan A, CD10 frequently positive
▶ Keratin and smooth muscle actin rarely positive

Ultrastructural Features

Sertoli Cells

▶ Basal lamina, tight junctions, abundant rough endoplasmic reticulum, lipid and microvilli
▶ Rarely noncrystalline parallel arrays of Charcot–Böttcher microfilaments

Leydig Cells

▶ Oval nuclei with regular contours and large nucleoli
▶ Abundant smooth endoplasmic reticulum, lipid droplets, mitochondria and secondary lysosomes containing lipochrome pigment
▶ Sometimes Reinke crystals and their filamentous precursors

Differential Diagnosis

▶ Endometrioid carcinoma with sex cord-like differentiation
▶ Sertoli cell tumor
▶ Tubular Krukenberg tumor
▶ Serous neoplasia (vs retiform variant)
▶ Yolk sac tumor (vs retiform variant)
▶ Immature teratoma (vs heterologous differentiation)
▶ Carcinosarcoma (vs heterologous differentiation)

and pathologic differences. These categories include: (1) well-differentiated (approximately 10%); (2) intermediately differentiated; (3) poorly differentiated; (4) retiform (10–15%); and (5) with heterologous elements. However, there is considerable overlap between the various categories, except in the category of well-differentiated SLCTs.

Well-differentiated SLCTs are composed of solid or hollow tubules lined by cuboidal to columnar Sertoli cells frequently separated into lobules by a stromal component that consists of fibromatous tissue containing Leydig cells (Reinke crystals present in 20% of cases and abundant lipochrome pigment only occasionally)

(Figure 12.31). Rarely, the tubules may resemble endometrioid-type glands. The Sertoli cells have abundant cytoplasm that may be eosinophilic or pale and vacuolated (due to lipid content) and round to oval basally located nuclei with small nucleoli, with no cytologic atypia and minimal to absent mitotic activity. These tumors are almost always pure and do not contain heterologous or retiform components.

Intermediately differentiated SLCTs often have a characteristic low-power appearance, displaying a lobulated growth with densely cellular areas separated by hypocellular edematous stroma (Figure 12.32). The cellular areas are composed of Sertoli cells arranged dif-

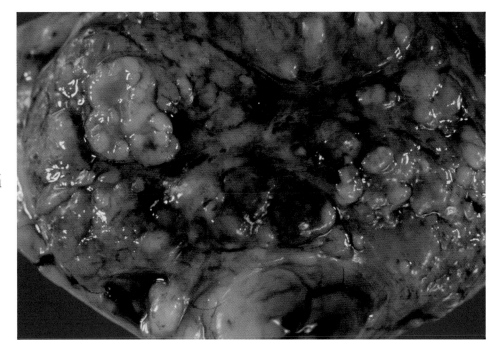

FIGURE 12.30

Sertoli–Leydig cell tumor. Solid, yellow to tan cut surface with focal cyst formation.

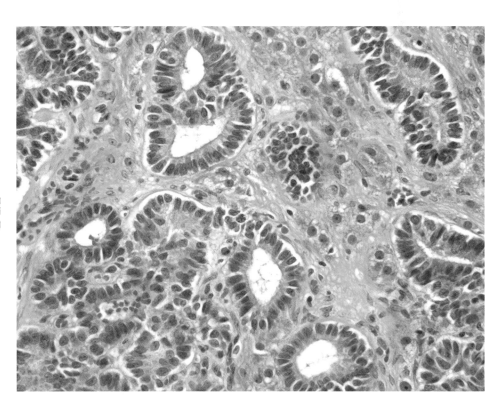

FIGURE 12.31

Well-differentiated Sertoli–Leydig cell tumor. Well-formed Sertoli tubules are intermixed with Leydig cells.

fusely or forming poorly developed tubules, nests, or cords (Figure 12.33). Occasionally, a microcystic pattern reminiscent of thyroid tissue secondary to striking edema may be present (Figure 12.34). The Sertoli cells are typically immature with scant cytoplasm, although occasionally it may be abundant, pale, or vacuolated. The nuclei are small and round to oval and sometimes bizarre nuclei may be seen. Leydig cells with abundant eosinophilic cytoplasm may be seen in the cellular areas admixed with the Sertoli cells, but they

are more often conspicuous at the periphery of the lobules, present within the edematous nonspecific stroma.

Poorly differentiated SLCTs are characterized by a diffuse or sarcomatoid growth of poorly differentiated Sertoli cells mimicking a pure sarcoma. The cells have scant cytoplasm, hyperchromatic nuclei, and brisk mitotic activity. Poorly formed tubules or cords of small Sertoli cells may be only focally present and Leydig cells are typically scant or absent (Figure 12.35).

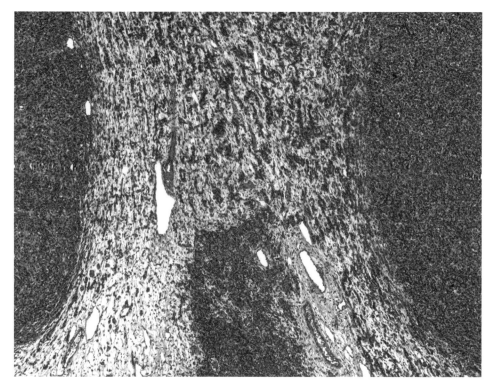

FIGURE 12.32

Intermediate-differentiated Sertoli–Leydig cell tumor. Cellular nodules and anastomosing cords are set in an edematous background.

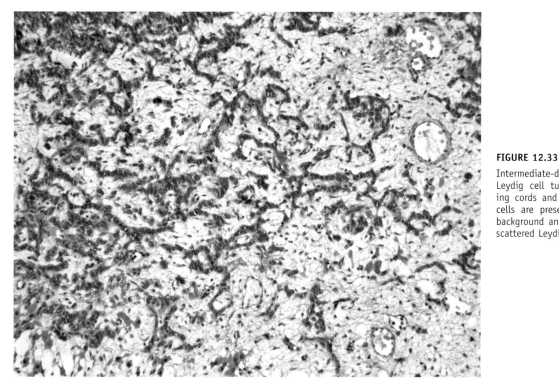

FIGURE 12.33

Intermediate-differentiated Sertoli–Leydig cell tumor. Interanastomosing cords and trabeculae of Sertoli cells are present in an edematous background and are associated with scattered Leydig cells.

Retiform component is seen in approximately 15 % of intermediate and poorly differentiated SLCTs. It is characterized by growth patterns that simulate those of the rete testis. There is an irregular network of elongated, often slit-like tubules and cysts containing papillae that may be short and rounded or blunt (Figure 12.36). The cysts may contain eosinophilic secretion resembling thyroid tissue. The papillary cores are often hyalinized, but may also be fibrous or edematous (Figure 12.36). The tubules, papillae, and cysts are typically lined by a single layer of cuboidal cells with scant cytoplasm, round to oval nuclei, and variable mitotic activity. The intervening stroma may be cellular and fibromatous with focal hyalinization, or may be composed of immature cellular mesenchyme. These tumors frequently show areas with the typical growth

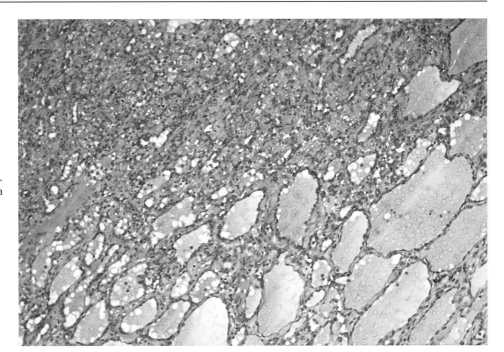

FIGURE 12.34

Intermediate-differentiated Sertoli–Leydig cell tumor. Marked edema produces a microcystic appearance.

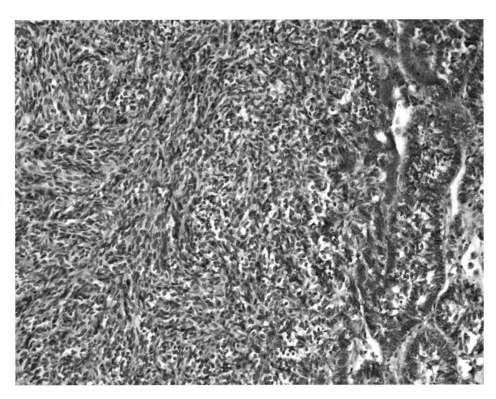

FIGURE 12.35

Poorly differentiated Sertoli–Leydig cell tumor. A diffuse sarcomatoid growth is focally associated with tubular formation.

patterns seen in intermediate and poorly differentiated SLCTs.

Heterologous elements occur in approximately 20 % of SLCTs, most commonly in the moderately differentiated category but they are also seen in poorly differentiated SLCTs. The most common heterologous element is mucinous epithelium of gastrointestinal type, which is present in almost 90 % of these tumors (Figure 12.37). The mucinous epithelium is usually morphologically benign, but occasionally has the appearance of a borderline tumor or a low-grade carcinoma. Typically, the glands and cysts show deeply eosinophilic secretion in their lumens. In approximately half of the cases with argentaffin cells, microscopic foci of carcinoid are present, with insular carcinoid being the most common type. Mesenchymal heterologous elements are usually found in tumors with a sarcomatoid background and may represent a large component of the tumor (up to 40 %). They include immature-appearing (fetal) cartilage and immature skeletal muscle, which may be either intimately admixed with the Sertoli–Leydig cell component or may be the sole element in large areas of the tumor (Figure 12.38).

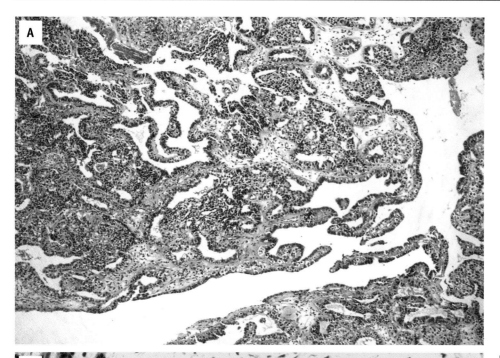

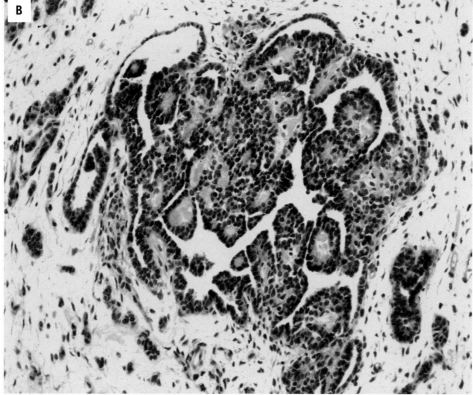

FIGURE 12.36

Retiform Sertoli–Leydig cell tumor. Prominent retiform growth (A). Papillae are small and rounded with hyalinized cores (B).

In 5 % of cases they may coexist with epithelial heterologous elements in the same tumor. Rarely, hepatic differentiation or foci of neuroblastoma may be seen.

Finally, as these patients are typically in their reproductive age, it is worth remembering that pregnancy may variably alter the architecture of these tumors secondary to prominent edema and the number of Leydig cells may be considerably increased.

ANCILLARY STUDIES

IMMUNOHISTOCHEMISTRY

The Sertoli cells are typically positive for vimentin and cytokeratin, but negative for EMA. They are also usually positive for CD99 and CD10, and may be posi-

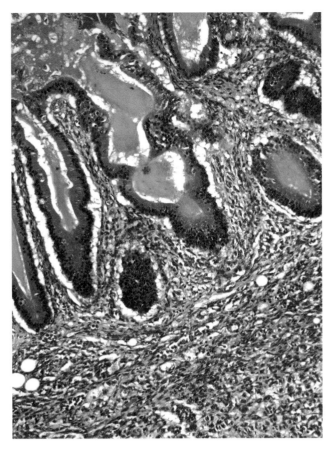

FIGURE 12.37
Sertoli–Leydig cell tumor with heterologous elements. Benign gastro-intestinal-type mucinous epithelium is seen next to poorly differentiated SCLT.

tive for WT-1, smooth muscle actin, and S-100. The Sertoli cells and the Leydig cells are both typically positive for inhibin, calretinin and CD56. Leydig cells are also typically positive for vimentin, frequently stain for melan-A and CD10.

ULTRASTRUCTURAL EXAMINATION

Diagnostic features include Sertoli cells forming tubules surrounded by basal lamina; cells with tight junctions, desmosomes, as well as abundant rough endoplasmic reticulum and lipid; microvilli; and junctional complexes. The Sertoli cells may contain noncrystalline parallel arrays of Charcot–Böttcher microfilaments. The Leydig cells have oval nuclei with regular contours and large nucleoli, abundant smooth endoplasmic reticulum, lipid droplets, mitochondria, and secondary lysosomes containing lipochrome pigment. Reinke crystals and their filamentous precursors may be seen.

DIFFERENTIAL DIAGNOSIS

Typical SLCTs should be differentiated from sertoli cell tumor (SCT), endometrioid carcinoma with sex cord-

like differentiation, and tubular Krukenberg tumor. The retiform variant may mimic serous neoplasia or yolk sac tumor, whereas SLCTs with heterologous differentiation should be distinguished from immature teratoma and carcinosarcoma. SLCTs are distinguished from *SCTs* by the presence of more than occasional Leydig cells or heterologous elements in SLCTs. In these cases, extensive sampling is very important. *Endometrioid carcinoma with sex cord features* may form cords and pseudotubules and the stroma is frequently fibromatous and may contain luteinized stromal cells, thus mimicking a SLCT. Typical areas of endometrioid carcinoma (e.g., areas showing squamous differentiation or luminal mucin) are almost always present, commonly in an adenofibromatous background or adjacent to endometriosis. In difficult cases, inhibin and EMA are the most helpful markers as endometrioid carcinomas are inhibin negative and EMA positive in contrast to SLCTs. *Krukenberg tumor* may mimic a SLCT as it is typically associated with stromal luteinization (and secondary virilization), may show tubular formation, and may have alternating hyper- and hypocellular areas. However, Krukenberg tumors are typically bilateral, and contain atypical cells, including signet-ring cells with mucin. Although the retiform variant of SLCT may mimic the growth of a *serous tumor*, conventional areas of intermediate differentiation associated with Leydig cells as well as the absence of tufting and ciliated cells in SLCT aid in this distinction. The retiform SLCT may also mimic a *yolk sac tumor*, as both occur in young patients, may have prominent hypocellular stroma, and share some architectural patterns, including microcystic and papillary. However, about one-third of patients with SLCTs have androgenic manifestations, which is in contrast to yolk sac tumors, which, although they may have peripheral stromal luteinization, do not usually have androgenic manifestations. Finally, the cells in yolk sac tumors are cytologically more primitive and stain with AFF. Sometimes SLCT with heterologous elements may mimic a *carcinosarcoma* especially when the stroma is cellular and primitive. However, carcinosarcomas occur in postmenopausal women, they are not virilizing and show high-grade müllerian-type epithelium. If cartilage is present, it is not of fetal type, but rather neoplastic in appearance. SLCTs with heterologous elements are most often misdiagnosed as *teratomas*, but the common constituents of teratomas, such as squamous epithelium, skin appendages, and respiratory epithelium, have not been reported in SLCTs. In addition, neuroectodermal tissues are very rare in these neoplasms, in contrast to their high frequency in teratomas. The diagnosis of SLCT with heterologous elements rests on finding a Sertoli–Leydig cell component, which is almost always of intermediate differentiation.

PROGNOSIS AND THERAPY

Stage, degree of differentiation, and presence of heterologous elements or retiform component are the most

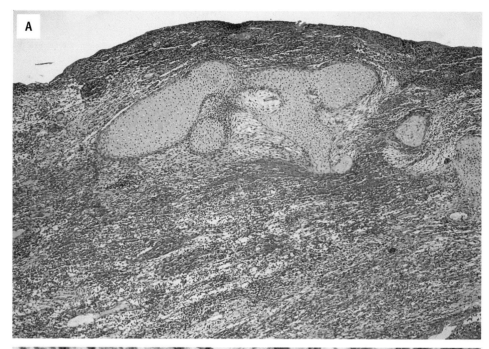

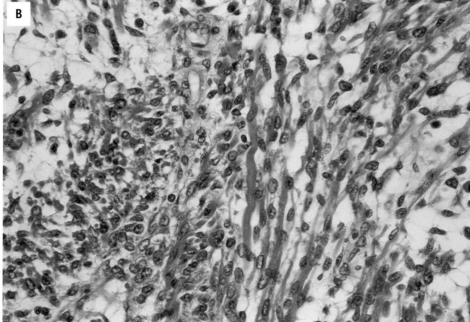

FIGURE 12.38

Sertoli–Leydig cell tumor with heterologous elements. Fetal cartilage (A) and skeletal muscle (B) are seen.

important prognostic factors in these tumors. Prognosis for patients with SLCT is generally good, as approximately 80 % of patients have stage Ia tumors at the time of diagnosis. Well-differentiated SLCTs are clinically benign and approximately 12 % of all SLCTs are clinically malignant. Almost all malignant tumors have been, alone or in combination, poorly differentiated or retiform, or contained heterologous mesenchymal elements. Therapy usually consists of salpingo-oophorectomy with consideration of chemotherapy for patients with less differentiated tumors, unusual variants and ruptured intermediate differentiated tumors. Early

recurrences may occur and are more often confined to pelvis and abdomen.

SERTOLI CELL TUMOR

Sertoli cell tumors are uncommon, accounting for approximately 4 % of Sertoli stromal cell tumors.

CLINICAL FEATURES

These tumors typically occur in reproductive-aged women (average 30 years), but may occur at any age. SCTs are usually nonfunctioning, but if they are associated with endocrine manifestations, they are more frequently estrogenic (~30%), and, less commonly, show evidence of androgen or, rarely, progesterone production. These tumors can be incidental findings, however, when associated with symptomatology, the most common are abdominal pain, swelling, or menstrual abnormalities, the latter associated with functioning tumors. Rare tumors, most of them of the lipid-rich type ("folliculome lipidique") have resulted in isosexual pseudoprecocity in children. Occasionally SCTs have been associated with renin production or with the Peutz–Jeghers syndrome (PJS).

SERTOLI CELL TUMOR – FACT SHEET

Definition

▶ Ovarian tumor characterized by a proliferation of hollow or solid tubules composed of Sertoli cells, which may simulate prepubertal testicular tubules or tubules of the adult testis; Leydig cells must be absent

Incidence and Location

▶ ~4% of Sertoli-stromal cell tumors
▶ Unilateral

Morbidity and Mortality

▶ If associated with Peutz–Jeghers syndrome, risk of other tumors

Age Distribution

▶ Reproductive-aged women (mean 30 years)

Clinical Features

▶ Abdominal pain, swelling, menstrual abnormalities, or incidental finding
▶ ~30% associated with estrogenic manifestations; in children, most commonly isosexual pseudoprecocity
▶ Occasional androgen and rarely progesterone production
▶ Association with Peutz–Jeghers syndrome (mucocutaneous pigmentation, hamartomatous polyps, and occasional carcinomas of the gastrointestinal tract, adenoma malignum of the cervix, and sex cord-stromal tumors of ovary)

Prognosis and Treatment

▶ Most tumors clinically benign
▶ Most helpful prognostic indicators of adverse outcome: cytologic atypia and ≥ 5 mitoses/10 HPFs, even in stage I tumors
▶ Treatment of choice unilateral salpingo-oophorectomy

PATHOLOGIC FEATURES

GROSS FINDINGS

Sertoli cell tumors are typically unilateral, averaging 9 cm in largest dimension, with most being between 4 and 12 cm. They are characteristically solid, lobulated masses with a yellow or, less commonly, brown, tan, or white cut surface (Figure 12.39). These tumors only rarely are predominantly cystic.

SERTOLI CELL TUMOR – PATHOLOGIC FEATURES

Gross Findings

▶ Typically unilateral
▶ Average 9 (usually between 4 and 12) cm
▶ Solid, lobulated yellow or, less frequently, brown, tan or white cut surface

Microscopic Findings

▶ Well demarcated from surrounding ovarian parenchyma
▶ Tubular, cord-like, trabecular, and diffuse patterns
▶ Tubular growth most common; either solid, hollow, endometrioid-like, or anastomosing
▶ Tubules lined by bland cuboidal to columnar cells
▶ Cells with moderate pink or pale vacuolated cytoplasm and round to oval nuclei ± grooves
▶ Lipid-rich variant: cells with abundant foamy cytoplasm (folliculome lipidique)
▶ Oxyphilic variant: cells with abundant and deeply eosinophilic cytoplasm
▶ Mild cytologic atypia and < 4 mitoses/10 HPFs in most tumors
▶ Variable amounts of stroma may impart a nodular appearance
▶ Unusual features:
  – Scattered bizarre nuclei
  – Marked stromal hyalinization (sclerosing variant)

Immunohistochemical Features

▶ Vimentin, keratin (AE1/3-Cam5.2), and inhibin positive
▶ Calretinin, CD99, CD56, CD10, and WT1 frequently positive
▶ Smooth muscle actin, NSE, and S100 may be positive
▶ EMA, CK7, and chromogranin negative

Ultrastructural Features

▶ Cells with tight junctions, desmosomes, rough endoplasmic reticulum, and lipid

Differential Diagnosis

▶ Endometrioid carcinoma with sex cord-like differentiation
▶ Female adnexal tumor of probable wolffian origin
▶ Well-differentiated Sertoli–Leydig cell tumor
▶ Carcinoid
▶ Tubular Krukenberg tumor

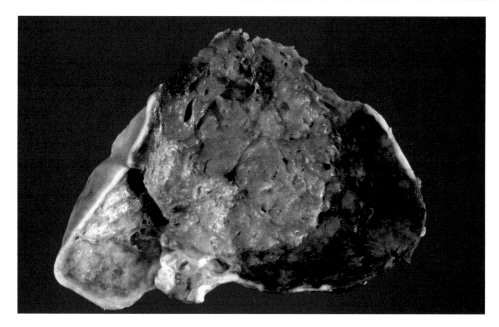

FIGURE 12.39
Sertoli cell tumor. This tumor has a solid and focally cystic, tan to brown cut surface.

MICROSCOPIC FINDINGS

On low-power examination, SCTs have either a diffuse or nodular growth. At high power, they show a tubular pattern, with the tubules ranging from hollow to solid, and round to elongated, sometimes with a complex branching architecture or with an endometrioid-like morphology (Figure 12.40). Tubular growth is the most common and predominant pattern; cord-like, trabecular, nested, and diffuse patterns are less common. The tubules are typically lined by cuboidal to columnar cells that have moderate to abundant cytoplasm that may be eosinophilic (oxyphilic) (Figure 12.41) or pale and vacuolated due to multiple small vacuoles that push the nucleus to the side. If vacuolated cells are diffusely present in the tumor, the term "lipid-rich" can be applied (Figure 12.42). Interestingly, this lipid-rich variant was originally thought to be a form of granulosa cell tumor and was termed "folliculome lipidique." The lumens of the tubules frequently contain eosinophilic material. Most of the cells have round to oval regular nuclei and nuclear grooves are common. Nuclear atypia is minimal in most tumors; however, some cells may contain scattered bizarre nuclei, such as those seen more often in granulosa cell tumors. Mitotic activity is typically low (< 4 mitoses/10 HPFs). The stroma is typically fibromatous, may be hyalinized (sclerosing variant; Figure 12.43) but varies from case to case. Areas of hemorrhage or necrosis are rare and more often seen in cytologically malignant tumors. In rare cases, minor foci of granulosa cell tumor or sex cord tumor with annular tubules may be seen.

ANCILLARY STUDIES

IMMUNOHISTOCHEMISTRY

Sertoli cell tumors are typically vimentin and keratin positive, but CK7 and EMA negative, although focal

EMA positivity has rarely been reported. They also typically stain for inhibin, they are frequently positive for CD99, CD56, and WT1, may also be positive for calretinin, CD10, and occasionally for SMA, NSE, and S-100.

ULTRASTRUCTURAL EXAMINATION

The tumor cells have tight junctions and desmosomes as well as abundant rough endoplasmic reticulum and lipid. Sertoli tubules are surrounded by basal lamina and the lumens contain microvilli. Some cells contain noncrystalline parallel arrays of Charcot–Böttcher microfilaments.

DIFFERENTIAL DIAGNOSIS

Sertoli cell tumors may be confused with a variety of primary and metastatic tumors to the ovary. The most common entities that fall into the differential diagnosis include endometrioid carcinoma, female adnexal tumor of probable wolffian origin (FATPWO), well-differentiated SLCT, and tubular Krukenberg tumor. *Endometrioid carcinoma* may have histologic features that resemble those of SCTs, including tubular and cord-like growth, fibromatous stroma and grooved nuclei. In addition, some endometrioid carcinomas may contain small clusters or isolated cells consistent with luteinized stromal cells surrounding the epithelial elements. Clinically, endometrioid carcinoma typically occurs at an older age. Morphologically, typical areas of endometrioid carcinoma, often with squamous or mucinous metaplasia, are almost always present, merging with the Sertoli-like areas. In some cases, there is an adenofibromatous background or associated endometriosis. In contrast to SCTs, endometrioid carcinomas are inhibin-negative and CK 7 and EMA positive, including those with sex cord-like

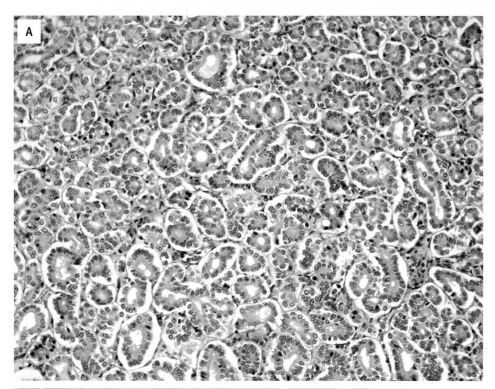

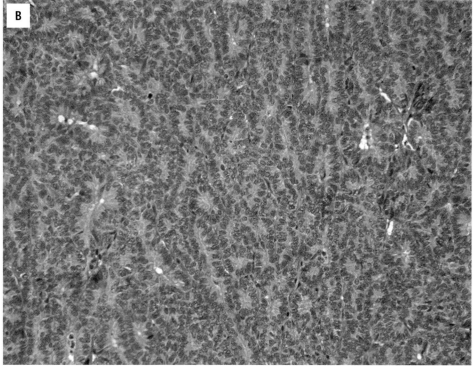

FIGURE 12.40
Sertoli cell tumor. The well-formed Sertoli tubules are frequently hollow (A) but may be solid (B).

features. *FATPWOs* more frequently occur in the broad ligament; however, they may predominantly involve the ovary and be mistaken for SCTs since they may form pseudotubular structures with cells that have a *slightly overlapping* cytologic appearance. In contrast to SCTs, FATPWO are characterized by an admixture of slit-like, cystic, and solid areas composed of small oval or spindle-shaped cells, which are not characteristic of SCTs. Although FATPWO may be positive for inhibin, staining is only weak and focal. SCTs are differentiated from *well-differentiated SLCTs* by the presence of abundant Leydig cells in between the lobules of Sertoli cells. Even though occasionally, SCTs can contain rare Leydig cells, the presence of Leydig cells should strongly raise the

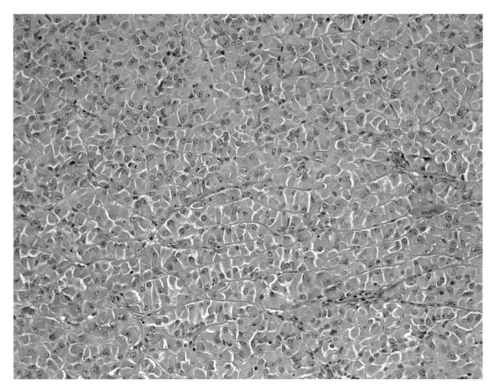

FIGURE 12.41

Sertoli cell tumor. The tumor is composed of cells with abundant eosinophilic cytoplasm (oxyphilic variant).

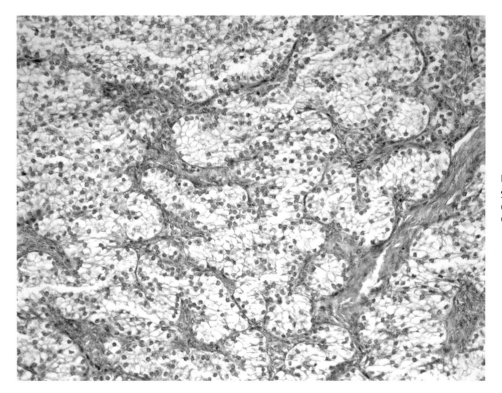

FIGURE 12.42

Sertoli cell tumor. The tumor consists of cells with abundant lipid-rich cytoplasm ("folliculome lipidique").

possibility of a well-differentiated SLCT and additional sampling should be considered. Furthermore, the presence of heterologous components also strongly supports the diagnosis of SLCT. Carcinoid tumor may be confused with SCT as both may have tubules and cords.

However, carcinoid shows distinctive nuclear features (e.g., salt and pepper chromatin), red cytoplasmic granules, frequent fibromatous background, and common association with a dermoid cyst. Immunohistochemistry for neuroendocrine markers is of limited value, with

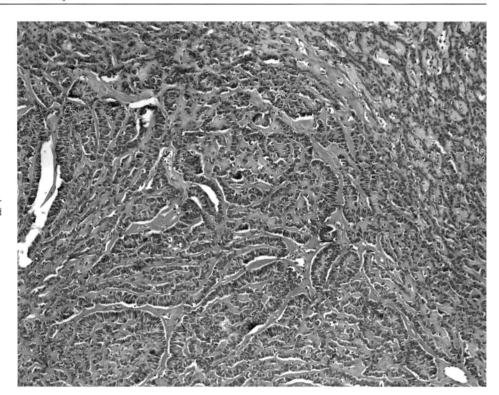

FIGURE 12.43
Sertoli cell tumor. Prominent sclerosis of the stroma compresses and distorts the neoplastic tubules.

inhibin and calretinin being may help. Occasionally, *Krukenberg tumors* may display striking tubular growth with prominent luteinized stroma and be associated with estrogenic manifestations, and therefore may be confused with a SCT. The presence of an extraovarian primary tumor, frequent bilateral ovarian involvement, spread of tumor elsewhere in the abdomen, typical microscopic features, including the presence of signet-ring cells, which stain positively for mucin, and some degree of cytologic atypia establish a diagnosis of Krukenberg tumor.

PROGNOSIS AND THERAPY

Sertoli cell tumors generally have a good prognosis which is related to tumor stage and degree of differentiation. The most useful histologic features that predict behavior include nuclear atypia and mitotic activity. Patients with adverse outcome have tumors with cytologic atypia and > 5 mitoses/10 HPFs. As most SCTs are clinically benign, they can be treated by salpingo-oophorectomy.

SEX CORD-STROMAL TUMORS OF MIXED OR UNCLASSIFIED TYPES

Sex cord-stromal tumors in the mixed category include gynandroblastoma (when there are > 10% of granulosa stromal and Sertoli stromal cell components) and SCTAT. Unclassified sex cord-stromal tumors account for < 10% of all sex cord-stromal tumors. This diagnosis should be considered when a tumor does not fulfill the morphologic features of the well-characterized sex cord-stromal tumors. In this section, only SCTAT will be discussed.

SEX CORD TUMOR WITH ANNULAR TUBULES

CLINICAL FEATURES

One-third of tumors are associated with PJS, a rare autosomal-dominant disorder characterized by gastrointestinal hamartomatous polyposis, mucocutaneous pigmentation, adenoma malignum of the cervix, and carcinoma of the gastrointestinal tract, pancreas, or breast. The clinical manifestations are different if the tumor is seen with or without the PJS. Patients range in age from 4 to 76 years. Patients with SCTAT in the setting of a PJS have an average age at diagnosis of 27 years and those without PJS average 34 years. Almost all SCTATs in patients with PJS are small and found incidentally. In contrast, patients without PJS often have a palpable pelvic mass and 40% have estrogenic manifestations, including isosexual pseudoprecocity. Rarely, progesterone production may occur.

SEX CORD TUMOR WITH ANNULAR TUBULES – FACT SHEET

Definition

▸ Sex cord tumor characterized by simple and complex ring-like tubules

Incidence and Location

▸ In Peutz–Jeghers syndrome (PJS):
  – Very common
  – Bilateral in two-thirds
▸ Without PJS:
  – Rare
  – 95% unilateral

Morbidity and Mortality

▸ Complications in patients with PJS secondary to adenoma malignum of cervix (15% of cases) or other tumors
▸ In the absence of PJS, 20% malignant with lymph node metastases
▸ Late recurrences and death from disease

Age Distribution

▸ 4–76 years
▸ If associated PJS, younger age at presentation (average 27 years)
▸ If no association with PJS, average age at presentation 34 years

Clinical Features

▸ Association with PJS in one-third of cases
▸ Typically incidental finding in patients with PJS
▸ Palpable mass if no PJS
▸ Estrogenic manifestations in 40%, including isosexual pseudoprecocity
▸ Rarely progesterone production

Prognosis and Treatment

▸ If associated with PJS, conservative management; however, significant risk of adenoma malignum
▸ Unilateral salpingo-oophorectomy with staging, including lymph nodes, for patients without PJS and stage Ia tumors
▸ Tumors with nuclear atypia and increased mitotic activity more likely to behave aggressively
▸ Cytoreductive surgery for recurrences

SEX CORD TUMOR WITH ANNULAR TUBULES – PATHOLOGIC FEATURES

Gross Findings

In Patients with Peutz–Jeghers Syndrome (PJS)
▸ Incidental finding
▸ Multiple and bilateral small ≤ 3 cm yellow nodules

In Patients without PJS
▸ 0.5–33 cm
▸ Solid yellow cut surface
▸ Cystic change, hemorrhage, or necrosis

Microscopic Findings

▸ Simple tubules or complex patterns with multiple anastomosing tubules
▸ Tubules surround central hyaline material, with nuclei oriented both peripherally and centrally, leaving an intervening pale anuclear zone
▸ In PJS, multiple tumorlets with scattered simple tubules or clusters of tubules associated with calcifications
▸ Nuclear pleomorphism and up to 10 mitoses/10 HPFs in malignant tumors
▸ Foci of typical Sertoli cell tumor or microfollicular granulosa cell tumor in some cases

Immunohistochemical Features

▸ Inhibin and calretinin positive

Differential Diagnosis

▸ Gonadoblastoma
▸ Sertoli cell tumor
▸ Granulosa cell tumor

PATHOLOGIC FEATURES

GROSS FINDINGS

In patients with PJS, the tumors are typically multiple and small (< 3 cm) but may be seen grossly as yellow nodules (25 %) and are frequently bilateral (two thirds). In patients without PJS, the tumors are typically unilateral, they range from 0.5 to 33 cm, and they usually have a solid yellow cut surface. Some tumors may show cyst formation, hemorrhage, or necrosis.

MICROSCOPIC FINDINGS

At low-power scrutiny, the tumor is characterized by simple and complex ring-shaped tubules (Figure 12.44A). The tubules encircle hyalinized basement membrane-like material with a round to oval shape. The simple pattern consists of a single tubule with central hyaline material, having nuclei located both at the periphery and centrally with intervening anuclear pale cytoplasm (ring-like appearance) (Figure 12.44B). In the complex pattern, there are anastomosing tubules around multiple deposits of hyaline material that in some cases are continuous with similar material surrounding the tubules. In patients with PJS, there are multiple little tumors composed of single or complex tubules throughout the ovarian parenchyma frequently associated with calcifications. The cells have abundant pale cytoplasm and the nuclei are round to oval with occasional grooves and single small nucleoli. Mitotic figures are absent to rare in most cases. Tumors that behave in a malignant fashion may have nuclear pleomorphism and up to 10 mitoses/10 HPFs. Some tumors, usually not associated with PJS, have foci of typical SCT or microfollicular granulosa cell tumor.

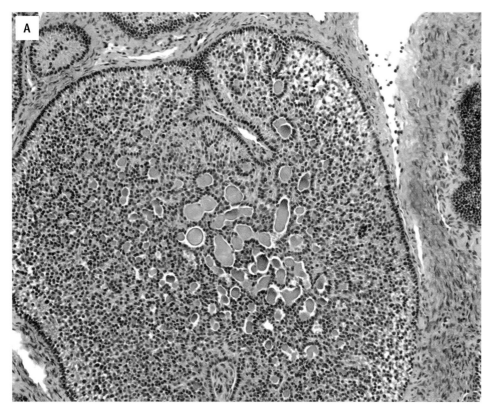

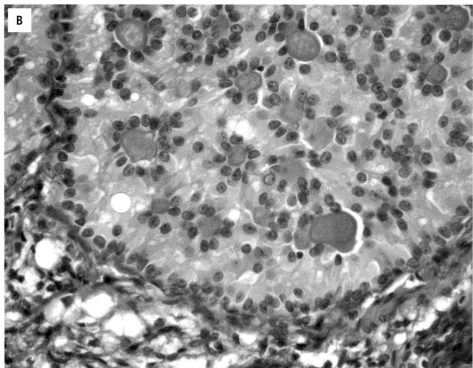

FIGURE 12.44

Sex cord-stromal tumor with annular tubules. The tumor is composed of simple and complex ring-shaped tubules (A) with nuclei located both at the periphery and centrally with intervening anuclear pale cytoplasm (B).

ANCILLARY STUDIES

IMMUNOHISTOCHEMISTRY

These tumors are typically positive for inhibin and calretinin.

ULTRASTRUCTURAL EXAMINATION

The tubules have basal lamina within and surrounding the lumens. The irregular and indented nuclei are located at the basal and luminal poles of the lining cells. Some of the tubules may have a close resemblance to seminiferous tubules lined by Sertoli cells, but they may also blend with cells resembling granulosa cells. Rarely, Charcot–Böttcher crystalloids are found.

DIFFERENTIAL DIAGNOSIS

Gonadoblastoma may resemble SCTAT, however, it has a germ cell component and is typically found in a setting of abnormal gonadal development (most often phenotypic females who are virilized). As in some instances SCTAT may have areas of *granulosa cell tumor or SCT*, and patients with PJS can also have SCTs, these tumors may also enter into the differential diagnosis. However, SCTAT areas are a minor component of SCTs or granulosa cell tumors with typical areas predominating.

PROGNOSIS AND THERAPY

In patients with PJS, SCTAT is almost always benign. However, a significant percentage of these patients also have adenoma malignum of the cervix (15 %), which may be responsible for a poor outcome. In patients without PJS, approximately 20 % of SCTATs behave in a malignant fashion. Unilateral salpingo-oophorectomy and staging are appropriate for young patients with stage Ia disease. These tumors have a greater tendency for lymph node metastases than other sex cord tumors; thus, lymph node dissection should be included as part of the staging operation. Recurrences are often late and cytoreductive surgery is indicated in these cases.

STEROID CELL TUMORS

Steroid cell tumors are composed entirely of hormone-producing cells that resemble lutein cells, Leydig cells, or adrenal cortical cells. These rare neoplasms comprising approximately 0.1 % of all ovarian tumors are divided into three groups: (1) stromal luteoma; (2) Leydig cell tumor; and (3) steroid cell tumor, not otherwise specified.

STROMAL LUTEOMA

These benign tumors account for 23 % of ovarian steroid cell tumors. They are thought to originate from the ovarian stroma as they are typically centered within the ovarian parenchyma and are associated with stromal hyperthecosis.

STROMAL LUTEOMA – FACT SHEET

Definition
- Benign steroid cell tumor lacking crystals of Reinke, frequently associated with stromal hyperthecosis

Incidence and Location
- ~ 20% of steroid cell tumors
- > 95% unilateral

Morbidity and Mortality
- Related to endometrial neoplasia

Age Distribution
- 80% of patients postmenopausal

Clinical Features
- Abnormal vaginal bleeding most common presentation
- Estrogenic manifestations in 60% of patients
- Virilization in 12% of patients
- Sometimes incidental finding

Prognosis and Treatment
- Excellent prognosis
- Excision/oophorectomy

CLINICAL FEATURES

Eighty percent of patients are postmenopausal, with a reported age range of 26–74 years. While some of the tumors are discovered incidentally, most patients present with abnormal vaginal bleeding thought to be related to estrogenic manifestations (endometrium showing variable degrees of hyperplasia or even carcinoma), and 12 % have androgenic manifestations. Rarely, stromal luteoma has been associated with acanthosis nigricans.

PATHOLOGIC FEATURES

GROSS FINDINGS

More than 95 % of tumors are unilateral. They range in size from 0.5 to 2.9 cm and are typically centered within the ovarian parenchyma. They are well circumscribed and have a gray-white to yellow-brown cut surface.

MICROSCOPIC FINDINGS

At low-power magnification, the tumors are well circumscribed but unencapsulated (Figure 12.45). They are composed of polygonal cells that are arranged diffusely, in nests and cords. Not infrequently, associated degenerative changes may produce pseudoglandular

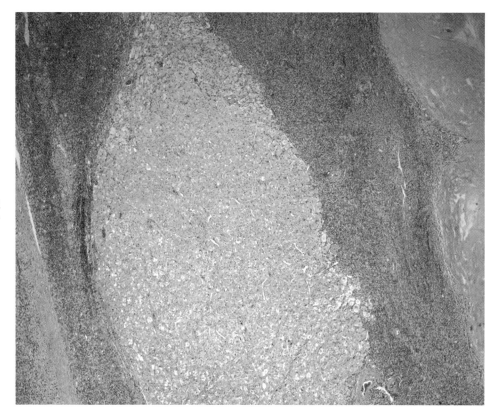

FIGURE 12.45
Stromal luteoma. The tumor is well circumscribed and completely embedded in the ovarian cortex.

STROMAL LUTEOMA – PATHOLOGIC FEATURES

Gross Findings

▶ Well-circumscribed, gray-white to yellow-brown nodule within the ovarian parenchyma
▶ Typically < 3 cm

Microscopic Findings

▶ Polygonal cells arranged diffusely or in nests and cords
▶ Degenerative changes may produce gland-like spaces
▶ Cells with abundant eosinophilic or pale slightly granular cytoplasm and small round nuclei with prominent nucleoli
▶ Absent or rare mitoses
▶ Lipochrome pigment but no Reinke crystals

Immunohistochemical Features

▶ Inhibin and calretinin positive
▶ Keratin focally positive

Differential Diagnosis

▶ Stromal hyperthecosis
▶ Nonhilar Leydig cell tumor
▶ Luteinized thecoma
▶ Granulosa cell tumor, luteinized
▶ Pregnancy luteoma

---

spaces (Figure 12.46). The cells have abundant eosinophilic to pale, slightly granular cytoplasm often containing lipochrome pigment, but no Reinke crystals. The nuclei are round and small, and often have prominent nucleoli; mitoses are rare. Stroma is sparse in most stromal luteomas, but in 20% it can be abundant and hyalinized. Most tumors are associated with stromal hyperthecosis in the same or opposite ovary, whereas slight hilus cell hyperplasia is uncommon.

ANCILLARY STUDIES

IMMUNOHISTOCHEMISTRY

The tumor cells are positive for inhibin and calretinin. Most tumor cells also express vimentin and some may have focal staining for keratin.

DIFFERENTIAL DIAGNOSIS

Stromal hyperthecosis can have nodular aggregates of lutein cells that verge on small luteomas; with a size of 0.5 cm being the arbitrary dividing line between the two lesions. *Leydig cell tumor of the nonhilar type* occurs in the same age group. However, these tumors are typically androgenic and on microscopic examination contain Reinke crystals. *Luteinized thecoma* also occurs more commonly in perimenopausal women and it can contain aggregates of luteinized cells, but the finding of fibromatous stroma in this tumor is not a feature of stromal luteoma. *Granulosa cell tumors* can be extensively

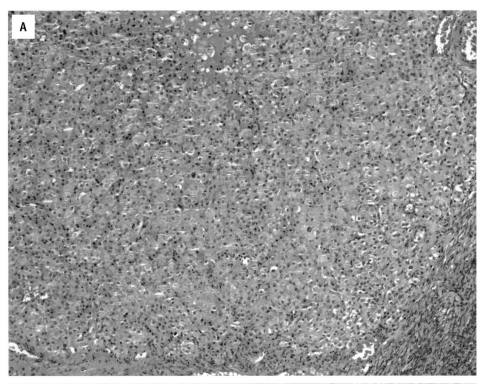

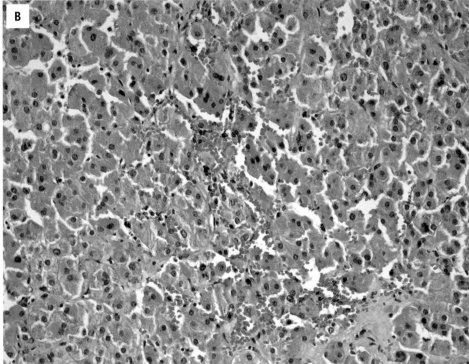

FIGURE 12.46

Stromal luteoma. The tumor is composed of sheets of cells with abundant eosinophilic cytoplasm (A) and contains irregularly shaped spaces filled with hemorrhage secondary to artifact (B).

luteinized, but more typical architectural and cytologic features should be present elsewhere in the tumor. *Pregnancy luteoma* can be histologically identical to stromal luteoma. The patient's young age, history of pregnancy, and multifocality of the pregnancy luteoma help in their

distinction. The spaces secondary to degeneration in some stromal luteomas may give rise to consideration of an adenocarcinoma or even a vascular tumor. However, luteoma cells lack atypia, are positive for inhibin and negative for CEA.

PROGNOSIS AND THERAPY

As stromal luteomas are benign, treatment is limited to unilateral oophorectomy or tumor excision if possible.

LEYDIG CELL TUMOR

This subtype of steroid cell tumor is characterized by the presence of Reinke crystals, identified either by light or electron microscopy, and comprises 19 % of all steroid cell tumors. They are divided into hilus cell tumor and nonhilar type (very rare), based on location and presumed cell of origin.

CLINICAL FEATURES

Patients range in age from 32 to 82 (average 58) years. They most often present with androgenic manifestations due to elevated levels of testosterone, while estrogenic effects are rare.

LEYDIG CELL TUMOR – FACT SHEET

Definition
▸ Steroid cell tumor characterized by presence of Reinke crystals

Incidence and Location
▸ 19% of steroid cell tumors
▸ If located in hilum (most common): hilus cell tumor
▸ If located within ovarian parenchyma: Leydig cell tumor, nonhilar type (very rare)

Morbidity and Mortality
▸ Secondary to androgenic manifestations

Age Distribution
▸ Average age 58 years

Clinical Features
▸ Most often androgenic manifestations
▸ Rarely, estrogenic manifestations

Prognosis and Treatment
▸ Unilateral oophorectomy as they are benign

PATHOLOGIC FEATURES

GROSS FINDINGS

Leydig cell tumors are circumscribed and small, with an average size of 2.4 cm, and only rarely are bilateral. Most tumors are centered in or adjacent to the ovarian hilus. They have a solid and soft, yellow-tan or red-brown cut surface (Figure 12.47).

MICROSCOPIC FINDINGS

On low-power examination, the tumors are well defined but unencapsulated, and the cells may show either a diffuse or lobulated growth (Figure 12.48). The stroma in between the lobules may be dense and hyalinized or edematous. Some tumors have a very characteristic arrangement of the cells consisting of cellular areas with clustering of nuclei separated by eosinophilic anuclear zones (Figure 12.49A). Another typical, but not constant, feature is the finding of fibrinoid replacement of blood vessel walls (Figure 12.49B). Degenerative changes can produce pseudoglands. The cells are round or polygonal in shape with moderate to abundant eosinophilic or vacuolated (lipid-filled) cytoplasm.

LEYDIG CELL TUMOR – PATHOLOGIC FEATURES

Gross Findings
▸ Typically unilateral and centered in the hilus
▸ Usually < 3 cm and well circumscribed
▸ Yellow-tan or red-brown solid and soft cut surface

Microscopic Findings
▸ Diffuse or lobular growth of round to polygonal cells
▸ Anuclear eosinophilic zones separated by areas of nuclear clustering
▸ Fibrinoid replacement of blood vessel walls
▸ Cells with abundant eosinophilic or vacuolated cytoplasm with Reinke crystals and lipochrome pigment
▸ Round nuclei with small nucleoli, nuclear pseudoinclusions; rarely, bizarre nuclei
▸ Rare mitoses

Immunohistochemical Features
▸ Inhibin, calretinin, CD56, and vimentin positive
▸ Occasionally keratin and actin positive

Ultrastructural Features
▸ Hexagonal shape of Reinke crystals on cross-section
▸ Cross-hatched appearance of interior of Reinke crystals
▸ Intracytoplasmic eosinophilic spheres (precursor of Reinke crystals)

Differential Diagnosis
▸ Stromal luteoma
▸ Stromal hyperthecosis

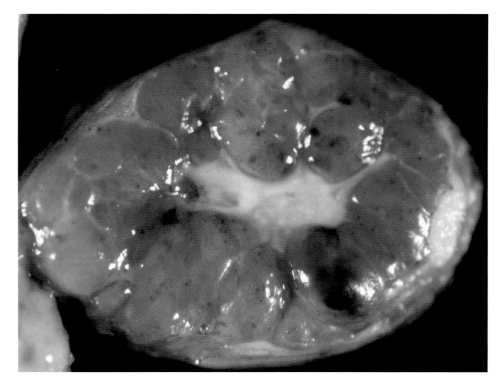

FIGURE 12.47

Leydig cell tumor. Solid tumor with a tan to yellow cut surface.

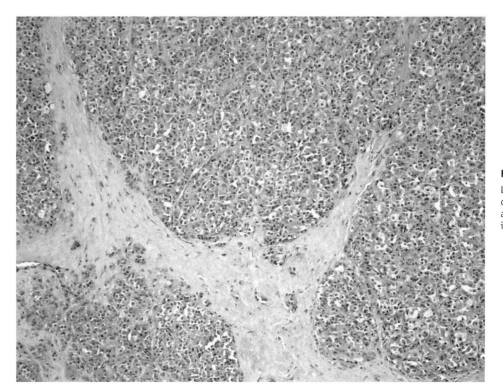

FIGURE 12.48

Leydig cell tumor. Lobules of tumor cells are separated by variable amounts of collagenous stroma imparting a nodular architecture.

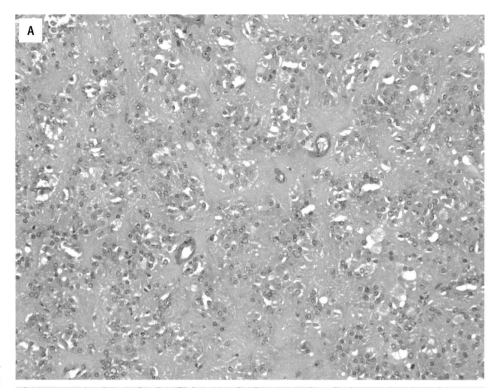

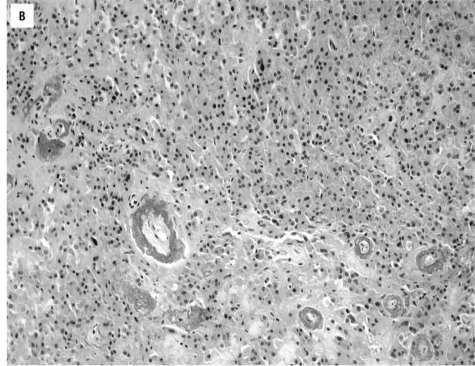

FIGURE 12.49

Leydig cell tumor. Eosinophilic anuclear zones are flanked by clustering of Leydig cell nuclei (A). Fibrinoid changes of vessel walls are striking (B).

Reinke crystals and lipochrome pigment are present in the cytoplasm in many tumor cells (Figure 12.50). The nuclei are round with small nucleoli, intranuclear cytoplasmic inclusions are often present, and bizarre nuclei are seen in a small number of tumors; mitotic figures are rare. Although Reinke crystals are required for a definitive diagnosis of a hilus cell tumor, the diagnosis is favored in a crystal-free tumor that is located in the hilus, juxtaposed to nonmedullated nerve fibers, and has a background of nodular hilar cell hyperplasia, cellular areas with nuclear clustering, and fibrinoid change in tumor vessels.

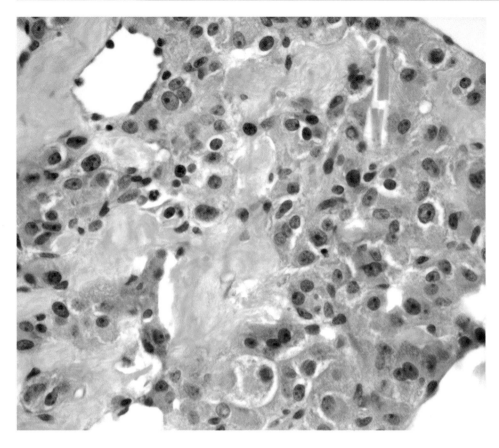

FIGURE 12.50
Leydig cell tumor. Reinke crystalloids are apparent.

ANCILLARY STUDIES

IMMUNOHISTOCHEMISTRY

Leydig cell tumors are positive for inhibin, calretinin, CD56, and vimentin. Keratin and actin can be positive in some cases.

ULTRASTRUCTURAL EXAMINATION

The tumor cells show abundant smooth endoplasmic reticulum, lipid, mitochondria, and lysozymes containing lipochrome pigment. Reinke crystals show a hexagonal shape on cross-section. The interior of the Reinke crystals have a cross-hatched appearance and intracytoplasmic eosinophilic spheres may be identified.

DIFFERENTIAL DIAGNOSIS

Leydig cell tumors are distinguished from *stromal luteomas* by the presence of Reinke crystals. Other considerations are similar to those discussed under stromal luteoma.

PROGNOSIS AND THERAPY

There are no well-documented cases of malignant behavior, therefore, unilateral oophorectomy is adequate therapy. Virilizing symptoms may regress following removal of the tumor.

STEROID CELL TUMOR, NOT OTHERWISE SPECIFIED

The category of steroid cell tumor, not otherwise specified consists of tumors that do not have diagnostic features of either stromal luteoma or Leydig cell tumor, and comprises 58% of all steroid cell tumors.

CLINICAL FEATURES

The patients range in age from 2 to 80 years, but tend to be younger than patients with other steroid cell tumors, with an average age of 43 years. Half of the

STEROID CELL TUMOR, NOT OTHERWISE SPECIFIED – FACT SHEET

Definition

▸ Steroid cell tumor that cannot be classified as stromal luteoma or Leydig cell tumor

Incidence and Location

▸ 58% of steroid cell tumors
▸ > 90% unilateral

Morbidity and Mortality

▸ Extraovarian spread at time of diagnosis in ~ 20%
▸ 43% clinically malignant

Age Distribution

▸ Average age 43 (range 2–80) years
▸ Younger age than patients with Leydig cell tumor or stromal luteoma

Clinical Features

▸ Androgenic manifestations in 50% of patients (virilization, hirsutism)
▸ Rarely, estrogenic manifestations
▸ Nonspecific symptoms; swelling and/or pain
▸ Occasionally Cushing syndrome
▸ Elevated serum levels of 17-ketosteroids, testosterone, and androstenedione

Prognosis and Treatment

▸ Extraovarian spread in 20% of tumors at diagnosis
▸ Extensive extraovarian spread in tumors with Cushing syndrome
▸ Clinically malignant tumors associated with > 2 mitoses/10 HPFs, necrosis, > 7 cm, hemorrhage, high-grade nuclear atypia
▸ Unilateral salpingo-oophorectomy in young patients with stage Ia disease
▸ Total abdominal hysterectomy and bilateral salpingo-oophorectomy if fertility not an issue or high-stage disease
▸ Late recurrences

STEROID CELL TUMOR, NOT OTHERWISE SPECIFIED – PATHOLOGIC FEATURES

Gross Findings

▸ Average size 8.4 cm
▸ Usually well circumscribed
▸ Lobulated or multinodular, solid, yellow to orange to brown cut surface
▸ Occasional hemorrhage and/or necrosis

Microscopic Findings

▸ Diffuse growth or clusters and cords
▸ Scant intervening stroma associated with a prominent vascular network
▸ Medium to large cells with distinct cell membranes
▸ Granular eosinophilic or vacuolated cytoplasm with frequent lipochrome pigment
▸ Round and centrally placed nucleus with single nucleolus
▸ Frequently no cytologic atypia and at most 2 mitoses/10 HPFs
▸ Grade 1 to 3 nuclear atypia ± mitotic rate ≤ 15/10 HPFs in 40% of tumors
▸ Occasionally foci of necrosis and hemorrhage

Immunohistochemical Features

▸ Inhibin and calretinin positive (calretinin more sensitive)
▸ Melan-A, CD10, CD56, and vimentin frequently positive
▸ S100 and HBM-45 positive in some cases
▸ MART-1 typically negative

Ultrastructural Features

▸ Cytoplasmic lipid droplets
▸ Microvilli covering most of the cell surface
▸ Basal lamina only on nonvillous portion of cell surface

Differential Diagnosis

▸ Stromal luteoma
▸ Leydig cell tumor
▸ Luteinized thecoma
▸ Luteinized granulosa cell tumor
▸ Pregnancy luteoma
▸ Clear cell carcinoma/ oxyphilic endometrioid carcinoma
▸ Sertoli cell tumor
▸ Metastatic neoplasm (renal clear cell, melanoma, and adrenocortical carcinoma)

patients present because of androgenic manifestations (virilization, hirsutism), while a minority have estrogenic manifestations (postmenopausal bleeding, menorrhagia) or Cushing syndrome due to hypercortisolemia. Some patients have nonspecific complaints such as abdominal swelling or pain and some tumors are discovered incidentally. Patients typically have elevated levels of 17-ketosteroids and testosterone and androstenedione levels are also frequently elevated.

PATHOLOGIC FEATURES

GROSS FINDINGS

Ninety-four percent of the tumors are unilateral. They range in size from 1.2 to 45 (average of 8.4) cm, and are well circumscribed. Most tumors are solid, although occasionally they may be solid and cystic or predominantly cystic. They frequently have a lobulated or multinodular, and yellow to orange to brown cut surface (Figure 12.51). Hemorrhage and necrosis are present in a minority of tumors.

MICROSCOPIC FINDINGS

Most tumors have a diffuse growth (Figure 12.52), but occasionally clusters and cords of cells are seen. The intervening stroma is scant but may be abundant and hyalinized, and associated with a prominent vascular network of thin compressed vessels. The cells are medium to large in size with distinct cell membranes, and have granular eosinophilic or vacuolated cytoplasm

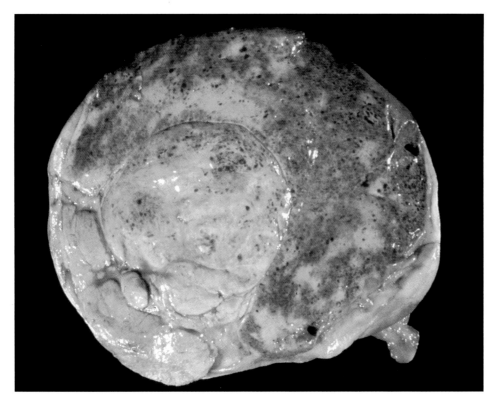

FIGURE 12.51
Steroid cell tumor, not otherwise specified. The tumor has a homogeneous tan to yellow cut surface and is focally lobulated.

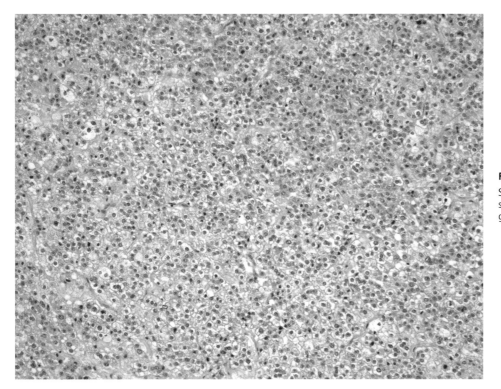

FIGURE 12.52
Steroid cell tumor, not otherwise specified. The tumor shows a diffuse growth pattern.

in various proportions (Figure 12.53); lipochrome pigment is frequently seen. The nuclei are usually round and centrally placed with a single nucleolus (Figure 12.54), although in vacuolated cells the nuclei have a more vesicular appearance. Most tumors have no cyto-

logic atypia and at most 2 mitoses/10 HPFs. However, in 40% of cases there is grade 1 to 3 nuclear atypia, which can be accompanied by an increased mitotic rate of up to 15/10 HPFs. Foci of necrosis and hemorrhage are present in a minority of tumors.

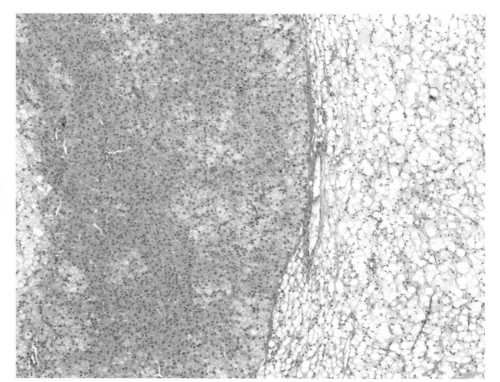

FIGURE 12.53

Steroid cell tumor, not otherwise specified. The tumor cells have abundant vacuolated or eosinophilic cytoplasm in varying proportions.

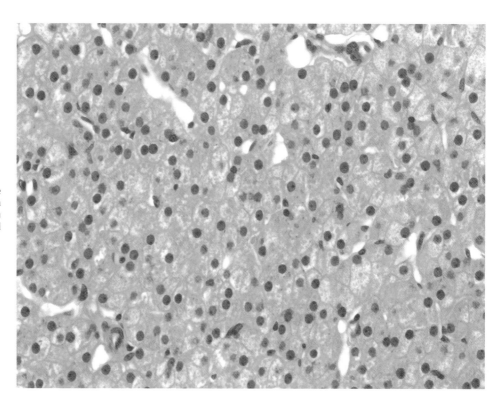

FIGURE 12.54

Steroid cell tumor, not otherwise specified. Most tumor cells have a uniform cytologic appearance with centrally located round nuclei and small nucleoli.

ANCILLARY STUDIES

HISTOCHEMISTRY AND IMMUNOHISTOCHEMISTRY

Fat stain demonstrates moderate to abundant lipid in most tumors. Inhibin and calretinin are characteristically positive, the latter being a more sensitive marker of steroid cell tumors. Vimentin, CD10 and CD56 are often positive and some tumors may stain for keratin or CD99. Melan-A (A103) is positive and focal staining for S-100 and HMB-45 has been reported. However, MART-1 (A63) is generally negative.

ULTRASTRUCTURAL EXAMINATION

The tumors show cytoplasmic droplets of lipid, abundant smooth endoplasmic reticulum, microvilli covering most of the cell surface, and basal lamina only covering the nonvillous portion of the cellular surface.

DIFFERENTIAL DIAGNOSIS

These tumors should be distinguished from the other steroid cell tumors, namely stromal luteoma and Leydig cell tumor. *Stromal luteoma* is typically confined within ovarian stroma and associated with stromal hyperthecosis whereas *Leydig cell tumor* shows a hilar location and the neoplastic cells contain Reinke crystals. Other tumors in the differential diagnosis in the stromal/sex cord-stromal category include *luteinized thecoma* and *luteinized granulosa cell tumor*. The former typically has a prominent spindle cell component and abundant reticulin fibers while the granulosa cell tumor usually shows more typical architectural and cytologic features in other areas. The nonneoplastic *pregnancy luteoma* can be difficult to separate microscopically from a steroid cell tumor, but is multifocal in half and bilateral in one-third of cases respectively, and typically regresses after delivery.

Other tumors with oxyphilic cells include *oxyphilic endometrioid adenocarcinoma* and *metastatic melanoma*. The former typically shows areas with gland formation, squamous and/or mucinous differentiation, and will stain with CK7 and EMA. Metastatic melanoma can histologically resemble a steroid cell tumor and the tumor cells also stain for melan-A, S-100, and HMB-45. Clinical history, focal presence of melanin pigment, and MART-1 positivity will facilitate the diagnosis of melanoma. When the tumor has abundant pale cytoplasm, the differential diagnosis includes clear cell carcinoma, metastatic renal cell carcinoma, and lipid-rich SCT. *Primary clear cell carcinoma* of the ovary, besides a diffuse growth, typically shows other characteristic architectural patterns, namely tubulocystic and papillary; hobnail cells are common, and the tumor diffusely expresses CK7 and EMA, but lacks inhibin and calretinin positivity. *Metastatic renal cell carcinoma* may have a diffuse growth as well as a prominent vascular network, and furthermore, both tumors frequently express CD10 and vimentin and have intracellular lipid contents. However, in renal cell carcinoma, the tumor cells also have abundant glycogen, the nuclei are frequently eccentric, and a known history of renal cell carcinoma will facilitate the diagnosis. *Lipid-rich SCT* may enter in the differential diagnosis, and in these cases, immunohistochemistry will not be of help. The diagnosis should rely upon finding more typical areas of Sertoli cell neoplasia. *Metastatic adrenocortical carcinoma* would be difficult to impossible to distinguish from a steroid cell tumor by microscopy, with clinical and radiographic correlation being required.

PROGNOSIS AND THERAPY

Nineteen percent of tumors are advanced-stage at presentation and overall approximately 43% are clinically malignant. Poor prognostic factors include ≥ 2 mitoses/10 HPFs (92% malignant), necrosis (86% malignant), size ≥ 7 cm (78% malignant), hemorrhage (77% malignant), and grade 2–3 nuclear atypia (64% malignant). Unilateral salpingo-oophorectomy and staging are the appropriate treatment in young women who have stage 1a tumors and wish to preserve fertility. For those in whom fertility is not an issue, total abdominal hysterectomy, bilateral salpingo-oophorectomy, and full staging should be performed. Patients with advanced-stage disease require cytoreductive surgery. Hirsutism and virilization may regress to some degree after resection. Although it is not always efficient, postoperative platinum-based chemotherapy is suggested for patients with advanced-stage disease. Recurrences develop more than 5 years after initial surgery in 10% of cases, and virilization may reappear with tumor recurrence.

SUGGESTED READING

Ovarian Sex Cord-Stromal Tumors – General

Clement PB, Young RH. Atlas of Gynecological Surgical Pathology. Philadelphia: WB Saunders, 2000.

Deavers MT, Malpica A, Liu J, et al. Ovarian sex cord-stromal tumors: an immunohistochemical study including a comparison of calretinin and inhibin. Mod Pathol 2003;16:584–590.

DeMay RM. The Art and Science of Cytopathology. Aspiration Cytology. Chicago: ASCP Press, 1996.

Kurman RJ (ed.) Blaustein's Pathology of the Female Genital Tract, 5th edn. New York: Springer-Verlag, 2002.

Roth LM. Recent advances in the pathology and classification of ovarian sex cord-stromal tumors. Int J Gynecol Pathol 2006;25:199–215.

Russo J, Sommers SC (eds) Tumor Diagnosis by Electron Microscopy, vol. 3. New York: Field and Wood, 1990.

Scully RE, Young RH, Clement PB. Atlas of Tumor Pathology. Tumors of the Ovary, Maldeveloped Gonads, Fallopian Tube, and Broad Ligament, third series. Washington, DC: Armed Forces Institute of Pathology, 1998.

Tavassoli FA, Devilee P (eds) Pathology and Genetics of Tumours of the Breast and Female Genital Organs. Lyon: IARC Press, 2003.

Young RH. Sex cord-stromal tumors of the ovary and testis: their similarities and differences with consideration of selected problems. Mod Pathol 2005;18:S81–S98.

Fibroma/Fibrosarcoma

Anderson B, Turner DA, Benda J. Ovarian sarcoma. Gynecol Oncol 1987;26:183–192.

Azoury RS, Woodruff JD. Primary ovarian sarcomas. Report of 43 cases from the Emil Novak Ovarian Tumor Registry. Obstet Gynecol 1971;37:920–941.

Dockerty MD, Masson JC. Ovarian fibromas: A clinical and pathologic study of two hundred and eighty-three cases. Am J Obstet Gynecol 1944;47:741–752.

Gorlin RJ. Nevoid basal-cell carcinoma (Gorlin) syndrome. Genet Med 2004;6:530–539.

Irving JA, Alkushi AM, Young RH, et al. Cellular fibromas of the ovary: a study of 75 cases including 40 mitotically active tumors emphasizing their distinction from fibrosarcoma. Am J Surg Pathol 2006;30:929–938.

Kraemer BB, Silva EG, Sniege N. Fibrosarcoma of ovary: a new component in the nevoid basal cell carcinoma syndrome. Am J Surg Pathol 1984;8:231–236.

Leung SW, Yuen PM. Ovarian fibroma: a review on the clinical characteristics, diagnostic difficulties, and management options of 23 patients. Gynecol Obstet Invest 2006;62:1–6.

Meigs JV. Fibroma of the ovary with ascites and hydrothorax: Meigs' syndrome. Am J Obstet Gynecol 1954;67:962–985.

Prat J, Scully RE. Cellular fibroma and fibrosarcomas of the ovary: a comparative clinicopathologic analysis of seventeen cases. Cancer 1981;47:2663–2670.

Singh SS, Chandra A, Majhi U. Primary fibrosarcoma of the ovary – report of two cases. Ind J Pathol Microbiol 2004;47:525–528.

Sood AK, Sorosky JI, Gelder MS, et al. Primary ovarian sarcoma: analysis of prognostic variables and the role of surgical cytoreduction. Cancer 1998;82:1731–1737.

Tsuji T, Catasus L, Prat J. Is loss of heterozygosity at 9q22.3 (PTCH geeb) and 19p13.3 (STK11 gene) involved in the pathogenesis of ovarian stromal tumors? Hum Pathol 2005;36:792–796.

Tsuji T, Kawauchi S, Utsunomiya T, et al. Fibrosarcoma versus cellular fibroma of the ovary: a comparative study of their proliferative activity and chromosome aberrations using MIB-1 immunostaining, DNA flow cytometry, and fluorescence in situ hybridization. Am J Surg Pathol 1997;21:52–59.

Thecoma

Bjorkholm E, Silfersward C. Theca-cell tumors. Clinical features and prognosis. Acta Radiol Oncol 1980;19:241–244.

McCluggage WG, Sloan JM, Boyle DD, et al. Malignant fibrothecomatous tumor of the ovary: diagnostic value of anti-inhibin immunostaining. J Clin Pathol 1998;51:868–871.

Waxman M, Vuletin JC, Urayo R, et al. Ovarian low-grade stromal sarcoma with thecomatous features: a critical reappraisal of the so-called "malignant thecoma." Cancer 1979;44:2206–2217.

Zhang J, Young RH, Arseneau J, et al. Ovarian stromal tumors containing lutein or Leydig cells (luteinized thecomas and stromal Leydig cell tumors) – a clinicopathological analysis of fifty cases. Int J Gynecol Pathol 1982;1:270–285.

Luteinized Thecoma Associated with Sclerosing Peritonitis

Bianco R, deRosa G, Staibano S, et al. Ovarian luteinized thecoma with sclerosing peritonitis in an adult woman treated with leuprolide and toremifene in complete remission at 5 years. Gynecol Oncol 2005;96:846–849.

Clement PB, Young RH, Hanna W, et al. Sclerosing peritonitis associated with luteinized thecomas of the ovary. A clinicopathological analysis of six cases. Am J Surg Pathol 1994;18:1–13.

Nishida T, Ushijima K, Watabane J, et al. Sclerosing peritonitis associated with luteinized thecoma of the ovary. Gynecol Oncol 1999;73:167–169.

Schweisguth O, Gerard-Marchant R, Plainfosse B. Bilateral nonfunctioning thecoma of the ovary in epileptic children under convulsivant therapy. Acta Pec Scand 1971;60:6–10.

Scurry J, Allen D, Dobson P. Ovarian fibromatosis, ascites and omental fibrosis. Histopathology 1996;28:81–84.

Staats PN, McCluggage WG, Clement PB, et al. Re-exploration of the distinctive ovarian lesion associated with sclerosing peritonitis: an analysis of 25 cases. Mod Pathol 2007;20:abstract 984.

Werness BA. Luteinized thecoma with sclerosing peritonitis. Arch Pathol Lab Med 1996;120:303–306.

Young RH, Scully RE. Fibromatosis and massive edema of the ovary possibly related entities: a report of 14 cases of fibromatosis and 11 cases of massive edema. Int J Gynecol Pathol 1984;3:153–178.

Sclerosing Stromal Tumor

Bildirici K, Yalcin OT, Ozalp SS, et al. Sclerosing stromal tumor of the ovary associated with Meigs' syndrome: a case report. Eur J Gynaecol Oncol 2004;25:528–529.

Chalvardjian A, Scully RE. Sclerosing stromal tumors of the ovary. Cancer 1973;31:664–670.

Kostopoulu E, Moulla A, Giakoustidis D, et al. Sclerosing stromal tumors of the ovary: a clinicopathologic, immunohistochemical and cytogenetic analysis of three cases. Eur J Gynaecol Oncol 2004;25:257–260.

Terauchi F, Onodera T, Nagashima T, et al. Sclerosing stromal tumor of the ovary with elevated CA125. J Obstet Gynaecol Res 2005;31:432–435.

Torricelli P, Caruso Lombardi A, Boselli F, et al. Sclerosing stromal tumor of the ovary: US, CT, and MRI findings. Abdom Imaging 2002;27:588–591.

Adult Granulosa Cell Tumor

Ahmed E, Young RH, Scully RE. Adult granulosa cell tumor of the ovary with foci of hepatic cell differentiation: a report of four cases and comparison with two cases of granulosa cell tumor with Leydig cells. Am J Surg Pathol 1999;23:1089–1093.

Fox H. Pathologic prognostic factors in early stage adult-type granulosa cell tumors of the ovary. Int J Gynecol Cancer 2003;13:1–4.

Freeman SA, Modesitt SC. Anastrozole therapy in recurrent ovarian adult granulosa cell tumors: a report of 2 cases. Gynecol Oncol 2006;103:755–758.

Lauszus FF, Petersen AC, Greisen J, et al. Granulosa cell tumor of the ovary: a population-based study of 37 women with stage 1 disease. Gynecol Oncol 2001;81:456–460.

Mom CH, Engelen MJA, Willemse PHB, et al. Granulosa cell tumors of the ovary: the clinical value of serum inhibin A and B levels in a large single center cohort. Gynecol Oncol. 2007;105:365–372.

Nakashima M, Young RH, Scully RE. Androgenic granulosa cell tumors of the ovary. A clinicopathologic analysis of 17 cases and review of the literature. Arch Pathol Lab Med 1984;108:786–791.

Pautier P, Lhomme C, Culine S, et al. Adult granulosa cell tumor of the ovary: a retrospective study of 45 cases. Int J Gynecol Cancer 1997;7:58–65.

Sehouli J, Drescher FS, Musted A, et al. Granulosa cell tumor of the ovary: 10 years follow-up data of 65 patients. Anticancer Res 2004;24:1223–1230.

Sharony R, Aviram R, Fisham A, et al. Granulosa cell tumors of the ovary: do they have any unique ultrastructural and color Doppler flow features? Int J Gynecol Cancer 2001;11:229–233.

Villella J, Herrmann FR, Kaul S, et al. Clinical and pathological predictive factors in women with adult-type granulosa cell tumor of the ovary. Int J Gynecol Pathol 2007;26:154–159.

Wolf JK, Mullen J, Eifel PJ, et al. Radiation treatment of advanced of recurrent granulosa cell tumor of the ovary. Gynecol Oncol 1999;73:35–41.

Young RH, Oliva E, Scully RE. Luteinized adult granulosa cell tumors of the ovary: a report of four cases. Int J Gynecol Pathol 1994;13:302–310.

Juvenile Granulosa Cell Tumor

Biscotti CV, Hart WR. Juvenile granulosa cell tumors of the ovary. Arch Pathol Lab Med 1989;113:40–46.

Calaminus G, Wessalowski R, Harms D, et al. Juvenile granulosa cell tumors of the ovary in children and adolescents: results from 33 patients registered in a prospective cooperative study. Gynecol Oncol 1997;65:447–452.

McCluggage WG. Immunoreactivity of ovarian juvenile granulosa cell tumours with epithelial membrane antigen. Histopathology 2005;46: 235–236.

Merros-Salmio L, Vettenranta K, Mottonen M, et al. Ovarian granulosa cell tumors in childhood. Pediatr Hematol Oncol 2002;19:145–156.

Young RH, Dickersin GR, Scully RE. Juvenile granulosa cell tumor of the ovary. A clinicopathological analysis of 125 cases. Am J Surg Pathol 1984;8:575–596.

Zaloudek C, Norris HJ. Granulosa tumors of the ovary in children: a clinical pathologic study of 32 cases. Am J Surg Pathol 1982;6:503–512.

Sertoli–Leydig Cell Tumor

Doussis-Anagnostopoulou IA, Remadi S, Czernobilsky B, Mucinous elements in Sertoli–Leydig and granulosa cell tumours: a reevaluation. Histopathology 1996;28:372–375.

Gagnon S, Tetu B, Silva E, et al. Frequency of alphafetoprotein production by Sertoli–Leydig cell tumors of the ovary: an immunohistochemical study of eight cases. Mod Pathol 1989;2:63–67.

Mooney EE, Nogales FF, Tavassoli FA. Hepatocytic differentiation in retiform Sertoli–Leydig cell tumors: distinguishing a heterologous element from Leydig cells. Hum Pathol 1999;30:611–617.

Prat J, Young RH, Scully RE. Ovarian Sertoli–Leydig cell tumors with heterologous elements. II. Cartilage and skeletal muscle: a clinicopathologic analysis of twelve cases. Cancer 1982;50:2465–2475.

Roth LM, Anderson MC, Govan AD, et al. Sertoli–Leydig cell tumors: a clinicopathologic study of 34 cases. Cancer 1981;48:187–197.

Roth LM, Slayton RE, Brady LW, et al. Retiform differentiation in ovarian Sertoli–Leydig cell tumors. A clinicopathologic study of six cases from a gynecologic oncology group study. Cancer 1985;55:1093–1098.

Talerman A. Ovarian Sertoli–Leydig cell tumor (androblastoma) with retiform pattern. A clinicopathologic study. Cancer 1987;60:3056–3064.

Tetu B, Ordoñez NG, Silva EG. Sertoli–Leydig cell tumor of the ovary with alpha-fetoprotein production. Arch Pathol Lab Med 1986;110:65–68.

Young RH. Sertoli–Leydig cell tumors of the ovary: review with emphasis on historical aspects and unusual variants. Int J Gynecol Pathol 1993;12:141–147.

Young RH, Scully RE. Ovarian sex cord-stromal tumors with bizarre nuclei: a clinicopathologic analysis of 17 cases. Int J Gynecol Pathol 1983;1:325–335.

Young RH, Scully RE. Ovarian Sertoli–Leydig cell tumors with a retiform pattern: a problem in histopathologic diagnosis. A report of 25 cases. Am J Surg Pathol 1983;7:755–771.

Young RH, Scully RE. Ovarian Sertoli–Leydig cell tumors. A clinicopathological analysis of 207 cases. Am J Surg Pathol 1985;9:543–569.

Young RH, Scully RE. Ovarian sex cord-stromal tumors. Problems in differential diagnosis. Pathol Annu 1988;23:237–296.

Young RH, Prat J, Scully RE. Ovarian Sertoli–Leydig cell tumors with heterologous elements. I. Gastrointestinal epithelium and carcinoid: a clinicopathologic analysis of thirty-six cases. Cancer 1982;50: 2448–2456.

Zaloudek C, Norris HJ. Sertoli–Leydig tumors of the ovary. A clinicopathologic study of 64 intermediate and poorly differentiated neoplasm. Am J Surg Pathol 1984;8:405–418.

Sertoli Cell Tumor

Aiba M, Hirayama A, Sakurada M, et al. Spironolactone bodylike structure in renin-producing Sertoli cell tumor of the ovary. Surg Pathol 1990;3:143–149.

Deavers M, Malpica A, Liu J, et al. Ovarian sex cord-stromal tumors: an immunohistochemical study including a comparison of calretinin with inhibin. Mod Pathol 2002;15:814.

Ferry JA, Young RH, Engel G, et al. Oxyphilic Sertoli cell tumor of the ovary: a report of three cases, two in patients with the Peutz–Jeghers syndrome. Int J Gynecol Pathol 1994;13:259–266.

Movahedi-Lankarani S, Kurman RJ. Calretinin, a more sensitive but less specific marker than inhibin for ovarian sex cord-stromal neoplasms: an immunohistochemical study of 215 cases. Am J Surg Pathol 2002;26:1477–1483.

Oliva E, Alvarez T, Young RH. Sertoli cell tumors of the ovary: a clinicopathologic and immunohistochemical study of 54 cases. Am J Surg Pathol 2005;29:143–156.

Shalev E, Zuckerman H, Risescu I. Estrogen-producing Sertoli cell tumor of the ovary – a case report. Gynecol Oncol 1984;19:348–354.

Solh HM, Azoury RS, Najjar SS. Peutz–Jeghers syndrome associated with precocious puberty. J Pediatr 1983;103:593–595.

Tavassoli FA, Norris HJ. Sertoli tumors of the ovary. A clinicopathologic study of 28 cases with ultrastructural observations. Cancer 1980;46: 2281–2297.

Tracy SL, Askin FB, Reddick RL, et al. Progesterone secreting Sertoli cell tumor of the ovary. Gynecol Oncol 1985;22:85–96.

Young RH, Scully RE. Ovarian Sertoli cell tumors: a report of 10 cases. Int J Gynecol Pathol 1984;2:349–363.

Zung A, Shoham Z, Open M, et al. Sertoli cell tumor causing precocious puberty in a girl with Peutz–Jeghers syndrome. Gynecol Oncol 1998;70: 421–424.

Sex Cord Tumor with Annular Tubules

Lele SM, Sawh RN, Zaharopoulos P, et al. Malignant ovarian sex cord tumor with annular tubules in a patient with Peutz–Jeghers syndrome: a case report. Mod Pathol 2000;13:466–470.

Shen K, Wu P-C, Lang J-H, et al. Ovarian sex cord tumor with annular tubules: a report of six cases. Gynecol Oncol 1993;48:180–184.

Young RH, Welch WR, Dickersin GR, et al. Ovarian sex cord tumor with annular tubules. Review of 74 cases including 27 with Peutz–Jeghers syndrome and four with adenoma malignum of the cervix. Cancer 1982;50:1384–1402.

Stromal Luteoma

Hayes MC, Scully RE. Stromal luteoma of the ovary: a clinicopathological analysis of 25 cases. Int J Gynecol Pathol 1987;6:313–321.

Scully RE. Stromal luteoma of the ovary. A distinctive type of lipoid-cell tumor. Cancer 1964;17:769–778.

Leydig Cell Tumor

Paraskevas M, Scully RE. Hillus cell tumor of the ovary. A clinicopathological analysis of 12 Reinke crystal-positive and nine crystal-negative cases. Int J Gynecol Pathol 1989;8:299–310.

Roth LM, Sternberg WH. Ovarian stromal tumors containing Leydig cells. II. Pure Leydig cell tumors, non-hilar type. Cancer 1973;32:952–960.

Steroid Cell Tumor, Not Otherwise Specified

Deavers MT, Malpica A, Ordoñez NG, et al. Ovarian steroid cell tumors: an immunohistochemical study including a comparison of calretinin with inhibin. Int J Gynecol Pathol 2003;22:162–167.

Hayes MC, Scully RE. Ovarian steroid cell tumors (not otherwise specified). A clinicopathological analysis of 63 cases. Am J Surg Pathol 1987;11:835–845.

Seidman JD, Abbondanzo SL, Bratthauer GL. Lipid cell (steroid cell) tumors of the ovary: immunophenotype with analysis of potential pitfall due to endogenous biotin-like activity. Int J Gynecol Pathol 1995;14: 331–338.

Taylor HB, Norris HJ. Lipid cell tumors of the ovary. Cancer 1967;20: 1953–1962.

Young RH, Scully RE. Oxyphilic tumors of the female and male genital tracts. Semin Diagn Pathol 1999;16:146–161.

13 Germ Cell Tumors of the Ovary

Patricia M Baker · Esther Oliva

This group of neoplasms consists of several histologically distinct tumors which arise from primordial germ cells that migrate from the yolk sac to the primitive gonadal ridge and become incorporated into the primary sex cords (Box 13.1). Germ cell tumors may occur anywhere along this midline pathway of germ cell migration, giving rise to histologically similar tumors in both females and males in gonadal and extragonadal sites. The morphological and structural heterogeneity of these tumors is secondary to the ability of germ cells to undergo divergent pathways of differentiation at various stages of development. Recent studies now suggest that dysgerminoma may be the precursor of at least some other germ cell tumors.

Germ cell tumors account for approximately 30% of primary ovarian tumors, with mature cystic teratoma (dermoid cyst) being the most common subtype (95%).

Malignant primitive germ cell tumors represent approximately 3–4% of all ovarian malignancies in western countries, with considerably higher rates in populations with a relatively lower frequency of surface epithelial carcinomas, such as Japan, where up to 20% of ovarian cancers are malignant germ cell tumors. Germ cell tumors comprise slightly more than one-half of ovarian tumors occurring in the first two decades of life and up to one-third in this age group are malignant.

Approximately 10% of the tumors show more than one cell type, dysgerminoma and yolk sac tumor being the most common combination. These tumors are classified as mixed germ cell tumors. Thus, careful gross inspection of the specimen is essential to identify all components. It is recommended that at least one section of tumor be submitted for each centimeter as measured in the greatest diameter, including additional sections of unusual areas. For example, the presence of even minor amounts of yolk sac tumor, embryonal carcinoma, or choriocarcinoma may significantly affect the patient's prognosis and therapy. Similarly, adequate sampling of teratomas is necessary to identify immature elements such as primitive neuroepithelium or the rare presence of malignant change.

Prior to modern combination chemotherapy, the prognosis of malignant germ cell tumors was very poor, with the exception of dysgerminoma. Multiagent chemotherapy has resulted in significant improvement in overall survival, allowing a conservative fertility-sparing approach, as the efficacy of cytoreductive surgery for advanced stage is not as clear as for malignant epithelial tumors of the ovary.

BOX 13.1

CLASSIFICATION OF OVARIAN GERM CELL TUMORS (WORLD HEALTH ORGANIZATION CLASSIFICATION 2003)

Dysgerminoma
Yolk sac tumor
Embryonal carcinoma
Polyembryoma
Choriocarcinoma
Teratomas
    Mature cystic (dermoid cyst)
        With secondary malignant tumor
    Mature solid
    Fetiform teratoma (homunculus)
    Immature
    Monodermal teratomas
        Struma ovarii
        Carcinoids
        Neuroectodermal tumors
        Sebaceous tumors
        Other
Mixed germ cell tumors
    Gonadoblastoma
    Germ cell-sex cord-stromal tumors, unclassified

DYSGERMINOMA

This is a primitive tumor that morphologically resembles primordial germ cells and shares structural features with seminoma and extragonadal germinomas. It is the most common malignant germ cell tumor of the ovary and accounts for approximately one-half of all primitive germ cell tumors and for 1% of all ovarian malignant tumors. Dysgerminomas are believed to arise from primordial germ cells and may be the precursor of other malignant germ cell tumors. Approximately 15% of ovarian dysgerminomas contain other malignant germ

DYSGERMINOMA – FACT SHEET

Definition

▶ Malignant germ cell tumor resembling primordial germ cells, morphologically identical to seminoma and extragonadal germinoma

Incidence

▶ Most common malignant ovarian germ cell tumor (50% of all malignant germ cell tumors)
▶ 1% of all malignant ovarian tumors

Age Distribution

▶ More common in second and third decades (median age 22 years)
▶ 10–20% diagnosed during pregnancy

Clinical Features

▶ Rapidly growing mass
▶ Rarely, estrogenic manifestations due to elevated β-HCG
▶ Elevated serum levels of lactate dehydrogenase (LDH) and placental alkaline phosphatase (PLAP)
▶ Serum AFP within normal limits
▶ Frequent occurrence in patients with gonadal dysgenesis

Radiologic Features

▶ Calcifications in a speckled pattern suggest underlying gonadoblastoma

Prognosis and Treatment

▶ Overall 5-year survival rate of 75–90%
▶ Survival as high as 90% for stage Ia tumors
▶ Conservative fertility-sparing surgery limited to unilateral salpingo-oophorectomy and staging biopsies
▶ Hysterectomy with bilateral salpingo-oophorectomy followed by multiagent chemotherapy (bleomycin, etoposide, and cisplatin) for advanced disease or patients in whom fertility is not desired
▶ Serum levels of LDH and PLAP to monitor recurrences

DYSGERMINOMA – PATHOLOGIC FEATURES

Gross Findings

▶ Solid tumor of variable size (median 15 cm)
▶ Homogeneous lobulated rubbery white to tan cut surface
▶ Calcifications may suggest an underlying gonadoblastoma
▶ 10–15% grossly bilateral and additional 5–10% bilateral involvement on microscopic examination

Microscopic Findings

▶ Typically, sheets and nests, and less commonly, trabeculae and cords
▶ Monotonous cells with large, polygonal, clear to eosinophilic granular cytoplasm and distinct cytoplasmic borders
▶ Large, round, central to slightly eccentric nuclei with a slightly squared-off contour, coarse chromatin, and prominent nucleoli
▶ Brisk mitotic activity
▶ Variable amount of stroma containing inflammatory cells (mainly lymphocytes), and in 20% epithelioid granulomas
▶ Syncytiotrophoblast cells in 2–3%
▶ Calcifications suggest underlying gonadoblastoma

Immunohistochemical Features

▶ Abundant PAS positive intracytoplasmic glycogen
▶ Placental alkaline phosphatase, OCT4, and c-kit (CD117) positive
▶ Scattered cytokeratin positivity in up to 30%

Cytology

▶ Loosely cohesive uniform tumor cells associated with reactive lymphocytes and epithelioid granulomas
▶ Tiger-striped or tigroid background due to a meshwork of PAS-positive material

Cytogenetics

▶ Abnormalities of chromosome 12, typically i(12p)

Differential Diagnosis

▶ Yolk sac tumor with solid pattern
▶ Embryonal carcinoma with solid pattern
▶ Large cell lymphoma
▶ Clear cell carcinoma with diffuse pattern
▶ Sertoli cell tumor

cell elements and these tumors are classified as malignant mixed germ cell tumors.

CLINICAL FEATURES

Dysgerminomas may occur at any age, with the vast majority (approximately 80%) occurring in the second and third decades (median 22 years). A significant number (10–20%) occur during pregnancy, some being discovered incidentally at the time of cesarean section. These tumors are very rare under the age of 5 years and after menopause. Patients usually present with signs and symptoms of a rapidly enlarging pelvic or abdominal mass (e.g., pain or pressure). Rarely, patients present with an acute abdomen or hemoperitoneum due to

torsion or rupture, and in advanced cases, ascites may develop. Uncommonly, they have been found incidentally during investigation of primary amenorrhea in phenotypic females with gonadal dysgenesis, either pure 46XY (bilateral streak gonads), mixed 45/45XY (unilateral streak gonads – contralateral testes) or the androgen insensitivity syndrome (46XY, testicular feminization). Estrogenic hormonal manifestations, including isosexual pseudoprecocity, menstrual irregularities, and vaginal bleeding or pregnancy-like symptoms, are usually due to elevated serum levels of beta β-hCG. Rarely, androgenic manifestations may also occur. Almost all patients with dysgerminoma have

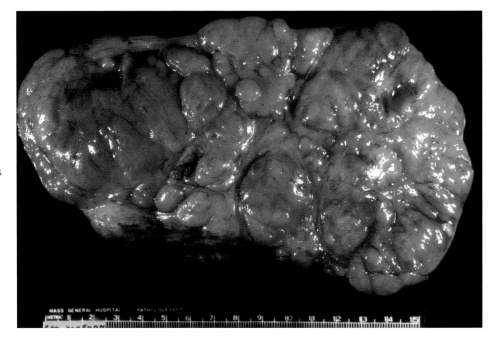

FIGURE 13.1
Dysgerminoma. The cut surface is tan, fleshy, and lobulated.

elevated serum lactate dehydrogenase (LDH) at presentation and in approximately 2–3% of cases, serum β-hCG is sufficiently elevated to suggest trophoblastic disease. Elevated serum levels of placental alkaline phosphatase (PLAP), CA-125, as well as inhibin have been reported. Alpha-fetoprotein is usually within normal limits, and if elevated, should suggest a yolk sac component. Although unusual, paraneoplastic hypercalcemia has been described.

RADIOLOGIC FEATURES

Imaging studies including ultrasound, CT-scan, and MRI show a solid mass with multiple nodules separated by fibrovascular septa. The presence of calcifications, particularly in a speckled pattern, suggests an underlying gonadoblastoma.

PATHOLOGIC FEATURES

GROSS FINDINGS

These tumors vary in size from microscopic (in the setting of dysgenetic gonads removed prophylactically) to large masses (median 15 cm). They are typically solid with a smooth bosselated intact capsule, and show a homogeneous, lobulated, rubbery white-tan to gray-pink cut surface (Figure 13.1); however, they may be soft and fleshy, and areas of hemorrhage or yellow necrotic areas may be seen, particularly in large tumors. Finally, approximately 10–15% of dysgermino-

mas are bilateral and, in another 5–10% of cases, tumor is microscopically identified in the contralateral ovary.

MICROSCOPIC FINDINGS

Dysgerminoma is composed of a rather monotonous population of cells resembling primordial germ cells that grow in islands and sheets (Figure 13.2) or, less often, trabeculae and cords (Figure 13.3). Rarely, solid tubular structures may be present and, on occasion, the tumor cells lack cohesion and form gland-like spaces. When adequately fixed, the tumor cells are large and polygonal with clear to lightly eosinophilic cytoplasm and distinct cytoplasmic borders. If the tumor is inadequately fixed, the cells show loss of cytologic detail with shrunken nuclei and compact eosinophilic cytoplasm. The nuclei are typically central or slightly eccentric and large with a round or slightly "squared off" contour, coarse chromatin and one or more prominent nucleoli (Figure 13.4). The mitotic rate is variable but is generally brisk. The accompanying stroma may be dense and hyalinized, but more often consists of loose fibrous bands containing a variable number of chronic inflammatory cells, mainly T-cell lymphocytes that if abundant, may form follicles with germinal centers (Figure 13.3). Plasma cells, eosinophils, histiocytes and, in 20% of cases, epithelioid granulomas may also be seen (Figure 13.5). Rarely, the inflammatory response is so pronounced that it obscures the identification of the tumor cells. Syncytiotrophoblast cells may be seen in 2–3% of dysgerminomas, often in a perivascular location or in hemorrhagic areas (Figure 13.6). In some cases, luteinized stromal cells, either admixed with the tumor cells or at the periphery of the tumor, can be found. Microcalcifications when present in dysgerminomas suggest

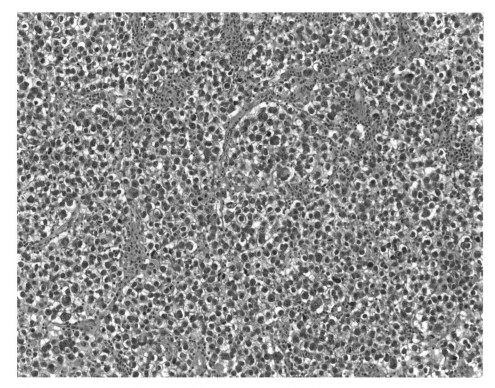

FIGURE 13.2
Dysgerminoma. Nests of tumor cells are separated by fibrous septa containing numerous lymphocytes.

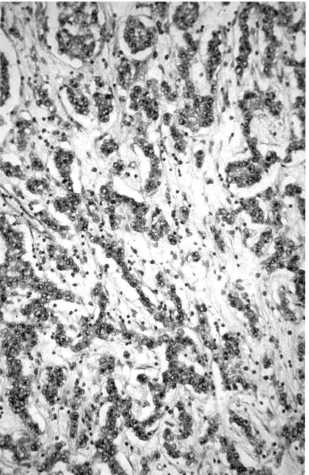

FIGURE 13.3
Dysgerminoma. The neoplastic cells are arranged in cords and separated by an edematous stroma containing scattered lymphocytes.

an underlying gonadoblastoma, which may have been overgrown by the dysgerminoma.

ANCILLARY STUDIES

IMMUNOHISTOCHEMISTRY

Dysgerminoma cells contain abundant intracytoplasmic glycogen that can be highlighted by PAS that disappears with diastase digestion. The cells typically show strong cytoplasmic membrane staining for PLAP. Recently, c-kit (CD117) and OCT4 positivity (Figure 13.7) has been reported in up to 92% and 100% of dysgerminomas respectively. Tumor cells are frequently positive for vimentin, LDH, and neuron-specific enolase (NSE). Approximately 30% of dysgerminomas contain scattered cells positive for cytokeratin. They are negative for EMA, CEA, S-100 protein, leukocyte common antigen (LCA), and AFP. Syncytiotrophoblast cells stain for β-hCG.

ULTRASTRUCTURAL EXAMINATION

Typical ultrastructural characteristics include cells with round to oval nuclei, nucleoli with "thread-like" dispersion of the nucleolonema, and abundant cytoplasm relatively poor in organelles containing ribosomes and glycogen. Intracytoplasmic lamellated structures (so-called "annulate lamellae") are characteristically present, and cell junctions are absent or poorly formed.

CYTOGENETICS

Dysgerminomas are associated with abnormalities of chromosome 12, in particular the presence of i(12p),

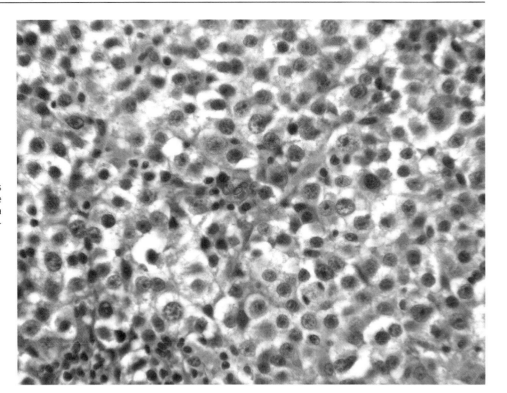

FIGURE 13.4

Dysgerminoma. The neoplastic cells have abundant clear cytoplasm, large central nuclei, sometimes with a "squared-off" contour, and prominent nucleoli.

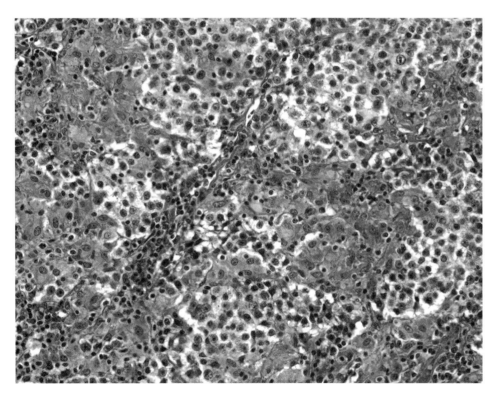

FIGURE 13.5

Dysgerminoma. Prominent epithelioid granulomatous inflammation is seen.

which is also a characteristic marker of these tumors in the testis.

CYTOLOGY

Fine-needle aspiration biopsy yields cellular smears with isolated or loosely cohesive uniform cells with round to oval vesicular nuclei having finely granular chromatin and large, sometimes multiple, nucleoli. Mitotic figures may be seen. A second population of cells consisting of reactive-appearing lymphocytes, plasma cells, eosinophils, and occasionally multinucleated epithelioid histiocytes may also be present. A tiger-striped or tigroid background consisting of a meshwork

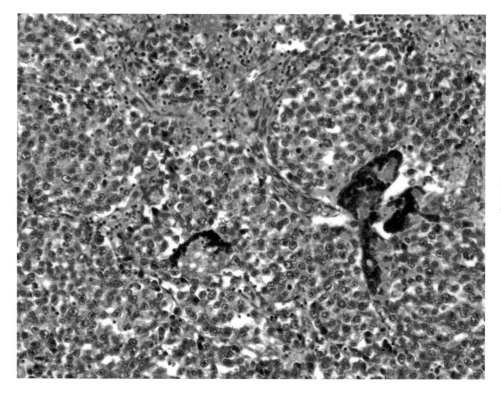

FIGURE 13.6
Dysgerminoma. Scattered syncytio-trophoblast cells are present.

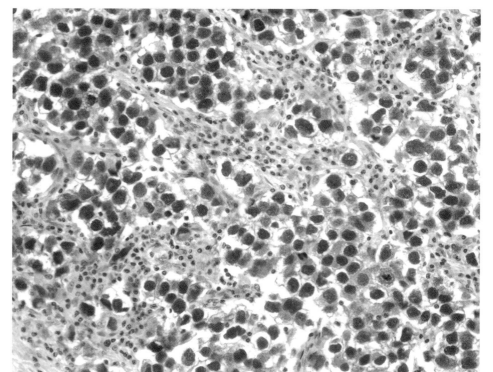

FIGURE 13.7
Dysgerminoma. The tumor cells show strong and diffuse nuclear positivity for OCT4.

of a PAS positive material is commonly seen on Diff-Quik-stained preparations.

DIFFERENTIAL DIAGNOSIS

Dysgerminomas must be distinguished from other malignant germ cell tumors, in particular yolk sac tumor and embryonal carcinoma with a predominantly solid pattern. *Yolk sac tumor* will show at least focally typical architectural patterns, more primitive-appearing nuclei, a relative absence of lymphocytes and other inflammatory cells, presence of hyaline bodies, and diffuse and strong immunoreactivity for cytokeratin and AFP. *Embryonal carcinoma* is extremely rare in the ovary and is generally composed of large cells, which are much more pleomorphic and hyperchromatic than those of dysgerminoma, and shows at least focal glandular or papillary patterns. Syncytiotrophoblast cells are more commonly seen in embryonal carcinoma and the characteristic inflammatory infiltrate seen in dysgerminoma is typically absent. Embryonal carcinoma is strongly and diffusely positive for cytokeratin and CD30. OCT4 is not helpful in this differential diagnosis as both tumors are strongly and diffusely positive for this marker. *Large cell lymphoma* may simulate dysgerminoma grossly and microscopically; however, lymphoma is at least twice more often bilateral and tends to involve the fallopian tube. The tumor cells in lymphoma typically grow in sheets and do not contain glycogen. Immunohistochemical stains including LCA (positive in lymphoma) as well as PLAP (negative in lymphoma) aid in this differential diagnosis. *Clear cell carcinoma* with a predominantly diffuse pattern may be confused with a dysgerminoma; however, it typically occurs in peri- or postmenopausal women. Furthermore, these tumors are frequently associated with endometriosis, and other architectural patterns typical of clear cell tumors are usually encountered. The inflammatory infiltrate is predominantly lymphocytic in dysgerminoma while clear cell carcinoma contains mainly plasma cells. PLAP is not helpful as it may also be positive in clear cell carcinoma. Cytokeratin and EMA are strongly and diffusely positive in clear cell carcinoma, but weakly positive and negative respectively in dysgerminoma. Rarely, dysgerminomas with pseudoglandular spaces or a solid tubular pattern may be confused with a *Sertoli cell tumor*. However, the characteristic nuclear features of dysgerminoma are lacking, and the immunohistochemical findings, particularly inhibin and calretinin (positive in Sertoli cell tumor) as well as OCT4 and PLAP, can be helpful in this differential diagnosis.

PROGNOSIS AND THERAPY

Dysgerminoma has an overall 5-year survival rate of 75–90%; survival for stage Ia patients is as high as 90%, decreasing to approximately 63% in patients with disease beyond the ovary. Tumors are frequently confined to the ovary, with approximately two-thirds of cases being stage Ia at presentation. The vast majority of recurrences occur in the first year after diagnosis. Metastatic disease usually occurs locally involving the peritoneum, but may involve pelvic, para-aortic, or retroperitoneal lymph nodes. Distant metastases typically occur with advanced disease and may involve bone, lung, liver, and kidney. Most patients can be safely treated with conservative fertility-sparing surgery limited to unilateral salpingo-oophorectomy and biopsy of the contralateral ovary as well as staging biopsies. In patients where fertility is not an issue, hysterectomy and bilateral salpingo-oophorectomy are performed followed by multiagent chemotherapy. Included in the staging procedure are peritoneal cavity washings and multiple biopsies, including retroperitoneal lymph nodes. Although dysgerminomas are very radiosensi-

tive, this form of therapy, even for large or high-stage tumors, has largely been replaced by chemotherapy. The most commonly used chemotherapy regime currently is BEP (bleomycin, etoposide, and cisplatin). Surveillance to detect early tumor recurrences includes close clinical follow-up and monitoring of LDH, PLAP, and β-hCG serum levels.

EMBRYONAL CARCINOMA

This is an extremely rare neoplasm of the ovary, which is morphologically identical to its counterpart in the testis. Embryonal carcinoma accounts for about 3% of primitive ovarian germ cell tumors. It is a very primitive tumor which is felt to be capable of differentiation along many pathways, including somatic structures or toward extra-embryonic components such as yolk sac or choriocarcinoma.

CLINICAL FEATURES

At least one-half of the patients are prepubertal, ranging from 4 to 28 (median 12) years. They usually present

---

EMBRYONAL CARCINOMA – FACT SHEET

Definition
▸ Primitive germ cell tumor morphologically identical to its counterpart in the testis, capable of somatic and extraembryonic differentiation

Incidence
▸ 3% of malignant germ cell tumors

Age Distribution
▸ Young females, 50% prepubertal (median age 12 years)

Clinical Features
▸ Abdominal or pelvic mass
▸ Frequent endocrine manifestations secondary to elevated levels of β-hCG, including isosexual precocity, changes in menstrual cycle, signs and symptoms of pseudopregnancy
▸ AFP within normal limits or slightly elevated

Prognosis and Treatment
▸ Spread beyond the ovary at time of presentation in approximately 50% of cases involving pelvic and abdominal viscera
▸ Unilateral salpingo-oophorectomy with surgical debulking followed by multiagent chemotherapy (bleomycin, etoposide, and cisplatin)
▸ Serum levels of β-hCG and AFP used to monitor recurrences

with a pelvic or abdominal mass. Approximately 50 % of cases have elevated levels of β-hCG due to the presence of syncytiotrophoblast cells which is responsible for endocrine manifestations, including isosexual precocity, changes in menstrual cycle or vaginal bleeding, signs and symptoms of pseudopregnancy, or virilizing signs such as hirsutism. Serum AFP has been found to be slightly elevated in a few patients in which an associated yolk sac tumor has not been found. Embryonal carcinoma may occasionally occur in association with a gonadoblastoma in a patient with dysgenetic gonads.

PATHOLOGIC FEATURES

GROSS FINDINGS

These tumors are typically unilateral and large, with a median size of 17 cm, and have a smooth external surface. On cut section, the tumor is generally solid and white to gray. Foci of hemorrhage and necrosis are common, particularly if the tumor is large or if a component such as choriocarcinoma is present.

MICROSCOPIC FINDINGS

In its most undifferentiated form, embryonal carcinoma is composed of very pleomorphic medium to large-sized cells that often grow in solid sheets or nests (Figure 13.8). In more differentiated tumors, the solid sheets

---

EMBRYONAL CARCINOMA – PATHOLOGIC FEATURES

Gross Findings
▶ Unilateral, large (median 17 cm) mass
▶ Solid, white to gray cut surface with areas of hemorrhage and necrosis

Microscopic Findings
▶ Typically solid sheets or nests
▶ More differentiated tumors have gland-like spaces and papillary structures
▶ Very pleomorphic medium to large-size cells with eosinophilic cytoplasm and centrally placed hyperchromatic or vesicular nuclei with prominent nucleoli
▶ Brisk mitotic activity with atypical mitoses
▶ Commonly single-cell necrosis (imparting a "dirty" background), discrete foci of necrosis, and hemorrhage
▶ Syncytiotrophoblast cells present

Immunohistochemical Features
▶ PLAP, OCT4, CD30, and cytokeratin positive
▶ May be positive for c-kit and AFP
▶ EMA, CEA, and vimentin negative

Differential Diagnosis
▶ Dysgerminoma with solid pattern
▶ Yolk sac tumor with solid pattern
▶ Poorly differentiated carcinoma

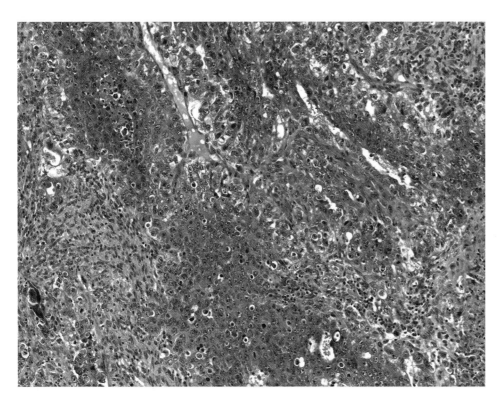

FIGURE 13.8
Embryonal carcinoma. A solid growth of primitive cells is surrounded by cellular stroma.

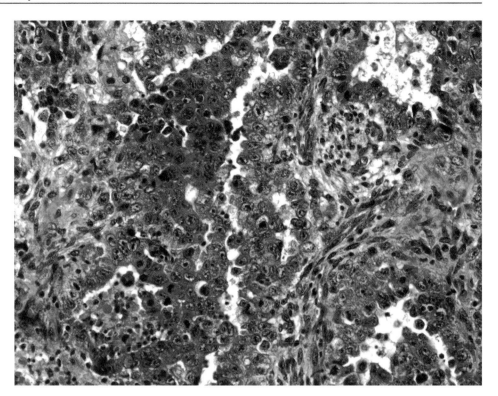

FIGURE 13.9

Embryonal carcinoma. Cells with a pseudoglandular pattern are associated with both single-cell and discrete foci of necrosis.

alternate with gland-like spaces (Figure 13.9) or papillary structures. The cells have centrally placed hyperchromatic or vesicular nuclei with one or more prominent nucleoli and irregular nuclear membranes. The cytoplasm is eosinophilic to amphophilic and often the cells have indistinct cytoplasmic borders (Figure 13.10). Mitotic activity is brisk and atypical mitoses are frequent. Hyaline globules may be present. Single-cell necrosis imparting a "dirty" background, as well as discrete foci of necrosis (Figure 13.11) and hemorrhage, are common. Syncytiotrophoblast cells may be present either at the periphery of tumor nests or in areas of hemorrhage (Figure 13.11).

ANCILLARY STUDIES

IMMUNOHISTOCHEMISTRY

Embryonal carcinoma is generally strongly and diffusely positive for cytokeratin, PLAP, CD30 (Figure 13.12), and OCT4. The tumor cells may be positive for c-kit and NSE, but are usually negative for EMA, CEA, and vimentin. Positive immunoreactivity for AFP can be found in up to one-third of cases, and the syncytiotrophoblast cells are positive for β-hCG.

ULTRASTRUCTURAL EXAMINATION

This primitive germ cell tumor shows a greater degree of differentiation than dysgerminoma, with nuclei more irregular in shape showing evenly dispersed chromatin, nucleoli with prominent nucleolonema, as well as an increased number of cytoplasmic organelles and sometimes glycogen. Occasional acinar formations containing microvilli, well-formed cell junctions with desmosomes, and occasional cells surrounded by basement membrane may also be seen. Cells showing differentiation intermediate to dysgerminoma and embryonal carcinoma can be found, which parallel the light microscopic appearance of dysgerminoma differentiating toward embryonal carcinoma.

DIFFERENTIAL DIAGNOSIS

Embryonal carcinoma may be confused with other germ cell tumors, particularly dysgerminoma and yolk sac tumor. Distinction from *dysgerminoma* is important due to differences in prognosis and treatment. The solid pattern of embryonal carcinoma may mimic dysgerminoma; however, the cells in embryonal carcinoma are more primitive, with higher mitotic rate, greater degree of nuclear irregularity, and less distinct cytoplasmic borders. In contrast, dysgerminoma contains a variable amount of fibrous stroma with striking lymphocytic and granulomatous infiltrate, features typically absent in embryonal carcinoma. Cytokeratin is strongly and diffusely positive in embryonal carcinoma whereas it is negative or only shows weak and focal positivity in dysgerminoma. Embryonal carcinoma lacks the distinc-

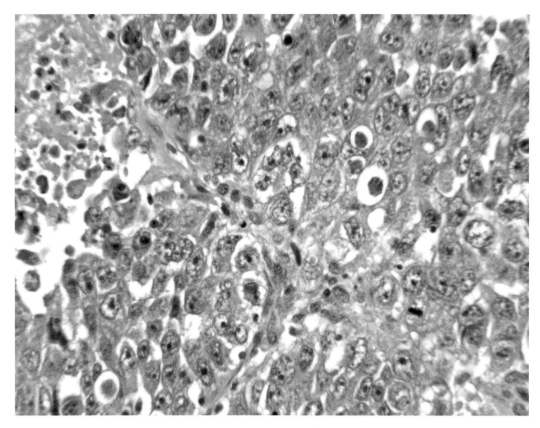

FIGURE 13.10
Embryonal carcinoma. Highly pleomorphic cells are associated with mitotic activity and single-cell necrosis as well as discrete foci of necrosis.

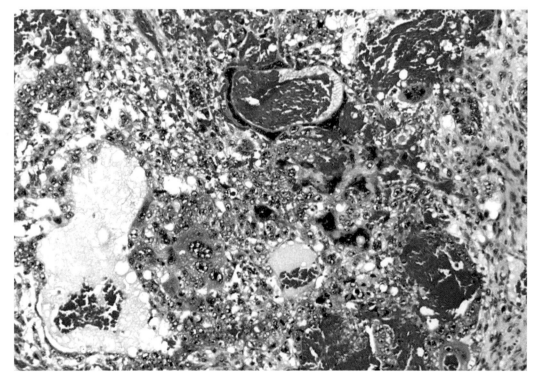

FIGURE 13.11
Embryonal carcinoma. Scattered syncytiotrophoblast cells are seen associated with hemorrhage.

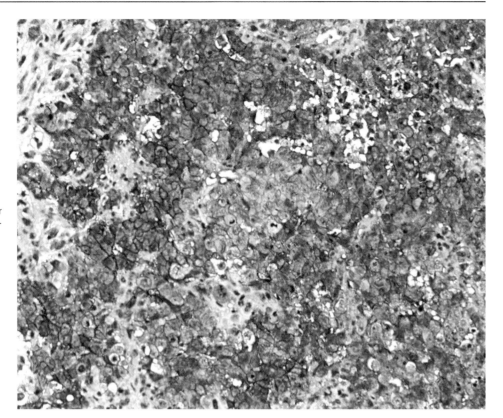

FIGURE 13.12
Embryonal carcinoma. The tumor cells show strong and diffuse membranous CD30 positivity.

tive patterns of *yolk sac tumor* displaying a more prominent necrotic background as well as cellular pleomorphism and often show more amphophilic cytoplasm. Helpful immunohistochemical stains include CD30 and OCT4, typically positive in embryonal carcinoma but negative in yolk sac tumor. Lastly, these tumors can be confused with *surface epithelial carcinomas*, either large cell carcinomas or poorly differentiated adenocarcinomas. The latter generally occur in an older age group and generally show neither AFP nor β-hCG production. In contrast to embryonal carcinoma, they are positive for EMA.

PROGNOSIS AND THERAPY

Prior to chemotherapy, the 5-year survival rate for stage I tumors was approximately 50%. With modern chemotherapy many patients are cured, including some patients with extraovarian spread. At the time of surgery, spread beyond the ovary, usually involving pelvic or intra-abdominal viscera, is present in slightly less than one-half of the patients.

Treatment consists of a unilateral salpingo-oophorectomy with surgical debulking of extraovarian tumor and postoperative multiagent chemotherapy (BEP). Serum β-hCG and AFP are followed to monitor tumor recurrence.

CHORIOCARCINOMA

Nongestational choriocarcinoma is a highly malignant tumor showing extraembryonic trophoblastic differentiation and accounts for < 1% of primitive germ cell tumors. It is more commonly found as a component of a mixed germ cell tumor. Gestational choriocarcinoma may also involve the ovary as metastatic disease from the uterus or from an ectopic pregnancy, and should be excluded before establishing the diagnosis of nongestational choriocarcinoma. In women of reproductive age, the distinction of gestational from nongestational choriocarcinoma cannot be made with absolute certainty on histology alone.

CLINICAL FEATURES

These tumors occur in females under 20 years of age. The clinical presentation and findings are similar to those of other malignant germ cell tumors. The consistently elevated serum β-hCG may lead to isosexual precocity in prepubertal girls, changes in menstrual cycle, breast enlargement, or features of pseudopregnancy in adult women. Extensive bleeding may occur in metastatic tumor deposits as well as within the tumor itself, which may result in hemoperitoneum.

RADIOLOGIC FEATURES

These tumors appear as a solid and cystic mass with areas of hemorrhage and necrosis and often have a prominent vascular pattern. Pulmonary deposits, similar to those seen in gestational choriocarcinoma, may create a "snowstorm" pattern on chest X-ray.

PATHOLOGIC FEATURES

GROSS FINDINGS

The tumors are usually large and frequently have a hemorrhagic and necrotic cut surface.

MICROSCOPIC FINDINGS

Choriocarcinoma is defined by the presence of syncytiotrophoblast cells intimately admixed with cytotrophoblast cells or, much less often, intermediate trophoblast cells. By definition, chorionic villi are absent.

The syncytiotrophoblast cells often appears "draped over" nests or sheets of cytotrophoblast cells in a so-called plexiform pattern (Figure 13.13). On occasion, sheets of cytotrophoblast or intermediate trophoblast may predominate, with only inconspicuous syncytiotrophoblast being present. The syncytiotrophoblast cells have abundant dense eosinophilic to basophilic cytoplasm, which may be vacuolated, and contain clusters of hyperchromatic or at times vesicular nuclei, often having smudged chromatin. These cells are terminally differentiated, incapable of cell division, and thus, mitotic figures are absent. Cytotrophoblasts are medium-sized, round to polygonal uniform cells with abundant clear to amphophilic cytoplasm and distinct cell membranes with a central vesicular nucleus and often a conspicuous nucleolus. Mitoses are frequent and often atypical. Intermediate trophoblast cell appear as large round to polygonal cells with amphophilic to eosino-philic cytoplasm. The cells are typically mononucleated or binucleated. They are often adjacent to dilated vessels and vascular invasion is common. Extensive areas of hemorrhage and necrosis are often seen, which may obscure the nature of the tumor.

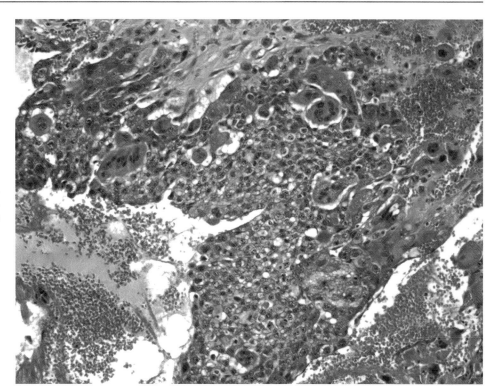

FIGURE 13.13
Choriocarcinoma. Sheets of cytotrophoblast cells are "draped" by multinucleated syncytiotrophoblast cells in a background of hemorrhage.

ANCILLARY STUDIES

Immunohistochemistry reveals strong cytokeratin staining in all three types of cells. Syncytiotrophoblast is strongly and diffusely positive for β-hCG and inhibin, and shows variable staining for human placental lactogen (HPL) and EMA. Cytotrophoblast is negative for β-hCG and HPL, whereas intermediate trophoblast shows strong staining for HPL and inhibin and variable weak staining for β-hCG. Approximately 50 % of choriocarcinomas are positive for PLAP.

DIFFERENTIAL DIAGNOSIS

The main diagnostic challenge is the distinction of a pure, nongestational choriocarcinoma from a *gestational choriocarcinoma* which cannot be established solely on morphological grounds. Flow cytometry or cytogenetic analysis to rule out paternal DNA is necessary to confirm a nongestational choriocarcinoma. The presence of syncytiotrophoblast cells in other malignant germ cell tumors such as dysgerminoma, embryonal carcinoma, or yolk sac tumor or in nongerm cell tumors does not justify a diagnosis of choriocarcinoma.

PROGNOSIS AND THERAPY

These tumors are rapidly fatal if not treated, usually with tumor spread throughout the abdomen as well as

distant lymphatic and hematogenous spread to lungs and brain. Gestational choriocarcinoma has been found to respond better to chemotherapy than nongestational choriocarcinoma. Survival is directly related to the stage at presentation and treatment consists of surgery which is usually unilateral salpingo-oophorectomy followed by chemotherapy. The β-hCG is monitored to evaluate treatment response or recurrence.

YOLK SAC TUMOR

Yolk sac tumor is the second most common malignant germ cell tumor among children and young females following dysgerminoma, representing approximately 20 % of malignant ovarian germ cell neoplasms.

CLINICAL FEATURES

The vast majority of patients are children or young females (mean age 19 years). Yolk sac tumor is almost as frequent as dysgerminoma during the two first decades of life. These tumors have rarely been reported in peri- or postmenopausal women and typically arise in association with surface epithelial tumors. Abdominal pain of short duration is the most common complaint, whereas the most common sign at the time of presentation is a rapidly enlarging abdomen. Rarely, patients develop endocrine-related manifestations, most commonly virilization. Occasional patients have been found to have gonadal dysgenesis and may present with primary amenorrhea. Patients have elevated serum levels of AFP (> 1000 ng/mL) and CA-125. Finally, in contrast to dysgerminoma, yolk sac tumor is much less frequently seen in association with pregnancy. In such a rare event, high levels of serum AFP in a young pregnant woman in the absence of fetal abdominal wall or neural defects should raise the possibility of a germ cell tumor.

RADIOLOGIC FEATURES

Ultrasound and CT-scan frequently show a complex mass which on occasion is predominantly cystic. As the cystic component of the tumor is better visualized with a CT-scan, this may be more helpful in characterizing the mass and staging the tumor.

PATHOLOGIC FEATURES

GROSS FINDINGS

These tumors are almost invariably unilateral and frequently large (median 15 cm), with a smooth external surface, and are solid, fleshy, gray to tan on cut section (Figure 13.14). Capsular rupture is not uncommon. Cysts are often seen and on occasion the tumor may be entirely cystic. The finding of diffuse small cysts imparting a "honeycomb appearance" is characteristic of the polyvesicular vitelline variant of yolk sac tumor. Extensive areas of hemorrhage and/or necrosis are frequent. Rupture secondary to torsion may occur, and in these cases, it may be difficult to identify viable tumor. If calcifications are encountered, they should raise the suspicion of another germ cell tumor component, typically a mature cystic teratoma (present in 15%). A

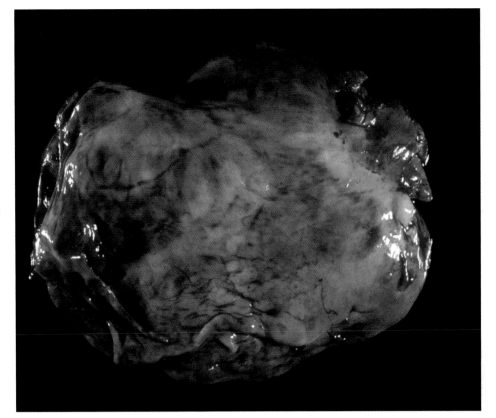

FIGURE 13.14

Yolk sac tumor. Fleshy cut surface with areas of hemorrhage are present.

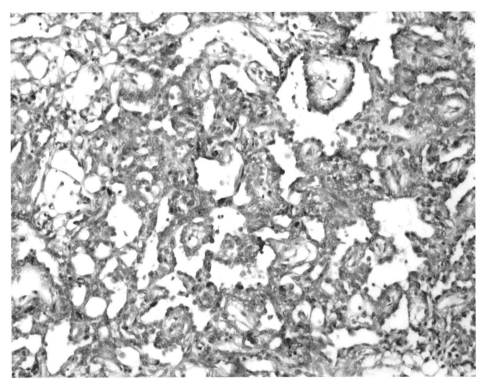

FIGURE 13.15

Yolk sac tumor. A reticular pattern is composed of interanastomosing channels.

streak gonad or mature cystic teratoma may sometimes be identified in the contralateral ovary.

MICROSCOPIC FINDINGS

These tumors typically display an admixture of different patterns. The most common is reticular, charac-terized by a loose meshwork of spaces or channels that frequently merge with a microcystic pattern (Figures 13.15 and 13.16). The spaces are lined by primitive cells that display clear cytoplasm, large hyperchromatic irreg-ular nuclei with prominent nucleoli, and brisk mitotic activity. The pseudopapillary or festoon pattern is the most distinctive of all patterns (Figure 13.17) and it is

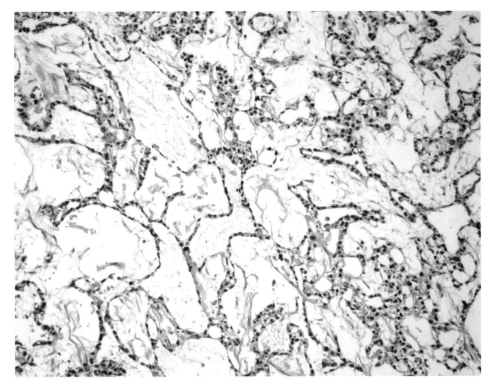

FIGURE 13.16

Yolk sac tumor. Thin cords of neoplastic cells are separated by loose stroma.

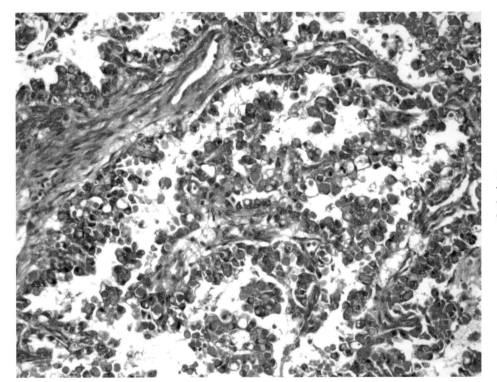

FIGURE 13.17

Yolk sac tumor. Papillary pattern with PAS diastase positive hyaline globules.

characterized by the presence of Schiller–Duval bodies (Figure 13.18). These papillary structures contain a central blood vessel surrounded by loose primitive stroma with an outer mantle of cuboidal to columnar neoplastic cells present in a space lined by flattened tumor cells. Although pathognomonic of this tumor, Schiller–Duval bodies are only found in one-third of cases. Parietal differentiation, although seen in up to 90% of yolk sac tumors, is only focally present and can be recognized by the finding of thick layers of basement membrane in the intercellular spaces. The polyvesicular pattern is composed of multiple cystic cavities, some showing an eccentric constriction with formation of a secondary vesicle reflecting differentiation toward

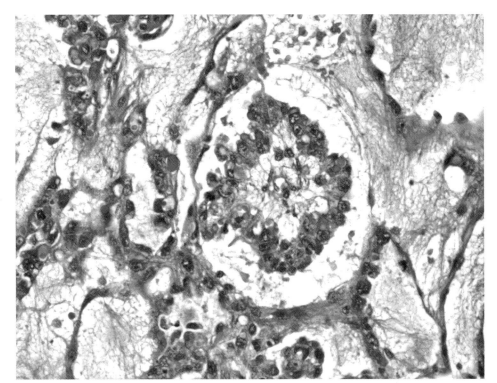

FIGURE 13.18

Yolk sac tumor. A typical Schiller–Duval body is present.

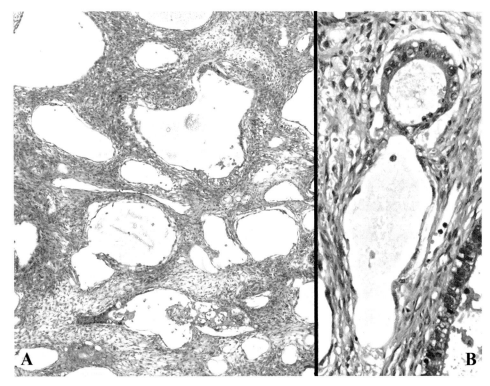

FIGURE 13.19

Yolk sac tumor, polyvesicular vitelline variant. Multiple vesicles, some showing the typical eccentric constriction are seen (A). Flattened cells lining the primary vesicle merge with taller epithelium characteristic of the secondary vesicle (B).

primitive gut (Figure 13.19). The larger vesicle is lined by flattened epithelium while the secondary vesicle is lined by tall epithelium resembling the secondary yolk sac (Figure 13.19). Thus, it is not infrequent to see this pattern of yolk sac tumor associated with hepatoid or glandular differentiation.

Other less frequent but more distinctive patterns of yolk sac tumor include hepatoid and glandular, both indicative of embryonic differentiation. Hepatoid differentiation is seen in up to 40% of yolk sac tumors. It is characterized by nests and cords of cells separated by fibrous bands imparting an appearance similar to that

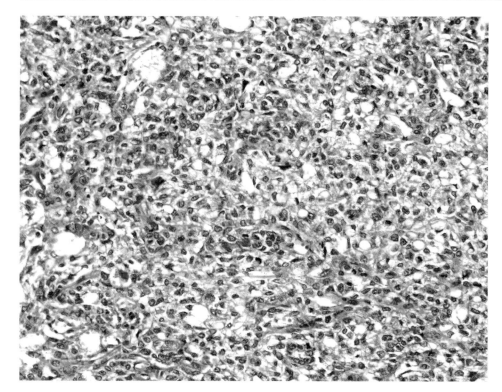

FIGURE 13.20
Yolk sac tumor. Solid pattern.

seen in the fibrolamellar variant of hepatocellular carcinoma. The cells are polygonal with abundant eosinophilic cytoplasm and a central round nucleus with a prominent single nucleolus. Glandular spaces containing mucin may be present, but there is no evidence of bile production. Glandular differentiation may be seen in the form of intestinal or endometrioid-like glands. The former has been reported in up to 54% of yolk sac tumors and is characterized by small glands containing pseudostratified columnar epithelium admixed with goblet cells and rarely, Paneth cells in single units or a cribriform pattern. Endometrioid-like glandular differentiation is characterized by glands or papillary structures lined by a single layer of columnar cells with prominent subnuclear or supranuclear vacuoles recapitulating secretory endometrium. The nuclei are pleomorphic with prominent nucleoli and show brisk mitotic activity, in contrast to the bland nuclear features seen in the intestinal-type glands. Finally, the solid pattern of yolk sac neoplasia is seen less frequently than in the testis; however, it may predominate, particularly in recurrences (Figure 13.20).

Hyaline bodies (Figure 13.18), often seen in yolk sac tumor and either intracellular or extracellular, are not pathognomonic of this tumor as they may be seen in a variety of ovarian neoplasms. The stroma, although typically loose and hypocellular, can be markedly myxomatous, densely fibrous, or very cellular with mitotically active primitive cells. Some investigators have reported a "mesenchyme-like" pattern of yolk sac tumor that is more often seen in patients who have received chemotherapy and it is postulated that this pattern may be the origin of sarcomas in post-chemotherapy patients. Stromal luteinization is seen in up to 25% of

the tumors and this finding is rarely associated with endocrine manifestations. Rarely syncytiotrophoblast cells may be found.

ANCILLARY STUDIES

IMMUNOHISTOCHEMISTRY

The tumor cells contain abundant glycogen and are PAS positive. They stain for AFP (Figure 13.21) and alpha-1-antitrypsin, although the intensity and extent of positivity are variable, and thus, not always helpful in the diagnosis. The tumors are also positive for cytokeratin, frequently stain for CD34 predominantly in reticular and solid areas, and can be positive for CD30 and PLAP. Leu-M1 may be weakly positive. The intestinal and endometrioid variants of yolk sac tumor stain for CEA, typically in the luminal border of the cells. Yolk sac tumors are usually negative for EMA and CK7. HepPar-1 is positive in hepatoid yolk sac tumors as well as in other tumors with hepatoid differentiation and therefore is not helpful in this differential diagnosis. Areas of parietal differentiation show collagen IV and laminin positivity. Hyaline globules are frequently PAS positive and diastase-resistant, but negative for AFP, albumin, prealbumin, and alpha-1-antitrypsin.

ULTRASTRUCTURAL EXAMINATION

Diagnostic features include epithelial-type cells arranged along a network of interconnecting spaces

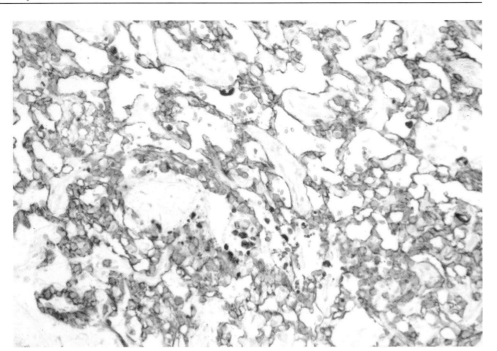

FIGURE 13.21

Yolk sac tumor. Diffuse immunopositivity for α-fetoprotein is seen.

(reticular pattern), profuse basal laminar material coating the cells, rough endoplastic reticulum, sometimes dilated and filled with material similar to basal lamina, microvilli in cells lining spaces, abundant cytoplasmic glycogen, and large irregular nuclei with prominent, multiple nucleoli and open nucleolonemas.

CYTOGENETICS

The most common chromosomal alteration associated with yolk sac tumor is gain of chromosome 12 i(12p) and parallels those reported in their testicular counterpart.

DIFFERENTIAL DIAGNOSIS

Clear cell carcinoma is the tumor most commonly confused with yolk sac tumor. These tumors share similar growth patterns, including tubular, cystic, and papillary architectures, and both may have clear and/or oxyphilic cells. Hyaline bodies, a common feature of yolk sac tumor, can also be seen in clear cell carcinoma. However, other typical patterns of yolk sac tumor are absent in clear cell carcinoma, which affects significantly older women. Furthermore, clear cell carcinoma is frequently associated with endometriosis or an adenofibromatous background. Of note, clear cell carcinoma may occasionally be positive for AFP and in these cases, CK7 and EMA are helpful in arriving at the correct diagnosis. The solid variant of yolk sac tumor may be misinterpreted as *dysgerminoma*; however, yolk sac tumor shows a greater degree of nuclear variability and generally an absence of lymphocytes. Hyaline globules and extracellular basement membrane are features not seen in dysgerminoma. Finally, yolk sac tumor is positive for cytokeratin and AFP whereas dysgerminoma is positive for OCT4.

When the endometrioid-like pattern of yolk sac tumor predominates it may closely mimic a *secretory endometrioid carcinoma* at low-power examination because of the presence of subnuclear or supranuclear vacuoles. However, in a yolk sac tumor, the nuclei have a primitive appearance and there is brisk mitotic activity, features that contrast with the well-differentiated appearance of the glands. These tumors occur in a younger age group and are not associated with squamous differentiation, a fibromatous background, or endometriosis. A complicating aspect of this differential diagnosis is the finding of yolk sac tumor in association with surface epithelial tumors, most commonly endometrioid carcinoma. These tumors occur in older women and areas of clear-cut carcinoma are identified. Cytokeratin, EMA, and AFP are helpful in this differential diagnosis.

The hepatoid variant of yolk sac tumor should be distinguished from *hepatoid carcinoma* as well as from *oxyphilic clear cell carcinoma*, both of which occur in older women. Hepatoid carcinoma is frequently associated with a conventional surface epithelial tumor while oxyphilic clear cell carcinoma frequently shows other conventional architectural patterns, an adenofibromatous background, and/or endometriosis. Lastly, *metastatic hepatoid carcinoma* may enter into the differential, but frequently shows bilateral ovarian involvement. Yolk sac tumor may be confused with the *retiform variant of Sertoli–Leydig cell tumor* as both tumors occur in young patients, may have a prominent loose hypocellular stroma with marked edema, and a papillary growth. However, approximately one-third of patients with Sertoli–Leydig cell tumors have androgenic manifestations, a feature rarely seen in yolk sac tumors. The retiform variant of Sertoli–Leydig cell tumor is typically seen in association with intermediate and poorly differentiated Sertoli–Leydig cell neoplasia. The papillae are small, containing hyalinized cores, or may be bulbous and edematous but do not form the typical Schiller–Duval bodies, and the cells are less primitive in appearance than in yolk sac tumors. Although Sertoli–Leydig cell tumors may have AFP elevation, they do not stain with AFP.

PROGNOSIS AND THERAPY

Two-thirds of patients with yolk sac tumors are stage I at the time of diagnosis. In the remainder, the pattern of spread is similar to that seen in surface epithelial tumors of the ovary, although lymphatic spread seems to be more prevalent than surface shedding. The most frequent sites of extraovarian involvement are liver, abdominal and pelvic peritoneum, as well as pelvic and para-aortic lymph nodes, with less frequent involvement of bowel and lungs. Patients with recurrent tumor frequently die within the first 2 years. However, late recurrences may occur, and for that reason, long-term follow-up is advised. Unilateral salpingo-oophorectomy combined with thorough staging provides adequate surgical management in patients with stage I disease who want to preserve fertility. Examination, but not excision, of the opposite ovary is necessary as these tumors are rarely bilateral. Patients with extraovarian spread should undergo unilateral adnexectomy and cytoreductive surgery. As the risk of recurrence after surgery alone is quite high, standard treatment includes surgery followed by chemotherapy. The use of cisplatin-based chemotherapy has dramatically improved the prognosis. The survival rate with this approach results in at least 95 % survival in patients with stage I tumors and 75 % survival for patients with advanced disease. Although no differences in survival have been noted among the different histologic patterns of yolk sac tumor, it is important to underscore that the prognosis of yolk sac tumors associated with a surface epithelial tumor is very poor and most patients die of disease independent of stage. Serial measurements of serum AFP are useful to monitor response to treatment and detect subclinical recurrences.

TERATOMAS

MATURE CYSTIC TERATOMA (DERMOID CYST)

This is the most common ovarian tumor (20–40 %) and the most prevalent germ cell tumor, accounting for the

vast majority of all germ cell neoplasms. It may be derived from any of the three embryonic layers and it is accepted that these tumors arise from parthenogenetic division of abnormal germ cells, either by fusion of the ovum with the second polar body or by suppression of the second meiotic division.

CLINICAL FEATURES

These tumors have a wide age distribution, with approximately 50 % occurring in women between 20 and 40 years of age. At least half of these patients are asymptomatic at the time of diagnosis. Abdominal pain is the most common symptom, followed by abnormal uterine bleeding. Complications include torsion, acute or subacute rupture (more common during pregnancy), infection, idiopathic autoimmune hemolytic anemia, virilization, and, rarely, malignant transformation. CA-125, CA19-9, and CEA may be elevated.

MATURE CYSTIC TERATOMA – FACT SHEET

Definition
▸ Benign cell germ tumor derived from any of the three germ cell layers that arises from parthenogenetic division of abnormal germ cells

Incidence
▸ 20–40% of all ovarian tumors
▸ Up to 95% of all germ cell tumors

Age Distribution
▸ Wide age range, with 50% occurring in women between 20 and 40 years

Clinical Features
▸ Asymptomatic in 50% of women
▸ Abdominal pain or abnormal bleeding
▸ May be associated with unusual clinical manifestations
▸ May undergo a variety of complications
▸ Elevated serum levels of CA-125, CA 19.9, and CEA

Prognosis and Treatment
▸ Survival rate of 100%
▸ Deaths occur secondary to malignant transformation
▸ Cystectomy in young women who wish to preserve fertility
▸ Salpingo-oophorectomy in older women

RADIOLOGIC FEATURES

Ultrasound most commonly shows a cystic lesion with a densely echogenic tubercle (Rokitansky nodule) protruding into the lumen. The presence of bone or teeth

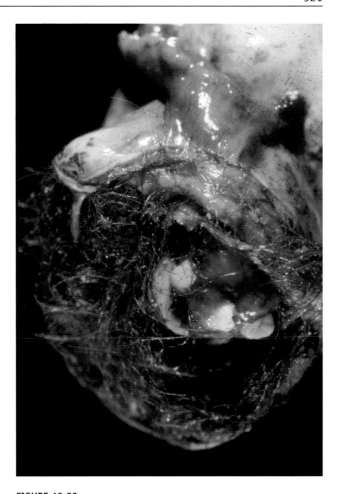

FIGURE 13.22

Mature cystic teratoma (dermoid cyst). Abundant hair is associated with a mural nodule containing teeth (Rokitansky protuberance).

facilitates the diagnosis. The second manifestation is a diffusely or partially echogenic mass with the echogenic area usually demonstrating sound attenuation owing to sebaceous material and hair, while the third manifestation consists of multiple thin, echogenic bands caused by hair in the cyst cavity. On CT-scan, mature cystic teratomas are seen as complex masses with dividing septa, internal debris, variable attenuation, distinct calcification, and presence of fat. If the tumor contains fat, it can also be distinguished by MRI.

PATHOLOGIC FEATURES

GROSS FINDINGS

These tumors are frequently < 10 cm in size, typically have a smooth external surface, and are cystic on cut section with abundant hair and sebaceous material. A rounded, white nodule containing bone or teeth is often noticed protruding from the cyst wall (Rokitansky protuberance) (Figure 13.22). In exceptional cases, a fetiform structure (homunculus) closely resembling a fetus may be seen attached to the wall of the cyst. In up to 10% of cases, mature cystic teratomas are bilateral.

MICROSCOPIC FINDINGS

The tumors are composed entirely of mature tissues with an organized arrangement that tends to simulate the composition of various normal organs. Skin and its appendages (Figure 13.23), glia, choroid plexus, peripheral nervous tissue, fat, cartilage (Figure 13.24), smooth muscle, respiratory (Figure 13.24) and gastrointestinal epithelium are the most common tissues. Other elements, including salivary gland (Figure 13.24), thyroid, or bone, are relatively common, while lung, liver, kidney, pancreas, breast, prostate, pituitary tissue, or gonads are rarely identified. Cytologic atypia is minimal and mitoses are absent or very rare. Not infrequently, a foreign body-type granulomatous reaction is seen in association with hair or the epithelial contents of the cyst. A "sieve-like pattern" characterized by a prominent lipogranulomatous response in the wall of the cyst and in the surrounding ovarian tissue is very characteristic, and sometimes the sole microscopic evidence of a dermoid cyst.

Unusual findings include:

1. The *fetiform teratoma* which closely resembles a fetus, showing the highest degree of tissue differentiation and organization in a teratoma.

2. *Prominent vascular proliferation* in the form of glomeruloid structures or confluent vessels forming

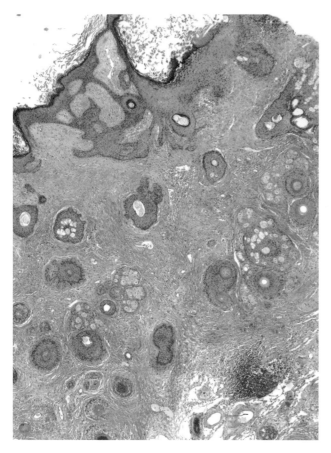

FIGURE 13.23

Mature cystic teratoma. Skin and pilosebaceous units are present in the cyst wall.

large aggregates typically associated with the neural tissue.

3. *Microscopic foci of immature neuroepithelial tissue* may be rarely found in the walls of a mature cystic teratoma. However, these microscopic foci do not affect the prognosis of the tumor.

4. *Granulomatous peritonitis* resulting from chronically leaking tumors. It is characterized by multiple granulomas with foreign-body giant cells associated with multiple adhesions, and may simulate a malignant process.

5. *Melanosis peritonei* consists of pigment-laden histiocytes within a fibrous stroma. The source of the pigment, although considered to be melanin in some cases, is not clear. This phenomenon is not always associated with a dermoid cyst. Its recognition as a benign process is extremely important.

6. *Benign tumors* and *secondary malignancies* may develop within mature cystic teratomas, the latter with a frequency of approximately 2%, more commonly invasive squamous cell carcinoma, followed by adenocarcinomas, small cell carcinoma, sarcomas, and malignant melanoma. They are typically seen in postmenopausal women and should be suspected when there is rapid growth of the dermoid cyst, the cyst wall is penetrated by tumor, multiple adhesions are present, or the tumor is solid and friable.

7. *Association with a malignant germ cell tumor*, more commonly yolk sac tumor or immature teratoma, either in the same or opposite ovary in 5–10% of mature cystic teratomas.

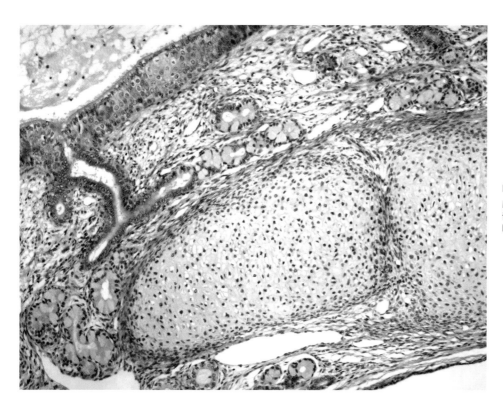

FIGURE 13.24

Mature cystic teratoma. Fetal cartilage is seen underlying respiratory epithelium and minor salivary glands.

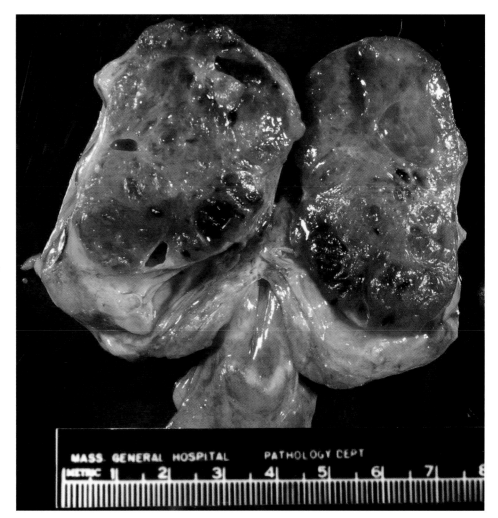

FIGURE 13.25
Struma ovarii. The cut surface is solid, green to brown, and gelatinous.

CYTOGENETICS

These tumors are diploid, and cytogenetic studies demonstrate that they almost always have a normal 46,XX karyotype. They are usually homozygous for polymorphic genetic markers.

DIFFERENTIAL DIAGNOSIS

See discussion of immature teratoma, below.

PROGNOSIS AND THERAPY

These are benign tumors and, as most patients are young at the time of diagnosis, a conservative surgical approach is recommended, with complete resection of the cyst to avoid recurrences. Management should include close examination of the opposite ovary to rule out bilateral ovarian involvement.

MONODERMAL TERATOMAS

These are rare forms of mature cystic teratoma composed exclusively of tissues derived from a single germ layer (Box 13.2).

STRUMA OVARII

This is the most common form of monodermal teratoma. Although thyroid tissue occurs in 5–15% of teratomas, the term "struma" should only be applied to those teratomas where the thyroid tissue represents the only or predominant component of the tumor. It represents approximately 3% of all ovarian teratomas.

CLINICAL FEATURES

Most patients are in their fifth decade and are asymptomatic; however, they may present with a palpable abdominal mass or rarely with ascites, Meigs syndrome, hyperthyroidism, or changes related to steroid hormone production. Elevated serum levels of CA-125 may also be detected.

BOX 13.2

MONODERMAL TERATOMAS

Struma ovarii
Carcinoids
   Insular
   Trabecular
   Strumal carcinoid
   Mucinous
   Mixed
Neuroectodermal tumors
   Ependymoma
   Glioblastoma multiforme
   Medulloblastoma
   Medulloepithelioma
   Central neurocytoma
   Neuroblastoma
Sebaceous tumors
Endodermal variant (respiratory epithelium only)
Others

STRUMA OVARII – FACT SHEET

Definition
▶ Rare form of mature cystic teratoma composed predominantly or solely of thyroid tissue

Incidence
▶ 3% of all ovarian teratomas

Age Distribution
▶ More common in the fifth decade

Clinical Features
▶ Usually asymptomatic
▶ Less common palpable mass and rarely ascites or Meigs syndrome
▶ Occasionally hyperthyroidism
▶ Elevated serum levels of CA-125

Prognosis and Treatment
▶ Oophorectomy and removal of extraovarian tumor if present
▶ Favorable outcome even with extraovarian tumor or with malignant transformation

---

RADIOLOGIC FEATURES

The ultrasound findings are nonspecific; however the presence of low-resistance blood flow in the central portion of the tumor or the finding of a well-vascularized solid component in the central part of a cystic teratoma is highly suggestive of struma ovarii. This component will also show strong enhancement on CT-scan, and on MRI, the cystic spaces will demonstrate both high and low signal intensities.

PATHOLOGIC FEATURES

GROSS FINDINGS

Struma ovarii frequently shows a solid to focally cystic, relatively soft and gelatinous, brown to green cut surface (Figure 13.25); however, some tumors may be predominantly cystic. An associated dermoid cyst or a mucinous tumor may be seen.

MICROSCOPIC FINDINGS

These tumors are composed of thyroid follicles that can undergo changes similar to those seen in normal thyroid (Figure 13.26) or in a thyroid adenoma (proliferating struma), including diffuse, trabecular, macro-

---

STRUMA OVARII – PATHOLOGIC FEATURES

Gross Findings
▶ Solid to focally cystic, soft and gelatinous, brown to green cut section
▶ On occasion, prominent cystic change
▶ Not infrequently associated with mature cystic teratoma or mucinous tumor

Microscopic Findings
▶ Thyroid follicles recapitulating normal thyroid
▶ May show features as seen in thyroid adenoma or goiter
▶ Follicles lined by cells with regular nuclei showing minimal cytologic atypia and rare mitotic figures
▶ Unusual forms with clear or oxyphilic cells
▶ Criteria for malignant transformation parallel those in thyroid
▶ Rarely cytologic and architectural features of papillary carcinoma

Immunohistochemistry
▶ Thyroglobulin and thyroid transcription factor-1-positive

Differential Diagnosis
▶ Clear cell carcinoma, primary or metastatic
▶ Sertoli cell tumor
▶ Steroid cell tumor
▶ Serous cystadenoma, cystic

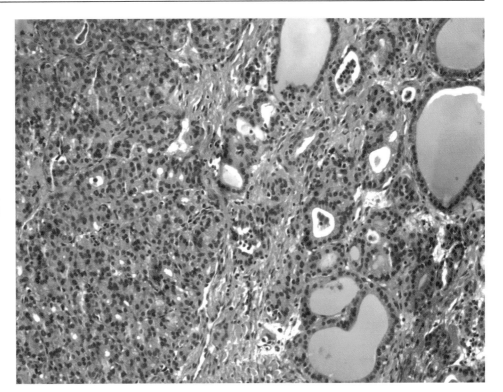

FIGURE 13.26

Struma ovarii. Typical thyroid follicles are juxtaposed with solid and microfollicular patterns.

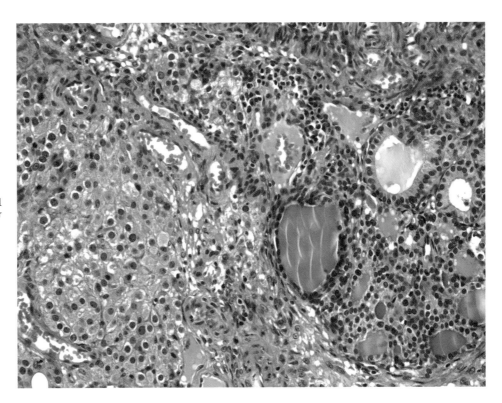

FIGURE 13.27

Struma ovarii. Prominent stromal luteinization is present in the lower left.

follicular, or microfollicular growth (Figure 13.26) or prominent cystic degeneration. The cells are usually cuboidal to columnar and may display a prominent component of cells with oxyphilic or clear cytoplasm. The follicles contain dense colloid with birefringent calcium oxalate crystals. The nuclei are typically round to oval with minimal cytologic atypia, and rare mitotic figures are seen. In general, these tumors have scant intervening stroma, but may show extensive edema or a fibrous background. One histologic feature frequently seen in monodermal teratomas, and specifically in struma ovarii, is peripheral stromal luteinization (Figure 13.27).

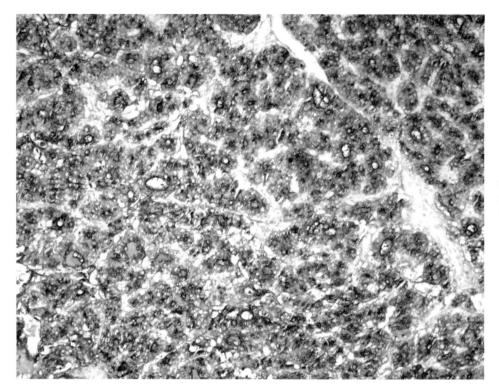

FIGURE 13.28
Struma ovarii. Strong and diffuse thyroglobulin positivity is seen.

The tumors are not infrequently associated with a dermoid cyst, a mucinous tumor, or a Brenner tumor.

Uniformly accepted criteria for malignant change in struma have not been established and strict criteria such as those used in the thyroid gland should be applied. A papillary or follicular growth with typical nuclear features is diagnostic of papillary thyroid carcinoma. Rarely, struma ovarii may be associated with peritoneal implants of thyroid tissue with benign cytologic features ("strumosis" or "strumatosis").

ANCILLARY STUDIES

IMMUNOHISTOCHEMISTRY

Thyroglobulin (Figure 13.28) and thyroid transcription factor-1 (TTF-1) positivity are helpful in establishing the diagnosis of struma.

DIFFERENTIAL DIAGNOSIS

Unusual forms of struma (clear cell or oxyphilic), especially when not associated with a dermoid cyst, should be distinguished from a *clear cell carcinoma, either primary or metastatic from the kidney,* a *Sertoli cell tumor,* a *steroid cell tumor,* or even *malignant*

melanoma. The presence of other histologic patterns characteristic of these tumors as well as immunohistochemical stains, including inhibin and calretinin positivity in. Sertoli cell tumors and steroid cell tumors, negative EMA in metastatic renal clear cell carcinoma, and S-100 and HMB-45 for melanoma, are helpful in this differential diagnosis. Cystic struma should be distinguished from a *serous cystadenoma*. In cases of struma, the finding of scattered adjacent follicles in the cyst wall as well as positive thyroglobulin staining are helpful.

PROGNOSIS AND THERAPY

The treatment of choice is oophorectomy; however, in malignant struma, oophorectomy should be accompanied by removal of any extraovarian tumor. Although 5–10% of strumas have been considered malignant, < half have been associated with extraovarian spread. Recently, some investigators have found that most strumas with atypical or malignant features on microscopic examination are not associated with a clinically malignant course. Even patients with malignant struma and extraovarian extension have had no clinical evidence of recurrent disease on follow-up. Another study has shown that factors predictive of recurrence in these tumors include tumor size, presence of adhesions or ascites, and a solid microscopic appearance. In general, long-term follow-up is advised.

CARCINOIDS

These are the second most common type of monodermal teratoma, but still represent < 1 % of ovarian teratomas and > 90 % of cases are associated with other teratomatous elements. Primary carcinoids have been classified into five different categories: (1) insular; (2) trabecular; (3) strumal; (4) mucinous; and (5) mixed types.

CLINICAL FEATURES

Most patients are postmenopausal. One-third of patients present with carcinoid syndrome, most frequently those with insular carcinoid (typically older women with tumors > 7 cm) and rarely, patients with mucinous carcinoid. Flushing and diarrhea are the most frequent clinical manifestations of the syndrome. Other symptoms include cardiac murmurs, pedal edema, and arterial hypertension. Five-hydroxyindole acetic acid (5-HIAA) levels in urine are frequently elevated. Since the blood supply from the ovary drains into the vena cava, bypassing the portal circulation, an ovarian carcinoid may produce the carcinoid syndrome in the absence of liver metastases. Rarely, these tumors may secrete neurohormonal peptides (PYY, insulin, and others) and cases of strumal carcinoid may be associated with thyroid symptoms.

RADIOLOGIC FEATURES

The findings are nonspecific as these tumors are solid, with the exception of mucinous carcinoids, which may show higher signal intensity on T2-weighted MRI as they contain high-signal-intensity mucin.

PATHOLOGIC FEATURES

GROSS FINDINGS

Carcinoids are solid, yellow to gray homogeneous masses of variable size if pure, or may typically form a

---

CARCINOIDS – FACT SHEET

Definition
▸ Monodermal teratoma composed of neuroendocrine cells morphologically similar to tumors arising in the gastrointestinal tract

Incidence
▸ < 1% of all ovarian teratomas
▸ Second most common type of monodermal teratoma

Age Distribution
▸ Postmenopausal patients

Clinical Features
▸ Carcinoid syndrome in one-third of patients (most commonly flushing and diarrhea)
▸ Elevated 5-HIAA serum levels

Prognosis and Treatment
▸ Vast majority benign
▸ Insular and mucinous carcinoids may be malignant, especially with extension beyond ovary

---

CARCINOIDS – PATHOLOGIC FEATURES

Gross Findings
▸ Solid, yellow to gray mass of variable size
▸ Solid nodule in the wall of a mature cystic teratoma
▸ Rarely, predominantly cystic

Microscopic Findings
▸ *Insular carcinoid (similar to midgut carcinoids)*
  ▸ Most common subtype
  ▸ Islands of cells with closely packed small acini at the periphery imparting a cribriform appearance
  ▸ Secretions may undergo psammomatous calcification
▸ *Trabecular (similar to midgut carcinoids)*
  ▸ Cords or trabeculae of cells
  ▸ Nuclei with perpendicular orientation to axis of cords or trabeculae
  ▸ 20% associated with insular carcinoid component
▸ *Strumal carcinoid*
  ▸ Carcinoid intermingled or juxtaposed with thyroid tissue
  ▸ More frequently, trabecular carcinoid
  ▸ Thyroid tissue resembling normal or abnormal thyroid tissue
  ▸ On occasion, component of mucinous carcinoid
▸ *Mucinous or goblet cell carcinoid (similar to appendiceal carcinoids)*
  ▸ Small glands with goblet cells floating within pools of acellular mucin
  ▸ Complex architecture with increasing cytologic atypia in atypical forms
▸ *Mixed (more than one cell type)*
▸ Shared features:
  ▸ Fibromatous or hyalinized stroma
  ▸ Cells containing brown to red granules and nuclei with "salt-and-pepper" chromatin
  ▸ Association with mature cystic teratoma, mucinous tumor, or Brenner tumor

Immunohistochemistry
▸ Chromogranin, synaptophysin and CD56 positive
▸ Cytokeratin, EMA, and CK7 positive; variable positivity for CK20

Differential Diagnosis
▸ Granulosa cell tumor
▸ Sertoli–Leydig or Sertoli cell tumor
▸ Metastatic carcinoid
▸ Metastatic carcinoma (Krukenberg tumor)

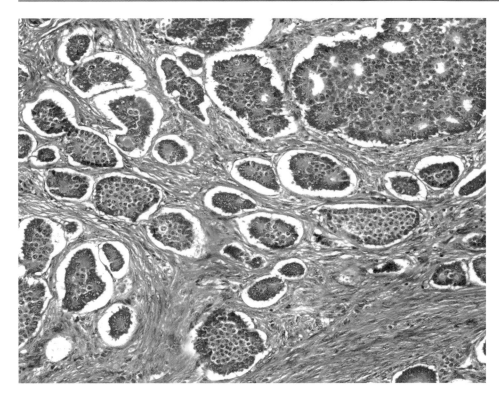

FIGURE 13.29

Insular carcinoid. Solid islands, some with a focal cribriform pattern. Prominent neuroendocrine granules are seen at the periphery of the islands.

solid nodule in the wall of the cyst if associated with a mature cystic teratoma. Rarely, carcinoid tumors are predominantly cystic. Insular carcinoids associated with carcinoid syndrome are often larger and predominantly solid. Foci of hemorrhage or necrosis are rare.

MICROSCOPIC FINDINGS

Insular carcinoid, the most common subtype, has an appearance reminiscent of midgut carcinoids and is composed of islands of tumor cells immersed in a variable amount of hyalinized or fibromatous stroma (Figure 13.29). Multiple closely packed small acini are typically seen at the periphery of the otherwise solid islands, imparting a cribriform appearance at low power (Figure 13.29), but single acini may also be seen. The acini contain cells with abundant eosinophilic cytoplasm and prominent red to brown granules frequently basally located, which tend to be more abundant in cells lining the periphery of the nests (Figure 13.29). The nuclei are round with "salt-and-pepper" chromatin and show very low mitotic activity. Dense eosinophilic secretions that may undergo psammomatous calcification are typically present in the lumen. Approximately 60 % of tumors are associated with a mature cystic teratoma, a mucinous tumor, or a Brenner tumor.

Trabecular carcinoid resembles the hindgut or foregut carcinoid. It is composed of long serpentine, parallel, or anastomosing cords or trabeculae in a fibromatous, frequently hyalinized or sometimes edematous stroma

(Figure 13.30). The cells have abundant eosinophilic cytoplasm, orange to red granules, and oval to round nuclei with a perpendicular orientation to the axis of the cords (Figure 13.30). The nuclei have a typical neuroendocrine appearance with minimal cytologic atypia. These tumors are almost always associated with a mature cystic teratoma and in approximately 20 % of cases a component of insular carcinoid can be seen.

Strumal carcinoid is characterized by the presence of carcinoid tumor, more often trabecular carcinoid, intermingled or juxtaposed with thyroid tissue (Figure 13.31). The latter commonly resembles normal thyroid tissue; however, features of a multinodular goiter, a macro- or microfollicular adenoma, or rarely papillary or follicular carcinoma may also be seen. The proportion of each element varies from tumor to tumor. Carcinoid cells replacing the cells lining the thyroid follicles are a common finding. The tumors are frequently associated with a mature cystic teratoma, less commonly a mucinous tumor, and in 40 % of these tumors a component of mucinous carcinoid.

Well-differentiated" mucinous (goblet cell) carcinoid resembles its appendiceal counterpart and is composed of small glands, many of them floating within pools of acellular mucin (Figure 13.32). The glands have small central lumens and are lined by goblet and columnar cells with eosinophilic cytoplasm, some of which contain coarse, red to orange argentaffin granules (Figure 13.32). There is absent or minimal cytologic atypia. In some instances, these typical areas may be associated with an atypical or even carcinomatous com-

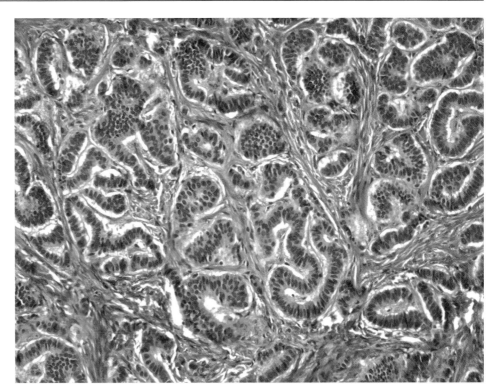

FIGURE 13.30

Trabecular carcinoid. Cords and trabeculae of uniform cells with perpendicular oriented nuclei are set in a fibrous stroma.

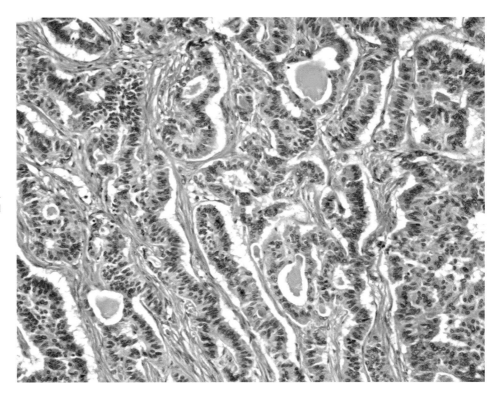

FIGURE 13.31

Strumal carcinoid. Intimate admixture of trabecular carcinoid and thyroid follicles.

ponent, which is characterized by an increased degree of architectural complexity, fewer goblet cells, and greater cytologic atypia. The stroma is often fibromatous. These tumors may be associated with a mature teratoma, a mucinous tumor, or a Brenner tumor.

It is not uncommon to see peripheral stromal luteinization in any of the monodermal teratomas.

ANCILLARY STUDIES

IMMUNOHISTOCHEMISTRY

These tumors show positivity for one or more neuroendocrine markers, including chromogranin,

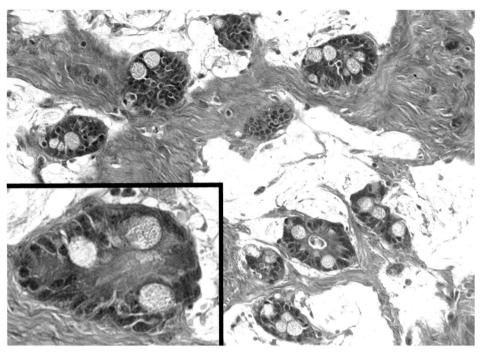

FIGURE 13.32
Mucinous carcinoid (goblet cell carcinoid). Nests of cells are floating in pools of mucin. Inset: the nests contain goblet cells and cells with neuroendocrine differentiation.

synaptophysin, and CD56. They also express cytokeratin, EMA, and CK7, and may be positive for CK20 when the cells are of intestinal derivation.

ULTRASTRUCTURAL EXAMINATION

Insular carcinoids contain abundant neurosecretory granules which show marked variation in size and shape, being round, ovoid, or elongated. The granules in trabecular carcinoids are round to oval, but typically uniform.

DIFFERENTIAL DIAGNOSIS

Insular carcinoid can be confused with other primary ovarian tumors, including granulosa cell tumor with a microfollicular arrangement or, less frequently, with Sertoli–Leydig or Sertoli cell tumors. *Granulosa cell tumors* with prominent Call–Exner bodies may closely simulate the acini seen in insular carcinoid. However, the latter the nuclei are not grooved but have the typical "salt-and-pepper" chromatin, and frequently have psammomatous calcifications in the lumen of the acini. The tubules of *Sertoli cell tumors* and *Sertoli Leydig cell tumors* may simulate the acini of insular carcinoid and those with heterologous elements may also contain a carcinoid component; however, other features typical of Sertoli–Leydig cell tumors should be identified. In difficult cases, a panel of immunohistochemical stains, including inhibin and neuroendocrine markers, may be of help.

Primary carcinoid of the ovary should be distinguished from *metastatic carcinoid*, more frequently insular and mucinous variants. The ileum is the most common site of origin for metastatic insular carcinoid, followed by other gastrointestinal sites and lung. The appendix is the most common origin for metastatic mucinous carcinoid. These tumors, in contrast to primary carcinoids, are more often associated with carcinoid syndrome, which persists after removal of the ovarian tumor. There is often bilateral ovarian involvement, and in 90% of cases, extraovarian metastases. On microscopic examination, these tumors differ from primary carcinoids in that they often show a multinodular growth, have prominent hyalinization of the stroma, and cystic change in the tumor nests as well as lymphovascular invasion. The tumors are not associated with a mature cystic teratoma or other primary ovarian tumor.

Mucinous carcinoid should be distinguished from a *Krukenberg tumor*, most commonly the tubular variant. Both tumors form tubules, have signet-ring cells, and may contain neurosecretory granules. However, the tubular Krukenberg tumor typically shows bilateral ovarian involvement, is associated with a conventional component with signet-ring cells, and does not have a component of mature cystic teratoma.

PROGNOSIS AND THERAPY

Approximately 95% of carcinoids are benign; however, insular and mucinous carcinoids may pursue a malignant course, especially when there is extension beyond the ovary.

IMMATURE TERATOMA

This represents the third most common malignant germ cell tumor of the ovary, accounting for 15–20 % of primitive germ cell tumors, although only 3 % of all teratomas are immature teratomas.

CLINICAL FEATURES

These tumors may occur at any age, but are more common in the first two decades of life. The symptoms are nonspecific and approximately 80 % of patients present with a painful abdominal mass. Elevated AFP serum level is seen in two-thirds of patients, although it is significantly lower than that encountered in patients with yolk sac tumors. CA-125 and CA19-9 are also elevated in about 90 % and 50 % of patients, respectively, whereas β-hCG and CEA are only rarely increased. Patients with immature teratomas may have a history of a mature cystic teratoma resected months to years earlier, typically multiple and ruptured.

IMMATURE TERATOMA – FACT SHEET

Definition
▸ Germ cell tumor showing variable amounts of immature tissues associated with mature elements

Incidence
▸ Third most common malignant germ cell tumor, accounting for 15–20% of all primitive germ cell tumors
▸ 3% of all ovarian teratomas

Age Distribution
▸ More common in first two decades

Clinical Features
▸ Painful abdominal mass
▸ Elevated AFP serum levels but significantly lower than in yolk sac tumor
▸ Serum levels of CA-125, CA 19-9, and CEA may be elevated
▸ If prior mature cystic teratoma, typically multiple and ruptured

Prognosis and Treatment
▸ Survival rate as high as 80% in stages I, II, and III when treated with chemotherapy
▸ Surgery for grade 1 tumors, including those associated with mature glial implants
▸ Surgery and chemotherapy for grade 2 and 3 tumors
▸ Small foci (< 2 mm) of other malignant germ cell tumors do not affect prognosis

---

IMMATURE TERATOMA – PATHOLOGIC FEATURES

Gross Findings
▸ Large tumors with ruptured capsule in approximately 50%
▸ Solid, soft, and fleshy cut section, often with a cystic component
▸ Dermoid cyst identified in one-quarter of tumors and in opposite ovary in 10%

Microscopic Findings
▸ Tissues from the three germ cell layers with a variable admixture of immature and mature tissues
▸ Amount of immature neuroepithelium used in grading:
  ▸ Grade 1: 1 low-power field in any one slide
  ▸ Grade 2: 1–3 low-power fields in any one slide
  ▸ Grade 3: exceeds 3 low-power fields in any one slide
▸ Unusual findings
  ▸ Prominent vascular proliferation
  ▸ Mature or immature glial implants (gliomatosis peritonei)
  ▸ Small foci of yolk sac tumor
  ▸ Scattered syncytiotrophoblast cells

Immunohistochemistry
▸ GFAP, S-100 and NSE in neuroectodermal elements

Differential Diagnosis
▸ Mature cystic teratoma with microscopic foci of immature elements
▸ Mature solid teratoma
▸ Yolk sac tumor
▸ Malignant neuroectodermal tumor
▸ Malignant mixed mesodermal tumor

RADIOLOGIC FEATURES

CT-scan and MRI show a heterogeneous large mass with aqueous fluid and solid areas with numerous cysts, scattered coarse calcifications, and punctate foci of fatty tissue.

PATHOLOGIC FEATURES

GROSS FINDINGS

These are large tumors with a ruptured capsule in approximately 50 % of cases. Most tumors are predominantly solid, soft, and fleshy on cut section, but often have a cystic component, in the form of small cysts (Figure 13.33). They are characterized by a multinodular brown to pink, gray to white cut surface with frequent areas of necrosis and hemorrhage. Hair and sebaceous material may be seen. A dermoid cyst may be grossly identified within the immature teratoma in up to 26 % of cases, or may be found in the opposite ovary (10 %).

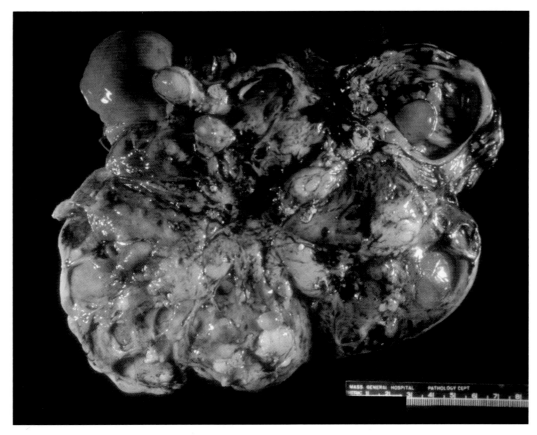

FIGURE 13.33
Immature teratoma. The solid and cystic cut surface is fleshy with areas of necrosis and hemorrhage.

MICROSCOPIC FINDINGS

Tissues from the three germ cell layers are identified with a variable admixture of mature and immature tissues, the latter resembling the normal embryo. However, it is the presence of immature tissue that establishes the diagnosis of immature teratoma. The most common immature element is neuroepithelium, with other common immature elements including immature epithelium or cartilage. The grading system of immature teratomas is based on the amount of immature neuroepithelium found in the tumor, which is evident as neuroepithelial rosettes and tubules (Figure 13.34), cellular foci of mitotically active glia (Figure 13.35), and in occasional cases, small areas resembling glioblastoma or neuroblastoma. In grade I tumors, the amount of immature neuroepithelium present on any one slide should not exceed 1 low-power field ($\times$ 40). In grade II tumors, the immature neuroepithelium occupies 1–3 low-power fields in any one slide, whereas in grade III tumors, the amount of immature neuroepithelium present exceeds 3 low-power fields in any one slide. More recently, O'Connor and Norris, after analyzing 244 immature teratomas, concluded that using a two-tiered system gave better interobserver reproducibility and was more useful from the clinical point of view. It is important that careful and extensive sampling be done (one section

per centimeter of viable tumor) in order to identify immature foci.

Unusual findings include:
1. *Prominent vascular proliferation* in the form of glomeruloid structures or confluent vessels forming large aggregates typically associated with neural tissue.
2. *Mature or immature glial implants in the peritoneum, omentum, or lymph nodes (gliomatosis peritonei)*. The implants typically appear as gray to white nodules, generally 1–3 mm, scattered throughout the peritoneum, but more frequently in the pelvis, omentum, or vicinity of the tumor, either an immature teratoma or rarely, a mature solid teratoma. They are exclusively or predominantly composed of mature glial tissue, often without an associated tissue response (Figure 13.36). On some occasions, the implants may be slightly immature. Other elements may rarely be present, or glial tissue may be found in lymph nodes. Although the origin of these lesions was initially assumed to relate to rupture and implantation of glial tissue in the peritoneum, recent studies have challenged this point of view, hypothesizing that glial implants represent in fact a metaplastic process of submesothelial cells. The finding of mature glial implants does not adversely affect the prognosis.

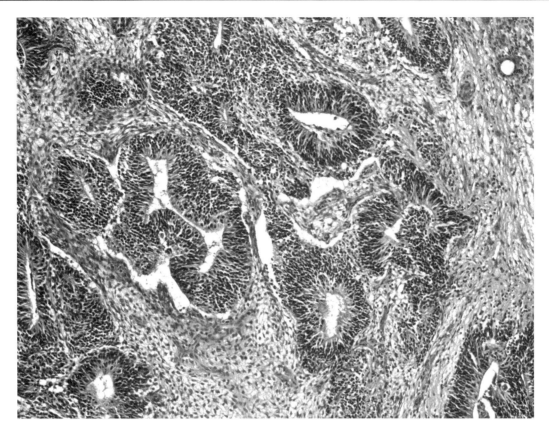

FIGURE 13.34
Immature teratoma. Multiple immature neuroepithelial rosettes are present in a glial fibrillary background.

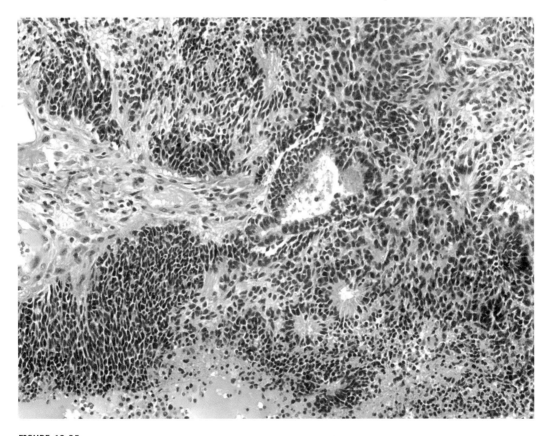

FIGURE 13.35
Immature teratoma. Immature neural elements include primitive neuroepithelial tubules and highly cellular atypical glial tissue.

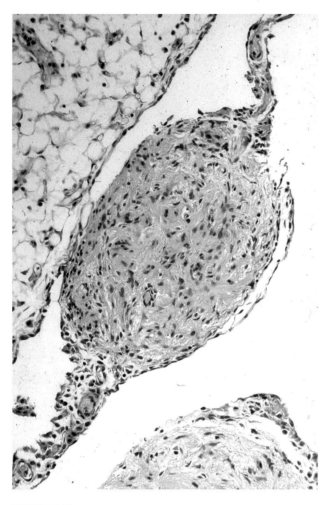

FIGURE 13.36
Peritoneal gliomatosis. The omental implant consists of mature glial tissue.

Exceptionally, malignant transformation of gliomatosis peritonei may occur. In immature teratomas, the finding of mature glial implants is associated with improved prognosis. However, mature glial implants may coexist with immature glial implants, thus extensive sampling is required.

3. The presence of *small foci of yolk sac tumor* measuring < 2 mm does not influence prognosis of the immature teratoma, thus the diagnosis of mixed germ cell tumor is not warranted.

4. *Syncytiotrophoblast cells* may be scattered throughout the tumor.

ANCILLARY STUDIES

IMMUNOHISTOCHEMISTRY

The neuroectodermal elements can be highlighted by neural markers, including glial fibrillary acid protein (GFAP), S-100 protein, and NSE. These markers may, on occasion, help to distinguish immature neural tissue – mainly neural rosettes – from other immature non-neural tissues with overlapping morphology.

CYTOGENETICS

A few immature teratomas have been associated with trisomy 12.

DIFFERENTIAL DIAGNOSIS

An important pitfall in the diagnosis of immature teratoma is the misinterpretation of cellular but fully differentiated neural tissue as immature tissue, such as the granular cell layer of the cerebellar cortex. Immature neural elements usually have nuclei with vesicular chromatin and show apoptosis and mitotic activity, in contrast to the fully differentiated neural elements which show nuclei with uniformly dense chromatin without mitotic activity or apoptosis. It is also important not to consider fetal-type tissue, such as cartilage, as evidence of immaturity. The diagnosis of immature teratoma requires the finding of tissue with an embryonic appearance, almost always neuroepithelium.

Mature solid teratomas, although exclusively composed of mature elements, may be confused with immature teratomas as they have similar age distribution and gross appearance, except for the absence of necrosis. On microscopic examination of mature solid teratomas, although neural tissue may predominate, it is always mature. *Yolk sac tumor* may enter in the differential diagnosis, as areas with endodermal differentiation in immature teratoma may contain embryonal hepatic or intestinal differentiation. The presence of these elements in a tumor with high AFP levels (> 1000 ng/mL) should strongly raise the suspicion of a yolk sac component in the tumor.

The presence of abundant immature mitotically active neuroectodermal tissue in an immature teratoma may bring a *malignant neuroectodermal tumor* into the differential diagnosis. However, the latter shows a monotonous growth of malignant cells without the admixture of other teratomatous elements. *Malignant mixed mesodermal tumors* may cause problems in the differential diagnosis as cartilage is present in both tumors. In contrast to immature teratomas, the cartilage in malignant mixed mesodermal tumors is highly malignant and resembles a chondrosarcoma. Furthermore, these tumors typically occur in postmenopausal women and are composed of high-grade carcinoma admixed with high-grade mesenchymal elements.

FIGURE 13.37

Gonadoblastoma. Large germ cells are surrounded by smaller sex cord-type cells with interspersed round spaces filled with basement membrane material.

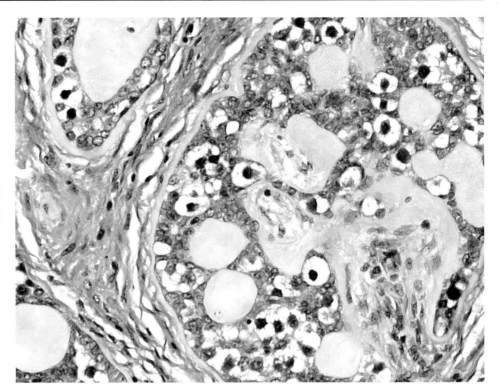

PROGNOSIS AND THERAPY

Treatment is based on histologic grade and clinicopathologic stage of the tumor. The presence of small foci (≤ 2 mm) of other germ cell elements does not adversely affect the prognosis of these tumors. Grade 1 immature teratomas are treated by surgery only. However, the metastatic rate of grade 2 or 3 immature teratomas without chemotherapy is as high as 80%. The majority of patients with stage I grade 2 or 3 immature teratoma treated with chemotherapy have 5- and 10-year survival rates > 80%. Consequently, these tumors should be treated with surgery and chemotherapy. Grade 1 immature teratomas associated with mature glial implants do not require further treatment. With chemotherapy, most peritoneal implants mature or regress; however, mature implants may continue to grow ("growing teratoma syndrome"). The treatment in these cases is surgical removal of the mass to prevent local mechanical complications.

OTHER RARE GERM CELL TUMORS

GONADOBLASTOMA

Most patients with gonadoblastoma are phenotypic females with a Y chromosome in their genotype. They have an associated contralateral gonadoblastoma in one-third of cases. This tumor is composed of nests of primordial germ cells intimately admixed with sex cord elements that resemble immature Sertoli and granulosa cells. The latter surrounds round spaces filled with eosinophilic basement material (Figure 13.37). Stromal lutein or Leydig cells are present at the periphery of the nodules, embedded in variable amounts of stroma. Calcifications are seen in the majority of these tumors. In approximately one-half of the cases, a dysgerminoma arises and frequently overgrows the underlying gonadoblastoma (Figure 13.38). Calcification may be the only clue to the diagnosis of the underlying gonadoblastoma in these cases.

POLYEMBRYOMA

This is an extremely rare form of malignant germ cell tumor, predominantly or exclusively composed of embryoid bodies. An embryoid body resembles an early embryo at different stages of development and is composed of an embryonic disk, the yolk sac, amniotic cavity, trophoblast, and extraembryonic mesenchyme (Figure 13.39). Hepatic and intestinal differentiation may be seen. The behavior of these tumors is similar to other malignant germ cell tumors.

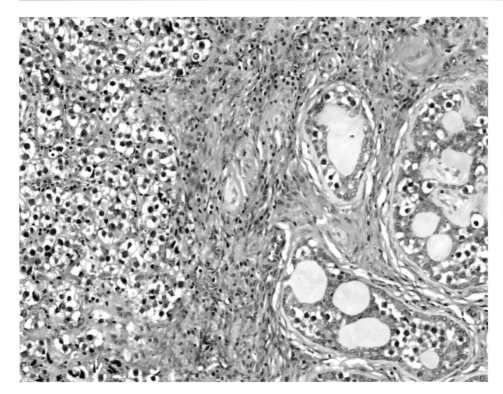

FIGURE 13.38
Dysgerminoma (left) arising in a gonad-oblastoma.

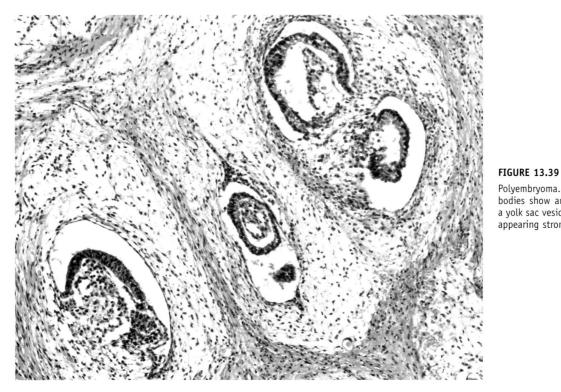

FIGURE 13.39
Polyembryoma. Several embryoid bodies show an embryonic disk and a yolk sac vesicle in loose, primitive-appearing stroma.

SUGGESTED READING

Akhtar M, al Dayel F. Is it feasible to diagnose germ cell tumors by fine-needle aspiration biopsy? Diagn Cytopathol 1997;16:72–77.

Baker PM, Oliva E. Immunohistochemistry as a tool in the differential diagnosis of ovarian tumors: an update. Int J Gynecol Pathol 2005;24:39–55.

Billmire D, Vinocur C, Rescorla F, et al. Outcome and staging evaluation in malignant germ cell tumors of the ovary in children and adolescents: an intergroup study. J Pediatr Surg 2004;39:424–429.

Brammer HM 3rd, Buck JL, Hayes WS, et al. From the archives of the AFIP. Malignant germ cell tumors of the ovary: radiologic–pathologic correlation. Radiographics 1990;10:715–724.

Clement PB, Young RH. Non-teratomatous germ cell tumors. Mini-symposium: germ cell tumours of the ovary (part I). Curr Diagn Pathol 1995;2:199–207.

Curtin JP, Morrow CP, D'Ablaing G, et al. Malignant germ cell tumors of the ovary: 20-year report of LAC-USC Women's Hospital. Int J Gynecol Cancer 1994;4:29–35.

Kurman RJ, Norris HJ. Malignant mixed germ cell tumors of the ovary. A clinical and pathologic analysis of 30 cases. Obstet Gynecol 1976;48:579–589.

Lu KH, Gershenson DM. Update on the management of ovarian germ cell tumors. J Reprod Med 2005;50:417–425.

Rodriguez E, Melamed J, Reuter V, et al. Chromosome 12 abnormalities in malignant ovarian germ cell tumors. Cancer Genet Cytogenet 1995;82:62–66.

Scully RE. Tumors of the ovary and maldeveloped gonads. In: Hartmann WH, Cowan WR (eds) Atlas of Tumor Pathology. second series, fascicle 16. Washington, DC: Armed Forces Institute of Pathology, 1979:239–312.

Ulbright TM. Germ cell tumors of the gonads: a selective review emphasizing problems in differential diagnosis, newly appreciated, and controversial issues. Mod Pathol 2005;18 (Suppl 2):S61–S79.

Ulbright TM, Goheen MP, Roth LM, et al. The differentiation of carcinomas of teratomatous origin from embryonal carcinoma. A light and electron microscopic study. Cancer 1986;57:257–263.

Dysgerminoma

Asadourian LA, Taylor HB. Dysgerminoma. An analysis of 105 cases. Obstet Gynecol 1969;33:370–379.

Cheng L, Thomas A, Roth LM, et al. OCT4: a novel biomarker for dysgerminoma of the ovary. Am J Surg Pathol 2004;28:1341–1346.

Gordon A, Lipton D, Woodruff JD. Dysgerminoma: a review of 158 cases from the Emil Novak Ovarian Tumor Registry. Obstet Gynecol 1981;58:497–504.

Parkash V, Carcangiu ML. Transformation of ovarian dysgerminoma to yolk sac tumor: evidence for a histogenetic continuum. Mod Pathol 1995;8:881–887.

Sayedur Rahman M, Al-Sibai MH, Rahman J, et al. Ovarian carcinoma associated with pregnancy. A review of 9 cases. Acta Obstet Gynecol Scand 2002;81:260–264.

Talerman A, Huyzinga WT, Kuipers T. Dysgerminoma. Clinocopathologic study of 22 cases. Obstet Gynecol 1973;41:137–147.

Zaloudek CJ, Tavassoli FA, Norris HJ. Dysgerminoma with syncytiotrophoblastic giant cells. A histologically and clinically distinctive subtype of dysgerminoma. Am J Surg Pathol 1981;5:361–367.

Embryonal Carcinoma

Davis KP, Hartmann LK, Keeney GL, et al. Primary ovarian carcinoid tumors. Gynecol Oncol 1996;61:259–265.

Kurman RJ, Norris HJ. Embryonal carcinoma of the ovary: a clinicopathologic entity distinct from endodermal sinus tumor resembling embryonal carcinoma of the adult testis. Cancer 1976;38:2420–2433.

Ueda G, Abe Y, Yoshida M, et al. Embryonal carcinoma of the ovary: a six-year survival. Int J Gynaecol Obstet 1990;31:287–292.

Choriocarcinoma

Axe SR, Klein VR, Woodruff JD. Choriocarcinoma of the ovary. Obstet Gynecol 1985;66:111–114.

Gerbie MV, Brewer JI, Tamimi H. Primary choriocarcinoma of the ovary. Obstet Gynecol 1975;46:720–723.

Oliva E, Andrada E, Pezzica E, et al. Ovarian carcinomas with choriocarcinomatous differentiation. Cancer 1993;72:2441–2446.

Tsujioka H, Hamada H, Miyakawa T, et al. A pure nongestational choriocarcinoma of the ovary diagnosed with DNA polymorphism analysis. Gynecol Oncol 2003;89:540–542.

Vance RP, Geisinger KR. Pure nongestational choriocarcinoma of the ovary. Report of a case. Cancer 1985;56:2321–2325.

Yolk Sac Tumor

Clement PB, Young RH, Scully RE. Endometrioid-like variant of ovarian yolk sac tumor. A clinicopathological analysis of eight cases. Am J Surg Pathol 1987;11:767–778.

Devouassoux-Shisheboran M, Schammel DP, Tavassoli FA. Ovarian hepatoid yolk sac tumours: morphological, immunohistochemical and ultrastructural features. Histopathology 1999;34:462–469.

Kurman RJ, Norris HJ. Endodermal sinus tumor of the ovary: a clinical and pathologic analysis of 71 cases. Cancer 1976;38:2404–2419.

Nawa A, Obata N, Kikkawa F, et al. Prognostic factors of patients with yolk sac tumors of the ovary. Am J Obstet Gynecol 2001;184:1182–1188.

Nogales FF Jr, Matilla A, Nogales O, et al. Yolk sac tumors with pure and mixed polyvesicular vitelline patterns. Hum Pathol 1978;9:553–566.

Nogales FF, Bergeron C, Carvia RE, et al. Ovarian endometrioid tumors with yolk sac tumor component, an unusual form of ovarian neoplasm. Analysis of six cases. Am J Surg Pathol 1996;20:1056–1066.

Ramalingam P, Malpica A, Silva EG, et al. The use of cytokeratin 7 and EMA in differentiating ovarian yolk sac tumors from endometrioid and clear cell carcinomas. Am J Surg Pathol 2004;28:1499–1505.

Ulbright TM, Roth LM, Brodhecker CA. Yolk sac differentiation in germ cell tumors. A morphologic study of 50 cases with emphasis on hepatic, enteric, and parietal yolk sac features. Am J Surg Pathol 1986;10:151–164.

Teratomas Excluding Monodermal Teratomas

Clement PB, Young RH. Teratomas excluding monodermal teratomas. Mini-symposium: germ cell tumours of the ovary (part II). Curr Diagn Pathol 1995;2:208–213.

Comerci JT Jr, Licciardi F, Bergh PA, et al. Mature cystic teratoma: a clinicopathologic evaluation of 517 cases and review of the literature. Obstet Gynecol 1994;84:22–28.

Cushing B, Giller R, Ablin A, et al. Surgical resection alone is effective treatment for ovarian immature teratoma in children and adolescents: a report of the pediatric oncology group and the children's cancer group. Am J Obstet Gynecol 1999;181:353–358.

Ferguson AW, Katabuchi H, Ronnett BM et al. Glial implants in gliomatosis peritonei arise from normal tissue, not from the associated teratoma. Am J Pathol 2001;159:51–55.

Kwan MY, Kalle W, Lau GT, et al. Is gliomatosis peritonei derived from the associated ovarian teratoma? Hum Pathol 2004;35:685–688.

Norris HJ, Zirkin HJ, Benson WL. Immature (malignant) teratoma of the ovary: a clinical and pathologic study of 58 cases. Cancer 1976;37:2359–2372.

O'Connor DM, Norris HJ. The influence of grade on the outcome of stage I ovarian immature (malignant) teratomas and the reproducibility of grading. Int J Gynecol Pathol 1994;13:283–289.

Pins MR, Young RH, Daly WJ, et al. Primary squamous cell carcinoma of the ovary. Report of 37 cases. Am J Surg Pathol 1996;20:823–833.

Robboy SJ, Scully RE. Ovarian teratoma with glial implants on the peritoneum. An analysis of 12 cases. Hum Pathol 1970;1:643–653.

Yanai-Inbar I, Scully RE. Relation of ovarian dermoid cysts and immature teratomas: an analysis of 350 cases of immature teratoma and 10 cases of dermoid cyst with microscopic foci of immature tissue. Int J Gynecol Pathol 1987;6:203–212.

Monodermal Teratomas

Baker PM, Oliva E, Young RH, et al. Ovarian mucinous carcinoids including some with a carcinomatous component: a report of 17 cases. Am J Surg Pathol 2001;25:557–568.

Clement PB, Young RH. Monodermal teratomas. Mini-symposium: germ cell tumours of the ovary (part III). Curr Diagn Pathol 1995;2:214–221.

Devaney K, Snyder R, Norris HJ, et al. Proliferative and histologically malignant struma ovarii: a clinicopathologic study of 54 cases. Int J Gynecol Pathol 1993;12:333–343.

Robboy SJ, Norris HJ, Scully RE. Insular carcinoid primary in the ovary. A clinicopathologic analysis of 48 cases. Cancer 1975;36:404–418.

Robboy SJ, Scully RE. Strumal carcinoid of the ovary: an analysis of 50 cases of a distinctive tumor composed of thyroid tissue and carcinoid. Cancer 1980;46:2019–2034.

Robboy SJ, Scully RE, Norris HJ. Primary trabecular carcinoid of the ovary. Obstet Gynecol 1977;49:202–207.

Szyfelbein WM, Young RH, Scully RE. Struma ovarii simulating ovarian tumors of other types. A report of 30 cases. Am J Surg Pathol 1995;19:21–29.

Talerman A, Evans MI. Primary trabecular carcinoid tumor of the ovary. Cancer 1982;50:1403–1407.

Gonadoblastoma

Gadducci A, Madrigali A, Simeone T, et al. The association of ovarian dysgerminoma and gonadoblastoma in a phenotypic female with 46 XY karyotype. Eur J Gynaecol Oncol 1994;15:125–131.

Kildal W, Kraggerud SM, Abeler VM, et al. Genome profiles of bilateral dysgerminomas, a unilateral gonadoblastoma, and a metastasis from a 46, XY phenotypic female. Hum Pathol 2003;34:946–949.

Scully RE. Gonadoblastoma. A review of 74 cases. Cancer 1970;25:1340–1356.

14

Metastatic and Miscellaneous Primary Tumors of the Ovary

Russell Vang · Brigitte M Ronnett

METASTATIC TUMORS INVOLVING THE OVARY

Metastases account for approximately 8% of malignant ovarian neoplasms in women undergoing surgery for an adnexal mass in the US. Metastases derived from nongynecologic sites are eleven times more common than those derived from female genital tract organs, with adenocarcinomas of gastrointestinal tract being most common. Ovarian metastases are not infrequently encountered in women with disseminated cancer, and when a nonovarian primary site has already been established, recognition of the ovarian tumors as metastatic is not difficult. Metastases to the ovaries are also usually readily recognized as such when they exhibit characteristic gross and microscopic features, even when another primary site has not been identified or is discovered concurrently with the ovarian tumor. However, not infrequently, metastases can share both gross and microscopic features with primary ovarian neoplasms, making recognition difficult, particularly when the primary site has not been identified. The distinction of primary and metastatic ovarian neoplasms is further complicated by the occurrence of synchronous independent ovarian and nonovarian (usually of other female genital tract organs) neoplasms having similar histologic features. In some cases, the tumors are independent but on occasion they may be metastatic, even when there is limited invasion in the nonovarian primary site.

GENERAL FEATURES OF METASTATIC CARCINOMA

A number of clinical, gross, and microscopic features are characteristic of metastatic involvement of the ovaries (Boxes 14.1–14.3). It should be emphasized, however, that none of these features are pathognomonic and metastases are most easily recognized when a combination of features is present. Moreover, some metastases lack all of the characteristic features and require ancillary techniques to establish a correct diagnosis.

CLINICAL FEATURES

Metastases to the ovaries can present synchronously or metachronously with the primary nonovarian neoplasm. Those presenting metachronously can do so subsequent to, or prior to, the diagnosis of the nonovarian primary tumor. In the former situation, the diagnosis of an ovarian metastasis is often not difficult, particularly when the history of a prior nonovarian malignant neoplasm is known to the pathologist and additional sites are involved by metastatic disease. In contrast, the latter scenario is often diagnostically challenging, particularly when metastatic disease appears to be confined to the ovaries and characteristic features of metastases are lacking. In exceptional cases, the primary site may not be identified until months or even years later. Finally, on occasion, metastatic neoplasms can cause virilization, simulating the clinical presentation of a primary ovarian sex cord-stromal neoplasm. Although relatively rare, this phenomenon is most frequently encountered with metastatic mucinous carcinomas, particularly Krukenberg tumors in young women during pregnancy.

PATHOLOGIC FEATURES

GROSS FINDINGS

Characteristic gross features of metastases in the ovaries include smaller size (often < 10 cm), bilateral involvement, nodular growth pattern, and presence of tumor on the ovarian surface and/or in the superficial cortex. Nodular tumors are typically solid and compress the surrounding ovarian stroma. Not infrequently, however, metastases can be large, unilateral, and cystic, simulating a primary ovarian neoplasm.

MICROSCOPIC FINDINGS

Characteristic histologic features of metastases include infiltrative growth with stromal desmoplasia, nodular architecture with involvement of the ovarian surface and superficial cortex, and hilar and lymphovascular space involvement. However, some metastatic carcinomas have a confluent glandular/expansile growth, simulating either primary ovarian atypical proliferative (borderline) tumors with intraepithelial carcinoma or well-differentiated carcinoma, usually of mucinous and endometrioid types. The presence of signet-ring cells almost invariably indicates metastatic carcinoma of gastrointestinal tract or breast origin. Certain other histologic features are characteristic of particular types of metastatic carcinomas, such as a garland pattern of epithelium surrounding so-called "dirty necrosis" in metastatic colorectal carcinoma. Some features that might suggest an ovarian origin are actually nonspecific and can be seen in metastatic carcinomas. These include the finding of histologically benign-appearing and low-grade proliferative (cystadenomatous and atypical prolifera-tive (borderline type)) mucinous epithelium in metastatic pancreatic mucinous carcinomas as well as stromal luteinization.

PROGNOSIS AND THERAPY

The prognosis and therapy of metastatic neoplasms to the ovary are highly dependent on the specific primary tumor diagnosis. Ovarian metastases derived from nongynecologic primary neoplasms qualify as stage IV disease and as such would generally be expected to have a poor outcome. Metastases of endometrial carcinoma reflect FIGO stage IIIA.

METASTASES FROM NONGYNECOLOGIC SITES

METASTASES FROM CARCINOMA OF THE LARGE INTESTINE/RECTUM

CLINICAL FEATURES

Metastases of colorectal adenocarcinoma most commonly occur in patients in the fifth to ninth decades but occasionally can be encountered in younger patients. The location within the large intestine is commonly the rectosigmoid, but all segments of the large bowel can be the site of origin. Some patients present with adnexal masses subsequent to the diagnosis of the primary colorectal carcinoma, but others present with an adnexal mass as the first manifestation of a synchronously or subsequently identified colorectal carcinoma; the latter situation can pose a diagnostic challenge at the time of frozen section diagnosis.

BOX 14.1

FEATURES CHARACTERISTIC OF METASTASES TO THE OVARY

Bilateral involvement
Size < 10 cm
Surface and/or superficial cortical involvement
Nodular growth
Infiltrative growth pattern with stromal desmoplasia
Signet-ring cell component
Hilar involvement or lymphovascular invasion
Known history of nonovarian primary tumor

BOX 14.2

FEATURES CHARACTERISTIC OF PRIMARY OVARIAN TUMORS

Unilateral involvement
Size > 10 cm
Lack of surface and/or superficial cortical involvement
Absence of nodularity

BOX 14.3

FEATURES SHARED BY PRIMARY OVARIAN TUMORS AND METASTASES TO THE OVARY

Cyst formation
Necrosis
Low-grade areas suggesting a primary ovarian precursor lesion
Stromal luteinization

METASTASES FROM CARCINOMA OF THE LARGE INTESTINE/RECTUM – FACT SHEET

Incidence and Location
▶ 37% of clinically apparent metastases from nongynecologic primaries
▶ 34% of all clinically apparent metastases
▶ Up to 10% of women with colonic carcinoma have ovarian metastases
▶ Rectosigmoid region most common location

Age Distribution
▶ Fifth to ninth decades

Clinical Features
▶ Symptoms related to ovarian mass(es)

PATHOLOGIC FEATURES

GROSS FINDINGS

Tumors are bilateral in 25–43% of cases, with median sizes ranging from 11 to 15 cm. The cut surfaces are frequently cystic but may be solid (Figure 14.1) and hemorrhage and necrosis are common.

MICROSCOPIC FINDINGS

Colorectal adenocarcinomas are composed of glands of variable size, ranging from small to large and cystically dilated (Figure 14.2), or can display complex architecture with cribriforming (Figure 14.3). The cells lining the glands are typically columnar, nonstratified or multilayered, with varying degrees of mucinous differentiation. Most commonly, there is minimal mucin and the epithelium has an "endometrioid" appearance, but not infrequently, there is some mucinous differentiation, imparting a hybrid morphology (Figure 14.4). Occasionally, the tumors can produce abundant extracellular mucin (colloid carcinoma) or can have a significant signet-ring cell component. The nuclei are oval to columnar showing cytologic atypia and brisk mitotic activity is seen. The tumors frequently have a characteristic appearance in which the epithelium is draped along the periphery of luminal eosinophilic necrotic material containing karyorrhectic debris ("garland pattern" of "dirty necrosis") (Figures 14.5 and 14.6). Segmental necrosis of the glands is also characteristic but not pathogno-

monic, of metastatic colonic carcinoma. Stromal condensation and luteinization around the neoplastic glands are frequent findings.

ANCILLARY STUDIES

IMMUNOHISTOCHEMISTRY

Metastatic colorectal adenocarcinomas are most commonly diffusely and strongly positive for CK20 and negative for CK7 (Figures 14.7 and 14.8). On occasion, CK7 expression is encountered but tends to be focal. Rectal and right sided colonic adenocarcinomas have a slight tendency to exhibit more extensive expression of CK7. CDX2, a marker of intestinal-type differentiation, is expressed in virtually all colorectal adenocarcinomas. Therefore, it has some utility in the distinction of metastatic colorectal carcinoma to the ovary (diffusely positive) from primary ovarian endometrioid carcinoma (often negative). However, its value in distinguishing metastatic colorectal carcinoma from primary ovarian mucinous tumors is limited due to frequent CDX2 expression in both tumor types.

DIFFERENTIAL DIAGNOSIS

Metastatic colorectal carcinomas can simulate primary endometrioid and mucinous tumors of the ovary. In general, the nuclear grade of metastatic colorectal carcinoma is higher than that of endometrioid carcinoma. Features favoring a *primary endometrioid tumor* include the presence of an adenofibromatous background, foci of squamous differentiation, and associated endometriosis. Primary mucinous ovarian carcinomas not infrequently show areas of benign or borderline morphology and features of metastases are typically

---

METASTASES FROM CARCINOMA OF THE LARGE INTESTINE/RECTUM – PATHOLOGIC FEATURES

Gross Findings
▶ 25–43% bilateral
▶ Mean/median size: 11–15 cm
▶ Cystic and necrotic or, less commonly, solid cut surface

Microscopic Findings
▶ Variably sized glands with frequent cribriform pattern
▶ Garland pattern, "dirty" and segmental necrosis
▶ Endometrioid-like, mucinous, or hybrid differentiation
▶ Less frequently, abundant extracellular mucin or signet-ring cells
▶ Columnar cells with notable nuclear atypia and mitotic activity
▶ Desmoplastic or edematous stroma
▶ Not infrequently, periglandular stromal condensation or luteinization

Immunohistochemical Features
▶ CK20 and CDX2 diffuse positivity
▶ CK7 usually negative except for rectal and right sided colonic carcinomas

Differential Diagnosis
▶ Endometrioid and mucinous tumors of ovary
▶ Independent synchronous colonic and ovarian tumors (Lynch syndrome, type II)

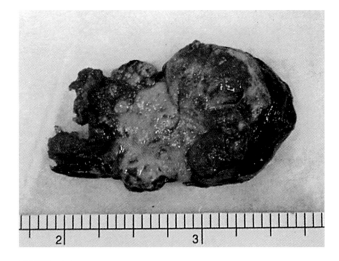

FIGURE 14.1

Metastatic large intestinal adenocarcinoma. The ovary is small and the cut surface has a nodular appearance.

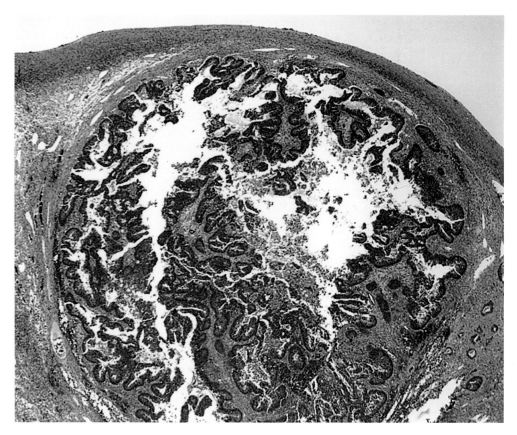

FIGURE 14.2
Metastatic large intestinal adenocarcinoma. Nodular growth in the superficial cortex is characteristic of metastatic carcinoma.

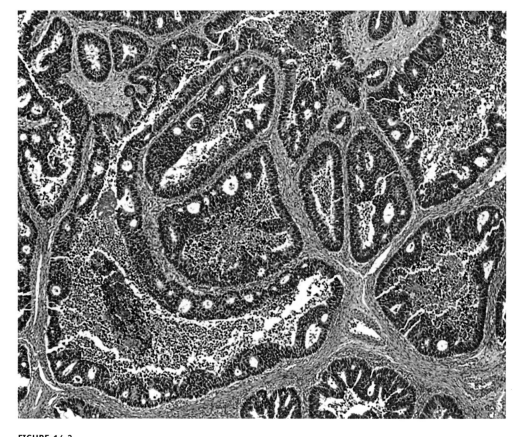

FIGURE 14.3
Metastatic large intestinal adenocarcinoma. Cribriform glands (garland pattern) are associated with abundant intraglandular necrotic material containing karyorrhectic debris ("dirty necrosis").

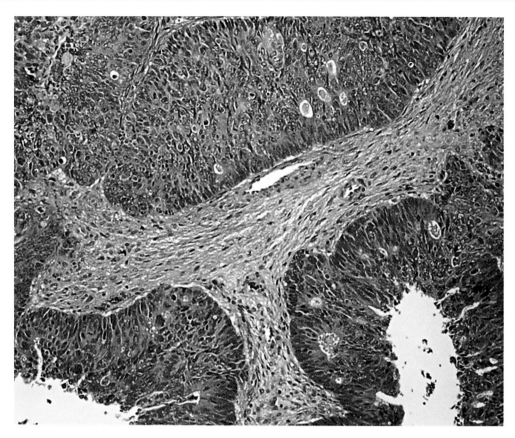

FIGURE 14.4

Metastatic large intestinal adenocarcinoma. The cribriform architecture and endometrioid-type differentiation simulate a primary endometrioid carcinoma of the ovary.

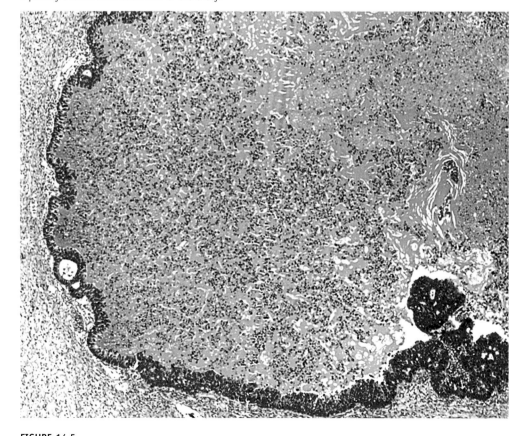

FIGURE 14.5

Metastatic large intestinal adenocarcinoma. Atypical epithelium is draped along the periphery of a cystic gland, which is filled with necrotic material containing cellular debris ("dirty necrosis").

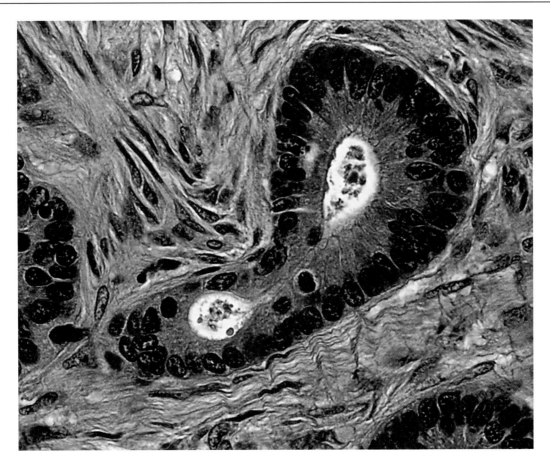

FIGURE 14.6
Metastatic large intestinal adenocarcinoma. Neoplastic glands are lined by atypical columnar cells.

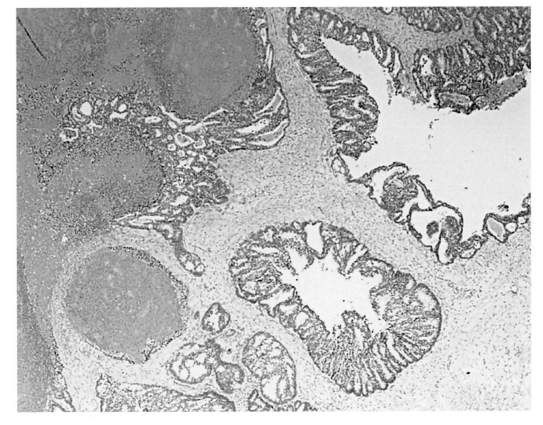

FIGURE 14.7
Metastatic large intestinal adenocarcinoma. The tumor lacks CK7 expression.

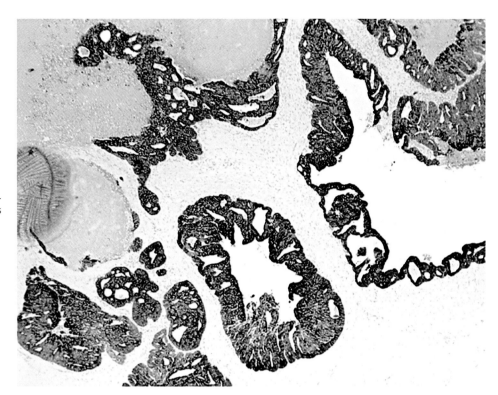

FIGURE 14.8
Metastatic large intestinal adenocarcinoma. The tumor diffusely expresses CK20.

absent. However, the finding of a large, unilateral tumor having a smooth surface and exhibiting a confluent glandular rather than infiltrative or nodular growth pattern does not guarantee that the tumor is primary in the ovary. CK7 and CK20 are useful in the distinction of metastatic colorectal carcinoma from primary ovarian endometrioid and mucinous tumors as these ovarian tumors are almost invariably diffusely positive for CK7 and often negative or only partially positive for CK20, whereas colorectal carcinomas typically have the reverse CK7/CK20 immunoprofile. Of note, rectal and right sided colonic adenocarcinomas may be CK7 positive.

METASTASES FROM CARCINOMA OF THE BREAST

CLINICAL FEATURES

Most patients range in age from 25 to 80 (mean 49) years and have a known history of primary breast carcinoma. However, the ovarian metastases may occasionally represent the initial manifestation of the disease.

PATHOLOGIC FEATURES

GROSS FINDINGS

In approximately two-thirds of cases, metastases are bilateral. The tumors are usually < 5 cm and they tend

---

METASTASES FROM CARCINOMA OF THE BREAST – FACT SHEET

Incidence
▸ 12% of clinically apparent metastases from nongynecologic primary tumors
▸ 11% of all clinically apparent metastases

Age Distribution
▸ 25–80 (mean 49) years

Clinical Features
▸ Adnexal mass(es), with or without prior history of breast carcinoma

---

to form identifiable solid nodules; cystic tumors are unusual. Occasionally, they cause diffuse enlargement of the ovary.

MICROSCOPIC FINDINGS

The metastatic deposits are from ductal and lobular carcinoma in 75 and 25 % of cases, respectively. A variety of growth patterns can be encountered, with ductal carcinomas often displaying glandular, papillary, cribriform, or diffuse growth, and lobular carcinomas exhibiting characteristic single-file, cords, trabeculae, insular and diffuse growth, occasionally with signet-ring cells (Krukenberg tumor) (Figures 14.9–14.14). The tumor

METASTASES FROM CARCINOMA OF THE BREAST – PATHOLOGIC FEATURES

Gross Findings

▸ Bilateral in 64% of cases
▸ Usually < 5 cm
▸ Nodular or, less commonly, diffuse ovarian involvement

Microscopic Findings

▸ Ductal carcinoma: glandular, papillary, cribriform, or diffuse growths
▸ Lobular carcinoma: single file, cords, trabeculae, insular and diffuse growths
▸ Signet-ring cells may be seen
▸ Cells with pale to eosinophilic cytoplasm and round to oval nuclei
▸ Minimal cytologic atypia and mitotic activity

Immunohistochemical Features

▸ CK7 positive
▸ Variable staining for ER, PR, and GCDFP-15 (more often in better-differentiated ductal carcinomas and approximately 50% of lobular carcinomas)
▸ CA-125 positivity in ~ 20%
▸ CK20 negative and WT1 usually negative

Differential Diagnosis

▸ Ovarian serous and endometrioid carcinoma
▸ Carcinoid tumor
▸ Adult granulosa cell tumor
▸ Lymphoma

cells tend to have pale to eosinophilic cytoplasm and display round to oval nuclei without prominent cytologic atypia. Necrosis is occasionally present.

ANCILLARY STUDIES

IMMUNOHISTOCHEMISTRY

Breast carcinomas are typically positive for CK7 and negative for CK20. Expression of ER, PR, and GCDFP-15 (BRST-2) is more often seen in better-differentiated ductal carcinomas and in a significant number of lobular carcinomas. GCDFP-15 positivity establishes the diagnosis of breast carcinoma, but a negative staining does not exclude this diagnosis. Approximately 23% of these tumors are positive for CA-125, but most do not express WT-1.

DIFFERENTIAL DIAGNOSIS

Metastatic breast carcinoma should be distinguished from primary ovarian carcinoma (most commonly serous and less commonly, endometrioid), carcinoid tumor, adult granulosa cell tumor, and lymphoma. It can be difficult to distinguish poorly differentiated ductal

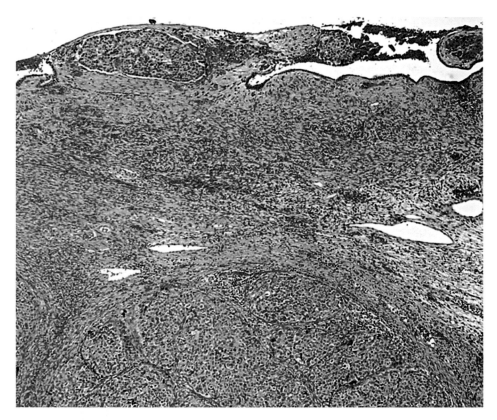

FIGURE 14.9

Metastatic breast carcinoma. A small nodule on the ovarian surface, separated from the main tumor in the parenchyma (lower half), suggests a metastasis.

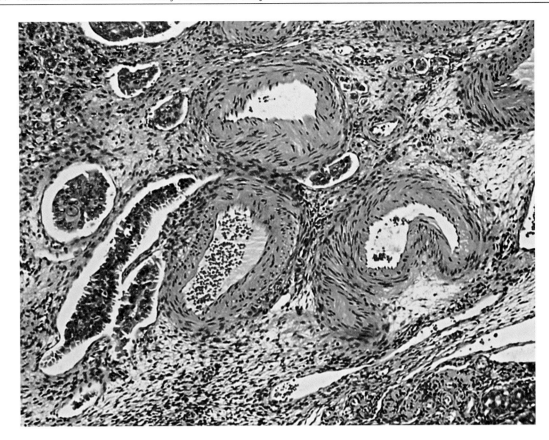

FIGURE 14.10
Metastatic breast carcinoma. Lymphovascular invasion in the hilus of the ovary suggests metastasis.

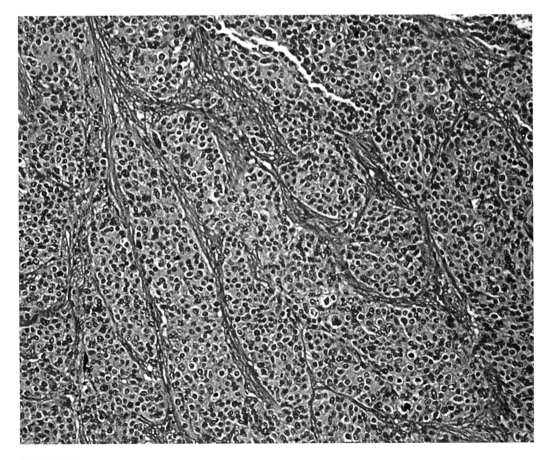

FIGURE 14.11
Metastatic breast carcinoma, ductal type. The neoplasm is composed of solid nests of monotonous tumor cells.

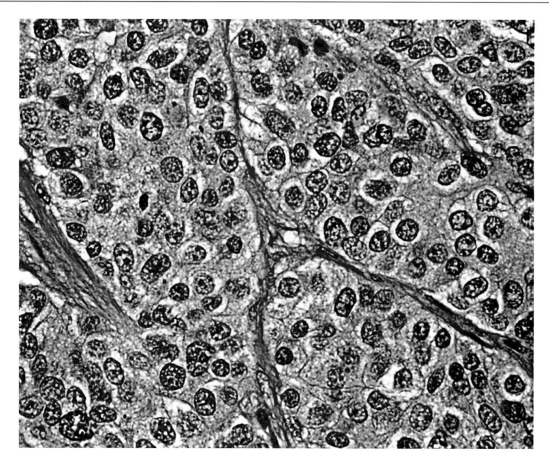

FIGURE 14.12

Metastatic breast carcinoma, ductal type. Tumor cells are cohesive and large with abundant eosinophilic cytoplasm and round nuclei.

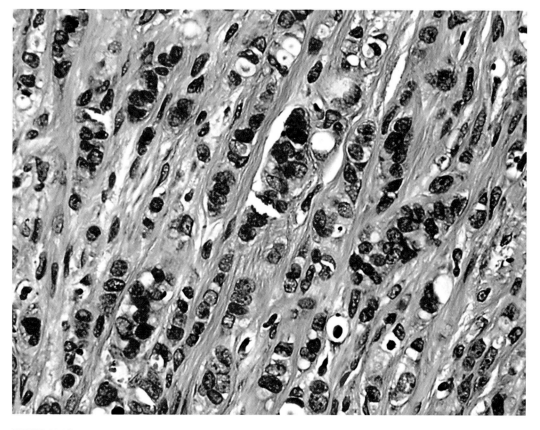

FIGURE 14.13

Metastatic breast carcinoma, lobular type. The tumor cells are arranged in single-file and cords.

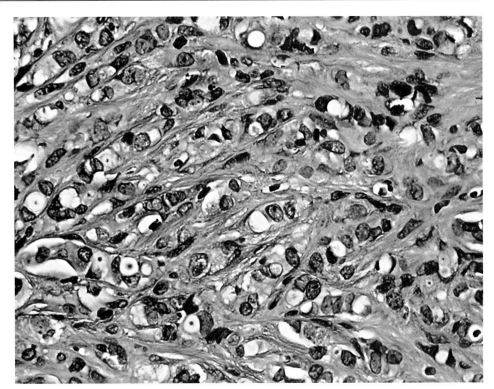

FIGURE 14.14
Metastatic breast carcinoma, lobular type. Note prominent signet-ring cell differentiation.

carcinomas from ovarian *high-grade serous carcinomas.* This is especially problematic in evaluating frozen sections for surgical management of adnexal masses in patients with a genetic susceptibility for breast and ovarian cancer who have known invasive breast cancer. Expression of ER and PR does not distinguish breast from ovarian carcinoma since both tumor types can be positive; however GCDFP-15 expression favors breast carcinoma. WT-1 (N-terminus) positivity generally favors ovarian serous carcinoma as almost all these tumor express this marker whereas most breast carcinomas do not. However, it does not distinguish between metastatic breast and endometrioid carcinoma. In addition to their characteristic nested growth pattern and nuclear features, *carcinoid tumors* are typically positive for chromogranin and synaptophysin. *Adult granulosa cell tumor* may mimic the growth pattern of a lobular carcinoma and also be positive for keratin; however, it shows characteristic nuclear features (grooves) and are typically diffusely positive for inhibin. *Lymphomas/leukemias* are typically keratin-negative.

METASTASES FROM CARCINOMA OF THE STOMACH

CLINICAL FEATURES

Patients range in age from 20 to 70 years but many are younger than 40 years. Most patients have symptoms related to an adnexal mass, with the remainder having gastrointestinal symptoms. Infrequently, virilization

---

METASTASES FROM CARCINOMA OF THE STOMACH – FACT SHEET

Incidence
▸ 9% of clinically apparent metastases from nongynecologic primary tumors
▸ 8% of all clinically apparent metastases

Age Distribution
▸ Mean 40–45 years

Clinical Features
▸ Symptoms related to ovarian mass(es) or gastrointestinal complaints
▸ History of prior carcinoma in only 25% of cases
▸ Infrequently virilization

may occur. A history of a prior gastric carcinoma is only present in about 25% of patients.

PATHOLOGIC FEATURES

GROSS FINDINGS

The tumors are bilateral in approximately 80% of cases. Sizes vary, and tumors as large as 18 cm have been reported. Most are solid and bosselated with a firm,

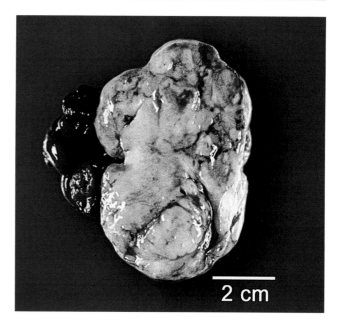

FIGURE 14.15
Metastatic gastric adenocarcinoma. Cut surface of the tumor reveals a lobulated appearance.

tively bland to highly atypical. Stromal luteinization is not infrequent.

ANCILLARY STUDIES

IMMUNOHISTOCHEMISTRY

Expression of CK7 and CK20 is variable, with expression of CK7 being somewhat more frequent than CK20. These tumors often express CDX2.

DIFFERENTIAL DIAGNOSIS

white or yellow cut surface (Figure 14.15); some may have a cystic component.

MICROSCOPIC FINDINGS

Carcinoma metastatic from the stomach is usually a signet-ring cell carcinoma (Krukenberg tumor). At low-power scrutiny, cellular and less cellular areas often alternate, imparting a pseudolobular architecture. The neoplastic cells predominate in the areas of hypercellular stroma (Figure 14.16). Classically, the signet-ring cells are arranged individually or in clusters (Figures 14.17 and 14.18); however, variations include formation of glands, hollow or solid tubules and trabeculae, and growth of tumor cells in sheets or lobules. Extracellular mucin is frequently conspicuous. Metastatic gastric carcinoma of the nonsignet-ring cell type contains intestinal-type glands with tubular, cribriform, cystic, and papillary architecture, including the finding of occasional goblet cells. In all cases, nuclei range from decep-

Metastatic gastric carcinoma to the ovary should be separated from signet-ring stromal tumor, "primary ovarian Krukenberg tumor," and primary mucinous carcinoid. When the signet-ring cells are not appreciated within the hypercellular stroma, *cellular fibroma, sclerosing stromal tumor, and fibrosarcoma* may be a consideration at low-power magnification. However, identification of signet ring cells is diagnostic and facilitated by mucin stains and cytokeratins. *Signet-ring stromal tumor* should neither stain for PAS/mucin nor express cytokeratins. *Primary Krukenberg tumor* is exceedingly rare (if it exists), should not be bilateral, and is a diagnosis of exclusion. Poorly differentiated areas in a *primary mucinous carcinoid* may closely mimic a Krukenberg tumor. However, well-differentiated areas show nests of tumor cells, frequently with goblet and Paneth cell differentiation, free floating in pools of mucin. Metastatic gastric carcinoma of the nonsignet-ring cell type should be distinguished from *primary endometrioid and mucinous carcinomas* of the

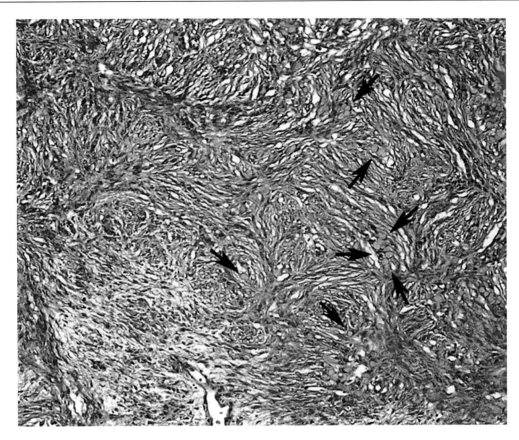

FIGURE 14.16
Metastatic gastric adenocarcinoma. The cellular fibromatous stroma obscures the neoplastic epithelial cells, simulating a primary ovarian fibroma. The signet-ring cells are barely evident at this magnification (arrows).

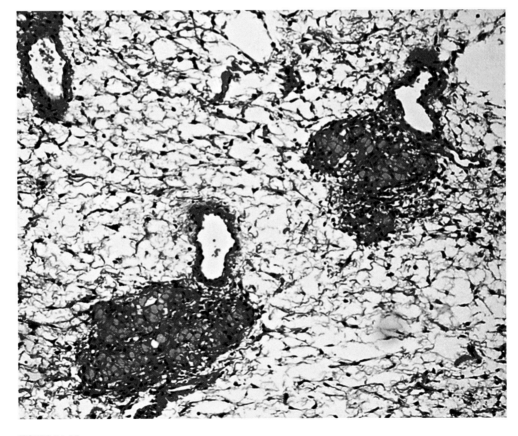

FIGURE 14.17
Metastatic gastric adenocarcinoma. An edematous area contains signet-ring cells arranged in a nested pattern.

ovary. In these cases, it is important to look for other morphologic features seen in metastatic carcinoma to the ovary.

METASTASES FROM CARCINOMA OF THE APPENDIX

CLINICAL FEATURES

Patients range in age from 32 to 70 (mean 52) years, and they often present with a pelvic/adnexal mass or generalized symptoms of abdominal disease.

METASTASES FROM CARCINOMA OF THE APPENDIX – FACT SHEET

Incidence
- 9% of clinically apparent metastases from nongynecologic primary tumors
- 8% of all clinically apparent metastases

Age Distribution
- 32–70 (mean 52) years

Clinical Features
- Pelvic/adnexal mass
- Generalized abdominal symptoms

PATHOLOGIC FEATURES

GROSS FINDINGS

The tumors are bilateral in 80% of cases. If unilateral, they have a predilection for the right side. The mean and median sizes are 10 cm, which is often larger than the primary tumor in the appendix. The cut surfaces are usually solid and firm, and may have a cystic component (Figure 14.19).

MICROSCOPIC FINDINGS

Metastases of appendiceal carcinomas most commonly display signet-ring cell differentiation and can have a variety of growth patterns ranging from individual cells within a cellular stroma (Krukenberg tumor) to tubules, nests, cords, and trabeculae resembling goblet cell (mucinous) carcinoid tumors. Others exhibit intestinal-type glandular differentiation ranging from well-differentiated mucinous glands to those resembling typical colorectal carcinomas with cribriform architecture and necrosis. Mixtures of any of these patterns can occur (Figures 14.20–14.23). Cytologic atypia and mitotic activity are common.

ANCILLARY FEATURES

IMMUNOHISTOCHEMISTRY

Appendiceal carcinomas invariably express CK20 diffusely. CK7 expression can be seen in approximately 40% and may be patchy or diffuse (it is generally some-

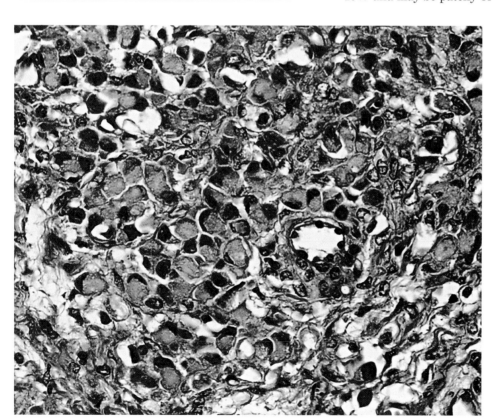

FIGURE 14.18
Metastatic gastric adenocarcinoma. The signet-ring cells are round and have hyperchromatic, eccentrically located, crescent-shaped nuclei deformed by a cytoplasmic mucin vacuole.

METASTASES FROM CARCINOMA OF THE APPENDIX – PATHOLOGIC FEATURES

Gross Findings

▸ 80% bilateral
▸ If unilateral, right ovary more commonly involved
▸ Mean/median size 10 cm
▸ Solid and firm cut surface

Microscopic Findings

▸ Individual signet-ring cells within a cellular stroma (Krukenberg tumor) (most common)
▸ Tubules, nests, cords, and trabeculae (goblet cell/mucinous carcinoid-like)
▸ Intestinal-type glands (well-differentiated mucinous or resembling typical colorectal carcinoma)
▸ Mixed patterns
▸ Cells with frequent cytologic atypia and brisk mitotic activity

Immunohistochemical Findings

▸ CK20 diffusely positive
▸ CK7 negative in 60% of tumors

Differential Diagnosis

▸ Primary goblet cell (mucinous) carcinoid tumor
▸ "Primary Krukenberg tumor"
▸ Endometrioid and mucinous tumors of ovary
▸ Metastases from stomach, colon, and pancreas/biliary tract

what weaker than CK20 expression) (Figures 14.21 and 14.25).

DIFFERENTIAL DIAGNOSIS

Tumors in the differential diagnosis include primary ovarian goblet cell (mucinous) carcinoid tumor, "primary ovarian Krukenberg tumor," primary ovarian mucinous and endometrioid tumors, and *metastases from the stomach, colon, and pancreas/biliary tract* (see individual sections). *Primary goblet cell (mucinous) carcinoid tumor* and *primary Krukenberg tumor* are both rare and

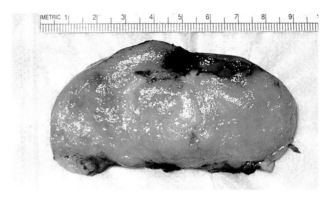

FIGURE 14.19
Metastatic appendiceal adenocarcinoma. The tumor has a tan-yellow, solid, and mucoid cut surface.

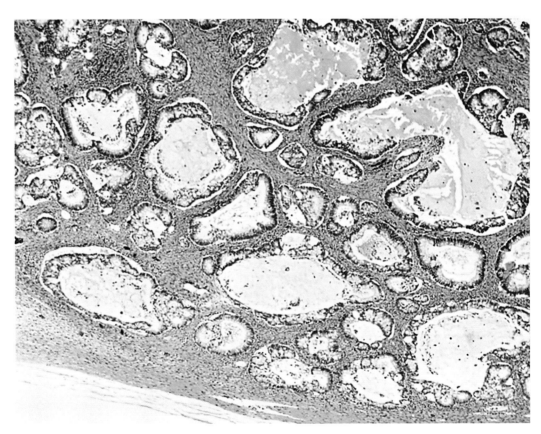

FIGURE 14.20
Metastatic appendiceal adenocarcinoma. The tumor is composed of cystic mucinous glands within a fibromatous stroma.

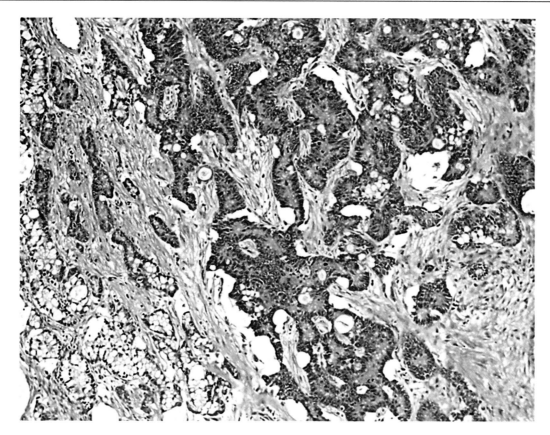

FIGURE 14.21
Metastatic appendiceal adenocarcinoma. The tumor has a trabecular growth and contains goblet cells (lower left).

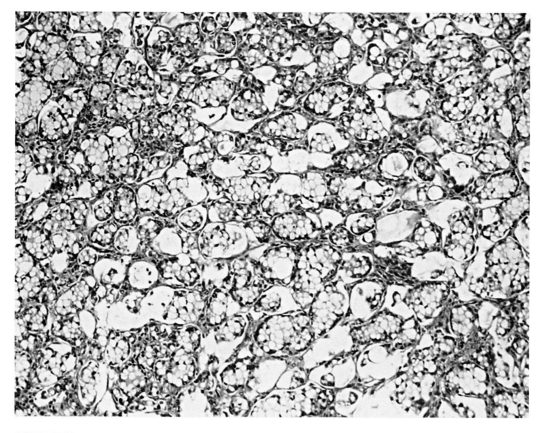

FIGURE 14.22
Metastatic appendiceal adenocarcinoma. Small back-to-back round nests of tumor are filled with signet-ring cells.

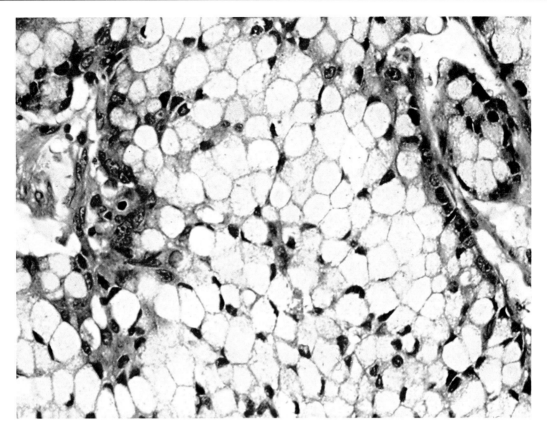

FIGURE 14.23
Metastatic appendiceal adenocarcinoma. Solid areas are composed of sheets of signet-ring cells.

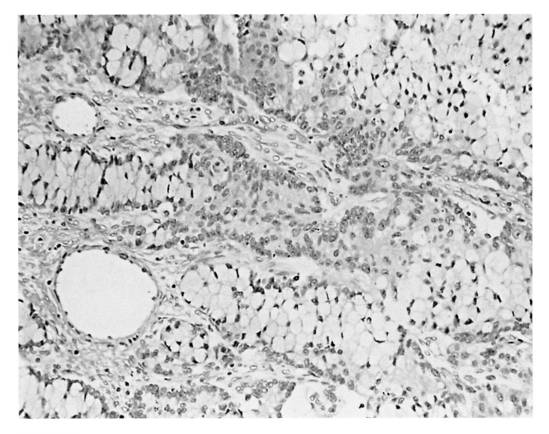

FIGURE 14.24
Metastatic appendiceal adenocarcinoma. The tumor cells lack CK7 expression.

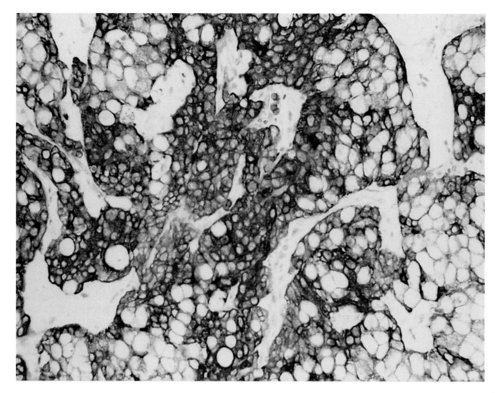

FIGURE 14.25
Metastatic appendiceal adenocarcinoma. The tumor exhibits diffuse CK20 expression.

typically unilateral. Moreover, primary Krukenberg tumor is a diagnosis of exclusion. The finding of a mature cystic teratoma supports a diagnosis of a primary ovarian goblet cell (mucinous) carcinoid. *Primary ovarian mucinous and endometrioid tumors* are more commonly unilateral and typically diffusely positive for CK7, a finding which is only occasionally seen in primary appendiceal carcinomas.

SECONDARY INVOLVEMENT BY LOW-GRADE ADENOMATOUS MUCINOUS NEOPLASM OF APPENDIX ASSOCIATED WITH PSEUDOMYXOMA PERITONEI

CLINICAL FEATURES

Patients range in age from 26 to 73 (mean 46) years. Most present with mucinous ascites (pseudomyxoma peritonei) and have diffuse peritoneal involvement. Still, many women present with adnexal masses and are thought to have an ovarian cancer; some patients have signs and symptoms of appendicitis. Rarely, they present with adnexal masses, a dilated appendix, and only limited peritoneal disease. The primary appendiceal neoplasm can be readily identified as a cystically dilated mass in some cases, but in others, rupture, extensive mucin, and fibrosis can obscure or obliterate the primary tumor.

SECONDARY INVOLVEMENT BY LOW-GRADE ADENOMATOUS MUCINOUS NEOPLASM OF APPENDIX ASSOCIATED WITH PSEUDOMYXOMA PERITONEI – FACT SHEET

Incidence
▶ Uncommon

Age Distribution
▶ 26–73 (mean 46) years

Clinical Features
▶ Mucinous ascites
▶ Adnexal mass(es)

PATHOLOGIC FEATURES

GROSS FINDINGS

The ovarian tumors are bilateral in approximately 80 % of cases. When unilateral, they tend to be right-sided. Tumors are typically < 10 cm in diameter and may be confined to the ovarian surface, but if larger, they involve the ovarian parenchyma and are often multicystic and mucoid.

MICROSCOPIC FINDINGS

Most tumors are associated with abundant dissecting extracellular mucin (pseudomyxoma ovarii) and relatively scant low-grade adenomatous mucinous epithelium. The epithelium can be hypermucinous and

SECONDARY INVOLVEMENT BY LOW-GRADE ADENOMATOUS MUCINOUS NEOPLASM OF APPENDIX ASSOCIATED WITH PSEUDOMYXOMA PERITONEI – PATHOLOGIC FEATURES

Gross Findings

▸ 80% bilateral
▸ If unilateral, right side more often involved
▸ Mean size < 10 cm
▸ Surface mucinous deposits ± multiloculated parenchymal mucinous cysts

Microscopic Findings

▸ Abundant dissecting mucin (pseudomyxoma ovarii)
▸ Scant haphazardly distributed incomplete glands embedded in pools of extracellular mucin
▸ If abundant epithelium may simulate a primary ovarian borderline mucinous tumor
▸ Often cells with very abundant (tall) mucinous cytoplasm (hypermucinous)
▸ Cells with low-grade cytologic features

Immunohistochemical Findings

▸ CK20 diffusely positive
▸ CK7 usually negative

Differential Diagnosis

▸ Atypical proliferative (borderline) mucinous tumor of gastrointestinal type
▸ Mucinous cystadenoma
▸ Mucinous carcinoma

typically forms haphazardly and irregularly distributed incomplete glands which are partially surrounded by pools of extracellular mucin, often with involvement of the ovarian surface. Occasionally, the mucinous epithelium is more abundant and may simulate a primary ovarian atypical proliferative (borderline) mucinous tumor (Figures 14.26–14.29). The ovarian tumors can be diagnosed as secondary involvement by disseminated peritoneal adenomucinosis of appendiceal origin or secondary involvement by low-grade (adenomatous) appendiceal mucinous neoplasm. Primary ovarian tumor nomenclature (cystadenoma, atypical proliferative/borderline tumor) is discouraged to avoid confusion regarding site of origin.

ANCILLARY STUDIES

IMMUNOHISTOCHEMISTRY

The ovarian tumors express CK20 diffusely, but are usually negative for CK7, similar to primary appendiceal mucinous tumors; on occasion, they can exhibit patchy CK7 expression (Figures 14.30 and 14.31).

DIFFERENTIAL DIAGNOSIS

The main differential diagnosis is with *primary ovarian atypical proliferative (borderline) mucinous tumors of gastrointestinal type*. These tumors are almost always unilateral and large (mean size 19 cm), lack surface

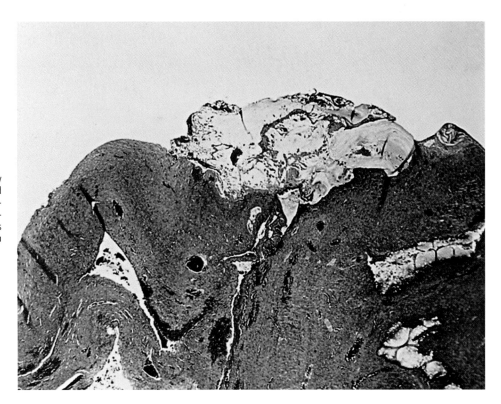

FIGURE 14.26

Secondary involvement of the ovary by low-grade mucinous tumor derived from the appendix. Mucinous epithelium is scant, is irregularly distributed in the ovarian stroma and it is associated with pools of mucin on the surface.

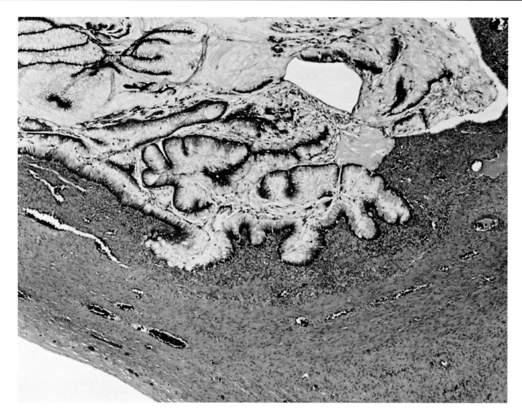

FIGURE 14.27
Secondary involvement of the ovary by low-grade mucinous tumor derived from the appendix. Undulating low-grade, hypermucinous epithelium simulates a primary ovarian tumor, but lacks the organization and true epithelial tufting of an atypical proliferative mucinous tumor.

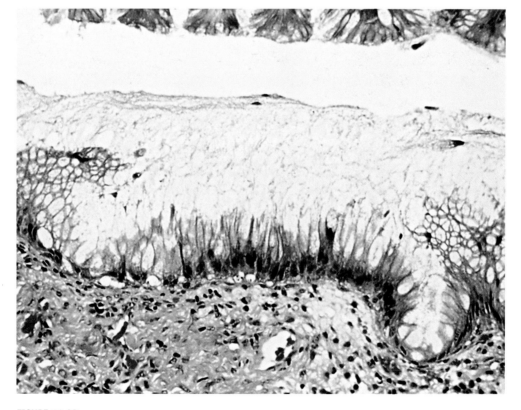

FIGURE 14.28
Secondary involvement of the ovary by low-grade mucinous tumor derived from the appendix. The epithelium has a "hypermucinous" appearance because the extracellular mucin merges with the intracellular mucin of the columnar cells.

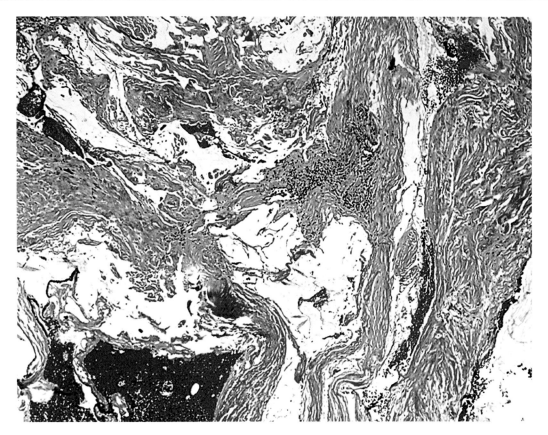

FIGURE 14.29

Secondary involvement of the ovary by low-grade mucinous tumor derived from the appendix. There is scant mucinous epithelium and abundant dissecting mucin (pseudomyxoma ovarii) associated with fibrosis.

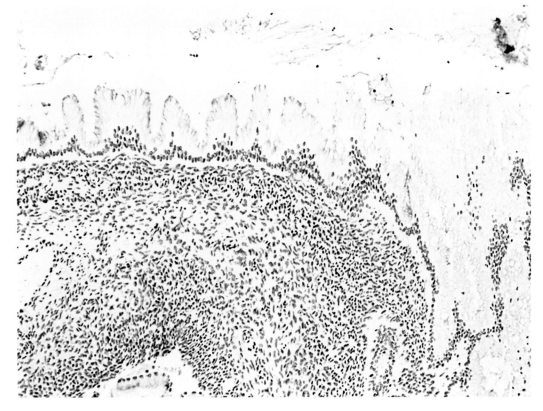

FIGURE 14.30

Secondary involvement of the ovary by low-grade mucinous tumor derived from the appendix. The tumor lacks CK7 expression.

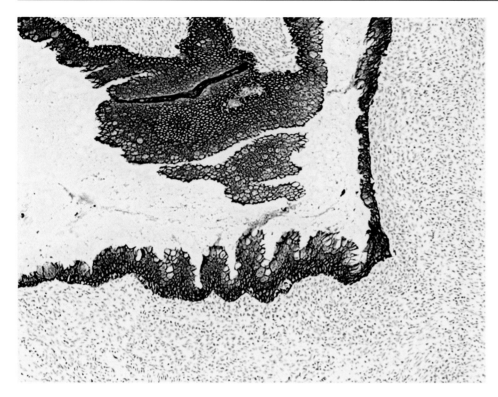

FIGURE 14.31
Secondary involvement of the ovary by low-grade mucinous tumor derived from the appendix. Tumor exhibits diffuse CK20 expression.

involvement, and have more abundant mucinous epithelium arranged in organized, evenly distributed cysts associated with minimal or absent pseudomyxoma ovarii. Rarely, *primary ovarian mucinous cystadenomas*, particularly when multicystic, may be considered in the differential diagnosis; however, they are invariably unilateral, lack surface involvement, may show cyst rupture but no pseudomyxoma peritonei, and cells have less abundant mucinous cytoplasm (lacking "hypermucinous" appearance). *Primary mucinous carcinomas* of the ovary are much less commonly bilateral, have a more complex architecture, and a greater degree of cytologic atypia. Moreover, they usually do not show features of secondary involvement. Immunohistochemistry can assist in the distinction of these primary ovarian mucinous tumors from secondary involvement by low-grade appendiceal mucinous tumors because the former are diffusely positive for CK7 and variably positive for CK20 (expression can be strong but is often patchy or incomplete), whereas the latter are diffusely positive for CK20 and usually negative for CK7 (focal CK7 expression is occasionally seen).

[handwritten annotation: Mucinous - CK20 | CK7; Ovary +/− | +; Appendix + | −/+]

METASTASES FROM CARCINOMA OF THE PANCREAS

CLINICAL FEATURES

Patients range in age from 29 to 87 (mean 63) years and usually present with symptoms related to bilateral

METASTASES FROM CARCINOMA OF THE PANCREAS – FACT SHEET

Incidence
▶ 6% of clinically apparent metastases from nongynecologic primary tumors
▶ 5% of all clinically apparent metastases

Age Distribution
▶ 29–87 (mean 63) years

Clinical Features
▶ Symptoms related to adnexal masses +/− diffuse carcinomatosis

adnexal masses, with or without diffuse abdominal disease. Often there is not an established diagnosis of pancreatic carcinoma; thus, in many patients the clinical impression is that of a primary ovarian carcinoma.

PATHOLOGIC FEATURES

GROSS FINDINGS

The tumors are typically bilateral (75–100%) and most often have a multiloculated, mucoid appearance, with or without surface involvement. The mean size ranges from 7 to 13 cm.

MICROSCOPIC FINDINGS

Metastatic pancreatic carcinoma most often displays mucinous differentiation but can have areas with a

METASTASES FROM CARCINOMA OF THE PANCREAS – PATHOLOGIC FEATURES

Gross Findings

▸ 75–100% bilateral

▸ Mean size 7–13 cm

▸ Multiloculated cystic and mucinous ± surface and cortical tumor nodules

Microscopic Findings

▸ Surface and cortical plaques or nodules

▸ Variable-sized, well-formed, small and tubular to large and cystic glands

▸ Haphazardly infiltrative, cribriform, cystic, villoglandular and papillary patterns

▸ Occasionally, poorly differentiated foci containing individual cells

▸ Glands with mucinous or endometrioid-like appearance

▸ Wide range of nuclear atypia from one area to another (bland to markedly atypical) very closely simulating primary ovarian mucinous tumors

▸ Desmoplastic stroma often present, but may be lacking

Immunohistochemical Findings

▸ CK7 diffusely positive

▸ CK20 often focally positive

▸ Dpc4 negative (~50%)

Differential Diagnosis

▸ Primary ovarian mucinous tumors (atypical proliferative, carcinoma)

▸ Metastatic gallbladder/bile duct carcinoma

pseudoendometrioid appearance, including secretory change. They are usually comprised of variably sized well-formed glands ranging from small and tubular to large and cystic; occasionally, more poorly differentiated foci containing individual cells can be seen. The glands may be infiltrative within a desmoplastic stroma or can form dilated cysts with simple or papillary architecture within a nonreactive stroma (Figures 14.32–14.34). Nuclear atypia can vary from minimal to marked (Figures 14.35 and 14.36).

ANCILLARY STUDIES

IMMUNOHISTOCHEMISTRY

Tumors are typically diffusely positive for CK7 and focally positive for CK20 (Figure 14.37). Expression of Dpc4 is lost in approximately 50% of these neoplastic (Figure 14.38).

DIFFERENTIAL DIAGNOSIS

The principal differential diagnostic consideration is distinction from *primary ovarian atypical proliferative (borderline) mucinous tumors and carcinomas*, as metastatic pancreatic tumors to the ovary may closely mimic the

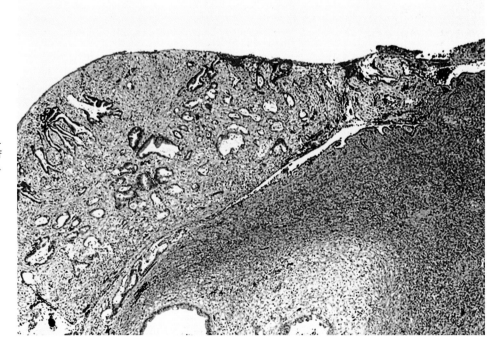

FIGURE 14.32

Metastatic pancreatic adenocarcinoma. There is a nodular plaque of carcinoma on the ovarian surface, characteristic of metastases.

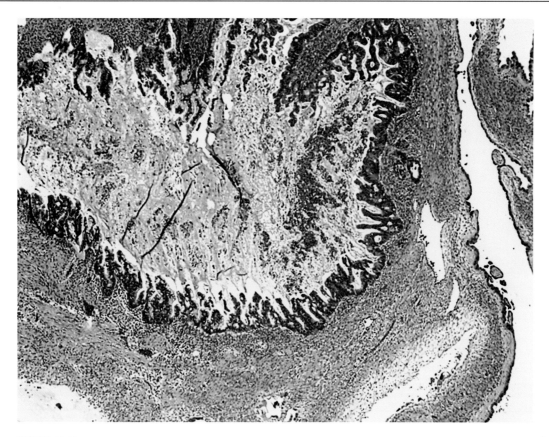

FIGURE 14.33

Metastatic pancreatic adenocarcinoma. A cystically dilated mucinous gland shows epithelial tufting and lacks infiltrative growth, simulating a primary ovarian atypical proliferative (borderline) mucinous tumor.

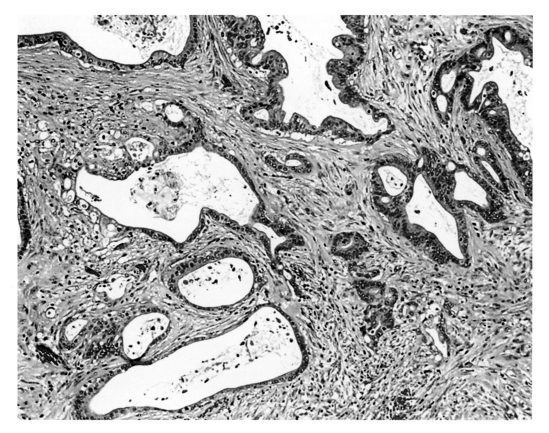

FIGURE 14.34

Metastatic pancreatic adenocarcinoma. Small to medium-sized haphazardly infiltrating glands in a desmoplastic stroma are characteristic of metastatic carcinoma.

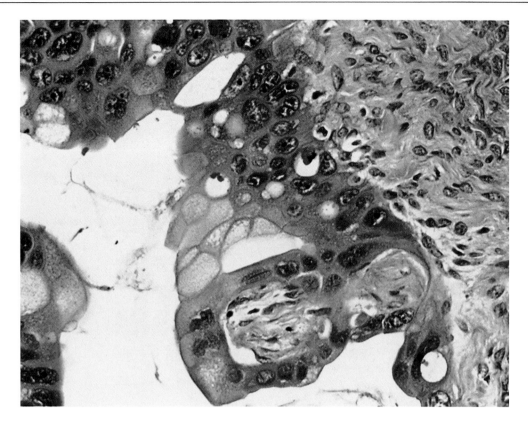

FIGURE 14.35
Metastatic pancreatic adenocarcinoma. The epithelium lining the glands displays significant nuclear atypia.

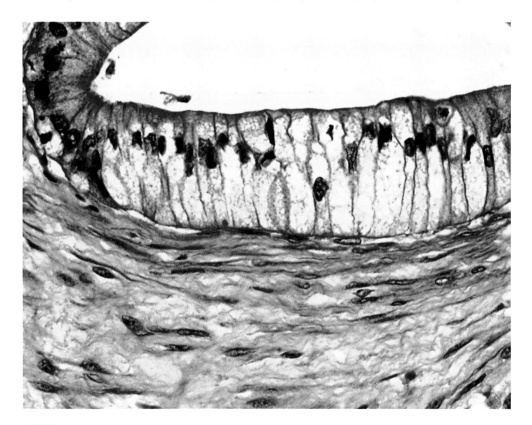

FIGURE 14.36
Metastatic pancreatic adenocarcinoma. The glandular epithelium is well differentiated and comprised of columnar cells having pale cytoplasm and small, round, minimally atypical nuclei, simulating a benign primary ovarian mucinous tumor. The luminal edge displays an eosinophilic "brush border-like" zone which can be seen in some primary pancreatic adenocarcinomas.

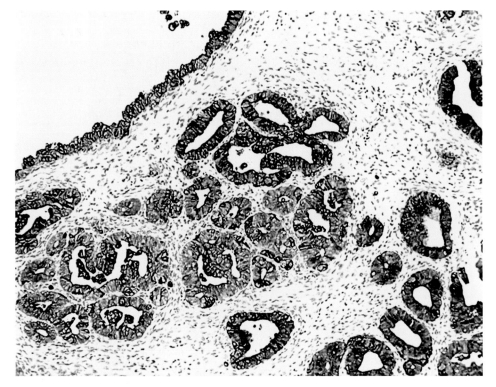

FIGURE 14.37
Metastatic pancreatic adenocarcinoma. The tumor exhibits diffuse CK7 expression.

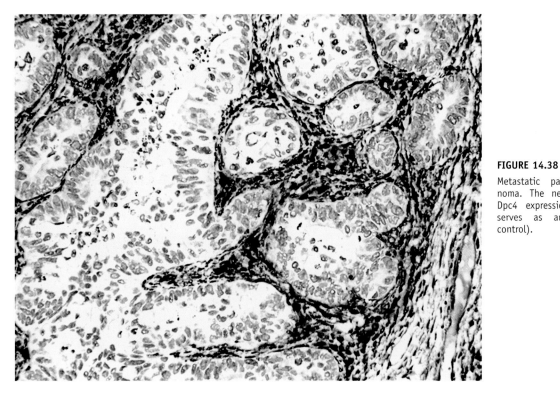

FIGURE 14.38
Metastatic pancreatic adenocarcinoma. The neoplastic glands lack Dpc4 expression. (Ovarian stroma serves as an internal positive control).

transition from benign to borderline to carcinoma, which may be seen in primary ovarian mucinous tumors. Features favoring metastatic pancreatic carcinoma include bilateral involvement, surface and superficial cortical tumor, nodular growth, and the finding of haphazard, irregularly distributed glands having variable sizes and shapes. Metastatic pancreatic carcinoma and primary ovarian mucinous tumors share the same CK7/CK20 immunoprofile. Loss of Dpc4 expression in an ovarian mucinous tumor is rather specific for metastatic pancreatic or biliary adenocarcinoma but retained expression of Dpc4 does not exclude a pancreatic origin. The distinction from primary gallbladder and bile duct carcinomas is almost impossible based on morphologic grounds.

SECONDARY INVOLVEMENT BY NON-HODGKIN LYMPHOMA

CLINICAL FEATURES

Patients with non-Hodgkin lymphoma involving the ovary are staged according to the Ann Arbor rather than the FIGO system. Ann Arbor stage III$_E$ or IV disease has been considered by some authors to represent secondary (disseminated) non-Hodgkin lymphoma involving the ovary, whereas Ann Arbor stage I$_E$ or II$_E$ disease has been considered to be primary (localized) in the ovary. Patients range in age from 21 to 69 (mean 43) years and may present with abdominal pain or bowel obstruction. A subset of patients has a history of leukemia.

PATHOLOGIC FEATURES

GROSS FINDINGS

Bilateral ovarian involvement is seen in half of cases with a mean size of 8 cm. Tumors are typically fleshy and tan to gray on cut section.

MICROSCOPIC FINDINGS

The most common lymphoma involving the ovary is diffuse large B-cell lymphoma. The tumor shows a diffuse architecture with large, usually noncohesive cells that have nuclei with round or irregular contours and moderate amount of pale cytoplasm. The chromatin is heterogeneous and nucleoli and mitotic figures are present. Other types of lymphoma that may be encountered include precursor B-cell lymphoblastic lymphoma, Burkitt lymphoma, blastoid natural killer (NK)-cell lymphoma/leukemia, peripheral T-cell lymphoma, and grade 1 follicular lymphoma (Figures 14.39 and 14.40).

ANCILLARY STUDIES

IMMUNOHISTOCHEMISTRY

B-cell tumors express CD45 and CD20 but lack CD3 expression (Figures 14.41 and 14.42). Peripheral T-cell lymphoma expresses CD3 and CD8 but lacks CD20 expression. Blastoid NK-cell lymphoma/leukemia expresses CD3, CD45, and CD56 but does not express CD20, CD30, CD45RO, CD79a, or myeloperoxidase.

DIFFERENTIAL DIAGNOSIS

Non-Hodgkin's lymphoma should be distinguished from *myeloid sarcoma (extramedullary myeloid cell tumor/ granulocytic sarcoma/chloroma), undifferentiated carcinoma, small cell carcinoma (hypercalcemic and pulmo-*

SECONDARY INVOLVEMENT BY NON-HODGKIN'S LYMPHOMA – PATHOLOGIC FEATURES

Gross Findings
- 50% bilateral
- Mean size 8 cm

Microscopic Findings
- Diffuse large B-cell lymphoma (most common):
  - Diffuse architecture
  - Large, usually noncohesive cells
  - Cells with moderate amount of pale cytoplasm and nuclei with round or irregular contours and nucleoli
  - Frequent mitotic figures
- Other types: precursor B-cell lymphoblastic lymphoma, Burkitt lymphoma, blastoid natural killer (NK)-cell lymphoma/leukemia, peripheral T-cell lymphoma, and grade 1 follicular lymphoma

Immunohistochemical Findings
- B-cell lymphoma: CD20(+) and CD3(−)
- Peripheral T-cell lymphoma: CD3(+), CD8(+), and CD20(−)
- Blastoid NK-cell lymphoma/leukemia: CD3, CD45, and CD56 (+); CD20, CD30, CD45RO, CD79a, and myeloperoxidase (−)

Differential Diagnosis
- Myeloid sarcoma (extramedullary myeloid cell tumor/granulocytic sarcoma/chloroma)
- Undifferentiated carcinoma
- Small cell carcinoma, hypercalcemic and pulmonary types
- Dysgerminoma
- Adult granulosa cell tumor
- Primary ovarian non-Hodgkin's lymphoma

---

nary), dysgerminoma, adult granulosa cell tumor, and other small round cell tumors. Use of conventional clinical, gross, histologic, and immunohistochemical features of each of these tumors in the differential diagnosis usually provides the correct diagnosis, particularly if an adequate panel of immunohistochemical markers is included. Secondary (disseminated) non-Hodgkin lymphoma should also be distinguished from primary (localized) disease. Although clinical/radiologic correlation is usually required, *primary non-Hodgkin lymphoma* has a lower prevalence of bilaterality (12% versus 50%) and a greater mean size (13 versus 8 cm) compared to secondary non-Hodgkin lymphoma.

METASTASES FROM CARCINOMA OF THE LUNG

CLINICAL FEATURES

Patients range in age from 26 to 63 (mean 43) years. Presentation may include pulmonary symptoms, a history of smoking, abdominal pain/enlargement, ascites, or an abdominal/pelvic mass. In one recent study, the ovarian tumor was detected after the lung

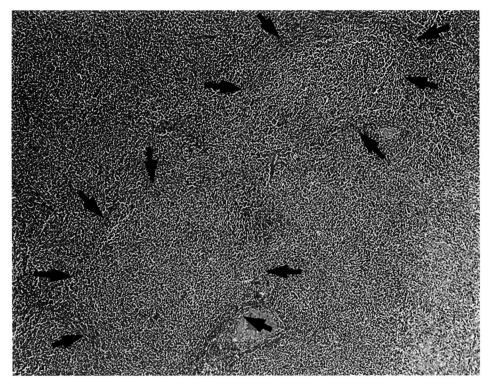

FIGURE 14.39
Secondary involvement of the ovary by follicular lymphoma. The tumor mostly shows a diffuse growth but ill-defined follicles are present (arrows).

METASTASES FROM CARCINOMA OF THE LUNG – FACT SHEET

Incidence
▸ 2% of clinically apparent metastases from nongynecologic primary tumors
▸ 2% of all clinically apparent metastases

Age Distribution
▸ Range 26–63 (mean 43) years

Clinical Features
▸ Pulmonary symptoms
▸ History of smoking
▸ Abdominal pain/distension or pelvic mass
▸ Ascites

METASTASES FROM CARCINOMA OF THE LUNG – PATHOLOGIC FEATURES

Gross Findings
▸ Commonly unilateral
▸ Mean size 8 cm
▸ Lobulated, white to yellow, hemorrhagic and necrotic

Microscopic Findings
▸ Small cell carcinoma (most common)
  ▸ Diffuse, trabecular, or nested growths
  ▸ Small to intermediate-sized cells
  ▸ High nuclear-to-cytoplasmic ratio, hyperchromatic nuclei, inconspicuous nucleoli, and brisk mitotic activity
  ▸ Conspicuous nuclear molding
▸ Other types: large cell carcinoma, adenocarcinoma, including bronchioloalveolar carcinoma, and very rarely, squamous cell carcinoma

Immunohistochemical Features
▸ Small cell carcinoma: Low-molecular-weight cytokeratin (CK8/18), TTF-1, chromogranin, synaptophysin, and CD56 positive
▸ TTF-1 also positive in 75% of adenocarcinomas and 45% of large cell carcinomas

Differential Diagnosis
▸ Ovarian small cell carcinoma, pulmonary type
▸ Small cell carcinoma, hypercalcemic type
▸ Metastases from extrapulmonary small cell carcinoma

---

cancer in 50% of cases (at a mean interval of 1 year), but in approximately 30% of patients, the lung and ovarian tumors occurred synchronously and in 15% the ovarian tumor was detected prior to the lung tumor.

PATHOLOGIC FEATURES

GROSS FINDINGS

The tumors are commonly unilateral, but some may be bilateral, with a mean size of 8 cm. The external

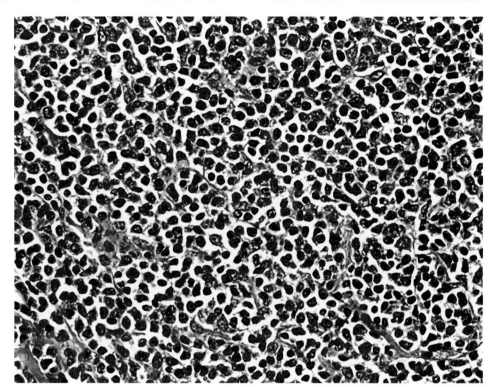

FIGURE 14.40

Secondary involvement of the ovary by follicular lymphoma. The tumor is predominantly composed of small cleaved lymphoid cells.

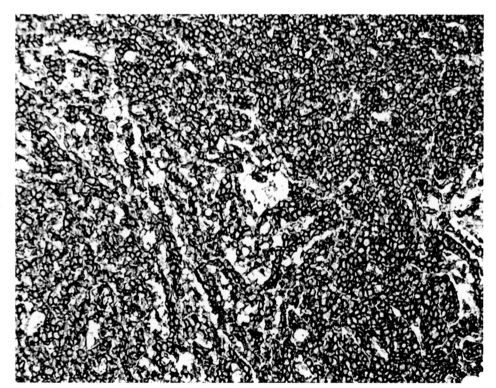

FIGURE 14.41

Secondary involvement of the ovary by follicular lymphoma. Tumor cells exhibit diffuse strong CD20 expression.

surface is typically smooth and intact whereas the cut surface is firm or soft, lobulated, white to yellow/tan, hemorrhagic, and/or necrotic with secondary cyst formation.

MICROSCOPIC FINDINGS

Among all histologic subtypes of lung carcinoma, small cell carcinoma most commonly metastasizes to the ovary.

The tumor cells may be arranged in sheets, trabeculae, or nests. They are small to intermediate in size and have a high nuclear-to-cytoplasmic ratio, hyperchromatic nuclei, nuclear molding, inconspicuous nucleoli and brisk mitotic activity. Other histologic types include large cell carcinoma, adenocarcinoma, including bronchioloalveolar carcinoma, and, very rarely, squamous cell carcinoma (Figures 14.43–14.45).

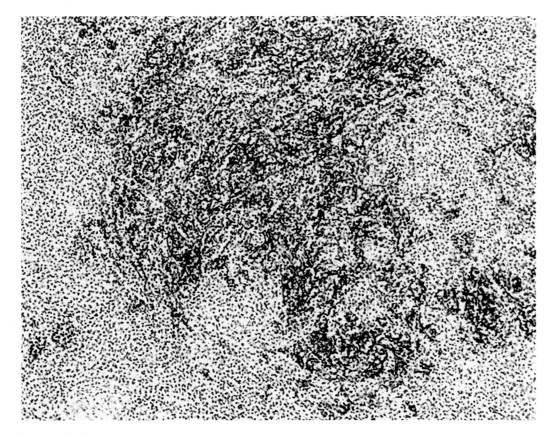

FIGURE 14.42
Secondary involvement of the ovary by follicular lymphoma. CD21 highlights the follicular dendritic cell network consistent with a follicle center cell origin.

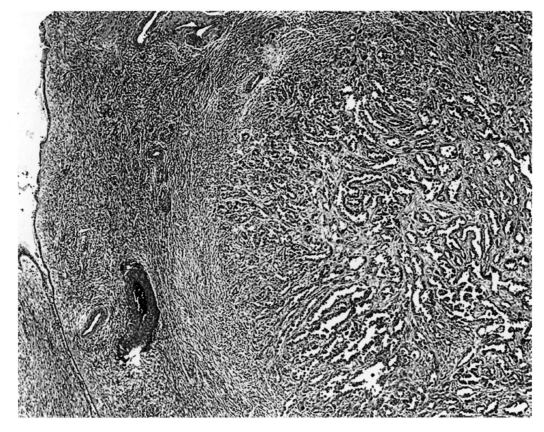

FIGURE 14.43
Metastatic pulmonary adenocarcinoma. The tumor has a nodular configuration and is located in the superficial cortex, features that suggest metastasis.

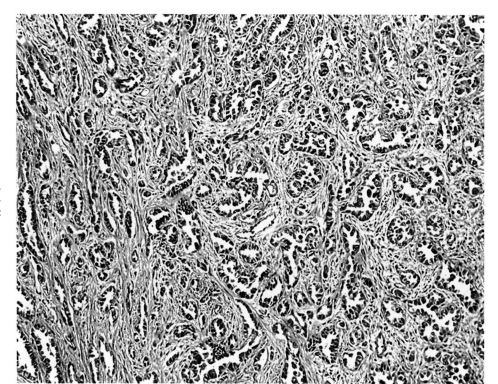

FIGURE 14.44

Metastatic pulmonary adenocarcinoma. The glands exhibit an infiltrative pattern within a desmoplastic stroma.

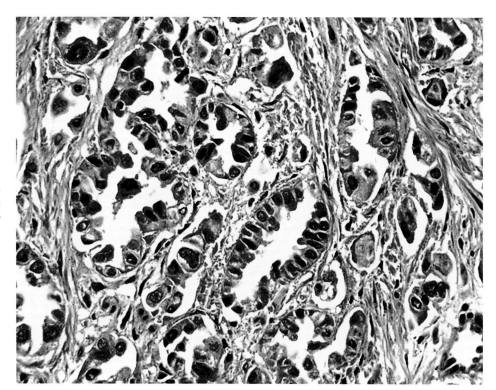

FIGURE 14.45

Metastatic pulmonary adenocarcinoma. The glands are lined by a single layer of atypical cuboidal cells.

ANCILLARY STUDIES

IMMUNOHISTOCHEMISTRY

Small cell carcinoma expresses low-molecular-weight cytokeratin (CK8/18), TTF-1, chromogranin, synaptophysin, and CD56 (Figures 14.46 and 14.47). TTF-1 is also expressed in 75% of adenocarcinomas and 45% of large cell carcinomas.

DIFFERENTIAL DIAGNOSIS

The main diagnostic consideration is a primary *ovarian pulmonary-type small cell carcinoma*. Laterality is not helpful; however the presence of a lung mass favors a pulmonary origin whereas the presence of another ovarian-surface epithelial tumor component supports an ovarian primary. Although the immunophenotype for both tumors overlaps, TTF-1 expression is much more

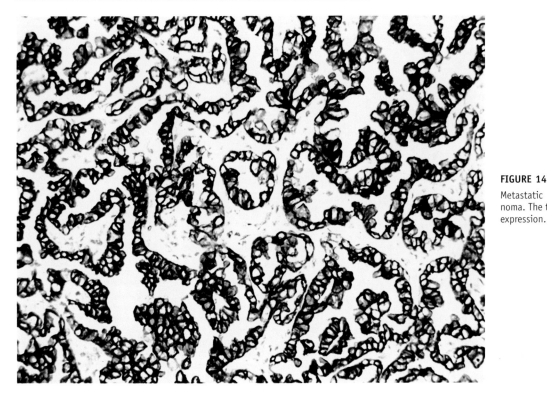

FIGURE 14.46

Metastatic pulmonary adenocarcinoma. The tumor exhibits diffuse CK7 expression.

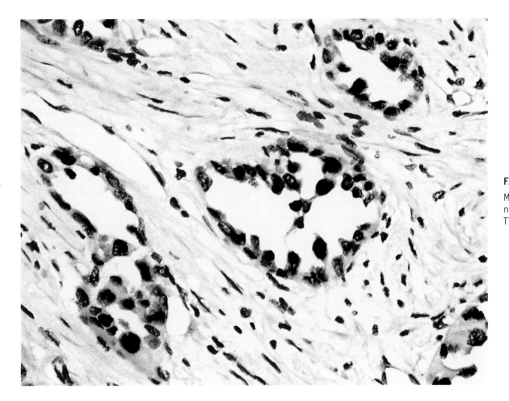

FIGURE 14.47

Metastatic pulmonary adenocarcinoma. The tumor exhibits nuclear TTF-1 expression.

common in small cell carcinoma of the lung (96% in small cell carcinoma of the lung versus 7% in extrapulmonary small cell carcinoma). In some cases, definitive distinction between a metastasis and an ovarian primary may not be possible. Less commonly, metastatic small cell carcinoma of the lung should be separated from *small cell carcinoma* *of the hypercalcemic type*, and rarely from other small round cell tumors. Small cell carcinoma of the hypercalcemic type occurs more frequently at a younger age, follicle-like spaces are common, nuclei have conspicuous nucleoli and clumped chromatin, and the tumors are typically negative for TTF-1.

METASTASES FROM MELANOMA

CLINICAL FEATURES

The primary site of the melanoma is the skin in most cases. Patients range in age from 14 to 60 (mean 37) years and may present with abdominal enlargement/pain, or an ovarian mass detected during follow-up of a prior cutaneous melanoma.

METASTASES FROM MELANOMA – FACT SHEET

Incidence
▶ 1% of clinically apparent metastases from nongynecologic primary tumors
▶ 1% of all clinically apparent metastases

Age Distribution
▶ Range 14–60 (mean 37) years

Clinical Features
▶ Abdominal distension/pain
▶ Pelvic mass

PATHOLOGIC FEATURES

GROSS FINDINGS

In one-third of patients ovarian involvement is bilateral, with mean sizes ranging from 10 to 11 cm. The external surface may be smooth or nodular, the cut surface is typically solid and cystic, and some tumors may have dark pigmentation.

MICROSCOPIC FINDINGS

The tumors have a nodular or diffuse architecture (Figure 14.48), but occasionally they may show round aggregates with a nevoid appearance, follicle-like spaces, and/or necrosis (Figure 14.49). The cells are commonly large and epithelioid with abundant eosinophilic cytoplasm, and may have a rhabdoid appearance (Figure 14.50), although small and spindled cells may also be seen. Some cells may contain melanin pigment. Prominent nucleoli and intranuclear pseudoinclusions are characteristic, and most tumors are mitotically active.

ANCILLARY STUDIES

IMMUNOHISTOCHEMISTRY

S-100 and HMB-45 are expressed in 95 and 80% of tumors, respectively, with most tumors displaying diffuse staining. They are also frequently positive for Melan-A (Mart-1).

DIFFERENTIAL DIAGNOSIS

Metastatic melanoma, particularly if it shows little or no melanin pigment deposition, must be distinguished from juvenile granulosa cell tumor, small cell carcinoma of the hypercalcemic type, lipid-poor steroid cell tumor, pregnancy luteoma, and primary ovarian melanoma. *Juvenile granulosa cell tumor* is usually unilateral, the background is frequently myxoid, and the cells generally have more cytoplasm than those of melanoma, and may show bizarre nuclei, a feature not seen in melanoma. In addition, juvenile granulosa cell tumor expresses inhibin and calretinin, but lacks HMB-45 expression. *Small cell carcinoma of the hypercalcemic type* may contain areas which have large cells with abundant cytoplasm mimicking melanoma; however, this tumor usually expresses keratin and EMA (although less frequently), but is negative for S-100 and HMB-45. *Lipid-poor steroid cell tumors* and *pregnancy luteoma* are also negative for melanoma markers. *Primary ovarian melanoma* is usually associated with teratomatous elements.

METASTASES FROM MELANOMA – PATHOLOGIC FEATURES

Gross Findings
▶ 33% bilateral
▶ Mean size 10–11 cm
▶ Solid and cystic and sometimes pigmented cut surface

Microscopic Findings
▶ Nodular or diffuse architecture
▶ Occasionally round aggregates with nevoid appearance
▶ Most frequently large epithelioid cells, small or spindled cells less common
▶ Cells with abundant eosinophilic cytoplasm, medium to large-sized nucleus with prominent nucleoli and brisk mitotic activity
▶ Not infrequently follicle-like spaces and intranuclear pseudoinclusions
▶ Rarely, melanin pigment

Immunohistochemical Features
▶ S-100, HMB-45, and Mart-1 positive

Differential Diagnosis
▶ Juvenile granulosa cell tumor
▶ Small cell carcinoma of the hypercalcemic type
▶ Lipid-poor steroid cell tumor
▶ Pregnancy luteoma
▶ Primary ovarian melanoma

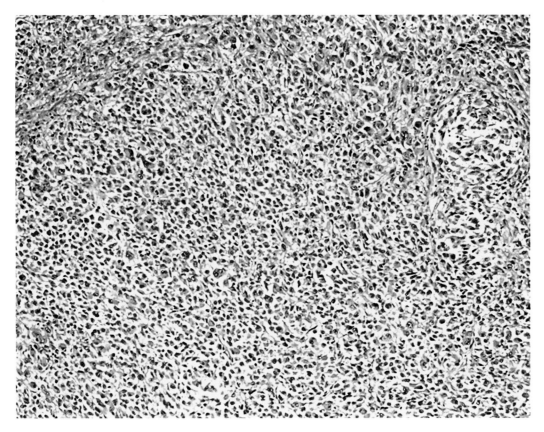

FIGURE 14.48
Metastatic melanoma. The tumor shows a diffuse growth pattern and is comprised of noncohesive cells.

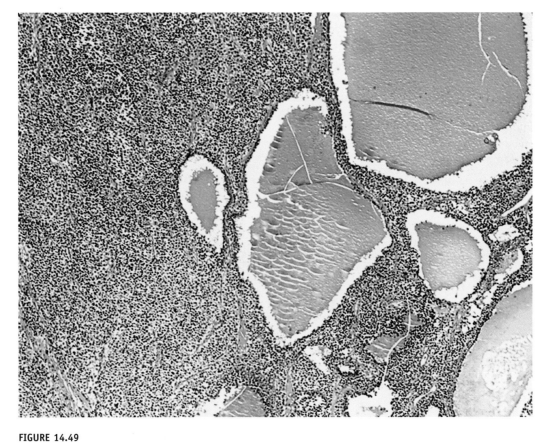

FIGURE 14.49
Metastatic melanoma. Follicle-like spaces resembling those seen in juvenile granulosa cell tumor and small cell carcinoma of the hypercalcemic type are present.

573

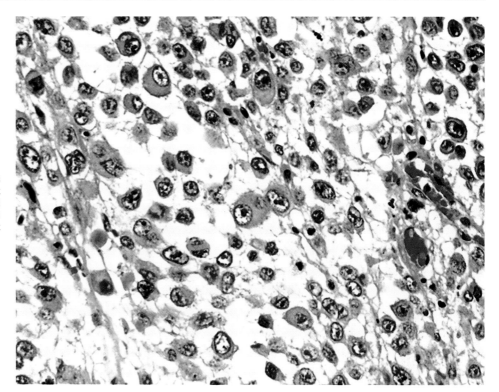

FIGURE 14.50
Metastatic melanoma. The tumor has large rhabdoid cells with abundant dense eosinophilic cytoplasm and large, eccentric, round nuclei with vesicular chromatin and prominent nucleoli.

METASTASES FROM CARCINOMA OF THE GALLBLADDER, BILE DUCTS, AND AMPULLA OF VATER

CLINICAL FEATURES

Patients range in age from 33 to 72 (mean 56) years. They may present with abdominal pain, abdominal discomfort, vomiting, fever, chills, jaundice, and/or weight loss. The majority of metastases from this anatomic region are derived from the gallbladder.

METASTASES FROM CARCINOMA OF THE GALLBLADDER AND BILE DUCTS – FACT SHEET

Incidence
▶ 1% of clinically apparent metastases from nongynecologic primary tumors
▶ 1% of all clinically apparent metastases

Age Distribution
▶ Range 33–72 (mean 56) years

Clinical Features
▶ Abdominal pain/discomfort, vomiting, fever, chills, or weight loss
▶ Adnexal mass(es)

METASTASES FROM CARCINOMA OF THE GALLBLADDER AND BILE DUCTS – PATHOLOGIC FEATURES

Gross Findings
▶ 75% bilateral
▶ Size up to 18 cm
▶ Nodular surface
▶ Solid and cystic cut surface

Microscopic Findings
▶ Surface implants sometimes forming nodules
▶ Glandular, cribriform, villoglandular, solid tubular, insular, and/or cystic patterns
▶ Overt infiltrative growth associated with desmoplastic stroma less common
▶ Cuboidal or flattened to tall or columnar cells
▶ Mucinous, goblet, and signet-ring cells may be seen
▶ Variable nuclear pseudostratification, nuclear atypia, and mitotic activity

Immunohistochemical Features
▶ CK7 positive
▶ CK20 variably positivite
▶ Dpc4 negative in 34%

Differential Diagnosis
▶ Endometrioid and mucinous ovarian tumors (atypical proliferative and carcinoma)
▶ Metastatic pancreatic carcinoma

PATHOLOGIC FEATURES

GROSS FINDINGS

Approximately 75% of cases are bilateral. Tumor size varies ranging up to 18 cm. The external surface is lobulated and may contain nodules, whereas the cut surface is frequently solid and cystic. The solid areas range from white to tan or red and may be firm or spongy.

MICROSCOPIC FINDINGS

Surface implants are seen in a majority of cases and in some, a nodular growth can be conspicuous. Tumors may exhibit a variety of growth patterns including glandular, cribriform, villoglandular, solid tubular, insular, and/or cystic. Minor areas may show overt infiltrative growth. The glands and papillae may be lined by cuboidal or flattened epithelium or by several layers of tall to columnar cells with eosinophilic cytoplasm showing atypical nuclei and mitotic activity. They may also show "dirty" necrosis, mucinous and goblet cell differentiation, (Figure 14.51–14.54), and/or a signet-ring cell component. As discussed with metastatic pancreatic carcinomas, these tumors may closely mimic the appearance of primary mucinous tumors of the ovary.

ANCILLARY STUDIES

IMMUNOHISTOCHEMISTRY

Although there may be minor differences between anatomic sites, adenocarcinoma of the gallbladder, extra- and intrahepatic bile ducts, and ampulla of Vater share similar immunophenotypes. Nearly all tumors diffusely express CK7 with variable expression of CK20. Gallbladder, extra- and intrahepatic bile duct, and ampulla of Vater adenocarcinomas combined show loss of Dpc4 expression in approximately 34% of cases but this frequency varies along the biliary system.

DIFFERENTIAL DIAGNOSIS

The main differential diagnostic considerations include *primary ovarian mucinous and endometrioid carcinomas*. In one recent series, neoplastic foci, often mimicking mucinous borderline tumors of typical type or with intraepithelial carcinoma and benign-appearing mucinous epithelium, were observed in 62% of tumors. Features favoring metastases include bilaterality, surface involvement, and nodularity. The CK7/CK20 immunoprofile is very similar for both metastatic biliary tract

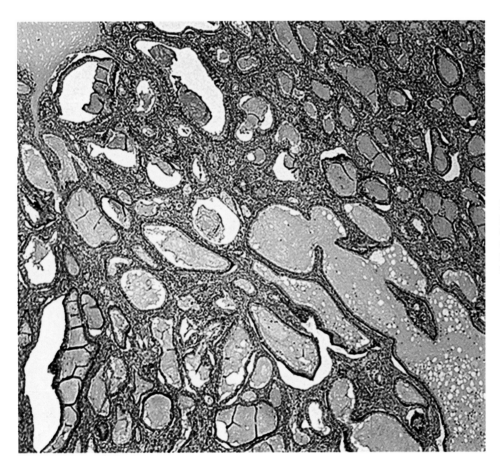

FIGURE 14.51
Metastatic gallbladder adenocarcinoma. The crowded mucinous glands do not appear overtly infiltrative and may simulate a primary ovarian mucinous tumor.

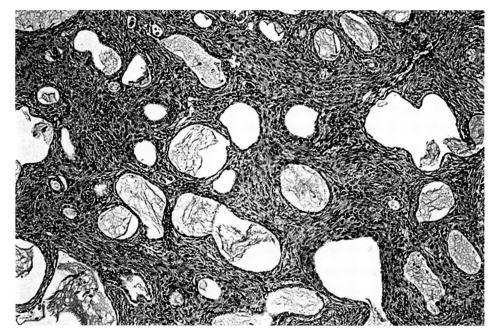

FIGURE 14.52

Metastatic gallbladder adenocarcinoma. Attenuated, dilated glands within a fibromatous stroma simulate a primary ovarian adenofibroma.

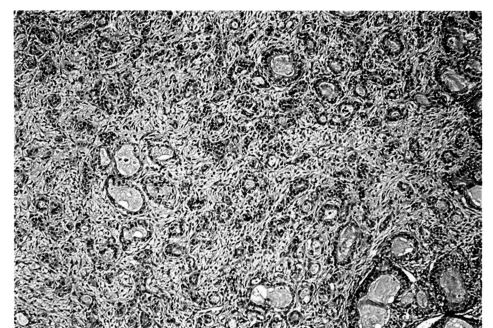

FIGURE 14.53

Metastatic gallbladder adenocarcinoma. Small tubular mucinous glands infiltrate an altered fibromyxoid stroma.

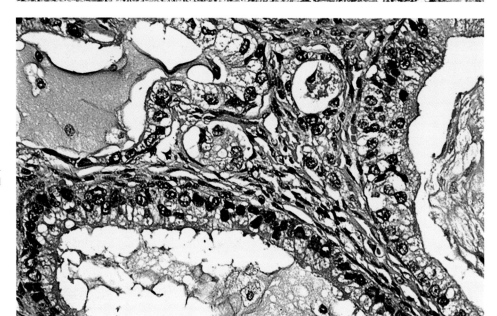

FIGURE 14.54

Metastatic gallbladder adenocarcinoma. The mucinous glands are lined by cells with nuclear atypia.

carcinoma and primary ovarian endometrioid and mucinous tumors. Loss of Dpc4 expression in an ovarian tumor is highly suggestive of metastatic pancreatico/biliary adenocarcinoma but Dpc4 expression does not exclude a biliary tract origin.

METASTASES FROM CARCINOMA OF THE URINARY BLADDER

CLINICAL FEATURES

Patients range in age from 34 to 73 (mean 55) years and typically present with abdominal distention/fullness, bowel obstruction, or an adnexal mass.

METASTASES FROM CARCINOMA OF THE URINARY BLADDER – FACT SHEET

Incidence
▶ 1% of clinically apparent metastases from nongynecologic primary tumors
▶ 1% of all clinically apparent metastases

Age Distribution
▶ Range 34–73 (mean 55) years

Clinical Features
▶ Abdominal distension/fullness
▶ Bowel obstruction
▶ Adnexal mass

PATHOLOGIC FEATURES

GROSS FINDINGS

The majority of tumors are unilateral (mean size 13 cm). They are frequently cystic but may have a solid component.

MICROSCOPIC FINDINGS

The most common histologic type is transitional cell carcinoma, which is characterized by large papillae lined by intermediate- to high-grade transitional cells projecting into cystic spaces. Infiltrating nests with central cystic change secondary to necrosis may also be seen (Figures 14.55–14.57). Other tumors have the appearance of usual high-grade transitional cell carcinoma, in which irregular nests of tumor cells are embedded in a desmoplastic stroma. These tumors may show squamous and/or glandular differentiation. The next most common histologic type is signet-ring cell carcinoma, in which the cells infiltrate individually, or form trabecu-

lae or sheets; a minor glandular component can also be seen. Finally, urachal adenocarcinoma rarely metastasizes to the ovaries and has the appearance of a mucinous cystadenocarcinoma.

ANCILLARY STUDIES

IMMUNOHISTOCHEMISTRY

Transitional cell carcinomas of the urinary bladder typically express CK7. The majority also stain for CK20 (Figure 14.58) and thrombomodulin, but they are negative for WT-1 (N-terminus).

DIFFERENTIAL DIAGNOSIS

It may be difficult to distinguish metastatic transitional cell carcinoma of the urinary bladder from an *atypical proliferative (borderline) Brenner tumor, malignant Brenner tumor,* or *primary ovarian transitional cell carcinoma.* Histologic features that favor a metastasis include ovarian surface involvement and lymphovascular invasion; laterality is not helpful. The presence of benign or borderline Brenner tumor or the coexistence of transitional cell carcinoma with serous carcinoma would favor an ovarian origin. CK20 and thrombomodulin expression combined with lack of WT-1 favors a urinary bladder origin whereas the converse expression

---

METASTASES FROM CARCINOMA OF THE URINARY BLADDER – PATHOLOGIC FEATURES

Gross Findings
▶ Most unilateral
▶ Mean size 13 cm
▶ Frequently cystic

Microscopic Findings
▶ Transitional cell carcinoma (most common type)
  ▶ Large papillae or irregularly shaped infiltrating nests
  ▶ Cystic change common
  ▶ Transitional cells with intermediate to high-grade nuclear atypia
▶ Other types: signet-ring cell carcinoma and mucinous cystadenocarcinoma (urachus)

Immunohistochemical Features
▶ CK7, CK20, and thrombomodulin positive
▶ WT-1 negative

Differential Diagnosis
▶ Transitional cell ovarian tumors (atypical proliferative, malignant Brenner, transitional cell carcinoma)

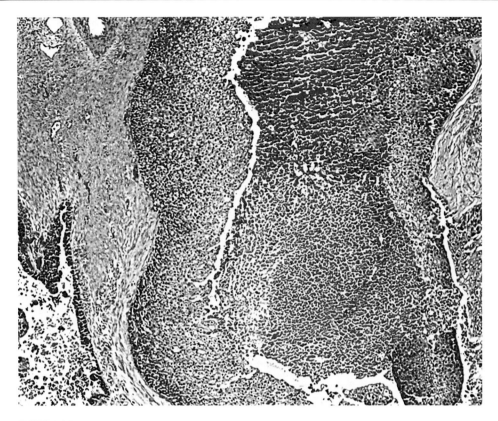

FIGURE 14.55

Metastatic transitional cell carcinoma of the urinary bladder. The tumor is composed of nests of transitional cells with central necrosis and secondary cystic change.

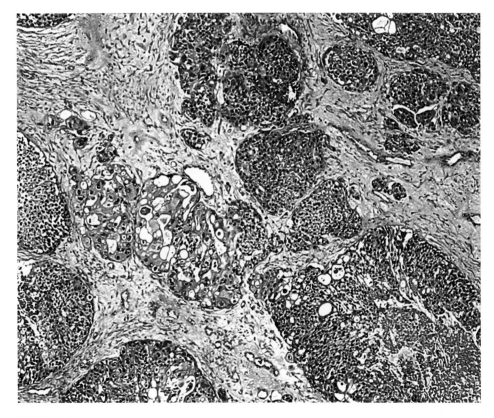

FIGURE 14.56

Metastatic transitional cell carcinoma of the urinary bladder. Nests of transitional cells with focal squamous differentiation are haphazardly arranged within a myxoid stroma. The tumor simulates a primary ovarian transitional cell carcinoma.

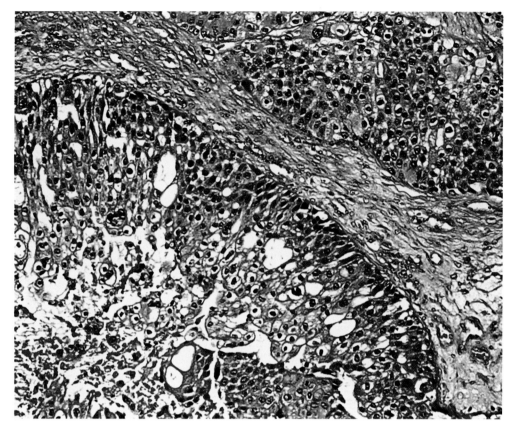

FIGURE 14.57
Metastatic transitional cell carcinoma of the urinary bladder. Low-grade transitional cell epithelium exhibits partial squamous differentiation.

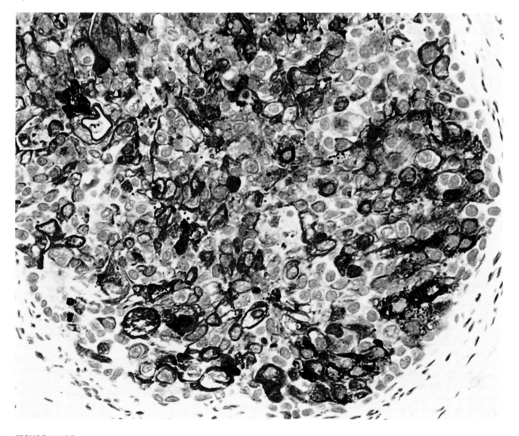

FIGURE 14.58
Metastatic transitional cell carcinoma of the urinary bladder. The tumor exhibits diffuse and strong CK20 expression.

profile favors an ovarian origin. It is important to seek for any history of previous urinary tract neoplasm.

METASTASES FROM CARCINOMA OF THE KIDNEY

CLINICAL FEATURES

Patients range in age from 17 to 64 (mean 49) years and they present with a pelvic/adnexal mass, abdominal mass, ascites, or vaginal bleeding.

METASTASES FROM CARCINOMA OF THE KIDNEY – FACT SHEET

Incidence
▶ < 1% of clinically apparent metastases from nongynecologic primary tumors
▶ < 1% of all clinically apparent metastases

Age Distribution
▶ Range: 17–64 (mean, 49) years

Clinical Features
▶ Pelvic/adnexal/abdominal mass
▶ Ascites
▶ Vaginal bleeding

PATHOLOGIC FEATURES

GROSS FINDINGS

Approximately 17% of tumors are bilateral with sizes ranging from 7 to 18 cm. They are typically solid, but may have a cystic component. The cut surface, which may be nodular and show areas of hemorrhage, ranges from gray to tan to yellow or brown.

MICROSCOPIC FINDINGS

Clear cell carcinoma is the most common histologic subtype of renal cell carcinoma that metastasizes to the ovary. This tumor is mainly composed of nests or tubules, some of which may be cystically dilated, but alveolar and solid growth patterns may also be seen. The tumor cells are polyhedral, cuboidal, and/or columnar with abundant clear cytoplasm and often low-grade nuclei (Figure 14.59 and 14.60). The tubules and cysts may contain colloid-like secretions or blood (Figure

14.59), and a conspicuous sinusoidal vasculature is seen (Figure 14.61).

ANCILLARY STUDIES

IMMUNOHISTOCHEMISTRY

Renal clear cell carcinoma expresses CD10, RCC marker, CA-125, and CK7 in 95%, 86%, 15%, and 14% of cases, respectively.

DIFFERENTIAL DIAGNOSIS

The principal differential diagnostic consideration is primary ovarian clear cell carcinoma. Features favoring *primary ovarian clear cell carcinoma* include an admixture of classic tubulocystic, papillary, and solid patterns; hobnail cells; hyalinized basement membrane-like material within the stroma; and intraluminal mucin. Features favoring metastatic renal clear cell carcinoma are the sinusoidal vasculature, intraluminal blood and colloid-like secretions. Immunohistochemical expression of CD10 and RCC marker, and negativity for CK7 and CA-125 support a diagnosis of metastatic renal clear cell carcinoma. Other tumors that rarely may enter into the differential diagnosis include *steroid cell tumor, dysgerminoma or yolk sac tumor* as they contain cells with clear cytoplasm. However, all these tumors have characteristic histologic features that allow for a correct diagnosis.

METASTASES FROM CARCINOMA OF THE KIDNEY – PATHOLOGIC FEATURES

Gross Findings
▶ 17% bilateral
▶ Size up to 18 cm
▶ Solid and occasionally cystic cut surface

Microscopic Findings
▶ Tubular, alveolar, and/or solid growth patterns
▶ Polyhedral, cuboidal, and/or columnar cells with abundant clear cytoplasm and variable nuclear atypia, although often low-grade
▶ Intraglandular colloid-like secretions or blood
▶ Delicate sinusoidal vasculature

Immunohistochemical Features
▶ RCC and CD10 positive
▶ CK7 and CA-125 usually negative

Differential Diagnosis
▶ Clear cell carcinoma of ovary
▶ Steroid cell tumor
▶ Dysgerminoma
▶ Yolk sac tumor

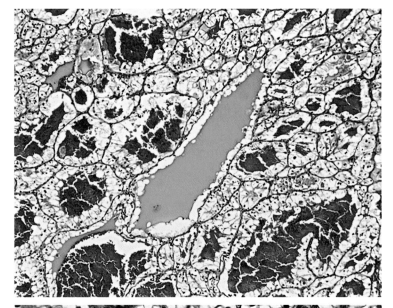

FIGURE 14.59

Metastatic renal clear cell carcinoma. Dilated tubules containing blood and colloid-like secretions are lined by cells with abundant clear cytoplasm.

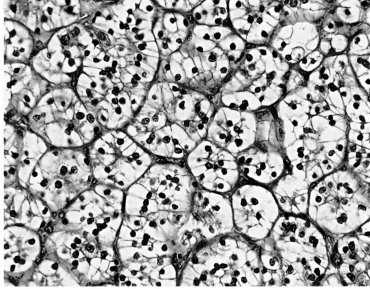

FIGURE 14.60

Metastatic renal clear cell carcinoma. The cells contain abundant clear cytoplasm and round low-grade nuclei.

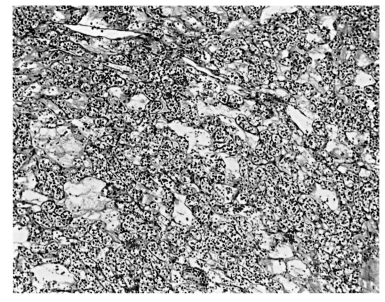

FIGURE 14.61

Metastatic renal clear cell carcinoma. Note the prominent sinusoidal vasculature.

SECONDARY INVOLVEMENT BY MALIGNANT MESOTHELIOMA

CLINICAL FEATURES

Patients range in age from 18 to 63 (mean 48) years and they present with abdominal/pelvic pain, abdominal/pelvic/adnexal mass, and/or ascites. They do not have a history of asbestos exposure.

SECONDARY INVOLVEMENT BY MALIGNANT MESOTHELIOMA – FACT SHEET

Incidence
▸ < 1% of clinically apparent metastases from nongynecologic primary tumors
▸ < 1% of all clinically apparent metastases

Age Distribution
▸ Range 18–63 (mean 48) years

Clinical Features
▸ No history of asbestos exposure
▸ Abdominal/pelvic pain, abdominal/pelvic/adnexal mass, and/or ascites
▸ Diffuse abdominal or pelvic peritoneal tumor/implants

PATHOLOGIC FEATURES

GROSS FINDINGS

Patients have diffuse abdominal or pelvic peritoneal tumor/implants with involvement of the omentum and diaphragmatic and liver surface. The ovaries are bilaterally involved in approximately 86% of cases. The tumors are solid but may have a minor cystic component with a mean size of 7 cm. The cut surface ranges from white to tan or yellow and may be nodular.

MICROSCOPIC FINDINGS

Malignant mesothelioma typically involves both the surface and parenchyma of the ovary. Tubulopapillary and solid patterns are typically seen; papillae are lined by a single layer of cells that focally may show detached cell tufts (Figures 14.62 and 14.63). Rarely, adenomatoid, retiform, trabecular, and cording patterns can be encountered. The cells are most frequently epithelioid with a polygonal, cuboidal, or flat appearance and have variable amounts of eosinophilic cytoplasm; cells may occasionally be vacuolated or have a deciduoid or spindled (sarcomatoid) morphology. The nuclei generally

show mild to moderate degree of cytologic atypia (Figure 14.64). Psammoma bodies may be present but are not numerous.

SECONDARY INVOLVEMENT BY MALIGNANT MESOTHELIOMA – PATHOLOGIC FEATURES

Gross Findings
▸ 86% bilateral
▸ Mean size 7 cm
▸ Solid and sometimes nodular cut surface

Microscopic Findings
▸ Typically tubulopapillary and/or solid patterns
▸ Retiform, adenomatoid, trabecular, and cording patterns occasionally
▸ Single layer or minor pseudostratification of cells with focal detached cell tufts
▸ Most commonly epithelioid cells with eosinophilic cytoplasm
▸ Hobnail vacuolated or spindled cells may be seen
▸ Mild to moderate degree of nuclear atypia
▸ Infrequent psammoma bodies

Immunohistochemical Features
▸ Calretinin, CK5/6 and h-caldesmon usually positive
▸ ER, MOC-31, Ber-EP4 and B72.3 typically negative

Differential Diagnosis
▸ Serous carcinoma of ovary
▸ Primary mesothelioma of ovary (very rare)

ANCILLARY STUDIES

IMMUNOHISTOCHEMISTRY

Peritoneal malignant mesothelioma usually expresses calretinin (91%) (Figure 14.65), CK5/6 and h-caldesmon, but it is usually negative for ER, Ber-EP4, MOC-31, and B72.3.

DIFFERENTIAL DIAGNOSIS

The principal differential diagnostic consideration is serous carcinoma. In contrast to mesothelioma, *serous carcinoma* tends to be bulkier and has a more cystic gross appearance (when involving the ovary), greater degree of cellular stratification lining the papillae with detached epithelial tufts, slit-like spaces, greater degree of cytologic atypia, more mitotic activity, and numerous psammoma bodies. Expression of calretinin and h-caldesmon combined with negativity for B72.3, MOC-31, ER, and Ber-EP4 supports a diagnosis of peritoneal malignant mesothelioma as serous carcinomas usually have the opposite immunoprofile (although they can be calretinin-positive).

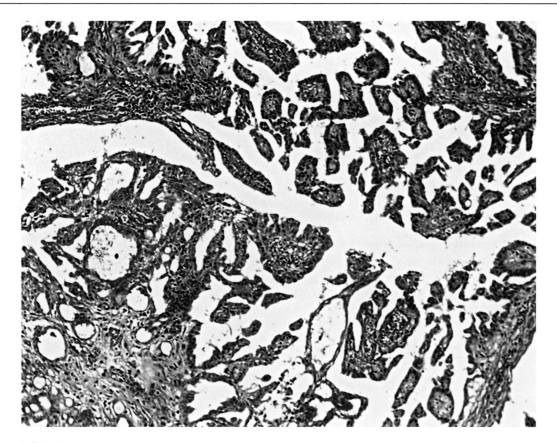

FIGURE 14.62
Secondary involvement of the ovary by malignant mesothelioma. The tumor has a papillary growth and lacks epithelial stratification and tufting characteristic of serous carcinoma.

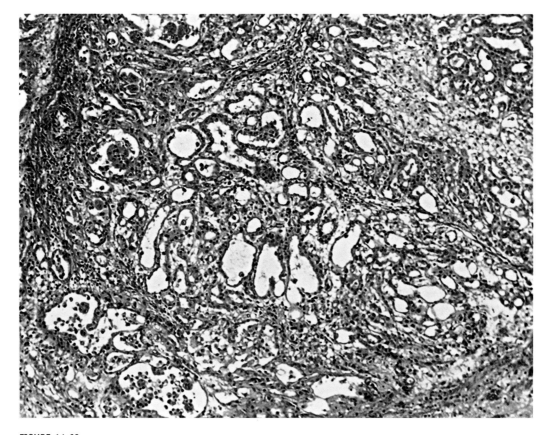

FIGURE 14.63
Secondary involvement of the ovary by malignant mesothelioma. The tumor is composed of closely packed tubules lined by cuboidal cells, which haphazardly infiltrate the stroma, simulating an adenomatoid tumor.

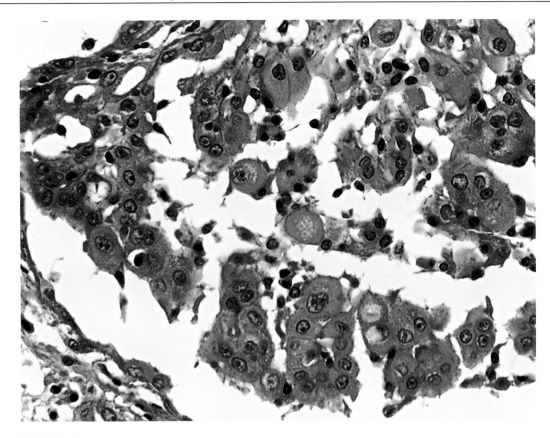

FIGURE 14.64
Secondary involvement of the ovary by malignant mesothelioma. The cells have abundant dense eosinophilic cytoplasm, round and vesicular nuclei, and prominent nucleoli.

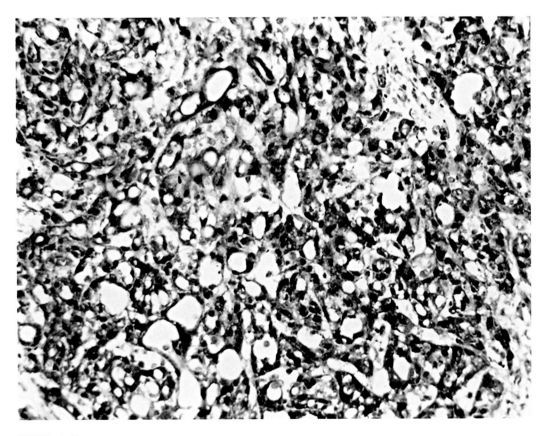

FIGURE 14.65
Secondary involvement of the ovary by malignant mesothelioma. The tumor cells exhibit diffuse strong calretinin expression (nuclear and cytoplasmic).

METASTASES FROM EXTRAOVARIAN CARCINOID TUMOR

CLINICAL FEATURES

Patients range in age from 21 to 82 (mean 57) years and may present with the carcinoid syndrome (40%), abdominal pain/enlargement, abdominal/pelvic mass, or prior history of an extraovarian carcinoid tumor. When the extraovarian primary tumor can be identified (80%), it is most commonly located in the ileum, followed by the cecum, pancreas, jejunum, appendix, and lung.

METASTASES FROM EXTRAOVARIAN CARCINOID TUMOR – FACT SHEET

Incidence
▶ 7% of clinically apparent metastases from nongynecologic primary tumors
▶ 4% of all clinically apparent metastases

Age Distribution
▶ Range 21–82 (mean 57) years

Clinical Features
▶ Abdominal pain/distension or abdominal/pelvic mass
▶ ± Carcinoid syndrome (40%)

PATHOLOGIC FEATURES

GROSS FINDINGS

In over 88% of patients there is bilateral ovarian involvement (mean size of 9 cm). The external surface is smooth, and the cut surface is firm, nodular, and ranges from tan to gray or yellow. Hemorrhage, necrosis, or a cystic component may be evident.

MICROSCOPIC FINDINGS

The tumors are histologically similar to primary ovarian carcinoids; however, other teratomatous elements are not present, and a nodular architecture may be quite prominent (Figure 14.66). The most common growth pattern is insular, but, trabecular, mixed insular–trabecular, and goblet cell (mucinous) growth can be seen (Figure 14.67–14.70). The cells have round and monotonous nuclei with "salt-and-pepper" chromatin; and red cytoplasmic granules can be present. The ovarian stroma is abundant and fibromatous, and frequently shows extensive hyalinization.

METASTASES FROM EXTRAOVARIAN CARCINOID TUMOR – PATHOLOGIC FEATURES

Gross Findings
▶ 88% bilateral
▶ Mean size 9 cm
▶ Firm and nodular cut surface

Microscopic Findings
▶ Nodular low-power architecture
▶ Insular (most common), trabecular, mixed insular–trabecular, and goblet cell (mucinous) growth patterns
▶ Cells with eosinophilic cytoplasm containing red granules and nuclei with "salt-and-pepper" chromatin
▶ Striking fibromatous/hyalinized stroma
▶ No teratomatous components

Immunohistochemical Features
▶ Chromogranin and synaptophysin usually positve
▶ Cytokeratin frequently positive
▶ Calretinin occasionally positive
▶ Inhibin, ER, and PR typically negative

Differential Diagnosis
▶ Primary ovarian carcinoid tumor
▶ Adult granulosa cell tumor
▶ Sertoli cell tumor
▶ Endometrioid carcinoma

ANCILLARY STUDIES

IMMUNOHISTOCHEMISTRY

Chromogranin and synaptophysin are expressed in 83 and 94% of these tumors, respectively. Cytokeratin is frequently positive, staining for calretinin is seen on occasion, and inhibin and ER/PR are almost always negative.

DIFFERENTIAL DIAGNOSIS

The chief differential diagnostic consideration of metastatic carcinoid tumor is a *primary ovarian carcinoid*, which is typically more common, practically always unilateral, and frequently associated with teratomatous components. In contrast, carcinoid tumors metastatic to the ovary are frequently bilateral, show a grossly nodular cut surface, and typically have abundant fibromatous/hyalinized stroma. Moreover, a prior history of a known extraovarian carcinoid tumor or the finding of extraovarian disease favors a metastatic origin. In some cases, thorough clinical/radiologic correlation may be necessary to determine the primary site. Rarely, other tumors in the differential diagnosis include *adult granulosa cell tumor, Sertoli cell tumor,* and *endometrioid carcinoma*, as all can show a trabecular/cord-like or even insular-like growth. However, they also display other characteristic growth patterns and are positive for calretinin and

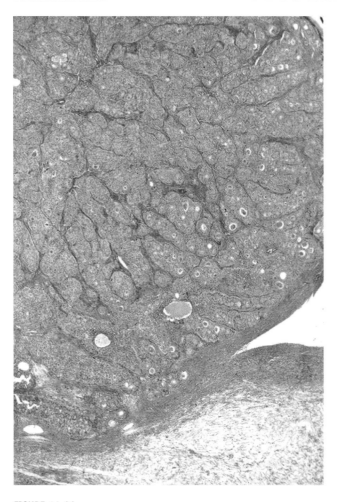

FIGURE 14.66
Metastatic carcinoid tumor. A discrete nodule is present on the ovarian surface.

inhibin (granulosa and Sertoli cell tumors) or ER and PR (endometrioid carcinoma).

SECONDARY INVOLVEMENT BY NONGYNECOLOGIC SMALL ROUND BLUE CELL SARCOMAS

CLINICAL FEATURES

Patients affected by this group of sarcomas are usually in the pediatric age range. The primary site varies depending on the type of sarcoma. Patients may present with abdominal distention/pain, or an abdominal/pelvic mass.

METASTASES FROM, OR SECONDARY INVOLVEMENT BY, OTHER TYPES OF NONGYNECOLOGIC SMALL ROUND BLUE CELL SARCOMAS – FACT SHEET

Incidence
▶ < 1% of clinically apparent metastases from nongynecologic primary tumors
▶ < 1% of all clinically apparent metastases

Age Distribution
▶ Usually pediatric age group

Clinical Features
▶ Abdominal distension, abdominal pain, or abdominal/pelvic mass

---

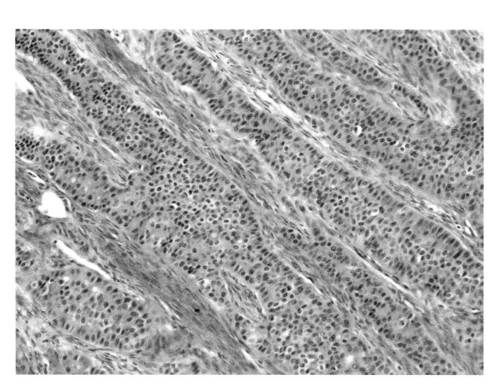

FIGURE 14.67
Metastatic carcinoid tumor. A prominent trabecular pattern is seen associated with focal acinar formation.

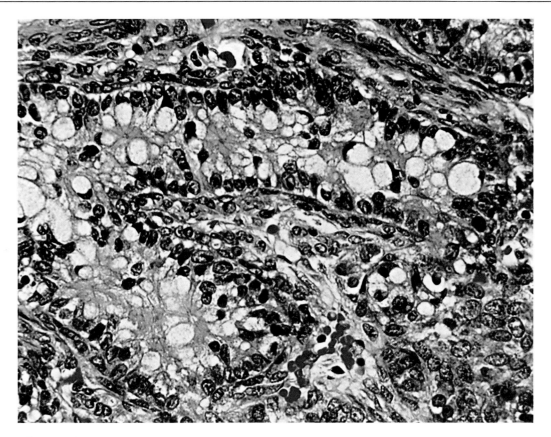

FIGURE 14.68
Metastatic mucinous (goblet cell) carcinoid. The tumor cells form trabeculae and contain goblet cells.

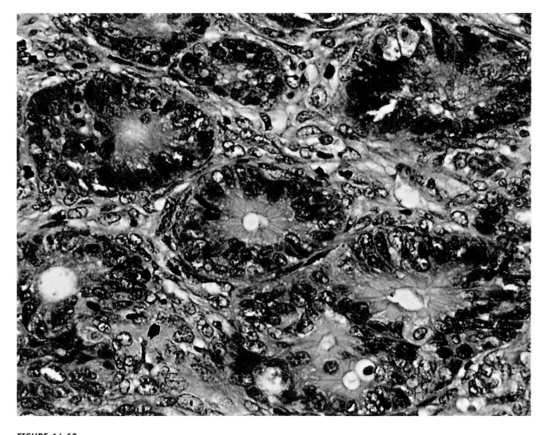

FIGURE 14.69
Metastatic mucinous (goblet cell) carcinoid. Some acini form small tubules and resemble colonic-type crypts but nuclei are notably atypical.

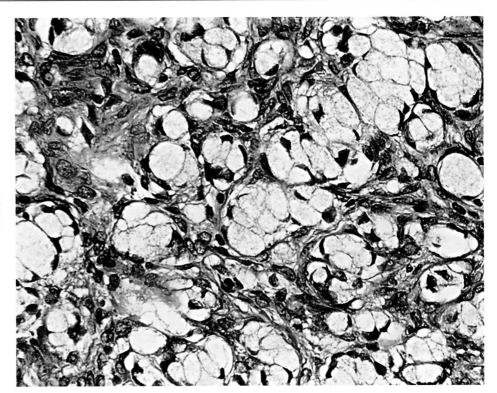

FIGURE 14.70
Metastatic mucinous (goblet cell) carcinoid. Tumor nests contain signet-ring cells, which have atypical, eccentric, crescent-shaped nuclei deformed by a cytoplasmic mucin vacuole.

PATHOLOGIC FEATURES

GROSS FINDINGS

The tumors may be unilateral or bilateral with a mean size of 11 cm. The cut surface may be solid or cystic, lobulated/nodular, and firm or soft. Color varies, ranging from red-purple, light tan, tan-brown, to gray or pink, and areas of hemorrhage may be present.

MICROSCOPIC FINDINGS

At low power, a nodular architecture is not uncommon. The histologic appearance is variable since the tumor may be one of a variety of sarcomas including rhabdomyosarcoma (Figures 14.71–14.72), neuroblastoma, Ewing's sarcoma, and desmoplastic small round cell tumor (Figures 14.73–14.75).

ANCILLARY STUDIES

IMMUNOHISTOCHEMISTRY

Rhabdomyosarcoma expresses desmin, myogenin, MyoD1, and myoglobin. Neuroblastoma is positive for CD56, neurofilaments, chromogranin, and synaptophysin. Primitive neuroectodermal tumor/Ewing's sarcoma immunoreacts with CD99 and Fli-1 and frequently shows the typical t(11;22)(q24;q12) chromosomal translocation. Desmoplastic small round cell tumor stains for pancytokeratin, EMA, desmin, and WT-1 (C-terminus).

METASTASES FROM, OR SECONDARY INVOLVEMENT BY, OTHER TYPES OF NONGYNECOLOGIC SMALL ROUND BLUE CELL SARCOMAS – PATHOLOGIC FEATURES

Gross Findings
▸ Unilateral or bilateral
▸ Mean size 11 cm
▸ Solid, lobulated, or nodular cut surface

Microscopic Findings
▸ Rhabdomyosarcoma
▸ Neuroblastoma
▸ Ewing's sarcoma
▸ Desmoplastic small round blue cell tumor

Immunohistochemical Features
▸ Rhabdomyosarcoma: Desmin, myogenin, Myo D1, and myoglobin positive
▸ Neuroblastoma: CD56, neurofilaments, chromogranin, and synaptophysin positive
▸ Primitive neuroectodermal tumor/extraosseous Ewing's sarcoma: CD99 and Fli-1 positive
▸ Desmoplastic small round blue cell tumor: pancytokeratin, EMA, desmin, and WT-1 positive

Differential Diagnosis
▸ Primary ovarian sarcomas
▸ Small cell carcinoma of the hypercalcemic type
▸ Lymphoma
▸ Metastatic melanoma
▸ Adult granulosa cell tumor

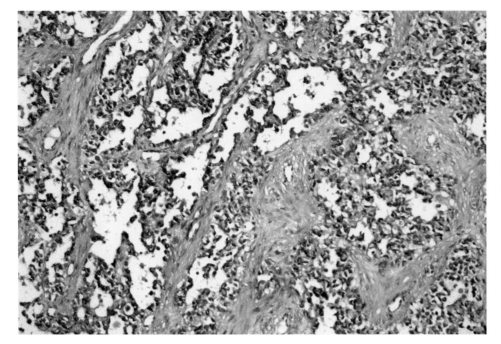

FIGURE 14.71
Metastatic alveolar rhabdomyosarcoma. The tumor cells line irregular spaces and some have abundant eosinophilic cytoplasm.

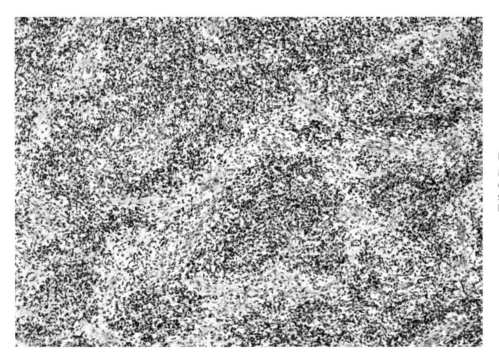

FIGURE 14.72
Metastatic embryonal rhabdomyosarcoma. Poorly formed aggregates of small cells alternate with hypocellular areas.

DIFFERENTIAL DIAGNOSIS

These groups of tumors should be distinguished from *primary ovarian sarcomas, small cell carcinoma of the hypercalcemic type, metastatic melanoma (if small cells)* and *lymphoma*. Bilaterality, nodularity, or a history of prior primary tumor of similar histologic type elsewhere are features favoring metastasis. In the setting of neuroblastoma, the presence of teratomatous components favors an ovarian origin. A panel of immunohistochemical markers is often necessary to establish the correct diagnosis.

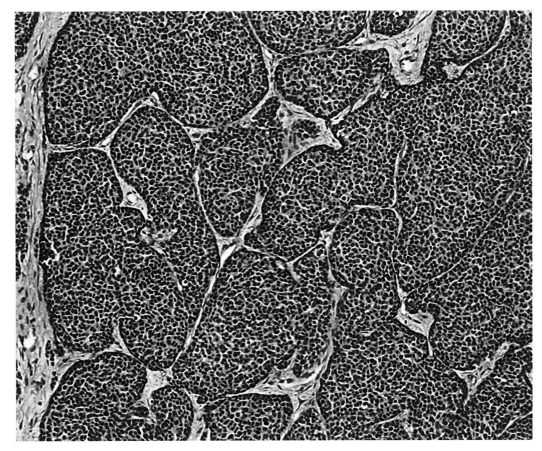

FIGURE 14.73
Secondary involvement of the ovary by desmoplastic small round cell tumor. Discrete nests of cells are separated by scant stroma.

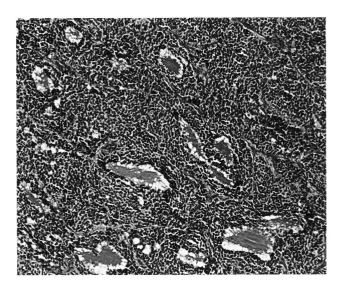

FIGURE 14.74
Secondary involvement of the ovary by desmoplastic small round cell tumor. The follicle-like spaces may falsely suggest an epithelial or sex cord-stromal tumor.

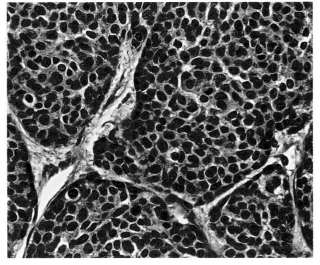

FIGURE 14.75
Secondary involvement of the ovary by desmoplastic small round cell tumor. The cells have nuclear atypia and moderate amount of eosinophilic cytoplasm.

METASTASES FROM CARCINOMA OF THE UTERINE CERVIX

CLINICAL FEATURES

Patients range in age from 23 to 73 (mean 46) years and may present with a pelvic/adnexal mass or abdominal distension/pain.

METASTASES FROM CARCINOMA OF THE UTERINE CERVIX – FACT SHEET

Incidence
▸ 78% of clinically apparent metastases from gynecologic primary tumors
▸ 6% of all clinically apparent metastases

Age Distribution
▸ Range 23–73 (mean 46) years

Clinical Features
▸ Pelvic/adnexal mass, abdominal distension or pain

PATHOLOGIC FEATURES

GROSS FINDINGS

Tumors are typically unilateral and sizes range from 5 to 30 cm. They tend to be multi- or unicystic, with or without a solid component, which when present may be white, tan, yellow, or focally hemorrhagic. The cut surface may have a nodular appearance.

MICROSCOPIC FINDINGS

The two most common histologic types of primary cervical tumors that metastasize to the ovary are squamous cell carcinoma and adenocarcinoma. The latter often exhibit noninfiltrative growth patterns (papillary, villoglandular, confluent glandular), thus simulating primary ovarian atypical proliferative (borderline) endometrioid and mucinous tumors with intraepithelial carcinoma (Figures 14.76 and 14.77). Enlarged, hyperchromatic atypical nuclei, basal apoptotic bodies, and numerous mitotic figures, as seen in endocervical adenocarcinoma in situ are characteristic of HPV-related endocervical adenocarcinoma (Figure 14.78). Rarely, the adenocarcinoma may be of the adenoma malignum type (minimal-deviation adenocarcinoma), which appears to be unrelated to HPV infection.

METASTASES FROM CARCINOMA OF THE UTERINE CERVIX – PATHOLOGIC FEATURES

Gross Findings
▸ Frequently unilateral
▸ Up to 30 cm
▸ Frequently cystic

Microscopic Findings
▸ Typical features of squamous cell carcinoma (well to poorly differentiated)
▸ Adenocarcinoma:
  ▸ Non-infiltrative papillary, villoglandular, confluent glandular growth patterns
  ▸ Mucinous, endometrioid, or hybrid cells
  ▸ Often hyperchromatic nuclei, numerous mitotic figures and apoptotic bodies
  ▸ HPV related
▸ Other types: small cell carcinoma, adenosquamous carcinoma, transitional cell carcinoma, and undifferentiated carcinoma

Immunohistochemical Features
▸ CK7 and p16 positive
▸ CK20 negative
▸ ER/PR often negative (adenocarcinoma)
▸ HPV (in situ hybridization) frequently positive

Differential Diagnosis
▸ Squamous cell carcinoma of ovary
▸ Mucinous and endometrioid tumors (atypical proliferative and carcinoma) of ovary

---

ANCILLARY STUDIES

IMMUNOHISTOCHEMISTRY

Both squamous cell carcinoma and adenocarcinoma of the cervix usually express CK7, are negative for CK20, and diffusely and strongly express p16 in association with high-risk HPV infection (Figure 14.79). In situ hybridization for HPV is useful as a more specific, definitive test than immunohistochemistry to establish that an adenocarcinoma in the ovary is metastatic from the endocervix (Figure 14.80).

DIFFERENTIAL DIAGNOSIS

Primary ovarian mucinous and endometrioid tumors and primary ovarian squamous cell carcinoma are the main diagnostic considerations. The characteristic microscopic features of HPV-related endocervical adenocarcinoma in conjunction with diffuse p16 expression, lack of hormone receptors, and detection of HPV DNA within the tumor are useful to exclude *primary ovarian endometrioid* and *mucinous tumors. Primary squamous cell carcinoma* may very closely mimic metastatic squamous cell carcinoma, but it tends to occur in an older population and it is frequently associated with a dermoid cyst.

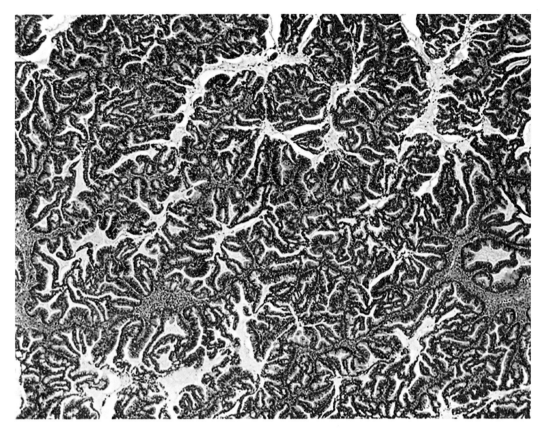

FIGURE 14.76

Metastatic endocervical adenocarcinoma. The tumor has a confluent glandular pattern that simulates a primary ovarian mucinous carcinoma.

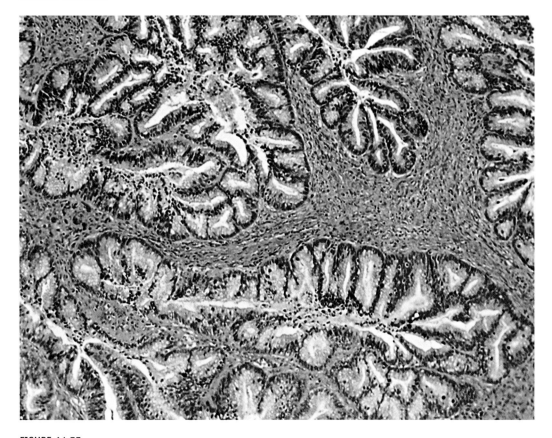

FIGURE 14.77

Metastatic endocervical adenocarcinoma. Mucinous glands displaying papillary infoldings, without infiltrative growth, simulate a primary ovarian atypical proliferative (borderline) mucinous tumor.

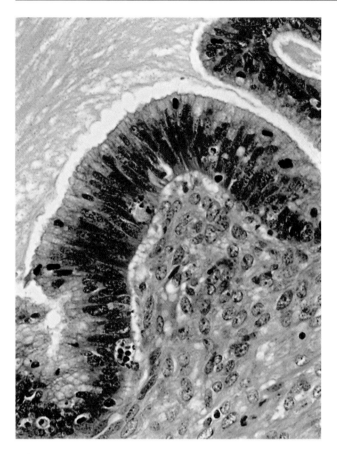

FIGURE 14.78
Metastatic endocervical adenocarcinoma. The mucinous epithelium is composed of pseudostratified columnar cells with hyperchromatic elongated nuclei. Numerous mitotic figures and apoptotic bodies are seen.

METASTASES FROM CARCINOMA OF THE UTERINE CORPUS

CLINICAL FEATURES

The mean age at presentation is 53 years. When the primary endometrial carcinoma does not produce symp-

METASTASES FROM CARCINOMA OF THE UTERINE CORPUS – FACT SHEET
Incidence
▸ 22% of clinically apparent metastases from gynecologic primary tumors
▸ 2% of all clinically apparent metastases
Age Distribution
▸ Mean 53 years
Clinical Features
▸ Adnexal mass(es), ± uterine bleeding

toms leading to its diagnosis prior to hysterectomy, patients can present with a pelvic mass suggesting a primary ovarian tumor.

PATHOLOGIC FEATURES

GROSS FINDINGS

Metastases to the ovary are usually < 5 cm and bilateral. They can be nodular and solid or have a mixture of solid and cystic components (Figure 14.81), with the solid areas being typically firm and tan-white to tan-yellow.

METASTASES FROM CARCINOMA OF THE UTERINE CORPUS – PATHOLOGIC FEATURES
Gross Findings
▸ Usually bilateral
▸ Size < 5 cm
Microscopic Findings
▸ Nodular growth
▸ Surface or superficial cortical tumor
▸ Lymphovascular invasion
▸ Types: endometrioid and serous carcinoma
Immunohistochemical Features
▸ Endometrioid carcinoma:
▸ ER/PR usually positive
▸ p53 and WT-1 usually negative
▸ Serous carcinoma:
▸ p53 usually strongly and diffusely positive
▸ ER/PR and WT-1 infrequently positive
Differential Diagnosis
▸ Synchronous primary ovarian and endometrial carcinoma

MICROSCOPIC FINDINGS

The tumors frequently show a nodular growth, surface involvement, and can demonstrate lymphovascular invasion (Figure 14.82). The two most common histologic types are endometrioid and serous carcinoma, resembling their uterine counterparts (Figures 14.83 and 14.84).

ANCILLARY STUDIES

IMMUNOHISTOCHEMISTRY

Endometrioid carcinoma usually expresses ER/PR and is negative for p53, whereas serous carcinoma shows infrequent expression of hormone receptors and WT-1, and displays diffuse and strong p53 expression.

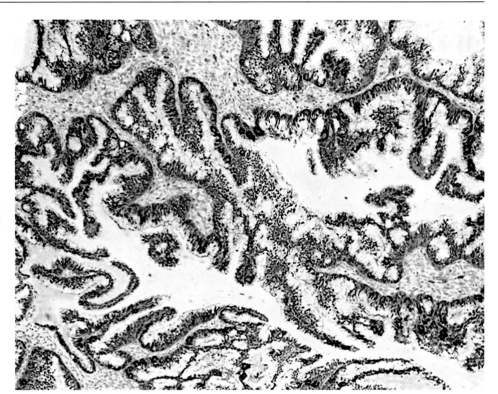

FIGURE 14.79

Metastatic endocervical adenocarcinoma. The tumor exhibits diffuse strong p16 expression (both nuclear and cytoplasmic).

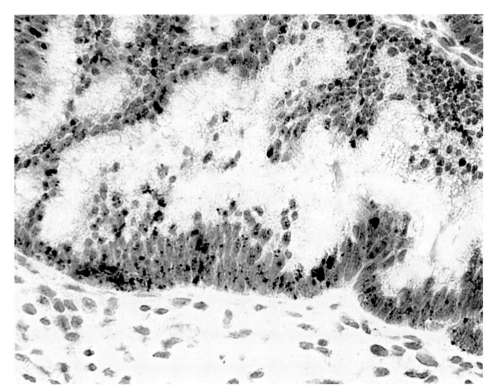

FIGURE 14.80

Metastatic endocervical adenocarcinoma. In situ hybridization for HPV 16 demonstrates numerous fine punctate reaction product signals within tumor nuclei.

DIFFERENTIAL DIAGNOSIS

The main diagnostic dilemma arises when *synchronous ovarian and endometrial tumors of similar histologic type* are present; in this setting distinction between synchronous tumors or metastasis can be difficult. For tumors with endometrioid histology, the presence of a primary endometrial endometrioid carcinoma with deep myometrial invasion, lymphovascular invasion, carcinoma within the fallopian tube or on the ovarian surface, bilateral ovarian tumors, multinodularity, and absence of endometriosis or adenofibroma within the ovary favor metastasis. In the setting of serous carcinoma, diffuse and strong WT-1 (N-terminus) expression in the ovary favors an ovarian primary as uterine serous carcinomas less frequently express this marker.

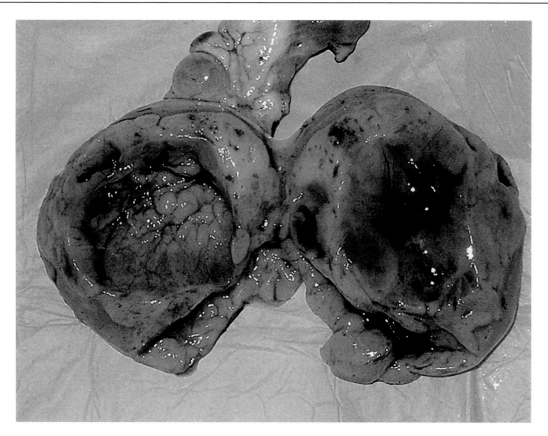

FIGURE 14.81

Metastatic endometrial endometrioid carcinoma. The cut surface is cystic and solid, as seen in primary ovarian endometrioid carcinomas.

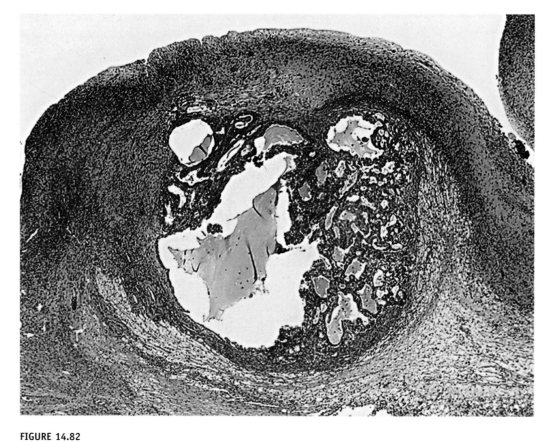

FIGURE 14.82

Metastatic endometrial endometrioid carcinoma. The tumor has a nodular growth in the superficial cortex suggesting metastasis.

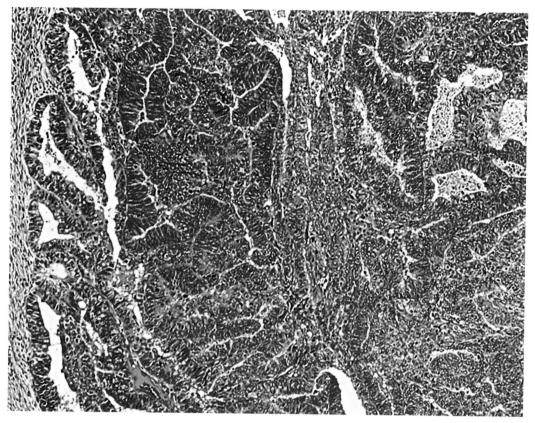

FIGURE 14.83

Metastatic endometrial endometrioid carcinoma. The tumor is composed of glands similar in appearance to a primary ovarian endometrioid carcinoma.

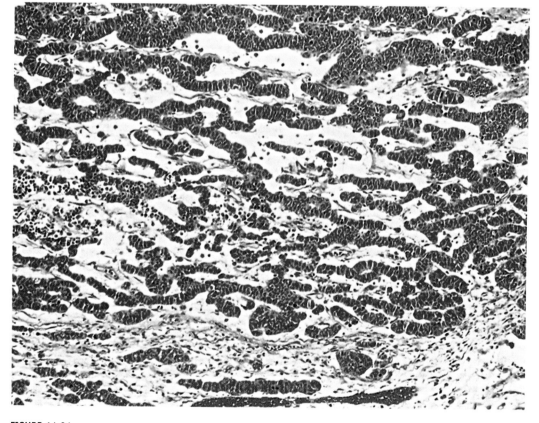

FIGURE 14.84

Metastatic endometrial endometrioid carcinoma. The tumor forms interanastomosing cords simulating a Sertoli cell or carcinoid tumor.

METASTASES FROM MESENCHYMAL TUMORS OF THE UTERINE CORPUS

CLINICAL FEATURES

Patients range in age from 33 to 79 (mean 47) years. They present with a pelvic/adnexal mass, abdominal distension, dysfunctional uterine bleeding, or pelvic/abdominal pain.

METASTASES FROM MESENCHYMAL TUMORS OF THE UTERINE CORPUS – FACT SHEET

Incidence
▸ Uncommon to rare

Age Distribution
▸ 33–79 (mean 47) years

Clinical Features
▸ Pelvic/abdominal mass, pelvic/abdominal pain or distension
▸ Dysfunctional uterine bleeding

PATHOLOGIC FEATURES

GROSS FINDINGS

Approximately 67% of cases are bilateral, with a mean size of 9 cm. The cut surface is solid (with or without a cystic component), lobulated or nodular, gray-white to yellow, frequently with areas of hemorrhage, and necrosis.

MICROSCOPIC FINDINGS

Endometrial stromal sarcoma appears to metastasize to the ovary more commonly than leiomyosarcoma. It grows in sheets and nodules (the characteristic permeative growth pattern may be inconspicuous), it has small arteriolar-type vessels, hyaline plaques, and frequent lymphovascular invasion (Figures 14.85–14.87). The tumor cells are small and monotonous, with scant cytoplasm, oval to round nuclei, and usually show low mitotic activity (Figure 14.88). Metastatic leiomyosarcoma resembles its uterine counterpart and shows fascicles of spindle cells frequently with significant nuclear atypia and mitotic activity; occasional myxoid change, and lymphovascular invasion may be seen.

ANCILLARY STUDIES

IMMUNOHISTOCHEMISTRY

Metastatic endometrial stromal sarcoma and leiomyosarcoma have immunophenotypes similar to those seen

---

METASTASES FROM MESENCHYMAL TUMORS OF THE UTERINE CORPUS – PATHOLOGIC FEATURES

Gross Findings
▸ 67% bilateral
▸ Mean size 9 cm
▸ Solid, lobulated, or nodular cut surface

Microscopic Findings
▸ Endometrial stromal sarcoma most common
▸ Leiomyosarcoma less common

Immunohistochemical Features
▸ Endometrial stromal sarcoma:
  ▸ CD10, ER and PR positive
  ▸ Smooth muscle actin often positive
  ▸ Desmin (especially if smooth-muscle differentiation) occasionally positive
▸ Leiomyosarcoma:
  ▸ Smooth muscle actin, desmin, and h-caldesmon positive
  ▸ ER/PR positive
  ▸ CD10 not infrequently positive

Differential Diagnosis
▸ Endometrioid stromal sarcoma of ovary
▸ Cellular fibroma (vs metastatic endometrial stromal sarcoma)
▸ Adult granulosa cell tumor (vs metastatic endometrial stromal sarcoma)
▸ Leiomyosarcoma of ovary
▸ Secondary involvement by gastrointestinal stromal tumor (vs leiomyoma/leiomyosarcoma)

---

in primary uterine tumors. Thus, endometrial stromal sarcoma typically expresses CD10 and leiomyosarcoma stains for desmin, h-caldesmon, and actin. However, there is some overlap in the expression of these markers, as endometrial stromal tumors can express actin and less frequently desmin and leiomyosarcoma can express CD10; both tumor types often positive for ER and PR.

DIFFERENTIAL DIAGNOSIS

The main differential diagnosis includes primary *ovarian endometrioid stromal sarcoma* and *primary ovarian leiomyosarcoma*. The presence of endometriosis (for tumors with endometrioid stromal histology) in the same ovary, absence of a uterine mass, or involvement of other pelvic or abdominal sites favor an ovarian primary. Finally, metastatic endometrial stromal sarcoma should be distinguished from *ovarian fibroma and granulosa cell tumor* (when endometrial stromal sarcoma shows sex cord-like differentiation). CD10 may be positive in sex cord tumors but not in fibromas. Searching for typical features of endometrial stromal tumor is most helpful. Clinical history and pathologic features of metastases help to distinguish metastatic leiomyosarcoma from primary ovarian leiomyosarcoma. Secondary involvement by a gastrointestinal stromal tumor will also typically exhibit involvement of the peritoneal organs/cavity and it is positive for CD117 and CD34.

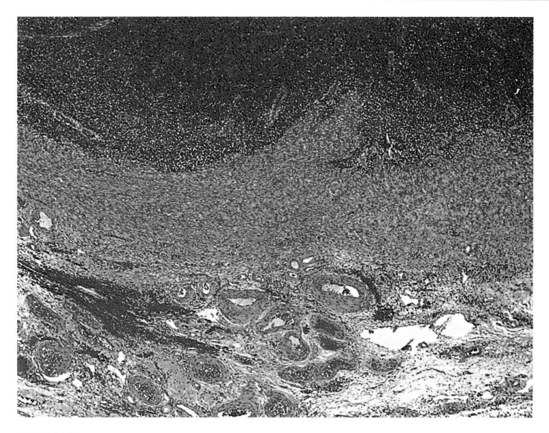

FIGURE 14.85
Metastatic endometrial stromal sarcoma. The tumor exhibits a diffuse growth comprised of small blue cells. The slight nodular configuration at the hilum suggests metastasis.

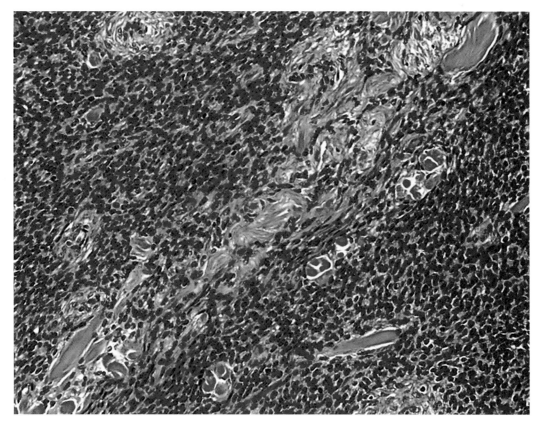

FIGURE 14.86
Metastatic endometrial stromal sarcoma. Collagen bands are present in between groups of small cells.

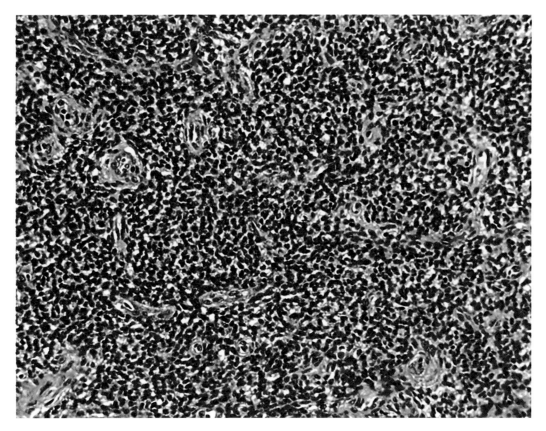

FIGURE 14.87
Metastatic endometrial stromal sarcoma. The tumor contains characteristic small arteriolar-type vessels.

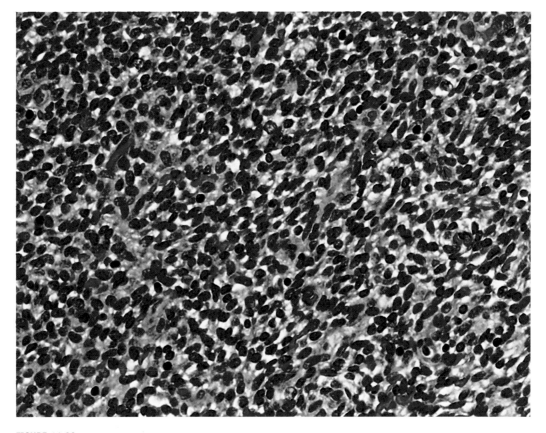

FIGURE 14.88
Metastatic endometrial stromal sarcoma. The tumor is composed of cells resembling proliferative-phase endometrial stroma. They are small, round to oval, and have scanty cytoplasm. The nuclei are small and uniformly bland.

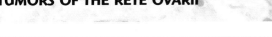

MISCELLANEOUS PRIMARY TUMORS OF THE OVARY

TUMORS OF THE RETE OVARII

CLINICAL FEATURES

In general, patients range in age from 23 to 80 (mean 59) years. They may present with abdominal discomfort, pelvic pressure, postmenopausal bleeding, and/or virilization.

PRIMARY TUMORS OF THE RETE OVARII – FACT SHEET

Definition
▸ Proliferations derived from the rete ovary

Incidence
▸ Rete cyst/cystadenoma ≃ 6% initially diagnosed as simple ovarian cyst or serous cystadenoma

Age Distribution
▸ Range 23–80 (mean 59) years

Clinical Features
▸ Abdominal discomfort or pelvic pressure
▸ Virilization
▸ Postmenopausal bleeding

Prognosis and Therapy
▸ Surgical excision for rete cysts/cystadenomas
▸ Very limited experience with adenoma and adenocarcinoma

PATHOLOGIC FEATURES

GROSS FINDINGS

Approximately 13% of tumors are bilateral with a mean size of 9 cm. They are uni- or mulitcystic and the internal lining is generally smooth.

MICROSCOPIC FINDINGS

All these lesions have in common a location within the hilus or an anatomic relationship with the rete ovarii (Figure 14.89). The different types of rete lesions include cyst, cystadenoma, adenoma, adenomatous hyperplasia, and adenocarcinoma. Among them, cyst/cystadenoma is most common, whereas adenocarcinoma is extremely rare. The distinction between cyst and cystadenoma is arbitrary; 1 cm has been proposed as the upper size limit for a cyst. Rete cyst/cystadenoma is lined by a simple, nonciliated, bland layer of epithelium, usually showing irregular crevices (Figure 14.90). Rete adenoma is well circumscribed and composed of closely spaced tubules that sometimes may contain papillae. They are lined by a single layer of bland epithelial cells. Adenomatous hyperplasia resembles an

adenoma but lacks circumscription. Adenocarcinoma has a complex tubular or papillary architecture and shows cytologic atypia and frequent mitoses. Additional characteristic features include fascicles of smooth muscle and hyperplastic hilus cells in the cyst wall as well as absence of ovarian-type stroma.

ANCILLARY STUDIES

IMMUNOHISTOCHEMISTRY

Rete lesions may stain for CA-125, CAM5.2, EMA, CD10, and PR, but may lack ER expression.

DIFFERENTIAL DIAGNOSIS

The most common issue (although of no clinical importance) is distinguishing rete cystadenoma from *serous cystadenoma*. The combination of location in the hilus or communication with the rete ovarii, cystic lining showing crevices, lack of ciliated cells, and cyst wall containing fascicles of smooth muscle and hyperplastic hilus cells suggests rete cystadenoma. A rete adenoma may be confused with a female adnexal tumor of probable wolffian origin; however, sieve-like and solid growths are lacking.

PROGNOSIS AND THERAPY

Rete cysts/cystadenomas are benign and treated surgically with excision, while experience with adenoma and adenocarcinoma is very limited.

PRIMARY TUMORS OF THE RETE OVARII – PATHOLOGIC FEATURES

Gross Findings
▸ 13% bilateral
▸ Mean size 9 cm
▸ Cystic

Microscopic Findings
▸ Located in the hilum/rete ovarii
▸ Cyst/cystadenoma:
  – Simple cystic lining with irregular crevices
  – Bland flat, cuboidal, or columnar cells without cilia
  – Smooth muscle fascicles, hyperplastic hilus cells but no ovarian stroma in cyst wall
▸ Adenoma/carcinoma:
  – Closely spaced tubules, some containing papillae (adenoma) to complex tubular or papillary architecture (carcinoma)
  – Variable degree of cytologic atypia

Immunohistochemical Features
▸ CA-125, CAM5.2, EMA, CD10, and PR variably positive

Differential Diagnosis
▸ Serous cystadenoma (vs rete cystadenoma)
▸ Adnexal tumor of probable wolffian origin (vs rete adenoma)

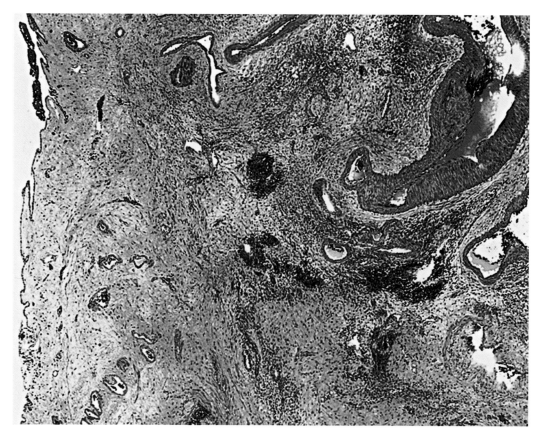

FIGURE 14.89
Primary ovarian rete cystadenoma. The tumor (left) is located adjacent to the ovarian hilum (right).

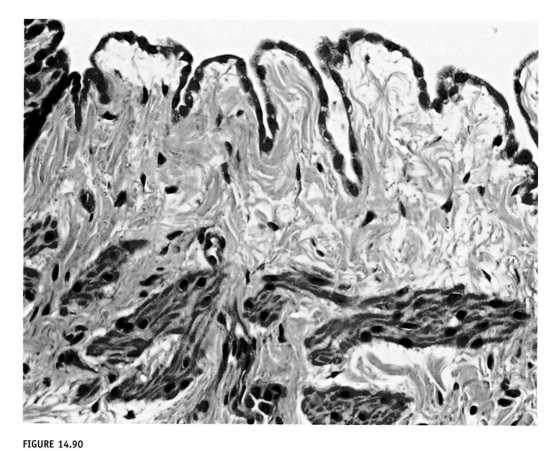

FIGURE 14.90
Primary ovarian rete cystadenoma. Flat bland cells without cilia are associated with smooth muscle bundles in the cyst wall.

SMALL CELL CARCINOMA, HYPERCALCEMIC TYPE

CLINICAL FEATURES

Patients range in age from 7 to 43 (mean 24) years and may present with paraneoplastic hypercalcemia (62%), abdominal distension or pain. Approximately 50% of patients present with advanced stage tumors.

**SMALL CELL CARCINOMA, HYPERCALCEMIC TYPE –
FACT SHEET**

Definition
▶ Poorly differentiated epithelial tumor usually composed of small blue cells with strong association with hypercalcemia

Incidence
▶ Uncommon to rare

Age Distribution
▶ 7–43 (mean 24) years

Clinical Features
▶ Abdominal distension/pain
▶ Hypercalcemia (62%)

Prognosis and Treatment
▶ Extraovarian spread at surgery in 50% of patients
▶ Prognosis closely related to tumor stage
▶ Overall survival rate < 10%
▶ 33% survival rate for patients with stage I tumors
▶ Favorable prognostic factors:
  ▶ Age > 30 years
  ▶ Normal preoperative calcium level
  ▶ Size < 10 cm
  ▶ Absence of large cells

PATHOLOGIC FEATURES

GROSS FINDINGS

Almost all tumors are unilateral and large (mean size 15 cm). The external surface is lobulated, nodular, or smooth, and the cut surface is typically solid, tan-gray, with frequent areas of hemorrhage and necrosis.

MICROSCOPIC FINDINGS

Tumor cells are closely packed and often grow in diffuse sheets, nests, and cords. Most tumors have follicle-like spaces, but they are rarely numerous. They are round to oval but may be irregular in shape, and often contain eosinophilic and less often basophilic secre-

tions. The tumor cells are small with scant cytoplasm and oval to round nuclei with one or two small nucleoli and are mitotically active. Necrosis and hemorrhage are common (Figures 14.91–14.93). Variable numbers of large cells with abundant eosinophilic cytoplasm, sometimes with a rhabdoid appearance, vesicular nuclei, and prominent nucleoli may be seen but rarely represent the predominant component (the so-called large cell variant). The intercellular stroma, typically scant, may be myxoid, a finding more frequently associated with the large cell variant.

ANCILLARY STUDIES

IMMUNOHISTOCHEMISTRY

These tumors frequently express cytokeratin and much less frequently are positive for EMA. They also frequently stain for CD10, WT-1, and calretinin and may express parathyroid-related hormone (but not parathyroid hormone). Occasional tumors stain for pancytokeratin (AE1/AE3), CD56, and synaptophysin. Inhibin, CK5/6, chromogranin, CD99, and TTF-1 are typically negative.

**SMALL CELL CARCINOMA, HYPERCALCEMIC TYPE –
PATHOLOGIC FEATURES**

Gross Findings
▶ Unilateral
▶ Mean size 15 cm
▶ Solid, tan, or gray with frequent areas of necrosis and hemorrhage

Microscopic Findings
▶ Diffuse sheets, nests, and cords
▶ Irregularly shaped follicle-like spaces with eosinophilic or basophilic secretion
▶ Small cells (most common) with scant cytoplasm and oval to round nuclei with one or two small nucleoli
▶ Variable numbers of large cells with abundant cytoplasm, large vesicular nuclei, and prominent nucleoli (sometimes rhabdoid)
▶ Brisk mitotic activity
▶ Scant myxoid intercellular stroma (more common with large cells)
▶ Frequent necrosis and hemorrhage

Immunohistochemical Features
▶ Low-molecular-weight cytokeratin (CK8/18) usually positive
▶ EMA, CD10, WT-1 and calretinin variably positive
▶ Parathyroid-related hormone, pancytokeratin, CD56, and synaptophysin occasionally positive
▶ Inhibin, CK5/6, chromogranin, CD99, and TTF-1 usually negative

Differential Diagnosis
▶ Juvenile granulosa cell tumor
▶ Small cell carcinoma, pulmonary type
▶ Small round blue cell tumors (lymphoma, rhabdomyosarcoma, others)
▶ Metastatic melanoma

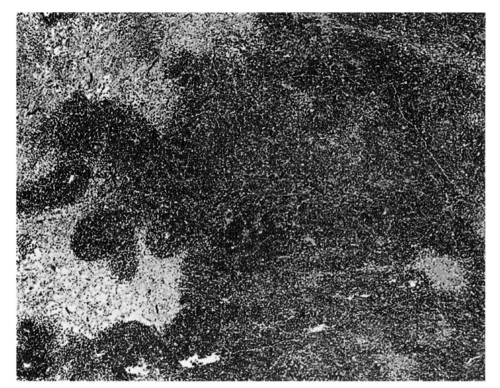

FIGURE 14.91
Primary ovarian small cell carcinoma, hypercalcemic type. Broad zones of geographic necrosis (left) are seen.

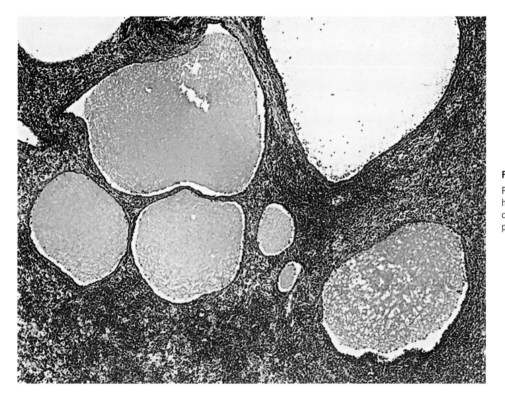

FIGURE 14.92
Primary ovarian small cell carcinoma, hypercalcemic type. Prominent follicle-like spaces filled with eosinophilic fluid are present.

DIFFERENTIAL DIAGNOSIS

The principal differential diagnosis is with granulosa cell tumors, most commonly the juvenile type, as this tumor also occurs at a young age, it forms follicles and it has brisk mitotic activity. However, unlike small cell carcinoma of the hypercalcemic type, *juvenile granulosa cell tumor* is usually associated with estrogenic manifestations and it occurs most commonly during the first decade of life. Furthermore, the tumor cells may have a nodular growth, follicles are more numerous and may be more irregular in shape than in the small cell carcinoma of the hypercalcemic type, and frequently there is a fibrothecomatous component. Immunohistochemically, granulosa cell tumors are positive for inhibin

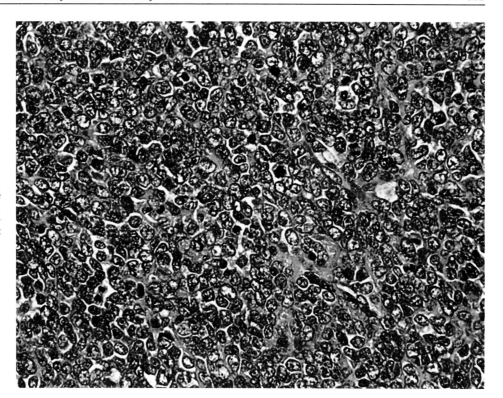

FIGURE 14.93
Primary ovarian small cell carcinoma, hypercalcemic type. The cells are round and have scant cytoplasm, resulting in a high nuclear-to-cytoplasmic ratio. Numerous mitotic figures are seen.

whereas small cell carcinoma, hypercalcemic type is typically negative. Other tumors in the differential diagnosis include small "blue" cell tumors, most commonly *small cell carcinoma of the pulmonary type*. The latter is not associated with hypercalcemia, it shows another surface epithelial component, lacks follicle-like spaces, nuclei have inconspicuous nucleoli and display molding, and they are typically positive for TTF-1.

PROGNOSIS AND THERAPY

Only one-third of patients with stage Ia tumors will have no evidence of disease at follow-up while outcome is very poor for all other stages. Favorable prognostic factors are age > 30 years, normal preoperative calcium level, size < 10 cm, and absence of large cells. Treatment has principally been surgical, and response to chemotherapy and radiation therapy is poor in general.

SMOOTH MUSCLE TUMORS

CLINICAL FEATURES

Patients range in age from 3 to 88 years, with leiomyoma occurring in younger patients (38–46 years) as compared to leiomyosarcoma (mean 58 years). Patients may present with a pelvic or adnexal mass. 62% of patients with leiomyosarcoma have stage I tumors at the time of initial diagnosis.

PRIMARY SMOOTH MUSCLE TUMORS – FACT SHEET

Definition
▶ Tumors composed of smooth muscle cells with variable degrees of cytologic atypia

Incidence
▶ Uncommon to rare

Age Distribution
▶ 3–88 years

Clinical Features
▶ Pelvic/adnexal mass

Prognosis and Treatment
▶ Excellent prognosis for leiomyomas with surgical excision
▶ Behavior of leiomyosarcoma correlates with tumor stage
▶ Metastasis, recurrence, or death secondary to disease occurs in 50% of patients with stage I leiomyosarcoma
▶ If advanced-stage leiomyosarcoma, death rate close to 100%
▶ Uncertain role of chemotherapy and radiation therapy

PATHOLOGIC FEATURES

GROSS FINDINGS

Most tumors are unilateral, with mean size ranging from 5 to 14 cm. The cut surface is typically tan-white, whorled, and firm, similar to their uterine counterparts. Areas of hemorrhage or necrosis may be seen.

MICROSCOPIC FINDINGS

These tumors show a similar range and combination of appearances as seen in primary uterine tumors (Figures 14.94 and 14.95). They are more often composed of long intersecting fascicles of spindled cells with eosinophilic fibrillary cytoplasm and elongated blunt-ended nuclei. Myxoid and epithelioid variants are very rare. Leiomyosarcoma should be diagnosed when at least two of the following features are present: significant nuclear atypia, mitotic index > 10/10 HPFs (40 × high-power field area = 0.237 mm²), and tumor cell necrosis. Some authors recommend that a smooth-muscle tumor with nuclear atypia be diagnosed as leiomyosarcoma if the mitotic index is > 5/10 HPFs, even in the absence of tumor cell necrosis. Rare tumors showing morphologic features intermediate between leiomyoma and leiomyosarcoma can be designated as "smooth muscle tumor of uncertain malignant potential."

PRIMARY SMOOTH MUSCLE TUMORS – PATHOLOGIC FEATURES

Gross Findings
- Usually unilateral
- Mean size 5–14 cm
- Solid, whorled, and tan-white cut surface ± hemorrhage or necrosis (more often if malignant)

Microscopic Findings
- Spectrum similar to uterine smooth muscle tumors

Immunohistochemical Features
- Smooth muscle actin, desmin, h-caldesmon positive
- CD10 variably positive

Differential Diagnosis
- Smooth muscle metoplasia
- Metastatic uterine leiomyosarcoma
- Ovarian fibroma/thecoma
- Gastrointestinal stromal tumor
- Secondary involvement by leiomyomatosis peritonealis disseminata or intravenous leiomyomatosis

---

ANCILLARY STUDIES

IMMUNOHISTOCHEMISTRY

Tumors are typically positive for smooth muscle actin, desmin, and h-caldesmon and may stain for CD10.

DIFFERENTIAL DIAGNOSIS

The principal differential diagnosis of primary ovarian leiomyoma is with *smooth muscle metaplasia*, which is typically a microscopic finding, and *ovarian fibroma/thecoma*, which lack a fascicular architecture and are typically negative for desmin and h-caldesmon. Uterine leiomyosarcoma should be distinguished from *metastatic uterine leiomyosarcoma*. A diagnosis of uterine leiomyosarcoma is supported by a prior clinical history, presence of a uterine mass, advanced-stage disease, bilaterality, nodularity, surface involvement, and/or

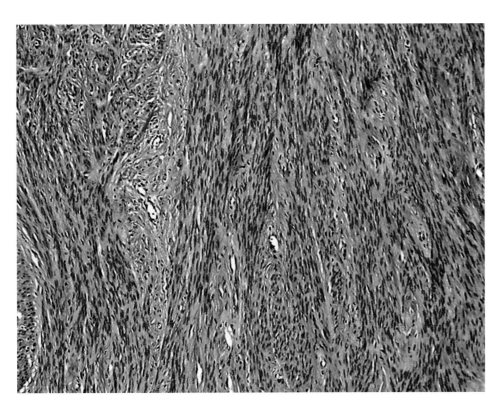

FIGURE 14.94
Primary ovarian leiomyoma. Intersecting fascicles contain bland, spindled smooth muscle cells.

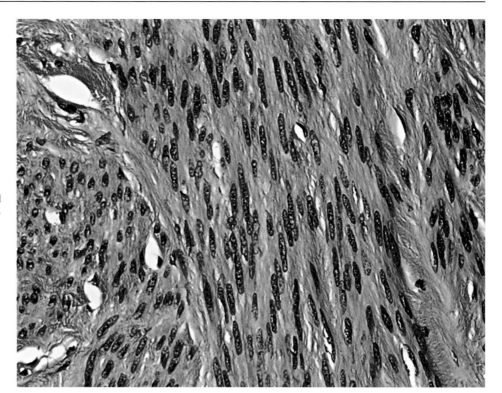

FIGURE 14.95
Primary ovarian leiomyoma. Spindled smooth muscle cells contain bland, boxcar-shaped, elongated nuclei.

lymphovascular invasion. Other tumors in the differential diagnosis include secondary involvement by a *gastrointestinal stromal tumor* (typically c-kit and CD34 positive) and secondary involvement by *leiomyomatosis peritonealis disseminata or intravenous leiomyomatosis.*

PROGNOSIS AND THERAPY

Leiomyoma has an excellent prognosis, whereas the behavior of leiomyosarcoma correlates with tumor stage. Approximately 50% of patients with disease confined to the ovary develop metastases, pelvic recurrence, or die of disease (as high as 100% with advanced-stage tumors). The role of chemotherapy and radiation therapy is uncertain.

ENDOMETRIOID STROMAL SARCOMA

CLINICAL FEATURES

Patients range in age from 20 to 76 (mean 54) years and they frequently present with abdominal distension or pain. Only 17% of patients have stage I tumors at presentation. In 39% of patients, there is either a prior history of endometrial stromal sarcoma or a synchronous uterine tumor.

PRIMARY ENDOMETRIOID STROMAL SARCOMA – FACT SHEET

Definition
‣ Low grade mesenchymal tumor composed of cells resembling proliferative-phase endometrial stroma

Incidence
‣ Uncommon to rare

Age Distribution
‣ 20–76 (mean 54) years

Clinical Features
‣ Abdominal distension/pain
‣ Only 17% stage I at time of presentation
‣ Prior history of endometrial stromal sarcoma or synchronous uterine tumor in 39% of patients

Prognosis and therapy
‣ Limited experience
‣ 63% of patients (all stages) with no evidence of disease with at least 1 year of follow-up

---

PATHOLOGIC FEATURES

GROSS FINDINGS

There is bilateral involvement (mean size 11 cm) in approximately 52% of cases. The tumors are solid or solid and cystic and only rarely predominantly cystic with a tan or yellow-white cut surface. Hemorrhage and/or necrosis may be present.

PRIMARY ENDOMETRIOID STROMAL SARCOMA – PATHOLOGIC FEATURES

Gross Findings

▸ 52% bilateral
▸ Mean size 11 cm
▸ Solid or solid and cystic with tan to yellow to white cut surface

Microscopic Findings

▸ Classic "tongue-like" growth pattern may not be obvious and only seen at the hilum
▸ Diffuse or nodular growth
▸ Tightly packed cells resembling proliferative-phase endometrial stroma
▸ Small cells with scant cytoplasm and round to oval bland nuclei
▸ Small arteriolar vessels
▸ Smooth muscle differentiation, fibromatous areas, and sex cord-like differentiation may be seen
▸ Endometriosis may be present

Immunohistochemical Features

▸ CD10 usually positive
▸ Smooth muscle actin may be positive
▸ Desmin and h-caldesmon usually negative if no smooth muscle differentiation
▸ Inhibin, calretinin, CD99, and Melan-A may be positive in areas of sex cord-like differentiation

Differential Diagnosis

▸ Metastatic uterine endometrial stromal sarcoma
▸ Fibroma/thecoma
▸ Adult granulosa cell tumor
▸ Poorly differentiated Sertoli–Leydig cell tumor

MICROSCOPIC FINDINGS

The histologic appearance resembles that seen in uterine endometrial stromal sarcoma. The tumors are composed of sheets of tightly packed blue cells resembling proliferative-phase endometrial stroma. Small arteriolar vessels are present, with occasional whorling of cells around the vessels. Focal nodularity, smooth muscle differentiation, fibromatous areas, and sex cord-like differentiation may be seen. The tongue-like pattern of infiltration typical of uterine endometrial stromal sarcoma can be seen in extraovarian sites of involvement or at the hilus of the ovary (Figures 14.96–14.98). The tumor cells are small with round to oval bland nuclei and scant cytoplasm (Figures 14.99 and 14.100). Foci of associated endometriosis may be present.

ANCILLARY STUDIES

IMMUNOHISTOCHEMISTRY

These tumors have an immunophenotype similar to their uterine counterparts. They are usually positive for CD10, occasionally positive for smooth muscle actin, and usually negative for desmin and h-caldesmon except when smooth muscle differentiation is present (Figures 14.101 and 14.102). Areas of sex cord-like differentiation may be positive for inhibin, calretinin, CD99, and Melan A.

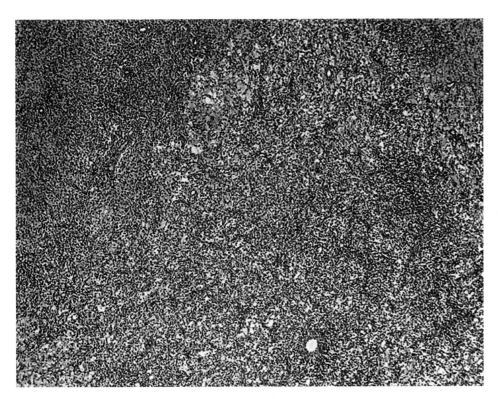

FIGURE 14.96
Primary ovarian endometrioid stromal sarcoma. The tumor exhibits a diffuse growth of monotonous cells.

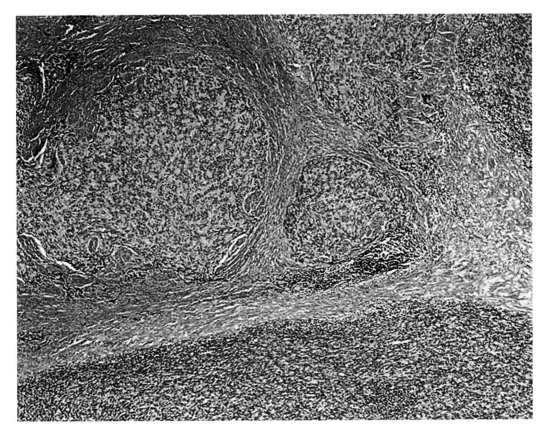

FIGURE 14.97
Primary ovarian endometrioid stromal sarcoma. Discrete tumor nodules, some with a tongue-like growth, are surrounded by collagenous stroma.

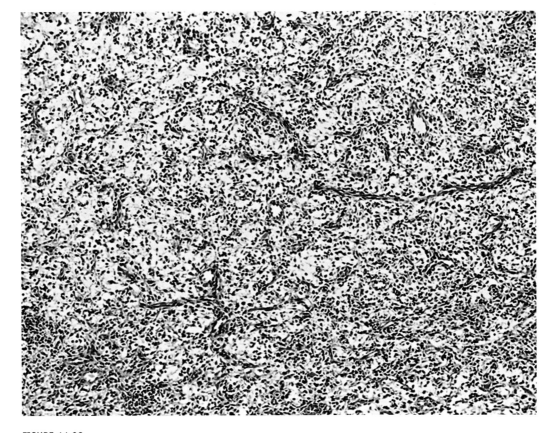

FIGURE 14.98
Primary ovarian endometrioid stromal sarcoma. The tumor is composed of small oval cells in an edematous background. Notice the prominent vasculature.

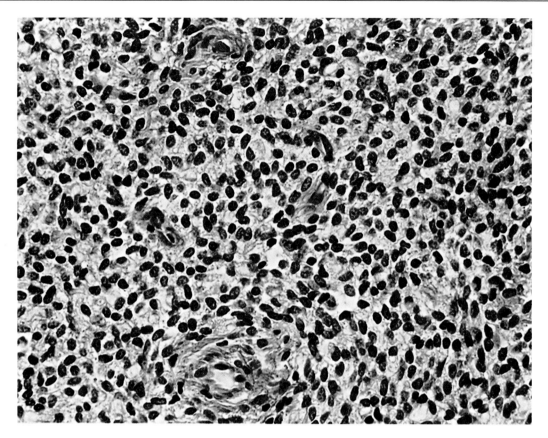

FIGURE 14.99
Primary ovarian endometrioid stromal sarcoma. The tumor cells resemble proliferative-phase endometrial stroma.

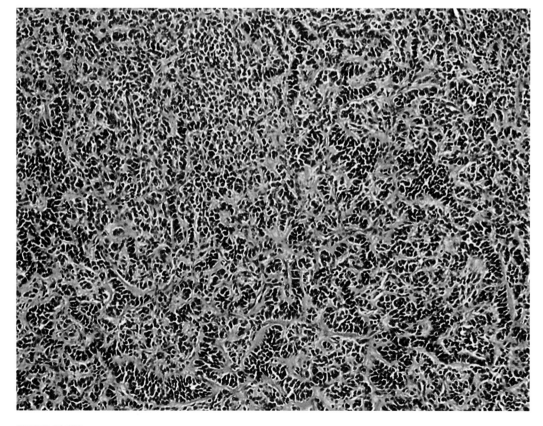

FIGURE 14.100
Primary ovarian endometrioid stromal sarcoma with sex cord-like differentiation. The tumor cells form anastomosing cords simulating an ovarian sex cord-stromal tumor.

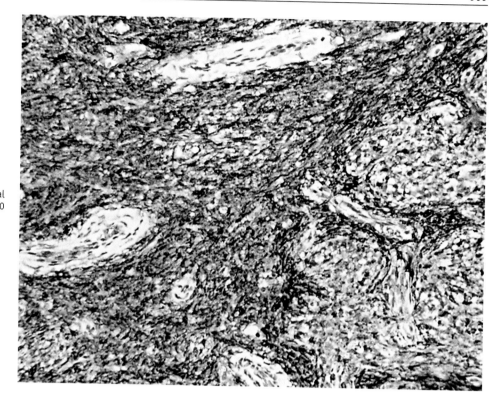

FIGURE 14.101

Primary ovarian endometrioid stromal sarcoma. Diffuse and strong CD10 expression is seen.

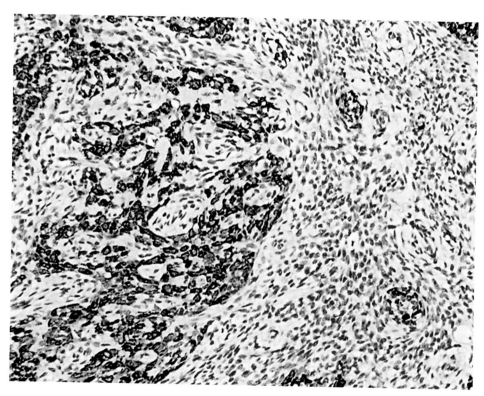

FIGURE 14.102

Primary ovarian endometrioid stromal sarcoma. Areas of smooth muscle differentiation show diffuse and strong h-caldesmon expression whereas the endometrioid stromal sarcoma cells are negative.

DIFFERENTIAL DIAGNOSIS

The principal consideration in the differential diagnosis is a *metastatic endometrial stromal sarcoma*. The presence of endometriosis associated with the ovarian tumor, absence of a uterine mass or involvement of other pelvic or abdominal sites support a diagnosis of primary ovarian endometrioid stromal sarcoma. Some primary tumors may be bilateral and have a synchronous endometrial stromal sarcoma; distinction between independent synchronous primaries in the ovary and uterus versus a metastasis from the uterus may not be possible in these cases. As primary endometrioid stromal sarcomas may show extensive fibromatous areas and sex cord-like differentiation, the differential diagnosis should include *fibroma, thecoma, and sex cord tumors* of the ovary. The finding of typical areas of endometrioid stromal neoplasia is most helpful to classify the tumor correctly and, thus, extensive sampling may be necessary.

PROGNOSIS AND THERAPY

Patients are treated with combinations of surgery, chemotherapy, and/or radiation therapy. In the only large series reported to date, 63% of patients with primary endometrioid stromal sarcoma (all stages) were alive with no evidence of disease with at least 1 year of follow-up.

SUGGESTED READING

General References for Metastases to the Ovary

Lee KR, Young RH. The distinction between primary and metastatic mucinous carcinomas of the ovary: gross and histologic findings in 50 cases. Am J Surg Pathol 2003;27:281–292.

Mazur MT, Hsueh S, Gersell DJ. Metastases to the female genital tract. Analysis of 325 cases. Cancer 1984;53:1978–1984.

McCluggage WG, Wilkinson N. Metastatic neoplasms involving the ovary: a review with an emphasis on morphological and immunohistochemical features. Histopathology 2005;47:231–247.

Moore RG, Chung M, Granai CO, et al. Incidence of metastasis to the ovaries from nongenital tract primary tumors. Gynecol Oncol 2004; 93:87–91.

Seidman JD, Kurman RJ, Ronnett BM. Primary and metastatic mucinous adenocarcinomas in the ovaries: incidence in routine practice with a new approach to improve intraoperative diagnosis. Am J Surg Pathol 2003;27:985–993.

Ulbright TM, Roth LM, Stehman FB. Secondary ovarian neoplasia. A clinicopathologic study of 35 cases. Cancer 1984;53:1164–1174.

Vang R, Gown AM, Barry TS, et al. Cytokeratins 7 and 20 in primary and secondary mucinous tumors of the ovary: analysis of coordinate immunohistochemical expression profiles and staining distribution in 179 cases. Am J Surg Pathol 2006;30:1130–1139.

Yazigi R, Sandstad J. Ovarian involvement in extragenital cancer. Gynecol Oncol 1989;34:84–87.

Yemelyanova AV, Vang R, Judson K, et al. Distinction of primary and metastatic mucinous tumors involving the ovary: analysis of size and laterality data by primary site with reevaluation of an algorithm for tumor classification. Am J Surg Pathol 2008;32:128–138.

Young RH. From Krukenberg to today: the ever present problems posed by metastatic tumors in the ovary: part I. Historical perspective, general principles, mucinous tumors including the Krukenberg tumor. Adv Anat Pathol 2006;13:205–227.

Young RH. From Krukenberg to today: the ever present problems posed by metastatic tumors in the ovary. Part II. Adv Anat Pathol 2007; 14:149–177.

Metastases from Carcinoma of the Large Intestine/Rectum

Cathro HP, Stoler MH. Expression of cytokeratins 7 and 20 in ovarian neoplasia. Am J Clin Pathol 2002;117:944–951.

Daya D, Nazerali L, Frank GL. Metastatic ovarian carcinoma of large intestinal origin simulating primary ovarian carcinoma. A clinicopathologic study of 25 cases. Am J Clin Pathol 1992;97:751–758.

Ji H, Isacson C, Seidman JD, et al. Cytokeratins 7 and 20, Dpc4, and MUC5AC in the distinction of metastatic mucinous carcinomas in the ovary from primary ovarian mucinous tumors: Dpc4 assists in identifying metastatic pancreatic carcinomas. Int J Gynecol Pathol 2002;21: 391–400.

Lash RH, Hart WR. Intestinal adenocarcinomas metastatic to the ovaries. A clinicopathologic evaluation of 22 cases. Am J Surg Pathol 1987; 11:114–121.

Vang R, Gown AM, Wu LS, et al. Immunohistochemical expression of CDX2 in primary ovarian mucinous tumors and metastatic mucinous carcino-

mas involving the ovary: comparison with CK20 and correlation with coordinate expression of CK7. Mod Pathol 2006;19:1421–1428.

Zhang PJ, Shah M, Spiegel GW, et al. Cytokeratin 7 immunoreactivity in rectal adenocarcinomas. Appl Immunohistochem Mol Morphol 2003; 11:306–310.

Metastases from Carcinoma of the Breast

Gagnon Y, Tetu B. Ovarian metastases of breast carcinoma. A clinicopathologic study of 59 cases. Cancer 1989;64:892–898.

Monteagudo C, Merino MJ, LaPorte N, et al. Value of gross cystic disease fluid protein-15 in distinguishing metastatic breast carcinomas among poorly differentiated neoplasms involving the ovary. Hum Pathol 1991;22:368–372.

Tornos C, Soslow R, Chen S, et al. Expression of WT1, CA 125, and GCDFP-15 as useful markers in the differential diagnosis of primary ovarian carcinomas versus metastatic breast cancer to the ovary. Am J Surg Pathol 2005;29:1482–1489.

Metastases from Carcinoma of the Stomach

Bullon A Jr, Arseneau J, Prat J, et al. Tubular Krukenberg tumor. A problem in histopathologic diagnosis. Am J Surg Pathol 1981;5:225–232.

Holtz F, Hart WR. Krukenberg tumors of the ovary: a clinicopathologic analysis of 27 cases. Cancer 1982;50:2438–2447.

Kiyokawa T, Young RH, Scully RE. Krukenberg tumors of the ovary: a clinicopathologic analysis of 120 cases with emphasis on their variable pathologic manifestations. Am J Surg Pathol 2006;30:277–299.

Lerwill MF, Young RH. Ovarian metastases of intestinal-type gastric carcinoma: a clinicopathologic study of 4 cases with contrasting features to those of the Krukenberg tumor. Am J Surg Pathol 2006; 30:1382–1388.

Vang R, Bague S, Tavassoli FA, et al. Signet-ring stromal tumor of the ovary: clinicopathologic analysis and comparison with Krukenberg tumor. Int J Gynecol Pathol 2004;23:45–51.

Yakushiji M, Tazaki T, Nishimura H, et al. Krukenberg tumors of the ovary: a clinicopathologic analysis of 112 cases. Nippon Sanka Fujinka Gakkai Zasshi 1987;39:479–485.

Metastases from Carcinoma of the Appendix

Ronnett BM, Kurman RJ, Shmookler BM, et al. The morphologic spectrum of ovarian metastases of appendiceal adenocarcinomas: a clinicopathologic and immunohistochemical analysis of tumors often misinterpreted as primary ovarian tumors or metastatic tumors from other gastrointestinal sites. Am J Surg Pathol 1997;21:1144–1155.

Secondary Involvement by Low-Grade Adenomatous Mucinous Neoplasm of Appendix Associated with Pseudomyxoma Peritonei

Cuatrecasas M, Matias-Guiu X, Prat J. Synchronous mucinous tumors of the appendix and the ovary associated with pseudomyxoma peritonei. A clinicopathologic study of six cases with comparative analysis of c-Ki-ras mutations. Am J Surg Pathol 1996;20:739–746.

Misdraji J, Yantiss RK, Graeme-Cook FM, et al. Appendiceal mucinous neoplasms: a clinicopathologic analysis of 107 cases. Am J Surg Pathol 2003;27:1089–1103.

Prayson RA, Hart WR, Petras RE. Pseudomyxoma peritonei. A clinicopathologic study of 19 cases with emphasis on site of origin and nature of associated ovarian tumors. Am J Surg Pathol 1994;18:591–603.

Ronnett BM, Seidman JD. Mucinous tumors arising in ovarian mature cystic teratomas: relationship to the clinical syndrome of pseudomyxoma peritonei. Am J Surg Pathol 2003;27:650–657.

Ronnett BM, Kurman RJ, Zahn CM, et al. Pseudomyxoma peritonei in women: a clinicopathologic analysis of 30 cases with emphasis on site of origin, prognosis, and relationship to ovarian mucinous tumors of low malignant potential. Hum Pathol 1995;26:509–524.

Ronnett BM, Zahn CM, Kurman RJ, et al. Disseminated peritoneal adenomucinosis and peritoneal mucinous carcinomatosis. A clinicopathologic analysis of 109 cases with emphasis on distinguishing pathologic features, site of origin, prognosis, and relationship to "pseudomyxoma peritonei." Am J Surg Pathol 1995;19:1390–1408.

Ronnett BM, Shmookler BM, Diener-West M, et al. Immunohistochemical evidence supporting the appendiceal origin of pseudomyxoma peritonei in women. Int J Gynecol Pathol 1997;16:1–9.

Ronnett BM, Yan H, Kurman RJ, et al. Patients with pseudomyxoma peritonei associated with disseminated peritoneal adenomucinosis have a significantly more favorable prognosis than patients with peritoneal mucinous carcinomatosis. Cancer 2001;92:85–91.

Szych C, Staebler A, Connolly DC, et al. Molecular genetic evidence supporting the clonality and appendiceal origin of pseudomyxoma peritonei in women. Am J Pathol 1999;154:1849–1855.

Young RH, Gilks CB, Scully RE. Mucinous tumors of the appendix associated with mucinous tumors of the ovary and pseudomyxoma peritonei. A clinicopathological analysis of 22 cases supporting an origin in the appendix. Am J Surg Pathol 1991;15:415–429.

Metastases from Carcinoma of the Pancreas

Duval JV, Savas L, Banner BF. Expression of cytokeratins 7 and 20 in carcinomas of the extrahepatic biliary tract, pancreas, and gallbladder. Arch Pathol Lab Med 2000;124:1196–1200.

Goldstein NS, Bassi D. Cytokeratins 7, 17, and 20 reactivity in pancreatic and ampulla of Vater adenocarcinomas. Percentage of positivity and distribution is affected by the cut-point threshold. Am J Clin Pathol 2001;115:695–702.

Ji H, Isacson C, Seidman JD, et al. Cytokeratins 7 and 20, Dpc4, and MUC5AC in the distinction of metastatic mucinous carcinomas in the ovary from primary ovarian mucinous tumors: Dpc4 assists in identifying metastatic pancreatic carcinomas. Int J Gynecol Pathol 2002;21: 391–400.

Young RH, Hart WR. Metastases from carcinomas of the pancreas simulating primary mucinous tumors of the ovary. A report of seven cases. Am J Surg Pathol 1989;13:748–756.

Metastases from Carcinoma of the Small Intestine

Andresen DM, Pedersen FH, Rasmussen KL. Adenocarcinoma of the small intestine mistaken as a primary ovarian cancer. Arch Gynecol Obstet 2001;265:214–215.

Lee MJ, Lee HS, Kim WH, et al. Expression of mucins and cytokeratins in primary carcinomas of the digestive system. Mod Pathol 2003;16: 403–410.

Young RH, Hart WR. Metastatic intestinal carcinomas simulating primary ovarian clear cell carcinoma and secretory endometrioid carcinoma: a clinicopathologic and immunohistochemical study of five cases. Am J Surg Pathol 1998;22:805–815.

Secondary Involvement by Non-Hodgkin's Lymphoma

Monterroso V, Jaffe ES, Merino MJ, et al. Malignant lymphomas involving the ovary. A clinicopathologic analysis of 39 cases. Am J Surg Pathol 1993;17:154–170.

Oliva E, Ferry JA, Young RH, et al. Granulocytic sarcoma of the female genital tract: a clinicopathologic study of 11 cases. Am J Surg Pathol 1997;21:1156–1165.

Vang R, Medeiros LJ, Fuller GN, et al. Non-Hodgkin's lymphoma involving the gynecologic tract: a review of 88 cases. Adv Anat Pathol 2001;8:200–217.

Vang R, Medeiros LJ, Warnke RA, et al. Ovarian non-Hodgkin's lymphoma: a clinicopathologic study of eight primary cases. Mod Pathol 2001; 14:1093–1099.

Metastases from Carcinoma of the Lung

Eichhorn JH, Young RH, Scully RE. Primary ovarian small cell carcinoma of pulmonary type. A clinicopathologic, immunohistologic, and flow cytometric analysis of 11 cases. Am J Surg Pathol 1992;16:926–938.

Irving JA, Young RH. Lung carcinoma metastatic to the ovary: a clinicopathologic study of 32 cases emphasizing their morphologic spectrum and problems in differential diagnosis. Am J Surg Pathol 2005; 29:997–1006.

Ordoñez NG. Value of thyroid transcription factor-1 immunostaining in distinguishing small cell lung carcinomas from other small cell carcinomas. Am J Surg Pathol 2000;24:1217–1223.

Young RH, Scully RE. Ovarian metastases from cancer of the lung: problems in interpretation – a report of seven cases. Gynecol Oncol 1985;21: 337–350.

Metastases from Melanoma

Gupta D, Deavers MT, Silva EG, et al. Malignant melanoma involving the ovary: a clinicopathologic and immunohistochemical study of 23 cases. Am J Surg Pathol 2004;28:771–780.

McCluggage WG, Bissonnette JP, Young RH. Primary malignant melanoma of the ovary: a report of 9 definite or probable cases with emphasis on their morphologic diversity and mimicry of other primary and secondary ovarian neoplasms. Int J Gynecol Pathol 2006;25:321–329.

Young RH, Scully RE. Malignant melanoma metastatic to the ovary. A clinicopathologic analysis of 20 cases. Am J Surg Pathol 1991;15: 849–860.

Metastases from Carcinoma of the Gallbladder and Bile Ducts

Duval JV, Savas L, Banner BF. Expression of cytokeratins 7 and 20 in carcinomas of the extrahepatic biliary tract, pancreas, and gallbladder. Arch Pathol Lab Med 2000;124:1196–1200.

Ji H, Isacson C, Seidman JD, et al. Cytokeratins 7 and 20, Dpc4, and MUC5AC in the distinction of metastatic mucinous carcinomas in the ovary from primary ovarian mucinous tumors: Dpc4 assists in identifying metastatic pancreatic carcinomas. Int J Gynecol Pathol 2002;21: 391–400.

Kang YK, Kim WH, Jang JJ. Expression of G1-S modulators (p53, p16, p27, cyclin D1, Rb) and Smad4/Dpc4 in intrahepatic cholangiocarcinoma. Hum Pathol 2002;33:877–883.

Khunamornpong S, Siriaunkgul S, Suprasert P, et al. Intrahepatic cholangiocarcinoma metastatic to the ovary: a report of 16 cases of an underemphasized form of secondary tumor in the ovary that may mimic primary neoplasia. Am J Surg Pathol 2007;31:1788–1799.

McCarthy DM, Hruban RH, Argani P, et al. Role of the DPC4 tumor suppressor gene in adenocarcinoma of the ampulla of Vater: analysis of 140 cases. Mod Pathol 2003;16:272–278.

Rullier A, Le Bail B, Fawaz R, et al. Cytokeratin 7 and 20 expression in cholangiocarcinomas varies along the biliary tract but still differs from that in colorectal carcinoma metastasis. Am J Surg Pathol 2000; 24:870–876.

Tang Z, Zou S, Hao Y, et al. Frequency of loss expression of the DPC4 protein in various locations of biliary tract carcinoma. Zhonghua Yu Fang Yi Xue Za Zhi 2002;36:481–484.

Young RH, Scully RE. Ovarian metastases from carcinoma of the gallbladder and extrahepatic bile ducts simulating primary tumors of the ovary. A report of six cases. Int J Gynecol Pathol 1990;9:60–72.

Metastases from Carcinoma of the Urinary Bladder

Eichhorn JH, Young RH. Transitional cell carcinoma of the ovary: a morphologic study of 100 cases with emphasis on differential diagnosis. Am J Surg Pathol 2004;28:453–463.

Logani S, Oliva E, Amin MB, et al. Immunoprofile of ovarian tumors with putative transitional cell (urothelial) differentiation using novel urothelial markers: histogenetic and diagnostic implications. Am J Surg Pathol 2003;27:1434–1441.

Ordoñez NG. Transitional cell carcinomas of the ovary and bladder are immunophenotypically different. Histopathology 2000;36:433–438.

Riedel I, Czernobilsky B, Lifschitz-Mercer B, et al. Brenner tumors but not transitional cell carcinomas of the ovary show urothelial differentiation: immunohistochemical staining of urothelial markers, including cytokeratins and uroplakins. Virchows Arch 2001;438:181–191.

Soslow RA, Rouse RV, Hendrickson MR, et al. Transitional cell neoplasms of the ovary and urinary bladder: a comparative immunohistochemical analysis. Int J Gynecol Pathol 1996;15:257–265.

Young RH. Urachal adenocarcinoma metastatic to the ovary simulating primary mucinous cystadenocarcinoma of the ovary: report of a case. Virchows Arch 1995;426:529–532.

Young RH, Scully RE. Urothelial and ovarian carcinomas of identical cell types: problems in interpretation. A report of three cases and review of the literature. Int J Gynecol Pathol 1988;7:197–211.

Metastases from Carcinoma of the Kidney

Cameron RI, Ashe P, O'Rourke DM, et al. A panel of immunohistochemical stains assists in the distinction between ovarian and renal clear cell carcinoma. Int J Gynecol Pathol 2003;22:272–276.

Insabato L, De Rosa G, Franco R, et al. Ovarian metastasis from renal cell carcinoma: a report of three cases. Int J Surg Pathol 2003;11: 309–312.

Nolan LP, Heatley MK. The value of immunocytochemistry in distinguishing between clear cell carcinoma of the kidney and ovary. Int J Gynecol Pathol 2001;20:155–159.

Vang R, Whitaker BP, Farhood AI, et al. Immunohistochemical analysis of clear cell carcinoma of the gynecologic tract. Int J Gynecol Pathol 2001;20:252–259.

Young RH, Hart WR. Renal cell carcinoma metastatic to the ovary: a report of three cases emphasizing possible confusion with ovarian clear cell adenocarcinoma. Int J Gynecol Pathol 1992;11:96–104.

Secondary Involvement by Malignant Mesothelioma

Attanoos RL, Webb R, Dojcinov SD, et al. Value of mesothelial and epithelial antibodies in distinguishing diffuse peritoneal mesothelioma in females from serous papillary carcinoma of the ovary and peritoneum. Histopathology 2002;40:237–244.

Clement PB, Young RH, Scully RE. Malignant mesotheliomas presenting as ovarian masses. A report of nine cases, including two primary ovarian mesotheliomas. Am J Surg Pathol 1996;20:1067–1080.

Comin CE, Saieva C, Messerini L. h-caldesmon, calretinin, estrogen receptor, and Ber-EP4: a useful combination of immunohistochemical markers for differentiating epithelioid peritoneal mesothelioma from serous papillary carcinoma of the ovary. Am J Surg Pathol 2007;31: 1139–1148.

Goldblum J, Hart WR. Localized and diffuse mesotheliomas of the genital tract and peritoneum in women. A clinicopathologic study of nineteen true mesothelial neoplasms, other than adenomatoid tumors, multicystic mesotheliomas, and localized fibrous tumors. Am J Surg Pathol 1995;19:1124–1137.

Ordoñez NG. Role of immunohistochemistry in distinguishing epithelial peritoneal mesotheliomas from peritoneal and ovarian serous carcinomas. Am J Surg Pathol 1998;22:1203–1214.

Trupiano JK, Geisinger KR, Willingham MC, et al. Diffuse malignant mesothelioma of the peritoneum and pleura, analysis of markers. Mod Pathol 2004;17:476–481.

Metastases from Carcinoma of Extraovarian Carcinoid Tumor

Baker PM, Oliva E, Young RH, et al. Ovarian mucinous carcinoids including some with a carcinomatous component: a report of 17 cases. Am J Surg Pathol 2001;25:557–568.

Robboy SJ, Scully RE, Norris HJ. Carcinoid metastatic to the ovary. A clinicopathologic analysis of 35 cases. Cancer 1974;33:798–811.

Robboy SJ, Norris HJ, Scully RE. Insular carcinoid primary in the ovary. A clinicopathologic analysis of 48 cases. Cancer 1975;36:404–418.

Robboy SJ, Scully RE, Norris HJ. Primary trabecular carcinoid of the ovary. Obstet Gynecol 1977;49:202–207.

Soga J, Osaka M, Yakuwa Y. Carcinoids of the ovary: an analysis of 329 reported cases. J Exp Clin Cancer Res 2000;19:271–280.

Secondary Involvement by Nongynecologic Small Round Blue Cell Sarcomas

Young RH, Scully RE. Alveolar rhabdomyosarcoma metastatic to the ovary. A report of two cases and a discussion of the differential diagnosis of small cell malignant tumors of the ovary. Cancer 1989;64:899–904.

Young RH, Scully RE. Sarcomas metastatic to the ovary: a report of 21 cases. Int J Gynecol Pathol 1990;9:231–252.

Young RH, Eichhorn JH, Dickersin GR, et al. Ovarian involvement by the intra-abdominal desmoplastic small round cell tumor with divergent differentiation: a report of three cases. Hum Pathol 1992;23: 454–464.

Young RH, Kozakewich HP, Scully RE. Metastatic ovarian tumors in children: a report of 14 cases and review of the literature. Int J Gynecol Pathol 1993;12:8–19.

Metastases from Carcinoma of the Uterine Cervix

Elishaev E, Gilks CB, Miller D, et al. Synchronous and metachronous endocervical and ovarian neoplasms: evidence supporting interpretation of the ovarian neoplasms as metastatic endocervical adenocarcinomas simulating primary ovarian surface epithelial neoplasms. Am J Surg Pathol 2005;29:281–294.

Kaminski PF, Norris HJ. Coexistence of ovarian neoplasms and endocervical adenocarcinoma. Obstet Gynecol 1984;64:553–556.

Kushima M, Fujii H, Murakami K, et al. Simultaneous squamous cell carcinomas of the uterine cervix and upper genital tract: loss of heterozygosity analysis demonstrates clonal neoplasms of cervical origin. Int J Gynecol Pathol 2001;20:353–358.

Nguyen L, Brewer CA, DiSaia PJ. Ovarian metastasis of stage IB1 squamous cell cancer of the cervix after radical parametrectomy and oophoropexy. Gynecol Oncol 1998;68:198–200.

Pins MR, Young RH, Crum CP, et al. Cervical squamous cell carcinoma in situ with intraepithelial extension to the upper genital tract and invasion of tubes and ovaries: report of a case with human papilloma virus analysis. Int J Gynecol Pathol 1997;16:272–278.

Sutton GP, Bundy BN, Delgado G, et al. Ovarian metastases in stage IB carcinoma of the cervix: a Gynecologic Oncology Group study. Am J Obstet Gynecol 1992;166:50–53.

Tabata M, Ichinoe K, Sakuragi N, et al. Incidence of ovarian metastasis in patients with cancer of the uterine cervix. Gynecol Oncol 1987; 28:255–261.

Vang R, Gown AM, Farinola M, et al. p16 expression in primary ovarian mucinous and endometrioid tumors and metastatic adenocarcinomas in the ovary: utility for identification of metastatic HPV-related endocervical adenocarcinomas. Am J Surg Pathol 2007;31:653–663.

Young RH, Scully RE. Mucinous ovarian tumors associated with mucinous adenocarcinomas of the cervix. A clinicopathological analysis of 16 cases. Int J Gynecol Pathol 1988;7:99–111.

Young RH, Gersell DJ, Roth LM, et al. Ovarian metastases from cervical carcinomas other than pure adenocarcinomas. A report of 12 cases. Cancer 1993;71:407–418.

Metastases from Carcinoma of the Uterine Corpus

Eifel P, Hendrickson M, Ross J, et al. Simultaneous presentation of carcinoma involving the ovary and the uterine corpus. Cancer 1982;50: 163–170.

Halperin R, Zehavi S, Hadas E, et al. Simultaneous carcinoma of the endometrium and ovary vs endometrial carcinoma with ovarian metastases: a clinical and immunohistochemical determination. Int J Gynecol Cancer 2003;13:32–37.

Irving JA, Catasús L, Gallardo A, et al. Synchronous endometrioid carcinomas of the uterine corpus and ovary: alterations in the beta-catenin (CTNNBI) pathway are associated with independent primary tumors and favorable prognosis. Hum Pathol 2005;36:605–619.

Prat J, Matias-Guiu X, Barreto J. Simultaneous carcinoma involving the endometrium and the ovary. A clinicopathologic, immunohistochemical, and DNA flow cytometric study of 18 cases. Cancer 1991;68:2455–2459.

Ulbright TM, Roth LM. Metastatic and independent cancers of the endometrium and ovary: a clinicopathologic study of 34 cases. Hum Pathol 1985;16:28–34.

Zaino R, Whitney C, Brady MF, et al. Simultaneously detected endometrial and ovarian carcinomas – a prospective clinicopathologic study of 74 cases: a gynecologic oncology group study. Gynecol Oncol 2001;83: 355–362.

Metastases from Mesenchymal Tumors of the Uterine Corpus

Lerwill MF, Sung R, Oliva E, et al. Smooth muscle tumors of the ovary: a clinicopathologic study of 54 cases emphasizing prognostic criteria, histologic variants, and differential diagnosis. Am J Surg Pathol 2004;28:1436–1451.

Oliva E, Garcia-Miralles N, Vu Q, et al. CD10 expression in pure stromal and sex cord-stromal tumors of the ovary: an immunohistochemical analysis of 101 cases. Int J Gynecol Pathol 2007;26:359–367.

Young RH, Scully RE. Sarcomas metastatic to the ovary: a report of 21 cases. Int J Gynecol Pathol 1990;9:231–252.

Young RH, Prat J, Scully RE. Endometrioid stromal sarcomas of the ovary. A clinicopathologic analysis of 23 cases. Cancer 1984;53:1143–1155.

Primary Tumors of the Rete Ovarii

Heatley MK. Adenomatous hyperplasia of the rete ovarii. Histopathology 2000;36:383–384.

Nogales FF, Carvia RE, Donne C, et al. Adenomas of the rete ovarii. Hum Pathol 1997;28:1428–1433.

Rutgers JL, Scully RE. Cysts (cystadenomas) and tumors of the rete ovarii. Int J Gynecol Pathol 1988;7:330–342.

Primary Small Cell Carcinoma of the Hypercalcemic Type

Aguirre P, Thor AD, Scully RE. Ovarian small cell carcinoma. Histogenetic considerations based on immunohistochemical and other findings. Am J Clin Pathol 1989;92:140–149.

McCluggage WG, Oliva E, Connolly LE, et al. An immunohistochemical analysis of ovarian small cell carcinoma of hypercalcemic type. Int J Gynecol Pathol 2004;23:330–336.

Young RH, Oliva E, Scully RE. Small cell carcinoma of the ovary, hypercalcemic type. A clinicopathological analysis of 150 cases. Am J Surg Pathol 1994;18:1102–1116.

Primary Smooth Muscle Tumors

Doss BJ, Wanek SM, Jacques SM, et al. Ovarian leiomyomas: clinicopathologic features in fifteen cases. Int J Gynecol Pathol 1999;18:63–68.

Doss BJ, Wanek SM, Jacques SM, et al. Ovarian smooth muscle metaplasia: an uncommon and possibly underrecognized entity. Int J Gynecol Pathol 1999;18:58–62.

Lerwill MF, Sung R, Oliva E, et al. Smooth-muscle tumors of the ovary: a clinicopathologic study of 54 cases emphasizing prognostic criteria, histologic variants, and differential diagnosis. Am J Surg Pathol 2004;28:1436–1451.

Nogales FF, Ayala A, Ruiz-Avila I, et al. Myxoid leiomyosarcoma of the ovary: analysis of three cases. Hum Pathol 1991;22:1268–1273.

Primary Endometrioid Stromal Sarcoma

Young RH, Scully RE. Sarcomas metastatic to the ovary: a report of 21 cases. Int J Gynecol Pathol 1990;9:231–252.

Young RH, Prat J, Scully RE. Endometrioid stromal sarcomas of the ovary. A clinicopathologic analysis of 23 cases. Cancer 1984;53:1143–1155.

15

Diseases of the Peritoneum

Robert A Soslow

Diseases affecting the peritoneum are diverse. They range from inflammatory and reactive to neoplastic, benign, borderline, and malignant. Many represent secondary (metastatic) tumors whereas others are examples of primary müllerian or mesothelial proliferations. Entities covered in detail in this chapter include endometriosis, primary peritoneal carcinoma (PPC), mesothelioma, pseudomyxoma peritonei, and a small group of unusual but interesting tumors such as desmoplastic small round cell tumor (DSRCT) and disseminated peritoneal leiomyomatosis (DPL). Lengthy lists of differential diagnostic entities will be discussed to aid practitioners in recognizing problematic lesions.

ENDOMETRIOSIS

CLINICAL FEATURES

Endometriosis is symptomatic and most commonly diagnosed in reproductive-age women, the mean age being 28 years. The estimated overall incidence is 300 cases per 100,000 person-years, but this varies widely with age, race, history of infertility, and perhaps, body mass index. The prevalence is highest in adolescents with severe dysmenorrhea (50%), other patients reporting pelvic pain (5–20%), and in infertile women (as high as 20–30%). The prevalence of endometriosis in asymptomatic patients diagnosed at tubal ligation ranges between 1% and 7%. Endometriotic deposits predominantly involve ovaries, uterine ligaments, rectovaginal septum, and less commonly, pelvic peritoneum, cervix, fallopian tube, vagina, vulva, urinary tract, lymph nodes, umbilicus, gastrointestinal tract, skin (particularly in scars) and lung, among others.

Endometriosis is the third leading gynecologic cause for hospitalization and is an important cause of infertility, dysmenorrhea, and pelvic pain. Less common presentations include cyclic dyspareunia, dysuria, and dyschezia; an extraordinarily rare manifestation is catamenial pneumothorax. The diagnosis is generally made by laparoscopic examination and biopsy.

ENDOMETRIOSIS – PATHOLOGIC FEATURES

Gross Findings

▶ Mass-forming, micronodular or plaque-like.
▶ Evidence of remote hemorrhage coupled with scarring
▶ Cysts, nodules, solid and polypoid masses, and dense fibrous tissue
▶ May form "chocolate" cyst, containing dark brown, sometimes viscous fluid
▶ Remote hemorrhage in noncystic tumors generally presents as "powder burn" spots or "mulberry lesions"
▶ Pelvic adhesions, including effacement of fimbriated ends of fallopian tubes, are common

Microscopic Findings

▶ Diagnostic triad: (1) endometrial glands; (2) endometrial stroma; (3) hemosiderin deposition
▶ Endometrial glands and stroma can display same range of metaplastic and hyperplastic changes seen in eutopic endometrium
▶ Carcinomas that develop in endometriosis are almost always either endometrioid or clear cell types
▶ Sarcomas that arise in association with endometriosis are generally either endometrioid stromal sarcomas or müllerian adenosarcomas
▶ Extensive hemorrhage and scarring over a prolonged period can give rise to necrosis with associated fibroblastic and inflammatory response (necrotic pseudoxanthomatous nodules) in which endometrial glands and stroma are not evident

Immunohistochemical Features

▶ Immunohistochemistry generally does not play an important role
▶ Immunophenotype mirrors that of eutopic endometrium
▶ CD10 marks endometrial stroma, which in some settings is useful

Differential Diagnosis

▶ Endosalpingiosis
▶ Granulomatous peritonitis
▶ Metastatic adenocarcinoma
▶ Endometrioid stromal sarcoma
▶ Low grade müllerian/mesodermal adenosarcoma

PATHOLOGIC FEATURES

It has been hypothesized that endometriosis can develop secondary to retrograde menstruation (transtubal dissemination of non-neoplastic endometrium), deportation of non-neoplastic endometrium to distant sites, or metaplasia. Recent work indicates that endometriosis associated with carcinomas is clonal. In addition, mouse models in which endometriosis results from manipulation of genes associated with ovarian carcinogenesis have also been described. This suggests that at least some types of endometriosis might be neoplastic.

Mass-forming, micronodular, or plaque-like endometriosis usually presents evidence of remote hemorrhage coupled with scarring. Cysts, nodules, solid or polypoid masses, and dense fibrous tissue may all occur. The most obvious manifestation of remote hemorrhage is the so-called chocolate cyst, a cyst containing dark brown,

sometimes viscous fluid. Pelvic adhesions, including effacement of the fimbriated ends of the fallopian tubes, are common.

Easily diagnosed endometriosis includes lesions with endometrial glands, endometrial stroma, and hemosiderin deposition (Figure 15.1). The endometrial glands can display the same range of changes seen in eutopic endometrium: squamous, tubal, eosinophilic, papillary syncytial, hobnail and mucinous metaplasia; hyperplasia; and carcinoma (Figures 15.2–15.6). The endometrial stroma can also display the same range of changes seen in eutopic endometrium: decidua, pseudodecidua, smooth-muscle metaplasia, fibroblastic metaplasia, and sarcoma (Figure 15.6). Uncommon manifestations of endometriosis are stromal-predominant lesions and intravascular examples, each of which can resemble endometrioid stromal sarcoma. Extensive hemorrhage and scarring over a prolonged period can give rise to necrosis with an associated fibroblastic and inflammatory response (necrotic pseudoxanthomatous nodules) in which endometrial glands and stroma are not evident (Figures 15.7 and 15.8).

Carcinomas that develop in endometriosis are almost always either endometrioid or clear cell carcinomas. Some arise in the setting of endometriosis with hyperplasia or in association with so-called atypical endometriosis – endometriosis containing cytologically atypical cells. Carcinosarcomas (malignant mixed müllerian/mesodermal tumors) have also been described. Sarcomas that arise in association with endometriosis are generally either endometrioid stromal sarcomas or müllerian adenosarcomas.

DIFFERENTIAL DIAGNOSIS

The differential diagnosis of endometriosis includes endosalpingiosis, metastatic adenocarcinoma, endometrioid stromal sarcoma, and müllerian/mesodermal adenosarcoma. *Endosalpingiosis* is composed of bland, ciliated cells resembling those of the fallopian tube. Endometrial stromal cells are lacking, thereby facilitating distinction with endometriosis. *Metastatic adenocarcinoma* is not associated with endometrial stroma and is generally substantially more cytologically atypical. If a metastatic adenocarcinoma is excluded, the possibility of a cancer arising within endometriosis should be considered. Such cancers have, by definition, associated areas of endometriosis frequently harboring hyperplastic and/or atypical areas.

Caution is advised in the examination of glandular tumors centered in the gastrointestinal tract, as mass forming endometriosis is not infrequently documented. Deeply placed mural examples with compensatory circumferential smooth muscle hyperplasia facilitate distinction from invasive colon carcinoma, but endometriosis can also present as a luminal polypoid lesion. The presence of associated endometrial stroma helps to establish the diagnosis. Endometrioid adenocarcinoma can also arise in association with endometriosis in the colon and rectum and can mimic a primary colorectal. Squamous

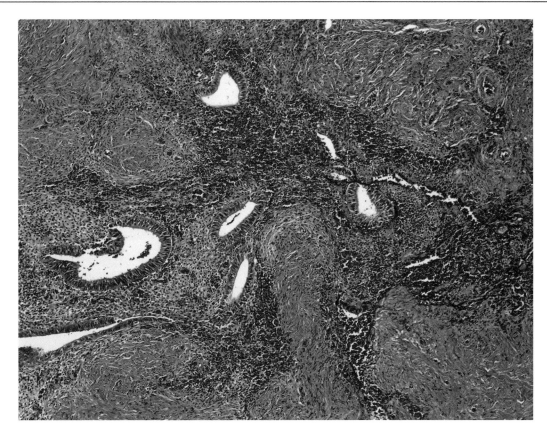

FIGURE 15.1
Endometriosis. Notice the presence of both endometrial-type glands and stroma.

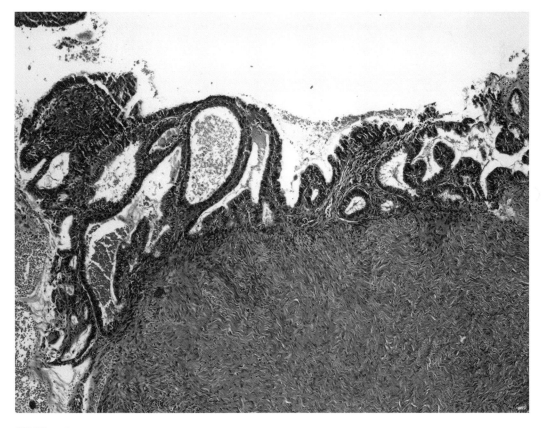

FIGURE 15.2
Endometriosis with hyperplasia. The glands exhibit architectural crowding and complexity.

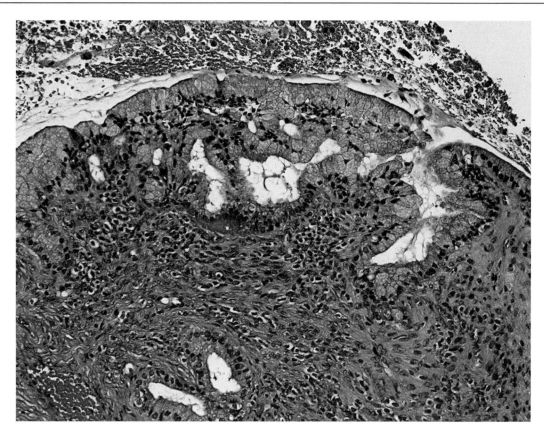

FIGURE 15.3

Endometriosis with mucinous metaplasia resembling endocervicosis. Endometrial stroma was recognizable elsewhere.

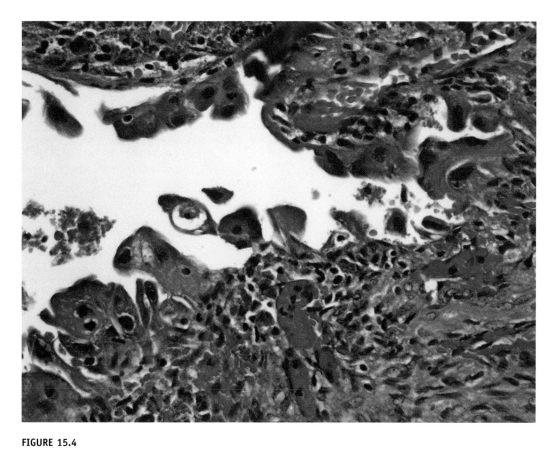

FIGURE 15.4

Atypical endometriosis with eosinophilic metaplasia. Note the presence of epithelial cells with abundant eosinophilic cytoplasm and focal cytoplasmic vacuolization.

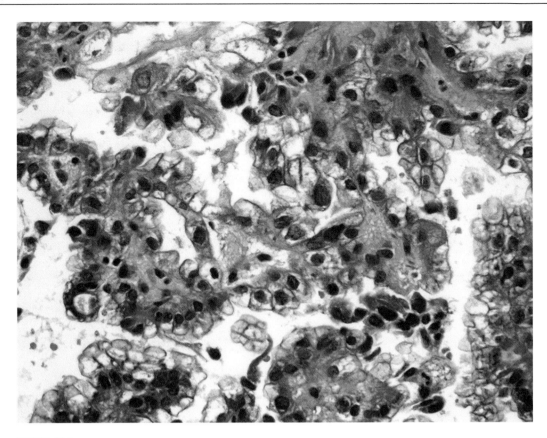

FIGURE 15.5
Clear cell carcinoma arising in an endometrioma (not shown). The papillary architecture and malignant cytologic features warrant a diagnosis of carcinoma.

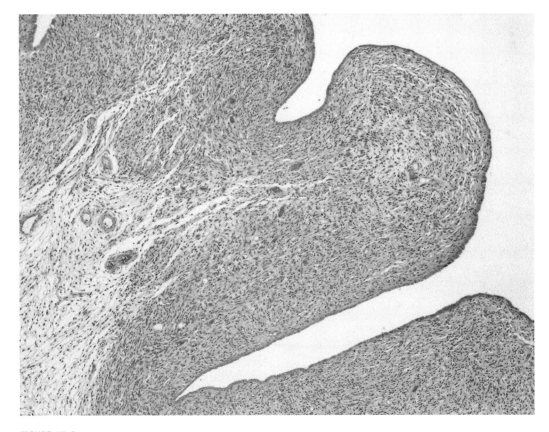

FIGURE 15.6
Low grade mesodermal adenosarcoma arising in endometriosis (not pictured). Note the leaf-like processes and stromal condensation beneath the epithelium.

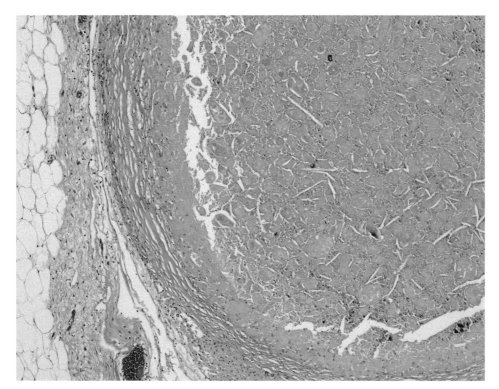

FIGURE 15.7
Necrotic pseudoxanthomatous nodule. This appearance may be seen in
long-standing lesions.

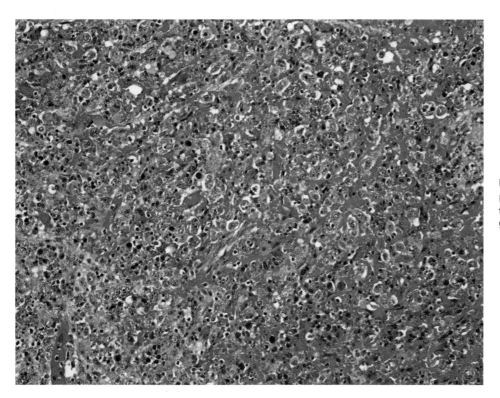

FIGURE 15.8
Hemosiderin deposition in endometriosis. Diagnostic endometrial-type
glands and/or stroma are absent.

metaplasia, a deep mural location, lack of CK20 expression, association with endometriosis, and absence of
an intestinal adenoma all favor an endometrioid
adenocarcinoma.

As noted previously, stromal-predominant and intravascular endometriosis can resemble *metastatic endometrial stromal sarcoma* or *primary endometrioid stromal
sarcoma arising in endometriosis*. Clinical history and

imaging can frequently aid in the separation of primary
versus metastatic lesions. Features favoring endometriosis include the presence of endometrioid glands
(although rare stromal sarcomas do contain endometrioid glands) and the absence of a stromal-predominant
mass with infiltrative margins. Polypoid variants of
endometriosis, gastrointestinal or otherwise, can mimic
primary or *metastatic müllerian/mesodermal adenosar-*

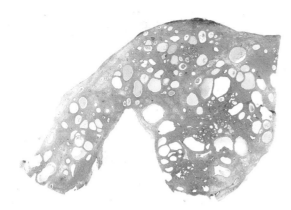

FIGURE 15.9

Polypoid endometriosis. In contrast with müllerian/mesodermal adenosarcoma, no intraglandular stromal protrusions or stromal condensation is seen.

coma (Figure 15.9). Features absent in polypoid endometriosis and essentially always found in adenosarcoma include intraglandular polypoid projections and prominent stromal cuffing around the epithelium. Many, but not all, adenosarcomas also contain mitotically active stroma with > 2 mitotic figures per 10 HPFs and at least mild cytologic atypia.

PROGNOSIS AND THERAPY

Endometriosis is a chronic disease; thus, complete regression short of hysterectomy/bilateral salpingo-oophorectomy or physiologic atrophy is hard to obtain. Medical treatment alone using oral contraceptives, androgenic agents, progestins, and GnRH analogs frequently reduces pain and the extent of lesions, but > half of patients experience recurrence following cessation of treatment. Side-effects from treatment are common. Surgical ablation of endometriotic lesions followed by medical therapy decreases recurrence rates and improves symptom-free intervals following therapy. Surgical ablation and pelvic anatomy restoration are recommended for infertile patients with mild to moderate endometriosis, as many as 30 % of these patients have become pregnant within 36 weeks of treatment. Reversal of infertility is extraordinarily difficult in patients with severe endometriosis.

PRIMARY PERITONEAL CARCINOMA

CLINICAL FEATURES

Primary peritoneal carcinoma (PPC) is almost always a serous carcinoma, arising from or within the peritoneal cavity.

PRIMARY PERITONEAL CARCINOMA – FACT SHEET

Definition

▶ Carcinoma of müllerian type, almost always serous carcinoma, arising from or within the peritoneal cavity
▶ Cervical, endometrial, tubal, and ovarian primaries as well as carcinomas arising in endometriosis should be excluded
▶ When tumor involves peritoneum and ovaries, the following guidelines are generally followed:
  ▶ Bulk of tumor is peritoneal, not ovarian
  ▶ Ovarian surface involvement predominates over parenchymal involvement
  ▶ Cortical ovarian parenchymal involvement, if present, should not exceed 5 mm

Incidence

▶ Uncommon; most cases thought to be primary peritoneal carcinomas are instead metastatic from ovaries, endometrium, or fallopian tube
▶ Lifetime incidence < 0.5%, but varies with *BRCA-1* status; patients with germline *BRCA-1* mutations have lifetime incidence of nearly 2%
▶ 5–10% of all primary peritoneal carcinomas are hereditary (due to inherited *BRCA-1* mutations)

Morbidity and Mortality

▶ Prognosis is probably close to or the same as ovarian carcinomas of similar histologic subtype, grade, and stage

Race and Age Distribution

▶ Caucasian women, particularly from industrialized countries, are at highest risk
▶ Women of African and Asian descent have lower risk
▶ Mean age at diagnosis 61 years

Clinical Features

▶ Identical presentation to ovarian cancer
▶ Most common complaints: fullness, bloating, increasing abdominal girth, and constipation
▶ Palpable abdominal and pelvic masses on physical exam, and ascites. Pleural effusions and palpable supraclavicular or inguinal lymphadenopathy much less common
▶ Serum CA-125 levels generally elevated
▶ Pelvic ultrasound and serial CA-125 levels relatively nonspecific screening tools

Prognosis and Treatment

▶ Most important prognostic features are stage (staged as ovarian cancer), tumor grade, surgeon's success in debulking visible tumor, and patient's response to chemotherapy
▶ Mean 5-year survival rate is roughly 40%, similar to that of high-stage, high-grade serous carcinoma of the ovary
▶ Primary therapeutic modalities include optimal tumor debulking followed by chemotherapy containing platinum- and taxane-based agents

---

It is uncommon; most cases thought to be PPC are instead metastatic from ovaries, endometrium, or fallopian tube, and these primary sites should be excluded prior to making the diagnosis of PPC. The lifetime incidence is < 0.5 %, but this varies with *BRCA-1* status;

PRIMARY PERITONEAL CARCINOMA – PATHOLOGIC FEATURES

Gross Findings

▸ Omental cake, miliary studding of peritoneal surfaces, discrete peritoneal masses
▸ Generally tan-white and may contain zones of necrosis
▸ Abundant psammoma bodies can feel gritty or even rock-hard

Microscopic Findings

▸ Most tumors are present on peritoneal surfaces and invade into underlying tissue, especially omental fat
▸ Histologic appearance identical to ovarian carcinomas of matched type and grade
▸ Nearly all are high-grade serous carcinomas
▸ Psammocarcinoma: very rare variant of low-grade serous carcinoma with abundant psammoma bodies

Immunohistochemical Features

▸ Pancytokeratins, CK7, WT1, CA-125, BerEP4, and B72.3 typically positive
▸ Most overexpress p53 protein and significant numbers express ER and PR
▸ Calretinin generally negative, although patchy expression can be seen

Differential Diagnosis

▸ Metastatic ovarian, tubal, endometrial, and cervical serous carcinoma
▸ Primary peritoneal serous borderline tumor (tumor of low malignant potential)
▸ Implants, both invasive and noninvasive, of ovarian serous borderline tumor
▸ Mesothelioma
▸ Metastatic papillary neoplasms, including:
  ▸ Metastatic papillary thyroid carcinoma, arising in struma ovarii
  ▸ Metastatic retiform Sertoli–Leydig cell tumor
  ▸ Metastatic yolk sac tumor with prominent Schiller–Duval bodies

---

patients with germline *BRCA-1* mutations have a lifetime incidence of nearly 2%.

The mean age at diagnosis is 61 years, which contrasts with that of ovarian carcinoma patients, in whom the mean age at diagnosis is 56 years; however, the clinical presentation is identical to that of ovarian cancer. The most common complaints, which are nonspecific, are feelings of fullness, bloating, increasing abdominal girth, and constipation. Patients frequently have palpable abdominal and pelvic masses on physical exam, and many have ascites. Fewer patients have pleural effusions and palpable supraclavicular or inguinal lymphadenopathy, and serum CA-125 levels are generally elevated.

Like ovarian cancer, PPC can be detected with pelvic ultrasound and serial CA-125 levels. These relatively nonspecific screening tools may help stratify patients who deserve further evaluation. Other manifestations of PPC include a hypercoagulable state, manifested by deep vein thrombosis, pelvic vein thrombosis, and pulmonary embolism.

PATHOLOGIC FEATURES

Primary peritoneal carcinomas present with an omental cake, miliary studding of peritoneal surfaces, and/or discrete peritoneal masses. Nearly all PPCs are high-grade serous carcinomas, but rare low-grade examples have been reported. Most tumors are present on peritoneal surfaces and invade into underlying tissue, especially omental fat; however a subset line peritoneal surfaces without invading underlying tissues. The histologic appearance of PPCs is identical to those of ovarian carcinomas of matched type and grade (Figures 15.10 and 15.11). A very rare variant of low-grade serous carcinoma with abundant psammoma bodies, so-called psammocarcinoma, has been described.

Primary peritoneal carcinoma is increasingly thought of as a diagnosis of exclusion. Meticulous examination of the fallopian tube fimbriae frequently shows occult carcinomas, including intraepithelial carcinoma, implicating the distal fallopian tube as the source of most peritoneal carcinomas.

ANCILLARY STUDIES

IMMUNOHISTOCHEMISTRY

Like ovarian serous carcinomas, PPCs express pancytokeratins, CK7, WT1, CA-125, BerEP4, and B72.3. The majority overexpress p53 protein and significant numbers express ER and PR. Calretinin is generally negative, although patchy expression has been reported.

DIFFERENTIAL DIAGNOSIS

The differential diagnosis includes metastatic ovarian, tubal, endometrial and cervical serous carcinoma, primary peritoneal serous borderline tumor (tumor of low malignant potential), implants of ovarian serous borderline tumor, mesothelioma, and metastatic papillary neoplasms.

WT1 expression in PPC contrasts with most examples of *endometrial serous carcinoma* that lack WT1 expression. However, since *ovarian* and *tubal serous carcinomas* also express WT1, immunohistochemistry is not helpful when the differential diagnosis includes these entities. *Primary peritoneal borderline tumors* (Figure 15.12) can be distinguished from ovarian borderline tumors when the ovaries are uninvolved or only minimally involved by tumor. By definition, borderline

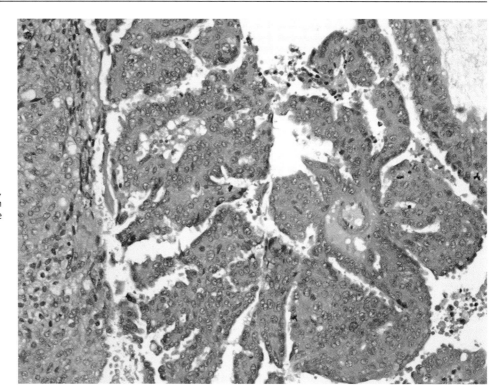

FIGURE 15.10

Primary peritoneal serous carcinoma, high-grade. Solid and papillary growth patterns are associate with high-grade cytologic features.

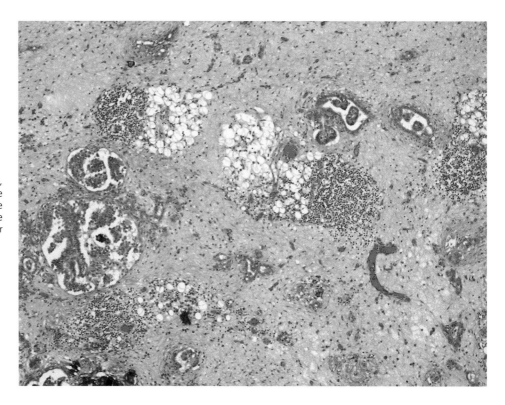

FIGURE 15.11

Primary peritoneal serous carcinoma, low-grade. Note similarity to invasive implant of ovarian serous borderline tumor. In contrast to high-grade tumors, there is uniform nuclear morphology.

tumors, whether ovarian or primary peritoneal, should show neither destructive tissue invasion nor high cytologic grade. Any of these two features should prompt a diagnosis of carcinoma. *Invasive implants of a serous borderline tumor* very closely resemble deposits of PPC and in many cases are indistinguishable. By convention, an invasive peritoneal tumor that coexists with an ovarian borderline tumor is considered to be of ovarian origin. Invasive implants that are not associated with either ovarian or peritoneal borderline tumors are considered low-grade PPC. Ongoing molecular studies will hopefully yield important insights into these issues.

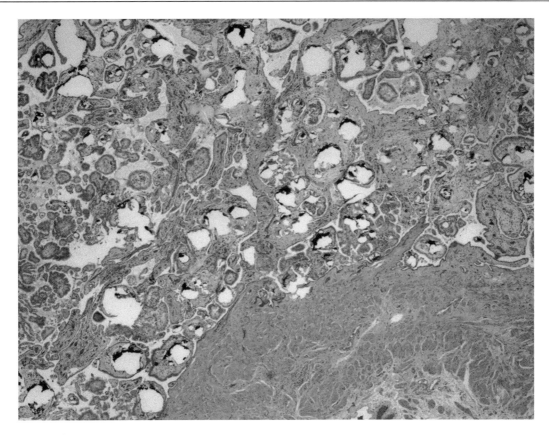

FIGURE 15.12

Primary peritoneal serous borderline tumor with numerous psammoma bodies. Note that the proliferation, although exuberant, is noninvasive; the underlying tubal smooth muscle is not invaded.

Mesotheliomas, particularly when papillary, can resemble PPCs. Primary peritoneal carcinomas, which are almost always cytologically high-grade tumors, usually exhibit a substantially greater degree of variation in nuclear size and shape. Mesothelioma cells, especially when components of well-differentiated papillary tumors, tend to be cuboidal instead of columnar and monolayered, in contrast to PPCs. Their immunophenotypes also differ as mesotheliomas express calretinin and CK5/6 whereas PPCs express BerEP4 and B72.3. Ultrastructurally, epithelial mesotheliomas show long, slender microvilli that are not seen in PPCs.

The differential diagnosis also includes papillary tumors metastatic to the peritoneal cavity. These include papillary thyroid carcinoma (originating in struma ovarii), metastatic retiform Sertoli–Leydig cell tumor, and metastatic yolk sac tumor with prominent Schiller–Duval bodies. Thyroglobulin and TTF-1 expression with a coincident struma ovarii are generally sufficient to suggest papillary thyroid carcinoma. *Retiform Sertoli–Leydig cell tumors* and *metastatic yolk sac tumors* occur in pediatric patients and in young adults, populations in which PPC is extremely rare. Each should be associated with an ovarian mass that is usually unilateral. In addition, inhibin expression would suggest a Sertoli–Leydig cell tumor; yolk sac tumor is characterized by expression of AFP without CK7, EMA, or LeuM1.

PROGNOSIS AND TREATMENT

The prognosis of PPC is probably close to, or the same as, ovarian carcinomas of similar histologic subtype, grade, and stage. The most important prognostic features are stage (staged as ovarian cancer), tumor grade, a surgeon's success in debulking visible tumor, and patient's response to chemotherapy. The mean 5-year survival rate is roughly 40%, similar to that of high-stage, high-grade serous carcinoma of the ovary. Primary therapeutic modalities include optimal tumor debulking followed by chemotherapy containing platinum- and taxane-based agents.

PERITONEAL MESOTHELIOMA

CLINICAL FEATURES

Approximately 40% of patients with peritoneal mesothelioma are women, but this varies with mesothelioma subtype. Women outnumber men with the well-differentiated papillary subtype and men outnumber women with the diffuse subtype, as is the case with

Definition

▸ Neoplasm arising from the peritoneum showing mesothelial differentiation; may be benign or malignant

Incidence and Location

▸ Extraordinarily rare tumors with an incidence of approximately 1 per 1,000,000; only about 20% of all mesotheliomas are peritoneal
▸ Localized or diffuse
▸ Both pelvic and abdominal peritoneum can be involved

Morbidity and Mortality

▸ Localized, noninvasive, and cytologically low-grade tumors are responsible for only limited morbidity and mortality
▸ Diffuse, invasive tumors are nearly always fatal, with a median survival time of < 1 year

Gender, Race, and Age Distribution

▸ Approximately 40% of patients with peritoneal mesothelioma are women, but varies with mesothelioma subtype (well-differentiated papillary subtype being more common in women)
▸ Reliable race distribution data not available; most reported in Caucasians
▸ 38–82 (mean age 53) years

Clinical Features

▸ Generally similar to that of ovarian and primary peritoneal carcinomas (nonspecific abdominal pain, fullness, bloating, and increasing abdominal girth)
▸ Serum CA-125 level can be elevated
▸ Asbestos exposure has been reported in men, but less commonly in women

Prognosis and Treatment

▸ Prognosis depends upon the type of mesothelioma:
  ▸ Diffuse, invasive, high-grade tumors are nearly always fatal, with a median survival time of < 1 year
  ▸ Diffuse, well-differentiated papillary mesotheliomas are probably difficult to cure, but their behavior is indolent with survival in the range of years and even decades
  ▸ Localized, well-differentiated papillary mesotheliomas cured with excision
▸ Primary treatment is tumor debulking

pleural mesothelioma. The age distribution is 38–82 years, with a mean age at diagnosis of 53 years. These are extraordinarily rare tumors, with an incidence of approximately 1 per 1,000,000. Only approximately 20 % of all mesotheliomas are peritoneal.

The clinical presentation of peritoneal mesothelioma is generally similar to that of ovarian and PPC i.e., non-specific abdominal pain, fullness, and bloating, and increasing abdominal girth. Dominant masses are also sometimes detected. Similar to ovarian carcinoma, serum CA-125 level can be elevated. There have been peritoneal mesotheliomas reported in men with a history

of asbestos exposure, but this association is less common in women.

PATHOLOGIC FEATURES

GROSS FINDINGS

Well-differentiated papillary mesotheliomas can be solitary or multiple, but they are, by definition, non-invasive. Mass-forming and solitary tumors are usually small (< 2 cm) with a nodular or papillary tan-white appearance. Diffuse malignant mesothelioma, on the other hand, often resembles disseminated ovarian carcinoma or PPC. These present as firm, tan to white plaques, nodules, and infiltrative masses. As an invasive tumor, diffuse malignant mesothelioma can involve parenchymal organs, the gastrointestinal tract, and pelvic structures, including ovaries.

MICROSCOPIC FINDINGS

Well-differentiated papillary mesotheliomas are non-invasive papillary tumors composed of a monolayer of cuboidal or flat mesothelial cells without significant cytologic atypia or mitotic activity (Figures 15.13 and 15.14). Diffuse malignant mesotheliomas (Figures 15.15–15.17) demonstrate the same range of histologic features as pleural mesothelioma: tubular, papillary and tubulopapillary pattern; solid sheets and nests; and sarcomatoid pattern. The cytoplasmic features are variable, but subtle circumferential paranuclear condensation can be seen, as well as fuzzy apical cytoplasmic membranes. The nuclear features range from mildly to severely atypical but, in general, tumor cell nuclei are more uniform than in high-grade serous carcinomas. Occasionally, psammoma bodies can be seen.

ANCILLARY STUDIES

IMMUNOHISTOCHEMISTRY

Mesotheliomas produce hyaluronic acid, which appears myxoid on routine histology. This material is positive with Alcian blue and colloidal iron stains, but it is mucicarmine-negative and the Alcian blue positivity can be removed with hyaluronidase pretreatment. A feature shared with many serous ovarian carcinomas is expression of pancytokeratins, EMA, CK7 and CA-125. Distinctive, but nonspecific, mesothelial-associated antigens include calretinin, WT1, CK5/6, and mesothelin. New relatively specific markers include D2-40 and h-caldesmon. Mesothelioma cells generally do not express CEA, B72.3, BerEP4, LeuM1, ER and PR. Because histologically similar ovarian carcinoma and PPC may lack CEA and LeuM1 expression (like mesotheliomas), B72.3 and BerEP4 are preferred components of an

PERITONEAL MESOTHELIOMA – PATHOLOGIC FEATURES

Gross Findings

Well-Differentiated Papillary Mesothelioma

▸ Solitary or multiple, by definition, noninvasive
▸ Usually small, < 2 cm, with tan-white nodular or papillary appearance

Diffuse Malignant Mesothelioma

▸ Often resembles disseminated ovarian or primary peritoneal carcinomas
▸ Plaques, nodules, and infiltrative masses of firm, tan-white tissue
▸ Can involve parenchymal organs, gastrointestinal tract, and pelvic structures, including ovaries

Microscopic Findings

Well-Differentiated Papillary Mesothelioma

▸ Noninvasive papillary tumors composed of a monolayer of cuboidal or flat mesothelial cells without significant cytologic atypia or mitotic activity

Diffuse Malignant Mesothelioma

▸ Same range of histologic features as pleural mesothelioma:
  ▸ Tubular pattern
  ▸ Papillary and tubulopapillary pattern
  ▸ Solid sheets and nests
  ▸ Sarcomatoid pattern
▸ Cytoplasmic features are variable, but subtle circumferential paranuclear condensation can be seen, as well as fuzzy, apical cytoplasmic membranes
▸ Nuclear features range from mildly to severely atypical
▸ Deciduoid malignant mesothelioma is composed of sheets of cells with abundant pink cytoplasm containing highly atypical nuclei

Immunohistochemical Features

▸ Pancytokeratins, EMA, CK7 and CA-125 frequently expressed
▸ Distinctive but nonspecific mesothelial-associated antigens include calretinin, WT1, CK5/6, and mesothelin
▸ CEA, B72.3, BerEP4, LeuM1, ER and PR usually negative
▸ D2-40 and h-caldesmon new promising markers

Ultrastructural Features

▸ Mesothelial cells possess long, slender microvilli
▸ Tumor cells lack intracytoplasmic mucin, but contain glycogen and have intercellular junctions
▸ Circumferential paranuclear condensation of intermediate filaments may be seen

Differential Diagnosis

▸ Mesothelial hyperplasia
▸ Adenomatoid tumor
▸ Multilocular peritoneal inclusion cysts
▸ Ovarian and primary peritoneal serous borderline tumor
▸ Ovarian, tubal, endometrial, cervical, and primary peritoneal serous carcinoma
▸ Metastatic neoplasms, including:
  ▸ Papillary thyroid carcinoma, arising in struma ovarii
  ▸ Retiform Sertoli–Leydig cell tumor
  ▸ Yolk sac tumor with prominent Schiller–Duval bodies
▸ Female adnexal tumor of probably wolffian origin
▸ Ependymoma
▸ Ectopic decidua
▸ Epithelioid angiosarcoma

immunohistochemical panel used for differential diagnosis.

ULTRASTRUCTURAL EXAMINATION

The characteristic mesothelial cell possesses long, slender microvilli that contrast with the short and simple microvilli of adenocarcinoma cells. Tumor cells lack intracytoplasmic mucin, but contain glycogen. Intercellular junctions and circumferential paranuclear condensation of intermediate filaments are present in a number of cases.

DIFFERENTIAL DIAGNOSIS

The differential diagnosis is extensive. A common challenge is distinguishing exuberant reactive mesothelial proliferations, hyperplasias, and benign mesothelial tumors from malignant mesothelioma. Equally important is the separation of mesothelioma from other primary and metastatic neoplasms.

Mesothelial hyperplasias take on a variety of morphologic appearances (Figures 15.18–15.20). These include loosely aggregated mesothelial cells, sometimes admixed with mononuclear and/or polymorphonuclear inflammatory cells, mesothelial cells arranged in papillae, and mesothelial cells that form small tubules. Many reactive mesothelial proliferations have associated spindle cell elements, the origin of which has been debated; possibilities include fibroblasts, myofibroblasts, submesothelial cells, and mesothelial cells with an altered morphology. Associated reactive mesothelial cells can also be encountered in lymph nodes (Figure 15.21). The gross appearance is frequently very informative. Almost all malignant mesotheliomas appear lesional to the surgeon and pathologist; in contrast, nearly all reactive mesothelial proliferations are identified incidentally or are clearly a component of an inflammatory, reactive, or reparative process. Any mesothelial proliferation that is unequivocally invasive into normal tissue (fat, smooth muscle) should be considered malignant. Also, severe cytologic atypia should make the pathologist consider a malignant diagnosis, but it should be noted that many reactive proliferations display at least moderate cyto-

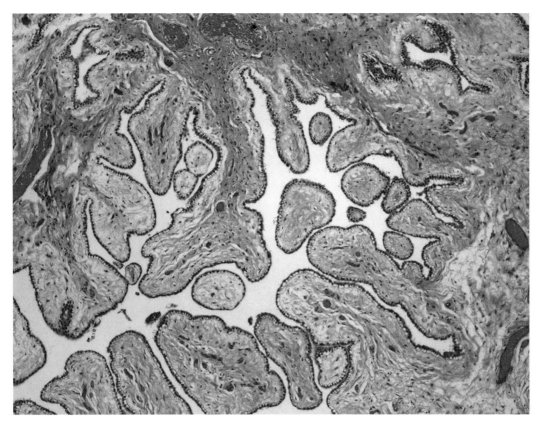

FIGURE 15.13
Well-differentiated papillary mesothelioma. The papillae are lined by a single layer of cells.

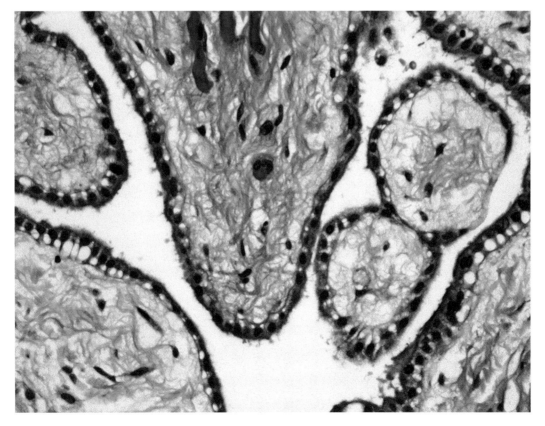

FIGURE 15.14
Well-differentiated papillary mesothelioma. Note low cuboidal cells without cytologic atypia.

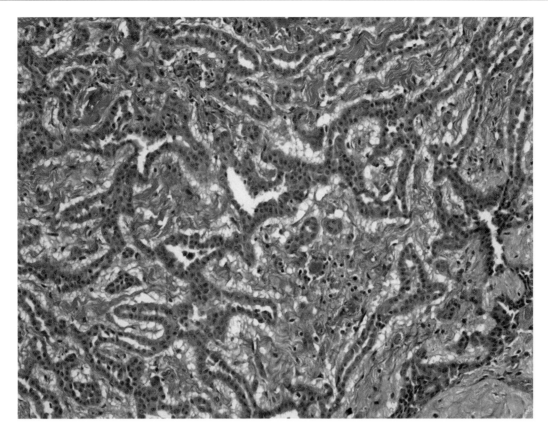

FIGURE 15.15
Diffuse malignant mesothelioma. Note low cytologic grade and myxoid stroma.

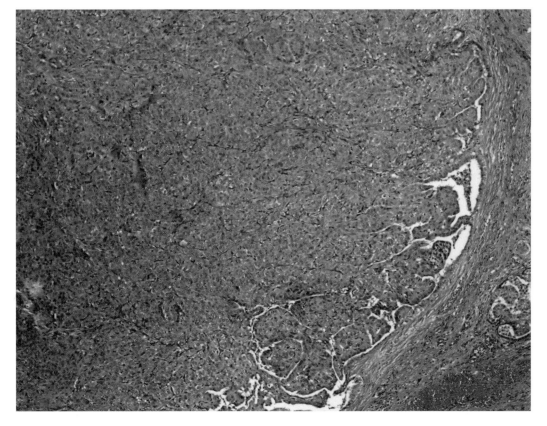

FIGURE 15.16
Diffuse malignant mesothelioma. The tumor shows a predominant solid growth with focal papillary formation.

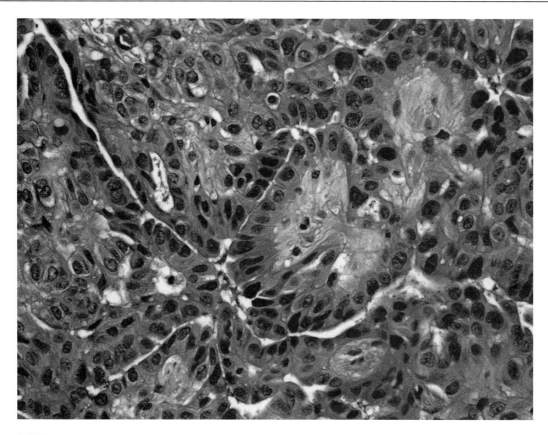

FIGURE 15.17
Diffuse malignant mesothelioma. The tumor cells exhibit moderate cytologic atypia.

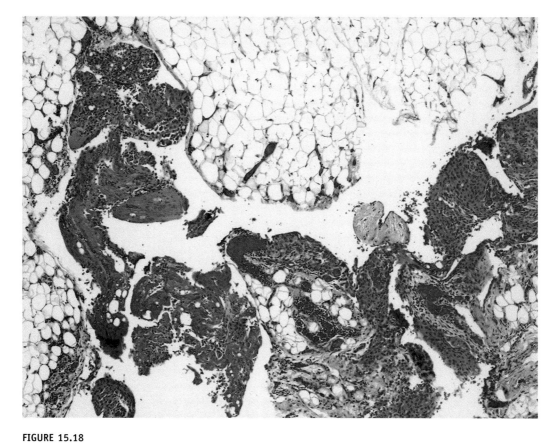

FIGURE 15.18
Mesothelial hyperplasia with papillary architecture. Note the low cytologic grade and lack of invasion into underlying tissue.

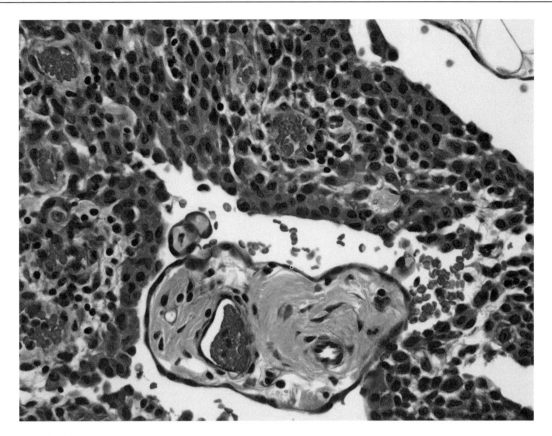

FIGURE 15.19
Mesothelial hyperplasia. Note the bland cytologic features.

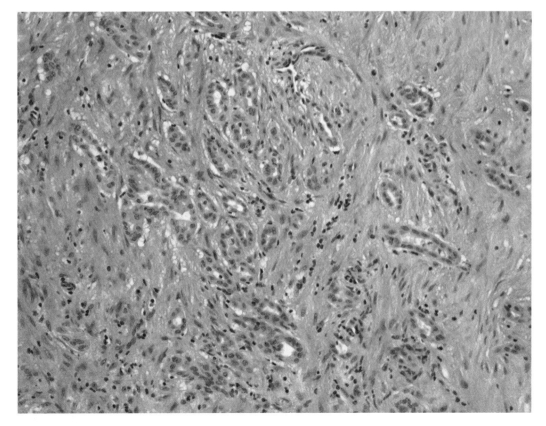

FIGURE 15.20
Mesothelial hyperplasia. Prominent tubule formation is associated with bland cytology.

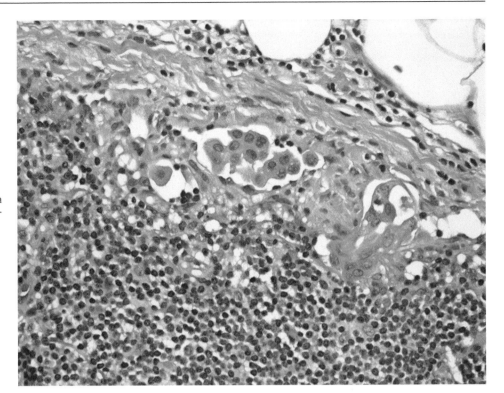

FIGURE 15.21

Reactive mesothelial cells in a regional lymph node (so-called mesothelial deportation).

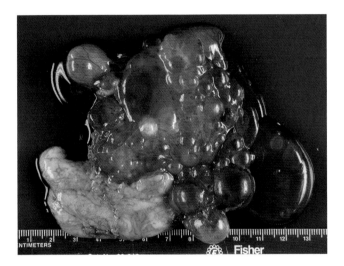

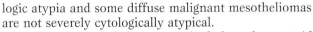

FIGURE 15.22

Multilocular peritoneal inclusion cysts.

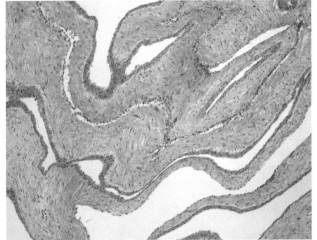

FIGURE 15.23

Multilocular peritoneal inclusion cysts. The cysts are lined by a bland, multilayered epithelium.

logic atypia and some diffuse malignant mesotheliomas are not severely cytologically atypical.

Benign mesothelial tumors include *adenomatoid tumor* and *multilocular peritoneal inclusion cysts* (also known as *benign multicystic mesothelioma* (Figures 15.22 and 15.23)). In women, adenomatoid tumors arise in the fallopian tubes, myometrium, and less commonly, on peritoneal surfaces. Although it appears infiltrative, adenomatoid tumor has a low-power lobulated configuration without destructive invasion at its edges. It is typically composed of irregular anastomosing, gland-like spaces and occasionally may contain signet ring cells (Chapter 9). The nuclei can be variably sized, but are

almost never obviously atypical. Multilocular peritoneal inclusion cysts although commonly symptomatic and large, are lined by cells with a bland appearance.

Several very uncommon entities merit consideration. The sieve-like pattern of the *female adnexal tumor of probable wolffian origin (FATWO)* and its occurrence in the broad ligament, might lead to the impression of a mesothelial neoplasm. There are other characteristic histologic patterns of FATWO that differ from mesothelioma (Chapter 9). In addition, FATWO frequently expresses keratin and calretinin, but almost always lacks EMA. *Ependymoma* has also been described in the broad ligament and may have a papillary architecture.

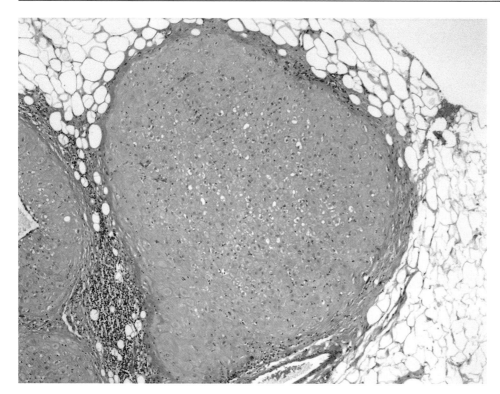

FIGURE 15.24

Ectopic decidua. A well demarcated nodule composed of cells with abundant pink cytoplasm is present in adipose tissue.

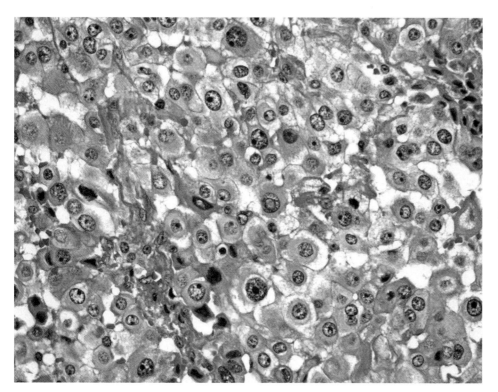

FIGURE 15.25

Deciduoid malignant mesothelioma. Note ample pink cytoplasm resembling decidua. The nuclear features, however, are clearly malignant.

Ependymal rosettes and pseudorosettes along with glial fibrillary acidic protein expression are characteristic of this entity.

Ectopic decidua (Figure 15.24) enters the differential diagnosis with the deciduoid variant of malignant mesothelioma (Figure 15.25). This mesothelioma variant forms a mass, in contrast to ectopic decidua, and has unequivocally malignant-appearing cytologic fea-
tures. In addition, decidualized cells do not express cytokeratins. Another tumor composed of epithelioid cells is *epithelioid angiosarcoma*, which differs from mesothelioma by virtue of its vasoformative nature and expression of endothelial antigens. Like mesothelioma, however, epithelioid angiosarcoma can express keratins and EMA and often grows in a sheet-like pattern without an obvious vascular component.

PROGNOSIS AND TREATMENT

The prognosis depends upon the type of mesothelioma. Diffuse, high-grade tumors are nearly always fatal, with a median survival time of < 1 year. Diffuse, well-differentiated papillary mesotheliomas are probably difficult to cure, but their behavior is indolent, especially when compared to diffuse, high-grade tumors; survival in the range of years and even decades has been reported. Localized, well-differentiated papillary mesotheliomas are cured by excision. The primary treatment for all mesothelioma subtypes is surgery. Several investigational protocols now provide chemotherapy as an adjuvant therapeutic option, but this tends to be reserved for diffuse, high-grade tumors.

PSEUDOMYXOMA PERITONEI

Pseudomyxoma peritonei is an imprecise clinical term that, more or less, describes mucinous ascites of various etiologies. Nearly all cases represent peritoneal dissemination from a gastrointestinal neoplasm, particularly of the appendix (90%). Colorectal mucinous carcinomas and rare gastric and pancreatobiliary tumors account for most of the remaining cases. Ovarian intestinal mucinous borderline tumors are no longer thought to give rise to pseudomyxoma peritonei, except when associated with a mature cystic teratoma. Pseudomyxoma peritonei should be distinguished from localized and organized collections of acellular mucin that can result from rupture of a primary mucinous ovarian neoplasm.

CLINICAL FEATURES

Overall, 60–75% of patients are female. The age range is 33–82 (mean 47) years. The symptoms of pseudomyxoma peritonei are nonspecific and include abdominal distension and pain. Other signs and symptoms include palpable abdominal or pelvic masses, nausea, vomiting, and fatigue. A proportion of patients are diagnosed incidentally during a surgical procedure for suspected appendicitis or herniorrhaphy.

Mucin tends to aggregate in dependent portions of the abdomen and pelvis, although loculation can give rise to accumulations in any part of the abdominopelvic cavity (Figure 15.26). Despite the fact that pseudomyxoma almost never derives from a primary ovarian tumor, there is a propensity for ovarian involvement.

PSEUDOMYXOMA PERITONEI – FACT SHEET

Definition
▶ Imprecise clinical term to describe mucinous ascites of various etiologies
▶ Nearly all cases represent peritoneal dissemination from an intestinal neoplasm, particularly of appendix, but rarely gastric, pancreatobiliary, and even ovarian origin
▶ Alternative pathologic diagnostic terms describing mucinous ascites containing epithelial cells include:
  ▶ Low-grade tumors – "disseminated peritoneal adenomucinosis"; "metastatic low-grade appendiceal mucinous neoplasm"; "metastatic well-differentiated mucinous adenocarcinoma"
  ▶ High-grade tumors – "peritoneal mucinous carcinomatosis"; "metastatic mucinous adenocarcinoma"
▶ Ovarian intestinal mucinous borderline tumors are no longer thought to give rise to pseudomyxoma peritonei except when associated with mature cystic teratoma
▶ Should be distinguished from localized and organized collections of acellular mucin

Incidence and Location
▶ Uncommon tumors arise from ruptured appendiceal mucinous neoplasms (approximately 90%)
▶ Mucin tends to aggregate in dependent portions of abdomen and pelvis
▶ Propensity for ovarian involvement

Morbidity and Mortality
▶ Gross abdominal distension, uncontrolled accumulations of mucin, and bowel obstruction

▶ Both low- and high-grade tumors frequently recurrent and fatal; however, the proportion of patients surviving typically substantially greater in low-grade group

Gender and Age Distribution
▶ 60–75% are female
▶ Age range is 33–82 (mean 47) years

Clinical Features
▶ Nonspecific symptoms including abdominal distension and abdominal pain.
▶ Occasionally incidental diagnosis during a surgical procedure for suspected appendicitis for herniorrhaphy

Radiographic Features
▶ Calcifications in abdomen, poorly defined soft-tissue masses and ascites on X-ray
▶ Scalloping of the hepatic margin, numerous multilocular cystic masses with rims of curvilinear calcifications, and compression of abdominal viscera without evidence of invasion on CT-scan

Prognosis and Treatment
▶ 5- and 10-year survival rates for low-grade tumors are 75% and 68%
▶ 5- and 10-year survival rates for intermediate-grade tumors are 84% and 38%
▶ 5- and 10-year survival rates for high-grade tumors are 14% and 3%
▶ Surgical debulking main treatment
▶ Systemic and intraperitoneal chemotherapy, including heated agents

Neoplasms resulting in pseudomyxoma peritonei commonly result in significant morbidity, particularly in the setting of gross abdominal distension, uncontrolled accumulations of mucin, and bowel obstruction. Although both low- and high-grade tumors are frequently recurrent and fatal, the proportion of patients surviving is typically substantially greater in the low-grade group.

PATHOLOGIC FEATURES

GROSS FINDINGS

Mucinous ascites is usually associated with bilaterally enlarged, cystic ovaries and surface mucin deposition. The appendix is commonly enlarged and distended by an appendiceal mucinous cystic neoplasm. The vast majority are either obviously ruptured or scarred, obscuring a site of previous rupture (Figures 15.27–15.28). Uncommonly, the appendix appears normal on gross examination. Peritoneal nodules and dominant masses are commonly encountered.

MICROSCOPIC FINDINGS

The appendix harbors a mucinous neoplasm composed of intestinal cells with a range of cytologic appear-ances, ranging from hyperplastic and low-grade to high-grade dysplastic (Figures 15.29 and 15.30). Extensive sectioning and complete submission of the appendix may be required to identify these abnormalities. Low-grade tumors generally disseminate via mucin dissection through the appendiceal wall, whereas high-grade tumors often display an invasive mucinous adenocarcinoma. Extra-appendiceal intestinal sources for pseudomyxoma peritonei are generally high-grade carcinomas with obvious destructive stromal invasion.

The appearance and amount of epithelium in pseudomyxoma peritonei varies. Low-grade tumors contain scant gastrointestinal-type mucinous epithelium floating in mucin (Figures 15.31 and 15.32). The cells generally resemble those of hyperplastic colonic polyps or, at most, low-grade adenomatous epithelium (so called "peritoneal adenomucinosis"). In this setting, peritoneal deposits may be accompanied by a striking fibroblastic response. Dissection of ovarian stroma by large acellular pools of mucin is common. Intermediate-grade tumors frequently resemble low-grade tumors, but they contain more abundant epithelium with at least focal moderate to severe cytologic atypia. High-grade tumors (Figures 15.33–15.35) usually contain abundant epithelium of high cytologic grade. Signet-ring cells and overt tissue invasion may be present.

Several different terms have been used to label peritoneal involvement by low-grade appendiceal

---

PSEUDOMYXOMA PERITONEI – PATHOLOGIC FEATURES

Gross Findings
▸ Mucinous ascites
▸ ± Enlarged, distended and ruptured appendix
▸ ± Peritoneal nodules and occasionally, a dominant mass
▸ ± Bilateral enlarged, cystic ovaries, with surface deposition of mucin

Microscopic Findings

Appendix
▸ Neoplasms composed of hyperplastic, low- to high-grade dysplastic mucinous cells ± invasive carcinoma
▸ Low-grade tumors generally disseminate by way of mucin dissection through appendiceal wall, whereas high-grade tumors often display stromal invasion

Pseudomyxoma peritonei
▸ Low-grade tumors contain scant mucinous epithelium floating in mucin. Cells generally resemble those of hyperplastic colonic polyps or, at most, low-grade adenomatous epithelium
▸ Peritoneal deposits, usually noninvasive, are often accompanied by prominent fibroblastic response
▸ Intermediate-grade tumors contain more abundant epithelium with at least focal moderate to severe cytologic atypia
▸ High-grade tumors usually contain abundant epithelium of higher cytologic grade; signet-ring cells and tissue invasion may be present
▸ Ovarian involvement is usually bilateral with common stromal mucin dissection and surface involvement

▸ Ovarian involvement may resemble mucinous cystadenoma, intestinal mucinous borderline tumor, or ovarian mucinous adenocarcinoma
▸ Rarely, ovarian teratomas containing mucinous cystic neoplasms may result in pseudomyxoma peritonei

Immunohistochemical Features
▸ Not usually needed for diagnosis (can be misleading)
▸ Appendiceal carcinomas express CK20 uniformly, frequently express DPC4 (90%), and less frequenty express MUC 5AC (33%) and CK 7 (33%)
▸ Primary ovarian mucinous carcinomas, in contrast, express patchy CK20 (68%), DPC4 uniformly, and typically MUC 5AC (98%) and CK7 (100%)

Differential Diagnosis
With involvement of ovary
▸ Ovarian mucinous cystadenoma
▸ Ovarian mucinous borderline tumor
▸ Ovarian mucinous adenocarcinoma
▸ Metastatic mucinous carcinoid
▸ Metastatic mucinous colorectal adenocarcinoma
▸ Metastatic mucinous pancreatic adenocarcinoma

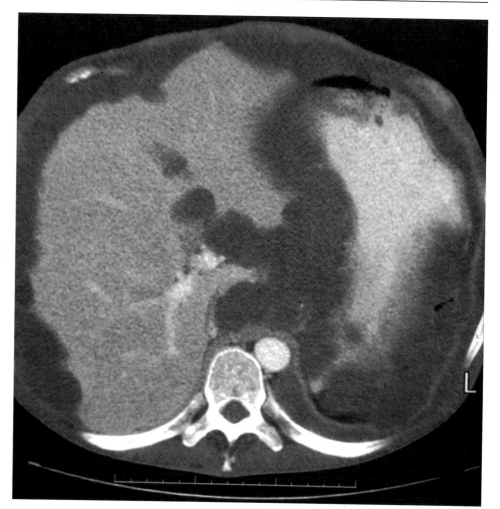

FIGURE 15.26

Pseudomyxoma peritonei. Abdominal CT scan shows scalloping of the hepatic surface without evidence of invasion (Courtesy of Teri Longacre, MD).

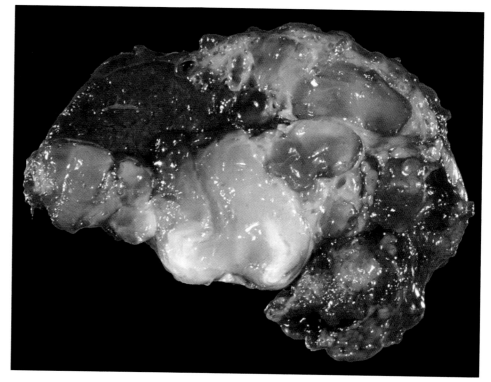

FIGURE 15.27

Pseudomyxoma peritonei. Mucinous locules replace and surround this distorted appendix (Courtesy of Teri Longacre, MD).

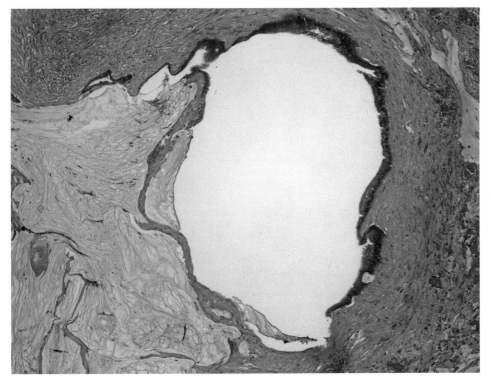

FIGURE 15.28
Appendiceal mucinous cystadenoma. There is rupture with transmural mucin dissection.

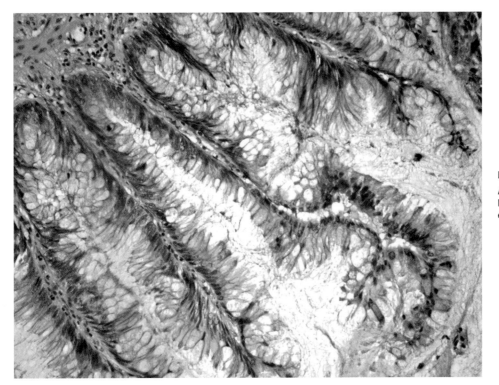

FIGURE 15.29
Appendiceal mucinous cystadenoma. Note the hyperplastic nature of the epithelium.

mucinous tumors including well-differentiated mucinous adenocarcinoma, disseminated peritoneal adenomucinosis, and metastatic low-grade appendiceal mucinous neoplasm. Peritoneal involvement by intermediate- and high-grade tumors is essentially always considered carcinoma, but the prognosis differs.

Ovarian involvement may resemble mucinous cystadenoma, intestinal mucinous borderline tumor, or ovarian mucinous carcinoma. In pseudomyxoma peritonei, ovarian involvement is usually bilateral and there is extensive mucin dissection, including ovarian surface involvement.

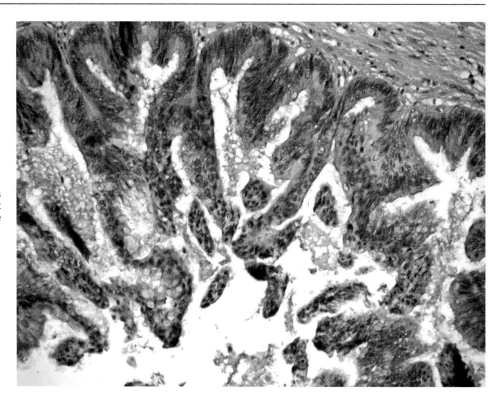

FIGURE 15.30

Low-grade appendiceal mucinous tumor. The tumor shows prominent papillary architecture and low-grade dysplastic features.

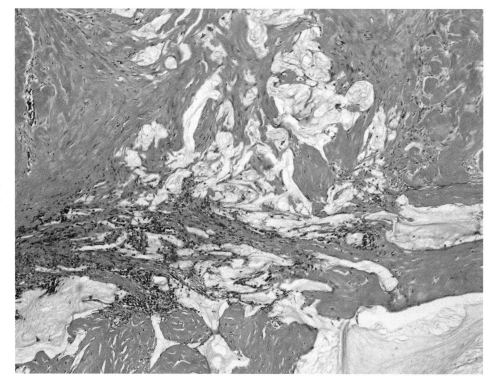

FIGURE 15.31

Pseudomyxoma peritonei. Acellular mucin dissection with prominent fibrous reaction is present.

ANCILLARY STUDIES

IMMUNOHISTOCHEMISTRY

Immunohistochemistry is not usually needed for diagnosis and may be misleading. Appendiceal carcino-mas express CK20 uniformly, DPC4 frequently (90%), and rarely MUC 5AC (33%) and CK7 (33%). However, this immunophenotype probably varies with the degree of cytologic atypia. In contrast, primary ovarian mucinous carcinomas show patchy CK20 positivity (68%), and typically express DPC4, MUC 5AC (98%), and CK7 (100%).

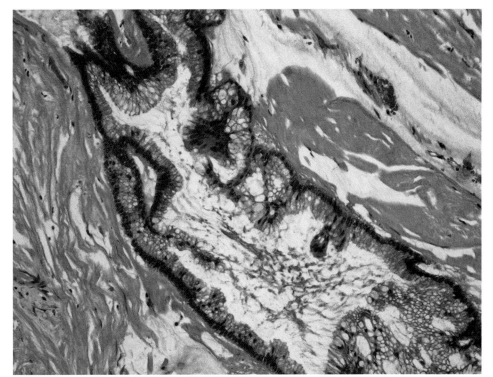

FIGURE 15.32
Pseudomyxoma peritonei. Bland-appearing intestinal epithelium is associated with mucin and is embedded in dense fibrous tissue ("peritoneal adenomucinosis).

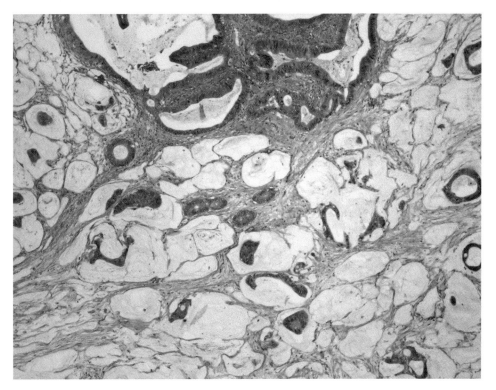

FIGURE 15.33
Pseudomyxoma peritonei. Abundant epithelium is present, some of which is free floating in mucin pools.

DIFFERENTIAL DIAGNOSIS

The first challenge in differential diagnosis is the distinction of *localized, acellular collections of mucin* from disseminated mucin deposits containing mucinous epithelium (pseudomyxoma peritonei). The operative findings, gross examination, and microscopic features are all contributory.

Once the process is recognized as pseudomyxoma peritonei, the source should be identified, being most commonly the appendix, despite the frequent intraoperative impression of an ovarian primary. Strategies for differentiating *primary mucinous borderline tumors* and *carcinomas* from metastases to the ovaries are detailed in Chapter 14. To summarize, it may be inappropriate to make a diagnosis of a primary ovarian mucinous borderline tumor or mucinous carcinoma if

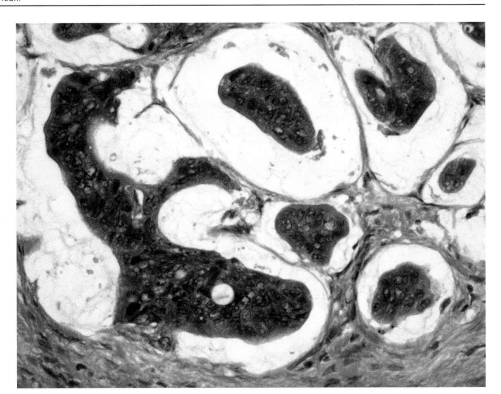

FIGURE 15.34

Pseudomyxoma peritonei. Cells with high-grade nuclear features are seen ("mucinous carcinoma").

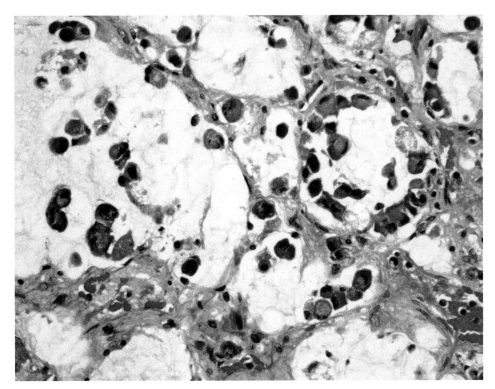

FIGURE 15.35

Pseudomyxoma peritonei. Metastatic mucinous carcinoma with signet-ring cells.

both ovaries are involved and the ovarian tumors measure < 10 cm in greatest dimension. Other characteristic features of metastatic mucinous carcinoma to the ovaries include ovarian surface involvement, hilar involvement, lymphovascular invasion, destructive stromal invasion, signet-ring cell morphology, and a nodular growth pattern.

PROGNOSIS AND TREATMENT

The 5- and 10-year survival rates for low-grade tumors are 75% and 68%, respectively, while the 5- and 10-year survival rates for intermediate-grade tumors are 84% and 38%, respectively. In contrast, the 5- and 10-

year survival rates for high-grade tumors are 14% and 3%, respectively. The treatment consists primarily of surgical debulking. Both systemic and intraperitoneal chemotherapy, including heated intraperitoneal agents, have been used.

DESMOPLASTIC SMALL ROUND CELL TUMOR AND DISSEMINATED PERITONEAL LEIOMYOMATOSIS

There are a potentially overwhelming number and variety of primary and metastatic neoplasms that can involve the peritoneal cavity. However, only two additional primary peritoneal conditions will be discussed: (1) desmoplastic small round cell tumor (DSRCT) and (2) diffuse peritoneal leiomyomatosis (DPL).

DESMOPLASTIC SMALL ROUND CELL TUMOR

Desmoplastic small round cell tumor is a rare tumor of adolescence that usually arises in the peritoneal cavity. Most affected individuals are boys, but presentation in the ovary and involvement of the abdomen and pelvis of girls and young women are now well recognized. Rarely, involvement of soft tissue, bone, and visceral organs may occur. The prognosis is dismal despite aggressive treatment with high-dose chemotherapy.

The tumor's name reflects its microscopic appearance (Figures 15.36–15.37) as it is typically composed of nests or sheets of small cells set in desmoplastic stroma. High-power examination reveals small round blue cells with scant cytoplasm. In addition, rhabdoid cells with eccentric nuclei featuring a nucleolus, and cytoplasm containing a paranuclear aggregate of eosinophilic material may be seen. The tumor is polyphenotypic; the cells express cytokeratin, desmin (Figure 15.38), neuron-specific enolase, and using antibodies that recognize its C-terminus, WT1 (Figure 15.39). Cytogenetic studies most commonly reveal a translocation between chromosomes 11 and 22, and molecular genetic analysis demonstrates a fusion of the *EWS* and *Wilms tumor suppressor* (*WT1*) genes. The differential diagnosis is extensive and includes all small round cell tumors that can involve the peritoneal cavity. A partial list includes the following: neuroblastoma, extraosseous Ewing sarcoma/primitive neuroectodermal tumor, immature teratoma, lymphoma, rhabdomyosarcoma, rhabdoid tumor, poorly differentiated Sertoli–Leydig cell tumor, adult and juvenile granulosa cell tumor, and small cell carcinoma of hypercalcemic type.

DISSEMINATED PERITONEAL LEIOMYOMATOSIS

Disseminated peritoneal leiomyomatosis is a rare disorder, usually diagnosed incidentally, particularly at cesarean section or tubal ligation. It is a benign condi-

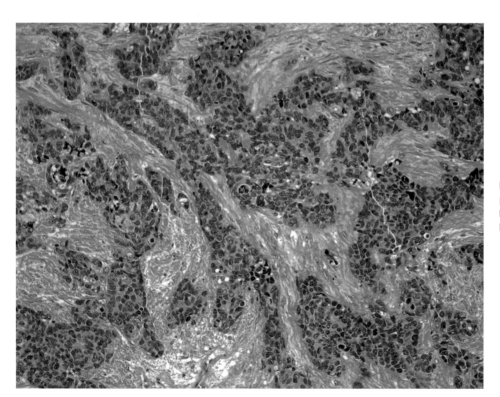

FIGURES 15.36

Desmoplastic small round cell tumor. Nests of small cells are present in a prominent desmoplastic stroma.

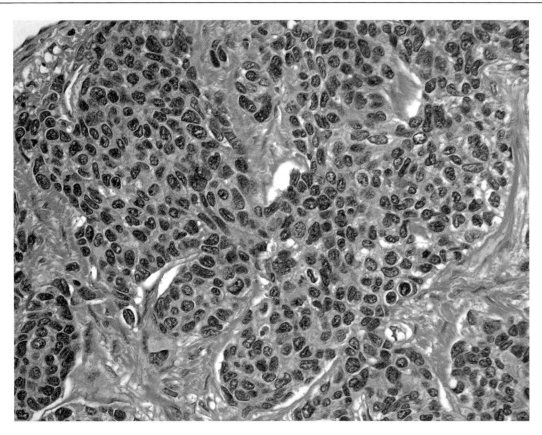

FIGURE 15.37
Desmoplastic small round cell tumor. Note scant amount of cytoplasm and small round to oval nuclei.

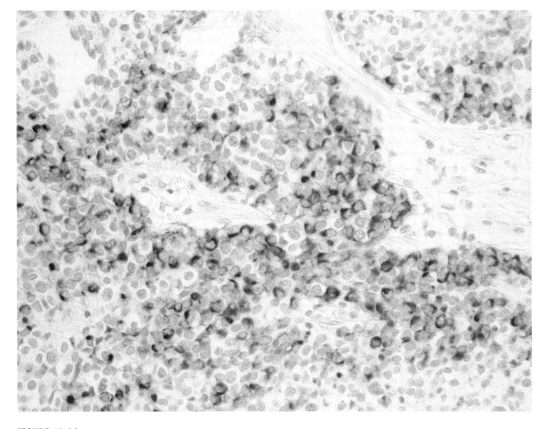

FIGURE 15.38
Desmoplastic small round cell tumor. Note perinuclear dot-like pattern of desmin immunoreactivity.

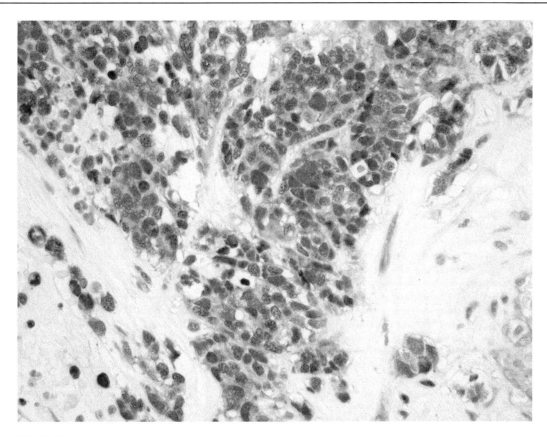

FIGURE 15.39
Desmoplastic small round cell tumor. Note nuclear WT-1 staining.

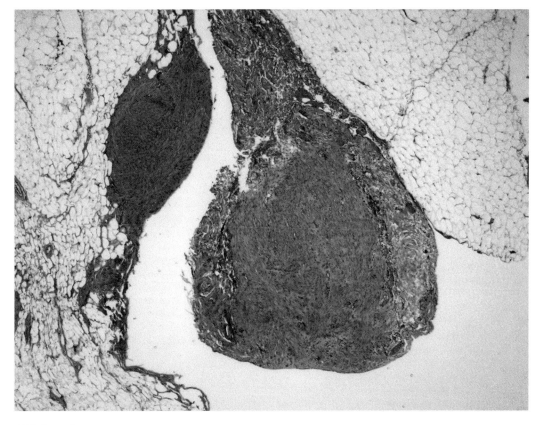

FIGURE 15.40
Disseminated peritoneal leiomyomatosis. A small, surface nodule resembles a leiomyoma.

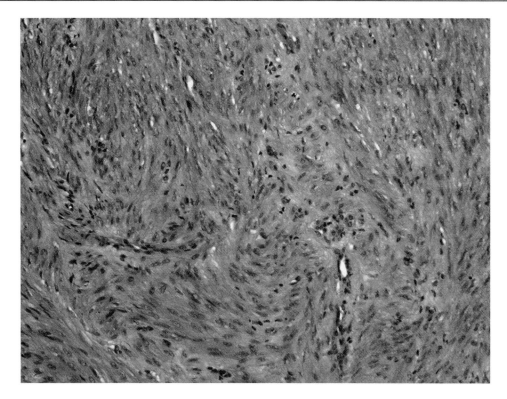

FIGURE 15.41
Disseminated peritoneal leiomyomatosis. Bland smooth muscle cells are arranged in fascicles.

tion that presents as miliary nodules on peritoneal surfaces usually measuring < 3 cm, but on occasion may be as large as 10 cm. Microscopic examination reveals small, rounded aggregates of bland smooth muscle cells (Figures 15.40 and 15.41). DPL should be distinguished from benign metastasizing leiomyoma, metastatic leiomyosarcoma, intravenous leiomyomatosis, lymphangioleiomyomatosis and gastrointestinal stromal tumors. However, the latter is usually centered in the bowel wall and is typically c-kit and CD34 positive.

SUGGESTED READING

Endometriosis

Clement PB, Young RH, Scully RE. Necrotic pseudoxanthomatous nodules of ovary and peritoneum in endometriosis. Am J Surg Pathol 1988;12:390–397.

Fukunaga M, Ushigome S. Epithelial metaplastic changes in ovarian endometriosis. Mod Pathol 1998;11:784–788.

Fukunaga M, Nomura K, Ishikawa E, et al. Ovarian atypical endometriosis: its close association with malignant epithelial tumours. Histopathology 1997;30:249–255.

Missmer SA, Hankinson SE, Spiegelman D, et al. Incidence of laparoscopically confirmed endometriosis by demographic, anthropometric, and lifestyle factors. Am J Epidemiol 2004;160:784–796.

Parker RL, Dadmanesh F, Young RH, et al. Polypoid endometriosis: a clinicopathologic analysis of 24 cases and a review of the literature. Am J Surg Pathol 2004;28:285–297.

Pritts EA, Taylor RN. An evidence-based evaluation of endometriosis-associated infertility. Endocrinol Metab Clin North Am 2003;32:653–667.

Seidman JD. Prognostic importance of hyperplasia and atypia in endometriosis. Int J Gynecol Pathol 1996;15:1–9.

Yantiss RK, Clement PB, Young RH. Neoplastic and pre-neoplastic changes in gastrointestinal endometriosis: a study of 17 cases. Am J Surg Pathol 2000;24:513–524.

Primary Peritoneal Carcinoma

Chu CS, Menzin AW, Leonard DG, et al. Primary peritoneal carcinoma: a review of the literature. Obstet Gynecol Surv 1999;54:323–335.

Eltabbakh GH, Piver MS, Natarajan N, et al. Epidemiologic differences between women with extraovarian primary peritoneal carcinoma and women with epithelial ovarian cancer. Obstet Gynecol 1998;91:254–259.

Eltabbakh GH, Werness BA, Piver S, et al. Prognostic factors in extraovarian primary peritoneal carcinoma. Gynecol Oncol 1998;71:230–239.

Levine DA, Argenta PA, Yee CJ, et al. Fallopian tube and primary peritoneal carcinomas associated with BRCA mutations. J Clin Oncol 2003;21:4222–4227.

Weir MM, Bell DA, Young RH. Grade 1 peritoneal serous carcinomas: a report of 14 cases and comparison with 7 peritoneal serous psammocarcinomas and 19 peritoneal serous borderline tumors. Am J Surg Pathol 1998;22:849–862.

Mesothelioma

Attanoos RL, Webb R, Dojcinov SD, et al. Value of mesothelial and epithelial antibodies in distinguishing diffuse peritoneal mesothelioma in females from serous papillary carcinoma of the ovary and peritoneum. Histopathology 2002;40:237–244.

Butnor KJ, Sporn TA, Hammar SP, et al. Well-differentiated papillary mesothelioma. Am J Surg Pathol 2001;25:1304–1309.

Daya D, McCaughey WT. Well-differentiated papillary mesothelioma of the peritoneum. A clinicopathologic study of 22 cases. Cancer 1990;65:292–296.

Goldblum J, Hart WR. Localized and diffuse mesotheliomas of the genital tract and peritoneum in women. A clinicopathologic study of nineteen true mesothelial neoplasms, other than adenomatoid tumors, multicystic mesotheliomas, and localized fibrous tumors. Am J Surg Pathol 1995;19:1124–1137.

Kerrigan SA, Turnnir RT, Clement PB, et al. Diffuse malignant epithelial mesotheliomas of the peritoneum in women: a clinicopathologic study of 25 patients. Cancer 2002;94:378–385.

Mohamed F, Sugarbaker PH. Peritoneal mesothelioma. Curr Treat Options Oncol 2002;3:375–386.

Ordonez NG. Role of immunohistochemistry in distinguishing epithelial peritoneal mesotheliomas from peritoneal and ovarian serous carcinomas. Am J Surg Pathol 1998;22:1203–1214.

Pisharodi LR, Bedrossian CW. Cytopathology of serous neoplasia of the ovary and the peritoneum: differential diagnosis from mesothelial proliferations. Diagn Cytopathol 1996;15:292–295.

Pseudomyxoma Peritonei

Galani E, Marx GM, Steer CB, et al. Pseudomyxoma peritonei: the "controversial" disease. Int J Gynecol Cancer 2003;13:413–418.

Ji H, Isacson C, Seidman JD, et al. Cytokeratins 7 and 20, Dpc4, and MUC5AC in the distinction of metastatic mucinous carcinomas in the ovary from primary ovarian mucinous tumors: Dpc4 assists in identifying metastatic pancreatic carcinomas. Int J Gynecol Pathol 2002;21:391–400.

Lee KR, Young RH. The distinction between primary and metastatic mucinous carcinomas of the ovary: gross and histologic findings in 50 cases. Am J Surg Pathol 2003;27:281–292.

Lee HH, Agha FP, Weatherbee L, et al. Pseudomyxoma peritonei. Radiologic features. J Clin Gastroenterol. 1986;8:312–316.

Misdraji J, Yantiss RK, Graeme-Cook FM, et al. Appendiceal mucinous neoplasms: a clinicopathologic analysis of 107 cases. Am J Surg Pathol 2003;27:1089–1103.

Ronnett BM, Kurman RJ, Zahn CM, et al. Pseudomyxoma peritonei in women: a clinicopathologic analysis of 30 cases with emphasis on site of origin, prognosis, and relationship to ovarian mucinous tumors of low malignant potential. Hum Pathol 1995;26:509–524.

Ronnett BM, Zahn CM, Kurman RJ, et al. Disseminated peritoneal adenomucinosis and peritoneal mucinous carcinomatosis. A clinicopathologic analysis of 109 cases with emphasis on distinguishing pathologic features, site of origin, prognosis, and relationship to "pseudomyxoma peritonei." Am J Surg Pathol 1995;19:1390–1408.

Ronnett BM, Kurman RJ, Shmookler BM, et al. The morphologic spectrum of ovarian metastases of appendiceal adenocarcinomas: a clinicopatho-

logic and immunohistochemical analysis of tumors often misinterpreted as primary ovarian tumors or metastatic tumors from other gastrointestinal sites. Am J Surg Pathol 1997;21:1144–1155.

Ronnett BM, Shmookler BM, Sugarbaker PH, et al. Pseudomyxoma peritonei: new concepts in diagnosis, origin, nomenclature, and relationship to mucinous borderline (low malignant potential) tumors of the ovary. Anat Pathol 1997;2:197–226.

Ronnett BM, Yan H, Kurman RJ, et al. Patients with pseudomyxoma peritonei associated with disseminated peritoneal adenomucinosis have a significantly more favorable prognosis than patients with peritoneal mucinous carcinomatosis. Cancer 2001;92:85–91.

Ronnett BM, Kajdacsy-Balla A, Gilks CB, et al. Mucinous borderline ovarian tumors: points of general agreement and persistent controversies regarding nomenclature, diagnostic criteria, and behavior. Hum Pathol 2004;35:949–960.

Seidman JD, Kurman RJ, Ronnett BM. Primary and metastatic mucinous adenocarcinomas in the ovaries: incidence in routine practice with a new approach to improve intraoperative diagnosis. Am J Surg Pathol 2003;27:985–993.

Desmoplastic Small Round Cell Tumor

Gerald WL, Miller HK, Battifora H, et al. Intra-abdominal desmoplastic small round-cell tumor. Report of 19 cases of a distinctive type of high-grade polyphenotypic malignancy affecting young individuals. Am J Surg Pathol 1991;15:499–513.

Gerald WL, Ladanyi M, de Alava E, et al. Clinical, pathologic, and molecular spectrum of tumors associated with t(11;22)(p13;q12): desmoplastic small round-cell tumor and its variants. J Clin Oncol 1998;16:3028–3036.

Zhang PJ, Goldblum JR, Pawel BR, et al. Immunophenotype of desmoplastic small round cell tumors as detected in cases with EWS-WT1 gene fusion product. Mod Pathol 2003;16:229–235.

Disseminated Peritoneal Leiomyomatosis

Tavassoli FA, Norris HJ. Peritoneal leiomyomatosis (leiomyomatosis peritonealis disseminata): a clinicopathologic study of 20 cases with ultrastructural observations. Int J Gynecol Pathol 1982;1:59–74.

16 Gestational Trophoblastic Lesions
Ie-Ming Shih

Gestational trophoblastic disease encompasses a diverse group of lesions that can be divided primarily into molar and nonmolar. Molar lesions include partial hydatidiform mole (PHM), complete hydatidiform mole (CHM), and invasive hydatidiform mole. They are lesions that represent abnormally developed placental tissue. Nonmolar lesions include placental-site nodule (PSN), epithelioid trophoblastic tumor (ETT), placental-site trophoblastic tumor (PSTT), and choriocarcinoma. They can be either nonneoplastic (PSN) or neoplastic (ETT, PSTT, and choriocarcinoma) proliferations of trophoblast not accompanied by chorionic villi. Correct classification of the different lesions is important, as each disease entity is characterized by distinctive clinical manifestations and therapeutic approaches. Furthermore, several nontrophoblastic tumors can resemble nonmolar trophoblastic lesions morphologically. Therefore, recognition of the distinct histologic features associated with these different trophoblastic entities is important to avoid such confusion.

HYDATIDIFORM MOLES

A hydatidiform mole, either partial or complete, represents an abnormally developed placenta and is characterized by marked enlargement of the chorionic villi. An invasive hydatidiform mole is defined by the presence of molar villi with associated trophoblastic cells in the myometrium and broad ligament, or at distant sites as the resulting sequela of a CHM or, less likely, a PHM. The overall incidence of hydatidiform moles has decreased remarkably in recent years. In the US, the incidence of molar pregnancies is approximately 1 in 1000 to 1 in 2000 pregnancies; however, the frequency of hydatidiform mole in Asian nations is 7–10 times > the reported frequency in North America and Europe. Most molar pregnancies (> 50 %) are CHM and 25–43 % are PHM, whereas invasive moles are rare. Although several etiologic factors have been linked to the development of molar pregnancies, it appears that multigravidity (> four pregnancies) and increased number of abortions are high-risk factors for the development of a molar pregnancy.

CLINICAL FEATURES

Molar pregnancies occur more frequently in women at the beginning and toward the end of child-bearing, with the highest incidence over 40 years of age. Patients with CHM typically present between the 11th and 25th week of pregnancy. They often have spontaneous abortions, presenting with vaginal bleeding or occasional passage of molar vesicles. There is excessive uterine enlargement for expected gestational age and typically absence of fetal heart sounds. Urine and serum beta-hCG levels are markedly elevated (> 1,000,000 mIU/mL) at the time of diagnosis, and approximately 10 % of patients have related symptoms, including severe hyperemesis, toxemia in early pregnancy, or hyperthyroidism. Patients may also present with ovarian enlargement secondary to multiple theca lutein cysts (hyperreactio luteinalis). On rare occasions, patients present with vaginal or lung metastases. Nowadays with routine use of ultrasound to monitor pregnancy, CHM are diagnosed much earlier (often below 12 weeks gestation). Therefore, many of the classic presenting signs and symptoms are absent, and they more commonly present as a missed abortion.

Patients with PHM usually present with abnormal uterine bleeding at the end of the first trimester that is clinically interpreted as a spontaneous or missed abortion. The uterus is typically normal or small in size for the gestational age, and fetal heart sounds may be present. Urine and serum beta-hCG levels are either normal or much lower than those observed in CHM. Toxemia of pregnancy may also occur, but much less frequently than with CHM.

Patients with invasive moles usually present with persistent vaginal bleeding, uterine subinvolution, or asymmetric uterine enlargement due to infiltration of the myometrium. Rarely, perforation or severe intraperitoneal or vaginal hemorrhage may occur.

RADIOLOGIC FEATURES

In a CHM, ultrasound exam often discloses a uterus that is enlarged for gestational age and filled with multiple small, hypoechoic areas 3–10 mm in diameter, typically described as "bunch-of-grapes" or "snowstorm" appearance. Transvaginal ultrasound with color Doppler demonstrates lack of vascularity within the mass. No fetal parts are identified. In a PHM, a transvaginal ultrasound shows only focal abnormalities but may detect the presence of fetal villous blood vessels and embryonic fetal tissues. Overall, the detection rate for PHM is much lower than for CHM.

The sonographic appearance in an invasive mole includes moderate uterine enlargement with focal increased echogenicity within the myometrium. CT-scan and MRI are useful in detecting myometrial invasion, parametrial extension, and metastases. A chest XRAY is useful to detect early pulmonary metastases, as well as providing a baseline for comparison should pulmonary disease ensue.

PATHOLOGIC FEATURES

GROSS FINDINGS

The cardinal features of a classic CHM mole include generalized villous edema accompanied by an increased amount of tissue (Figure 16.1). Enlarged villi form grape-like, transparent vesicles measuring up to 1–2 cm across. In florid cases, the uterus is enlarged and filled with vesicles that may protrude through the cervical os. However, the vesicles may be more difficult to identify due to partial or extensive collapse in a curettage specimen. In contrast, an early complete mole may show no recognizable gross abnormalities. Typically, no fetus or gestational sac is identified, although in rare cases evidence of fetal development has been reported.

In a PHM, the amount of tissue is typically less abundant than in a CHM (< 200 mL). Grossly, large vesicles are less striking and admixed with nonmolar placental tissue, this being an important distinguishing feature. A fetus is more commonly associated with a PHM, frequently showing developmental abnormalities, particularly syndactyly.

An invasive mole typically appears as a small area of hemorrhage or multiple vesicles in the myometrium or, in florid cases, as hemorrhagic cavities deeply and extensively invading the myometrial wall. The diagnosis of invasive mole can only be made in a hysterectomy specimen.

MICROSCOPIC FINDINGS

In a typical CHM, abnormally formed chorionic villi show generalized hydropic change (cystic swelling) associated with extensive circumferential villous trophoblastic hyperplasia (Figure 16.2). Most villi show striking edema and many contain cisterns, which are

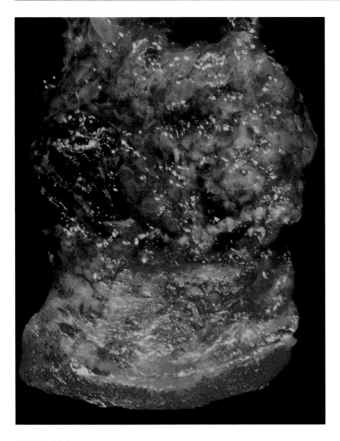

FIGURE 16.1
Complete hydatidiform mole. Enlarged, transparent, and cystically dilated villi fill the uterine cavity.

acellular, fluid-filled spaces within the center of villi. The proliferating cytotrophoblast and syncytiotrophoblast show circumferential growth from the villous surface. This is in marked contrast to the orderly growth of normal trophoblastic cells, which only proliferate from the end of anchoring villi in early nonmolar placentas. There is also hyperplasia and cytologic atypia of the intervillous trophoblast (Figure 16.3) as well as the implantation-site trophoblast (intermediate trophoblast), the latter frequently associated with an exaggerated implantation site. In addition to being hyperplastic, the villous trophoblastic cells often show considerable cytologic atypia. In contrast, the typical morphologic features of a CHM may be absent or very subtle in molar specimens evacuated during first-trimester pregnancies. Early complete moles are characterized by the following histologic features: (1) redundant bulbous "club-shaped" terminal villi; (2) hypercellular villous stroma with primitive stellate cells associated with myxoid background and karyorrhexis; (3) a labyrinthine network of villous stromal canaliculi; (4) focal hyperplasia of cytotrophoblast and syncytiotrophoblast on both villi and the undersurface of the chorionic plate; and (5) relatively atypical trophoblast lining the villi and in the implantation site (Figure 16.4). Thus, any villous tissue with abnormal bulbous tips, blue stroma, degenerating "empty" stromal vessels, or somewhat increased amount of villous tissue (typically 3 × 3 × 0.5 cm in the normal first-trimester loss) in a perimenopausal woman should be scrutinized for the diagnosis of early CHM.

The hallmark of a PHM is a mixture of two populations of chorionic villi, one large and edematous, and

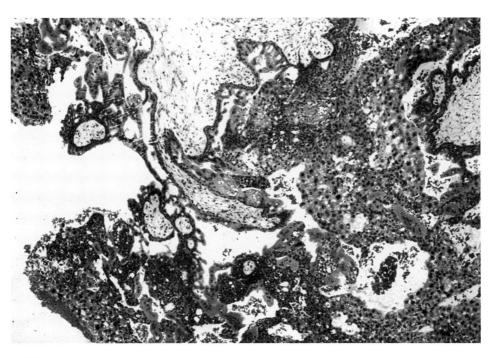

FIGURE 16.2
Complete hydatidiform mole. Enlarged hydropic chorionic villi are surrounded by exuberant circumferential cyto- and syncytiotrophoblast proliferation.

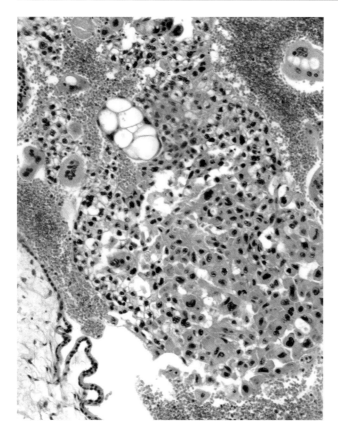

FIGURE 16.3
Complete hydatidiform mole. The hyperplastic nonvillous trophoblast shows striking cytologic atypia.

the other small or normal-sized with stromal fibrosis. At least some of the hydropic villi show a central, acellular cistern as seen in CHM. The enlarged villi show irregular, scalloped outlines and may contain "trophoblast inclusions" as a result of tangentially sectioned infoldings of the surface trophoblast cells into the villous stroma. Trophoblastic hyperplasia is limited to the syncytiotrophoblast cells (Figure 16.5). They form worm-like slender projections emanating from the villous surface, frequently with prominent cytoplasmic lacunar development, resulting in a "lacy" or "moth-eaten" appearance. Nucleated red blood cells may be seen in the villous capillaries. Other histologic evidence of fetal development includes the findings of chorionic plate, amnion, cord, and fetal tissues.

An invasive mole is characterized by invasion of the myometrium or its vascular spaces by molar villi with proliferating cytotrophoblast and syncytiotrophoblast without intervening decidua. As mentioned earlier, an invasive mole is more frequently a CHM.

ANCILLARY STUDIES

IMMUNOHISTOCHEMISTRY

The immunohistochemical phenotype of hydatidiform moles is similar to that of normal placenta with

---

HYDATIDIFORM MOLES – PATHOLOGIC FEATURES

Gross Findings

Complete Hydatidiform Mole
▸ Uniformly large grape-like, transparent vesicles (if classic)
▸ No fetus or gestational sac in most cases

Partial Hydatidiform Mole
▸ Large hydropic vesicles admixed with nonmolar placental tissue
▸ Fetus frequently with developmental abnormalities, particularly syndactyly

Microscopic Findings

Complete Hydatidiform Mole
▸ Generalized hydropic change in villi with central cisterns
▸ Marked hyperplasia of villous cytotrophoblast and syncytiotrophoblast
▸ Hyperplasia of the intervillous and implantation trophoblast
▸ Striking cytologic atypia
▸ Absence of fetal tissues

Early Complete Hydatidiform Mole
▸ Bulbous "club-shaped" terminal villi
▸ Hypercellular myxoid villous stroma with karyorrhexis
▸ Labyrinthine network of villous stromal canaliculi
▸ Focal hyperplasia of cytotrophoblast and syncytiotrophoblast

Partial Hydatidiform Mole
▸ Enlarged villi admixed with small and normal-sized villi
▸ Enlarged villi with scalloped borders and trophoblast inclusions
▸ Less frequent or prominent cavitation than in CHM
▸ Mild and focal syncytiotrophoblast hyperplasia with "lacy" or "moth-eaten" appearance
▸ Evidence of fetal development including nucleated red blood cells in villous capillaries, chorionic plate, amnion, cord, or fetal tissues

Immunohistochemical Features
▸ p57 positive in normal placenta and PHM
▸ p57 negative in CHM

Cytogenetics
▸ Complete hydatidiform mole: 46,XX (fertilization of an empty egg by a single sperm)
▸ Partial hydatidiform mole: 69XXX, XXY, or rarely XYY (fertilization of an egg by two sperm)

Differential Diagnosis

Complete Hydatidiform Mole
▸ Hydropic abortion
▸ Choriocarcinoma

Partial Hydatidiform Mole
▸ Hydropic abortion
▸ Non triploid chromosomal abnormalities (trisomy 18, Beckwith–Weidemann syndrome, others)
▸ Triploid nonmolar gestation
▸ Twin placenta with a normal placenta and CHM
▸ Early complete mole

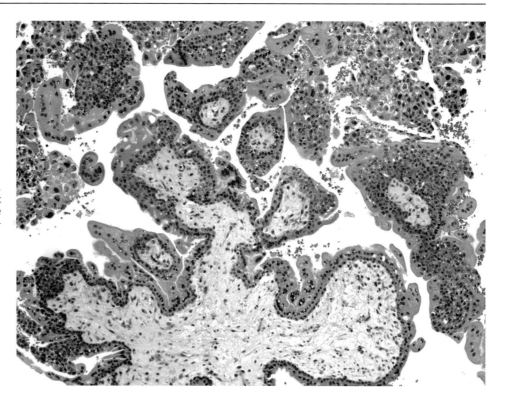

FIGURE 16.4

Early complete hydatidiform mole. Mildly hydropic villi show only slight trophoblastic hyperplasia. Note the myxoid background and the "club-like" outline of the villi.

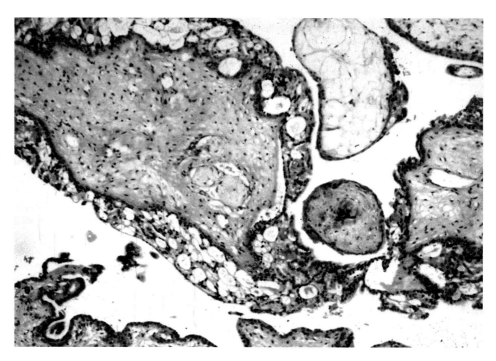

FIGURE 16.5

Partial hydatidiform mole. Enlarged villi are surrounded by a "lacy" proliferation of syncytiotrophoblast. Note the irregular outline of some villi (bottom).

distinctive expression patterns of markers in different trophoblastic cell types. Cytotrophoblast is typically positive for keratins and CD10, but negative for hCG, inhibin, and HPL, while syncytiotrophoblast cells are strongly positive for hCG, placental lactogen alkaline phosphatase (PLAP), inhibin, and CD10, but weakly positive for hPL. p57 is a paternally imprinted, maternally expressed gene for which immunohistochemistry has recently become available. As CHM are androgenetic in origin, this paternally derived gene is not expressed in stromal villous cells and cytotrophoblast, in contrast to positive staining in cytotrophoblast and stromal cells of PHM. Thus, p57 can serve as a reliable marker for the diagnosis of CHM.

CYTOGENETICS

Distinct mechanisms of origin have been shown by cytogenetic analysis for CHM and PHM. CHM are typically diploid with a 46,XX karyotype as a result of haploid genome duplication (fertilization of an empty egg by a single sperm) (23X). This chromosomal composition is known as androgenetic, implying that the genetic material is exclusively derived from paternal DNA. PHM, on the other hand, are generally triploid (fertilization of an egg by two sperm) (frequently 69XXX or XXY) with a haploid set of maternal DNA and two sets of paternal DNA (i.e., diandric). Therefore, the ratio of paternal to maternal chromosomes is 2:0 in a CHM and 2:1 in a PHM. It has been shown that paternal DNA plays a significant role in the development of placental tissues and that an excess of paternal DNA leads to overgrowth of trophoblast, while maternal DNA is more important for fetal development. Thus, a difference in the contribution of paternal or maternal DNA explains differences between the two types of hydatidiform mole.

DIFFERENTIAL DIAGNOSIS

The differential diagnosis of a hydatidiform mole, whether complete or partial, includes gestations with other genetic abnormalities. *Spontaneous abortions* are often associated with failure of embryonic development or early embryonic demise, so-called blighted ovum or hydropic abortus. *Chromosomal abnormalities* may include autosomal trisomies and monosomy X and some other genetic syndromes (Beckwith–Weidemann syndrome) which may display hydropic changes and abnormal villous morphology mimicking a PHM. These cases are not associated with an increased risk of developing gestational trophoblastic disease, and therefore, establishing the correct diagnosis is very important. The volume of tissue obtained in a hydropic abortus is typically much less than in a molar placenta. On microscopic examination, the villi are only slightly enlarged/edematous without true cisternae, there is no extratrophoblast proliferation, and the trophoblast demonstrates a polar distribution characterized by trophoblastic columns that face the basal plate at the distal end of the villous.

Even though traditionally the diagnosis of PHM has been based on morphologic features, *triploid nonmolar pregnancies* may show some overlapping histologic features. However, a triploid gestation with two complete maternal sets of genes gives rise to a fetus with intrauterine growth retardation with dysmorphic features and a small placenta. As mentioned earlier, PHM usually display at least three of the following histologic features: two discrete populations of villi; trophoblastic hyperplasia that may be circumferential; trophoblastic inclusions; prominent scalloping of villi; and cistern formation. In contrast, nontriploid abortuses display at most two of these features. However, it may not be pos-

sible to distinguish an early partial mole from a hydropic abortus based only on morphological features. Therefore, a note in the pathology report recommending the monitoring of serum beta-hCG levels is advisable for difficult cases or those in which cytogenetics studies are not available.

Although isolated fragments of trophoblastic hyperplasia in a CHM resemble the biphasic growth of *choriocarcinoma*, the presence of chorionic villi excludes this diagnosis, except rarely when associated with an otherwise normal gestation (a nonmolar third-trimester placenta). Furthermore, the diagnosis of gestational choriocarcinoma requires evidence of destructive infiltrative growth in addition to the absence of chorionic villi, and should be made with caution before 8–12 weeks after evacuation of a confirmed hydatidiform mole.

As previously mentioned, the differential diagnosis between CHM and PHM is based primarily on histologic features. However, an *early complete mole* may be difficult to distinguish from a PHM, and a *twin placenta with one normal placenta and a complete mole* may be misinterpreted as a PHM because of the finding of two populations of villi. p57 immunohistochemical staining can be helpful in this setting. In CHM, nuclear p57 expression is absent in cytotrophoblast and stromal cells, which differs from the diffuse staining seen in PHM and nonmolar placentas.

PROGNOSIS AND THERAPY

The most serious complications of a molar pregnancy include persistent gestational trophoblastic disease and choriocarcinoma.

Persistent gestational trophoblastic disease is a clinical term describing a plateau or continual rise of serum beta-hCG levels in the presence or absence of extrauterine trophoblastic disease. Pathologically, it may represent a persistent mole with no invasion, an invasive mole, or a choriocarcinoma. Persistent gestational trophoblastic disease occurs in approximately 17–20% of women who have undergone evacuation of a CHM and in 3–5% of women who have undergone hysterectomy. The risk of developing choriocarcinoma following a CHM is about 2–5% in the US. Recent studies have demonstrated that PHM are rarely followed by persistent or metastatic gestational trophoblastic disease, with risk estimates ranging from 0.5 to 4%.

Early and complete evacuation of a mole is the treatment of choice. Monitoring of serum beta-hCG levels after treatment of a molar pregnancy has become routine in the management of patients with trophoblastic disease. Patients with a CHM are followed for 6–12 months or until serum hCG falls to normal levels. If the serum hCG levels do not normalize, the diagnosis of persistent trophoblastic disease is made and chemotherapy is initiated. Modern chemotherapy has led to a cure rate approaching 100% in persistent trophoblastic disease.

PLACENTAL SITE NODULE

This is a nonneoplastic lesion thought to represent extravillous intermediate trophoblast of chorionic type retained in the uterus after pregnancy. It is considered the benign counterpart of epithelioid trophoblastic tumor.

CLINICAL FEATURES

Typically, PSN is an incidental finding in uterine curettages, cervical biopsies, and occasionally hysterectomy specimens in patients of reproductive age and rarely, in postmenopausal women. The diagnosis of PSN has been made in a variety of clinical settings, including evaluation of cervical intraepithelial neoplasm following an abnormal cervical smear (35%), dysmenorrhea and metromenorrhagia (30%), recurrent spontaneous abortion (5%), retained products of conception (5%), postcoital bleeding (2.5%), and infertility (2.5%). A previous pregnancy has been reported to occur up to 108 months before the diagnosis of PSN. PSNs have been reported in tubal ligation specimens.

PATHOLOGIC FEATURES

GROSS FINDINGS

Most often, PSNs are small, microscopic lesions. When grossly visible, they present as yellow, tan, or hemorrhagic nodules measuring up to 1 cm in diameter. They may be located in the endocervix–lower uterine segment, endometrium, or superficial myometrium.

PLACENTAL SITE NODULE – FACT SHEET

Definition
▶ Nonneoplastic lesion of intermediate trophoblast derived from the chorion laeve (fetal membrane) that represents the benign counterpart of epithelioid trophoblastic tumor

Age Distribution
▶ Reproductive age, and rarely, postmenopausal women

Clinical Features
▶ Incidental finding
▶ Previous pregnancy up to 108 months before

Prognosis and Treatment
▶ No treatment or follow-up necessary
▶ No association with local recurrence or progression to other types of trophoblastic tumors

---

MICROSCOPIC FINDINGS

Placental site nodule(s) can be seen on low-power examination as single or multiple nodules or plaques, characterized by a well-circumscribed and lobulated border (Figures 16.6 and 16.7). The nodules and plaques are composed of intermediate trophoblast cells arranged in nests, cords, or singly, and embedded in abundant dense eosinophilic extracellular matrix (Figure 16.8) that may undergo secondary cystic degeneration or even calcification. In some nodules, the center is hyalinized while the periphery appears more cellular. It is not infrequent to find, focally, at the periphery of the nodules, small rounded extensions imparting a pseudoinfiltrative growth (Figure 16.9). The cells vary in size, they have abundant eosinophilic or vacuolated cytoplasm, and the nuclei range from relatively small and vesicular to large and irregular with a degenerative chromatin pattern (Figure 16.8). Occasionally, scattered binucleated or multinucleated cells are present. Mitoses are rare to absent. A thin band of chronic inflammatory cells often surrounds the lesion.

ANCILLARY STUDIES

IMMUNOHISTOCHEMISTRY

Intermediate trophoblast cells in PSNs exhibit an immunophenotype similar to that of intermediate trophoblast cells in the chorion laeve (fetal membrane) but

---

PLACENTAL SITE NODULE – PATHOLOGIC FEATURES

Gross Findings
▶ Small to up to 1 cm
▶ Yellow, tan, or hemorrhagic cut surface if visible
▶ Endocervix–lower uterine segment, endometrium, or superficial myometrium

Microscopic Findings
▶ Well-circumscribed, lobulated border
▶ Nests, cords, or single cells embedded in abundant dense eosinophilic extracellular matrix
▶ Small rounded extensions with pseudoinfiltrative growth sometimes present at the periphery
▶ Abundant eosinophilic or vacuolated cytoplasm, small and vesicular, or large and irregular nuclei with degenerative chromatin pattern
▶ No mitotic activity

Immunohistochemical Features
▶ p63, human leukocyte antigen (HLA)-G, AE1/AE3, cytokeratin 18, EMA, inhibin diffusely positive
▶ HPL and CD146 focally positive or negative
▶ Ki-67 labeling index ≤ 10% (usually around 5%)

Differential Diagnosis
▶ Epithelioid trophoblastic tumor
▶ Placental site trophoblastic tumor
▶ Invasive squamous cell carcinoma of cervix

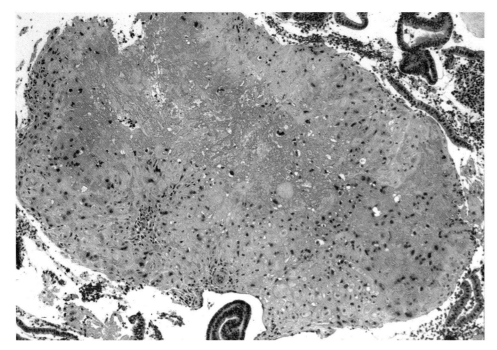

FIGURE 16.6
Placental site nodule. An incidental nodule found in an endometrial curettage shows a hyalinized center with a peripheral cellular rim.

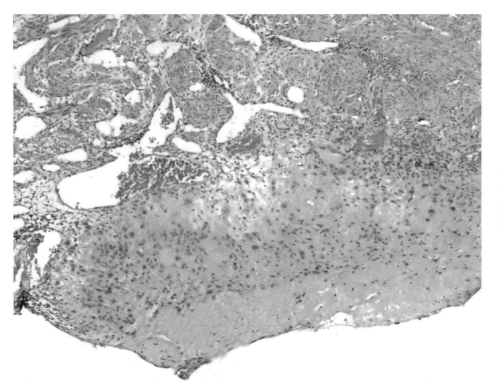

FIGURE 16.7
Placental site plaque. An elongated pink plaque replaces the endometrium and is separated from the myometrium by a rim of inflammation.

distinct from the intermediate trophoblast in the implantation site. They react diffusely with antibodies against AE1/AE3, cytokeratin 18, EMA, PLAP, human leukocyte antigen (HLA)-G, inhibin, and p63. Most PSNs also express the "classical" intermediate trophoblast markers, including hPL, hCG, and Mel-CAM (CD146), although in only a small number of cells (Figure 16.10). The Ki-67 labeling index is ≤ 10% but usually around 5%, which contrasts with the absence of Ki-67-labeled trophoblast cells in the normal implantation site.

DIFFERENTIAL DIAGNOSIS

The most important differential diagnoses include ETT, PSTT, and invasive squamous carcinoma of the cervix. Microscopic size and circumscription of the lesion, extensive hyalinization, and low cellularity are features that distinguish PSN from *ETT* and *PSTT*.

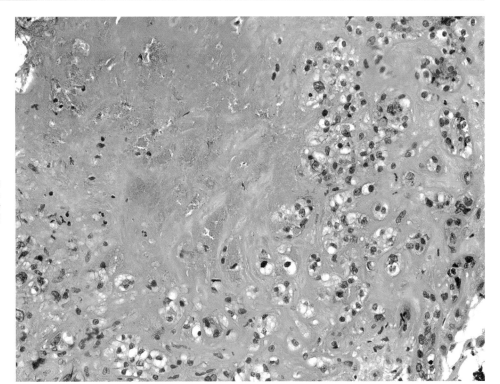

FIGURE 16.8

Placental site nodule. Intermediate trophoblast cells with clear or vacuolated cytoplasm and vesicular or hyperchromatic nuclei are embedded in a hyaline matrix.

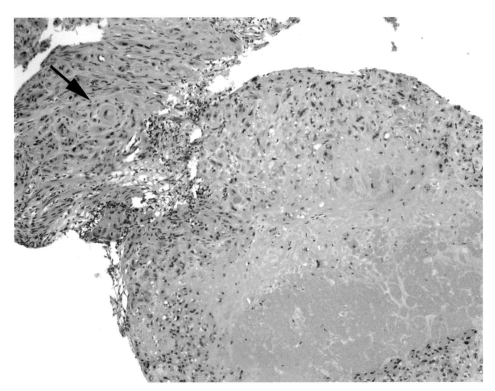

FIGURE 16.9

Placental site nodule. Small round nests at the periphery of the main nodule with a pseudoinfiltrative appearance simulate an invasive squamous cell carcinoma (arrow).

Differentiating between PSN and *cervical squamous cell carcinoma* can be challenging, as PSN is frequently an incidental finding in cervical biopsies and curettage specimens from patients who are evaluated for a possible cervical squamous intraepithelial lesion. Circumscription of the lesion, abundant eosinophilic extracellular material, and lack of mitotic activity favor the diagnosis of PSN. Immunoreactivity for HLA-G, inhibin, cytokeratin 18 and a low (≤ 10%) Ki-67 labeling index also support the diagnosis of PSN and exclude cervical squamous cell carcinoma (Figure 16.10).

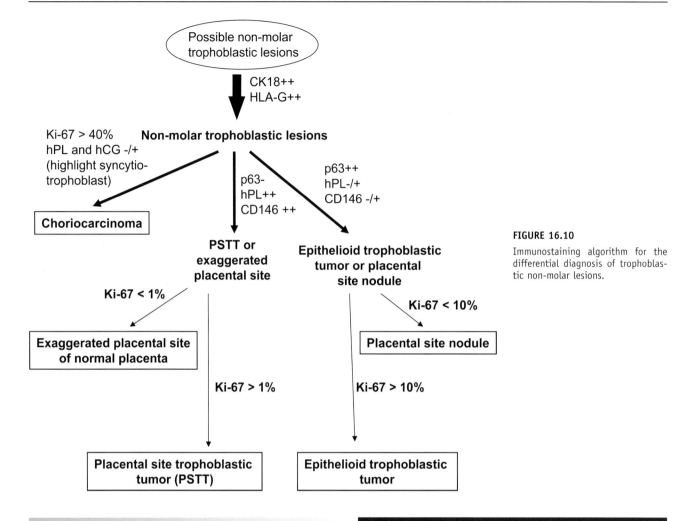

FIGURE 16.10

Immunostaining algorithm for the differential diagnosis of trophoblastic non-molar lesions.

PROGNOSIS AND THERAPY

Placental site nodules are benign. Because of their small size and circumscription, they are usually completely removed by the surgical procedure that led to their discovery. Neither local recurrence nor progression to persistent gestational trophoblastic disease has been documented. Therefore, no specific treatment or follow-up is necessary.

EPITHELIOID TROPHOBLASTIC TUMOR

This is a rare gestational trophoblastic tumor composed of neoplastic intermediate trophoblast cells that are related to cells in the chorion laeve (fetal membrane). It is thought to represent the malignant counterpart of PSN.

CLINICAL FEATURES

This tumor typically occurs in women of reproductive age. It can be diagnosed more than 10 years after the

---

EPITHELIOID TROPHOBLASTIC TUMOR – FACT SHEET

Definition
▶ Neoplasm of intermediate trophoblast derived from the chorion laeve (fetal membrane) thought to represent the malignant counterpart of placental site nodule

Incidence and Age Distribution
▶ Rare
▶ Reproductive age; may occur in postmenopausal women

Clinical Features
▶ Abnormal uterine bleeding
▶ Serum beta hCG level only mildly elevated
▶ Recent or remote antecedent pregnancy

Prognosis and Treatment
▶ Malignant behavior in 10–20%
▶ Distant metastases and death in approximately 10–20% and 10% of patients, respectively
▶ Treatment of choice hysterectomy or local resection
▶ Partially responsive to chemotherapy
▶ Serum hCG level to monitor response to treatment

last known pregnancy or in postmenopausal women. This is in contrast to choriocarcinoma, which is usually more closely associated with an identifiable gestational event. Epithelioid trophoblastic tumor can occur following a term pregnancy, an elective abortion, or a hydatidiform mole. Abnormal vaginal bleeding is the most common clinical presentation and serum beta-hCG levels are always elevated, although at a much lower level than choriocarcinoma. At times, ETT is initially diagnosed in the lungs with or without evidence of prior gestational trophoblastic disease in the uterus.

PATHOLOGIC FEATURES

GROSS FINDINGS

Epithelioid trophoblastic tumor almost always presents as a discrete, expansile nodule up to 5 cm in the endomyometrium, lower uterine segment, cervix, or lung. The cut surface is solid, tan to brown, often with cystic degeneration and areas of hemorrhage and necrosis (Figure 16.11).

MICROSCOPIC FINDINGS

At low magnification, ETTs typically show a well-circumscribed, expansile growth in relation to the surrounding tissues (Figure 16.12), although small groups of infiltrating tumor cells may be seen at the periphery. The tumors exhibit several histologic growth patterns, including sheets, cords, nests, and islands or nodules (Figures 16.12 and 16.13). The nests, islands, and nodules of tumor cells have centrally located blood vessels and are surrounded by extensive areas of geographic necrosis (Figure 16.13). The tumors are composed of a relatively uniform population of mononucleated cells that are intimately associated with an eosinophilic, fibrillar, hyaline-like material and necrotic debris which can mimic keratin (Figure 16.14). These cells have round, uniform nuclei and eosinophilic or clear cytoplasm surrounded by a well-defined cell membrane, features similar to those encountered in the intermediate trophoblast cells of the chorion laeve. The mitotic index varies from 0 to 9/10 HPFs ($\times$ 40), with an average of 2 mitoses/10 HPFs. A lymphocytic infiltrate often surrounds the tumor, and calcification is a characteristic feature of ETT.

EPITHELIOID TROPHOBLASTIC TUMOR – PATHOLOGIC FEATURES

Gross Findings

▶ Discrete, expansile nodule up to 5 cm
▶ Solid, tan to brown cut surface, often with areas of hemorrhage and necrosis
▶ Endomyometrium, lower uterine segment, cervix, or lung

Microscopic Findings

▶ Well-circumscribed, expansile margin
▶ Sheets, cords, nests, islands, or nodules
▶ Blood vessels present in the center of nests, islands, and nodules
▶ Extensive geographic necrosis in between nests, islands, and nodules
▶ Intimate association of cells with eosinophilic, hyaline-like material and necrotic debris
▶ Mononucleated cells with uniform nuclei and eosinophilic or clear cytoplasm
▶ Average mitotic index 2/10 HPFs (range 0–9)

Immunohistochemical Features

▶ p63, HLA-G, AE1/AE3, cytokeratin 18, and inhibin diffusely positive
▶ HPL, HCG, and Mel-CAM focally positive or negative
▶ Ki-67 labeling index between 10–25% (mean 18%)

Differential Diagnosis

▶ Placental site nodule
▶ Placental site trophoblastic tumor
▶ Choriocarcinoma
▶ Keratinizing squamous cell carcinoma of cervix
▶ Epithelioid smooth muscle tumor

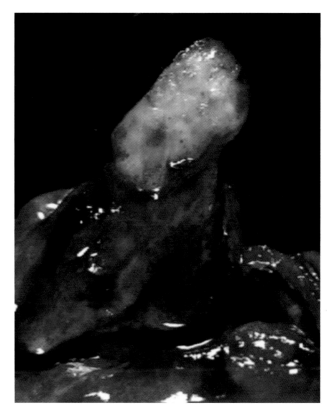

FIGURE 16.11

Metastatic epithelioid trophoblastic tumor to the lung. A well-circumscribed nodule shows a tan, solid cut surface with multiple small cysts and discrete areas of hemorrhage.

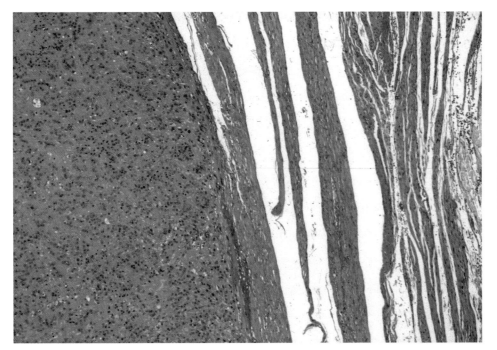

FIGURE 16.12

Epithelioid trophoblastic tumor. The tumor has a well defined margin and is composed of mononucleated cells forming discrete nests and cords.

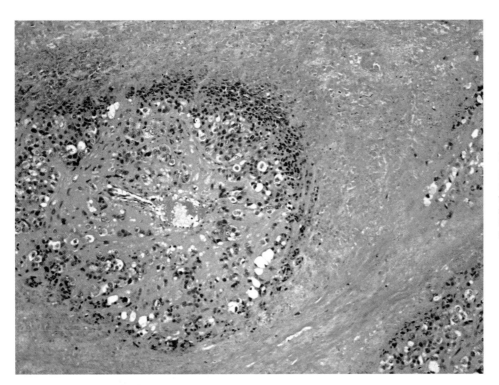

FIGURE 16.13

Epithelioid trophoblastic tumor. A nodule of tumor cells with a central vessel is surrounded by extensive hyaline necrosis. Uniform cells have either eosinophilic or clear cytoplasm.

ANCILLARY STUDIES

IMMUNOHISTOCHEMISTRY

The immunohistochemical profile of ETT is similar to that of chorionic-type intermediate trophoblast. In addition to cytokeratin (AE1/AE3 and cytokeratin 18) and HLA-G, ETT is positive for p63 and inhibin. The "classic" trophoblast markers, including hPL, hCG, and Mel-CAM (CD146), which are diffusely expressed in normal implantation-site intermediate trophoblast and PSTT, are focally expressed in ETT. The mean Ki-67 labeling index is 18%, ranging from 10 to 25%.

DIFFERENTIAL DIAGNOSIS

Although most ETTs display a uniform and characteristic architecture, focal areas resembling PSN, PSTT, and choriocarcinoma can occasionally be identified within the tumor. In contrast to ETT, *PSN* is typically an incidental finding and the cells show overt nuclear size variation but no mitotic activity. Nodular growth with an expansile border and the presence of geographic necrosis and calcification favor the diagnosis of ETT versus *PSTT* or *choriocarcinoma*. Furthermore, invasion and colonization of vessel walls, as seen normally in the implantation site and also very characteristic of PSTT, are not seen in ETT. The monophasic growth of ETT contrasts with the biphasic pattern of cytotrophoblast and syncytiotrophoblast seen in choriocarcinoma. A panel of antibodies, including p63, CD-146, hCG, hPL, and Ki-67, is a useful adjunctive tool to aid in establishing the final diagnosis (Figure 16.10).

Epithelioid trophoblastic tumor may mimic a *cervical keratinizing squamous cell carcinoma*, especially in biopsy and curettage specimens, because of its frequent localization in the cervix and the presence of cells with abundant eosinophilic cytoplasm associated with hyaline-like material that may mimic keratin (Figure 16.14). Immunohistochemistry for cytokeratin 18, inhibin, and HLA-G are very helpful in this differential diagnosis, since these three markers are typically expressed in ETTs but not in squamous carcinoma of the cervix (Figure 16.10). p63 is not helpful as both tumors are typically positive.

Epithelioid smooth muscle tumors may enter into the differential diagnosis of ETT; however, they usually contain conventional spindled areas in addition to epithelioid areas. Furthermore, although epithelioid smooth muscle tumors may be positive for keratin and EMA, they are also positive for muscle markers and conversely, ETTs are positive for cytokeratin 18, HLA-G, p63, and inhibin, but negative for smooth muscle markers.

PROGNOSIS AND THERAPY

The behavior of ETT is still unclear, as it has only recently been recognized as a form of trophoblastic disease, and long-term follow-up is not available. Collected data indicate that ETT, like PSTT, is less aggressive than choriocarcinoma. These tumors are associated with distant metastases and death in approximately 10–20% and 10% of cases, respectively. However, as the number of reported cases is small, features predictive of outcome have not been identified. Unlike choriocarcinoma, ETT appears to be only partially responsive to chemotherapy, and tumors may recur or metastasize despite intensive chemotherapy. Hysterectomy is the main treatment for these tumors, with resection of the lung nodule(s) if there is pulmonary involvement. Although the serum hCG level is only mildly elevated in most ETTs, as with PSTTs, it appears to be useful in monitoring response to treatment.

PLACENTAL SITE TROPHOBLASTIC TUMOR

This is a relatively uncommon form of gestational trophoblast lesion. The tumor is composed of neoplastic intermediate trophoblast cells that arise from the placental site and represents the malignant counterpart of the exaggerated placental site.

CLINICAL FEATURES

These tumors typically occur in women of reproductive age, but they can also occur during early menopause. Patients present with either amenorrhea or abnormal bleeding, often accompanied by uterine enlargement. Serum beta-hCG levels are either low or moderately elevated. The latter, in conjunction with the finding of uterine enlargement or abnormal bleeding and/or amenorrhea, may lead to the erroneous diagnosis of normal pregnancy, missed abortion, or ectopic pregnancy. In contrast to choriocarcinoma, which is preferentially associated with a CHM, PSTT occurs most commonly following a normal pregnancy or a nonmolar abortion, and may be present after a latency period of 10 years.

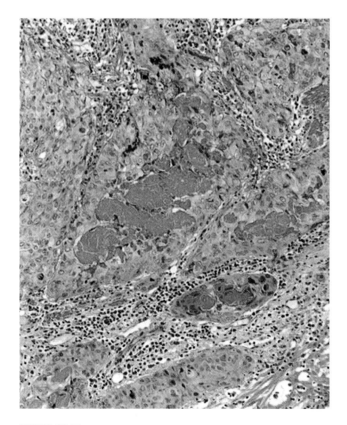

FIGURE 16.14
Epithelioid trophoblastic tumor. Large nests of tumor cells are intimately associated with eosinophilic, hyaline-like material and necrotic debris mimicking keratinizing squamous cell carcinoma.

Rare patients may present with disseminated intravascular coagulation associated with nephrotic syndrome.

RADIOLOGIC FEATURES

The radiologic findings associated with PSTT are mostly nonspecific. Imaging can identify either a hypervascular or a hypovascular uterine mass. In the former, ultrasonography shows a mass with multiple cystic (vascular) spaces and MRI shows a mass with multiple flow voids. On ultrasonography, the hypovascular type shows a solid mass without prominent vascularity or no abnormalities. The main roles of diagnostic imaging are to determine tumor vascularity and extent, the latter being useful information for planning a strategy for surgical management.

PATHOLOGIC FEATURES

GROSS FINDINGS

Most PSTTs are well circumscribed with an average size of 5 cm. They may be polypoid and project into the uterine cavity, or predominantly invade the myometrium. The sectioned surface is soft, tan to yellow, and contains only focal areas of hemorrhage or necrosis. Invasion frequently extends to the uterine serosa, in which case it may be complicated by uterine perforation, and rarely may extend to adnexal structures (10%).

MICROSCOPIC FINDINGS

Placental site trophoblastic tumor typically infiltrates deep into the myometrium with the neoplastic cells "splitting" smooth muscle fibers. The morphology of the neoplastic intermediate trophoblast cells is similar to that of cells in a normal placental site. The large and polygonal tumor cells grow in sheets (Figure 16.15), but at the periphery, the tumor cells infiltrate between the muscle fibers in sheets, nests, cords, or singly. The cells are typically mononucleated or less frequently, binucle-

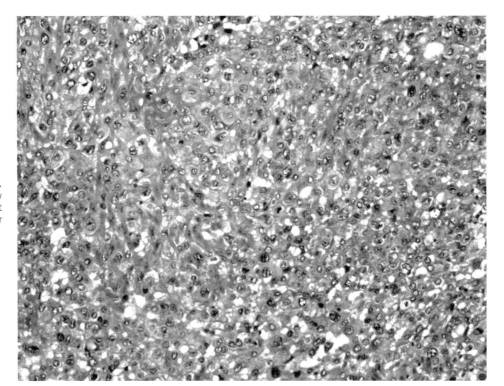

FIGURE 16.15

Placental site trophoblastic tumor. Intermediate trophoblast cells grow in sheets and have abundant eosinophilic cytoplasm with vesicular nuclei.

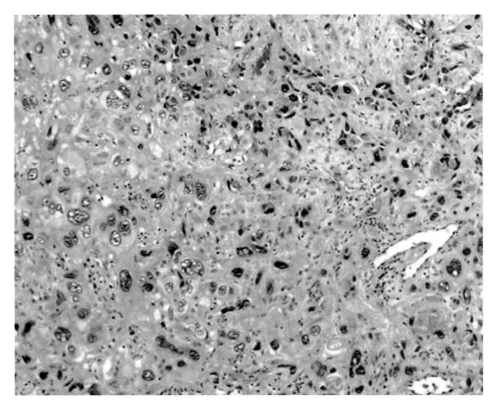

FIGURE 16.16

Placental site trophoblastic tumor. Confluent growth of mononucleated and occasionally binucleated cells. The nuclei have irregular contours with either vesicular or dense chromatin.

ated or multinucleated, and rarely, syncytiotrophoblast cells may be seen. The cytoplasm is amphophilic, eosinophilic (Figure 16.16), or less frequently clear, and the nuclei vary from small and uniform to large, irregular, and hyperchromatic with smudgy chromatin showing variable degrees of nuclear pleomorphism. PSTT is characterized by a unique pattern of vascular invasion reminiscent of that seen in normal implantation site. Invasion and replacement of the vascular walls by intermediate trophoblast cells are followed by fibrinoid material deposition, with the vessel typically maintaining a central lumen (Figure 16.17). These transformed vessels appear as pink or eosinophilic rings at lower-power scrutiny. The same fibrinoid material is also found sur-

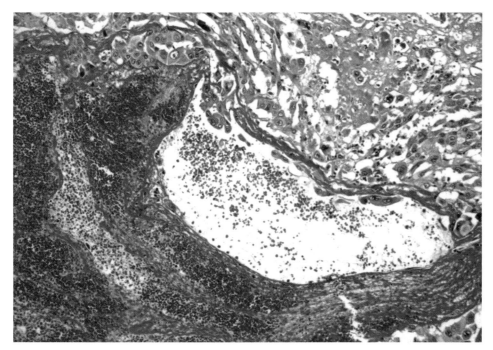

FIGURE 16.17
Placental site trophoblastic tumor. The neoplastic intermediate trophoblast cells infiltrate and replace the vascular wall and are associated with extensive fibrinoid deposition.

rounding groups of cells in most cases, a finding particularly characteristic of this tumor. Mitotic activity averages 2–5/10 HPFs, but some PSTTs may have up to 20 mitoses/10 HPFs. PSTT is not generally associated with the presence of chorionic villi.

ANCILLARY STUDIES

IMMUNOHISTOCHEMISTRY

Similar to implantation site intermediate trophoblast cells, PSTT is diffusely positive for cytokeratin (AE1/AE3 and cytokeratin 18), EMA, inhibin, HLA-G, hPL, and Mel-CAM (CD146), but rarely positive for beta-hCG and p63.

ULTRASTRUCTURAL EXAMINATION

Electron microscopy has very limited utility in the diagnosis of PSTT. The tumor cells are large and contain abundant cytoplasm. When closely apposed, their outlines are polygonal and joined by well-formed desmosomes. Free surfaces reveal microvilli that are less numerous and more blunt than the microvilli of syncytiotrophoblast cells. The cytoplasm of the intermediate trophoblast cells contains numerous organelles, although it lacks the overall complexity of the cytoplasm seen in syncytiotrophoblast cells. One frequently described feature is the presence of large paranuclear intermediate filament bundles that are apparently unique to implantation site intermediate trophoblasts in comparison with syncytiotrophoblast or cytotrophoblast cells.

DIFFERENTIAL DIAGNOSIS

Placental site trophoblastic tumor should be distinguished from exaggerated placental site, ETT, choriocarcinoma, and epithelioid smooth muscle tumor.

The differential diagnosis with an *exaggerated placental site*, a variation of normal implantation site, may be difficult, especially in curettage specimens. Both lesions are characterized by an exuberant infiltration of intermediate trophoblastic cells between the smooth muscle fibers, and they share the same immunohistochemical profile. However, an exaggerated placental site does not form a mass grossly, does not show destructive invasion of the myometrium, or form confluent sheets of cells; mitotic activity is minimal, and it is typically associated with chorionic villi. In addition, an exaggerated placental site contains larger numbers of multinucleated trophoblast cells (Figure 16.18). Ki-67 staining has been shown to be superior to mitotic index as a diagnostic adjunct is in this distinction as it is significantly elevated (> 10%) in PSTT but is almost absent in exaggerated implantation site. A diagnosis of PSTT should be strongly considered if the Ki-67 index in implantation site intermediate trophoblast cells is > 5%. If assessment of the Ki-67 index turns out to be problematic due to difficulty in recognizing intermediate trophoblast cells on immunostained slides, a double-staining technique using MIB-1 antibody to determine the Ki-67 proliferative index and Mel-CAM (CD146) or HLA-G to identify implantation site intermediate trophoblast cells has been shown to be useful (Figure 16.10).

Helpful features in the differential diagnosis between a PSTT and an *ETT* include the expansile border, alternating cellular areas and geographic areas of necrosis, prominent nested-nodular architecture, and striking

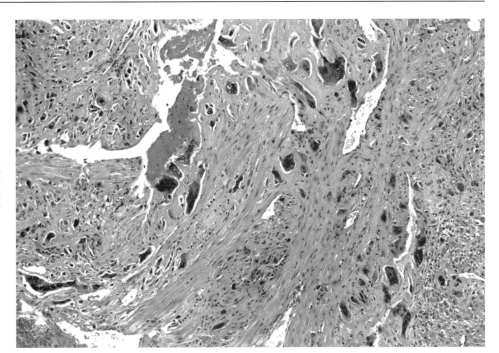

FIGURE 16.18

Exaggerated placental site. Exuberant intermediate trophoblast cells associated with syncytiotrophoblast cells infiltrate the myometrium. Notice the absence of mitoses.

hyalinization seen in an ETT. Finally, PSTT is p63 negative in contrast to ETT.

The finding of multinucleated trophoblast cells in PSTT may raise concern for *choriocarcinoma*. The characteristic biphasic growth of cyto- and syncytiotrophoblast of choriocarcinoma is absent in PSTT, which is typically composed of a relatively monomorphic population of intermediate trophoblast cells. Furthermore, in contrast to the interlacing pattern of elongated syncytiotrophoblast in choriocarcinoma, the multinucleated intermediate trophoblastic cells in PSTT are usually polygonal or round. Finally, an extensive necrotic and hemorrhagic background is more commonly seen in choriocarcinoma than in PSTT.

The differential diagnosis between a PSTT and an *epithelioid smooth muscle tumor, poorly differentiated carcinoma,* and *metastatic melanoma* can occasionally be problematic. The distinctive pattern of vascular invasion and the deposition of fibrinoid material in PSTT are helpful morphologic clues.

PROGNOSIS AND THERAPY

Most PSTTs behave in a benign fashion, whereas malignant PSTT (manifested by metastases) occurs in approximately 10–15 % of cases. Metastases can occur in the lungs (most common), liver, vagina, gastrointestinal tract, pelvis, and elsewhere. Although it is difficult to predict the behavior of these tumors with certainty, factors reported to be predictive of prognosis include tumor stage, older age (> 35 years), tumor size, depth of myometrial invasion, mitotic rate (> 5 mitoses/10 HPFs), clear cytoplasm (even when only focal), necrosis, elevated serum hCG levels, previous term pregnancy, and

increased interval from previous pregnancy (> 2 years). Among these clinicopathologic features, stage has been reported as the strongest predictor of outcome.

Hysterectomy is the treatment of choice for patients with disease confined to the uterus. In patients with stage I tumors and no adverse prognostic factors who desire preservation of fertility, more conservative surgical therapy may be considered. This may include dilatation and curettage or other uterine-sparing surgery, followed by monitoring of serum hCG levels and radiologic studies.

For patients with more extensive or metastatic disease, chemotherapy is indicated, although the clinical outcome is variable, since chemotherapy, as used for other gestational trophoblastic tumors, is usually ineffective. Thus, multiagent chemotherapy is recommended over a single agent, with complete responses reported in approximately 38 % of patients.

Because these tumors are composed of neoplastic intermediate trophoblast cells that produce only small amounts of beta-hCG, serum beta-hCG levels are usually low (100–2000 mIL/mL) in comparison to choriocarcinoma (> 10 000 mIL/mL). Despite these low serum levels, beta-hCG remains the best available marker to monitor the course of the disease, as a marked rise in serum hCG levels often occurs at the time of metastasis.

CHORIOCARCINOMA

Choriocarcinoma is a rare but highly malignant neoplasm with an incidence of 1 in 25,000–40,000 pregnancies. These tumors occur in patients with a previous history of molar pregnancy (50 %), commonly a CHM,

CHORIOCARCINOMA – FACT SHEET

Definition

▶ Malignant trophoblastic neoplasm most commonly derived from a molar pregnancy

Incidence and Age Distribution

▶ 1 in 25,000–40,000 pregnancies
▶ Previous history of molar pregnancy (50%), more commonly CHM; abortion (25%), normal pregnancy (22%), rarely ectopic pregnancy

Clinical Features

▶ Vaginal bleeding or symptoms related to distant metastases
▶ Markedly elevated serum beta-hCG level
▶ Recent pregnancy
▶ Secondary hemorrhage more commonly in lungs

Prognosis and Treatment

▶ Hematogenous metastases, more frequently to lungs, followed by vagina, liver, and brain
▶ Methotrexate-based chemotherapy
▶ Serum beta-hCG levels to monitor treatment response
▶ Almost 100% survival rate with chemotherapy

CHORIOCARCINOMA – PATHOLOGIC FEATURES

Gross Findings

Gestational Choriocarcinoma

▶ Dark-red, hemorrhagic masses with friable cut surface and variable necrosis
▶ Ill-defined infiltrative borders

Choriocarcinoma in Term Placenta

▶ Central, ill-defined, hard and often pale lesion frequently interpreted as a placental infarct

Microscopic Findings

▶ Biphasic growth with syncytiotrophoblast cells surrounding groups of cytotrophoblast cells
▶ Syncytiotrophoblast cells with abundant deeply basophilic cytoplasm and multiple large irregular and hyperchromatic nuclei
▶ Cytotrophoblast cells with clear cytoplasm and large, atypical and vesicular nuclei with clumped chromatin and prominent nucleoli
▶ Frequent mitoses in cytotrophoblast cells
▶ Minor component of intermediate trophoblast cells
▶ Prominent vascular invasion with hemorrhagic lakes and extensive necrosis
▶ No chorionic villi (in gestational choriocarcinoma)

Immunohistochemical Features

▶ HLA-G, cytokeratin 18, and inhibin diffusely positive
▶ HPL, beta-hCG, CD146, and p63 diffusely or focally positive

Differential Diagnosis

▶ Very early gestation
▶ Complete hydatidiform mole
▶ Placental site trophoblastic tumor
▶ Epithelioid trophoblastic tumor
▶ Poorly differentiated carcinoma

---

abortion (25%), normal pregnancy (22%), and rarely, an ectopic pregnancy. Choriocarcinoma may also be diagnosed concurrently with a pregnancy, usually term or nearly term, although this is a much rarer event.

CLINICAL FEATURES

Patients present with abnormal uterine bleeding and elevated serum beta-hCG levels developing several months following a pregnancy. However, symptoms may sometimes be related to metastases. In such cases, patients present with hemorrhagic events, the lungs being the most frequent metastatic site (90%).

PATHOLOGIC FEATURES

GROSS FINDINGS

Both uterine and metastatic choriocarcinomas typically form dark-red, hemorrhagic masses with a friable cut surface associated with variable amounts of necrosis and have ill-defined infiltrative borders (Figure 16.19). Occasionally, they may lack significant hemorrhage and appear as a fleshy, tan-gray mass. The tumors may vary greatly in size, ranging from tiny to large bulky masses.

Choriocarcinoma associated with a third-trimester placenta is frequently interpreted as a placental infarct. It appears as an ill-defined, hard, and often pale lesion found in an unusual site for a placental infarct (often central).

MICROSCOPIC FINDINGS

The classic pattern of choriocarcinoma has been described as bilaminar, dimorphic, or biphasic (Figure 16.20). These different terms refer to the distinctive arrangement of alternating multinucleated syncytiotrophoblast cells and mononucleate cytotrophoblast cells, where the syncytiotrophoblast cells appear to surround groups of cytotrophoblast cells (Figure 16.21). This architecture recapitulates the normal arrangement of the two types of trophoblast in the chorionic villi. The tumor may also have a minor component of intermediate trophoblast cells. Due to the extensive necrosis associated with choriocarcinoma, the neoplastic trophoblast may be scant and is likely to appear at the tumor border.

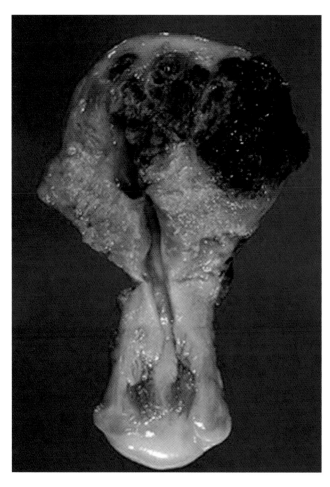

FIGURE 16.19

Choriocarcinoma. A dark-red, hemorrhagic mass with a shaggy, irregular cut surface diffusely infiltrates the myometrium.

Thus, extensive sampling may be necessary to visualize the diagnostic biphasic growth. Rarely, if the syncytiotrophoblast cells are inconspicuous, the tumor may be predominantly composed of mononucleated cells. Although vascular invasion is often striking, choriocarcinoma lacks intrinsic endothelium-lined vascular channels, making it a unique malignant solid tumor without associated angiogenesis. Instead, the tumors receive their blood supply from invasion of pre-existing vessels with secondary formation of hemorrhagic lakes. At higher power, the syncytiotrophoblast cells have abundant deeply eosinophilic cytoplasm and multiple large irregular and hyperchromatic nuclei. The cytotrophoblast cells are polygonal with clear cytoplasm and large, atypical, and vesicular nuclei with clumped chromatin, prominent nucleoli, and frequent mitoses.

By definition, chorionic villi are not seen in choriocarcinoma, except when the tumor arises in a third-trimester placenta. In these instances, the typical biphasic growth of cytotrophoblast and syncytiotrophoblast is seen in a background of normally developed placenta (Figure 16.22).

ANCILLARY STUDIES

IMMUNOHISTOCHEMISTRY

Syncytiotrophoblast cells are strongly reactive to cytokeratin 18, beta-hCG, and hPL, while the cytotrophoblast cells are only reactive to cytokeratin 18. The minor component of intermediate trophoblast cells is

FIGURE 16.20

Gestational choriocarcinoma. Biphasic growth of cyto- and syncytiotrophoblast cells.

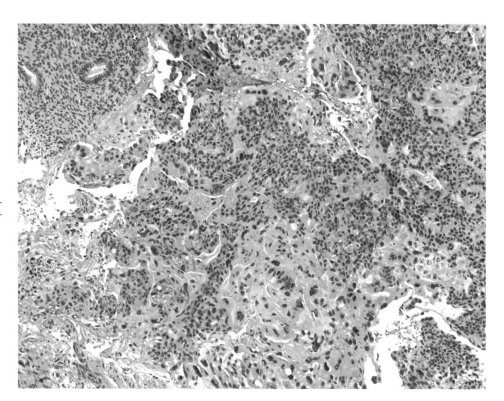

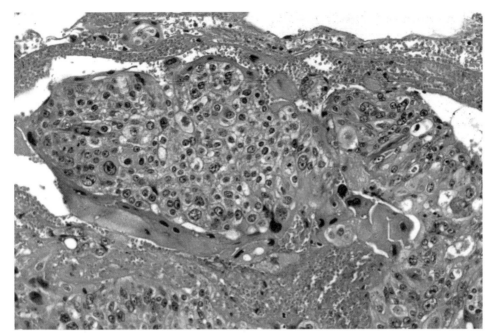

FIGURE 16.21

Gestational choriocarcinoma. Cytotrophoblast cells are "hugged" by elongated syncytiotrophoblast cells showing deeply eosinophilic cytoplasm. Notice the hemorrhagic background.

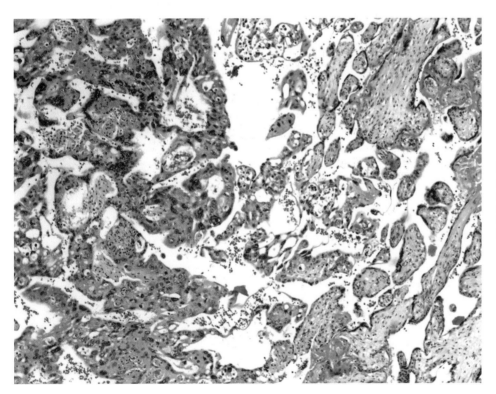

FIGURE 16.22

Choriocarcinoma in a term placenta. A biphasic growth of cyto- and syncytiotrophoblast is juxtaposed to mature terminal villi of a term placenta.

positive for hPL, Mel-CAM (CD146), HLA-G, inhibin, and cytokeratin 18.

ULTRASTRUCTURAL EXAMINATION

The tumor cells in choriocarcinoma have features similar to trophoblast in normal placenta and hydatidiform mole. Cytotrophoblast cells are characterized by numerous free cytoplasmic ribosomes and aggregates of particulate glycogen. Interestingly, other organelles are

sparse, including mitochondria, rough endoplasmic reticulum, and Golgi complexes. The cells are joined by widely separated, well-formed desmosomes. In contrast, syncytiotrophoblast cells have complex cytoplasmic contents and cell membrane structure. Thick bundles of tonofilaments are scattered throughout, while the cell surface is covered with many long microvilli. They are joined directly to cytotrophoblast cells by desmosomes. In addition to multiple nuclei that tend to have highly irregular outlines and coarsely clumped chromatin, syncytiotrophoblast cells demonstrate an electron-dense cytoplasm due to the presence of multiple organelles.

DIFFERENTIAL DIAGNOSIS

Choriocarcinoma should be distinguished from normal trophoblast of early gestation, molar pregnancies, PSTT, and other malignancies with an epithelioid phenotype.

Although infrequent, normal trophoblast of *very early gestation* (before the villi are fully developed) can be found in curettage specimens in the absence of associated chorionic villi. In this circumstance, trophoblast should only be present in small amounts. Trophoblast of early gestation does not show the atypical cellular features found in choriocarcinoma. Furthermore, fragments of normal trophoblast are not associated with necrosis or destructive invasion. Thus, large amounts of trophoblast showing atypia should be considered highly suspicious for choriocarcinoma.

Distinguishing choriocarcinoma from *poorly differentiated carcinoma*, within or outside the uterus, is not usually a problem. Occasionally, however, a small sample of a lesion may contain few syncytiotrophoblast cells or be composed entirely of mononucleate trophoblast cells, a pattern that can mimic a poorly differentiated carcinoma. When this diagnostic quandary arises, a clinical history of previous molar pregnancy or other suspicious gestational event can assist in the diagnosis. Serum beta-hCG levels and immunohistochemical localization of beta-hCG, hPL, and inhibin in the syncytiotrophoblast cells can also be useful.

The differential diagnoses of choriocarcinoma with *ETT* and *PSTT* have been discussed in previous sections.

PROGNOSIS AND THERAPY

Choriocarcinoma disseminates hematogenously, most frequently metastasizing to the lungs, followed by vagina, liver, and brain. Prior to the development of effective cytotoxic chemotherapy, gestational choriocarcinoma was often fatal. Survival rates have dramatically improved since the use of cytotoxic chemotherapy combined with accurate and sensitive assays for beta-hCG to monitor the course of this disease. With the introduction of chemotherapy regimens, choriocarcinoma is now one of the few potentially curable cancers, with an overall survival at the present time that approaches 100%.

SUGGESTED READING

Hydatidiform Moles

Fukunaga M, Katabuchi H, Nagasaka T, et al. Interobserver and intraobserver variability in the diagnosis of hydatidiform mole. Am J Surg Pathol 2005;29:942–947.

Hui P, Martel M, Parkash V. Gestational trophoblastic diseases: recent advances in histopathologic diagnosis and related genetic aspects. Adv Anat Pathol 2005;12:116–125.

Keep D, Zaragoza MV, Hassold T, et al. Very early complete hydatidiform mole. Hum Pathol 1996;27:708–713.

Mosher R, Goldstein DP, Berkowitz R, et al. Complete hydatidiform mole. Comparison of clinicopathologic features, current and past. J Reprod Med 1998;43:21–27.

Nonmolar Trophoblastic Lesions

Baergen RN, Rutgers JL, Young RH, et al. Placental site trophoblastic tumor: a study of 55 cases and review of the literature emphasizing factors of prognostic significance. Gynecol Oncol 2006;100:511–520.

Fadare O, Parkash V, Carcangiu ML, et al. Epithelioid trophoblastic tumor: clinicopathological features with an emphasis on uterine cervical involvement. Mod Pathol 2006;19:75–82.

Feltmate CM, Genest DR, Goldstein DP, et al. Advances in the understanding of placental site trophoblastic tumor. J Reprod Med 2002;47:337–341.

Oldt RJ, 3rd, Kurman RJ, Shih Ie M. Molecular genetic analysis of placental site trophoblastic tumors and epithelioid trophoblastic tumors confirms their trophoblastic origin. Am J Pathol 2002;161:1033–1037.

Shih I-M, Kurman RJ. Epithelioid trophoblastic tumor – a neoplasm distinct from choriocarcinoma and placental site trophoblastic tumor simulating carcinoma. Am J Surg Pathol 1998;22:1393–1403.

Shih IM, Kurman RJ. The pathology of intermediate trophoblastic tumors and tumor-like lesions. Int J Gynecol Pathol 2001;20:31–47.

Shih IM, Seidman JD, Kurman RJ. Placental site nodule and characterization of distinctive types of intermediate trophoblast. Hum Pathol 1999;30:687–694.

Young RH, Kurman RJ, Scully RE. Placental site nodules and plaques. A clinicopathologic analysis of 20 cases. Am J Surg Pathol 1990;14:1001–1009.

Immunohistochemistry

Castrillon DH, Sun D, Weremowicz S, et al. Discrimination of complete hydatidiform mole from its mimics by immunohistochemistry of the paternally imprinted gene product p57KIP2. Am J Surg Pathol 2001;25:1225–1230.

Shih IM, Kurman RJ. Ki-67 labeling index in the differential diagnosis of exaggerated placental site, placental site trophoblastic tumor, and choriocarcinoma: a double immunohistochemical staining technique using Ki-67 and Mel-CAM antibodies. Hum Pathol 1998;29:27–33.

Shih IM, Kurman RJ. Immunohistochemical localization of inhibin-alpha in the placenta and gestational trophoblastic lesions. Int J Gynecol Pathol 1999;18:144–150.

Shih IM, Kurman RJ. p63 Expression is useful in the distinction of epithelioid trophoblastic and placental site trophoblastic tumors by profiling trophoblastic subpopulations. Am J Surg Pathol 2004;28:1177–1183.

Singer G, Kurman RJ, McMaster M, et al. HLA-G immunoreactivity is specific for intermediate trophoblast in gestational trophoblastic disease and can serve as a useful marker in differential diagnosis. Am J Surg Pathol 2002;26:914–920.

Immunohistochemistry in the Differential Diagnosis of Female Genital Tract Pathology

W Glenn McCluggage

Until recently, immunohistochemistry was rarely used as a diagnostic aid in gynecological pathology. However, lately there has been a marked expansion of the literature regarding the utility of immunohistochemical markers in the diagnosis of lesions of the female genital tract. In this chapter, the value of these markers is detailed. Markers of prognostic significance are not covered since these are few and, in general, offer no advantage over careful pathological examination. The uses of immunohistochemistry are covered by site within the female genital tract with an emphasis on the most useful panels of markers in various diagnostic situations.

VULVA AND VAGINA

PREINVASIVE VULVAL SQUAMOUS LESIONS

In the vulva, the morphological hallmarks of HPV infection, such as koilocytosis, may not be as well developed as in the cervix and therefore, it may be difficult to diagnose a viral-induced lesion. In equivocal cases, in which the diagnosis of condyloma is suspected, immunohistochemical staining with the proliferation marker MIB-1 may be of value as low-risk HPV infection of the vulva is associated with the presence of MIB-1-positive nuclei in the middle and upper thirds of the epithelium, which is in contrast to reactive epithelium, in which the

positivity is typically confined to the basal and parabasal area. MIB-1 staining is also useful in confirming a high-grade VIN as the cells of high-grade VIN (VIN II–III) express MIB-1 throughout much of the full epithelial thickness (Figure 17.1) which is useful in the separation of high-grade VIN from atrophic squamous epithelium. Another marker that may be helpful in supporting the diagnosis of VIN associated with high-risk HPV subtypes, i.e., high-grade VIN, is p16 as this marker is typically positive (both in the nucleus and the cytoplasm) in these HPV-related lesions (Figure 17.1). In contrast, HPV-negative VIN, i.e., differentiated VIN, is p16-negative. Immunohistochemistry may also assist in the diagnosis of differentiated VIN, which may be a difficult diagnosis since its morphological features may be subtle. Intense nuclear staining for p53 in the basal and suprabasal cells is characteristic of differentiated VIN and may help distinguish it from nonneoplastic squamous epithelium.

VULVAL PAGET DISEASE

Immunohistochemistry may be of value in the diagnosis of Paget disease involving the vulva and in the distinction of primary Paget disease (which is not usually associated with an underlying malignancy) from Paget disease secondary to spread from an internal organ such

---

PREINVASIVE VULVAL SQUAMOUS LESIONS – FACT SHEET

▶ MIB-1 positivity in upper epithelial layers supports the histologic impression of vulvar condyloma
▶ High-grade VIN exhibits full-thickness MIB-1 positivity and is useful in its distinction from atrophic epithelium
▶ p16 positivity supports diagnosis of HPV related high-grade VIN
▶ Nuclear positivity for p53 in basal and suprabasal squamous cells is characteristic of HPV-negative VIN ("differentiated VIN")

VULVAL PAGET DISEASE – FACT SHEET

▶ Primary vulval Paget disease typically CAM 5.2, CK7, G-CDFP-15, and CEA positive
▶ Pagetoid Bowen disease typically CK 7, CAM 5.2, G-CDFP-15, and CEA negative
▶ Pagetoid urothelial carcinoma typically uroplakin-III positive; variably CK20 and CEA positive; and CK7 and G-CDFP-15 negative
▶ Paget disease secondary to spread from a colorectal primary typically CK20 and CEA positive; CK7 and GCDFP negative

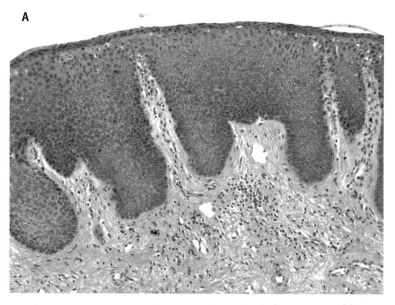

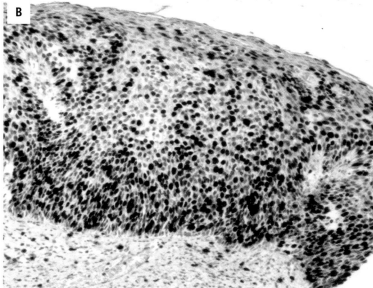

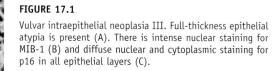

FIGURE 17.1

Vulvar intraepithelial neoplasia III. Full-thickness epithelial atypia is present (A). There is intense nuclear staining for MIB-1 (B) and diffuse nuclear and cytoplasmic staining for p16 in all epithelial layers (C).

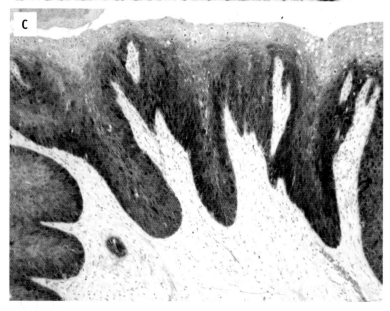

as the colorectum or urinary bladder. Positivity of Paget cells with CAM5.2 (Figure 17.2) and CEA helps to exclude pagetoid Bowen disease, melanocytic lesions, and mycosis fungoides, which would be negative for this marker. The cells of primary vulval Paget disease are also positive for CK7 (Figure 17.2) and GCDFP-15. These markers not only confirm the diagnosis, but are also useful in the determination of margin status and in identifying small foci of dermal invasion. In contrast to primary Paget disease, most cases of pagetoid Bowen disease are CK7 negative, although CK7 positivity has been described in pagetoid Bowen disease of the external genitalia in both males and females. While primary Paget disease may show focal CK20 positivity, diffuse positivity for this marker strongly raises the possibility of spread from an internal organ such as the colorectum or urinary bladder, as primary carcinomas in these sites are commonly CK20 positive. Paget disease secondary to spread from a urinary bladder carcinoma is also commonly positive for uroplakin-III whereas those secondary to a colorectal adenocarcinoma stain with MUC2. In addition, secondary Paget disease is usually negative for GCDFP-15. Positive p53 staining of the intraepithelial cells of primary vulval Paget disease may be associated with an increased likelihood of dermal invasion.

VULVOVAGINAL MESENCHYMAL LESIONS

Since many of the relatively site-specific vulvovaginal mesenchymal lesions are positive for ER (Figure 17.3), PR, desmin (Figure 17.4), and α-SMA, immunohistochemistry is of limited value in distinguishing between the various entities. However, it may be useful in the diagnosis of cellular angiofibroma since this tumor is usually, although not always, negative for smooth muscle markers, whereas most of the other vulvovaginal mesenchymal lesions are at least focally positive for desmin, α-SMA, or h-caldesmon.

Immunohistochemical staining with HMGA2 (formerly HMGIC) may also be of value in the diagnosis of aggressive angiomyxoma, which usually exhibits nuclear positivity, as most of the other vulvovaginal mesenchymal lesions are typically negative. Staining with HMGA2

may also be of value in the assessment of margins in resection specimens and in the determination of the presence or absence of residual disease in wider excision specimens, since nonneo-plastic vulvovaginal mesenchyme is negative for this marker.

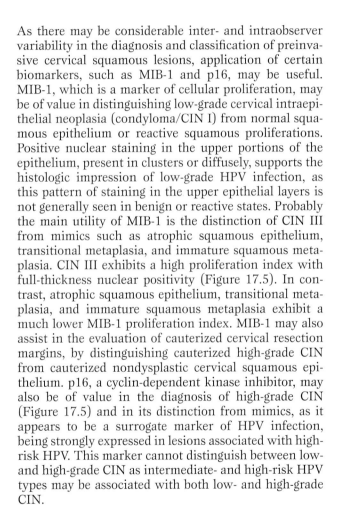

UTERINE CERVIX

PREINVASIVE CERVICAL SQUAMOUS LESIONS

As there may be considerable inter- and intraobserver variability in the diagnosis and classification of preinvasive cervical squamous lesions, application of certain biomarkers, such as MIB-1 and p16, may be useful. MIB-1, which is a marker of cellular proliferation, may be of value in distinguishing low-grade cervical intraepithelial neoplasia (condyloma/CIN I) from normal squamous epithelium or reactive squamous proliferations. Positive nuclear staining in the upper portions of the epithelium, present in clusters or diffusely, supports the histologic impression of low-grade HPV infection, as this pattern of staining in the upper epithelial layers is not generally seen in benign or reactive states. Probably the main utility of MIB-1 is the distinction of CIN III from mimics such as atrophic squamous epithelium, transitional metaplasia, and immature squamous metaplasia. CIN III exhibits a high proliferation index with full-thickness nuclear positivity (Figure 17.5). In contrast, atrophic squamous epithelium, transitional metaplasia, and immature squamous metaplasia exhibit a much lower MIB-1 proliferation index. MIB-1 may also assist in the evaluation of cauterized cervical resection margins, by distinguishing cauterized high-grade CIN from cauterized nondysplastic cervical squamous epithelium. p16, a cyclin-dependent kinase inhibitor, may also be of value in the diagnosis of high-grade CIN (Figure 17.5) and in its distinction from mimics, as it appears to be a surrogate marker of HPV infection, being strongly expressed in lesions associated with high-risk HPV. This marker cannot distinguish between low- and high-grade CIN as intermediate- and high-risk HPV types may be associated with both low- and high-grade CIN.

VULVOVAGINAL MESENCHYMAL LESIONS – FACT SHEET

▶ Most vulvovaginal mesenchymal lesions share immunohistochemical profiles, being positive for α-SMA, desmin, ER, and PR
▶ Cellular angiofibroma, unlike other mesenchymal tumors at this site, is usually negative for smooth muscle markers
▶ HMGA2 may be useful in the distinction of aggressive angiomyxoma from other mesenchymal tumors

---

PREINVASIVE CERVICAL SQUAMOUS LESIONS – FACT SHEET

▶ MIB-1-positive cell clusters in the upper epithelial layers can help discriminate condyloma/CIN I from reactive squamous epithelium
▶ MIB-1 positivity in the upper epithelial cell layers can help discriminate CIN III from atrophic squamous epithelium and immature squamous metaplasia
▶ p16 positivity is a surrogate marker for high-risk HPV

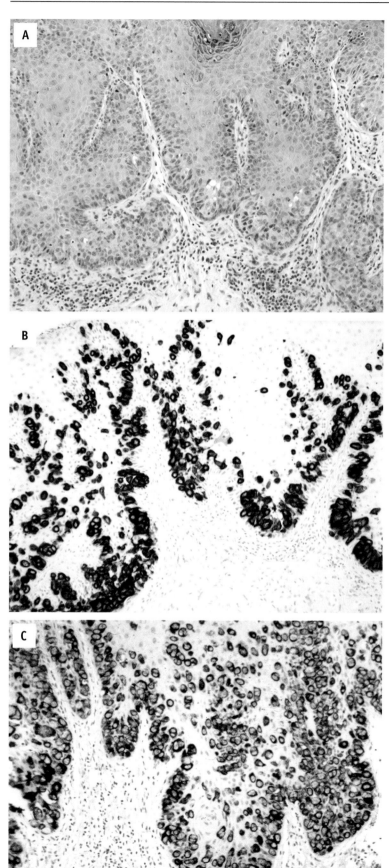

FIGURE 17.2

Vulval Paget disease. Large epithelioid cells are present singly and in clusters within the epidermis, most often in the parabasal area (A). Tumor cells typically exhibit CAM5.2 (B) and diffuse CK7 positivity (C). Note that the nonneoplastic squamous epithelium is negative for these markers.

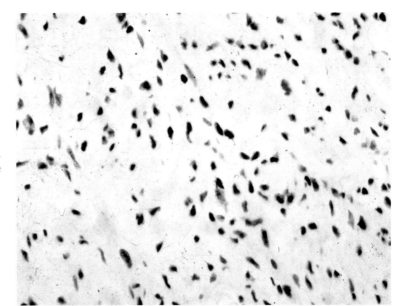

FIGURE 17.3

Vulval aggressive angiomyxoma. Diffuse nuclear ER positivity is present. Most vulval mesenchymal tumors are positive for this marker.

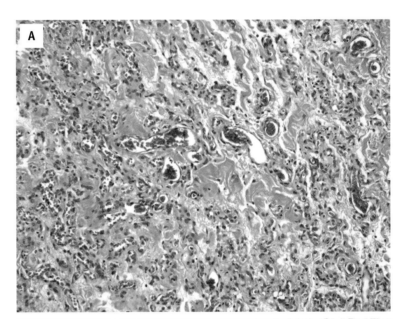

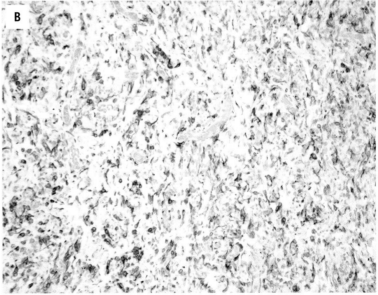

FIGURE 17.4

Vulval angiomyofibroblastoma. A highly vascular tumor shows variably cellular stroma (A) and exhibits diffuse desmin positivity (B). Many vulval mesenchymal tumors are positive for this marker.

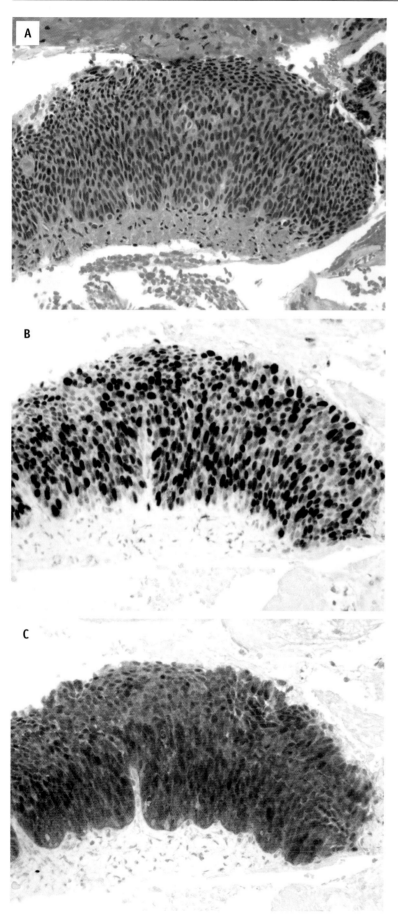

FIGURE 17.5

Cervical intraepithelial neoplasia III. Crowded monomorphic proliferation of cells with hyperchromatic nuclei lack maturation (A). The presence of diffuse nuclear staining for MIB-1 (B) and diffuse nuclear and cytoplasmic p16 staining throughout the full epithelial thickness (C) supports this diagnosis.

PREINVASIVE CERVICAL GLANDULAR LESIONS

The distinction between cervical adenocarcinoma in situ (AIS) and benign mimics, including tuboendometrial metaplasia (TEM), endometriosis, and microglandular hyperplasia (MGH), may be problematic. A panel of markers, including MIB-1, bcl-2, and p16, may assist in difficult cases. AIS generally exhibits a high MIB-1 proliferation index, usually > 30% and often much higher (Figure 17.6). In contrast, most benign endocervical glandular lesions exhibit a low proliferation index < 30%. However, sometimes there is overlap, with occasional cases of AIS exhibiting a low MIB-1 proliferation index and some benign endocervical glandular lesions exhibiting a proliferation index > 30%. Almost all AIS exhibit diffuse nuclear and cytoplasmic p16 positivity (Figure 17.6), while MGH is typically negative. TEM and endometriosis are often positive for p16, usually focal in distribution (Figure 17.7), contrasting with the diffuse positivity in AIS; similarly, MIB-1 index is also typically much lower (Figure 17.7). TEM and endometriosis also exhibit diffuse cytoplasmic positivity for bcl-2 (Figure 17.8), whereas AIS is generally negative. CEA may also be of value in the distinction of AIS (usually cytoplasmic positivity) and benign mimics (negative or luminal positivity), although there is significant overlap and in an individual case, it may not be discriminatory. TEM and endometriosis are also generally vimentin-positive while AIS is negative.

PREINVASIVE CERVICAL GLANDULAR LESIONS AND MIMICS – FACT SHEET

▸ Adenocarcinoma in situ usually exhibits a high MIB-1 proliferation index, diffuse p16 nuclear and cytoplasmic positivity, shows cytoplasmic positivity for CEA, and is negative for bcl-2 and vimentin

▸ Tuboendometrioid metaplasia usually exhibits a low MIB-1 proliferation index, is bcl-2 and vimentin positive, but p16 and CEA negative

▸ Microglandular hyperplasia usually p16 and bcl-2 negative and has a low MIB-1 proliferation index

---

CERVICAL MESONEPHRIC LESIONS

Mesonephric remnants are common within the cervix and especially when hyperplastic, may be confused with other benign endocervical glandular lesions. Rarely, a mesonephric adenocarcinoma arises within the cervix. CD10 is a useful immunohistochemical marker of cervical mesonephric lesions, both benign and malignant,

---

CERVICAL MESONEPHRIC LESIONS – FACT SHEET

▸ Mesonephric remnants, hyperplasia, and, to a lesser extent, carcinoma exhibit luminal staining for CD10

▸ Mesonephric lesions may be positive for vimentin, calretinin, and AR

---

although mesonephric adenocarcinomas are less likely to be positive. CD10 characteristically exhibits luminal positivity in cervical mesonephric remnants (Figure 17.9) and is therefore a good indicator of mesonephric origin. However, some usual endocervical adenocarcinomas are CD10 positive and thus, this marker is of limited value in confirmation of a mesonephric origin of an adenocarcinoma. Other markers that may be positive in cervical mesonephric lesions are vimentin, calretinin, and AR. These markers are also often positive in benign and malignant mesonephric lesions elsewhere within the female genital tract.

CERVICAL MINIMAL-DEVIATION ADENOCARCINOMA OF MUCINOUS TYPE (ADENOMA MALIGNUM)

The mucinous variant of cervical minimal-deviation adenocarcinoma (adenoma malignum) often exhibits a gastric or pyloric immunophenotype, which may be useful in its distinction from well-differentiated endocervical adenocarcinoma, not otherwise specified (NOS), and other benign mimics. In most cases, there is positivity for HIK1083, an antibody directed against pyloric gland mucin, whereas most usual endocervical adenocarcinomas and benign endocervical glandular lesions are negative. Adenoma malignum is also usually p16 negative, in contrast to the diffuse positivity seen in most usual endocervical adenocarcinomas. The benign endocervical glandular lesion termed lobular endocervical glandular hyperplasia, NOS may also exhibit a pyloric phenotype and be positive for HIK1083; therefore, one must rely on the differences in morphologic appearance to make the distinction between these two entities. It has been suggested that in some cases this is a precursor lesion of cervical adenoma malignum.

CERVICAL MINIMAL-DEVIATION ADENOCARCINOMA – FACT SHEET

▸ Cervical minimal-deviation adenocarcinoma is characteristically HIK1083 positive.

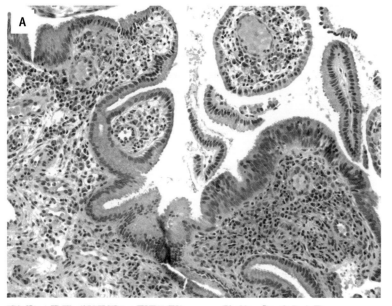

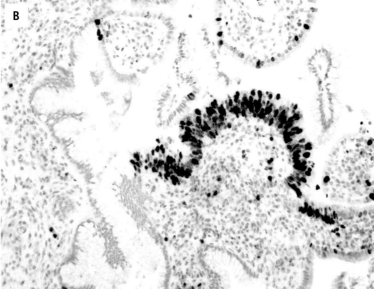

FIGURE 17.6

Cervical adenocarcinoma in situ (AIS). A subtle focus of AIS (A) shows high MIB-1 proliferation index (B) and diffuse nuclear and cytoplasmic positivity for p16 (C).

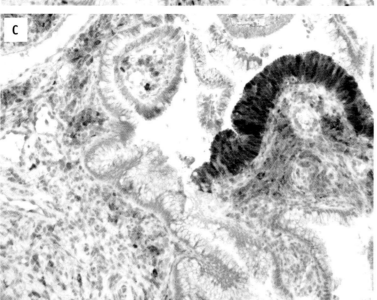

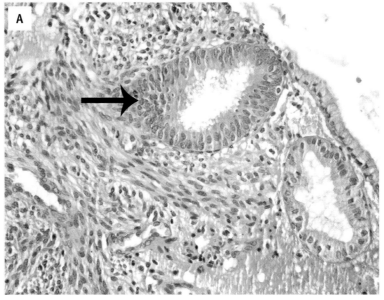

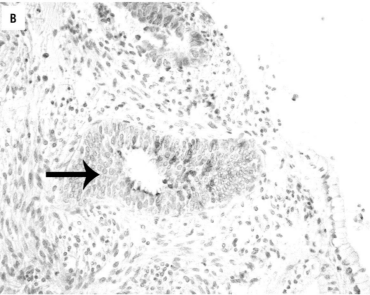

FIGURE 17.7

Cervical tuboendometrioid metaplasia. A gland showing tuboendometrioid metaplasia (A) exhibiting weak staining for p16 (B) and a low MIB-1 proliferation index (C).

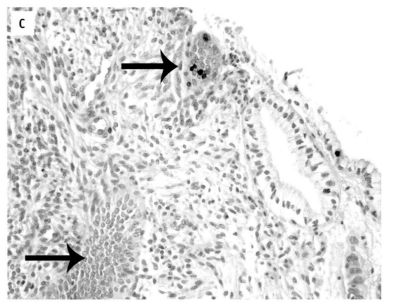

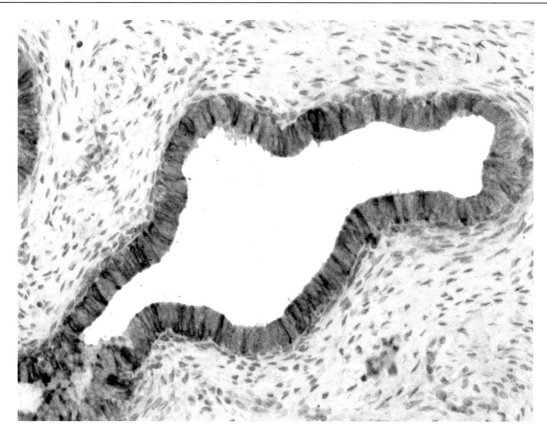

FIGURE 17.8
Cervical tuboendometrioid metaplasia. There is diffuse bcl-2 staining.

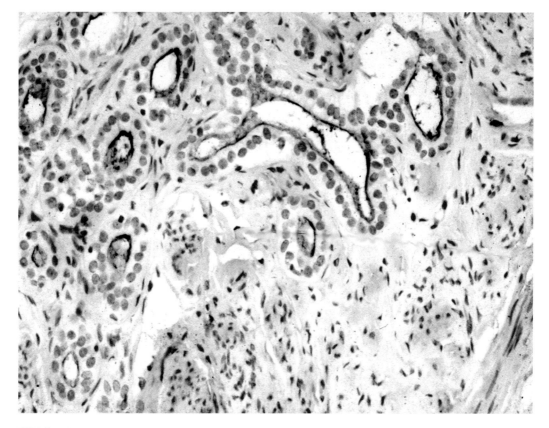

FIGURE 17.9
Cervical mesonephric remnants. Characteristic CD10 luminal staining is seen.

DISTINCTION BETWEEN ENDOMETRIAL AND ENDOCERVICAL ADENOCARCINOMA

On occasion, it is difficult to distinguish an endometrial versus an endocervical origin of an adenocarcinoma in biopsy/curettage material. In such cases, a panel of antibodies comprising ER, vimentin, monoclonal CEA, and p16 is of value in distinguishing between a usual cervical adenocarcinoma and an endometrioid adenocarcinoma of the endometrium. Endometrial adenocarcinomas of endometrioid type usually exhibit diffuse nuclear positivity for ER (Figure 17.10) and diffuse cytoplasmic positivity for vimentin (Figure 17.11). CEA and p16 are usually negative or only focally positive, although occasionally p16 may be diffusely positive in endometrial

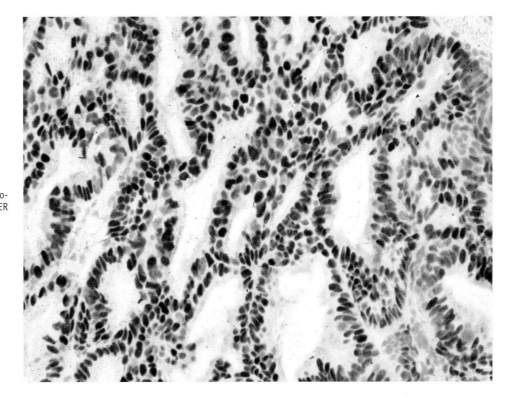

FIGURE 17.10

Endometrial adenocarcinoma, endometrioid type. Diffuse nuclear ER positivity is characteristic.

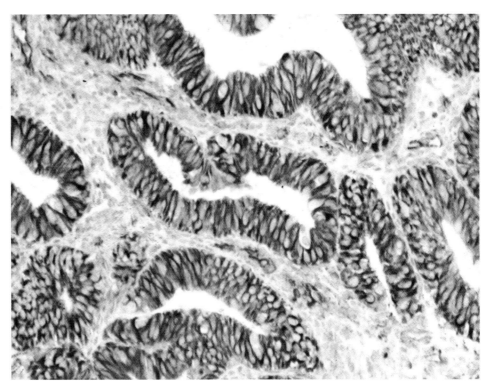

FIGURE 17.11

Endometrial adenocarcinoma, endometrioid type. Diffuse cytoplasmic vimentin positivity is typically seen.

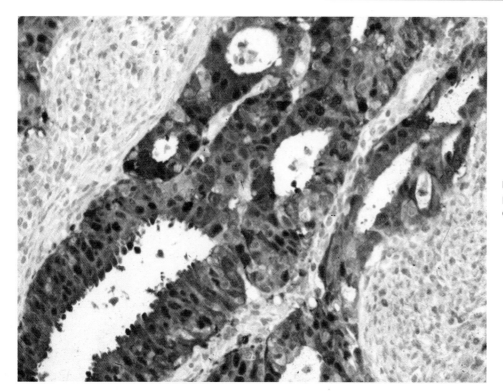

FIGURE 17.12
Endocervical adenocarcinoma. Diffuse cytoplasmic CEA positivity is seen.

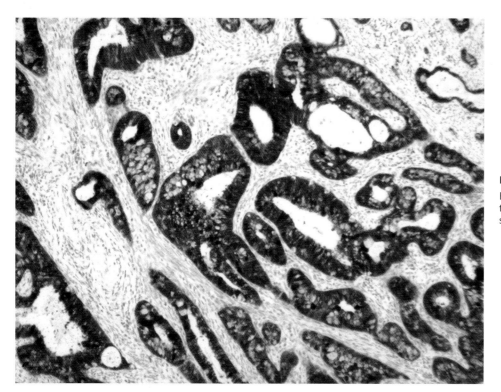

FIGURE 17.13
Endocervical adenocarcinoma. The tumor cells show strong and extensive p16 positivity is present.

endometrioid adenocarcinoma and is thus a potential pitfall in immunostain interpretation. Furthermore, squamoid elements, which are common in endometrial adenocarcinomas of endometrioid type, are often positive for both CEA and p16, and should not be included in the interpretation of the final results. In contrast most, but not all, endocervical adenocarcinomas are positive for CEA (Figure 17.12) and exhibit diffuse nuclear and cytoplasmic positivity for p16 (Figure 17.13), but ER and vimentin are generally negative or only focally positive. Immunohistochemistry is also helpful to distinguish a mucinous carcinoma of the endometrium and an endometrioid endocervical adenocarcinoma. If the tumor shows diffuse positivity for both ER and vimentin, the tumor is almost certainly of endometrial origin. The aforementioned panel of antibodies may be combined with molecular methods, such as in situ hybridization, to detect HPV, which is demonstrable in almost all cervical adenocarcinomas, whereas endometrial adenocarcinomas are negative.

CERVICAL NEUROENDOCRINE CARCINOMAS

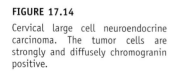

Establishing a diagnosis of a cervical neuroendocrine carcinoma is important since these are highly aggressive neoplasms that are treated with different chemotherapeutic regimens. It may be difficult to distinguish a small cell neuroendocrine carcinoma from a small cell nonkeratinizing squamous carcinoma as both are composed of small cells with scant amounts of cytoplasm and the latter may not exhibit obvious morphologic features of squamous differentiation. Similarly, the distinction between a large cell neuroendocrine carcinoma and an undifferentiated carcinoma or a poorly differentiated squamous or adenocarcinoma may be difficult. In problematic cases, neuroendocrine markers, such as chromogranin A, synaptophysin, PGP9.5, and CD56, may be useful. However, positivity for these markers is not required for the diagnosis of cervical small cell neuroendocrine carcinomas as these tumors are commonly only focally positive (and in some cases negative). Positive staining with neuroendocrine markers, however, is a prerequisite to diagnose a cervical large cell neuroendocrine carcinoma (Figure 17.14). p63 may also be of value since most squamous carcinomas are diffusely positive while neuroendocrine carcinomas, including small cell neuroendocrine carcinoma, are negative or only focally positive.

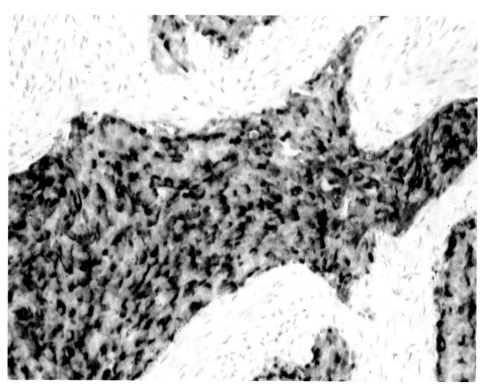

FIGURE 17.14
Cervical large cell neuroendocrine carcinoma. The tumor cells are strongly and diffusely chromogranin positive.

UTERINE CORPUS

TYPE I VERSUS TYPE II ENDOMETRIAL CARCINOMA

A dualistic model of endometrial carcinogenesis is well established. The prototype type 1 endometrial carcinoma is endometrioid-type whereas the most common type 2 carcinoma is serous (papillary) carcinoma. The distinction between an endometrioid and serous carcinoma is usually straightforward. However, many endometrioid adenocarcinomas have a papillary architecture and may be confused with serous carcinoma. Conversely, a glandular variant of serous carcinoma exists with little or no papillary formation and this may be misdiagnosed as an endometrioid adenocarcinoma. In difficult cases, immunohistochemical staining with ER, PR, and p53 may assist in this distinction. Endometrioid adenocarcinomas (especially low-grade) usually exhibit diffuse nuclear positivity for ER and PR whereas p53 is negative or only focally positive. Conversely, most serous carcinomas exhibit diffuse nuclear p53 positivity (Figure 17.15), while ER and PR are negative or only focally positive, a profile useful in the diagnosis of the glandular variant of serous carcinoma. However, immunophenotypic overlap may occur, therefore, correlation with morphology is essential as some endometrioid carcinomas (predominantly but not exclusively high grade) exhibit p53 positivity. Moreover, a small number of serous carcinomas are p53 negative and some are positive for ER and PR. Additionally, mixed serous and endometrioid adenocarcinomas are not uncommon and these also may have an overlapping immunophenotype.

DISTINCTION BETWEEN UTERINE SEROUS CARCINOMA (USC) AND OVARIAN SEROUS CARCINOMA (OSC)

When disseminated serous carcinoma involves the uterus, ovaries, and peritoneum, it may be difficult to ascertain the primary site of origin. Immunohistochemical staining with an antibody against the N-terminal of

TYPE I VERSUS TYPE II ENDOMETRIAL CARCINOMA – FACT SHEET

‣ Endometrioid adenocarcinoma (type 1) usually diffusely positive for ER and PR, and negative for p53 (especially low grade)
‣ Serous carcinoma (type 2) is usually diffusely positive for p53, and negative for ER and PR

UTERINE SEROUS CARCINOMA VERSUS OVARIAN SEROUS CARCINOMA – FACT SHEET

‣ WT1 (antibody against N-terminal) generally diffusely positive in ovarian serous carcinoma whereas most, but not all, uterine serous carcinomas negative (or only focally positive)

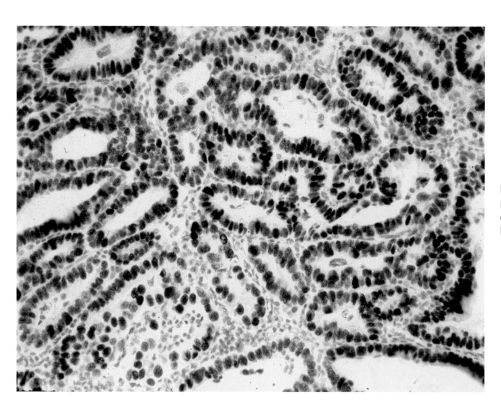

FIGURE 17.15
Uterine serous carcinoma. The tumor cells exhibit strong nuclear p53 positivity.

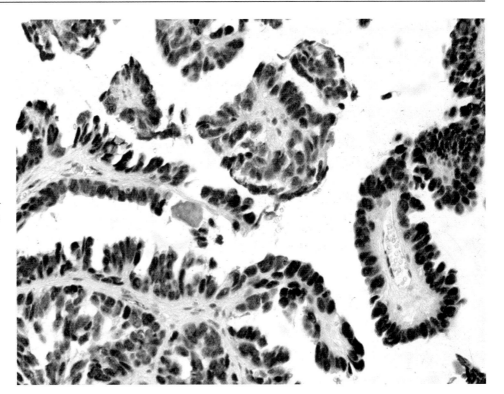

FIGURE 17.16

Ovarian serous carcinoma. The tumor shows strong nuclear WT1 positivity.

WT1 may assist in the distinction between OSC and USC. Most OSCs (and primary peritoneal and tubal serous carcinomas) exhibit diffuse nuclear positivity (Figure 17.16) while most, but not all, USCs are negative or only focally positive; therefore, diffuse nuclear WT1 positivity argues against a uterine primary. However, there is some immunohistochemical overlap as a very small proportion of OSCs are WT1-negative while some USCs exhibit focal positivity (and occasional cases are diffusely positive). Thus, the results of WT1 staining should always be correlated with clinical, morphologic, and radiologic features.

ENDOMETRIAL STROMAL VERSUS SMOOTH MUSCLE NEOPLASM – FACT SHEET

▶ Endometrial stromal neoplasms typically diffusely positive for CD10 but many cellular and highly cellular leiomyomas also diffusely positive

▶ Desmin diffusely positive in most smooth muscle neoplasms; most endometrial stromal neoplasms negative or only focally positive

▶ Uterine smooth muscle neoplasms typically diffusely positive for h-caldesmon; endometrial stromal neoplasms usually negative

DISTINCTION BETWEEN ENDOMETRIAL STROMAL AND SMOOTH MUSCLE NEOPLASMS

A panel of immunohistochemical stains, including CD10, desmin, and h-caldesmon may be useful in distinguishing between an endometrial stromal and a smooth muscle neoplasm, as these tumors may exhibit morphologic overlap. Most endometrial stromal neoplasms exhibit diffuse positivity for CD10 (Figure 17.17); however, some uterine smooth muscle neoplasms are also positive, and cellular and highly cellular leiomyomas (which are most likely to be misdiagnosed as endometrial stromal neoplasms) may exhibit diffuse positivity. Desmin is of value in that most smooth muscle neoplasms exhibit diffuse positivity (Figure 17.18), whereas although some endometrial stromal neoplasms are positive, diffuse staining is uncommon. In addition, most uterine smooth muscle neoplasms exhibit diffuse positivity for h-caldesmon whereas most endometrial stromal neoplasms are negative (positivity being confined to areas of smooth muscle differentiation). α-SMA is of limited value since, although most smooth muscle neoplasms are diffusely positive, many endometrial stromal neoplasms are also positive, including some with diffuse reactivity.

Other antibodies, which may be positive in both uterine endometrial stromal and smooth muscle neoplasms, include ER, PR, cytokeratin, and WT1. Oxytocin receptor, however, is positive in uterine smooth muscle but not endometrial stromal neoplasms.

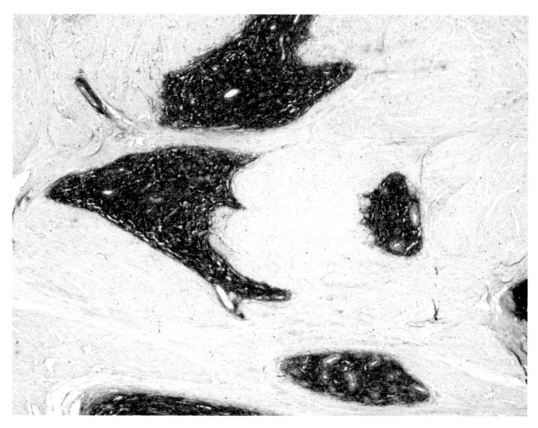

FIGURE 17.17
Endometrial stromal sarcoma. Diffuse CD10 positivity highlights the tumor cells.

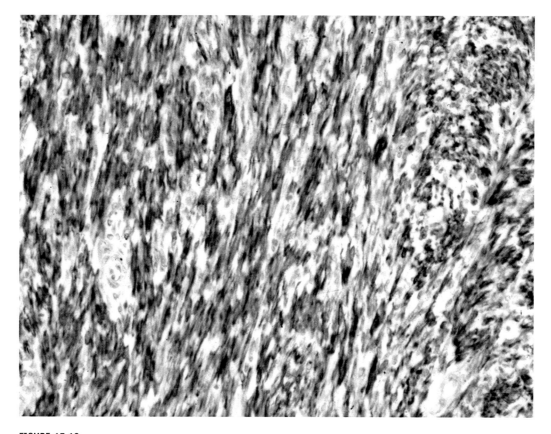

FIGURE 17.18
Highly cellular leiomyoma. The tumor exhibits diffuse desmin positivity.

UTERINE TUMOR RESEMBLING OVARIAN SEX CORD TUMOR (UTROSCT)

These unusual uterine tumors morphologically resemble ovarian sex cord tumors. Minor foci of sex cord differentiation may be found in otherwise typical endo-metrial stromal neoplasms, but the term "UTROSCT" is reserved for tumors in which the sex cord-like areas predominate or are exclusive. UTROSCT (and sex cord-like areas in endometrial stromal neoplasms) may be positive for a variety of markers, including smooth muscle antibodies, cytokeratins, and hormone receptors. Some are positive for inhibin (Figure 17.19), calretinin, and CD99, perhaps indicating true sex cord differentiation.

FIGURE 17.19

Uterine tumor resembling ovarian sex cord tumor. The tumor forms cords and nests (A) and exhibits positive staining with α-inhibin (B).

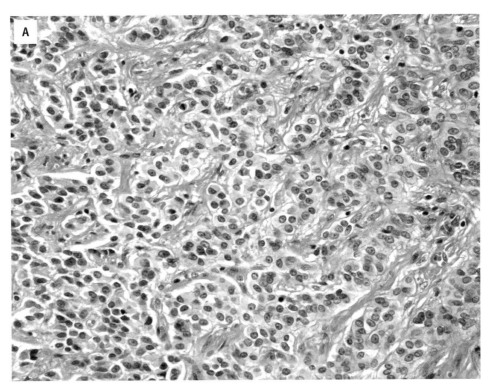

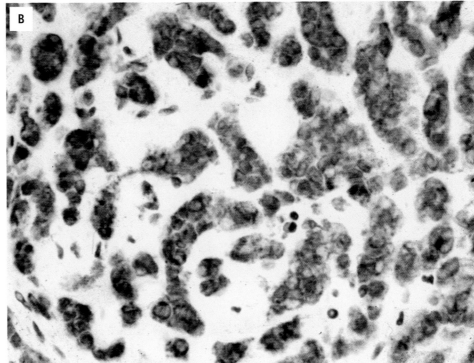

OVARY

UTERINE TUMOR RESEMBLING OVARIAN SEX CORD TUMOR (UTROSCT) – FACT SHEET

▸ May be positive for smooth muscle markers, cytokeratins, hormone receptors, and markers of sex cord differentiation

---

UTERINE PERIVASCULAR EPITHELIOID CELL TUMOR (PECOMA)

These rare uterine neoplasms exhibit coexpression of HMB-45 (Figure 17.20) and smooth muscle markers. However, HMB-45 staining may also be seen in morphologically unequivocal uterine leiomyosarcomas with clear cell areas; therefore, interpretation of HMB-45 should always be made in light of the morphologic appearance.

UTERINE PERIVASCULAR EPITHELIOID CELL TUMOR (PECOMA) – FACT SHEET

▸ Exhibits coexpression of HMB-45 and smooth muscle markers

PRIMARY VERSUS SECONDARY OVARIAN ADENOCARCINOMA

Differential cytokeratin staining (CK7 and CK20) may be useful in the distinction between a primary ovarian endometrioid or mucinous adenocarcinoma and a metastatic colorectal adenocarcinoma. These antibodies, in conjunction with CEA and CA-125, are especially useful in the distinction between an ovarian endometrioid adenocarcinoma and a metastatic colorectal adenocarcinoma

---

PRIMARY VERSUS SECONDARY OVARIAN ADENOCARCINOMA – FACT SHEET

▸ CK7 and CK20 are of value in the distinction between a primary ovarian endometrioid adenocarcinoma (CK7-positive, CK20-negative) and a metastatic colorectal adenocarcinoma (CK20-positive, CK7-negative)
▸ Primary ovarian mucinous carcinomas may exhibit focal CK20 positivity but are usually diffusely positive for CK7
▸ Nuclear CDX2 positivity is helpful in the distinction between a colorectal adenocarcinoma (positive) and a primary ovarian adenocarcinoma (negative)
▸ Loss of Dpc4 immunoreactivity is seen in approximately 50% of pancreatic adenocarcinomas

---

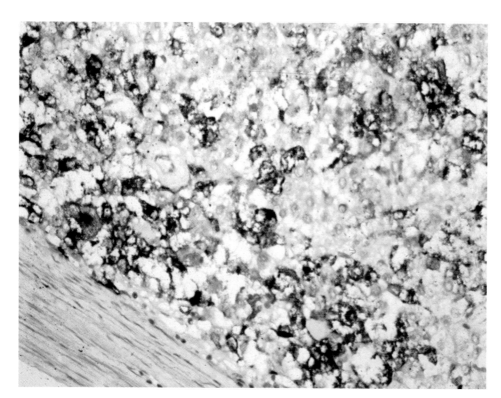

FIGURE 17.20
Perivascular epithelioid cell tumor (PEComa). The tumor shows cytoplasmic HMB-45 positivity.

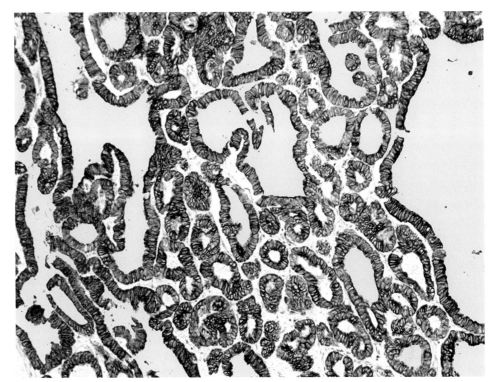

FIGURE 17.21

Primary ovarian endometrioid adenocarcinoma. There is diffuse cytoplasmic CK7 positivity.

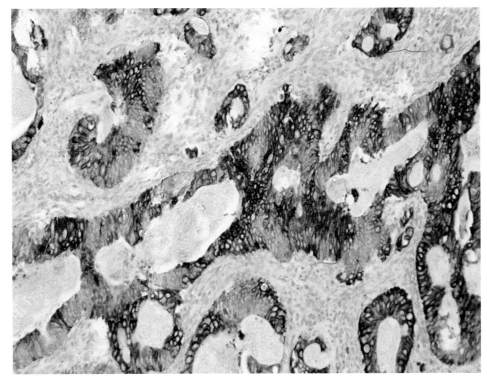

FIGURE 17.22

Metastatic colorectal adenocarcinoma to the ovary. The neoplastic glands exhibit diffuse cytoplasmic CK20 positivity.

with an endometrioid appearance. Primary ovarian endometrioid adenocarcinomas usually exhibit diffuse positivity for CK7 (Figure 17.21) and CA-125, and are negative for CK20 and CEA. Conversely, metastatic colorectal adenocarcinomas with an endometrioid appearance generally exhibit diffuse CK20 (Figure 17.22) and CEA positivity, and are negative for CK7 and CA-125. This panel of antibodies is of less value in the distinction between a

primary ovarian mucinous carcinoma and a metastatic colorectal adenocarcinoma with a mucinous appearance, since many colorectal adenocarcinomas with a mucinous appearance exhibit focal CK7 positivity and conversely, some ovarian mucinous tumors that exhibit intestinal differentiation are focally positive for CK20 and CEA. Nevertheless, diffuse CK7 and focal CK20 positivity favors a primary ovarian mucinous neoplasm whereas diffuse CK20 and focal CK7 positivity favors a metastatic colorectal adenocarcinoma. As there is considerable immunohistochemical overlap, these results should be interpreted in light of the morphologic findings in the ovary as well as pertinent clinical and radiologic information.

Differential cytokeratin staining is also of value in the setting of coexistent mucinous tumors of the ovary and appendix in association with pseudomyxoma peritonei. In most cases, the ovarian and appendiceal lesions and the mucinous epithelium present in the peritoneum are CK20 positive and CK7 negative, supporting an appendiceal origin.

Other antibodies that may be useful in the distinction between a primary ovarian adenocarcinoma and a metastatic colorectal adenocarcinoma include CDX2, β-catenin, villin, MUC2, and MUC5AC. Diffuse nuclear CDX2 positivity is characteristic of metastatic colorectal adenocarcinoma whereas most primary ovarian carcinomas are negative. β-catenin nuclear positivity is present in approximately half of metastatic colorectal adenocarcinomas, while most ovarian mucinous neoplasms exhibit no nuclear staining; however, ovarian endometrioid adenocarcinomas may exhibit patchy nuclear β-catenin positivity. Villin may also be of value in the confirmation of a metastatic colorectal adenocarcinoma as it is typically expressed by this tumor. Finally, MUC5AC is usually expressed in ovarian mucinous tumors, but is typically absent in colorectal carcinomas.

Differential cytokeratin staining is of no value in distinguishing between a primary ovarian adenocarcinoma and a metastatic adenocarcinoma from the pancreas, biliary tree, or stomach. Secondary tumors from the aforementioned organs are usually positive for CK7 whereas CK20 is usually negative (or focally positive). Dpc4 staining, however, may be helpful in diagnosing a metastatic pancreatic adenocarcinoma since primary ovarian mucinous neoplasms are Dpc4-positive while approximately 50% of pancreatic adenocarcinomas are negative.

Other markers, which may be of value in the diagnosis of rare metastatic tumors in the ovary, include RCC marker and CD10 (positive in metastatic renal cell carcinoma), TTF-1 (positive in metastatic lung carcinoma), uroplakin-III (positive in metastatic urinary transitional cell carcinoma) and S-100, HMB-45, and melan-A (positive in metastatic malignant melanoma). However, it should be noted that ovarian sex cord-stromal tumors may be positive for S-100 and melan-A and rarely for HMB-45.

OVARIAN SEROUS VERSUS OVARIAN ENDOMETRIOID ADENOCARCINOMA – FACT SHEET

▸ Ovarian serous carcinoma usually exhibits nuclear WT1 positivity while most ovarian endometrioid adenocarcinomas are negative

---

neoplasms this distinction may be difficult. Most ovarian serous carcinomas exhibit diffuse nuclear WT1 positivity whereas almost all ovarian endometrioid adenocarcinomas are negative. WT1 is also commonly positive in ovarian transitional cell carcinomas, but clear cell and mucinous carcinomas are generally negative.

OVARIAN SEX CORD-STROMAL TUMORS

Ovarian sex cord-stromal tumors are a heterogeneous group of lesions that may be mistaken for a variety of neoplasms. A number of markers may be helpful in their diagnosis, including α-inhibin and calretinin (most useful), as well as melan-A, CD99, müllerian-inhibiting substance, and relaxin-like factor. Calretinin is slightly more sensitive for an ovarian sex cord-stromal neoplasm whereas α-inhibin is more specific, the latter staining most ovarian sex cord-stromal tumors, with the exception of fibromatous neoplasms (Figure 17.23). These antibodies also stain nonneoplastic luteinized ovarian stromal cells, which can occur as a nonspecific response in the ovary. In the distinction between an ovarian sex cord-stromal and an epithelial neoplasm, α-inhibin and calretinin should be used as part of a panel that includes EMA, since this latter marker is rarely positive in ovarian sex cord-stromal neoplasms, in contrast to cytokeratin, which is not infrequently positive in these tumors. Positive staining for α-inhibin and calretinin may also assist in confirming a metastatic ovarian granulosa cell tumor, including the sarcomatous variant.

OVARIAN SEX CORD-STROMAL TUMORS – FACT SHEET

▸ Calretinin is slightly more sensitive marker than α-inhibin whereas α-inhibin is more specific
▸ EMA is rarely positive, in contrast to cytokeratins, which are not infrequently positive

---

DISTINCTION BETWEEN OVARIAN SEROUS AND OVARIAN ENDOMETRIOID ADENOCARCINOMA

The distinction between a well-differentiated ovarian serous and endometrioid adenocarcinoma is usually straightforward. However, with poorly differentiated

SMALL ROUND CELL TUMORS OF THE OVARY

The differential diagnosis of ovarian small round cell tumors may be wide and immunohistochemistry typically plays an important role in their diagnosis. Ovarian small cell carcinoma of hypercalcemic type

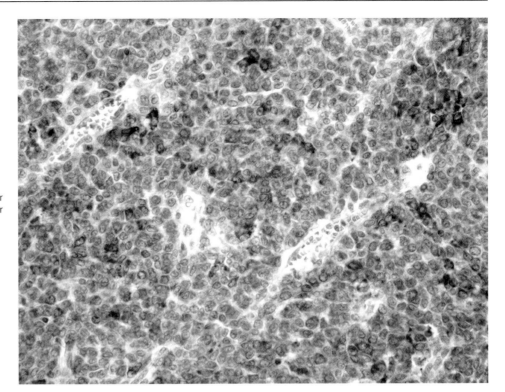

FIGURE 17.23
Granulosa cell tumor. The tumor cells exhibit diffuse positivity for α-inhibin.

SMALL ROUND CELL TUMORS OF THE OVARY – FACT SHEET

▶ Ovarian small cell carcinoma, hypercalcemic type, generally exhibits diffuse nuclear positivity for an antibody against the N-terminal of WT1
▶ Intraabdominal desmoplastic small round cell tumor exhibits cytoplasmic positivity for desmin and is positive for an antibody against the C-terminal of WT1
▶ Ovarian peripheral neuroectodermal tumors are positive for CD99 and FLI-1

EPITHELIAL VERSUS MESOTHELIAL PROLIFERATIONS – FACT SHEET

▶ Epithelial proliferations are BerEP4-positive while mesothelial proliferations are generally positive for calretinin, CK5/6, and thrombomodulin
▶ WT1 is positive in serous and mesothelial proliferations

---

generally exhibits diffuse nuclear positivity for an antibody against the N-terminal of WT1 (Figure 17.24). EMA, cytokeratins, CD10, calretinin, and p53 may also be positive. Intraabdominal desmoplastic small round cell tumor, which in females may mimic an ovarian neoplasm, is characterized by positivity for a variety of epithelial, mesenchymal, and neural markers. Most tumors exhibit punctate cytoplasmic positivity for desmin and are positive for an antibody against the C-terminal of WT1. Ovarian primitive neuroectodermal tumors may be positive for CD99 and FLI-1.

EPITHELIAL VERSUS MESOTHELIAL PROLIFERATIONS

A panel of antibodies may assist in the sometimes difficult distinction between serous epithelial and mesothe-lial proliferations involving the ovary or peritoneum. Epithelial proliferations are BerEP4-positive (Figure 17.25) whereas mesothelial proliferations may be positive for calretinin (Figure 17.26), CK5/6, thrombomodulin, and HBME1. WT1 nuclear positivity is characteristic of both serous and mesothelial proliferations. The best combination of markers therefore to distinguish between a serous and a mesothelial proliferation is BerEP4 (positive in serous proliferations; negative in mesothelial proliferations) and calretinin (positive in mesothelial proliferations; most often negative in serous proliferations).

OVARIAN GERM CELL TUMORS

The most useful markers in the diagnosis of ovarian germ cell tumors include placental alkaline phosphatase, OCT4 (positive in dysgerminoma), AFP (positive in yolk sac tumor) and beta-HCG (positive in trophoblastic tumor components).

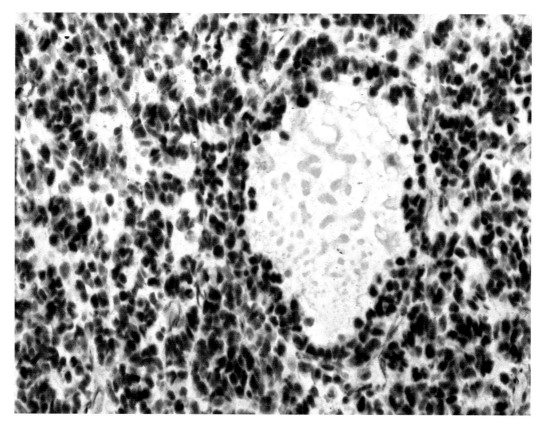

FIGURE 17.24
Small cell carcinoma of hypercalcemic type. Diffuse nuclear positivity for antibody against N-terminal of WT1 is present.

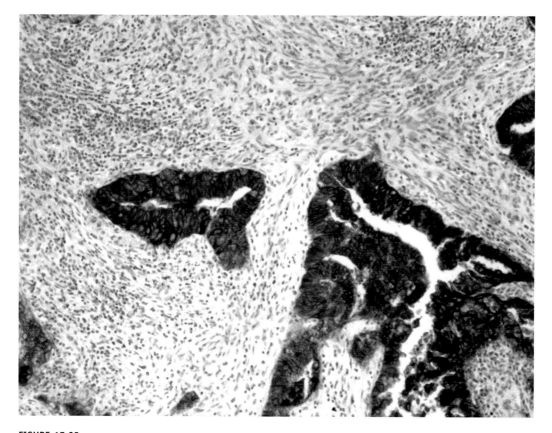

FIGURE 17.25
Ovarian serous carcinoma. The tumor cells exhibit cytoplasmic positivity for BerEP4.

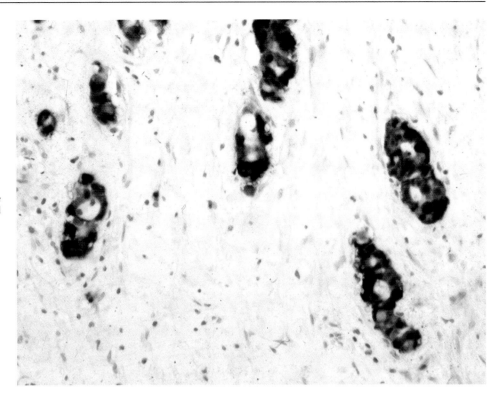

FIGURE 17.26
Mesothelial proliferation. Reactive mesothelial cells exhibit nuclear and cytoplasmic calretinin positivity.

OVARIAN GERM CELL TUMORS – FACT SHEET

▸ Placental alkaline phosphatase and OCT4 are characteristically positive in dysgerminoma

TROPHOBLASTIC DISEASES

RECENTLY CHARACTERIZED MARKERS OF TROPHOBLASTIC CELLS

Established markers of trophoblastic cell populations include beta-HCG and HPL. More recent markers shown to be positive in trophoblastic cell populations include α-inhibin, mel-CAM (CD146), HLA-G, CD10, and p63. α-inhibin stains syncytiotrophoblast and some intermediate trophoblastic cells, but not cytotrophoblast cells. Mel-CAM stains implantation-site intermediate trophoblastic cells, HLA-G stains intermediate trophoblastic cells, and CD10 is positive in most trophoblastic cell populations. Different p63 isoforms stain different trophoblastic populations. These markers may be of value in the diagnosis of a trophoblastic neoplasm and lesions such as placental site nodule or exaggerated placental site reaction.

TROPHOBLASTIC DISEASES – FACT SHEET

▸ Recently described markers of trophoblastic cell populations include α-inhibin, mel-CAM, HLA-G, CD10, and p63
▸ p57 is useful in the distinction between PHM or hydropic abortus (nuclear staining of cytotrophoblast and villous mesenchyme) and CHM (no staining of cytotrophoblast and villous mesenchyme)

P57 IN THE CLASSIFICATION OF HYDATIDIFORM MOLES

The histologic distinction between hydropic abortion, PHM, and CHM may be difficult as they all may have enlarged, swollen villi. p57, which is a paternally imprinted, maternally expressed gene, is particularly useful in distinguishing between a CHM mole and a PHM or hydropic abortus. Since complete moles contain no maternal DNA, the cytotrophoblast and villous mesenchyme are negative for p57 (Figure 17.27). In contrast, PHMs, hydropic abortions, and normal placenta, which contain maternal DNA, show positive nuclear staining of cytotrophoblast and villous mesenchyme for this marker. In CHMs, positive staining of decidua and

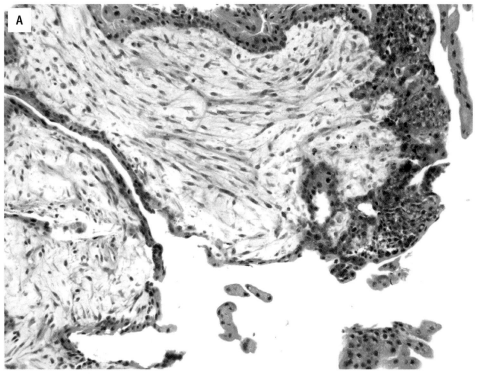

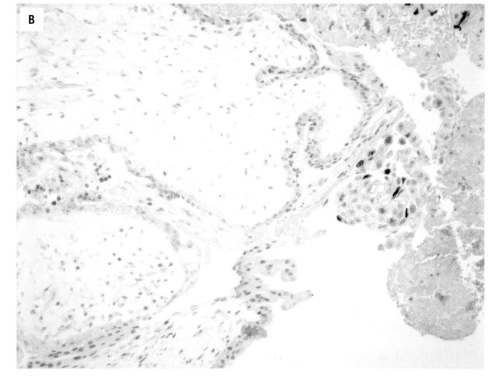

FIGURE 17.27
Early complete hydatidiform mole. Villi with irregular outlines and stromal karyorrhexis but no cavitation (A) exhibit loss of nuclear positivity of cytotrophoblast and villous mesenchyme with p57 (B). Extravillous trophoblast serves as an internal positive control.

implantation-site intermediate trophoblast acts as a positive internal control.

MISCELLANEOUS

CD10 may be useful in confirming the presence of endometrial stroma and establishing the diagnosis of endometriosis. However, this is of limited value in

MISCELLANEOUS – FACT SHEET

▶ Outside the cervix, CD10 may be of value in demonstrating endometrial-type stroma and confirming a diagnosis of endometriosis
▶ FATWO may be positive for cytokeratins, α-inhibin (focal and weak), vimentin, calretinin, and CD10

the cervix where a rim of CD10 positive stromal cells surrounds normal endocervical glands.

Female adnexal tumor of probable wolffian origin (FATWO) is often positive for α-inhibin (usually focal and weak), in contrast to the diffuse positivity generally, but not always, seen in ovarian sex cord-stromal neoplasms, which is the main differential diagnostic consideration. FATWO generally expresses cytokeratins and vimentin, and may be positive for calretinin and CD10. EMA and CEA are generally negative. This immunophenotype is similar to that of mesonephric remnants and provides evidence for a mesonephric origin of FATWO.

Other applications of α-inhibin staining in gynecological pathology include the identification of luteinized stromal cells. Staining with α-inhibin assists in confirming the presence of granulosa cells in cytological specimens and indicates a functional rather than an epithelial lined cyst.

WT1 and calretinin staining may assist in the diagnosis of an adenomatoid tumor and help confirm its mesothelial derivation.

SUGGESTED READING

General

Baker PM, Olwa E. Immunohistochemistry as a tool in the differential diagnosis of ovarian tumors: an update. Int J Gynecol Pathol 2005;24: 39–55.

Marjoniemi VM. Immunohistochemistry in gynaecological pathology: a review. Pathology 2004;36:109–119.

McCluggage WG. Recent advances in immunohistochemistry in the diagnosis of ovarian neoplasms. J Clin Pathol 2000;53:327–334.

McCluggage WG. Recent advances in immunohistochemistry in gynaecological pathology. Histopathology 2002;40:309–326.

Nucci MR, Castillon DH, Bai H, et al. Biomarkers in diagnostic obstetric and gynecologic pathology: a review. Adv Anat Pathol 2003;10:55–68.

Preinvasive Vulval Squamous Lesions

Logani S, Cu D, Quint WGV, et al. Low-grade vulvar and vaginal intraepithelial neoplasia: correlation of histologic features with human papillomavirus DNA detection and MIB-1 immunostaining. Mod Pathol 2003;16:735–741.

Pirog EC, Chen Y-T, Isacson C. MIB-1 immunostaining is a beneficial adjunct test for accurate diagnosis of vulvar condyloma acuminatum. Am J Surg Pathol 2000;24:1393–1399.

Santos M, Montagut C, Mellado B, et al. Immunohistochemical staining for p16 and p53 in premalignant and malignant epithelial lesions of the vulva. Int J Gynecol Pathol 2004;23:206–214.

Yang B, Hart WR. Vulvar intraepithelial neoplasia of the simplex (differentiated) type : a clinicopathologic study including analysis of HPV and p53 expression. Am J Surg Pathol 2000;24:429–441.

Vulval Paget Disease

Brown HM, Wilkinson EJ. Uroplakin-III to distinguish primary vulvar Paget disease from Paget disease secondary to urothelial carcinoma. Hum Pathol 2002;33:545–548.

Goldblum JR, Hart WR. Perianal Paget's disease – a histologic and immunohistochemical study of 11 cases with and without associated rectal adenocarcinoma. Am J Surg Pathol 1998;2:170–171.

Kuan S-F, Montag AG, Hart J, et al. Differential expression of mucin genes in mammary and extramammary Paget's disease. Am J Surg Pathol 2001;25:1469–1477.

Raju RR, Goldblum JR, Hart WR. Pagetoid squamous cell carcinoma in situ (pagetoid Bowen's disease) of the external genitalia. Int J Gynecol Pathol 2003;22:127–135.

Zhang C, Zhang P, Sung J, et al. Overexpression of p53 is correlated with stromal invasion in extramammary Paget's disease of the vulva. Hum Pathol 2003;34:880–885.

Vulvovaginal Mesenchymal Lesions

Iwasa Y, Fletcher CD. Cellular angiofibroma: clinicopathologic and immunohistochemical analysis of 51 cases. Am J Surg Pathol 2004;28: 1426–1435.

McCluggage WG. A review and update of morphologically bland vulvovaginal mesenchymal lesions. Int J Gynecol Pathol 2005;24:26–38.

McCluggage WG, Patterson A, Maxwell P. Aggressive angiomyxoma of pelvic parts exhibits oestrogen and progesterone receptor positivity. J Clin Pathol 2000;53:603–605.

McCluggage WG, Ganesan R, Hirschowitz L, et al. Cellular angiofibroma and related fibromatous lesions of the vulva: report of a series of cases with a morphological spectrum wider than previously described. Histopathology 2004;45:360–368.

Nucci MR, Tallini G, Quade BJ. HMGIC expression as a diagnostic marker for vulvar aggressive angiomyxoma. Mod Pathol 2001;14:829(A).

Nucci MR, Weremonicz S, Neskey DM, et al. Chromosomal translocation t (8, 12) induced aberrant HMGIC expression in aggressive angiomyxoma of the vulva. Genes Chromosomes Cancer 2001;32:172–176.

Preinvasive Cervical Squamous Lesions

Agoff SN, Lin P, Morihara J, et al. p16 INK4A expression correlates with degree of cervical neoplasia: a comparison with Ki-67 expression and detection of high-risk HPV types. Mod Pathol 2003;16:665–673.

Klaes R, Benner A, Freidrich T, et al. p16 (INK4A) immunohistochemistry improves interobserver agreement in the diagnosis of cervical intraepithelial neoplasia. Am J Surg Pathol 2002;26:1387–1399.

Klaes R, Friedrich T, Spitkovsky D, et al. Overexpression of p16 (INK4A) as a specific marker for dysplastic and neoplastic epithelial cells of the cervix uteri. Int J Cancer 2002;92:276–284.

Kruse A-J, Baak JPA, Helliesen T, et al. Evaluation of MIB-1 positive cell clusters as a diagnostic marker for cervical intraepithelial neoplasia. Am J Surg Pathol 2002;26:1501–1507.

McCluggage WG, Tang L, Maxwell P, et al. Monoclonal antibody MIB-1 in the assessment of cervical squamous intraepithelial lesions. Int J Gynecol Pathol 1996;15:131–136.

Mittal K. Utility of MIB-1 in evaluating cauterized cervical cone biopsy margins. Int J Gynecol Pathol 1999;18:211–214.

Mittal K, Mesia A, Demopoulos RL. MIB-1 expression is useful in distinguishing dysplasia from atrophy in elderly women. Int J Gynecol Pathol 1999;18:122–124.

Pirog EC, Baergen RN, Soslow RA, et al. Diagnostic accuracy of cervical low-grade squamous intraepithelial lesions is improved with MIB-1 immunostaining. Am J Surg Pathol 2002;26:70–75.

Preinvasive Cervical Glandular Lesions

Cameron RI, Maxwell P, Jenkins, D, et al. Immunohistochemical staining with MIB-1, bcl2 and p16 assists in the distinction of cervical glandular intraepithelial neoplasia from tubo-endometrial metaplasia, endometriosis and microglandular hyperplasia. Histopathology 2002;41: 313–321.

Cina SJ, Richardson MS, Austin RM, et al. Immunohistochemical staining for Ki-67 antigen, carcinoembryonic antigen, and p53 in the differential diagnosis of glandular lesions of the cervix. Mod Pathol 1997;10: 176–180.

Ishikawa M, Fujii T, Nasumoto N, et al. Correlation of p16 INK4A overexpression with human papillomavirus infection in cervical adenocarcinomas. Int J Gynecol Pathol 2003;22:378–385.

Lee KR, Sun D, Crum CP. Endocervical intraepithelial glandular atypia (dysplasia): a histopathologic, human papillomavirus, and MIB-1 analysis of 25 cases. Hum Pathol 2000;31:656–664.

McCluggage WG, Maxwell P, McBride HA, et al. Monoclonal antibodies Ki-67 and MIB-1 in the distinction of tuboendometrial metaplasia from endocervical adenocarcinoma and adenocarcinoma in situ in formalin fixed material. Int J Gynecol Pathol 1995;14:209–216.

McCluggage WG, Maxwell P. Bcl-2 and p21 staining of cervical tuboendometrial metaplasia. Histopathology 2002;40:107.

Negri G, Egarter–Vigi E, Kasal A, et al. p16 (INK4a) is a useful marker for the diagnosis of adenocarcinoma of the cervix uteri and its precursors. Am J Surg Pathol 2003;27:187–193.

Pirog EC, Isacson C, Szabolcs MJ, et al. Proliferative activity of benign and neoplastic endocervical epithelium and correlation with HPV DNA detection. Int J Gynecol Pathol 2002;21:22–26.

Riethdorf L, Riethdorf S, Lee KR, et al. Human papillomaviruses, expression of p16 INK4A, and early endocervical glandular neoplasia. Hum Pathol 2002;33:899–904.

Cervical Mesonephric Lesions

McCluggage WG, Oliva E, Herrington CS, et al. CD10 and calretinin staining of endocervical glandular lesions, endocervical stroma and endometrioid adenocarcinoma of the uterine corpus: CD10 positivity is characteristic of, but not specific for, mesonephric lesions and is not specific for endometrioid stroma. Histopathology 2003;43:144–150.

Ordi J, Nogales FF, Palacin A, et al. Mesonephric adenocarcinoma of the uterine corpus: CD10 expression as evidence of mesonephric differentiation. Am J Surg Pathol 2001;25:1540–1545.

Ordi J, Romagosa C, Tavasson FA, et al. CD10 expression in epithelial tissues and tumors of the gynecologic tract; a useful marker in the diagnosis of mesonephric, trophoblastic and clear cell tumors. Am J Surg Pathol 2003;27:178–186.

Silver SA, Devouassoux-Shisheboran M, Mezetti TP, et al. Mesonephric adenocarcinomas of the uterine cervix: a study of 11 cases with immunohistochemical findings. Am J Surg Pathol 2001;25:379–387.

Cervical Minimal Deviation Adenocarcinoma of Mucinous Type (Adenoma Malignum)

Mikami Y, Hata S, Melamed J, et al. Lobular endocervical glandular hyperplasia is a metaplastic process with a pyloric gland phenotype. Histopathology 2001;39:364–372.

Mikami Y, Kiyokawa T, Hata S, et al. Gastrointestinal immunophenotype in adenocarcinomas of the uterine cervix and related glandular lesions: a possible link between lobular endocervical glandular hyperplasia/pyloric gland metaplasia and adenoma malignum. Mod Pathol 2004;17:962–972.

Utsugi K, Hira Y, Takeshima N, et al. Utility of the monoclonal antibody HIK1083 in the diagnosis of adenoma malignum of the uterine cervix. Gynecol Oncol 1999;75:345–348.

Distinction Between Endometrial and Endocervical Adenocarcinoma

Ansari-Lari MA, Staebler A, Zaino RJ, et al. Distinction of endocervical and endometrial adenocarcinomas: immunohistochemical p16 expression correlated with human papillomavirus (HPV) DNA detection. Am J Surg Pathol 2004;28:160–167.

Castrillon DH, Lee KR, Nucci MR. Distinction between endometrial and endocervical adenocarcinoma: an immunohistochemical study. Int J Gynecol Pathol 2002;21:4–10.

Kamoi S, Al Juboury ML, Akin MR, et al. Immunohistochemical staining in the distinction between endometrial and endocervical adenocarcinomas: another viewpoint. Int J Gynecol Pathol 2002;21:217–223.

McCluggage WG, Jenkins D. Immunohistochemical staining with p16 may assist in the distinction between endometrial and endocervical adenocarcinoma. Int J Gynecol Pathol 2003;2:231–235.

McCluggage WG, Sumathi VP, McBride HA, et al. A panel of immunohistochemical stains, including carcinoembryonic antigen, vimentin and estrogen receptor aids the distinction between primary endometrial and endocervical adenocarcinomas. Int J Gynecol Pathol 2002;21:11–15.

Staebler A, Sherman ME, Zaino RJ, et al. Hormone receptor immunohistochemistry and human papillomavirus in situ hybridization are useful for distinguishing endocervical and endometrial adenocarcinomas. Am J Surg Pathol 2002;26:998–1006.

Zaino RJ. The fruits of our labours: distinguishing endometrial from endocervical adenocarcinoma: Int J Gynecol Pathol 2002;21:1–3.

Cervical Neuroendocrine Carcinomas

Gilks CB, Young RH, Gersell DJ, et al. Large cell neuroendocrine carcinoma of the uterine cervix: a clinicopathologic study of 12 cases. Am J Surg Pathol 1997;21:905–914.

Type I Versus Type II Endometrial Adenocarcinoma

Demopoulos RL, Mesia AF, Mittal K, et al. Immunohistochemical comparison of uterine papillary serous and papillary endometrioid carcinoma: clues to pathogenesis. Int J Gynecol Pathol 1999;18:233–237.

Lax SF, Kendall B, Tashiro H, et al. The frequency of p53, K-ras mutations, and microsatellite instability differs in uterine endometrioid and serous carcinoma: evidence of distinct molecular genetic pathways. Cancer 2000;88:814–825.

Schlosshauer PW, Hedrick Ellenson L, Soslow RA. β-cateinin and E-cadherin expression patterns in high-grade endometrial carcinoma are associated with histological subtype. Mod Pathol 2002;15:1032–1037.

Vang R, Barner R, Wheeler DT, et al. Immunohistochemical staining for Ki-67 and p53 helps distinguish endometrial Arias–Stella reaction from high grade carcinoma, including clear cell carcinoma. Int J Gynecol Pathol 2004;23:223–233.

Wang TY, Chen BF, Yang YC, et al. Histologic and immnophenotypic classification of cervical carcinomas by expression of the p53 homologue p63: a study of 250 cases. Hum Pathol 2001;32:479–486.

Distinction Between Uterine Serous Carcinoma and Ovarian Serous Carcinoma

Al-Hussaini M, Stockman A, Foster H, et al. WT-1 assists in distinguishing ovarian from uterine serous carcinoma and in distinguishing serous and ovarian endometrioid carcinoma. Histopathology 2004;44:109–115.

Egan JA, Ionescu ML, Eapen E, et al. Differential expression of WT1 and p53 in serous and endometrioid carcinoma of the endometrium. Int J Gynecol Pathol 2004;23:119–122.

Goldstein NS, Uzieblo A. WT-1 immunoreactivity in uterine papillary serous carcinoma is different from ovarian serous carcinomas. Am J Clin Pathol 2002;117:541–545.

Hashi A, Yuminamochi T, Murata S-I, et al. Wilms tumor gene immunoreactivity in primary serous carcinomas of the fallopian tube, ovary, endometrium and peritoneum. Int J Gynecol Pathol 2003;22:374–377.

Hwang H, Quenneville L, Yaziji H, et al. Wilms tumor gene product. Sensitive and contextually specific marker of serous carcinomas of ovarian surface epithelial origin. Appl Immunohistochem Mol Morphol 2004;12:122–126.

McCluggage WG. WT1 is of value in ascertaining the site of origin of serous carcinomas within the female genital tract. Int J Gynecol Pathol 2004;23:97–99.

Distinction Between Stromal and Smooth Muscle Neoplasms

Chu PG, Arber PA, Weiss LM, et al. Utility of CD10 in distinguishing between endometrial stromal sarcoma and uterine smooth muscle tumors: an immunohistochemical comparison of 34 cases. Mod Pathol 2001;14:465–471.

Loddenkemper C, Mechsner S, Foss H-D, et al. Use of oxytocin receptor expression in distinguishing between uterine smooth muscle tumors and endometrial stromal sarcoma. Am J Surg Pathol 2003;27:1458–1462.

McCluggage WG, Sumathi VP, Maxwell P. CD10 is a sensitive and diagnostically useful immunohistochemical marker of normal endometrial stroma and of endometrial stromal neoplasms. Histopathology 2001;39:273–278.

Nucci MR, O'Connell JT, Huettner PC, et al. h-caldesmon expression effectively distinguishes endometrial stromal tumors from uterine smooth muscle tumors. Am J Surg Pathol 2001;25:253–258.

Oliva E, Young RH, Amin MB, et al. An immunohistochemical analysis of endometrial stromal and smooth muscle tumors of the uterus: a study of 54 cases emphasising the importance of using a panel because of overlap in immunoreactivity for individual antibodies. Am J Surg Pathol 2002;26:403–412.

Rush DS, Tan JY, Baergen RN, et al. h-caldesmon, a novel smooth muscle-specific antibody, distinguishes between cellular leiomyoma and endometrial stromal sarcoma. Am J Surg Pathol 2001;25:253–258.

Sumathi VP, Al-Hussaini M, Connolly LE, et al. Endometrial neo-plasms are immunoreactive with WT-1 antibody. Int J Gynecol Pathol 2004;23:241–247.

Uterine Tumor Resembling Ovarian Sex Cord Tumor

Baker RJ, Hildebrandt RH, Rouse RV, et al. Inhibin and CD99 (MIC2) expression in uterine stromal neoplasms with sex cord-like elements. Hum Pathol 1999;30:671–679.

Irving JA, Carinelli S, Part J. Uterine tumors resembling ovarian sex cord tumors are polyphenotypic neoplasms with true sex-cord differentiation. Mod Pathol 2006;19:17–24.

Krishnamurthy S, Jungbloth AA, Busam KJ, et al. Uterine tumors resembling ovarian sex cord tumors have an immunophenotype consistent with true sex cord differentiation. Am J Surg Pathol 1998;22:1078–1082.

McCluggage WG. Uterine tumours resembling ovarian sex cord tumours: immunohistochemical evidence for true sex cord differentiation. Histopathology 1999;34:373–380.

Uterine Perivascular Epithelioid Cell Tumor

Silva EG, Deavers MT, Bodurka DC, et al. Uterine epithelioid leiomyosarcomas with clear cells: reactivity with HMB-45 and the concept of PEComa. Am J Surg Pathol 2004;28:244–249.

Sumpson KW, Albores-Saavedra J. HMB-45 reactivity in conventional uterine leiomyosaromas. Am J Surg Pathol 2007;31:95–8.

Vang R, Kempson RL. Perivascular epithelioid cell tumour (PEComa) of the uterus: a subset of HMB-45 positive epithelioid mesenchymal neoplasms with an uncertain relationship to pure smooth muscle tumors. Am J Surg Pathol 2002;26:1–13.

Primary Versus Secondary Ovarian Adenocarcinoma

Albarracin CT, Jafri J, Montag AG, et al. Differential expression of MUC2 and MUC5AC mucin genes in primary ovarian and metastatic colonic carcinoma. Hum Pathol 2000;31:672–677.

Berezowski K, Stasny JF, Kornstein MJ. Cytokeratins 7 and 20 and carcinoembryonic antigen in ovarian and colonic carcinoma. Mod Pathol 1996;9:426–429.

Cameron RI, Ashe P, O'Rourke DM, et al. A panel of immunohistochemical stains assists in the distinction between ovarian and renal clear cell carcinoma. Int J Gynecol Pathol 2003;22:272–276.

Chou YY, Jeng YM, Kao HL, et al. Differentiation of ovarian mucinous carcinoma and metastatic colorectal adenocarcinoma by immunostaining with β-catenin. Histopathology 2003;43:151–156.

Groisman GM, Meir A, Sabo E. The value of cdx2 immunostaining in differentiating primary ovarian carcinomas from colonic carcinomas metastatic to the ovaries. Int J Gynecol Pathol 2003;23:52–57.

Ji H, Isacson C, Seidman JD, et al. Cytokeratins 7 and 20, Dpc4, and MUC5AC in the distinction of metastatic mucinous carcinomas in the ovary from primary ovarian mucinous tumors : Dpc 4 assists in identifying metastatic pancreatic carcinomas. Int J Gynecol Pathol 2002;21:391–400.

Ladendijk JA, Mullink EH, van Diest PJ, et al. Tracing the origin of adenocarcinomas with unknown primary using immunohistochemistry. Differential diagnosis between colonic and ovarian carcinomas as primary sites. Hum Pathol 1998;29:491–497.

Logani S, Oliva E, Arnell PM, et al. Use of novel immunohistochemical markers expressed in colonic adenocarcinoma to distinguish primary ovarian tumors from metastatic colorectal carcinoma. Mod Pathol 2005;18:19–25.

McCluggage WG. Recent advances in immunohistochemistry in the diagnosis of ovarian neoplasms. J Clin Pathol 2000;3:327–334.

Park SY, Kim HS, Hong EK, et al. Expression of cytokeratins 7 and 20 in primary carcinomas of the stomach and colorectum and their value in the differential diagnosis of metastatic carcinomas to the ovary. Hum Pathol 2002;33:1078–1085.

Raspollini MR, Amunni G, Villanucci A, et al. Utility of CDX-2 in distinguishing between primary and secondary (intestinal) mucinous ovarian carcinoma. Appl Immunohistochem Mol Morphol 2004;12:127–131.

Tornillo L, Moch H, Diener PA, et al. CDX-2 immunostaining in primary and secondary ovarian carcinomas. J Clin Pathol 2004;57:641–643.

Wauters CCAP, Smedts F, Gerrits LGM, et al. Keratins 7 and 20 as diagnostic markers of carcinomas metastatic to the ovary. Hum Pathol 1995;26:852–855.

Werling RW, Yaziji H, Bacchi CE, et al. CDX2, a highly sensitive and specific marker of adenocarcinomas of intestinal origin: an immunohistochemical survey of 476 primary and metastatic carcinomas. Am J Surg Pathol 2003;27:303–310.

Distinction Between Ovarian Serous and Ovarian Endometrioid Adenocarcinoma

Al-Hussaini M, Stockman A, Foster H, et al. WT-1 assists in distinguishing ovarian from uterine serous carcinoma and in distinguishing serous and endometrioid ovarian carcinoma. Histopathology 2004;44:109–115.

Shimizu M, Toki T, Takagi Y, et al. Immunohistochemical detection of the Wilms' tumor gene (WT1) in epithelial ovarian tumors. Int J Gynecol Pathol 2000;19:158–163.

Ovarian Sex Cord-Stromal Tumors

Bamberger AM, Ivell R, Balvers M. Relaxin-like factor (RLF): a new specific marker for Leydig cells in the ovary. Int J Gynecol Pathol 1998;18:163–168.

Cao QJ, Jones JG, Li M. Expression of calretinin in human ovary, testis and ovarian sex cord-stromal tumors. Int J Gynecol Pathol 2001;20:346–352.

Costa MJ, Ames PF, Walls J, et al. Inhibin immunohistochemistry applied to ovarian neoplasms: a novel, effective diagnostic tool. Hum Pathol 1997;28:1247–1254.

Deavers MT, Malpica A, Liu J, et al. Ovarian sex cord-stromal tumors: an immunohistochemical study including a comparison of calretinin and inhibin. Mod Pathol 2003;16:584–590.

Guerrieri C, Franlund B, Malmstrom H, et al. Ovarian endometrioid carcinomas simulating sex cord-stromal tumors: a study using inhibin and cytokeratin 7. Int J Gynecol Pathol 1998;17:266–271.

Kommoss F, Oliva E, Bhan AK, et al. Inhibin expression in ovarian tumors and tumor-like lesions: an immunohistochemical study. Mod Pathol 1998;11:656–664.

Loo KT, Leung AKF, Chan JKC. Immunohistochemical staining of ovarian granulosa cell tumours with MIC2 antibody. Histopathology 1995;27:388–390.

Matias-Guiu X, Pons C, Prat J. Mullerian inhibiting substance, alpha-inhibin, and CD99 expression in sex cord-stromal tumors and endometrioid ovarian carcinomas resembling sex cord-stromal tumors. Hum Pathol 1998;29:840–845.

McCluggage WG, Maxwell P. Adenocarcinomas of various sites may exhibit immunoreactivity with anti-inhibin antibodies. Histopathology 1999;35:216–220.

McCluggage WG, Maxwell P. Immunohistochemical staining for calretinin is useful in the diagnosis of ovarian sex cord-stromal tumours. Histopathology 2001;38:403–408.

McCluggage WG, Maxwell P, Sloan JM. Immunohistochemical staining of ovarian granulosa cell tumors with monoclonal antibody against inhibin. Hum Pathol 1997;28:1034–1038.

Movahedi-Lankarani S, Kurman RJ. Calretinin, a more sensitive but less specific marker than α-inhibin for ovarian sex cord-stromal neoplasms. An immunohistochemical study of 215 cases. Am J Surg Pathol 2002;26:1477–1483.

Pelkey TJ, Frierson HF Jr, Mills SE, et al. The diagnostic value of inhibin staining in ovarian neoplasms. Int J Gynecol Pathol 1998;17:97–105.

Riopel MA, Perlman EJ, Seidman JD, et al. Inhibin and epithelial membrane antigen immunohistochemistry assist in the diagnosis of sex cord-stromal tumors and provide clues to the histogenesis of hypercalcemic small cell carcinoma. Int J Gynecol Pathol 1998;17:46–53.

Rishi M, Howard LN, Bratthauer GL, et al. Use of monoclonal antibody against human inhibin as a marker for sex cord-stromal tumors of the ovary. Am J Surg Pathol 1997;21:583–589.

Stewart CJR, Jeffers MD, Kennedy A. Diagnostic value of inhibin immunoreactivity in ovarian gonadal stromal tumours and their histological mimics. Histopathology 1997;31:67–74.

Stewart CJR, Nandini CL, Richmond JA. Value of A103 (melan-A) immunostaining in the differential diagnosis of ovarian sex cord tumours. J Clin Pathol 2000;53:206–211.

Yao DX, Soslow RA, Hedvat CV, et al. Melan-A (A103) and inhibin expression in ovarian neoplasms. Appl Immunohistochem Mol Morphol 2003;11:244–249.

Small Round Cell Tumors of the Ovary

Eichhorn JH, Young RH, Scully RE. Primary ovarian small cell carcinoma of pulmonary type. A clinicopathologic, immunohistologic, and flow cytometric analysis of 11 cases. Am J Surg Pathol 1992;16:926–938.

Kawrachi S, Fukuda T, Miyamoto S, et al. Peripheral primitive neuroectodermal tumor of the ovary confirmed by CD99 immunostaining, karyotypic analysis and RT-PCR for EWS/FLI-1 chimeric mRNA. Am J Surg Pathol 1998;22:1417–1422.

Matias-Guiu X, Prat J, Young RH, et al. Human parathyroid hormone-related protein in ovarian small cell carcinoma. An immunohistochemical study. Cancer 1994;73:1878–1881.

McCluggage WG. Ovarian neoplasms composed of small round cells. A review. Adv Anat Pathol 2004;11:288–296.

McCluggage WG, Oliva E, Connolly LE, et al. An immunohistochemical analysis of ovarian small cell carcinoma of hypercalcemic type. Int J Gynecol Pathol 2004;23:330–336.

Ordoñez NG. Desmoplastic small round cell tumour, II: An ultrastructural and immunohistochemical study with emphasis on new immunohistochemical markers. Am J Surg Pathol 1998;22:1314–1327.

Riopel MA, Perlman PJ, Seidman JD, et al. Inhibin and epithelial membrane antigen immunohistochemistry assist in the diagnosis of sex cord-stromal tumors and provide clues to the histogenesis of hypercalcemic small cell carcinomas. Int J Gynecol Pathol 1988;17:46–53.

Epithelial Versus Mesothelial Proliferations

Attanoos RL, Webb R, Dojcinov SD, et al. Value of mesothelial and epithelial antibodies in distinguishing diffuse peritoneal mesothelioma in females from serous papillary carcinoma of the ovary and peritoneum. Histopathology 2002;40:237–244.

Khoury N, Raju U, Crissman JD, et al. A comparative immunohistochemical study of peritoneal and ovarian serous tumors and mesotheliomas. Hum Pathol 1990;21:811–819.

Ordoñez NG. Role of immunohistochemistry in distinguishing epithelial peritoneal mesothelioma from peritoneal and ovarian serous carcinomas. Am J Surg Pathol 1998;22:1203–1214.

Ovarian Germ Cell Tumors

Cheng L, Thomas A, Roth CM, et al. OCT4. A novel biomarker for dysgerminoma of the ovary. Am J Surg Pathol 2004;18:1341–1346.

Trophoblastic Disease

Castrillon DH, Sun DQ, Weremowicz S, et al. Discrimination of complete hydatidiform mole from its mimics by immunohistochemistry of the paternally imprinted gene product p57 (KIP2). Am J Surg Pathol 2001;25:1225–1230.

Crisp H, Burton JL, Stewart R, et al. Refining the diagnosis of hydatidiform mole: image ploidy analysis and p57 KIP2 immunohistochemistry. Histopathology 2003;43:363–373.

Fukunaga M. Immunohistochemical characterization of p57 KIP2 expression in early hydatiform moles. Hum Pathol 2002;33:1188–1192.

Genest DR, Dorfman DM, Castrillon DH. Ploidy and imprinting in hydatidiform moles. Complementary use of flow cytometry and immunohistochemistry of the imprinted gene product p57 KIP2 to assist molar classification. J Reprod Med 2002;47:342–346.

Jun S-Y, Ro JY, Kim K-R. p57 KIP2 is useful in the classification and differential diagnosis of complete and partial hydatidiform moles. Histopathology 2003;43:17–25.

McCluggage WG, Ashe P, McBride H, et al. Localization of the cellular expression of inhibin in trophoblastic tissue. Histopathology 1998;32:252–256.

Ordi J, Romagosa C, Tavassoli FA, et al. CD10 expression in epithelial tissues and tumors of the gynecologic tract: a useful marker in the diagnosis of mesonephric, trophoblastic and clear cell tumors. Am J Surg Pathol 2003;27:178–186.

Shih IM, Kurman RJ. Ki-67 labelling index in the differential diagnosis of exaggerated placental site, placental site trophoblastic tumor and choriocarcinoma. A double immunohistochemical staining technique using Ki-67 and mel CAM antibodies. Hum Pathol 1998;29:27–33.

Shih IM, Kurman RJ. Immunohistochemical localization of inhibin-alpha in the placenta and gestational trophoblastic lesions. Int J Gynecol Pathol 1999;18:144–150.

Shih IM, Kurman RJ. p63 expression is useful in the distinction of epithelioid trophoblastic and placental site trophoblastic tumors by profiling trophoblastic subpopulations. Am J Surg Pathol 2004;28:1177–1183.

Shih IM, Kurman RJ. The pathology of intermediate trophoblastic tumors and tumor-like lesions. Int J Gynecol Pathol 2001;20:31–47.

Shih IM, Seidman JD, Kurman RJ. Placental site nodule and characterization of distinctive types of intermediate trophoblast. Hum Pathol 1999;30:687–694.

Singer G, Kurman RJ, McMaster MT, et al. HLA-G immunoreactivity is specific for intermediate trophoblast in gestational trophoblastic disease and can serve as a useful marker in differential diagnosis. Am J Surg Pathol 2002;26:914–920.

Xue W-C, Khoo U-S, Ngan HYS, et al. c-mos immunoreactivity aids in the diagnosis of gestational trophoblastic lesions. Int J Gynecol Pathol 2004;23:145–150.

Miscellaneous

Devouassoux-Shisheboran M, Silver SA, Tavassoli FA. Wolffian adnexal tumor, so-called female adnexal tumor of probable wolffian origin (FATWO): immunohistochemical evidence in support of a wolffian origin. Hum Pathol 1999;30:856–863.

Groisman GM, Meir A. CD10 is helpful in detecting occult or inconspicuous endometrial stromal cells in cases of presumptive endometriosis. Arch Pathol Lab Med 2003;127:1003–1006.

McCluggage WG. The value of inhibin staining in gynecological pathology. Int J Gynecol Pathol 2001;20:79–85.

McCluggage WG, Patterson A, White J, et al. Immunocytochemical staining of ovarian cyst aspirates with monoclonal antibody against inhibin. Cytopathology 1998;9:336–342.

Schwartz EJ, Longacre TA. Adenomatoid tumors of the female and male genital tract express WT1. Int J Gynecol Pathol 2004;23:123–128.

Sumathi VP, McCluggage WG. CD10 is useful in demonstrating endometrial stroma at ectopic sites and in confirming a diagnosis of endometriosis. J Clin Pathol 2002;55:391–392.

Tiltman AJ, Allard U. Female adnexal tumours of probable wolffian origin: an immunohistochemical study comparing tumours, mesonephric remnants and para-mesonephric derivatives. Histopathology 2001;38:237–242.

Index

Indexer: Dr Laurence Errington

Figures and tables are comprehensively referred to from the text. Therefore, significant material in figures and tables have only been given a page reference in the absence of their concomitant mention in the text referring to that figure. "vs" indicates the differential diagnosis of conditions. With reference to adenocarcinomas, some main entries have been constructed in the form 'mucinous (adeno)carcinoma'. The brackets have been used as the text sometimes refers to these adenocarcinomas as carcinomas.